HANDBOOK OF

Neonatal Intensive Care

FIFTH EDITION

HANDBOOK OF
Neonatal Intensive Care

GERALD B. MERENSTEIN, MD, FAAP
Professor of Pediatrics,
Senior Associate Dean, Education,
University of Colorado School of Medicine
Denver, Colorado

SANDRA L. GARDNER, RN, MS, CNS, PNP
Neonatal/Perinatal/Pediatric Consultant
Director, Professional Outreach Consultation
Aurora, Colorado

with 285 illustrations

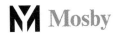

An Imprint of Elsevier Science

St. Louis   London   Philadelphia   Sydney   Toronto

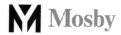

An Imprint of Elsevier Science

Vice President, Publishing Director: Sally Schrefer
Executive Editor: Barbara Nelson Cullen
Senior Developmental Editor: Cindi Anderson
Developmental Editor: Eric Ham
Publication Services Manager: John Rogers
Project Manager: Beth Hayes
Senior Designer: Kathi Gosche
Cover Photo: © Corbis Corporation/Lester Lefkowitz

FIFTH EDITION
Copyright © 2002 by Mosby, Inc.

Previous editions copyrighted 1985, 1989, 1993, and 1998.

NOTICE

Pharmacology is an ever-changing field. Standard safety precautions must be followed, but as new research and clinical experience broaden our knowledge, changes in treatment and drug therapy may become necessary or appropriate. Readers are advised to check the most current product information provided by the manufacturer of each drug to be administered to verify the recommended dose, the method and duration of administration, and contraindications. It is the responsibility of the treating physician, relying on experience and knowledge of the patient, to determine dosages and the best treatment for each individual patient. Neither the publisher nor the editor assumes any liability for any injury and/or damage to persons or property arising from this publication.

Mosby, Inc.
An Imprint of Elsevier Science
11830 Westline Industrial Drive
St. Louis, Missouri 63146

ISBN 0-323-014712

Library of Congress Cataloging in Publication Data

Handbook of neonatal intensive care / [edited by] Gerald B. Merenstein, Sandra L. Gardner.—5th ed.
    p.   ; cm.
  Includes bibliographical references and index.
  ISBN 0-323-01471-2
    1. Neonatal intensive care—Handbooks, manuals, etc.   I. Merenstein, Gerald B.   II. Gardner, Sandra L.
    [DNLM: 1. Intensive Care, Neonatal.   2. Infant, Newborn, Diseases—therapy.   WS 421   H236 2002]
  RJ253.5 .H36   2002
618.92'01—dc 21
                                                                                    2002025078

Contributors

Steven H. Abman, MD
Professor of Pediatrics
Department of Pediatrics—Pulmonary Medicine
Director, Pediatric Heart Lung Center
Department of Pulmonary Medicine
University of Colorado Health Sciences Center
School of Medicine

Karen M. Adams, BSN
Registered Nurse—Head Research Coordinator,
Nursing
Baylor College of Medicine,
Houston, Texas

Eugene W. Adcock III, MD
Professor of Pediatrics, Emeritus
Wake Forest School of Medicine
Winston Salem, North Carolina

Rita Agarwal, MD
Associate Professor
Department of Anesthesiology
University of Colorado Health Sciences Center
Denver, Colorado

Marilee C. Allen, MD
Professor of Pediatrics
Associate Director of Neonatology,
Johns Hopkins University School of Medicine;
Co-Director of the Maryland Regional Neonatal
Transport Program
Co-Director of the NICU Developmental Clinic
Kennedy-Kriger Institute
Baltimore, Maryland

Nancy H. Allen, MS, RD, CNSD
Neonatal Nutritionist
Children's Mercy Hospital and Clinics
Kansas City, Missouri

Marianne S. Anderson, MD
Assistant Professor
Section of Neonatology
University of Colorado Health Sciences Center
Denver, Colorado

Denis D. Bensard, BA, MD
Associate Professor of Surgery and Pediatrics
University of Colorado
Denver, Colorado

David D. Berry, MD
Former Professor, Pediatrics
Wake Forest School of Medicine
Winston-Salem North Carolina

W. Woods Blake, MD
Associate Professor of Pediatrics, Chattanooga
Unit
University of Tennessee College of Medicine
Chattanooga, Tennessee

Melvin Bonilla-Felix, MD
Associate Professor
Department of Pediatrics and Physiology
University of Puerto Rico—Medical Sciences
Campus
San Juan, Puerto Rico

Casey M. Calkins, BA, MD
Instructor of Surgery
University of Colorado
Denver, Colorado

Paul R. Carney, BS, MD
Assistant Professor of Pediatrics and Neurology
Director, University of Florida Health Science
  Center
Comprehensive Pediatric Epilepsy Program
University of Florida
Gainesville, Florida

Brian S. Carter, MD, FAAP
Associate Professor of Pediatrics, Division of
  Neonatology
Vanderbilt University Medical Center
Associate Director of Neonatology
Gateway Medical Center
Nashville, Tennessee

Ruby D Cerda, RN
Clinical Coordinator, Pediatric Nephrology and
  Hypertension
Hermann Hospital
Houston, Texas

Susan B. Clarke, MS, RN C
Clinical Nurse Specialist, Education Services
The Children's Hospital
Denver, Colorado

Shannon Collins, BSN, MSCIS
Professional Research Assistant
Pediatric General Clinical Research Center
University of Colorado Health Sciences Center
Denver, Colorado

Sharla C. Cooper, RNC, NNP, ND
Assistant Professor
Radford University, School of Nursing
Radford, Virginia

C. Michael Cotton, MD
Clinical Associate, Department of Pediatrics
Duke University Medical Center
Durham, North Carolina

Pamela K. Donohue, ScD, PA-C
Assistant Professor of Pediatrics
Department of Pediatrics
Johns Hopkins University School of Medicine
Baltimore, Maryland

David J. Durand, MD
Neonatologist
Children's Hospital and Research Center
Oakland, California

Nancy K. English, PhD, RN
Coordinator, The Supportive Care Network
The Children's Hospital
Denver, Colorado

Loretta P. Finnegan, MD
Medical Advisor to the Director
Office of Research on Women's Health
National Institutes of Health
Bethesda, Maryland
Professor of Pediatrics
Professor of Psychiatry and Human Behavior
Jefferson Medical College
Thomas Jefferson University
Philadelphia, Pennsylvania

C. Gilbert Frank, MD
Neonatologist
Pediatrix Medical Group
Carilion Roanoke Community Hospital

Sandra L. Gardner, RN, MS, CNS, PNP
Neonatal/Perinatal/Pediatric Consultant
Director, Professional Outreach Consultation
Aurora, Colorado

Anita Duhl Glicken, MSW
Associate Professor of Pediatrics
Physician Assistant Program
Department of Pediatrics
University of Colorado Health Sciences Center
Denver, Colorado

Edward Goldson, MD
Professor of Pediatrics
Staff Pediatrician
Child Development Unit
Section of Developmental and Behavioral
  Pediatrics
The Children's Hospital
Denver, Colorado

Mary I. Enzman Hagedorn, PhD, RN, HNC, CNS, CPNP
Associate Professor
Beth El College of Nursing
University of Colorado at Colorado Springs
Colorado Springs, Colorado

Margaret M. (Peggy) Hauser, BA, MSW, LCSW
Licensed Social Worker
Swedish Medical Center
Englewood, Colorado

William W. Hay, Jr, MD
Professor
Department of Neonatology
University of Colorado Health Sciences Center
Denver, Colorado

Carolyn Houska-Lund, RN, MSN, FAAN
Assistant Clinical Professor, WOS
Department of Family Health Care Nursing
University of California San Francisco

Gary M. Joffe, MD
Private Practice
Maternal Fetal Medicine
Perinatal Associates of New Mexico
Albuquerque, New Mexico

Cynthia Boyer Johnson, RNC, MS, NNP
Neonatal Nurse Practitioner
Department of Neonatology
The Children's Hospital
Denver, Colorado

Janis L. Johnson, MD
Neonatologist
Pediatrix Medical Group
Englewood, Colorado

Marilyn Manco-Johnson, MD
Professor, Pediatrics
University of Colorado School of Medicine
Denver, Colorado

Rita T. Keuten, BSN, RN
Nursing Clinical Coordinator
Department of Radiology
The Children's Hospital
Denver, Colorado

Howard W. Kilbride, MD
Professor of Pediatrics
University of Missouri–Kansas City
Chief, Section of Neonatal Medicine
Children's Mercy Hospital
Kansas City, Missouri

Ruth A. Lawrence, MD, FAAP, FACT
Professor of Pediatrics, Obstetrics & Gynecology
Department of Pediatrics
University of Rochester
Rochester, New York

Mary Kay Leick-Rude, RNC, MSN
Clinical Nurse Specialist
Children's Mercy Hospital and Clinics
Kansas City, Missouri

†Lula O. Lubchenco
Professor Emerita
School of Medicine
University of Colorado
Denver, Colorado

Anne L. Matthews, RN, PhD, FACMG
Associate Professor of Genetics
Director, Genetic Counseling Training
Department of Genetics
Case Western Reserve University

Jane E. McGowan, MD
Associate Professor of Pediatrics
The Johns Hopkins University School of Medicine
Baltimore, Maryland

Gerald B. Merenstein, MD, FAAP
Professor of Pediatrics
Senior Associate Dean, Education
University of Colorado School of Medicine
Denver, Colorado

†Deceased.

Mary Miller-Bell, PharmD
Clinical Pharmacologist
Neonatal Nurse Practitioner Program
Duke University Hospital
Durham, North Carolina

Kimberly D. Montoya, RN, BSN
Pediatric Cardiovascular Nurse
Department of Pediatric Cardiology
Western Cardiology, Pediatric Division
Denver, Colorado

Judith A. Murray, RNC, MSN, NNP
Neonatal Nurse Practitioner
TC Thomson Children's Hospital
Chattanooga, Tennessee

Susan Niermeyer, MD
Associate Professor of Pediatrics
University of Colorado
Denver, Colorado

Miriam Orleans, PhD
Professor Emerita
Department of Preventive Medicine and
    Biometrics
University of Colorado School of Medicine

Patti L. Paige, BSN, MSN
Assistant Professor, ASN Program
Santa Fe Community College, Nursing Programs
Gainesville, FL

William H. Parry, MD, PhD, FAAP
Medical Director
Christus Santa Rosa Health
San Antonio, Texas

David Partrick, MD
Assistant Professor of Surgery
The Children's Hospital
University of Colorado
Denver, Colorado

Gary Petett, MD
Associate Dean for Academic Affairs
University of Missouri
Kansas City School of Medicine
Professor, Pediatrics and Neonatology
Children's Mercy Hospital
Kansas City, Missouri

John R. Pierce, MD
Director, Patient Safety
Walter Reed Army Medical Center
Washington, DC

Margaret J. Porter, MS, RNC
Case Manager
Neonatal Intensive Care Unit
Johns Hopkins University Hospital
Baltimore, Maryland

Ronald J. Portman, MD
Professor and Director,
Division of Pediatric Nephrology and
    Hypertension
Department of Pediatrics
University of Texas-Houston, Medical School
Houston, Texas

Frances N. Price, RN, MSN, CPNP
Pediatric Nurse Practitioner
Department of Pediatric Surgery
The Children's Hospital
Denver, Colorado

Donna Rodden, RN, BSN
Assistant Nursing Director
Pediatric General Clinical Research Center
University of Colorado Health Sciences Center
Denver, Colorado

Nathaniel H. Robin, MD
Associate Professor of Genetics and Pediatrics
Center for Human Genetics
Case Western Reserve University School of
    Medicine
Cleveland, Ohio

Sally Sewell, RN
Staff Nurse
Emergency Department
Saint Elizabeth's Medical Center
Edgewood, Kentucky

Roberta E. Siegel, MSW, LCSW
Perinatal Social Worker
Department of Pediatrics
The Children's Hospital
Denver, Colorado

B. J. Snell, PhD, CNM, WHCNP
Assistant Professor
Director, Midwifery and Women's Health Care
Department of Nursing
University of Southern California
Los Angeles, California

Alisa Starbuck, RNC, NNP, MSN
Neonatal Nurse Practitioner
Wake Forest University Baptist Medical Center
Winston-Salem, North Carolina

John D. Strain, MD, FACR
Professor of Radiology
University of Colorado Health Science Center
Chairman, Department of Radiology
The Children's Hospital
Denver, Colorado

Julie R. Swaney, MDiv
Coordinator, Department of Pastoral Care
Clinical Faculty, Department of Medicine
Clinical Faculty, Department of Psychiatry
University of Colorado Hospital
Denver, Colorado

Rita D Swinford, MD
Assistant Professor, Pediatrics
Medical Director, End Stage and Transplantation
Department of Pediatrics
University of Texas at Houston
Houston, Texas

Ellen Tappero, RNC, MN, NNP
Neonatal Nurse Practitioner
Special Care Nursery
Exampla Lutheran Medical Center
Wheat Ridge, Colorado

Susan F. Townsend, MD
Associate Professor
Section of Neonatology
University of Colorado Health Sciences Center
The Children's Hospital
Denver, Colorado

Barbara S. Turner, RN, DNSc, FAAN
Associate Dean for Research
Duke University School Nursing
Durham, North Carolina

Reginald Washington, MD
Chief of Staff
Mother and Child Hospital at Presbyterian/
    St. Luke Hospital
Western Cardiology, Pediatric Division
Denver, Colorado

**Susan M. Weiner, RN, C, MSN, PhD
(ABD)**
Nurse Manager, Postpartum/Newborn Nursery
Thomas Jefferson University Hospital
Philadelphia, Pennsylvania

Leonard E. Weisman, MD
Professor of Pediatrics
Head, Section of Neonatology
Baylor College of Medicine
Houston, Texas

Mary Wright, MSN, RNC
Instructor/Maternity Nursing
University of New Mexico, College of Nursing
Albuquerque, New Mexico

Jan Zimmer, RN, MSN
Vice President,
Patient Care Services
Christus Santa Rosa Health
San Antonio, Texas

To Bonnie, and our children and grandchildren with love
GBM

In memory of Stephanie Marie Garder, whose three days
of life did have a purpose
SLG

In Memoriam
L. Joseph Butterfield, MD
Lula O. Lubchenco, MD

Preface

The concept of the team approach is important in neonatal intensive care. Each health care professional must not only perform the duties of his or her own role but must also understand the roles of other involved professionals. Nurses, physicians, other health care professionals, and parents must work together in a coordinated and efficient manner to achieve optimal results for patients in the neonatal intensive care unit (NICU).

Because this team approach is so important in the field of neonatal intensive care, we believe it is necessary that this book contain input from both major fields of health care—medicine and nursing. Therefore a physician and a registered nurse have coedited it. In addition, both physicians and nurses and other health care professionals have contributed the chapters.

The book is divided into six parts, all of which have been reviewed, revised, and updated for the fifth edition. Part I presents evidence-based practice and the need to scientifically evaluate neonatal therapies, emphasizing randomized controlled trials as the ideal approach. Parts II through V are the clinical sections, and this edition contains several additions, including a new chapter on follow-up care and imaging of the neonate.

The combination of physiology and pathophysiology and separate emphasis on clinical application in this text is designed for neonatal intensive care nurses, nursing students, medical students, and pediatric, surgical, and family practice housestaff. This text is comprehensive enough for physicians and nurses, yet basic enough to be useful to all ancillary personnel.

Part VI presents the psychosocial aspects of neonatal care. It includes a new chapter on follow-up care. The medical, psychologic, and social aspects of providing care for the ill neonate and family are discussed. This section, in particular, will benefit social workers and clergy who frequently deal with family members of patients in the NICU. Of course, it will also be a valuable resource for all other involved health care professionals.

In this handbook we present physiologic principles and practical applications and point out areas as yet unresolved. Material that is clinically applicable is set in boldface type so that it can be easily identified.

Gerald B. Merenstein
Sandra L. Gardner

Contents

Introduction

THE GOALS OF NEONATAL INTENSIVE CARE

"What are the goals of neonatal intensive care for this patient?"

Most fundamental to the inquiry of what is best for an individual baby in the NICU, however the question may be phrased, is the ability to speak to the goals of care for the particular patient. These goals, although individualized for the patient's needs, must reach beyond the isolated clinical considerations of the health care professionals at work in the NICU environment. They must reflect a discernment and incorporation of those values and goals sought by the family on behalf of their newborn child, and they must be pursued within the context of more broadly held, but perhaps poorly expressed, societal goals for the provision of health care for women and infants.

Daily we may ask ourselves, or hear others around us asking, "Are we doing the right thing for this baby?" "What else can we do for this patient?" "Why are we doing this?" "Should we stop?" "What do the parents want?" "What are we trying to accomplish here?"

These questions raise issues that are central to our individual perception as valued health care professionals trying to serve patients, families, and a broader society. They call on us to address the values of our profession, ourselves, and those we serve. To ignore these issues is to fail to recognize their significance in shaping our professional lives and affecting our human interactions. But beyond that, failing to answer these questions will perpetrate our inability, or unwillingness, to responsibly address the value-laden charge we have to each other. **It is no small thing to profess the willingness to help a vulnerable and sick newborn; to devote our lives toward service; and to be educated and trained to practice our art with scientific rigor, technologic skill, and human caring, even in the face of medical uncertainty.** Ignoring these questions, however, will lead to moral uncertainty and quite possibly moral angst, causing us to do things against our own better judgement.

Despite well over a quarter of a century of providing "modern" neonatal intensive care, it is difficult to answer the questions regarding the goals of neonatal intensive care. This lies at the root of many of our problems in working through challenging cases and situations, as well as addressing parental and societal concerns. I do not believe that we can simply state our goals as "to save all babies" or "to reduce infant mortality."

Throughout the interactions of every health care professional in dealing with issues in the NICU, consideration should be given at all times to the goals of specific monitoring, diagnostic tests, therapies, or even research protocols that are part of what we do. **The goals of care should be patient- and family-centered. It is the patient we treat, but it is the family, of whatever construct, with whom the baby will go home. Indeed, it is the family who must live with the long-term consequences of our daily decisions in caring for their baby.**

The goals of neonatal intensive care include more than simple application of critical care technology (such as ventilators, monitors, medications, invasive devices, a multiplicity of laboratory measurements, etc.) to sick and premature newborn infants. **These goals include the provision of skilled professional care. An effective neonatal intensive care team consists of trained professionals of many disciplines—no one of us can do it alone. This care is, however, to be extended over a necessarily limited, rather than endless, period of time.**

The ends to which this care is provided include the initial stabilization of the newborn, and, ultimately, the facilitation of transition to normal, extrauterine, neonatal physiology. Obviously, this transition takes longer for some infants than others and my require significant intervention and support. Similarly, the reversal of acute disease processes such as infection and respiratory distress is a recognized end. Minimizing chronic or debilitating outcomes (including iatrogenic sequelae of applied neonatal intensive care) also falls within these goals. We need to recognize the potential impact of iatrogenic effects that include (1) the environment in which the baby is managed; (2) the mode of ventilation; (3) the types, doses, and effect of medications used; (4) the short- and long-term effects of certain procedures, foreign bodies, or devices used; and (5) ways to meet the baby's nutritional needs.

All of this care should be provided with a reasonable expectation of steady improvement. Care should proceed with the absence of excruciating pain and unnecessary suffering and develop toward a capacity for the newborn to enjoy and participate in the human experience over a life prolonged beyond infancy.

These goals seek to maintain a focus upon the best interests of the child. In determining the best interests of the child, the parents are generally considered to be the spokespersons. Hence, their opinions should be sought, values discerned, and goals considered.

Shared decision making should be the commonly employed process, requiring shared information among relevant health care professionals and a willingness and capability to effectively and regularly communicate with parents. This process also suggests the need for outcome data. Such data should be relevant to the population seeking care at a given institution. It is not always valid to rely on nationally reported data outside the local practice setting because both population and practices may neither be constituted no controlled in the same fashion that yours may be. Both the provision of care, decided upon by local clinical and population data, and determination of best interests—or what can be viewed as either effective, beneficial, and appropriate care versus ineffective, burdensome, or inappropriate care—demand the availability of data from which to make the determinations with parents. Until such data are available, we should be frank in recognizing and communicating some uncertainty in our decision-making process with parents.

From inquiries into "What are we doing?" let's move toward defining our goals for our patients. **Each patient's care should be based on his or her best interests, consonant with professional goals, societal norms, and institutional mission, through a process of mutually derived goals with the parents and/or family.** This requires time, thoughtful reflection, communication with families, and advocation for our patients' benefit. In so doing, the good with which we all seek to provide for our patients hopefully will become apparent to all concerned.

Brian S. Carter, MD

PART I

Evidence-Based Practice

1

Evidence-Based Clinical Practice Decisions

Miriam Orleans, Ellen Tappero, Anita Glicken, Gerald B. Merenstein

The rapid spread and high cost of new technologies have led practitioners to question the benefits of many clinical practices. As neonatal advocates, physicians, nurses, therapists, and parents hope that treatments will improve the health and future development of newborns. When clinical practices are widely diffused and accepted, it is difficult to raise challenging questions. Practitioners often assume that traditional clinical practices have been studied in appropriately selected populations of sufficient size to accurately inform clinicians of their efficacy, benefits, safety, side effects, and costs. Silverman has described how painfully slow the development of skepticism and the use of the scientific method and experimentation were until we reached our present views of how to ask and answer clinical questions[39]:

> Spectacular therapeutic disasters have made it clear that informal let's-try-it-and-see methods of testing new proposals are more risky now than ever before in history. Since there are no certainties in medicine, it must be understood that every clinical test of a new treatment is, by definition, a step into the unknown.

QUALITY OF EVIDENCE

As new therapies reach the marketplace and are quickly integrated into state-of-the-art practice, we must continue to increase our knowledge of the health and health problems of newborn infants. We must learn to overcome our impatience with uncertainty and ask questions about the quality of the evidence regarding the use and benefit of these new clinical practices. Questions arise with careful reading of our own research literature—questions that can best be answered by the careful design and conduct of clinical studies.

It is not the purpose of this chapter to review the various research designs that allow strong scientific inference. Rather, it is our purpose to (1) challenge our clinical observations and wisdom by subjecting them to systematic study and (2) encourage careful assessment of the research that supports or argues against the use of both new and older clinical practices.

Sinclair and Bracken[41] suggested four levels of clinical research used to evaluate safety and efficacy, based on their ability to provide an unbiased answer. In ascending order, these include (1) single case or case series reports without controls, (2) nonrandomized studies with historic controls, (3) nonrandomized studies with concurrent controls, and (4) randomized controlled trials (RCTs). An RCT is considered to be the strongest design for evaluating the effect of therapy. An RCT tests a hypothesis by using randomly assigned treatment and control groups of adequate size to test the efficacy and safety of the new treatment. Tyson[45] has suggested criteria for proven therapies (Box 1-1).

Clinical observations, although valuable in sharpening our questions, often are limited by selective perception—our wish to see a strategy work or fail to work. We also know that although in some situations we can learn a great deal from carefully maintained databases, such knowledge is gained only when we have formed these databases with clear intentions and have collected the necessary data. For a variety of good reasons, case-controlled and prospective studies with historic controls are sometimes the only feasible way to answer clinical questions.[20,26]

1

Box 1-1	PROVEN THERAPIES

Reported to be beneficial in a well-performed metaanalysis of all trials

or

Beneficial in at least one multicenter trial or two single-center trials

Modified from Tyson JE: Use of unproven therapies in clinical practice and research: how can we better serve our patients and their families? *Semin Perinatol* 19:98, 1995.

Commercial interests
Fee-for-service payment
Status protection
Fear of litigation
Need to use equipment or drugs
Need to fill beds, use techniques, fill buildings, or use personnel

Decision to intervene

"NEED"
Culture
Clinical experience
Client experience
Scientific evidence
Risk assessment
Tradition
Fashion
Place of care
Care provider

FIGURE 1-1   Pressures to intervene. (From Chalmers I: Scientific inquiry and authoritarianism in perinatal care and education, *Birth* 10:3, 1983.)

Although there is a rapidly growing point of view that RCTs provide the best scientific evidence on which to base clinical decisions, these investigations take time, and it is often difficult to overcome our impatience with delays in the introduction of promising innovative therapies.

PRESSURES TO INTERVENE

The pressure to intervene before studies are conducted or completed has many sources. Ian Chalmers,[10] in considering the struggle to gather scientific evidence in a climate of firmly held beliefs, has illustrated some of the pressures facing the scientific investigator (Figure 1-1). Unfortunately, the pressure to intervene often becomes an overriding reason not to conduct scientific studies.

Other authors have described various attitudes about controlled trials that have also inhibited their development. Bryce and Enkin[9] discussed myths about RCTs, which become reasons not to conduct such trials. Among such myths is the belief, often heard in clinical circles, that randomization is unethical. This may be true in some instances but not if there is poor evidence for adopting the commonly used strategy in the first place. To alternate a strategy whose benefit is not scientifically supported (but widely acclaimed) with one that is openly called "experimental" is not unethical; in fact, both are "experimental." It is the use of an unstudied intervention that might more readily be labeled "unethical."

The pressure to intervene is often overpowering. Believing that an infant is in trouble, we intervene; sometimes a cascade of interventions may follow,[32,35] one leading to the next, each carrying its own risk as well as benefit. One of the most frequently cited examples of this cascade is the epidemic of blindness associated with the use of oxygen in newborns. Silverman[38,39] detailed our experience with this therapy in two of his books. Oxygen, used since the early 1900s for resuscitation and treatment of cyanotic episodes, was noted in the 1940s to "correct" periodic breathing in premature infants. After World War II and the introduction of new gas-tight incubators, an epidemic of blindness occurred, resulting from retrolental fibroplasia (RLF). Silverman pointed out that although many causes were suspected, it was not until 1954 that a multicenter controlled trial confirmed the association between high oxygen concentration and RLF. Frequently forgotten, however, is that in subsequent years there was increased mortality in infants cared for in restricted oxygen environments, and many survivors had spastic diplegia. In the middle to late 1960s the introduction of microtechniques for measuring arterial oxygen permitted more rational monitoring of oxygen therapy, with a reduction in mortality, spastic diplegia, and RLF, now called *retinopathy of prematurity* (ROP). ROP is now usually limited to extremely low-birth-weight (ELBW) infants, and although ROP may not be preventable,[38] current research continues to explore other causes, preventive measures, and treatments (see Chapter 23).

The desire to see an intervention "work" permeates much of health care and research, encouraging both practitioners and investigators to seek early signs of improvement of problems. Neonatology is not alone in focusing on the short-term effects of an intervention immediately after its introduction. Long-term effects of treatment are rarely sought for several reasons. The ultimate results of our interventions and studies may not have been foreseen.

Consider the unfortunate effects of diethylstilbestrol (DES). For many years, hormones such as DES were given to pregnant women to prevent mis-

Table 1-1	EFFECTS OF DIETHYLSTILBESTROL (DES) ON PREGNANCY OUTCOMES	
	TYPICAL ODDS RATIO*	95% CONFIDENCE LIMITS
Miscarriage	1.20	0.89-1.62
Stillbirth	0.95	0.50-1.83
Neonatal death	1.31	0.74-2.34
All three	1.38	0.99-1.92
Prematurity	1.47	1.08-2.00

Modified from Goldstein PA, Sacks HS, Chalmers TC: Hormone administration for the maintenance of pregnancy. In Chalmers I, Enkin M, Kerse M, eds: *Effective care in pregnancy and childbirth*, New York, 1989, Oxford University Press.

*An odds ratio is an estimate of the likelihood (or odds) of being affected by an exposure (e.g., a drug or treatment), compared with the odds of having that outcome without having been exposed. Women receiving DES did not have fewer stillbirths or miscarriages than women who were untreated. The only statistically significant improvement that was seen was in the reduction of prematurity.

carriage, fetal death, preterm delivery, and other adverse outcomes of pregnancy. In the 1950s the use of DES in pregnant women was thought to be effective after several uncontrolled studies. Controlled trials conducted during that same time period were the subject of an overview (metaanalysis) by Goldstein, Sacks, and Chalmers[21] (Table 1-1). Clearly, DES was not effective, but it continued to be offered to pregnant women until the 1970s, when the FDA finally disapproved its use. Children of mothers who were given DES have been found to have genital tract abnormalities, including vaginal adenosis; vaginal adenocarcinoma; decreased female fertility; and structural abnormalities of the cervix, vagina, uterus, and ovaries. Male children have epididymal cysts, hypotrophic testes, and relative infertility.

Chalmers[14] noted that this was not the only time that physicians have ignored the evidence and continued to use therapies that have been shown in RCTs to be of no benefit. The costs of long-term studies or of follow-up surveillance are greater than those of short-term investigations. However, when delayed effects or effects that are measurable only later in the life of the child (psychologic problems, inability to function well in school, and so on) are likely, cost should not be the determining factor in selection of a study design.

Even when practitioners are assured that randomized trials show successful outcomes, often unanswered questions remain: Will a technology or treatment have the same effect in all settings? Has an "appropriate" target population been selected? Are there short-term side effects? Are there long-term foreseeable consequences?

EVALUATION OF THERAPIES

The major cause of death in premature infants is respiratory failure resulting from RDS (see Chapter 23). Previously called *idiopathic respiratory distress syndrome* (IRDS) or *hyaline membrane disease* (HMD), this syndrome was a mystery only 25 years ago. The patient with IRDS was a premature infant in respiratory distress with expiratory grunting, nasal flaring, chest wall retractions, and cyanosis that could or could not be ameliorated with high oxygen concentrations.[39] The evaluation of various therapies for respiratory distress syndrome (RDS) contrasts the value of controlled and uncontrolled trials.

Sinclair[40] evaluated the popular methods of treatment of these patients in 1966. He noted that the most popular treatments were more frequently thought to be beneficial in uncontrolled studies than in controlled trials. In 19 uncontrolled studies, 17 showed "benefit." In 18 controlled studies only 9 demonstrated benefit. An untrained reviewer of the research may have based clinical practice on the faulty conclusions of the uncontrolled trials, thereby jeopardizing patient outcome.

Surfactant Therapy

In contrast to many of the proposed treatments, surfactant therapy in premature infants has been well studied in randomized controlled trials. These studies have evaluated the use of surfactant in the treatment of RDS, including the optimal source and composition of surfactant and prophylactic versus rescue treatment. Within these studies, premature infant morbidity (including pneumothorax, periventricular and/or intraventricular hemorrhage, bronchopulmonary dysplasia [BPD], and patent ductus arteriosus) and mortality rates in the treatment and control groups have been compared. In an overview of surfactant RCTs, Soll[42] noted increased survival rates, improved oxygenation and ventilation, and a decrease in the incidence of pneumothorax. Effects on BPD were unclear. There appeared to be no difference in outcomes when rescue and prophylactic treatments were compared (Table 1-2).

RCTs involving thousands of newborns have clearly demonstrated the benefits of surfactant

Table 1-2	MORTALITY AFTER PROPHYLACTIC SURFACTANT COMPARED WITH SURFACTANT TREATMENTS			
AUTHOR	PROPHYLACTIC	TREATMENT	RELATIVE RISK*	95% CONFIDENCE INTERVAL
Dunn	9/62	8/60	1.09	0.45,2.65
Kendig	29/235	49/244	0.62	0.62,0.94
Merritt	29/102	23/101	1.25	0.78,2.00
Typical Effect			0.85	0.63,1.14

Modified from Soll RF, McQueen MC: Respiratory distress syndrome. In Sinclair JC, Bracken MB, eds: *Effective care of the newborn infant,* Oxford, England, 1992, Oxford University Press.

*In this table it can be seen that mortality was not different when the results of the two treatments were compared. None of the relative risk estimates were statistically significant.

therapy in RDS. However, some unanswered questions remain, and further research is needed to define the optimal dose, optimal number of treatments, and most efficacious formulation.

Thyrotropin-Releasing Hormone Therapy

To further reduce the incidence of RDS and chronic lung disease in very low–birth-weight (VLBW) infants, investigators sought to determine the efficacy and safety of thyrotropin-releasing hormone (TRH) as an additional prenatal treatment. Several early studies concluded that antenatal TRH and corticosteroid administration reduced the risk of neonatal respiratory distress.[1,6,29,33] However, one of the largest randomized controlled trials conducted in Australia found that the TRH-treated group had an increased risk of RDS and a need for ventilation. TRH administration was also associated with maternal nausea, vomiting, and a rise in maternal blood pressure.[4] Why the sharp contrast in findings between these clinical trials? When examining the treatment procedures used in these studies, one notes that the Australian investigators administered a lower dose of TRH (200 µg rather than 400 µg) and gave it less frequently than in the other trials (every 12 hours rather than every 8 hours). Could this account for the discrepancies in efficacy and safety of the drug? Further clinical studies have searched for an answer to this question. In two recent double-blind, placebo-controlled trials, TRH was given intravenously in four doses of 400 µg each at 8-hour intervals to women in preterm labor; investigators found no differences in efficacy between the treatment groups and placebo groups. There were no differences in the incidence of respiratory distress

syndrome, chronic lung disease, or neonatal mortality.[5,16] In an overview of prenatal TRH by Crowther, Alfirevic, and Haslam,[18] data were reviewed from 11 clinical trials that included 4500 women. These authors concluded that "prenatal TRH, in addition to corticosteroids, did not reduce the risk of neonatal respiratory disease, chronic oxygen dependency or improve fetal, neonatal, or childhood outcome in any outcomes assessed by intention-to-treat analysis." Based on currently available evidence, administration of prenatal TRH is not recommended for clinical use to reduce the severity of RDS and the risk of neonatal mortality.

Corticosteroid Therapy

Does the benefit outweigh the risks? The use of corticosteroids in perinatal medicine illustrates potential failures in the practice of evidence-based medicine. Historically, antenatal steroids were rarely used to prevent RDS despite strong evidence to support this use, demonstrating **a failure to use a proven therapy.**[30] More recently, repeated doses of antenatal steroids have been widely used despite a lack of evidence for efficacy and questions about safety.[3] **This represents the unproven use of a proven therapy.** Administration of postnatal steroids has also been widely prescribed, despite evidence that questions their efficacy and suggests significant harm, illustrating **the use of an uncertain therapy.**

Antenatal Corticosteroid Therapy: Single Course

Not only have treatment methods for RDS been examined, but also methods to prevent RDS have come under close scrutiny. Antenatal administration of corticosteroids to pregnant women who threatened to deliver prematurely was first shown in 1972 to decrease the neonatal mortality rate and the incidence of RDS and intraventricular hemorrhage (IVH) in premature infants.[30] In 1990 Crowley, Chambers, and Keirse[17] used metaanalysis to evaluate 12 randomized controlled trials of maternal corticosteroid administration involving more than 3000 women. Their data showed that maternal corticosteroid treatment significantly reduced the risk of neonatal mortality, RDS, and IVH. After two decades of published clinical trials[15,17,26] and the consensus development conference statement on "Effects of Corticosteroids for Fetal Maturation on Perinatal Outcomes" (1994), antenatal steroids have been shown to be effective and safe in enhancing fetal lung maturity and reducing neonatal mortality.[34]

Antenatal Corticosteroid Therapy: Repeated Courses

Repeat courses of antenatal corticosteroids have been administered to both humans and animals. Findings in animals include improved surfactant pools and lung function but adverse effects on lung structure, somatic growth, and adrenocorticoid function.[22] An NIH Consensus Development Conference revisited the use of antenatal steroids in humans and found that there were limited quality studies on the use of repeated courses of antenatal steroids. The report noted a possible decrease in the incidence and severity of RDS and patent ductus arteriosus but also noted an increase in maternal infection and suppressed hypothalamic pituitary adrenal function. Fetal risks included decreased somatic and brain growth, adrenal suppression, increased neonatal sepsis, and increased chronic lung disease and mortality.[3] From these findings it is clear that repeated courses of antenatal corticosteroids should be limited at this point to well-designed randomized controlled trials.

Postnatal Steroid Therapy

Although administration of postnatal steroids has been shown in some studies to improve survival and decrease ventilator time, PDA, and chronic lung disease, there are also significant problems with their use.[23-25,43,44] In RCTs they have been shown to lead to short-term problems, such as gastrointestinal (GI) perforation, sepsis, periventricular leukomalacia (PVL), and long-term problems, including decreased somatic and head growth, and abnormal neurodevelopmental outcome, including cerebral palsy (CP).[19,28]

A recent RCT has documented the increased risk of sepsis.[44] This should have been anticipated as this risk was first identified in an RCT by Reese et al[37] nearly 50 years ago. If postnatal steroids are to be used, studies must be done to determine dose, timing, duration, type of steroid, benefits, and risks, including long-term neurodevelopmental outcome.

Extracorporeal Membrane Oxygenation Therapy

Although extracorporeal membrane oxygenation (ECMO) was first reported for use in infants in 1976, it was not until 1984 that a randomized trial was reported.[7,8] Another "controlled" trial was reported in 1989.[36] Some care providers questioned the results of these trials based on sample size and study design. In 1990 the Committee on Fetus and Newborn of the American Academy of Pediatrics noted the expansion of ECMO centers and cautioned that its use should be limited to research centers.[2] Neither those who believed in the benefits nor those who argued against its use could turn to clear, sufficient evidence to support their views. In 1993 a multicenter trial was organized in 83 collaborating British hospitals with the help of the Clinical Trial Service Unit at Oxford.[46] Mature infants with severe respiratory failure were randomly assigned either to one of five treatment centers or to continuing conventional care in the hospital in which they were born. Each treatment center was experienced in the provision of long-term ventilatory support and capable of conducting cardiologic assessment, echocardiography, cranial ultrasonography, ECMO, and the care required for infants with severe respiratory failure. The benefit of ECMO was so clear that the external committee monitoring the data recommended that the trial be halted. Of the 93 infants assigned to ECMO, 30 died, compared with 52 of the 92 neonates receiving conventional care. This difference in outcome meant that there was one extra survivor for every three or four infants assigned to ECMO care. This well-conducted single study was able to diminish the uncertainty regarding the use of ECMO. The example illustrates the way in which good studies resolve knotty problems.

SYSTEMATIC REVIEW IN PERINATAL MEDICINE

Chalmers and Sinclair[12] conducted a rather disconcerting analysis of the perinatal literature many years ago. When they considered perinatal trials as a proportion of all publications in selected obstetric, pediatric, anesthetic, and general journals published between 1966 and 1980, they found that reports of randomized trials were remarkably infrequent when compared with the attention given to other forms of study and commentary (Table 1-3).

Believing that the results of perinatal controlled trials had to be summarized in a manner useful to practitioners, Chalmers et al[13] and other perinatal professionals from various countries developed a registry of randomized controlled trials. They reviewed a vast amount of literature for published trials, sought out unpublished trials, and encouraged those who had begun, but not completed, studies to make them known to the registry. Once gathered, the studies' findings were summarized in "overviews."

A systematic review (or metaanalysis) pools the results of independently conducted RCTs whose study methods are reasonably similar, both in the selection and characteristics of participants and in the treatments that are offered. The results produce unbiased estimates of the effect of an intervention on clinical outcomes and are distinguished from nonsystematic reviews, in which author opinions are often reported along with the evidence. Tables 1-1 and 1-2 were developed after pooling the results of different studies.

From these systematic reviews, practitioners can learn of the strength or weakness of support for a claim of benefit or ill effect of a strategy. The result of Chalmers', Enkin's, and Keirse's efforts was a remarkably useful book, *Effective Care in Pregnancy and Childbirth*.[13] At the end of this book, Chalmers, Enkin, and Keirse reported their own views of the treatments reviewed based on conclusions formed in the preceding articles. They found that although some strategies and forms of care were very useful, others were of questionable value. Some interventions believed to be useful are in fact not useful— sometimes of little benefit, or, in fact, even harmful. In 1992 a companion publication, *Effective Care of the Newborn Infant*,[41] compiled and reviewed neonatal RCTs.

About the same time the Cochrane Collaboration was established, again largely through the efforts of Ian Chalmers. The Cochrane Collaboration is a worldwide group with about 30 Collaborative Review Groups who prepare, maintain, and disseminate systematic reviews mainly based on the results of randomized controlled trials. These reviews are published electronically in the Cochrane Library, which contains the Cochrane Database of Systematic Reviews, along with editorial comments on these reviews. In addition to the Collaborative Review Groups, there are now 12 Cochrane Centers in the world. These centers provide support for the review groups. The Perinatal Medicine Neonatal Review Group is based at McMaster University in Hamilton, Ontario, Canada, and the Pregnancy and Childbirth Review Group is based at Liverpool Women's Hospital, Liverpool, England. The Cochrane Neonatal reviews are available at the NICHD Cochrane Neonatal Internet home page; more than 100 overviews are currently listed.[31]

Multiple networks have been developed to perform multicenter RCTs. This is particularly useful, providing an opportunity to see whether treatments have similar effects in different practice settings. It is also useful in that practitioners in individual settings may not always see enough cases to reach robust conclusions. Rare conditions and rare outcomes are better understood when trials are replicated or their findings are pooled. Systematic reviews provide the opportunity to understand these findings in the context of clinical practice. To use these resources, individuals must become familiar with the principles and value of evidence-based patient care. Although evidence-based medicine can be practiced successfully at the individual level, an individual clinician can also act as a change agent and advocate for evidence-based institutional practice.

As stated by Silverman,[39] "Since ours is the only species on the planet that has achieved rates of newborn survival which exceed 90 percent, it seems to me we must demand the highest order of evidence possible before undertaking widespread actions that may affect the full lifetimes of individuals in the present as well as in future generations. Here a

Table 1-3	CONTROLLED TRIALS IN PERINATAL MEDICINE AS A PERCENTAGE OF ALL PUBLICATIONS IN SELECTED JOURNALS: 1966-1980		
JOURNALS	1966-1970	1971-1975	1976-1980
5 Obstetric	1.7	1.6	3.0
5 Pediatric	0.9	1.0	1.6
5 Anesthetic	0.5	0.8	0.8
6 General	0.2	0.1	0.2

Modified from Chalmers I, Sinclair JC: Promoting perinatal health: is it time for a change of emphasis in research? *Early Hum Dev* 10:171, 1985.

strong case can be made for a slow and measured pace of medical innovations."

REFERENCES

1. Althabe F, Fustinana C, Athabe O et al: Controlled trial of prenatal betamethosone plus TRH vs betamethasone plus placebo for prevention of RDS in preterm infants, *Pediatr Res* 29:200, 1991 (abstract 1186).
2. American Academy of Pediatrics, Committee on Fetus and Newborn: Recommendations on extracorporeal membrane oxygenation, *Pediatrics* 85:618, 1990.
3. Antenatal corticosteroids revisited: repeat courses, NIH Consensus Statement 2000 August 17:1, 2000.
4. Australian collaborative trial of antenatal thyrotropin-releasing hormone (ACTOBAT) for prevention of neonatal respiratory disease, *Lancet* 345:877, 1995.
5. Ballard RA, Ballard PL, Cnaan A et al: Antenatal thyrotropin-releasing hormone to prevent lung disease in preterm infants. North American Thyrotropin-Releasing Hormone Study Group, *N Engl J Med* 338:493, 1998.
6. Ballard RA, Ballard PL, Creasy RK et al: Respiratory disease in very-low-birthweight infants after prenatal thyrotopin-releasing hormone and glucocorticoid, *Lancet* 339:510, 1992.
7. Bartlett RH, Gazzaniga AB, Jeffries MR et al: Extracorporeal membrane oxygenation (ECMO) cardiopulmonary support in infancy, *Trans Am Soc Artif Intern Organs* 22:80, 1976.
8. Bartlett RH, Roloff DW, Cornell RG et al: Extracorporeal circulation in neonatal respiratory failure: a prospective randomized study, *Pediatrics* 76:479, 1985.
9. Bryce RL, Enkin MW: Six months about controlled trials in perinatal medicine, *Am J Obstet Gynecol* 151:6, 1985.
10. Chalmers I: Scientific inquiry and authoritarianism in perinatal care and education, *Birth* 10:3, 1983.
11. Chalmers I, ed: *Oxford database of perinatal trials,* Oxford, England, 1988, Oxford University Press.
12. Chalmers I, Sinclair JC: Promoting perinatal health: is it time for a change of emphasis in research? *Early Hum Dev* 10:171, 1985.
13. Chalmers I, Enkin M, Keirse M: *Effective care in pregnancy and childbirth,* New York, 1989, Oxford University Press.
14. Chalmers T: The impact of controlled trials on the practice of medicine, *Mt Sinai J Med* 41:753, 1974.
15. Collaborative Group on Antenatal Steroid Therapy: Effect of antenatal dexamethasone administration on the prevention of respiratory distress syndrome, *Am J Obstet Gynecol* 141:276, 1981.
16. Collaborative trial of prenatal thyrotropin-releasing hormone and corticosteroids for prevention of respiratory distress syndrome. Collaborative Santiago Surfactant group, *Am J Obstet Gynecol* 178(1 Pt 1):33, 1998
17. Crowley P, Chambers I, Keirse MJNC: The effects of corticosteroid administration before preterm delivery: an overview of the evidence from controlled trials, *Br J Obstet Gynaecol* 97:11, 1990.
18. Crowther CA, Alfirevic Z, Haslam RR: Prenatal thyrotropin-releasing hormone for preterm birth (Cochrane Review). In The Cochrane Library, Issue 3, Oxford, England, 2000, Update Software.
19. Finer NN, Craft A, Vaucher YE et al: Postnatal steroids: short-term gain, long-term pain? *J Pediatr* 137:9, 2000.
20. Fletcher RH, Fletcher SW, Wagner EH: *Clinical epidemiology,* ed 2, Baltimore, 1988, Williams & Wilkins.
21. Goldstein PA, Sacks HS, Chalmers TC: Hormone administration for the maintenance of pregnancy. In Chalmers I, Enkin M, Keirse M, eds: *Effective care in pregnancy and childbirth,* New York, 1989, Oxford University Press.
22. Grover TR, Ackerman KG, LeCras TD et al: Repetitive prenatal glucocorticoids increase lung endothelial nitric oxide synthase expression in ovine fetuses delivered at term, *Pediatr Res* 48:75, 2000.
23. Halliday HL, Ehrenkranz RA: Early postnatal (<96 hours) corticosteroids for preventing chronic lung disease in preterm infants, update 11/2000. http://www.nichd.nih.gov/cochrane/Halliday3/Halliday.htm
24. Halliday HL, Ehrenkranz RA: Moderately early (7-14 days) postnatal corticosteroids for preventing chronic lung disease in preterm infants, update 11/2000. http://www.nichd.nih.gov/cochrane/Halliday2/Halliday.htm
25. Halliday HL, Ehrenkranz RA: Delayed (>3 weeks) postnatal corticosteroids for preventing chronic lung disease in preterm infants, update 2/2001. http://www.nichd.nih.gov/cochrane/Halliday4/Halliday.htm
26. Hulley SB, Cummings SB: *Designing clinical research,* Baltimore, 1988, Williams & Wilkins.
27. Jobe AH: Glucocorticoids in perinatal medicine: misguided rockets? *J Pediatr* 137:1, 2000.
28. Jobe AH, Mitchell BR, Gunkel JH: Beneficial effects of the combined use of prenatal corticosteroids and postnatal surfactant on preterm infants, *Am J Obstet Gynecol* 168:508, 1993.
29. Knight DB, Liggins GC, Wealthall SR: A randomized controlled trial of antepartum thyrotropin-releasing hormone and betamethasone in the prevention of respiratory disease in preterm infants, *Am J Obstet Gynecol* 171:11, 1994.
30. Liggins GC, Howie RN: A controlled trial of antepartum glucocorticoid treatment for prevention of the respiratory distress syndrome in premature infants, *Pediatrics* 50:515, 1972.

31. Mold JW, Stein HF: The cascade effect in the clinical care of patients, *N Engl J Med* 314:512, 1986.
32. National Institute of Child Health and Human Development: Cochrane Neonatal home page. http://www.nichd.nig.gov/cochrane.
33. National Institutes of Health Consensus Development Conference Statement: Effects of corticosteroids for fetal maturation on perinatal outcomes, *JAMA* 273:413, 1995.
34. Morales WI, O'Brien WF, Angel JL et al: Fetal lung maturation: the combined use of corticosteroids and thyrotropin-releasing hormone, *Obstet Gynecol* 73:111, 1989.
35. Orleans M, Haverkamp AD: Are there health risks in using risking systems? The case of perinatal risk assessment, *Health Policy* 7:297, 1987.
36. O'Rourke PP, Crone RK, Vacanti JP et al: Extracorporeal membrane oxygenation and conventional medical therapy in neonates with persistent pulmonary hypertension of the newborn: a prospective randomized study, *Pediatrics* 84:957, 1989.
37. Reese AB, Blodi FC, Locke JC et al: Results of use of corticotropin (ACTH) in treatment of retrolental fibroplasia, *AMA Arch Ophthalmol* 47:551, 1952.
38. Silverman WA: *RLF: a modern parable,* New York, 1980, Grune & Stratton.
39. Silverman WA: *Human experimentation: a guided step into the unknown,* New York, 1985, Oxford University Press.
40. Sinclair JC: Preventions and treatment of respiratory distress syndrome, *Pediatr Clin North Am* 13:711, 1966.
41. Sinclair JC, Bracken MB: *Effective care of the newborn infant,* New York, 1992, Oxford University Press.
42. Soll RF: Overviews of surfactant treatment. In Chalmers I, ed: *Oxford database of perinatal trials,* version 1.2, records 5206, 5207, 5252, 5253, 5664, 5675, Oxford, England, 1991, Oxford University Press.
43. Stark AR, Carlo WA, Tyson JE et al: Adverse effects of early dexamethasone treatment on extremely low-birth-weight infants, *N Engl J Med* 344:95, 2001
44. Stoll BJ, Temprosa M, Tyson JE et al: Dexamethasone therapy increases infection in very low birth weight infants, *Pediatrics* 104:63, 1999
45. Tyson JE: Use of unproven therapies in clinical practice and research: how can we better serve our patients and their families? *Semin Perinatol* 19:98, 1995.
46. UK Collaborative ECMO Trial Group: UK Collaborative trial of neonatal extracorporeal membrane oxygenation, *Lancet* 348:75, 1996.

EVIDENCE-BASED MEDICINE RESOURCES

WEB SITES

Centers for Health Evidence
    http://www.cche.net/ebm/userguid/
Directory of EBM sites
    http://www.shef.ac.uk/uni/academic/R-Z/scharr/ir/netting.html
EBM Toolbox
    http://cebm.jur2.ox.ac.uk/docs/toolbox.html
Evidence-Based Medicine: What It Is and What It Isn't
    http://cebm.jr2.ox.ac.uk/embisisnt.html
Health Information Research Unit (HIRU)
    http://hiru.mcmaster.ca/default.htm
User's Guide to Evidence Based Practice
    http://www.cche.net/principles/content_all.asp
User's Guide to the Medical Literature Bibliography
    http://medicine.ucsf.edu/resources/guidelines/users.html

TEXTS

Friedland DJ, Go AS, Davoren JB, et al: *Evidence-based medicine: a framework for clinical practice,* Stamford, Conn, 1998, Appleton-Lange.
Greenhalgh, T: *How to read a paper: the basics of evidence based medicine,* London, 1997, BMJ Publishing Group.
Riegelman RK: Studying a study and testing a test: how to read the medical evidence, Boston, 1999, Little, Brown.
Sackett DL, Richardson WS, Rosenberg W et al: *Evidence-based medicine: how to practice and teach EBM,* Edinburgh, 2000, Churchill Livingstone.

ARTICLES

Bergman DA: Section 1: Evidence-based quality improvement, principles and perspectives; Evidence-based guidelines and critical pathways for quality improvement *Pediatrics* 103:225, 1999.
Halliday HL: Systematic reviews in perinatal medicine, *J Perinat Med* 27:41, 1999.
Soll RF, Andruscavage LA: Section 1: Evidence-based quality improvement, principles, and perspectives; The principles and practice of evidence-based neonatology, *Pediatrics* 103:215, 1999.

PART II

SUPPORT OF THE NEONATE

2 | Prenatal Environment: Effect on Neonatal Outcome

Gary M. Joffe, Mary Wright

The human fetus develops within a complex setting. Structurally defined by the intrauterine/intraamniotic compartment, the character of the prenatal environment is largely determined by maternal variables. The fetus is absolutely dependent on the maternal host for respiratory and nutritive support and is significantly influenced by maternal metabolic, cardiovascular, and environmental factors. In addition, the fetus is limited in its ability to adapt to stress or modify its surroundings. This creates a situation in which the prenatal environment exerts a tremendous influence on fetal development and well-being. This influence lasts well beyond the period of gestation, often affecting the newborn in ways that have profound significance for both immediate and long-term outcome.

There is great utility in identifying maternal factors that adversely affect the condition of the fetus. Providers of obstetric care have long used this information to identify the "at-risk" population and to design interventions that prevent or reduce the occurrence of fetal and neonatal complications. It is equally important that neonatal care providers obtain a clear picture of the prenatal environment and use this information before delivery to anticipate the newborn's immediate needs and make appropriate preparations for resuscitation and initial nursery care. After delivery, an awareness of the likely sequelae of environmental compromise helps to focus ongoing assessment and aids in clinical problem solving.

The purpose of this chapter is to help neonatal care providers to evaluate maternal influences on the prenatal environment, identify significant environmental compromise, and anticipate the associated neonatal problems. Information on the assessment and treatment of specific neonatal problems is provided throughout this text and is not repeated here. For a more extensive discussion of perinatal physiology and complicated pregnancies, refer to the references cited within this chapter.

PHYSIOLOGY

Two variables have a critical influence on fetal well-being throughout gestation: placental function and the inherent maternal resources. The interplay of these factors is a major determinant of fetal oxygenation, metabolism, and growth.

The placenta has a dual role in providing nutrients and metabolic "fuels" to the fetus. First, placental secretion of endocrine hormones, chiefly human chorionic somatomammotropin (HCS), increases throughout pregnancy, causing progressive changes in maternal metabolism. The net effect of these changes is an increase in maternal glucose and amino acids available to the fetus, especially in the second half of pregnancy. Second, the placenta is instrumental in the transfer of these (and other) essential nutrients from the maternal to the fetal circulation and, conversely, of metabolic wastes from the fetal to the maternal system.

Fetal "respiration" also depends on adequate placental function. Respiratory gases (oxygen and carbon dioxide) readily cross the placental membrane by simple diffusion, with the rate of diffusion determined by the P_{O_2} (or P_{CO_2}) differential between maternal and fetal blood.

Although the placenta mediates the transport of respiratory gases, carbohydrates, lipids, vitamins, minerals, and amino acids, it is the maternal "reservoir" that is their source. Maternal-fetal transfer depends on the characteristics and absolute content of substances within the maternal circulation, the relative efficiency of the maternal cardiovascular system in perfusing the placenta, and the function of the placenta itself.[148] The fetal environment can be disrupted by inappropriate types or amounts of substances in the maternal circulation, decreases or interruptions in placental blood flow, or abnormalities in placental function.

COMPROMISED FETAL ENVIRONMENT

Maternal Disease
Diabetes
The prevalence of diabetes mellitus and gestational diabetes mellitus (GDM) is increasing worldwide. Approximately 1.4% to 12.3% of pregnant women in the United States are diagnosed with GDM annually.[7,8] Despite major reductions in mortality over the past several decades, the infant of a diabetic mother (IDM) continues to have a considerable perinatal disadvantage. The physiologic changes in maternal glucose utilization that accompany pregnancy, coupled with either a preexisting hyperglycemia (as found in types I and II diabetes) or an inability to mount an appropriate insulin response (as seen in patients with gestational diabetes) results in a fetal environment that is significantly abnormal as a result of the increased level of maternal glucose, often in concert with episodic hypoglycemia and ketone exposure. Early in pregnancy this environment may have a teratogenic effect on the embryo, accounting for the dramatic increase in congenital malformations in the offspring of diabetic women with poor metabolic control.[52,67,137] During the second and third trimesters the mechanics of placental transport dictate that fetal glucose levels depend on, but are slightly less than, maternal levels.[8,118] Assuming adequate placental function and perfusion, elevations in maternal glucose lead to fetal hyperglycemia and increased fetal insulin production. Repeated or continued elevations in blood glucose result in fetal hyperinsulinism, alterations in the utilization of glucose and other nutrients, and altered patterns of growth and development.[8,67,118] **Fetal macrosomia (greater than the 90th percentile for weight) occurs in 25% to 42% of pregnancies in diabetic women.** Macrosomic infants of diabetic women suf-

fer increased morbidity and mortality from unexplained death in utero, birth trauma, hypertrophic cardiomyopathy, vascular thrombosis, neonatal hypoglycemia, hyperbilirubinemia, erythrocytosis, and respiratory distress.[73] In macrosomic infants, shoulder dystocia during vaginal birth is associated with increased incidence of brachial plexus injury. However, brachial plexus injury does have other causes in addition to shoulder dystocia and may result from an abnormality during the antepartum or intrapartum period.[55]

In addition to the basic metabolic disturbances, diabetes predisposes the woman to several other complications, including hypertension, preeclampsia, renal disease, and vascular compromise.[9] Various complications of diabetes are also associated with fetal and neonatal problems, including prematurity, growth restriction, chronic hypoxia, cardiovascular problems, RDS, and intrauterine demise. In terms of predicting perinatal morbidity and mortality, the "prognostically bad signs of pregnancy," first identified by Pedersen in the 1960s, are especially significant. **The occurrence of any of these signs, which include diabetic ketoacidosis, pregnancy-induced hypertension, pyelonephritis, and maternal noncompliance, continue to be useful predictors of increased fetal and neonatal risk.**[35,118]

In preparing for the delivery of an IDM, the neonatal team should consider the classification of maternal diabetes (type I or II, or a gestational diabetic mother), the quality of metabolic control throughout the pregnancy and labor, maternal complications, and the duration of the pregnancy, along with indicators of fetal growth and well-being. Table 2-1 summarizes key maternal factors, their environmental implications, and the fetal and neonatal outcomes associated with diabetes in pregnancy.

Thyroid Disease
The thyroid hormones triiodothyronine (T_3) and thyroxine (T_4) cross the placenta in small amounts only. The significance of this transfer is unclear. Iodine is readily transferred from mother to fetus. The fetal thyroid gland concentrates iodine and synthesizes its own hormones as early as 10 to 12 weeks' gestation; this is independent of maternal thyroid function. Severe maternal hypothyroidism often results in infertility. Mild maternal hypothyroidism has been associated with decreased IQ in the offspring and so must be treated during pregnancy. More severe hypothyroidism has been linked to ges-

Table 2-1	**MATERNAL DIABETES, THE PRENATAL ENVIRONMENT, AND PERINATAL OUTCOME**	
MATERNAL FACTORS	**ENVIRONMENTAL IMPLICATIONS**	**FETAL AND NEONATAL CONSEQUENCES**
Hyperglycemia		
Early	Exposure to elevated glucose levels during organogenesis	Increased incidence of congenital anomalies
Late	Availability of excess glucose, which leads to fetal hyperinsulinism, abnormal growth, and delayed surfactant production	Macrosomia, organomegaly, trauma during delivery, neonatal hypoglycemia, increased incidence of respiratory distress syndrome (RDS), polycythemia secondary to hypoxemia
Ketoacidosis	Fetal exposure to excess glucose and ketones, which can result in fetal diabetic ketoacidosis[67]	Fetal hypoxemia, intrauterine fetal demise
Hypertension, cardio-vascular, and renal disease	Placental insufficiency secondary to vascular compromise, which results in diminished fetal oxygenation and nutrition	Growth restriction, fetal asphyxia, intrauterine fetal demise, prematurity
	Increased incidence of maternal urinary tract infections	Prematurity, RDS, sepsis

tational hypertension, prematurity, and low birth weight.[82] Treatment with replacement hormone is well tolerated by the fetus and reduces these risks.[99,103,119]

Maternal hyperthyroidism presents a different situation. Thyroid-stimulating antibodies, commonly found in patients with Graves' disease, as well as many of the drugs used to treat hyperthyroidism, cross the placenta and can have a significant effect on the fetus. Antibodies, including long-acting thyroid stimulant (LATS) and thyroid-stimulating immunoglobulin (TSI), can cause an increase in fetal thyroid hormone production. High levels are associated with fetal and neonatal hyperthyroidism.[99,157] Untreated maternal thyrotoxicosis has been linked to preterm delivery, low birth weight, and stillbirths.[32] In rare cases the offspring of women with Graves' disease may themselves have this condition. In fetuses and newborns, this is evidenced by elevations in heart rate, growth restriction, goiter, and congestive heart failure. Perinatal mortality is high.[118] Administration of antithyroid medication to the mother can decrease thyroid hormone production in both the mother and the fetus but may result in fetal hypothyroidism and goiter.[32]

Another maternal antibody, thyroid-stimulating hormone (TSH)–binding inhibitor immunoglobulin, also crosses the placenta and can prevent the expected fetal thyroid response to TSH. The result is a transient fetal and neonatal hypothyroidism.[94,99,157] Iodine deficiency in the mother is another cause of fetal and neonatal hypothyroidism and, in its severe form, leads to cretinism because of the fetus's dependence on maternal iodine reserves.[64]

Phenylketonuria

Phenylketonuria (PKU) is a genetic disorder in which an enzymatic defect precludes conversion of the essential amino acid phenylalanine to tyrosine. This metabolic derangement is evidenced by an accumulation of excessive amounts of phenylalanine in the blood and its subsequent excretion in the urine of affected persons. Historically, PKU resulted in virtually certain mental retardation; affected individuals were often institutionalized and rarely reproduced. With the advent of widespread neonatal screening and effective dietary treatment to prevent hyperphenylalaninemia during infancy and early childhood, genetically affected persons may now avoid the devastating effects of this disease, have relatively normal development, and become pregnant. However, even in women who were treated in childhood and are developmentally normal, maternal PKU poses a significant environmental risk for their fetuses. The care of these women and their infants presents a unique perinatal challenge.

The offspring of women with PKU are frequently microcephalic and mentally retarded. They also have an increased incidence of growth restriction and congenital cardiac defects regardless of whether they are themselves affected with PKU.[79,80] The problem arises because although current recommendations are to maintain a low phenylalanine diet for life to avoid progressive deterioration and an increased risk of blindness, many phenylketonuric individuals remain on this diet only through early childhood. However, during pregnancy elevated levels of phenylalanine in the mother are associated with fetal hyperphenylalaninemia. This prenatal exposure to excessive phenylalanine appears to be the primary mechanism of fetal injury. Maternal diet therapy offers the best hope for an unimpaired infant. Phenylalanine levels drop quickly once dietary restrictions are instituted, and there is a strong correlation between maternal blood levels and neonatal outcome.[83,132] As with diabetes, control is ideally achieved before conception. Several studies have identified improved long-term outcomes when desirable phenylalanine levels (less than 2 to 8 mg/dl) are achieved before or early in pregnancy and maintained throughout.[30,80,124,133]

Renal Disease

Maternal adaptation to pregnancy involves significant changes in renal function and structure. Plasma volume increases 40% to 50%, with an associated increase in renal blood flow and a 50% increase in glomerular filtration rate (GFR).[95] There is increased retention of sodium and water. These changes place unique demands on the urinary tract; women with preexisting renal disease are often unable to tolerate this stress and may experience a deterioration in function. Furthermore, renal dysfunction complicates pregnancy and increases fetal risk.

Renal disease in pregnancy may occur as a result of urinary tract infections, glomerular disease, or as a complication of systemic diseases including diabetes and systemic lupus erythematosus (SLE). Regardless of the underlying etiologic factors, pregnancy outcome relates most closely to two factors: the presence of hypertension and the degree of renal insufficiency that existed before the pregnancy.[75,114,144,145] Many women with renal disorders are hypertensive before pregnancy, and they often develop a superimposed pregnancy-induced hypertension leading to preeclampsia. Even those with previously normal blood pressures run an increased risk of developing hypertension during pregnancy.[63,68,114] The presence of hypertension in these pregnancies represents a significant risk to the fetus and is strongly associated with intrauterine growth restriction (IUGR), preterm delivery, and perinatal loss. Drug therapy to control chronic hypertension has been shown to have a beneficial effect on fetal outcome and is generally continued throughout pregnancy. Renal insufficiency,

as measured by creatinine clearance or serum creatinine level, also has implications for fetal outcome. Mild to moderate renal insufficiency (serum creatinine less than 1.5 mg/dl) is associated with a generally favorable outcome, whereas severe insufficiency (serum creatinine greater than 1.6 mg/dl) often carries an increased risk for perinatal death.[68,75,114] As a rule, the number of preterm deliveries and growth restricted infants increases with increasing blood pressure and decreasing renal function.[33,69,114]

Two special circumstances are dialysis during pregnancy and pregnancy after renal transplantation. Women undergoing dialysis rarely become pregnant. When pregnancy does occur, it is associated with significant perinatal morbidity and mortality with spontaneous abortions reaching 50%. Hemodialysis is also associated with numerous complications including placental abruption, polyhydramnios, IUGR, preterm labor, and pregnancy loss.[39,53,63,69,95] The risk may be lower with ambulatory peritoneal dialysis.[39,128] Pregnancy after transplantation is more common and has a better prognosis than pregnancy managed by dialysis.[31,114] Infants born after maternal transplantation are commonly preterm. Other complications may include growth restriction, RDS, congenital anomalies, adrenocortical insufficiency, hyperviscosity, seizures, and neonatal sepsis.[31,120,145] The criteria used to predict fetal outcome with other renal patients (i.e., hypertension and renal insufficiency) also have predictive value in posttransplantation pregnancies.

Neurologic Disorders

Neurologic disorders such as epilepsy, multiple sclerosis (MS), and myasthenia gravis generally have little effect on fertility; pregnancy can, and does, occur. The risks that accompany such pregnancies vary according to the individual disease entity and pertain to both the course of the mother's disease and the pregnancy outcome.

Maternal seizure disorders have been associated with increased fetal and neonatal risks, including prematurity, congenital defects, intrauterine demise, neonatal depression, and hemorrhage. These risks are in part attributable to the alterations in the fetal environment that occur as a result of either the seizure disorder itself or the administration of anticonvulsant drugs to the mother. An epilepsy-related genetic predisposition to certain major congenital defects may also be a factor.[72,112] Significant numbers of women experience an increase in seizure activity during pregnancy. This is most likely because of decreased compliance with medication regimens, physiologic changes associated with pregnancy, and gestational changes in plasma levels of anticonvulsant drugs.[13,72] There is evidence that maternal seizures compromise fetal oxygenation, possibly because of diminished placental blood flow or maternal hypoxemia resulting from postseizure apnea.[147] There are also data linking seizure activity during pregnancy to an increased incidence of poor pregnancy outcome.[109] For these reasons, control of maternal seizure activity with anticonvulsants is one of the primary goals of prenatal care.

Placental transport of anticonvulsants does occur, resulting in fetal levels that approximate or in some cases exceed maternal levels.[13,108] Many studies have demonstrated an increased incidence of congenital defects in the offspring of epileptic women treated with anticonvulsants.[13,72,109,112] These anomalies are most likely attributable in part to drug teratogenicity, but the influence of the seizure disorder itself, as well as genetic makeup, may also be a factor. **Trimethadione is considered to be a potent teratogen, and its use is contraindicated in pregnancy.** It is associated with spontaneous abortion, craniofacial anomalies, intrauterine growth restriction, hypoplasia of the fingers and nails, congenital heart defects, and mental retardation.[13,106,156] **Valproic acid is associated with neural tube defects, craniofacial abnormalities, and several minor malformations.**[106,146] Carbamazepine has also been linked to neural tube defects.[134] Other anticonvulsants, including hydantoins, primidone, and barbiturates, have been implicated in minor birth defects; specific syndromes have been associated with their use.

Infants born to mothers treated with anticonvulsants, especially barbiturates, may exhibit signs of generalized depression, including decreased respiratory effort, poor muscle tone, and feeding difficulties. They may also have symptoms indicative of drug withdrawal (see Chapter 10). These symptoms usually present in the first week of life and include tremors, restlessness, hypertonia, and hyperventilation.[9] **In addition, there have been reports of abnormal clotting and hemorrhage in the offspring of women treated with phenytoin, phenobarbital, and primidone. This appears to be caused by a decrease in vitamin K–dependent clotting factors. Hemorrhage usually starts within the first 24 hours, is often severe, and may result in death. Infants born to** these mothers should have cord blood clotting studies done, vitamin K prophylaxis on admission to the nursery, and close observation.[13,112]

Multiple sclerosis (MS) frequently strikes women during their reproductive years. The onset of MS is usually insidious; the course is marked by a seemingly capricious cycle of exacerbation and remission. A wide range of sensory, motor, and functional changes is associated with this disease; the type and severity of symptoms vary dramatically from one individual to another and in any one patient over time. The etiologic factors associated with the disease are not well understood. Genetic, environmental, and immunologic mechanisms have been implicated; viral factors have also been suggested.[136] Pregnancy is usually well tolerated; however, a higher than expected number of relapses has been identified in the first 6 months after delivery.[126,136]

In women with MS, the disease process itself is not a threat to fetal or neonatal well-being. No increases in perinatal morbidity, mortality, or in the incidence of congenital defects have been demonstrated.[126,136] **The priority for neonatal care providers is to determine the extent of the mother's disability, including her level of fatigue and her ability to care for her infant. The availability of appropriate support systems, both personal and professional, should be assessed, and needed follow-up and referrals should be made.**

Even though the prognosis for these infants is excellent, there are some factors associated with MS that are potentially problematic. Bladder dysfunction, common in women with MS, often results in urinary tract infections during pregnancy. Associated fetal and neonatal problems include preterm delivery and sepsis. Early identification and prompt treatment with appropriate antibiotics should minimize these risks. An additional area of concern is the variety of drugs administered to MS patients. Immunosuppressants are frequently used during severe exacerbations. The placental transport and fetal risk vary with the individual agent used. Prednisone is generally considered safe for use in pregnancy; the safety of azathioprine is still in question.[12] Although there have been reports of healthy infants born after maternal azathioprine therapy, there have also been reports of fetal complications, including hypoplasia of the thymus, immunoglobulin deficiency, decreases in cortisol levels, and transient chromosomal abnormalities. Cyclophosphamide has been associated with skeletal defects, growth retardation, and preterm labor.[12,41] Both azathioprine and cyclophosphamide are best avoided during pregnancy. A final consideration is a long-term one: the incidence of MS in the offspring of a parent with the disease is somewhat higher than the incidence in the general population.

Myasthenia gravis is an autoimmune disorder in which a dearth of acetylcholine receptor (AChR) results in neuromuscular dysfunction.[129] Antibodies to AChRs have been found in most affected persons.[85] Distinguishing features include generalized weakness and muscle fatigue with activity. Persons with myasthenia gravis may also experience respiratory compromise and difficulty swallowing. In some cases pregnancy leads to deterioration; maternal deaths related to postdelivery myasthenic crisis have occurred.[125] Infants born to myasthenic mothers may be affected by maternal drug therapy; an increased rate of preterm delivery has also been reported.[125] **An additional risk stems from transplacentally acquired antiacetylcholine receptor antibodies, which cause approximately 12% of these newborns to experience a transient, self-limited course of myasthenia gravis.[36,129] It is difficult to predict which pregnancies will result in an affected infant, although infants born to women with very high AChR antibody titers may be at highest risk. Affected infants usually present at birth or within the first 24 hours of life with generalized weakness, diminished suck and swallow, and a decreased respiratory effort that may require mechanical support.**

Systemic Lupus Erythematosus

SLE is an autoimmune disease that primarily presents in women of childbearing age. The clinical effects of lupus range from mild or subclinical disease to serious illness affecting multiple organ systems. In pregnancy, SLE is associated with increased rates of spontaneous abortion, preterm delivery, and stillbirths.[121] Outcome is best when renal disease or hypertension does not complicate pregnancy.[34,121]

The neonatal manifestations of SLE are attributed to the placental transfer of maternal antibodies to the fetus. Findings in the newborn include a transient lupus-like rash, thrombocytopenia, and cardiac abnormalities.[152] A strong association has been established between maternal antiRo (SS-A) antibodies and congenital heart block in the offspring of women with SLE.[152] The heart block is often identified prenatally; infants are treated with cardiac pacemakers after delivery.

Heart Disease

Significant changes in cardiovascular function accompany normal pregnancy. Plasma and red blood cell volumes rise, heart rate and cardiac output increase, and peripheral vascular resistance falls. These changes facilitate increased uterine blood flow, placental perfusion, and fetal oxygenation and growth; they also increase maternal oxygen consumption and cardiovascular workload and can further compromise the cardiovascular status of women with preexisting serious heart disease.[100] Pregnancy also creates a risk for maternal cardiovascular complications, including an increased incidence of thromboembolism and sudden death.[96] In some cases, such as Eisenmenger's syndrome and primary pulmonary hypertension, the risk to maternal survival is so great that pregnancy is contraindicated.[97] In general, how well the woman with heart disease tolerates pregnancy depends on the specific disease process and the degree to which her cardiac status is compromised.[16,76,100,153]

Maternal heart disease also affects the fetus. Fetal risks are the result of genetic factors, alterations in placental perfusion and exchange, and the effect of maternally administered drugs. **The genetic risk is demonstrated by the increased incidence of congenital heart defects that occur in the offspring of parents who have such a defect.** The exact risk depends on the specific parental lesion, mode of inheritance, and exposure to environmental triggers.[15]

Alterations in placental perfusion and gas exchange occur when the mother's condition involves chronic hypoxemia or a significant decrease in cardiac output. These factors increase the threat to the fetus, with fetal risk increasing as maternal cardiac status declines.[100] Chronic maternal hypoxemia results in a decrease in oxygen available to the fetus and is associated with fetal loss, prematurity, and IUGR.[153] Significant reductions in maternal cardiac output create decreased uterine blood flow and diminished placental perfusion with a resulting impairment in the exchange of nutrients, oxygen, and metabolic wastes.[5,100] **Possible fetal and neonatal consequences include spontaneous abortion, IUGR, neonatal asphyxia, central nervous system (CNS) damage, and intrauterine death.**

A wide variety of drugs are used in the management of maternal cardiovascular disease. Although it is sometimes difficult to differentiate drug effects from the effects of the underlying disease, some associations between drug administration and fetal outcomes can be made. Anticoagulants are used to decrease the risk of thromboembolism, especially in women with artificial valves, a history of thrombophlebitis, or rheumatic heart disease. **Oral anticoagulants, specifically warfarin sodium (Coumadin), have been associated with fetal malformations, including nasal hypoplasia and epiphyseal stippling, when administered during the first trimester. They have also been associated with eye and CNS abnormalities when administered later in pregnancy.**[61] **The incidence of warfarin embryopathy is estimated to be 15% to 25%. Warfarin is also associated with maternal and fetal hemorrhage. Heparin is generally considered the preferable agent for anticoagulation therapy during pregnancy. Heparin does not cross the placenta and therefore does not result in fetal anticoagulation or neonatal hemorrhage (although maternal hemorrhage may still occur), nor has it been associated with congenital defects.**[149]

Antiarrhythmic medications and cardiac glycosides used during pregnancy cross the placenta to varying degrees. They have not been implicated in fetal malformations and, although several have been associated with minor complications, are generally considered safe for use in pregnancy.[135,149] Reported complications include uterine contractions (quinidine, disopyramide), decreased birth weights (digoxin, disopyramide), and maternal hypotension with a sudden decrease in placental perfusion (verapamil).

Antihypertensives and diuretics have also been used in the treatment of cardiovascular disease during pregnancy. Propranolol, a beta-blocker commonly used to treat both hypertension and arrhythmias, acts as a uterine stimulant; its administration is a possible cause of preterm labor.[100] Propranolol is also associated with neonatal depression, including decreased respiratory effort and bradycardia at the time of delivery, as well as with hypoglycemia, polycythemia, and hyperbilirubinemia in the newborn period.[100,135,154] Atenolol and metoprolol, selective beta-blockers that can also be used to treat chronic hypertension, appear to have fewer adverse consequences for the neonate and are preferable agents.[135,149] Diuretic use in pregnancy remains an area of some controversy. Fetal and neonatal compromise can result from diuretic-induced electrolyte and glucose imbalance and decreased placental perfusion caused by maternal hypovolemia. The use of thiazide diuretics has been linked to neonatal liver damage and thrombocytopenia. In general, diuretic use is restricted to women with pulmonary edema

or acute cardiac or renal failure.[100,149] Although a great number of possible complications have been listed here, it is important to remember that with few exceptions most of the drugs used in the treatment of maternal heart disease can be used in pregnancy if the maternal condition warrants it.

Respiratory Disease

Respiratory function is altered even in normal pregnancy. Changes include a decrease in lung volume and increases in both oxygen consumption and minute ventilation. Significant decreases in maternal respiratory function and oxygenation could have a negative effect on the fetus, but careful management of respiratory disease during pregnancy generally results in a favorable outcome.

Asthma is the most commonly occurring respiratory disease in pregnancy. Infants born to women whose asthma is well controlled usually do well; unstable or worsening disease, especially status asthmaticus, increases fetal risk. Commonly used asthma medications, including corticosteroids, adrenergic bronchodilators (terbutaline, albuterol, and epinephrine), and aminophylline, are considered safe for use in pregnancy.[29] No teratogenic effects have been clearly demonstrated. Although avoidance of any drug is a good rule, especially in the first weeks of pregnancy, the first priority in asthma is to maintain control of the disease throughout pregnancy. Asthma medications are used as needed to maintain control and avoid (or treat) acute episodes.[29] **Fetal risks related to maternal asthma include low birth weight and/or prematurity. However, with good control the occurrence rate of these problems is essentially the same as in pregnancies in women who do not have asthma.**[143]

Cystic fibrosis (CF) was once considered a lethal childhood disease, but the life expectancy of a person with CF has increased, with more women surviving to conceive pregnancies. Pregnancy is not recommended for women with severe disease, because they often experience a significant deterioration during gestation. Patients with less severe disease and careful prenatal care may tolerate pregnancy well and achieve good neonatal outcomes. **Fetal risks include prematurity, IUGR, and perinatal death, caused primarily by maternal hypoxemia and infection.** Women with CF frequently require treatment with antibiotics during pregnancy. Several antibiotics have been associated with fetal abnormalities and neonatal complications.[78] These include tetracycline (tooth discoloration and abnormal bone development), aminoglycosides (ototoxicity), and sulfonamides (hyperbilirubinemia). Trimethoprim is a folic acid antagonist, and its use should be avoided because of the association between folic acid deficiency and neural tube defects. **Penicillins and cephalosporins are generally considered safer for use in pregnancy. All infants born to mothers with CF will be, at least, heterozygous carriers for CF.**

Maternal Behavior

Smoking

It is well established that maternal smoking is associated with reductions in both birth weight and length, as well as with an increase in the incidence of birth weights below 2500 g. The exact mechanism by which fetal growth is retarded is not entirely clear, but reduced placental blood flow resulting from vasoconstriction, elevated carbon monoxide levels, and chronic fetal hypoxia may all play a role.[14,66,102] Maternal smoking is also associated with placental dysfunction, an increased incidence of placental abruptions and previas, premature rupture of the membranes, preterm labor, and intrauterine fetal death. Fetal risk increases with the number of cigarettes smoked, maternal anemia, and poor nutrition.[60,101] Eliminating or reducing smoking can improve fetal growth; women should be counseled to do so even relatively late in pregnancy.[139] The use of nicotine patches (instead of smoking during pregnancy) reduces the absorption of nicotine and other potentially harmful substances in tobacco smoke, which may result in increased birth weight of the fetus.[155]

Substance Abuse

Drug and alcohol abuse by the mother places the fetus and newborn at risk for a plethora of structural, functional, and developmental problems. Perinatal morbidity is related to the direct effects of the abused substance on the developing fetus, its sudden withdrawal, the interactions of multiple abused substances, the nutritional effects of addiction on the mother, and/or the social and health care implications of substance abuse. Alcohol is one of the most commonly abused substances during pregnancy. Alcohol in the maternal circulation crosses the placenta, resulting in direct fetal exposure to alcohol and its metabolites.[1] **There may be a wide range of effects on the exposed fetus; these include craniofacial malformations, growth restriction, CNS dysfunction, and organ or joint abnormalities.**[1,70] The mechanism of fetal injury is not entirely clear but is likely related to three main factors: a teratogenic effect, hypoxia as a result of increased oxygen consumption, and a diminished ability to use amino acids in protein synthesis.[1] **The expression of fetal alcohol effects ranges from subtle to extreme and depends on the timing of exposure, the dose, and the genetic response of the mother and fetus to the effects of alcohol. Secondary factors, such as maternal age, nutritional status, general health, and the effects of other abused substances may also influence outcome. When the more severe effects are exhibited, the condition is known as *fetal alcohol syndrome* (FAS). FAS occurs in the offspring of chronic alcoholics and is defined by a triad of defects: IUGR with microcephaly, facial anomalies (small palpebral fissures, low nasal bridge, indistinct philtrum, thin upper lip, shortened lower jaw), and CNS dysfunction, including mental restriction.**[70] **These infants may also exhibit tremors, irritability, and hypertonus related to alcohol withdrawal. The effects of prenatal alcohol exposure may be seen in postnatal life as continued abnormalities in motor, behavioral, and intellectual development.**

Drug use and addiction in pregnancy is a complex problem. The mother's reporting of drug use is often unreliable; frequently more than one substance is involved, and there may be a cycle of drug use and periodic abstinence during pregnancy. In addition, a host of medical and social problems are associated with maternal drug abuse. Substance abusers have generally poor health: infectious diseases, including pneumonia, sexually transmitted disease, urinary tract infections, and hepatitis are common. Anemia is frequently seen, and nutrition and prenatal care are often inadequate. These factors contribute to a poor pregnancy outcome and make it difficult to isolate the effects of any individual drug on the fetus. However, several generalizations can be made. The majority of drugs used by the mother, including narcotics, stimulants, and depressants, cross the placenta and have an effect on the fetus. **Fetal risks include IUGR, malformations, intrauterine demise, prematurity, asphyxia, and CNS dysfunction; fetal addiction does occur and is associated with neonatal abstinence syndrome.**[43,70,98,158]

Cocaine use by the mother merits special attention. **Cocaine is a CNS stimulant that produces vasoconstriction, tachycardia, and hypertension** in both the mother and fetus. Its use during pregnancy has been linked to IUGR, genitourinary (GU) tract anomalies, placental abruption, stillbirths, and cerebral infarcts, as well as impaired performance as measured with the Brazelton behavioral assessment tool.[21,22] (See Chapter 10 for a more complete discussion of complications in drug-exposed neonates.)

Maternal Malnutrition

Fetal nutrition is linked to maternal intake during pregnancy and to the existent maternal stores of various nutrients, as well as to placental function. In general, poorly nourished mothers have more perinatal losses, preterm births, lower Apgar scores, and low birth weight (LBW) babies; this is especially true of significantly underweight women who fail to gain adequate weight during pregnancy.[81,90,151] Women with eating disorders such as anorexia and bulimia are reluctant to disclose symptoms to health care providers; hence the first clue may be a small for gestational age (SGA) newborn associated with poor or no maternal weight gain.[47] However, it is difficult to draw direct correlations between poor maternal diet and fetal growth unless the nutritional disturbances are severe. Many fetuses grow well despite suboptimal maternal nutrition, in part because of the complexities of placental transport and the ability of the fetus to be preferentially supplied with some nutrients.

Although reduced birth weight is associated with inadequate carbohydrate, protein, and total caloric intake, inappropriate amounts of other nutrients may also affect the fetus. Vitamin and mineral deficiencies have been linked to spontaneous abortion (vitamin C), congestive heart failure (thiamine), megaloblastic anemia (folic acid, B_{12}), congenital anomalies including neural tube defects (folic acid, zinc, copper), and skeletal abnormalities (vitamin D, calcium).[151] Vitamin overdosage, especially of the fat-soluble vitamins, has also been implicated in fetal abnormalities; vitamin A overdose has been associated with kidney malformations, neural tube defects, and hydrocephalus and vitamin D overdose with cardiac, neurologic, and renal defects.[88,89,151]

Nutritional deficiencies (or excesses) should be identified before or early in pregnancy, and both weight gain and fetal growth should be monitored throughout gestation. When problems are identified, individualized intervention strategies should be implemented in an attempt to increase birth weights and improve perinatal outcome.

Obstetric Complications
Antepartum Bleeding

Maternal cardiovascular support is crucial to fetal well-being. Chronic blood loss can lead to maternal anemia and a related decrease in oxygen-carrying capacity. Uncompensated acute bleeding results in diminished blood volume, decreased systolic pressure, decreased cardiac output, and ultimately decreased placental perfusion. The net effect on the fetus is decreased oxygenation and impaired nutrient delivery.

Gestational bleeding in the first or second trimesters of pregnancy has been linked to increased risks of preterm labor, preterm birth, premature rupture of membranes (PROM), and low birth weight (LBW).[50] The most common causes of hemorrhage late in pregnancy include placental abruption and placenta previa. In an abruption, a normally implanted placenta separates from the uterine wall before the time of delivery, resulting in maternal bleeding and a functional decrease in uteroplacental size. A relationship between cocaine use and an increase incidence of abruptions has been reported.[44] There is also an increased risk for placental abruption with both cigarette smoking and hypertensive disorders.[4] The separation may be partial or complete, involving peripheral and/or central portions of the placenta. Fetal compromise relates to the extent of the separation and to the frequent need for preterm delivery. When the abruption is small and bleeding is minimal, the pregnancy may continue without significant fetal compromise; however, it is important to remember that the decrease in uteroplacental surface area is irreversible and reduces the absolute placental capability. As the fetus grows or experiences additional stressors, its ability to tolerate the abruption may change. Extensive abruptions are poorly tolerated by both fetus and mother; the resulting maternal hemorrhage and decreased placental function lead to fetal asphyxia and, without immediate intervention, to intrauterine demise.[26,59]

A placenta previa exists when the placenta lies abnormally low in the uterus and to some extent covers or encroaches on the internal cervical os. In the latter part of pregnancy, the normal elongation of the lower uterine segment and changes in the cervix disrupt the attachment of the overlying placenta. This generally presents as episodic, painless, maternal bleeding, often accompanied by preterm labor. To avoid active labor with resulting maternal hemorrhage, fetal lung maturity is assessed at 35 to

36 weeks. If the lungs are sufficiently mature, a cesarean section is scheduled before the onset of labor.[130] **Fetal compromise relates to the extent of the previa, severity of maternal hemorrhage, degree of the resulting fetal hypoxia, and gestational age at delivery.**

Chronic Hypertension

Chronic hypertension in pregnancy, defined as hypertension diagnosed before pregnancy or before 20 weeks' gestation, complicates 1% to 6% of births in the United States each year. **Chronic hypertension is associated with IUGR, preterm birth, placental abruption, and stillbirth.[42] The degree of fetal compromise is related to the degree and control of maternal hypertension.**

Preeclampsia

Preeclampsia, a type of pregnancy-induced hypertension, is a condition in which hypertension, accompanied by proteinuria and edema, develops during the second half of pregnancy in women with or without preexisting hypertensive disease. It is most common in primigravidas, in women younger than 16 or older than 35, in multiple gestations and molar pregnancies, and in women with a family history of this disorder.[23] As a perinatal complication, preeclampsia is significant because of its high toll in terms of both maternal and fetal well-being.

Pregnancy is normally associated with vasodilation and decreased peripheral vascular resistance. The net effect is that even though there is a significant increase in blood volume, maternal blood pressure does not increase during pregnancy. In contrast, pregnancy-induced hypertension is associated with vasoconstriction and an increase in vascular resistance and arterial pressure. The result is a reduction in blood flow to the vital organs, including the kidney, liver, brain, and uterus; reduced maternal blood volume; and a host of maternal hepatic, CNS, and coagulation abnormalities. The major effect on the intrauterine environment is placental insufficiency caused by significant reductions in uteroplacental blood flow and the development of placental vascular abnormalities.[93,132] **Associated fetal and neonatal risks include IUGR, prematurity with all of its attendant problems, perinatal asphyxia, and perinatal death.* The risk to the infant increases with earlier onset and increasingly severe mater-**

nal disease, such as chronic hypertension with superimposed preeclampsia.[91] **Maternal seizures (eclampsia) further compromise the fetus by promoting hypoxemia and acidosis, which can result in intrauterine demise.**[132]

HELLP syndrome, a severe form of pregnancy-induced hypertension manifested by *h*emolysis, *el*evated *l*iver enzymes, *l*ow *p*latelets, and renal function abnormalities, carries a high risk of fetal and maternal death. In milder cases of HELLP syndrome, conservative management may facilitate improvements in condition before delivery, but the risk of IUGR remains. However, in most cases of HELLP syndrome, immediate delivery is indicated regardless of the gestational age of the fetus.[140]

Drugs commonly used to treat pregnancy-induced hypertension include magnesium sulfate, hydralazine (Apresoline), labetalol, nifedipine, and other antihypertensive agents. Magnesium sulfate is the most commonly used agent in the United States for the prevention of maternal seizures. **Hypotonia and CNS depression have been reported as neonatal side effects, yet no correlation has been found between neonatal magnesium level and Apgar score.**[132] **These effects are more likely the result of coexisting complications, such as prematurity and asphyxia.**[61,138] Hydralazine and other antihypertensives are used in the treatment of severe maternal hypertension; actions include relaxation of the arterial bed, decreased vascular resistance, and decreased blood pressure. Maternal response to antihypertensives must be carefully monitored, because precipitous decreases in blood pressure reduce placental perfusion and further compromise the fetus.[116]

Preterm Labor

Preterm birth, defined as any birth before 37 or 38 weeks' gestation, poses an unparalleled threat to neonatal survival and well-being. Its cost, both human and economic, is staggering, and its prevention is a primary focus of modern obstetric care. Prevention is best accomplished through an aggressive effort to identify women at risk and close follow-up to achieve early recognition and appropriate intervention should preterm labor occur.[65,87] Unfortunately, many women continue to receive inadequate prenatal care or no care at all. Even women who obtain early and ongoing care often fail to recognize the signs of preterm labor and delay reporting symptoms until intervention is difficult if not impossible.[25,50]

---

*References 10, 40, 93, 113, 131, 141.

Although in many specific instances a definitive cause cannot be identified, it is possible to identify several factors that are generally associated with preterm labor and delivery.[57,65,74] These factors are summarized in Box 2-1. When preterm labor cannot be halted, it culminates in the delivery of a physiologically immature infant. The result is a host of neonatal problems that relate largely to the degree of immaturity, but also to compounding problems such as infant anomalies or maternal disease, as well as to the events that led to the preterm delivery (e.g., asphyxia resulting from a bleeding placenta previa). **Problems commonly encountered in preterm infants include respiratory distress, asphyxia, hyperbilirubinemia, metabolic disturbances, fluid and electrolyte imbalance, neurologic and behavioral problems, infection, nu-**

tritional deficits and feeding problems, ineffective thermoregulation, cardiovascular disturbances, chronic respiratory disease, and hematologic disturbances.

Beta-sympathomimetic agents, such as ritodrine hydrochloride and terbutaline sulfate, are commonly used as a means of interrupting preterm labor. They achieve their tocolytic action by maximizing the beta$_2$-adrenergic effects on the uterus, with a resulting decrease in uterine smooth muscle contractility.[28,87] Although these drugs are effective in prolonging gestation, they are also associated with maternal, fetal, and neonatal complications.* Mothers may experience tachycardia and dysrhythmias, hyperglycemia, hypokalemia, anxiety, nausea, and vomiting. Myocardial ischemia and pulmonary edema are rare but serious maternal side effects. The fetus may also develop tachycardia and hyperglycemia. **Neonates born after beta-sympathomimetic therapy may develop a rebound hypoglycemia in response to in utero hyperglycemia and overproduction of insulin. Beta-sympathomimetic tocolytic agents increase fetal aortic blood flow and fetal cardiac output that might increase fetal systolic pressure and cerebral blood flow which can lead to an increased incidence of intracranial bleeding in immature fetal brains.**[115]

Magnesium sulfate has also been employed as a tocolytic. Magnesium sulfate decreases muscle contractility, thereby inhibiting uterine activity and effectively interrupting preterm labor.[28,122,138] **Neonatal consequences of maternal magnesium administration include decreased muscle tone and drowsiness, as well as decreases in serum calcium levels.**[59,117,122]

Prostaglandins play an important role in the onset of labor. Prostaglandin synthetase inhibitors, such as indomethacin, are a class of pharmacologic agents that interfere with the body's synthesis of prostaglandin, thereby inhibiting prostaglandin-mediated uterine contractions. These drugs have been used to treat preterm labor. They can cause in utero constriction, or closure, of the ductus arteriosus with resulting development of fetal pulmonary hypertension and congestive heart failure.[6,83,109,110] They may also lead to oligohydramnios and must be used with caution, especially late in the third trimester.[6,18,77] Other neonatal risks include decreased platelet activity and gastrointestinal irritation.[109]

Box 2-1	**FACTORS ASSOCIATED WITH PRETERM LABOR AND DELIVERY**

Maternal History

Chronic disease
Diabetes
Renal disease
Cardiovascular disease
Respiratory disease
In utero exposure to diethylstilbestrol
Reproductive tract anomalies
Underweight (before pregnancy)
Smoking
Age extremes (below 18, above 40)
Previous preterm labor
African-American race
Low socioeconomic status

This Pregnancy

Inadequate weight gain
Acute maternal illness
   Pregnancy-induced hypertension
   Urinary tract infection
   Chorioamnionitis, vaginal infection
Antepartum hemorrhage
Isoimmunization
Premature rupture of membranes
Multiple gestation
Polyhydramnios
Retained intrauterine device

Fetal Factors

Fetal anomalies
Intrauterine fetal demise
Infection

---

*References 11, 19, 28, 86, 87, 127.

Calcium antagonists, such as nifedipine, also have a demonstrated ability to interfere with the labor process. Uterine contractility is directly related to the presence of free calcium; increased calcium concentration enhances muscle contractility, whereas decreased calcium levels inhibit contractility.[28,45] Calcium antagonists block the entry of calcium into cells and inhibit uterine muscle contraction. In animal studies, these drugs have been associated with fetal acidosis.[38,62] However, lower umbilical artery pH values or lower Apgar scores have not been associated with nifedipine.[115]

Corticosteroid treatment of pregnant women who deliver prematurely was first introduced in 1972 to enhance fetal lung maturity. In 1994, the National Institutes of Health sponsored a Consensus Development Conference on the Effect of Corticosteroids for Fetal Maturation on Perinatal Outcomes. **The consensus panel concluded that giving a single course of corticosteroids to pregnant women at risk for preterm birth reduced the risk of death, respiratory distress syndrome, and intraventricular hemorrhage in preterm infants.** The 1994 panel noted that the optimal benefit of antenatal corticosteroid therapy lasts seven days. Since then the use of repeat courses of antenatal corticosteroids became widespread in the United States, England, and Australia. In 2000 the National Institutes of Health reconvened to present research of repeat courses of antenatal corticosteroid therapy. In studies in preterm animals, multiple doses of antenatal corticosteroids improve lung function when compared with a single dose. Human studies suggested possible benefits in reduction of the incidence and severity of respiratory distress syndrome and in the incidence of patent ductus arteriosus. **There was little or no evidence to support a reduction in mortality rate or reductions in the incidence of intraventricular hemorrhage, chronic lung disease, sepsis, necrotizing enterocolitis, or retinopathy of prematurity with repeated antenatal corticosteroid therapy. Some of the suggested fetal risks of repeated antenatal corticosteroid therapy include decreased somatic and brain growth, adrenal suppression, neonatal sepsis, chronic lung disease, and mortality. The current clinical recommendations based on the 2000 NIH Consensus Statement are:**

- **All pregnant women between 24 and 34 weeks' gestation who are at risk of preterm delivery within 7 days should be considered candidates for antenatal treatment with a single course of corticosteroids.**
- **Treatment consists of two doses of 12 mg of betamethasone given intramuscularly 24 hours apart or four doses of 6 mg of dexamethasone given intramuscularly 12 hours apart.**
- **Repeat courses of corticosteroids should not be used routinely. In general, it should be reserved for patients enrolled in randomized controlled trials.**[107]

ENVIRONMENTAL EFFECTS OF LABOR ON THE FETUS

Effects of Contractions

During labor the dynamics of uterine contractions alter the intrauterine environment and influence the fetus. A "healthy" fetus is equipped to withstand the challenge of labor, but when the fetus is compromised or the labor is dysfunctional, the fetus can be taxed beyond its capacity, placing it at risk for further compromise, asphyxia, or intrauterine death.

Strong uterine contractions are characterized by decreased blood flow through the intervillous spaces in the placenta.[24,49,105] As blood flow decreases, there is a corresponding decline in placental gas exchange, and the fetus must depend on its existing reserves to maintain oxygenation until placental blood flow is reestablished. The net effect is that fetal PaO_2 decreases as the consequence of uterine contraction. In the fetus with adequate reserves, the fall in PaO_2 is not drastic; the fetus remains adequately oxygenated and so is able to tolerate the stress of labor.

Fetal Reserve

The factors that influence fetal reserve fall into two general categories: those that diminish reserves and those that exhaust reserves. When fetal oxygen reserves are diminished, the fetus has less than optimal oxygenation at the onset of a contraction. This may occur as a consequence of any condition that decreases placental exchange, including reduced placental surface area caused by abruption, previa, an abnormally small placenta, decreased placental perfusion caused by maternal hypotension or hypertension, or maternal hypoxemia.[2,13,105] Oxygen reserves can also be diminished as a result of a reduction in fetal oxygen-carrying capacity, as in severe anemia or acute fetal hemorrhage.

A fetal reserve that is adequate at the onset of labor can be exhausted by factors that place unusual demands on the fetus. Exhaustion of reserves occurs with contractions that last for a prolonged period of time, that are of extremely high intensity, or that occur with increased frequency and without an adequate recovery period between individual contractions.[2,13,105] This is often a consequence of the use of oxytocics to induce or augment labor.

Fetal Response to Contraction-Induced Hypoxia

When the fetal oxygen reserve is diminished or exhausted, uterine contractions can precipitate a significant fall in PaO_2. The fetus is quite limited in its ability to compensate for this hypoxemia. The adult mechanism, which involves increasing total cardiac output by increasing heart rate, does not play a major role in the fetal response.[56] Instead, the fetus responds with a redistribution of cardiac output as a means of maintaining critical function; blood flow to the brain and heart increases, whereas perfusion of less critical organs is reduced.[2,5,56,105] This mechanism enables the fetus to survive brief episodes of hypoxia, but severe and prolonged hypoxic episodes are poorly tolerated.

Acute hypoxemia leads to the development of acidosis and also produces a reflex bradycardia as a result of vagal stimulation, both of which further compromise fetal oxygenation. In addition, myocardial hypoxia has a direct bradycardic effect.[5,49] These mechanisms give rise to one of the classic signs of fetal distress, the late deceleration, in which the peak of uterine pressure, which also represents the nadir of intervillous blood flow and the onset of fetal hypoxemia, is followed by a decline in fetal heart rate.[2,24,49,56] Late decelerations are significant in that they help to identify the fetus unable to tolerate labor because of inadequate oxygen reserves, and they allow for the implementation of measures to enhance fetal reserve, improve placental perfusion, or interrupt labor.

Late decelerations are particularly ominous when accompanied by loss of fetal heart rate variability and/or fetal baseline tachycardia, because these findings are indicative of fetal acidosis. In the preterm infant, the findings of decreased variability and tachycardia, with or without late decelerations, correlate highly with acidosis, depression, and low Apgar scores.[3,49,105]

Other Factors That Evoke a Fetal Response During Labor

Head Compression

Pressure on the fetal head during labor, especially with pushing efforts in the second stage, also produces a vagal response and a reflex slowing of the fetal heart rate.[2,24,49,105] In general, this does not indicate hypoxia or fetal compromise and is often seen in a healthy fetus. The deceleration that accompanies head compression, also called an *early deceleration,* is differentiated from the late deceleration of fetal asphyxia by its timing in relation to a contraction. In early deceleration the heart rate begins to fall as a contraction builds, reaching its lowest point as the contraction peaks. As the contraction subsides, the heart rate returns to baseline. The result is a uniformly shaped dip that mirrors the shape of the contraction. In comparison, a late deceleration also has a uniform shape but lags behind the contraction, with the fall in heart rate beginning at or slightly after the contraction peak and continuing to fall as the contraction subsides. With a late deceleration the heart rate does not return to baseline until well after the contraction has ended.

Cord Compression

Compression of the umbilical cord occurs when the cord is looped around fetal body parts, when the cord is knotted, when the cord prolapses, or when there is scant amniotic fluid (oligohydramnios). During labor, cord compression may be exacerbated by contractions and by descent of the fetus, resulting in varying degrees of occlusion of the umbilical vessels and diminutions of blood flow. Partial venous occlusion may be manifested by fetal heart rate acceleration, whereas significant occlusion precipitates a rapid fall in heart rate, caused at least in part by vagal reflex.[2,24,49,71,105] Variable decelerations can be spontaneous, occurring at any time, or periodic, occurring with contractions. They typically have an abrupt descent in heart rate and may be V, U, or W shaped; hence the term *variable deceleration.* Periodic variable decelerations are identified by a decline in heart rate that generally begins before the contraction peaks but, unlike early decelerations, falls rapidly and does not mirror the shape of the contraction. Typically, recovery of the heart rate is also rapid. However, when the occlusion is severe or of long duration, or the fetus has diminished oxygen reserves, recovery may be slow, indicating fetal hypoxia and in essence incorporating a component of late deceleration within the variable deceleration.[24]

When variable decelerations are persistent and worsening during labor in the presence of oligohydramnios, intrapartum amnioinfusions have significantly decreased FHR abnormalities, acidemia at birth, and rates of cesarean birth.[123] **An amnioinfusion involves infusion of fluid into the uterine cavity via an intrauterine pressure catheter (IUPC). This fluid provides cushioning of the**

Table 2-2	FETAL AND NEONATAL EFFECTS OF MATERNAL ANALGESIA AND ANESTHESIA DURING LABOR
DRUG	**POSSIBLE FETAL AND NEONATAL SIDE EFFECTS**
Narcotics	Fetal and neonatal effects are related to the dose, route, and timing of maternal administration and may be reversed by the administration of a narcotic antagonist (naloxone); they include the following: CNS depression / Fetal bradycardia / Depressed respiratory effort / Decreased muscle tone and reflexes / Decreased responsiveness
Paracervical block	Fetal bradycardia and asphyxia related to decreased uterine blood flow and direct fetal myocardial depression
Epidural and spinal block	Fetal bradycardia and asphyxia related to maternal hypotension / Fetal neonatal toxicity
General (inhalation) anesthesia	Fetal and newborn effects related to the duration and depth of maternal anesthesia include the following: CNS depression / Respiratory depression / Decreased responsiveness

CNS, Central nervous system.

umbilical cord, which may reduce the frequency and severity of the cord compression. Amnioinfusions may also be used when thick meconium is present in amniotic fluid providing a diluting effect that can reduce the amount of meconium present in the infant's trachea and hence the incidence and severity of meconium aspiration at birth.

Maternal Pain Medication

Maternal anesthesia and/or analgesia have the potential to affect the infant, either during labor and delivery or in the newborn period. The risk is increased if the fetus is preterm or is otherwise compromised. This is not to say that there is no place for these drugs in obstetric care—only that they must be used judiciously and with a clear understanding of the risks and benefits involved. Table 2-2 summarizes the effects of commonly used analgesic and anesthetic agents on the fetus and the newborn.[51]

ASSESSMENT OF FETAL WELL-BEING

Over the past 20 to 30 years the ability to assess fetal well-being has advanced from simple auscultation of the fetal heart to direct physiologic and biochemical measurement of fetal status. With these advances, an appreciation of the similarities between the fetus and the newborn, as well as a more complete understanding of the unique features of fetal life, has been gained. This knowledge reinforces the importance of viewing fetal physiology as a precursor of neonatal function, and especially as a significant influence on the success with which the fetus will complete the adaptations required by the birth process.

The goal of antepartum fetal surveillance is to answer the following questions: What is the safest environment for a fetus at the gestational age at which the testing is taking place? Is the fetus more likely to survive in utero for the week after testing, or does the fetus have a significant risk of in utero death based on the degree of environmental or intrinsic intolerance demonstrated through testing? In the case of preterm infants, this may mean delivery at a gestational age at which there is a high likelihood for respiratory, neurologic, cardiac, gastrointestinal, and immunologic immaturity that will require neonatal intensive care.

The obstetric practitioner has several tools available to help answer the above questions. First and foremost is the **identification of maternal conditions that may predispose the fetus to in utero compromise. Examples of such conditions include type I diabetes mellitus, chronic hyperten-**

sion, collagen vascular disease, antiphospholipid antibody disease, maternal cardiac or pulmonary disease, preeclampsia, blood group isoimmunization, in utero infection, preterm rupture of membranes, and maternal substance abuse. This list is not all inclusive but demonstrates several commonly encountered conditions for which antepartum fetal surveillance is warranted.

Once the decision is made to assess fetal well-being, there are four modalities available in general practice to help the practitioner and client answer the questions regarding the optimal environment for the fetus at any given time. These include fetal movement counts, the contraction stress test, the nonstress test, and the fetal biophysical profile. Two additional tools often used by maternal fetal medicine specialists in certain clinical situations are Doppler flow studies and percutaneous umbilical cord sampling. None of these tools is used as the sole determinant for delivery; rather, each is used in conjunction with the entire clinical picture. The choice of testing method is also clinically driven; each method is useful in certain clinical settings, but no one method is the correct choice in all situations.

Although most of the procedures used to monitor fetal well-being are decidedly high-tech, the simple "kick count," or fetal movement survey, is a low-tech, low-cost screening tool. Many women with an intrauterine fetal demise have no identifiable risk factors that would place them in a fetal testing protocol. Fetal motor activity reflects the fetal condition in utero, and a decrease in or absence of fetal movements often presages fetal death. This is one reason that many institutions ask their patients to begin a fetal movement counting protocol at 26 to 32 weeks' gestation. Although there are continuing study results, some centers have demonstrated a significant decrease in the incidence of fetal mortality after the institution of a fetal movement counting protocol.

There are several different approaches to fetal movement counting. None has been shown to be superior.[3] One approach is to have the client choose a certain time every day to rest in the lateral position and count fetal movements. The perception of ten distinct fetal movements within two hours constitutes a reassuring session. The most important aspect of this type of testing is to emphasize to the client the importance of notifying her practitioner immediately if the fetal movement counting has not met the established criteria. A system must be in place where patients have immediate access to health care personnel 24 hours per day.

The contraction stress test (CST) is used in an attempt to evaluate fetal response to uterine contractions. The principle behind CST is that uterine contractions cause a transient interruption in utero placental perfusion. With normal fetal reserve, this intermittent interruption is well tolerated. With inadequate or exhausted reserve, late fetal heart rate decelerations appear.[48] Because late decelerations during labor had been associated with fetal hypoxia and acidosis, it was reasoned that similar interpretations could be applied to contractions induced in the antepartum client. Thus the CST is considered a test of uteroplacental reserve.

During a CST, uterine contraction activity is evoked with either the use of maternal nipple stimulation or an intravenous infusion of oxytocin. The fetal heart rate is charted using graph paper attached to a monitor that uses a continuous wave ultrasound transducer placed on the maternal abdomen over the uterus. The minimum number of spontaneous or evoked contractions is necessary for adequate testing is three contractions of 40 seconds' duration in a 10-minute period. The results are interpreted as follows: a negative CST result is one in which no late fetal heart rate decelerations occur during the examination. In a positive CST result, late decelerations occur after 50% or more of the contractions, even if contraction frequency is less than three in 10 minutes.

A suspicious or equivocal finding is one in which intermittent late or significant variable decelerations occur. A CST result is considered unsatisfactory if fewer than three contractions occur per 10 minutes or a poor-quality tracing is obtained. In many clinical situations a positive CST warrants delivery of the fetus because of suspected in utero hypoxemia during periods of uterine contraction. However, there are numerous exceptions to this rule. For example, if a positive CST is noted in the presence of maternal diabetic ketoacidosis, a correction of the underlying metabolic process may reverse the fetal acidosis, and a negative CST may be subsequently obtained. Thus the delivery of a neonate who has metabolic acidosis and is preterm can be avoided.

The nonstress test (NST) is a tool used to indirectly assess the integrity of the fetal autonomic nervous system. The fetal heart is under the dual influences of the sympathetic and parasympathetic nervous systems. By approximately 28 weeks' gestation, 85% of fetuses will demonstrate fetal heart rate accelerations in response to fetal movement. Lack of these intermittent fetal heart rate accelerations usually indicates a fetal sleep cycle. However, there are many other intrinsic and extrinsic factors, including fetal acidosis, which may lead to an absence of these intermittent accelerations in heart rate. Examples include but are not limited to medication exposure, maternal smoking, uteroplacental insufficiency, and fetal structural or chromosomal anomaly. Factors leading to maternal acidosis (severe anemia, congenital heart disease, and sepsis) can also result in fetal acidosis and a nonreactive NST.

The NST is performed with the client in a semi-Fowler's or lateral tilt position. As in the CST, the fetal heart rate is monitored with an external transducer. NSTs are interpreted as either reactive or nonreactive. An accepted definition of a reactive NST is an increase in fetal heart rate of 15 beats/min above the baseline heart rate occurring twice in a 20-minute period.[3] Some centers require that the fetal heart rate accelerations be associated with fetal movements as well as perceived by the maternal client.[37] A nonreactive test is defined as lacking the required fetal heart rate accelerations during a 40-minute period. The following may be candidates for nonstress testing:

- Women with diabetes that must be controlled with insulin
- Women who have pregnancy-induced hypertension or intrinsic renal disease
- Women in whom fetal IUGR or postdate pregnancy has been determined
- Women who have reported decreased fetal movement

The NST has certain advantages over the CST. It does not entail the production of uterine contractions, and so there are fewer potential problems or contraindications to the NST. Because the NST is quicker and easier to conduct, it is often the first-line screening test of fetal well-being. Its disadvantages are that it does not evaluate uteroplacental reserve and that it has a higher false positive rate than the CST.

When the NST is nonreactive, an option that is often used in lieu of the CST or delivery of the fetus is the biophysical profile (Table 2-3). This test combines the NST with real-time ultrasound evaluation of the fetus. Although there are several different BPP scoring systems, the one most generally accepted assigns a numerical score of 0 or 2 for the absence or presence of five different parameters. These include fetal movement, tone, "breathing" movements, amniotic fluid volume, and the NST. One advantage to evaluation of several different fetal biophysical variables is enhanced specificity of testing with a diminished incidence of delivery for false-positive results. The presence or absence of acute markers (movement, tone, breathing, and NST) help reflect fetal status at the time of testing. Evaluation of amniotic fluid volume as a marker is indirect evidence that the portions of the fetal CNS that control that activity are intact and functioning and therefore not acidotic. However, the absence of a given marker may be difficult to interpret, because it may simply reflect normal periodicity.

The biophysical activities that mature first in fetal development disappear last as acidosis worsens. Fetal tone (flexion and extension) is present at 7.5 to 8.5 weeks after the last menstrual period. This activity, as well as gross body movement, is mediated in the cortex and nuclei of the CNS. Fetal movement is present by 9 weeks. Fetal breathing movements (rhythmic breathing movements of 35 seconds or more) are generally seen by 20 weeks'

Table 2-3 BIOPHYSICAL PROFILE SCORING		
BIOPHYSICAL VARIABLE	**NORMAL (2)**	**ABNORMAL (0)**
Fetal breathing—At least one episode of at least 30 seconds during 30-minute observation	Present	Absent
Gross body movement—At least three body or limb movements during 30-minute observation	≥3	≤2
Fetal tone—One episode of extension or flexion of limbs or trunk during 30-minute observation	Present	Absent or sluggish movements
Reactive nonstress test—At least two episodes of 15 beats/min fetal heart rate accelerations during 30-minute observation	Yes	No
Amniotic fluid volume—At least one pocket of at least 1 cm × 1 cm in two directions	Present	Absent

Normal score: 8-10.

gestation. The CNS center responsible for control of this activity is the ventral surface of the fourth ventricle. The final acute marker to mature is fetal heart rate acceleration in response to movement (reactive NST) seen in the later second trimester. The posterior hypothalamus and medulla control this activity. Given that the first marker to appear in development is the last to disappear with worsening fetal acidosis, the absence of fetal tone has been found to be associated with high perinatal morbidity and mortality.[150] Chronic sustained fetal hypoxia or acidosis may produce a protective redistribution of cardiac output away from less vital fetal organs (e.g., kidney and lung) toward the essential organs (e.g., brain, heart, and adrenal glands). Redistribution of fetal blood flow may be so profound that renal perfusion decreases to the point that oligohydramnios is established. When the largest vertical amniotic fluid pocket within the uterus is less than 1 cm, the perinatal mortality rate is as high as 110/1000.[20]

A BPP score of 8 or 10 is normal; a score of 6 is equivocal, and the profile should be repeated in 12 to 24 hours. A score of 4 or less is abnormal. Management in the presence of an abnormal BPP depends on the gestational age and the maternal and/or fetal factors contributing to the altered state.

The BPP employs the advantages of real-time ultrasonography to observe fetal behavior.[92] One of its major advantages is as an intermediate step in the evaluation of a fetus with a nonreactive NST before a time-consuming CST is performed. It is also a useful tool for patients with contraindications to the CST, such as premature labor, premature rupture of membranes, unexplained vaginal bleeding, or multiple gestation. The modified BPP, which combines an acute marker (NST) with the chronic marker of fetal well-being (amniotic fluid index [AFI]), has been shown by some centers to be as predictive of fetal well-being as the full BPP. Because evaluation of the AFI is less time consuming and requires less technical skill, this may be an acceptable alternative for many centers.

No matter which of these testing modalities is used, the client should be counseled as to the predictive value of a "normal" test. The incidence of stillbirth within 1 week of a reactive NST is 1.4/1000; for a negative CST it is 0.4/1000, and for a normal BPP 0.6/1000.[3] Although some investigators have reported a decreased incidence of fetal mortality after initiation of a fetal movement counting program for "low risk" patients, there is not yet enough data available to apply these numbers to the general population.[104]

The role of Doppler flow assessment of the fetal arterial and venous systems in the prediction of in utero well-being remains controversial. At the present time, Doppler velocimetry is not required.[3] However, if Doppler is used to assess umbilical arterial waveform, the absence of end-diastolic velocity may appear days before conventional antenatal tests become abnormal. In cases such as these, at a minimum, intensive fetal surveillance is advised.[46] Reversal of diastolic flow is highly predictive of in utero fetal demise within 24 hours and warrants immediate intense investigation or delivery.

The dramatic improvement in ultrasound image quality over the past 15 years has also made it possible to directly sample fetal blood and tissue. The technique of percutaneous umbilical blood sampling (PUBS) has given the obstetrician access to the fetal circulation with relative safety for both the fetus and the mother. In this procedure, real-time ultrasonography is used to guide the insertion of a needle into the umbilical vein or artery. Samples of fetal blood can be obtained or, as in the case of red cell isoimmunization, transfusions can be carried out. The fetal loss rate is generally quoted as 1% to 2%.[142] PUBS is now frequently used in specialized perinatal centers for assessment of fetal well-being.

REFERENCES

1. Abel EL: Consumption of alcohol during pregnancy: a review of effects on growth and development of offspring, *Hum Biol* 54:421, 1982.
2. Adelsperger D, Carr J, Davis D et al: *Fetal heart monitoring principles and practice,* Washington, DC, 1993, Association of Women's Health, Obstetric and Neonatal Nurses.
3. American College of Obstetricians and Gynecologists: Technical bulletin No. 188, Chicago, 1994, The College.
4. Ananth CV, Smulian JC, Vintzileos AM: Incidence of placental abruption in relation to cigarette smoking and hypertensive disorder during pregnancy: a meta-analysis of observational studies, *Obstet Gynecol* 93:622, 1999.
5. Battaglia FC, Meschia G: *An introduction to fetal physiology,* Orlando, 1986, Academic Press.
6. Besinger R, Niebyl JR, Keyes WG et al: Randomized comparative trial of indomethacin for the long term treatment of preterm labor, *Am J Obstet Gynecol* 164:981, 1991.
7. Bevier WC, Jovanovic-Peterson L, Peterson CM: Pancreatic disorders of pregnancy: diagnosis, management, and outcome of gestational diabetes, *Endocrinol Metab Clin North Am* 24:103, 1995.

8. Blank A, Grave GD, Metzger BE et al: Effects of gestational diabetes on perinatal morbidity reassessed, *Diabetes Care* 18:127, 1995.

9. Bossi L, Assael BM, Avanzini G et al: Plasma levels and clinical effects of antiepileptic drugs in pregnant epileptic patients and their newborns. In Johannessen SI, Morselli PL, Pippinger CE et al, eds: *Antiepileptic therapy; advances in drug monitoring,* New York, 1980, Raven Press.

10. Brazy JE, Grimm JK, Little VA: Neonatal manifestations of severe maternal hypertension occurring before the thirty-sixth week of pregnancy, *J Pediatr* 100:256, 1982.

11. Brazy JE, Little VA, Grimm JK: Isoxsuprine in the perinatal period. II. Relationships between neonatal symptoms, drug exposure, and drug concentration at the time of birth, *J Pediatr* 98:146, 1981.

12. Briggs G: *Drugs in pregnancy and lactation: a reference guide to fetal and neonatal risk,* Baltimore, 1983, Williams & Wilkins.

13. Buehler BA, Stempel LE: Anticonvulsant therapy during pregnancy. In Rayburn WF, Zuspan FP, eds: *Drug therapy in obstetrics and gynecology,* ed 3, St Louis, 1992, Mosby.

14. Bureau MA, Shapcott D, Berthiaume Y et al: Maternal cigarette smoking and fetal oxygen transport: a study of P50,2,3-diphosphoglycerate, total hemoglobin, hematocrit, and type F hemoglobin in fetal blood, *Pediatrics* 72:22, 1983.

15. Burns J: Congenital heart disease: risk to offspring, *Arch Dis Child* 58:947, 1983.

16. Cannobbio MM: Reproductive issues for the woman with congenital heart disease, *Nurs Clin North Am* 29:285, 1994.

17. Canny GJ, Correy M, Livingstone RA et al: Pregnancy and cystic fibrosis, *Obstet Gynecol* 77:850, 1991.

18. Cantor B, Tyler T, Nelson RM et al: Oligohydramnios and transient neonatal anuria, a possible association with the maternal use of prostaglandin synthetase inhibitors, *J Reprod Med* 24:220, 1980.

19. Caritis SN, Lin LS, Toig G et al: Pharmacodynamics of ritodrine in pregnant women during preterm labor, *Am J Obstet Gynecol* 147:752, 1983.

20. Chamberlin PFC Manning FA, Morrison I et al: Ultrasound evaluation of amniotic fluid volumes. I. The relationship of marginal and decreased amniotic fluid volumes to perinatal outcome, *Am J Obstet Gynecol* 118:327, 1984.

21. Chasnoff IJ, Bussey ME, Savich R et al: Perinatal cerebral infarction and maternal cocaine use, *J Pediatr* 108:456, 1986.

22. Chasnoff IJ, Griffith DR, MacGregor DS et al: Temporal patterns of cocaine use in pregnancy: perinatal outcome, *JAMA* 261:1741, 1989.

23. Chesley LC: Hypertensive disorders in pregnancy, *J Nurse Midwifery* 30:99, 1985.

24. Cibils LA: *Electronic fetal-maternal monitoring,* Littleton, Mass, 1981, PSG Publishing.

25. Cohen LF, di Sant'Agnese PA, Friedlander J: Cystic fibrosis and pregnancy, *Lancet* 2:842 1980.

26. Crane JM, Armson BA, Dodds L et al: Risk scoring, fetal fibronectin, and bacterial vaginosis to predict preterm delivery, *Obstet Gynecol* 93:517, 1999.

27. Crane JM, van der Hof MC, Dodds L et al: Neonatal outcomes with placenta previa, *Obstet Gynecol* 93:541, 1999.

28. Creasy RK: Preterm labor and delivery. In Creasy RK, Resnick R: *Maternal fetal medicine principles and practices,* ed 3, Philadelphia, 1994, WB Saunders.

29. D'Alonzo GE: The pregnant asthmatic patient, *Semin Perinatol* 14:119, 1990.

30. Davidson DC, Isherwood DM, Ireland JT et al: Outcome of pregnancy in a phenylketonuric mother after low phenylalanine diet introduced from the ninth week of pregnancy, *Eur J Pediatr* 137:45, 1981.

31. Davidson JM: Renal transplantation in pregnancy, *Am J Kidney Dis* 9:374, 1987.

32. Davis LE, Lucas MJ, Hankins GD et al: Thyrotoxicosis complicating pregnancy, *Am J Obstet Gynecol* 160:63, 1989.

33. Davison JM, Katz AL, Lindheimer MD: Kidney disease and pregnancy: obstetric outcome and long-term renal prognosis, *Clin Perinatol* 12:497, 1985.

34. De Swiet M: Systemic lupus erythamatosus and other connective tissue disorders. In De Swiet, ed: *Medical disorders in obstetric practice,* ed 3, Oxford, England, 1995, Blackwell Scientific.

35. Diamond MP, Salyer SL, Vaughn WK et al: Reassessment of White's classification and Pedersen's prognostically bad signs of diabetic pregnancies in insulin-dependent diabetic pregnancies, *Am J Obstet Gynecol* 156:599, 1987.

36. Donaldson JO, Penn AS, Lisak RP et al: Antiacetylcholine receptor anti-body in neonatal myasthenia gravis, *Am J Dis Child* 135:222, 1981.

37. Druzin ML: Antepartum fetal heart rate monitoring, state of the art, *Clin Perinatol* 16:627, 1989.

38. Ducsay CA, Thompson JS, Wu AT et al: Effects of calcium entry blocker (nicardipine) tocolysis in rhesus macaques: fetal plasma concentrations and cardiorespiratory changes, *Am J Obstet Gynecol* 157:1482, 1987.

39. Elliott JP, O'Keefe DF, Schon DA et al: Dialysis in pregnancy: a critical review, *Obstet Gynecol Surv* 46:319, 1991.

40. Eskenazi B, Fenster L, Sidney S et al: Fetal growth retardation in infants or multiparous and nulliparous women with preeclampsia, *Am J Obstet Gynecol* 169:1112, 1993.

41. Evans OB, Subramoney SH, Hanson R et al: Neurologic diseases. In Sweet AY, Brown EG, eds: *Fetal and neonatal effects of maternal disease,* St Louis, 1991, Mosby.

42. Ferrer RL, Sibai BM, Mulrow CD et al: Management of mild chronic hypertension during pregnancy: a review, *Obstet Gynecol* 96:849, 2000.

43. Finnegan LP: Drugs and other substance abuse in pregnancy. In Stern L, ed: *Drug use in pregnancy,* Balgowlah, NSW, Australia, 1984, Adis Health Science Press.

44. Fleming AD: Abruptio placentae, *Crit Care Clin* 7:865, 1991.

45. Forman A, Anderson KE, Ulmsten U: Inhibition of myometrical activity by calcium antagonists, *Semin Perinatol* 5:288, 1981.

46. Forouzan I: Absence of end-diastolic flow velocity in the umbilical artery: a review, *Obstet Gynecol Surv* 50:219, 1995.

47. Franko DL, Spurrell EB: Detection and management of eating disorders during pregnancy, *Obstet Gynecol* 95:942, 2000.

48. Freeman R: Contraction stress testing for primary fetal surveillance in patients at high risk for uteroplacental insufficiency, *Clin Perinatol* 9:265, 1982.

49. Freeman RK, Garite TJ, Nageotte MP: *Fetal heart rate monitoring,* ed 2, Baltimore, 1991, Williams & Wilkins.

50. French JI, McGregor JA, Draper D et al: Gestational bleeding, bacterial vaginosis, and common reproductive tract infections: risk for preterm birth and benefit of treatment, *Obstet Gynecol* 93:715, 1999.

51. Frigoletto FD, Little GA: *Guidelines for perinatal care,* ed 2, Chicago, 1988, American Academy of Pediatrics and American College of Obstetricians and Gynecologists.

52. Fuhrmann K, Reiher H, Semmler K et al: Prevention of congenital malformations in infants of insulin-dependent diabetic mothers, *Diabetes Care* 6:219, 1983.

53. Gabert HA, Miller JM: Renal disease in pregnancy, *Obstet Gynecol Surv* 40:449, 1985.

54. Gandhi FA, Zhang XY, Maidman JE et al: Fetal cardiac hypertrophy and cardiac function in diabetic pregnancies, *Am J Ostet Gynecol* 173:1132, 1995.

55. Gilbert WM, Nesbitt TS, Danielsen B: Associated factors in 1611 cases of brachial plexus injury, *Obstet Gynecol* 93:536, 1999.

56. Gimovsky ML, Caritis SN: Diagnosis and management of hypoxic fetal heart rate patterns, *Clin Perinatol* 9:313, 1982.

57. Gravett MG: Causes of preterm delivery, *Semin Perinatol* 8:246, 1984.

58. Green J: Placenta previa and abrupto placentae. In Creasy RK, Resnick R, eds: *Maternal fetal medicine principles and practices,* ed 3, Philadelphia, 1994, WB Saunders.

59. Green KW, Key TC, Coen R et al: The effects of maternally administered magnesium sulfate in the neonate, *Am J Obstet Gynecol* 142:29, 1983.

60. Gruslin A, Perkins SL, Manchanda R et al: Maternal smoking and fetal erythropoietin levels, *Obstet Gynecol* 95:561, 2000.

61. Hall JG, Pauli RM, Wilson KM: Maternal and fetal sequelae of anticoagulation during pregnancy, *Am J Med* 68:122, 1980.

62. Harake B, Gilbert RD, Ashwal S et al: Nifedipine: effects on fetal and maternal hemodynamics in pregnant sheep, *Am J Obstet Gynecol* 157:1003, 1987.

63. Hayslett JP: Interaction of renal disease and pregnancy, *Kidney Int* 25:579, 1984.

64. Hetzel BS: Iodine deficiency disorders (IDD) and their eradication, *Lancet* 2:1126, 1983.

65. Hillier SL, Nugent RP, Eschenbach DA et al: Association between bacterial vaginosis and preterm delivery of a low birth weight infant, *N Engl J Med* 333:1737, 1995.

66. Hoff C, Wertelecki W, Blackburn WR et al: Trend associations of smoking with maternal, fetal, and neonatal morbidity, *Obstet Gynecol* 68:317, 1986.

67. Hollingsworth DR: *Pregnancy, diabetes and birth: a management guide,* ed 2, Baltimore, 1992, Williams & Wilkins.

68. Hou SH, Grosman SD, Madias NE: Pregnancy in women with renal disease and moderate renal insufficiency, *Am J Med* 78:185, 1985.

69. Hsieh TT, Chen KC, Cheng BJ et al: Pregnancy outcome in patients undergoing longterm hemodialysis, *Acta Obstet Gynecol Scand* 70:299, 1991.

70. Hutchings DE: Drug abuse during pregnancy: embropathic and neurobehavioral effects. In Braude MC, Zimmerman AM: *Genetic and perinatal effects of abused substances,* Orlando, 1987, Academic Press.

71. James LS, Yeh MN, Morishima HO: Umbilical vein occlusion and transient acceleration of the fetal heart rate, *Am J Obstet Gynecol* 126:276, 1976.

72. Janz D: Antiepileptic drugs and pregnancy: altered utilization patterns and teratogenesis, *Epilepsia* 23(suppl):53, 1982.

73. Jovanovic-Peterson L, Peterson CM, Reed GF et al: Maternal postprandial glucose levels and infant birth weight: the diabetes in early pregnancy study, *Am J Obstet Gynecol,* 164:103, 1991.

74. Kaltreider DF, Kohl S: Epidemiology of preterm delivery, *Clin Obstet Gynecol* 23:17, 1980.

75. Katz AI, Davison JM, Hayslett JP et al: Pregnancy in women with kidney disease, *Kidney Int* 18:192, 1980.

76. Katz M, Pinko A, Lurio S et al: Outcome of pregnancy in 110 patients with organic heart disease, *J Reprod Med* 31:343, 1986.

77. Kirshon B, Moise KJ Jr, Mari G et al: Long-term indomethacin therapy decreases fetal urine output and results in oligohydramnios, *Am J Perinatol* 8:86, 1991.

78. Kotloff RM, Fitzsimmons SC, Fiel SB: Fertility and pregnancy with cystic fibrosis, *Clin Chest Med* 13:623, 1992.

79. Lenke RR, Levy HL: Maternal phenylketonuria and hyperphenylalaninemia: an international survey of the outcome of untreated and treated pregnancies, *N Engl J Med* 303:1202, 1980.

80. Lenke RR, Levy HL: Maternal phenylketonuria: results of dietary therapy, *Am J Obstet Gynecol* 142:548, 1982.

81. Leonard LG: Pregnancy and the underweight woman, *Am J Matern Child Nurs* 9:331, 1984.

82. Leung AS, Millar LK, Koonings PP et al: Perinatal outcome in hypothyroid pregnancies, *Obstet Gynecol* 81:349, 1993.

83. Levin DL: Effects of inhibition of prostaglandin synthesis in fetal development, oxygenation and the fetal circulation, *Semin Perinatol* 4:35, 1980.

84. Levy HL, Waisbren SE: Effects of untreated maternal phenylketonuria and hyperphenylalaninemia on the fetus, *N Engl J Med* 309:1269, 1983.

85. Lindstrom JM, Seybold ME, Lennon VA et al: Antibody to acetylcholine receptor in myasthenia gravis, *Neurology* 26:1054, 1976.

86. Lipshitz J: Beta-adrenergic agonists, *Semin Perinatol* 5:252, 1981.

87. Lirette M, Holbrook RH, Creasy RK: Management of the woman in preterm labor, *Perinatol Neonatol* 10:30, 1986.

88. Luke B: Megavitamins and pregnancy: a dangerous combination, *Mat Child Nurs* 10:18, 1985.

89. Luke B: Maternal fetal nutrition, *Clin Obstet Gynecol* 37:93, 1994.

90. Luke B: Nutritional influences on fetal growth, *Clin Obstet Gynecol* 37:538, 1994.

91. Mandeville LK, Trojano NH: *High risk intrapartum nursing,* Philadelphia, 1992, JB Lippincott.

92. Manning FA, Morrison I, Lange IR et al: Fetal assessment based on fetal biophysical profile scoring: experience in 12,620 referred high risk pregnancies. I. Perinatal mortality by frequency and etiology, *Am J Obstet Gynecol* 151:343, 1985.

93. Martin JN Jr, Perry KG Jr: Hypertension and preeclampsia. In Sweet AY, Brown EG, eds: *Fetal and neonatal effects of maternal disease,* St Louis, 1991, Mosby.

94. Matsuura N, Yamada Y, Nohara Y et al: Familial neonatal transient hypothyroidism due to maternal TSH-binding inhibitor immunoglobulins, *N Engl J Med* 303:738, 1980.

95. Maurer G, Ambriola D: Pregnancy following renal transplant, *J Perinat Neonat Nurs* 8:28, 1994.

96. McAnulty JH, Metcalfe J, Ueland K: General guidelines in the management of cardiac disease, *Clin Obstet Gynecol* 24:773, 1981.

97. McAnulty JH, Morton MH, Ueland, K: The heart and pregnancy, *Curr Prob Cardiol* 13:589, 1988.

98. Merker L, Higgins P, Kinnard E: Assessing narcotic addiction in neonates, *Pediatr Nurs* 11:177, 1985.

99. Mestman JH: Thyroid disease in pregnancy, *Clin Perinatol* 12:651, 1985.

100. Metcalfe J, McAnulty JH, Ueland K: *Heart disease and pregnancy: physiology and management,* ed 2, Boston, 1986, Little, Brown.

101. Meyer MB, Jonas BS, Tonascia JA: Perinatal events associated with maternal smoking during pregnancy, *Am J Epidemiol* 103:464, 1976.

102. Mochizuki M et al: Effects of smoking on fetoplacental-maternal system during pregnancy, *Am J Obstet Gynecol* 149:413, 1984.

103. Montoro M, Collea JV, Frasier SD et al: Successful outcome of pregnancy in women with hypothyroidism, *Ann Intern Med* 94:31, 1981.

104. Moore TR, Piacquadio K: A prospective evaluation of fetal movement screening to reduce the incidences of antepartum fetal death, *Am J Obstet Gynecol* 160:1075, 1989.

105. Murray M: *Antepartal and intrapartal fetal monitoring,* Albuquerque, 1997, Learning Resources International.

106. Nakane Y, Okuma T, Takahashi R et al: Multi-institutional study in the teratogenicity and fetal toxicity of antiepileptic drugs: a report of a collaborative study group in Japan, *Epilepsia* 21:663, 1980.

107. National Institutes of Health Consensus Development Statement: Antenatal corticosteroids revisited: repeat courses, 2000.

108. Nau H, Rating D, Koch S et al: Valproic acid and its metabolites: placental transfer, neonatal pharmacokinetics, transfer via mother's milk and clinical status in neonates of epileptic mothers, *J Pharmacol Exp Ther* 219:768, 1981.

109. Nelson KB, Ellenberg JH: Maternal seizure disorder, outcome of pregnancy and neurologic abnormalities in the children, *Neurology* 32:1247, 1982.

110. Niebyl JR: Prostaglandin synthetase inhibitors, *Semin Perinatol* 5:274, 1981.

111. Niebyl JR, Johnson JWC: Inhibition of preterm labor, *Clin Obstet Gynecol* 23:115, 1980.

112. Noronha A: Neurological disorders during pregnancy and the puerperium, *Clin Perinatol* 12:695, 1985.

113. Odegard RA, Vatten LJ, Nilsen ST et al: Preeclampsia and fetal growth, *Obstet Gynecol* 96:950, 2000.

114. Paller MS: Renal diseases. In Burrows GN, Ferris TF, eds: *Medical complications during pregnancy,* ed 2, Philadelphia, 1995, WB Saunders.

115. Papatsonis DNM, Kok JH, van Geijn HP et al: Neonatal effects of nifedipine and ritodrine for preterm labor, *Obstet Gynecol* 95:477, 2000.

116. Patterson-Brown S, Robson S, Redfern N et al: Hydralazine boluses for the treatment of severe hypertension in preeclampsia, *Brit J Obstet Gynaecol* 101:409, 1994.

117. Peaceman AM, Meyer BA, Thorp JA et al: The effect of magnesium sulfate tocolysis on the fetal biophysical profile, *Am J Obstet Gynecol* 161:771, 1989.

118. Pedersen J: *The pregnant diabetic and her newborn,* ed 2, Baltimore, 1977, Williams & Wilkins.

119. Pekonen F, Teramo K, Ikonen E et al: Women on thyroid hormone therapy, pregnancy course, fetal outcome, and amniotic fluid thyroid hormone level, *Obstet Gynecol* 63:635, 1984.

120. Penn I, Makowski EL, Harris P: Parenthood following renal transplantation, *Kidney Int* 18:221, 1980.

121. Petri M, Allbritton J: Fetal outcomes of lupus pregnancy: a retrospective case-control study of the Hopkins Lupus Cohort, *Rheumatology* 20:650, 1993.

122. Petrie RH: Tocolysis using magnesium sulfate, *Semin Perinatol* 5:266, 1981.

123. Pitt C, Sanchez-Ramos L, Kaunitz AM, et al: Prophylactic amnioinfusion for intrapartum oligohydramnios: a meta-analysis of randomized controlled trials, *Obstet Gynecol* 96:861, 2000.

124. Platt LD, Koch R, Azen C et al: Maternal phenylketonuria collaborative study, obstetric aspects and outcome: the first 6 years, *Am J Obstet Gynecol* 166:1150, 1992.

125. Plauche WC: Myasthenia gravis, *Clin Obstet Gynecol* 26:592, 1983.

126. Poser S, Poser W: Multiple sclerosis and gestation, *Neurology* 33:1422, 1983.

127. Procianoy RS, Pinheiro CEA: Neonatal hyperinsulinism after short term maternal beta sympathomimetic therapy, *J Pediatr* 101:612, 1982.

128. Redrow M, Cherem L, Elliott J et al: Dialysis in the management of pregnant patients with renal insufficiency, *Medicine* 67:199, 1988.

129. Repke JT: Myasthenia gravis in pregnancy. In Goldstein PJ, Stern BJ, eds: *Neurological disorders of pregnancy,* ed 2, Mt Kisco, NY, 1992, Futura Publishing.

130. Resnick R, Morre TR: Obstetric management of the high risk patient. In Burrows GN, Ferris TF, eds: *Medical complications during pregnancy,* ed 4, Philadelphia, 1995, WB Saunders.

131. Rey E, Couturier A: The prognosis of pregnancy in women with chronic hypertension, *Am J Obstet Gynecol* 171:410, 1994.

132. Roberts J: Pregnancy-related hypertension. In Creasy RK, Resnick R, eds: *Maternal fetal medicine principles and practices,* ed 3, Philadelphia, 1994, WB Saunders.

133. Rohr FJ, Doherty LB, Waisbren SE et al: New England Maternal PKU Project: prospective study of untreated and treated pregnancies and their outcomes, *J Pediatr* 110:391, 1987.

134. Rosa FW: Spina bifida in infants of women treated with carbamazepine during pregnancy, *N Engl J Med* 324:674, 1991.

135. Rotmensch HH, Elkayam U, Frishman W: Antiarrhythmic drug therapy during pregnancy, *Ann Intern Med* 98:487, 1983.

136. Rudnick RA, Birk KA: Multiple sclerosis and pregnancy. In Goldstein PJ, Stern BJ, eds: *Neurological disorders of pregnancy,* ed 2, Mt Kisco, NY, 1992, Futura Publishing.

137. Sadler TW, Hunter ES III, Wynn RE et al: Evidence for multifactorial origin of diabetes induced embryopathies, *Diabetes* 38:70, 1989.

138. Scardo JA, Hogg BB, Newman RB et al: Favorable hemodynamic effects of magnesium sulfate in preeclampsia, *Am J Obstet Gynecol* 174:1249, 1995.

139. Sexton M, Hebel JR: Clinical trial of change in maternal smoking and its effect on birth weight, *JAMA* 251:911, 1984.

140. Sibai BM: The HELLP syndrome (hemolysis, elevated liver enzymes, and low platelets): much ado about nothing? *Am J Obstet Gynecol* 162:311, 1990.

141. Sibai BM, Watson GL, Hill DA et al: Maternal-fetal correlations in patients with severe preeclampsia/eclampsia, *Obstet Gynecol* 62:745, 1983.

142. Skupski DW, Wolf CFW, Bussel JB: Fetal transfusion therapy, *Obstet Gynecol Surv* 51:181, 1996.

143. Stenius-Aarniala B, Piirila P, Teramo K: Asthma and pregnancy: a prospective study of 198 pregnancies, *Thorax* 43:12, 1988.

144. Surian M, Imbasciati E, Cosci P et al: Glomerular disease and pregnancy, *Nephron* 36:101, 1984.

145. Sweet AY: Diseases of the kidneys and urinary tract. In Sweet AY, Brown EG, eds: *Fetal and neonatal effects of maternal disease,* St Louis, 1991, Mosby.

146. Tein I, MacGregory DL: Possible valproate teratogenicity, *Arch Neurol* 42:291, 1985.

147. Teramo K, Hiilesmaa V, Bardy A et al: Fetal heart rate during a maternal grand mal epileptic seizure, *J Perinat Med* 7:3, 1979.

148. Tropper PJ, Petrie RH: Placental exchange. In Lavery JP, ed: *The human placenta: clinical perspectives,* Rockville, Md, 1987, Aspen.

149. Ueland K, McAnulty JH, Ueland FR et al: Special considerations in the use of cardiovascular drugs, *Clin Obstet Gynecol* 24:809, 1981.

150. Vintzileos AM, Campbell WA, Rodes JF: Fetal biophysical profile scoring: current status, *Clin Perinatol* 16:661, 1989.

151. Wall RE: Nutritional problems during pregnancy. In Abrams RS, Wexler P, eds: *Medical care of the pregnant patient,* Boston, 1983, Little, Brown.

152. Watson RM, Lane AT, Barnett NK: Neonatal lupus erythematosus, *Medicine* 63:362, 1984.

153. Whittemore R: Congenital heart disease: its impact on pregnancy, *Hosp Pract* 18:65, 1983.

154. Witter FR, King TM, Blake DA: Adverse effects of cardiovascular drug therapy on the fetus and neonate, *Obstet Gynecol* 58(suppl):100, 1981.

155. Wisborg K, Henriksen TB, Jespersen LB, Secher NJ: Nicotine patches for pregnant smokes: a randomized controlled study, *Obstet Gynecol* 96:967, 2000.

156. Zackai EJ, Mellman WJ, Neiderer B et al: The fetal trimethadione syndrome, *J Pediatr* 87:280, 1975.

157. Zakarija M, McKenzie M: Pregnancy-associated changes in the thyroid-stimulating antibody of Graves' disease and the relationship to neonatal hyperthyroidism, *J Clin Endocrinol Metab* 57:1036, 1983.

158. Zuspan FP, Rayburn WF: Drug abuse during pregnancy. In Rayburn FP, Zuspan FP, eds: *Drug therapy in obstetrics and gynecology,* ed 3, St Louis, 1992, Mosby.

3

Regionalization and Transport in Perinatal Care

Gary Pettett, Sally Sewell, Gerald B. Merenstein

REGIONALIZATION

Regionalization can be defined as a process of resource allocation or service delivery based on geographic boundaries.[13,19] Frequently employed in the business and industrial sectors, regionalization improves service delivery and efficiency by reducing costly duplication of operations. Advocates have urged its implementation in a variety of health care settings for more than 60 years.[32] As the result of a series of legislative, professional, and local community efforts, regionalization emerged in the 1960s as the organizational model for efforts to improve the reproductive outcome of pregnant women.

In 1966 the American Medical Association (AMA) Committee on Maternal and Child Care focused attention on the relatively stagnant trend in infant mortality in the United States.[12] Despite the United States' role as a leader in the industrialized world, reduction of infant mortality in the United States lagged significantly behind that of other industrialized countries. The committee emphasized the need for identifying risk factors and problems associated with prematurity; finding more efficient use of human resources; developing research in perinatal biology; and educating obstetricians, pediatricians, and expectant parents on appropriate health care. The Eighty-ninth Congress passed two major pieces of federal legislation related to regionalized health care. Public Law 89-239, Regional Medical Programs (RMPs), concentrated on delivery of service by disease category, and Public Law 89-749, Comprehensive Health Planning (CHP), dealt with plans for using resources. Unfortunately, neither act carried any significant administrative or fiscal authority.

In 1971 the AMA[2] policy statement, "Centralized Community or Regionalized Perinatal Intensive Care," pressed for the development of centrally operated special care facilities. It encouraged the training of personnel, formulation of guidelines and evaluations, and development of adequate facilities. The AMA Maternal and Child Care Committee was directed to establish the necessary guidelines for regional perinatal programs.[3] In 1972, in conjunction with the National Foundation–March of Dimes, representatives of the American Academy of Pediatrics, the American College of Obstetricians and Gynecologists, the American Academy of Family Physicians, and the AMA met to draft these guidelines. Operating as the Committee on Perinatal Health, their recommendations were published in 1975.[55] In 1990, at the request of the American Academy of Pediatrics and the American College of Obstetricians and Gynecologists, the March of Dimes convened a new committee on perinatal health. Their recommendations were published in 1993.[33] In addition to continued support for regionalization, the committee emphasized the need for (1) health promotion and health awareness, (2) reproductive awareness, (3) perinatal regional structure and accountability, and (4) preconception and interconception care. Additional recommendations were also included. Federal expansion of Title V (Social Security Act of 1935) by Public Law 92-345 required each state to develop programs in intensive infant care that addressed the location of perinatal centers, type of care offered, type of transport systems used, and plans for regionalization.

Administrative and financial authority for regionalization was given new strength with the passage of Public Law 93-641, the National Health Planning and Resource Development Act. The intent of this legislation was to standardize effective methods of delivering health care, redistribute health care facilities, and offset the increasing costs of health care. Planning was facilitated by establishing Health Systems Agencies (HSA) or State Health Planning Agencies. Regional goals were to

31

be developed by joint efforts of health care professionals and local citizenry working within a health department or HSA subunit. By 1979 there were approximately 200 regional neonatal centers in the United States.[53] Only four states had not developed a regional plan for perinatal care.[12] The success of regional programs in reducing neonatal mortality is well documented.*

The American Academy of Pediatrics and the American College of Obstetricians and Gynecologists have developed guidelines for the regional organization of perinatal services.[23] A conceptual model based on these recommendations is shown in Figure 3-1. Level I facilities (basic care) provide continuing care for neonates with relatively minor

---

*References 9, 11, 37, 42, 47, 52, 56, 57, 60-62.

problems not requiring advanced diagnostic or therapeutic support. Most level I units can also provide convalescent care for infants from level II and level III facilities. Level II facilities (specialty care) primarily provide neonatal expertise for moderately low-birth-weight babies (1500 to 2500 g, 32 to 36 weeks' gestation) from relatively healthy participants. Level III units (subspecialty care) provide a combination of neonatal and maternal fetal services to those at the highest risk (less than 1500 g birth weight or less than 32 weeks' gestation). Included in this latter category are women who require specialized medical care and/or fetuses with identified serious malformations. Unfortunately, regionalization has not fared well in the current economic environment. Traditional concepts of regionalization have frequently given way to the economic forces of a more competitive health care market.[38] The in-

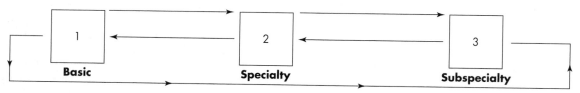

Level 1 to level 2
Complicated cases not requiring intensive care

Level 1 to level 3
Complicated cases requiring intensive care

Level 1 (responsibilities)
1. Uncomplicated maternity and neonatal care for areas not served by other units
2. Emergency management of unexpected complications

Special services
1. Early identification of high-risk patients
2. Preventive and social services

Level 2 to level 3
Complicated cases requiring intensive care
1. Labor less than 34 weeks' gestation
2. Severe isoimmune disease
3. Severe medical complications
4. Anticipated need for neonatal surgery

Level 2 (responsibilities)
1. Complete maternity and neonatal care for uncomplicated and most high-risk patients

Special services
1. 15-minute start-up time for cesarean section
2. 24-hour in-house anesthesia for obstetrics
3. Short-term assisted ventilation of newborn
4. 24-hour clinical laboratory services
5. 24-hour radiology services
6. 24-hour blood bank services
7. Fetal monitoring
8. Special care nursery

Level 3 or level 2 to hospital of origin
For growth and development of infants no longer requiring intensive care

Level 3 (responsibilities)
1. Complete maternity and neonatal care plus intensive care of intrapartum and neonatal high-risk patients

Special services
1. 24-hour consultation service for region
2. Coordination of transport system
3. Development and coordination of educational program for region
4. Data analysis for region

FIGURE 3-1 Consultation and possible transfer patterns in regional system. (From Ryan GM: Toward improving the outcome of pregnancy, *Am J Obstet Gynecol* 46:375, 1975.)

creasing availability of trained neonatal-perinatal specialists, wider dissemination of new technologies, and the growth of managed health care have encouraged many hospitals to expand their perinatal services, primarily in response to patient care activities.[40] Integration of services within many of these new health care plans and rapidly merging hospital systems has fostered the duplication of perinatal services in the guise of providing a "more competitive" market. Ironically, the result has often been a greater fragmentation of perinatal services. As the complexity of health care needs increases, access to specialized services within many plans and/or delivery systems actually becomes more restrictive and difficult to obtain. Within the same hospital there is often a wide disparity in the level of care for obstetric, neonatal, surgical, and other critical support services.[15] Whether managed care programs can provide critical care services as efficiently as they provide preventive services remains a serious and unanswered question.

Although this growing "deregionalization" of perinatal services may provide immediate benefits to local hospitals and perinatal professionals, the long-term advantage to the patient and community is less clear.[54] Cost control and universal access are two of the most important issues affecting perinatal health care today. Despite the recent advances in perinatal care, neonatal mortality in the United States remains higher than in many European and Asian countries. In part this disparity reflects the uneven effect of improved perinatal care on the population. Racial and ethnic minorities continue to have neonatal mortality rates 1.5 to 2.0 times that of whites. Excess mortality is related to the persistent high rates of premature and low-birth-weight infants in the United States, particularly among disadvantaged minorities. Evidence suggests that this gap may be widening, with the burden of poor pregnancy outcome falling more acutely on those women or families least likely to have adequate financial resources or access to comprehensive care.

Rapidly increasing costs are an important problem for those who underwrite perinatal care. Newborn intensive care units are currently among the most expensive hospital services.[26,36,50,51] The development of specialized high-risk obstetric and neonatal units requires a substantial capital investment in both personnel and high-tech equipment. Continuing improvements in diagnostic and therapeutic techniques, such as high-resolution ultrasonography, magnetic resonance imaging, high-frequency ventilation, ECMO, and surfactant replacement therapy, add to the rising costs of neonatal-perinatal care. The central role of specialized perinatal facilities in lowering the infant and neonatal mortality rate has, to some extent, exempted them from cost-containment efforts. However, as the bill for these services continues to increase, many federal, state, and commercial insurers may feel more compelled to consider methods for controlling perinatal costs.

How successfully we address these issues may largely determine the nature of neonatal and maternal-fetal medicine in the not-too-distant future. The need for more cost-effective utilization of resources and improved access to perinatal care is a strong argument for the continued support of regional organization. Perhaps as Merkatz and Johnson[42] suggested in 1976, it is time to more forcefully explore the incorporation of regional perinatal programs into our pluralistic system of health care.

Despite current economic pressures, regionalization of perinatal care continues to provide a framework for ensuring that the relatively small number of perinatal patients at the highest risk for a poor outcome have timely access to the appropriate medical facilities, equipment, and personnel. As recently as 1990 through 1994, the changing patterns of (deregionalized) perinatal care have not improved the outcome of infants less than 1500 g birth weight unless they were born in a level III center.[64] The ultimate objective is to improve reproductive outcome by reducing perinatal morbidity and mortality in the most cost-effective and care-efficient manner.

Transport

Because of the increasing complexity of perinatal care and the emphasis on early access, triage of perinatal patients has assumed growing importance. High-risk perinatal patients need to be identified during the early prenatal, intrapartum, and neonatal periods. Participating hospitals must establish criteria for the transfer of patients within the region and develop support systems for consultation, laboratory services, education, and patient transport.

An interhospital transport service is an essential component of a regional perinatal program. Based on established referral criteria, the transport service gives high-risk patients timely access to the appropriate services without interrupting their care. Return or "back" transports move recovering patients from tertiary centers to local community hospitals for completion of convalescent care in preparation for discharge from the hospital. The transport service is an important factor in the efficient management of regional bed space.

Maternal (Obstetric) Referrals

The identification of high-risk perinatal patients begins with antepartum surveillance. During the first prenatal visits the physician or nurse obtains medical, social, and demographic information pertinent to the mother's health and fetal well-being.[21,25,27] Early identification of factors that can affect pregnancy outcome is important in developing appropriate diagnostic and treatment plans to minimize potential maternal and neonatal morbidity.[23,39,43,45,48]

A list of factors derived from the history and physical examination that may increase pregnancy and neonatal risk is included in Box 3-1.

Although there is a strong correlation between antenatal risk factors and subsequent outcome in large population studies, risk assessment does not reliably predict the outcome of an individual pregnancy.[23,56] Women who are found to be at high risk during the antepartum period should be considered candidates for further evaluation and closer surveillance. Where a risk of uteroplacental insufficiency exists, evaluation of fetal well-being (e.g., BPP, CST, NST) may be indicated (see Chapter 2). Consultation and referral decisions will have to be made based on the results of a thorough evaluation of each individual patient.[10]

Box 3-1 MATERNAL RISK FACTORS FREQUENTLY ELICITED FROM HIGH-RISK PREGNANCIES

I. Prenatal
  A. History
    1. Sociodemographic
      a. Low socioeconomic status
      b. Ethnic minority
      c. Low educational level
      d. Emotional instability
      e. Substance abuse
        (1) Alcohol
        (2) Drugs
        (3) Cigarettes
      f. Age <15, >35
    2. Medical-obstetric
      a. Moderate to severe renal disease
      b. Chronic hypertension
      c. Moderate to severe toxemia
      d. Organic heart disease, class 2-4
      e. Prior Rh sensitization, prior erythroblastosis fetalis
      f. Previous stillbirth
      g. Previous premature infant
      h. Previous neonatal death
      i. Previous cesarean section
      j. Habitual abortion
      k. Prior birth >10 lb
      l. Sickle cell disease
      m. History of tuberculosis (TB) or purified protein derivative (PPD) +
      n. History of genital herpes
  B. Physical examination/prenatal follow-up
    1. Severe toxemia, hypertension
    2. Severe renal disease
    3. Severe heart disease, classes 2-4
    4. Acute pyelonephritis
    5. Diabetes mellitus
    6. Uterine malformation
    7. Incompetent cervix
    8. Abnormal fetal position
    9. Polyhydramnios, oligohydramnios
    10. Abnormal cervical cytology
      a. Dysplasia
      b. Herpes
    11. Multiple pregnancy
    12. Rh sensitization
    13. Positive serology
    14. Vaginal bleeding
II. Intrapartum
  A. Maternal
    1. Moderate to severe toxemia
    2. Polyhydramnios, oligohydramnios
    3. Amnionitis
    4. Uterine rupture
    5. Premature rupture of membranes
    6. Premature labor
    7. Labor lasting >20 hr
    8. Second stage of labor >2 hr
    9. Precipitous labor (<3 hr)
    10. Prolonged latent phase of labor
    11. Uterine tetany
  B. Placenta
    1. Placenta previa
    2. Abruptio placentae
    3. Postdates (>42 weeks' gestation)
    4. Meconium-stained amniotic fluid
  C. Fetal
    1. Abnormal presentation
    2. Multiple pregnancy
    3. Fetal bradycardia
    4. Prolapsed cord
    5. Fetal weight <2500 g
    6. Fetal acidosis, pH <7.25
    7. Fetal tachycardia
    8. Operative/vacuum delivery
    9. Difficult forceps delivery

On the other hand, certain maternal conditions more predictably require specialized care in a perinatal center (Box 3-2).[8] Evidence of these disorders should prompt a more timely consultation and consideration for referral. Transfer to a combined obstetric-neonatal intensive care facility may be especially necessary when these conditions are accompanied by the potential for delivery of an infant before 34 weeks' gestation and/or at an estimated weight of less than 2000 g.

One of the increasingly frequent barriers to referral of high-risk mothers is the federal legislation of the Emergency Medical Treatment and Labor Act (EMTALA). Originally designed to prevent the transfer of patients solely for financial reasons (dumping), the assurances required for transport often make physicians less likely to transfer mothers in early labor, regardless of the risk for poor pregnancy outcome.

Neonatal Referrals

Despite efforts to identify high-risk perinatal patients during the antepartum period, as many as 30% to 50% of infants who ultimately require additional neonatal care will not be recognized until the late intrapartum or early neonatal periods.[31] The critically ill neonate must have immediate care and stabilization at the time of delivery. Supportive care needs to be maintained until either the infant is out of danger or the transport team has arrived and assumed care.

For high-risk infants who do not require immediate resuscitation, potential problems can be identified from a systematic assessment of birth weight and gestational age.[4,5,7,16,44] Additional problems may be identified through systematic observation of the newborn infant. Stabilization and intervention procedures should be directed toward the prevention or treatment of the most likely complications.[34,35]

The decision to transfer a high-risk neonate should be based on predetermined criteria. Premature infants of less than 32 weeks' gestation will generally need specialized physiologic support and should be cared for in a well-equipped intensive care unit. Between 33 and 37 weeks' gestation, premature infants can frequently be managed in a less complicated environment. Attention to thermal support, glucose levels, fluid therapy, hematocrit, bilirubin, ventilation, and perfusion is important but may frequently be of a lower order of magnitude than in the very small infant.

Communication and Consultation

The communication system is an important factor in any regional perinatal program. The rapidly advancing field of telecommunications offers a wide variety of opportunities for transmitting medical information.

A central dedicated telephone line can provide direct and immediate access to the regional center and should be staffed 24 hours a day, 7 days a week. The line must be unencumbered by other requirements of the center. Access should be made as easy as possible. Use of a single telephone number to contact the center with subsequent distribution of calls simplifies the process for the referring community. Toll-free numbers can be employed. Appropriate consultants must be available at all times. The use of mobile phones, the ability to transfer calls or set up conference calls, and the ready availability of fax technology enhance access to consultants.

The success of the initial call may be crucial to the infant's intact survival. Ongoing stabilization of the infant before the arrival of the transport team is critical, particularly in those regions where service areas are large and transport times are long. The ability to assess the infant's condition accurately and to provide management can be facilitated by the use of a standard list of questions and information that should be obtained.

Box 3-2	MATERNAL CONDITIONS REQUIRING SPECIALIZED PERINATAL CARE

I. Obstetric complications
  A. Premature rupture of the fetal membranes
  B. Premature onset of labor
  C. Severe preeclampsia or hypertension
  D. Multiple gestation
  E. Intrauterine growth restriction with evidence of fetal distress
  F. Third-trimester bleeding
  G. Rh isoimmunization
  H. Premature cervical dilation
II. Medical complications
  A. Maternal infection that may affect the fetus or lead to premature birth
  B. Severe organic heart disease, classes 3-4
  C. Thyrotoxicosis
  D. Renal disease with deteriorating function or hypertension
  E. Drug overdose
III. Surgical complications
  A. Trauma requiring intensive care
  B. Acute abdominal emergency
  C. Thoracic emergency requiring intensive care

Whether the calls are received by a physician, a transport team member, or a professionally (medically) trained dispatcher will vary with different regional programs. Junior personnel (trainees) and staff members who are not active in newborn or maternal transport should not perform this function.

A final and frequently overlooked priority in communication occurs at the conclusion of a transport. Once the patient has arrived at the receiving center, a call should be placed to the referring physician, parents, and spouse. The purpose of the call is to relay information regarding the patient's condition and to indicate the scope of immediate care plans. Ideally, staff at the receiving center would make frequent calls to the parents and referring staff, keeping them informed on both progress and problems. At all times a line of immediate contact must be available in case the patient's condition suddenly changes.

Preparation for Transport

The goal of every transport is to bring a high-risk or critically ill patient to the tertiary center in stable condition. Federal guidelines enacted through Congressional Budget Reconciliation Act (COBRA) legislation now specify certain activities that must occur as part of the transport of any patient from one facility to another. Included in these guidelines are definitions of stable patients and a description of the types of communication that must occur to ensure the proper availability of services at the receiving hospital. Stabilization of patients for transport should actually begin before the transport team arrives. Specific areas of attention may be determined in initial communications between the referring physician and hospital and the transport team or its medical control officer.

The most common reasons for antenatal maternal referral include premature rupture of the membranes, premature onset of labor, and pregnancy-associated hypertension. Factors that require a thorough assessment before transport include fetal well-being, stage or likelihood of labor, and the probability of delivery en route. A good physical and obstetric examination, prenatal record review, and evaluation of fetal heart rate and activity would constitute a minimum evaluation. After consultation with the receiving hospital, further measures may be indicated before transport, depending on the referring hospital's capabilities. These may include an ultrasonographic examination, NST, fetal scalp pH, or amniocentesis. If indicated, magnesium sulfate,

tocolytic agents, antibiotic agents, or antihypertensive agents may be administered. **Although the reasons for neonatal referral may be quite diverse, the most common indications include respiratory distress, prematurity, congenital anomalies (surgical and nonsurgical), and suspected congenital heart disease. Stabilization and support of these infants may require frequent interhospital communication (referring physician and transport medical officer) to identify specific interventions. When the transport team arrives, the receiving hospital will generally assume control of the infant's care, although a certain degree of flexibility and cooperation with the referring staff will be maintained. A complete copy of the patient's records (hospital and prenatal), results of any laboratory tests, heart rate monitor strips, x-ray examination, and notation of all medications (with the times and doses given) should be ready to accompany the patient.**

A properly fixed placenta should be sent to the receiving hospital for pathologic examination. The mother or infant should always remain at the hospital until the transport team arrives. It is never wise to send the patient ahead with plans to meet the transport team at an alternate location, however expedient it may seem.

Whenever possible the transport team should make contact with the parents (in a neonatal transport) or spouse (in a maternal transport) before departing for the center. This offers the parents or spouse the opportunity to meet the interim care team, ask questions, and receive information about where and how the patient will be cared for. The transport team leader can explain how the transport will occur, approximately how long it will take, and what will be done en route.

Information regarding the tertiary center should be left with the parents. This should include the following:

- **Exact location of the unit—address, map**
- **Visiting hours and hospital rules**
- **Telephone numbers**
- **Names of individuals likely to be involved with the patient's care**
- **Information on the special care unit—what it is, what it does**
- **Location of parking facilities, nearby lodging, and rules regarding young children (siblings)**
- **Any particular rules or regulations regarding the special care unit**

Transport Team

Transport teams may be composed of a variety of medical personnel, including neonatologists, neonatal nurse practitioners, registered nurses, respiratory therapists, paramedics, and emergency medical technicians.[41,55] There are two general categories of transport teams: dedicated and nondedicated. The decision of which type of team to use largely depends on institutional factors. These factors often include the unit's acuity of care level, annual volume of transports, financial support, and state or local laws regarding the expanded role of nurses in health care. **Regardless of the team composition, the team must have the cumulative expertise to resuscitate, stabilize, and provide critical care throughout the transport.**[5]

Nondedicated teams are usually made up of staff nurses within the neonatal intensive care unit (NICU).[7,13] The advantage to having a unit-based, nondedicated transport team is the large pool of trained personnel available around the clock. Qualifications of team members can be based on their daily bedside critical care experience and supplemental education, such as certification as a neonatal resuscitation provider. When a neonate is critically ill and more advanced procedures may be anticipated, a physician or nurse practitioner may be added to the team.[20] The primary disadvantage to this team design is that the transport nurse's patient assignments must be absorbed by the unit until he or she returns. However, unit-based teams are usually very cost effective, because critical care skills are maintained during regular patient care, advanced skill training may be more focused, and administrative oversight duties are diminished.

Dedicated transport teams originated in the 1980s when large metropolitan hospitals began to experience an increase in the demand for neonatal transports. These teams are often composed of a nurse designated as team leader and a second nurse or a respiratory therapist as a partner. Nurse-led teams have been shown to provide better continuity of care, improved documentation, better maintenance of transport equipment, improved team availability, and stronger liaisons with referring hospitals and reduce overall operating costs.[15] The principal advantage to dedicated teams includes their immediate around-the-clock availability and their advanced training in neonatal resuscitation and stabilization procedures. However, the additional personnel required for dedicated teams may make these teams expensive to maintain.

Participation on a transport team requires leadership qualities, an ability to prioritize and organize care, and skill in handling stressful situations. A minimum of 2 years of neonatal experience with 1 year of NICU experience is a basic requirement of most transport services. **Nurses who specialize in neonatal transport should have a basic understanding of neonatal pathophysiology, stabilization and resuscitation techniques, ventilatory management, and x-ray film interpretation. Nurses who function as team leaders should have advanced training in endotracheal intubation, umbilical vessel catheterization, and thoracentesis.** When transport by aircraft is a service component, an understanding of flight physiology and flight safety is often required. Specific standards of care for neonatal transport have been developed by the National Association of Neonatal Nurses Practice Committee.[47] Written treatment protocols should be developed by each transport service. These protocols should be directed and authorized by the team's medical director and should be updated or expanded on a regular basis.

Because of the large volume of transports involving respiratory distress, respiratory therapists have been involved in a growing number of neonatal transports. Our service uses a nurse and a respiratory therapist as the basic dedicated transport team. The respiratory therapist has proved to be a valuable asset in pulmonary stabilization and airway or ventilatory management. Respiratory therapists possess a more detailed knowledge of transport respiratory equipment, ventilators, and oxygen delivery systems, obviating the need for additional technical training of nurses. The respiratory therapist must acquire the same knowledge base as the nurse counterpart. Joint training and review sessions have allowed us to standardize our instructional programs and have provided the opportunity to engender a cohesive team attitude.

Continuing education is essential for all team members. Procedural skills training should be performed on a regular (annual, semiannual, quarterly, etc.) basis to maintain competency. Educational opportunities are also provided through periodic case reviews, topic-specific lectures, outreach teaching activities, and operational (clinical) research projects.

Equipment

The equipment and medications required for neonatal transport are similar to those used in the NICU. **Box 3-3 provides a list of common transport**

Box 3-3	NEONATAL TRANSPORT EQUIPMENT

Equipment

Transport incubator*
Cardiorespiratory monitor*
Blood pressure monitor*
Suction apparatus*
Thermometer with skin probe*
Oxygen analyzer*
IV infusion pump*
Laryngoscope (various sizes)*
Transcutaneous oxygen monitor*
Pulse oximeter*
Oxygen hood
Nebulizer
Light source*
Oxygen/air cylinders
Stethoscope
Blood pressure transducers

Supplies

Suction catheters (6, 8, 10 Fr)
Bulb/ear syringe
Feeding tubes (5, 8 Fr)
Umbilical artery catheters (3.5, 5, 8 Fr)
Thoracostomy tubes
DeLee suction catheter
Three-way stopcocks
Blunt needle catheter adapter (18- and 20-gauge)
Scalp vein needles (21-, 23-, 25-gauge)
Intracaths (22- and 24-gauge)
IV pump tubing
Alcohol swabs
Skin prep swabs
Povidone-iodine (swabs and solution)
Umbilical ligature
4-0 silk suture with needle
Tape (½-inch, 1-inch)
Glucose screening strips
Lancets
Capillary tubes
Culture bottles (aerobic/anaerobic)
Syringes (various sizes)
Needles (various sizes)
Gauze pad (2 × 2, 4 × 4)
Monitor leads
IV filters
Sterile water vials
Bacteriostatic saline
Endotracheal tubes (2.5, 3, 3.5, 4 mm)

Supplies—cont'd

Endotracheal tube stylets
Heimlich valves
Flashlight batteries
Laryngoscope bulbs
Y-connectors
Oxygen tubing
Diapers
Blanket
Umbilical catheter tray
Plastic bag
Oxygen face mask (0, 1, 2 sizes)
Resuscitation bag
Chemical warming blanket

Drugs

Albumin 5%
Atropine multidose vial
10% Calcium gluconate solution
$D_{10}W$, 250-ml IV bags
D_5W, 250-ml IV bags
Digoxin, 0.5-mg ampule
Heparin, 1000 U/ml
Isuprel, 0.5-mg ampule
Tolazoline, 25 mg/ml
Lasix, 20-mg ampule
Lidocaine multidose vial
Narcan, 0.4-mg ampule
Sodium bicarbonate, 0.5 mEq/ml
Valium, 10-mg vial
Phenobarbital, 120-mg vial
Fentanyl
Ampicillin
Gentamicin
Aquamephyton, 10-mg ampule
Dopamine
Dobutamine
Pavulon
Epinepherine 1:10,000
Ringer's lactate solution, 250 ml
Prostaglandin, 500 µg/ml
Heparinized flush solution
Surfactant
Adenosine, 2 mg
Cefotaxime
Decadron, 4 mg/ml
Morphine, 2 mg/ml
Vecuronium, 10 mg

*Battery-operated/backup system.

equipment and medications. Essential items are those for physiologic (heart rate, respiratory rate, blood pressure, pulse oximetry) monitoring, temperature support, infusion therapy, and ventilatory support. Because much of the major equipment is electronic, these units must be easily adaptable to the types of power supply used in transport. All electronic equipment used in transport should be supplied with battery-operated capability. The batteries should be able to support the equipment for the entire transport if no other power source is available. Conversion devices are often needed to adapt equipment to various ambulance and aircraft power supplies. Adequate grounding of electrical equipment is as important during transport as it is in the special care unit. Equipment used in air transport must also meet Federal Aviation Administration (FAA) requirements. Some of the monitoring devices on the market today may interfere with aircraft navigational equipment. Equipment of this type should not be taken on air transport, particularly where instrument flying may be necessary.

The transport incubator is the central piece of neonatal equipment. It must be capable of controlling an infant's immediate environmental condition and allowing sufficient access to manage a critically ill patient. If extremes in environmental temperature may be encountered, the transport team should understand the incubator's capabilities and limits. Transport incubators should be of double-wall design to assist with thermal wall support. Where extremely low temperatures might be encountered, additional equipment or insulation devices (thermal incubator hood, warming blanket and Plexiglas, cellophane, and plastic "bubble" heat shields) may be necessary. The incubator should be mounted on or built into an easily movable stand that can be locked into position during transport. Some transport modules are designed with incubator and ancillary monitoring equipment in a single configuration. Because the incubator and monitoring equipment will need to be lifted on and off the transport vehicle, total weight becomes an important factor in selecting these units. The unit must be light enough to be easily lifted by the crew or transport team.

Because many neonates are transported for reasons of respiratory distress, oxygen and air-blended mixtures are essential. The most convenient gas container for transport is the compressed gas cylinder. The FAA has strict regulations about compressed gas cylinders in aircraft. The transport team should be familiar with these regulations and use appropriately designed cylinders.[18,54] The capacity of standard gas cylinders and expected life of the cylinder at various flow rates are listed in Table 3-1. Table 3-2 gives the flow rates of oxygen and air required to produce various oxygen concentrations (Fio_2).

Table 3-1	VOLUME AND FLOW DURATION OF OXYGEN IN TWO SIZES OF CYLINDERS							
	FULL		**¾ FULL**		**½ FULL**		**¼ FULL**	
Reading on Cylinder Pressure Gauge								
Pressure (lb/in²)	244		183		122		61	
Cylinder type	E	H	E	H	E	H	E	H
Contents (ft³)	22	244	16.5	183	11	122	5.5	61
(liters)	622	6900	466	5175	311	3450	155	1725
Approximate Number of Hours of Flow								
Cylinder type	E	H	E	H	E	H	E	H
Flow rate (liters/min)								
2	5.1	56	3.8	42	2.5	28	1.3	14
4	2.5	28	1.8	21	1.2	14	0.6	7
6	1.7	18.5	1.3	13.7	0.9	9.2	0.4	4.5
8	1.2	14	0.9	10.5	0.6	7	0.3	3.5
10	1.0	11	0.7	8.2	0.5	5.5	0.2	2.7
12	0.8	9.2	0.6	6.7	0.4	4.5	0.2	2.2
15	0.6	7.2	0.4	5.5	0.3	3.5	0.1	1.7

From Segal S: *Transport of high risk newborn infants,* 1972, Canadian Pediatric Society.

Table 3-2 EFFECTIVE FiO_2 DELIVERY FROM VARIOUS COMBINATIONS OF AIR AND OXYGEN FLOW*

V_{air} (AIR FLOW IN LITERS/MIN)	VIO_2 V (OXYGEN FLOW IN LITERS/MIN) 1	2	3	4	5	6	7	8	9
10	0.93	0.87	0.82	0.77	0.74	0.70	0.67	0.65	0.63
9	0.92	0.86	0.80	0.76	0.72	0.68	0.65	0.63	0.61
8	0.91	0.84	0.76	0.74	0.70	0.66	0.63	0.61	0.58
7	0.90	0.82	0.76	0.71	0.67	0.64	0.61	0.58	0.56
6	0.89	0.80	0.74	0.68	0.64	0.61	0.57	0.55	0.53
5	0.87	0.77	0.70	0.65	0.61	0.57	0.54	0.51	0.49
4	0.84	0.74	0.66	0.61	0.56	0.53	0.50	0.47	0.45
3	0.80	0.68	0.61	0.55	0.51	0.47	0.45	0.43	0.41
2	0.74	0.61	0.53	0.47	0.44	0.41	0.39	0.37	0.35
1	0.61	0.47	0.41	0.37	0.34	0.32	0.30	0.30	0.29

$$*FiO_2 = \frac{0.21\ VIO_2 + V_{air}}{V_{air} + VIO_2}$$

From Ferrara H, Harin A: *Emergency transfer of the high-risk neonate,* St Louis, 1980, Mosby.

Box 3-4 MATERNAL TRANSPORT EQUIPMENT

Equipment

IV infusion pump*
IV stand/poles
Blood pressure monitor*
Fetal heart rate monitor*
Portable light source*
Stainless steel buckets and basins
Speculum
Scissors

Supplies

Kelly clamps (4)
Cord clamps
Sponges (4 × 4)
Tape
Surgeon's gloves
Suture set
Assorted suture material
Pudendal block set
Tourniquet
Suction bulb
Adult oxygen masks and nasal cannula
Red-topped blood collection tubes
Povidone-iodine sticks
0.5 normal saline (NS) solution, 1000 ml
D_5W, 1000 ml

Supplies—cont'd

Ringer's lactate solution, 1000 ml
Blood administration set
Assorted syringes
Assorted needles
Assorted angiocaths
Adult arm boards

Drugs

Demerol, 50- and 75-mg ampules
Apresoline, 20-mg ampule
Narcan, adult, 0.4-mg ampule
Magnesium sulfate, 10% IV solution, 50% IM solution
Phenobarbital, 120-mg vial
Phenergan, 25 mg/ml
Diazoxide, 300-mg ampule
Lasix, 20 or 40 mg
Vistaril, 50 mg/ml
Pitocin, 10 U/ml
Calcium gluconate, 1 g/10 ml
Methergine, 0.2 mg/ml
Lidocaine, 1%, without epinephrine
Isoxsuprine, 10 mg/ml
Terbutaline, 80 mg in 500 ml $D_5\frac{1}{4}NS$
Ritodrine, 150 mg/500 ml
Betamethasone

*Battery-operated/backup system.

Regardless of the type of equipment purchased, maintenance and servicing are important considerations:

- Replacement parts should be readily available.
- Hospital biomedical engineers should be familiar with the equipment and provide routine preventive and reparative maintenance.
- Local equipment representatives should be available to service the equipment and provide technical updates to the transport team.
- Warranty and maintenance contracts should be easily obtained.
- Loan equipment should be available when major equipment is being repaired.

Maternal transports may require additional equipment to monitor and support both the mother and fetus. A list of additional items is provided in Box 3-4. At the completion of each transport, the equipment should be checked, batteries charged, and supplies restocked. A checklist of these functions kept with the transport equipment can help ensure timely completion and preparation for the next call. As the equipment used in the NICU has become more sophisticated, so has that in the transport environment. Portable, hand-held analysis instruments are now being used by several transport systems. Depending on the device used, these instruments provide the capability of measuring blood gases, glucose, hemoglobin, hematocrit, and electrolytes on small samples of blood obtained during transport. However, the opportunity to measure blood chemistries en route also raises the problems of standardization and quality control. We have enlisted the assistance of our hospital to provide analytic standards and quality control monitoring to fulfill current Clinical Laboratory Improvement Act (CLIA) requirements. In addition, results obtained during transport can be downloaded directly to our laboratory computer and printed to the patient's medical record upon arrival.

During the last 10 years, advances in respiratory support have included the development of patient-triggered ventilators, high-frequency ventilation, and ECMO. Although these devices have been specifically adapted to the transport setting, anecdotal reports of the use of high-frequency ventilation[1] and ECMO[14,17] during transport have appeared. As the need for these services becomes more apparent and interest in their use during transport increases, it is possible that specific transport equipment may be made available.

SPECIFIC THERAPEUTIC MODALITIES

Surfactant

The endotracheal administration of exogenous surfactant, either prophylactically or as a rescue therapy, has been shown to significantly reduce morbidity and mortality from RDS (see Chapter 23). Its use in other neonatal respiratory disorders such as meconium aspiration and prolonged mechanical ventilation, though as yet unproven, is receiving increasing attention. Because respiratory disorders continue to account for the majority of neonatal transports, the use of surfactant in the transport setting deserves careful evaluation. Techniques for the administration of surfactant must be closely observed. Whether given by transport personnel or the referring hospital staff, experience with the method of administration is important. The endotracheal tube must be in proper location to ensure a uniform distribution of the surface active material as possible. Confirmation of proper tube placement by chest x-ray examination is an important safety check. In VLBW infants (less than 1500 g), surfactant may need to be administered in small aliquots to prevent airway occlusion and further respiratory compromise. After treatment, it is important to reestablish ventilatory stabilization. Effective therapy may produce fairly rapid changes in lung compliance. Failure to recognize clinical improvement with appropriate ventilatory adjustments increases the risk of alveolar overdistention and pulmonary airleaks (e.g., pneumothorax and/or pneumomediastinum). As a result, surfactant therapy may increase stabilization time at the referring hospital. However, if respiratory control is improved, it may be time well spent.

Pulmonary hemorrhage as a result of improved lung compliance, reduced pulmonary vascular resistance, and increased left-to-right blood flow (patent ductus arteriosus [PDA], persistent foramen ovale [PFO]) is a significant, though infrequent, complication. Pretreatment with indomethacin to promote constriction of the ductus arteriosus has been suggested, but evidence of a true beneficial effect is as yet lacking.

In deciding to use or withhold surfactant, the transport team must carefully weigh the risks and benefits. At present we make decisions on a case-by-case basis. Surfactant is an expensive therapeutic agent. Once it is constituted, the manufacturer currently recommends only a single course per vial, even though most small infants require much less than the full vial. Neither keeping a sufficient stock of surfactant for transport use nor preparing surfactant in anticipation of its use seems to be a practical alternative. Our transport service restricts surfactant use to infants in whom the medical control officer feels its use would be essential. Before leaving the receiving hospital, the transport team obtains surfactant from the hospital pharmacy but does not reconstitute the drug until the infant has been properly evaluated or an order to do so is obtained from the transport physician. At the completion of the transport, unused surfactant is returned to the hospital pharmacy, where its utilization is closely monitored.

Prostaglandin E1

After respiratory distress, suspected congenital heart disease (see Chapter 24) represents one of the next most common reasons for neonatal transport. Prostaglandin E1 is an effective drug for maintaining patency of the ductus arteriosus and in important palliative therapy for infants with ductal dependent heart lesions. Indications include cyanotic lesions, such as pulmonary atresia, transposition with intact septum, tricuspid atresia, and tetralogy of Fallot, as well as acyanotic lesions including interrupted aortic arch, coarctation of the aorta, and hypoplastic left ventricle.

Unfortunately, confirmation of a defect or a description of the anatomy is often not available in the pretransport setting. Clinical indicators of congenital heart disease include persistent cyanosis (particularly cyanosis that is unresponsive to oxygen enrichment or ventilatory support), diminished peripheral pulses (weak or thready quality), poor perfusion and delayed capillary refill time, persistent metabolic acidosis, and hypotension. The absence of a heart murmur is not particularly reassuring, although its presence may be further suggestive of a heart defect. We have not found that the administration of prostaglandin on clinical grounds has significantly compromised the clinical course of infants even when no heart lesion is found on subsequent evaluation.

Prostaglandin must be given intravenously to be effective. Although this may include either a peripheral or central intravenous (IV) line, we prefer the central (umbilical vein) route to ensure proper distribution and to provide central venous access for further therapy and support. The most common side effects of prostaglandin are bradycardia, cutaneous flushing, splotchy cutaneous rash, hyperthermia, hypotension, and apnea. Apnea tends to be most frequent in those infants who also have an elevated Pco_2. The transport team should be prepared to intubate or to provide additional inotropic support should serious complications occur.

Sedation and Paralysis

The use of sedative and paralyzing agents may be required to achieve adequate oxygenation, pain control and improve stability of vital signs (see Chapter 12). Most frequently this occurs in larger infants with meconium aspiration syndrome and/or persistant pulmonary hypertension. Many of these infants have only marginal respiratory gas exchange that is further compromised by agitation and asynchronous ventilation.

Among the most commonly used agents are fentanyl and morphine for sedation and pancuronium or vecuronium for paralysis. Fentanyl is a rapid-acting drug that may be administered by either intravenous bolus or continuous infusion. It is a short-acting agent that can be reversed by discontinuing its use and by the administration of naloxone (Narcan). It does not increase intracranial pressure but can produce bradycardia, hypotension, apnea, and muscle rigidity as side effects. Morphine, although similar to fentanyl, has a longer duration of action. Side effects include increasing intracranial pressure, decreased intestinal motility, respiratory depression, and peripheral vasodilation.

Pancuronium and vencuronium are neuromuscular blocking agents that act as cholinergic antagonists at the neuromuscular endplate. Both have a near-immediate onset of action. Several clinical states not uncommon to the transported infant may either potentiate or antagonize the effects of these medications. Although preterm infants may be particularly sensitive to neuromuscular blockade, acidosis, hypothermia, hypokalemia, and renal insufficiency may potentiate the effect of these agents even further. Antagonists include alkalosis, hyperkalemia, and the use of epinephrine. Paralyzing agents should not be used in the absence of sedation and/or analgesia, because neither of these agents materially alters pain or pain perception. With the loss of spontaneous respiratory effort and chest wall stability, ventilatory support may need to be significantly increased after paralyzation. As with surfactant, restabilization of ventilatory support is often necessary before transporting paralyzed infants.

Nitric Oxide

The addition of small amounts (5 to 20 ppm) of nitric oxide (NO) to inspired gases of infants with pulmonary hypertension has been found to lower pulmonary vascular resistance and improve gas exchange (oxygenation)[28,29] (see Chapter 23). Inhaled NO is a particularly attractive therapy because of its selective action on the pulmonary vasculature. Previously used therapeutic agents such as tolazoline (Priscoline) were of limited efficacy because of their generalized systemic and pulmonary vasodilatory actions.

The use of inhaled NO in the transport setting has received very little attention. A single anecdotal report involving six patients would indicate that this therapy may be adaptable to transport systems.[30] Because NO is a recognized noxious pollutant, its use during transport also requires adherence to safety considerations. The primary side effect of NO administration is the development of methemoglobinemia. However, the small quantities used and the relatively short duration of most neonatal transports would suggest that this will not be a major deterrent.

Mode of Transport

Selecting the proper mode of transport (ambulance, helicopter, or fixed-wing aircraft) may not always be a straightforward decision. Factors to consider include distance (round-trip), the severity of the illness, immediacy of specialty intervention (e.g., surgery, cardiac evaluation) and costs to the patient. As a general rule we have used ambulances for distances of up to 100 miles (one way), a helicopter for those from 100 to 200 miles, and fixed-wing aircraft for distances of greater than 200 miles. Weather becomes an important determinant for air transport. These decisions rest primarily with the pilot, as well they should. In some settings different modes may be indicated for each leg of the transport. Nonavailability of aircraft or rapidly changing weather patterns may require a change in plans before the transport is completed.

Regardless of the mode of transport, there must be ample room to care for the patient. Smaller aircraft and low-topped ambulances frequently do not afford this capability. Helicopters have a major disadvantage. Once aboard a helicopter, the team and patient are exposed to an unusual amount of noise, vibration, and rotational forces. Many of these factors may have a direct effect on a critically ill infant. Evaluation and monitoring of a patient may be almost impossible. On flights after dusk, lighting in the patient area may interfere with the pilot's night vision. If the mother or infant is not adequately stabilized before lift-off, the patient will not likely become so in flight. For patients whose condition is tenuous or who require constant attention, another mode of transport may be advisable.

Finally, there are a few miscellaneous cautions about selecting the transport vehicle. Never initiate a transfer with a crew that is unfamiliar with the craft. The FAA and many state or county health agencies have certifying procedures for ambulance or aircraft personnel. The regional center should always be sure that the patient and transport team are in the best possible hands for travel.

For each transport alternative referral sites or temporary stops should be identified. Regardless of the amount of preparation, the possibility of vehicle malfunction or patient deterioration always exists. It may be necessary to stop temporarily for equipment or vehicle repair or for stabilization of the patient.

By whatever means the team is traveling, they should always have access to communication with the center. The center should be kept informed of their progress, the estimated time of arrival, any changes in the patient's condition, and the patient's anticipated needs on arrival.

CARE OF THE PARENTS

The birth of a critically ill infant can be a devastating event for the mother and the family (see Chapter 29). Transferring the infant to a distant hospital adds an element of physical separation that disrupts the normal process of maternal and family bonding. Parents often feel as though they have lost control of the situation and continually fear their infant will die. Parental attachment and family interactions may become dysfunctional. There are several things that the transport team can do to help parents cope with their infant's illness. Before leaving the referring hospital, the parents should be encouraged to see and touch their infant. As soon as conditions permit, the parents need to be informed of their infant's condition in an honest and forthright manner. As soon as possible, the parents should be allowed to visit their child. Physical contact between parents and infant should be encouraged. Seeing, touching, and talking to their baby can be very therapeutic for the parents. If the parents cannot visit, snapshots, and/or a videotape of their baby can provide alternative contact for the parents.

When both mother and infant have been transported, the normal family support mechanisms for dealing with crisis are disrupted. The center should provide alternate mechanisms by involving the hospital's chaplains, social workers, and parent support groups.

Depending on the distance from the parents' home to the center, lodging and financial assistance may be needed. The referral hospital should maintain a listing and provide information about local support groups. Every attempt should be made to keep the parents informed, available, and involved in their child's care.

REFERENCES

1. Allen PD, Turner DT, Brinck MJ: Ground transport of an infant on high-frequency ventilation: a case presentation, *Neonatal Net* 14:39, 1995.
2. American Medical Association: Centralized community or regionalized perinatal intensive care (Report J). Adopted by the AMA House of Delegates, June 1971.
3. American Medical Association Committee on Maternal and Child Care: *Action guide for maternal and child care committees,* Chicago, 1974, The Association.
4. Amil-Tison C: Neurologic evaluation of the maturity of newborn infants, *Arch Dis Child* 43:89, 1969.
5. Ballard JL: A simplified assessment of gestational age, *Pediatr Res* 11:374, 1977.
6. Barth J: Staff preparation and training for high-risk neonatal transport. In Graven S, ed: *Newborn air transport,* Evansville, Ind, 1978, Mead Johnson.
7. Battaglia FC, Lubchenco LO: A practical classification of newborn infants by birth weight and gestational age, *J Pediatr* 71:159, 1967.
8. Bowes WA, Merenstein GB: Recommendations and guidelines for the transport of high risk obstetrical patients, Colorado Perinatal Care Council Transport Committee, March 1978.
9. Brann AW: Perinatal health care in Mississippi 1973. In Sunshine P, ed: *Regionalization of perinatal care: report of the Sixty-sixth Ross Conference on Pediatric Research,* Columbus, Ohio, 1974, Ross Laboratories.
10. Brown FB: The management of high-risk obstetric transfer patients, *Obstet Gynecol* 51:674, 1978.
11. Butterfield LJ: Newborn country U.S.A., *Clin Perinatol* 3:281, 1976.
12. Butterfield LJ: Organization of regional perinatal programs, *Semin Perinatol* 1:217, 1977.
13. Butterfield LJ: The impact of regionalization on neonatal outcome. In Smith JF, Vidyasagar D, eds: *Neonatal and perinatal medicine,* New Delhi, 1985, Inberprint.
14. Clarke TA, Zmora E, Chen JH et al: Transcutaneous oxygen monitoring during neonatal transport, *Pediatrics* 65:884, 1980.
15. Cornish JD, Carter JM, Gerstmann DR et al: Extracorporeal membrane oxygenation as a means of stabilizing and transporting high risk neonates, *ASAIO Trans* 37:564, 1991.
16. Danzig D: Neonatal transport teams: a survey of functions and roles, *Neonatal Netw,* Oct 1984, p 41.
17. Dubowitz LMS, Dubowitz V, Goldberg C: Clinical assessment of gestational age in the newborn infant, *J Pediatr* 77:1, 1970.
18. Faulkner SC, Taylor BJ, Chipman CW et al: Mobile extracorporeal membrane oxygenation, *Am Thorac Surg* 55:1244, 1993.
19. Ferrara A, Harin A: *Emergency transfer of the high-risk neonate,* St Louis, 1980, Mosby.
20. Ginsberg E: The meaning of regionalization in health, Regionalization and Health Policy, Department of Health, Education, and Welfare, Pub No (HRA) 77-263, 1977.
21. Gomez M: Hiring, staffing, and team composition. In McClosky K, Orr R, eds: *Pediatric transport medicine,* St Louis, 1995, Mosby.
22. Goodwin JW, Dunne JT, Thomas BW: Antepartum identification of the fetus at risk, *Can Med Assoc J* 101:458, 1969.
23. Harris TR, Isaman J, Giles HR: Improved survival in very low birth weight premature and postmature neonates through maternal transport, *Clin Perinatol* 26:180, 1976.
24. Hauth J, Merenstein G, eds: *Guidelines for perinatal care,* ed 4, Elk Grove Village, Ill, 1997, American Academy of Pediatrics and American College of Obstetricians and Gynecologists.
25. Hobel CJ: Perinatal health care in Mississippi 1973. In Sunshine P, ed: *Regionalization of perinatal care: report of Sixty-sixth Ross Conference on Pediatric Research,* Columbus, Ohio, 1974, Ross Laboratories.
26. Hobel CJ, Hyvarinen MA, Okada, DM et al: Prenatal and intrapartum high-risk screening: prediction of the high-risk neonate, *Am J Obstet Gynecol* 117:1, 1973.
27. Imershein AW, Turner C, Wells JG et al: Covering the costs of care in neonatal intensive care units, *Pediatrics* 89:56, 1992.
28. *Infant death: an analysis by maternal risk and health care,* Washington, DC, 1973, Institute of Medicine, National Academy of Sciences.
29. Kinsella JP, Abman S: Inhalational nitric oxide therapy for persistant pulmonary hypertension of the newborn, *Pediatrics* 91:997, 1993.
30. Kinsella JP, Neish SR, Ivy DD et al: Clinical responses to prolonged treatment of persistant pulmonary hypertension of the newborn with low doses of inhaled nitric oxide, *J Pediatr* 123:103, 1993.

31. Kinsella JP, Schmidt JM, Abman SH: Inhaled nitric oxide treatment for stabilization and emergency medical transport of critically ill newborns and infants, *Pediatrics* 92:773, 1995.
32. Ledger WJ: Identification of the high risk mother and fetus: does it work? *Clin Perinatol* 7:125, 1980.
33. Lewis CE: *Improved access through regionalization,* Regionalization and Health Care Policy 71-84, Department of Health, Education, and Welfare, Washington, DC, Pub No (HRA) 77-263, 1977.
34. Little GA, Merenstein GB: *Toward improving the outcome of pregnancy, the 90s and beyond,* White Plains, NY, 1993, March of Dimes.
35. Lubchenco LO, Hansman C, Boyd E: Intrauterine growth in length and head circumference as estimated from live births from 26-42 weeks, *Pediatrics* 47:831, 1971.
36. Lubchenco LO, Searls DT, Brazie JV: Neonatal mortality rate: relationship to birth weight and gestational age, *J Pediatr* 81:814, 1972.
37. McCarthy JT, Koops BL, Honeyfield PR et al: Who pays the bill for neonatal intensive care? *J Pediatr* 95:755, 1979.
38. McCormick MC, Richardson DK: Access to neonatal intensive care, *Future Child* 5:162, 1995.
39. McCormick MC, Shapiro S, Starfield BH: The regionalization of perinatal services, *JAMA* 253:799, 1985.
40. Mehta S, Atherton HD, Schoettker PJ et al: Differential markers for regionalization, *J Perinatol* 20:366, 2000.
41. Merenstein GB, Pettett G, Woodall J et al: An analysis of air transport results in the sick newborn. II. Antenatal and neonatal referrals, *Am J Obstet Gynecol* 128:520, 1977.
42. Merkatz IR, Johnson KG: Regionalization of perinatal care for the United States, *Clin Perinatol* 3:271, 1976.
43. Meyer HBP: Transportation of high risk infants in Arizona. In Sunshine P, ed: *Regionalization of perinatal care: report of the Sixty-sixth Ross Conference on Pediatric Research,* Columbus, Ohio, 1974, Ross Laboratories.
44. Meyer HBP: Regional care for mothers and their infants, *Clin Perinatol* 7:205, 1980.
45. Mitchell RG, Farr V: The meaning of maturity and the assessment of maturity at birth. In Dawkins M, MacGregor WG, eds: *Gestational age, size, and maturity,* London, 1965, William Heineman.
46. Modenlow HD: Antenatal versus neonatal transport to a regional perinatal center: a comparison between matched pairs, *Obstet Gynecol* 53:725, 1979.
47. National Association of Neonatal Nurses, Practice Committee: *Neonatal transport standards and guidelines,* Petaluna, Calif, 1992, The Association.
48. Paneth N, Kiely JL, Wallenstein S et al: Newborn intensive care and neonatal mortality in low-birth-weight infants, *N Engl J Med* 307:149, 1982.
49. Pettett G: Outcome of maternal air transport. In Graven S, ed: *Maternal air transport,* Evansville, Ind, 1979, Mead Johnson.
50. Pettett G, Merenstein G, Battaglia FC et al: An analysis of air transport results in the sick newborn infant. I. The transport team, *Pediatrics* 55:774, 1975.
51. Phibbs CS, Williams RL, Phibbs RH: Newborn risk factors and costs of neonatal intensive care, *Pediatrics* 68:313, 1981.
52. Pomerance JJ, Ukrainski CT, Ukra T et al: Cost of living for infants weighing 1,000 grams or less at birth, *Pediatrics* 61:908, 1978.
53. Reynolds EOR, Taghizadeh A: Improved prognoses of infants mechanically ventilated for hyaline membrane disease, *Arch Dis Child* 49:505, 1974.
54. Richardson DK, Reed K, Cutler JC et al: Perinatal regionalization versus hospital competition: the Hartford example, *Pediatrics* 96:417, 1995.
55. Ross Planning Associates: *Referral centers providing perinatal and neonatal care,* Columbus, Ohio, 1979, Ross Laboratories.
56. Ryan GM Jr: Toward improving the outcome of pregnancy, *Am J Obstet Gynecol* 46:375, 1975.
57. Ryan GM Jr: Regional planning for maternal and perinatal health services, *Semin Perinatol* 1:255, 1977.
58. Segal S: *Transport of high risk newborn infants,* 1972, Canadian Pediatric Society.
59. Shenai J: Neonatal transport outreach educational program, *Pediatr Clin North Am* 40:275, 1993.
60. Sobol RJ, Rosen MG, Stojkov J et al: Clinical application of high-risk scoring on an obstetric service, *Am J Obstet Gynecol* 128:652, 1977.
61. Stahlman MT, Hedvall G, Dolanski E et al: A six-year follow-up of clinical hyaline membrane disease, *Pediatr Clin North Am* 20:433, 1973.
62. Stewart AL, Reynolds EOR: Improved prognosis for infants of very low birth weight, *Pediatrics* 54:724, 1974.
63. Usher RH: Clinical implications of perinatal mortality statistics, *Clin Obstet Gynecol* 14:885, 1976.
64. Yeast JD, Poskin M, Stockbauer MA, et al: Changing patterns in regionalization of perinatal care and the impact on neonatal mortality, *Am J Obstet Gynecol* 178:131, 1998.

4

Delivery Room Care

Susan Niermeyer, Susan B. Clarke

The purpose of immediate delivery room care is to support the newborn's respiratory and circulatory systems during the transition from fetal to neonatal life. Normal physiologic changes at birth include expansion of the lungs with air, initiation of gas exchange across the alveolar membrane, and closure of circulatory shunts that were necessary during intrauterine life. When delivery is complicated by perinatal conditions leading to asphyxia, resuscitation aims to reverse hypoxia, hypercarbia, and acidosis. The survival and outcome of distressed newborns depend on timely and effective intervention in the first few minutes after birth.

Information in this chapter will provide the reader with a clearer understanding of the physiologic events that take place in a distressed neonate and the evidence behind the techniques used in delivery room resuscitation. The basic techniques of thermal control and airway management constitute the initial steps in all resuscitations.[32] Indications are discussed for supplemental oxygen administration, bag and mask ventilation, endotracheal intubation, chest compressions, and use of medications and volume expansion. A discussion of delivery room emergencies integrates the basic elements of resuscitation as well as more advanced procedures sometimes called for during stabilization in the delivery room and transitional nursery. Finally, guidelines for care of the family and perinatal decision-making are presented.

PHYSIOLOGY

Rapid physiologic transition from intrauterine to extrauterine environments must be made at birth. Effective, regular respirations should be initiated within 30 to 45 seconds of delivery. Environmental factors such as a relatively cool ambient temperature and tactile stimulation assist in initiating respiration. The changes in Pao_2 and $Paco_2$ resulting from clamping the umbilical cord affect chemoreceptors and aid in the reflexive initiation of respira-

tion. The initial breath may generate from 20 to 70 cm H_2O of negative intrathoracic pressure to replace lung liquid with air inside the alveoli.[51] A rapid decrease in pulmonary vascular resistance and an increase in pulmonary blood flow occur after expansion of the lung with air, resulting in increased pulmonary perfusion and oxygenation.[49] Removal and absorption of intrauterine lung fluid is also necessary. Resorption of fetal lung liquid across the respiratory epithelium accelerates during labor, resulting in net clearance of liquid from the potential airspaces.[6] Colloid osmotic pressure and the relatively lower postnatal hydrostatic pressure of blood within the pulmonary circuit assist in absorbing alveolar fluid after delivery. Fetal right-to-left shunts through the ductus arteriosus and foramen ovale gradually close during this process[19] (Figure 4-1 and Table 4-1).

ASPHYXIA AND APNEA

Asphyxia is defined as inadequate tissue perfusion that fails to meet the metabolic demands of the tissues for oxygen and waste removal. **Asphyxia is characterized by progressive hypoxemia ($\downarrow Po_2$), hypercarbia ($\uparrow Pco_2$), and acidosis ($\downarrow pH$).** Hypoxic tissues begin anaerobic metabolism, producing metabolic acids that are initially buffered by bicarbonate. When the bicarbonate supply fails, acidosis occurs. Initially acidosis and hypoxemia result in reflexive, compensatory changes. After an initial tachycardic response, cardiac output decreases and a generalized peripheral vasoconstriction occurs to maintain a blood pressure that is adequate for perfusion of vital organs. Conversion from aerobic to anaerobic glycolysis takes place with the accumulation of lactate and the development of metabolic acidosis.[17]

Asphyxia may occur in utero or postnatally. In either circumstance, a well-defined series of events follows (Figure 4-2). After a brief period of rapid breathing, respiratory movements cease

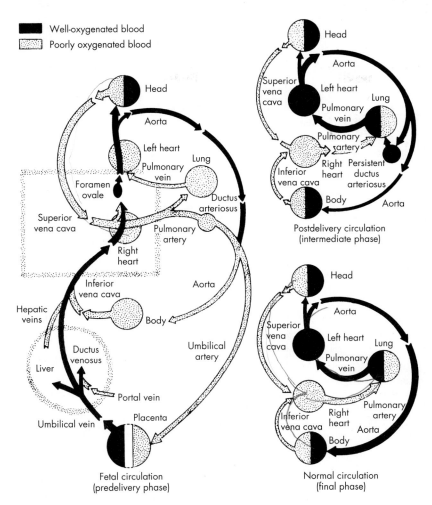

FIGURE 4-1 Blood circulation before and after birth. (From Babson SG, Pernoll ML, Benda GL: *Diagnosis and management of the fetus and neonate at risk: a guide for team care,* ed 4, St. Louis, 1980, Mosby.)

Table 4-1	COMPARISON OF VASCULAR AND PULMONARY FUNCTIONS BEFORE AND AFTER BIRTH	
FETAL FUNCTION	**BODY STRUCTURE**	**EXTRAUTERINE FUNCTION**
Carries oxygenated blood from left ventricle and deoxygenated blood from pulmonary arteries to fetal organs and placenta	Aorta	Carries oxygenated blood from left ventricle into systemic circulation
Shunts most of the oxygenated blood from placenta to inferior vena cava	Ductus venosus	Disappears within 2 weeks after birth; becomes ligamentum venosum
Connects right and left atria; permits oxygenated blood from right atrium to bypass right ventricle and pulmonary circuit and go directly into left atrium	Foramen ovale	Functionally closes soon after birth; anatomically seals during childhood
Shunts blood from pulmonary artery directly into aorta	Ductus arteriosus	Functionally closes soon after birth; eventually becomes ligamentum arteriosum
Carries blood to and from placenta, the organ of respiration before birth	Umbilical arteries and vein	Clamped at birth, obliterating placental connections; become ligaments
Distended with fluid; minimal pulmonary circulation; fetal respiratory movements	Lungs	Expanded and aerated; pulmonary circulation allows CO_2 and O_2 exchange; organ of respiration

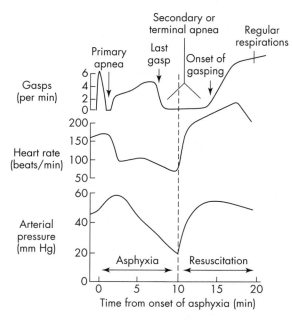

FIGURE 4-2 Changes in physiologic parameters during asphyxiation and resuscitation of Rhesus monkey fetus at birth. (From Dawes G: *Foetal and neonatal physiology,* St. Louis, 1968, Mosby.)

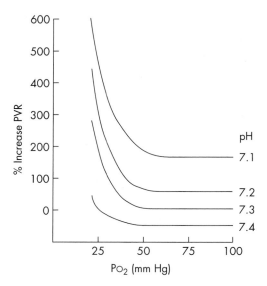

FIGURE 4-3 Pulmonary vascular resistance in calf. *PVR,* Pulmonary vascular resistance. (From Rudolph AM, Yuan S: *J Clin Invest* 45:399, 1966.)

and a period of apnea called *primary apnea* follows. At the same time heart rate falls and neuromuscular tone diminishes. Intrauterine asphyxia may result in the passage of meconium before birth. If the asphyxial insult continues, the heart rate falls further, blood pressure falls, hypotonia worsens, and a series of spontaneous deep gasps occurs. Gasping continues but becomes weaker, more irregular, and finally ceases. After the last gasp occurs, a period of apnea begins; this is known as *secondary apnea.*[17,32]

Delivery may occur at any point in the progression of an asphyxial insult. If an infant is born during the primary apnea phase, exposure to oxygen and stimulation will usually induce respirations. If delivery occurs during secondary apnea, the infant will not respond to stimulation. Spontaneous respirations will not resume until resuscitation is initiated with assisted ventilation and oxygen.[1,17,32] **In the clinical setting, primary and secondary apnea are essentially indistinguishable from one another. In both the infant is not breathing, the heart rate may be below 100 beats/min, and the infant is hypotonic. Thus any infant who is apneic at delivery must be assumed to be in secondary apnea, and resuscitation should begin immediately.**

The longer artificial ventilation is delayed after an infant's last gasp in secondary apnea, the longer the time required for the infant's first spontaneous gasp after resuscitation. For every 1-minute delay, the time to the first gasp increases by about 2 minutes, and the time to the onset of spontaneous breathing is prolonged by more than 4 minutes.[1] In the absence of effective resuscitation after delivery, apnea and decreased cardiac output will result in progressive biochemical deterioration.[1,17]

Severe fetal and neonatal asphyxia impair the physiologic transitions to extrauterine life. The normally high fetal pulmonary vascular resistance may not decrease in the presence of persistent acidosis and hypoxemia; consequently the pulmonary circuit continues to carry low volumes of blood and oxygen transfer is impeded, perpetuating the hypoxemia (Figure 4-3).[49] As part of persistent pulmonary hypertension of the newborn, normal closure of fetal shunts is delayed by high pulmonary vascular resistance, pulmonary hypoperfusion, hypoexpansion, and hypoxemia, thus resulting in persistent right-to-left shunting through the ductus arteriosus and foramen ovale. Lung fluid clearance may also be delayed because of poor lung inflation and/or pulmonary hypoperfusion and hypoxemia. Additionally, intraalveolar fluid may accumulate as a result of leakage from damaged pulmonary capillaries, resulting in pulmonary edema. With worsening hypoxemia and acidosis, myocardial function begins to fail, cardiac output falls, and perfusion to vital body organs including the brain, kidney, and intestine decreases, setting the stage for postasphyxial injury of these organs.[13]

RESUSCITATION OF THE NEWBORN

Preparation for Resuscitation

Immediate, effective resuscitation of the newborn infant can reduce or prevent morbidity and mortality. **Much of neonatal resuscitation focuses on oxygenation, ventilation, and reversal of perinatal asphyxia.** Application of basic procedures is often all that is necessary to successfully resuscitate a depressed infant.[44] **Additionally, effective resuscitation requires anticipation and adequate preparation of equipment and personnel.**[4,46,56]

Elements of the antepartum and intrapartum histories may identify the infant at risk for perinatal asphyxia (Box 4-1). Any normal pregnancy, however, may become high-risk with the onset of previously unexpected or undetected complications during the intrapartum phase. Examples include maternal hemorrhage, prolapsed cord, and meconium staining of the amniotic fluid.

Prevention, detection, and treatment of fetal asphyxia is the responsibility of the obstetric team. Once fetal asphyxia is diagnosed, therapeutic intervention should be coordinated between obstetric and neonatal services to allow for a timely delivery and effective, coordinated resuscitation.

In the mid-1980s the need for a national training program for neonatal resuscitation in the United States was addressed by the American Heart Association (AHA) and the American Academy of Pediatrics (AAP) through development of the Neonatal Resuscitation Program (NRP). The goal of the NRP is to provide the materials and training necessary for health care professionals to follow guidelines established and updated periodically at the International Guidelines Conference on Cardiopulmonary Resuscitation and Emergency Cardiovascular Care. In 2000 new guidelines based on rigorous evidence evaluation were adopted.[39] These changes have been

---

| **Box 4-1** | **CONDITIONS THAT MAY REQUIRE AVAILABILITY OF SKILLED RESUSCITATION AT DELIVERY** |

Intrapartum Problems

- Fetal distress
  Persistent late decelerations
  Severe variable decelerations without baseline variability
  Bradycardia
  Meconium-stained amniotic fluid
  Cord prolapse
- Prolonged, unusual, or difficult labor
- Emergency operative or assisted delivery
- Breech presentation with vaginal delivery
- Narcotic administration to mother within 4 hours of delivery

Medical/Obstetric/Genetic Problems

- Diabetes mellitus
- Suspected or confirmed maternal infection
- Substance abuse
- Third trimester bleeding
- Pregnancy-induced hypertension
- Abnormal amniotic fluid volume
- Prolonged rupture of membranes
- Multiple gestation
- Low-birth-weight infant
- Prematurity
- Isoimmunization
- Fetal congenital anomalies

---

incorporated into the fourth edition of the NRP textbook. The program's widespread acceptance ensures consistent use of current guidelines, awareness of proper equipment, and preparation of personnel to work as a team using shared cognitive knowledge and performance skills.

The NRP recommends that **"At every delivery there should be at least one person whose primary responsibility is the baby and who is capable of initiating resuscitation. Either that person or someone else who is immediately available should have the skills required to perform a complete resuscitation, including endotracheal intubation and administration of medications."** When a high-risk delivery is anticipated, two persons whose sole responsibility is resuscitation of the infant should be present, and their roles should be designated in advance. Multiple births require a full team of personnel with complete equipment for each infant.[32]

The pediatric staff should be familiar with the prenatal and intrapartum history of the mother and fetus (see Box 4-1), because this information will affect the initial level of resuscitation preparation.

Resuscitation equipment (Box 4-2) and drugs (Table 4-2) should always be readily available, functional, and assembled for immediate use in a designated location, ideally in a specific area of the delivery/birthing room. Consumable supplies and small equipment can be stored on specially constructed wall shelves or on a radiant warmer/intensive-care bed equipped with easily accessible storage (Figures 4-4 and 4-5).

Prepare for neonatal resuscitation by performing the following:
- Preheat the radiant warmer.
- Assemble consumable supplies: warm linens, bulb syringe, suction catheter, cord clamp, and appropriate personal protection.
- Check suction equipment for function and set the wall vacuum regulator control not to exceed 100 mm Hg.
- Turn on the oxygen flow to the ventilation bag and check all connections, flow-control valves, pressure release valve, and manometer function to enable the ventilation bag to inflate to 30 to 40 cm H_2O pressure. Ensure an appropriate size face mask is available.
- Check the laryngoscope for a bright light source and appropriate blades (size 0 for premature infants and size 1 for term infants); tighten the bulb.
- Check the availability of appropriately sized endotracheal tubes (2.5 to 4.0).
- Locate a stethoscope of appropriate size and confirm that it is functioning properly.
- Check the ancillary equipment (i.e., umbilical catheter supplies, intravenous [IV] solutions, nonexpired resuscitation drugs).
- If the clinical situation warrants, draw up and label emergency medications for ready administration, using the estimated fetal weight, and obtain O-negative packed red blood cells for emergency transfusion.

The steps of neonatal resuscitation follow the standard ABCs of resuscitation:
    A—Airway
    B—Breathing
    C—Circulation

Box 4-2	EQUIPMENT USED DURING NEONATAL RESUSCITATION
Thermal Management	**Breathing—cont'd**
Radiant warmer	Endotracheal tubes 2.5, 3.0, 3.5, 4.0 mm ID
Warmed blankets or towels	Stylet
Infant stocking caps	Tape, skin preparation
	Scissors
Airway	(CO₂ detector)
Bulb syringe	**Circulation**
Mechanical suction	
Suction catheters 5, 6, 8, 10 Fr	Stethoscope
8 Fr feeding tube and 20 ml syringe	Wall clock or stopwatch
Meconium aspirator/suction device	Cord clamp
Shoulder roll	Medications (see Table 4-2)
	Sterile gloves
Breathing	Alcohol sponges, povidone-iodine solution
Bag and mask ventilation	Umbilical vessel catheterization tray
Oxygen source with flowmeter and tubing	Umbilical catheters 3.5 and 5 Fr
Neonatal resuscitation bag with 100% oxygen capability	Three-way stopcocks
and manometer or pressure release valve	Umbilical tape
Face masks, newborn and premature sizes	Suture material
Oral airways, newborn and premature sizes	Intravenous catheters, tubing, fluid
(Pulse oximeter)	Needles 25-, 23-, 22-, 20-, 18-gauge
Intubation	Syringes 1-, 3-, 5-, 10-, 20-, 50-ml
Laryngoscope with extra batteries	(Cardiorespiratory monitor)
Straight blades No. 0 and No. 1 with extra bulbs	(Procedure light)

Table 4-2 MEDICATIONS FOR NEONATAL RESUSCITATION

MEDICATION	CONCENTRATION TO ADMINISTER	DOSAGE/ROUTE*	TOTAL DOSE/INFANT	RATE/PRECAUTIONS	INDICATIONS FOR USE
Epinephrine	1:10,000	0.1-0.3 ml/kg (0.01-0.03 mg/kg) IV or ET	**Weight (kg)** / **Total ml** 1 / 0.1-0.3 2 / 0.2-0.6 3 / 0.3-0.9 4 / 0.4-1.2	Give rapidly May dilute with 1 ml normal saline solution if giving ET	Heart rate <60 after 30 sec of adequate ventilation and chest compressions
Volume expanders	Normal saline solution Ringer's lactate solution Whole blood	10 ml/kg IV	**Weight (kg)** / **Total ml** 1 / 10 2 / 20 3 / 30 4 / 40	Give over 5-10 min	Evidence of acute bleeding with signs of hypovolemia; poor response to resuscitation
Sodium bicarbonate	0.5 mEq/ml (4.2% solution)	4 ml/kg (2 mEq/kg) IV	**Weight (kg)** / **Total dose (mEq)** / **Total ml** 1 / 2 / 4 2 / 4 / 8 3 / 6 / 12 4 / 8 / 16	Give slowly over at least 2 min Give only if infant is being effectively ventilated	Severe metabolic acidosis is suspected or proved by blood gas analysis
Naloxone hydrochloride	0.4 mg/ml	0.25 ml/kg (0.1 mg/kg) IV, ET IM, SC	**Weight (kg)** / **Total dose (mg)** / **Total ml** 1 / 0.1 / 0.25 2 / 0.2 / 0.50 3 / 0.3 / 0.75 4 / 0.4 / 1.00	Give rapidly IV, ET preferred IM, SC acceptable	Severe respiratory depression and history of maternal narcotic administration within past 4 hr
	1.0 mg/ml	0.1 ml/kg (0.1 mg/kg) IV, ET IM, SC	1 / 0.1 / 0.1 2 / 0.2 / 0.2 3 / 0.3 / 0.3 4 / 0.4 / 0.4		

ET, Endotracheal; *IM,* intramuscular; *IV,* intravenous; *SC,* subcutaneous.

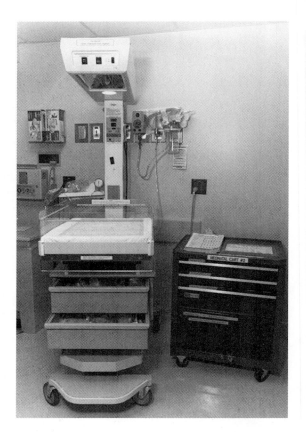

FIGURE 4-4 Labor/delivery/recovery (LDR) room resuscitation area consisting of radiant warmer with flow-inflating bag and manometer and wall oxygen and suction outlets. Other supplies for airway suctioning and intubation are stored in the drawers of the radiant warmer. Resuscitation drugs and umbilical catheterization trays are kept in a separate resuscitation cart accessible from all LDR rooms.

A 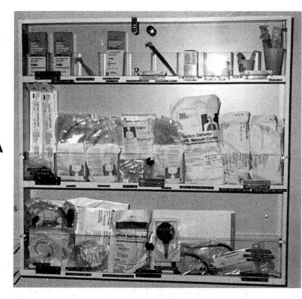 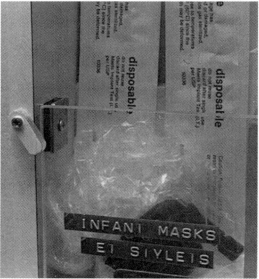 B

FIGURE 4-5 **A,** Wall-mounted storage bin. Unit consists of three Plexiglas shelves; each shelf is divided by Plexiglas into smaller compartments. Each compartment is labeled. Shelves can be opened for cleaning. Each shelf is held in place by hinge and magnet. **B,** Hinge and magnet device used to ensure closure of Plexiglas shelves.

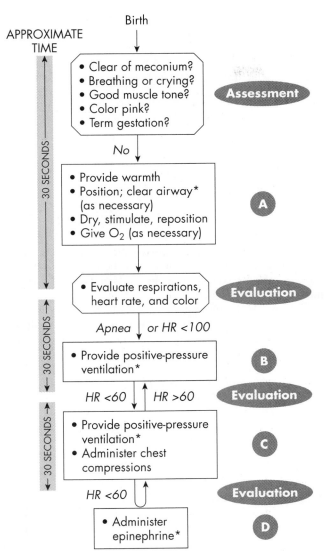

Birth

APPROXIMATE
TIME

- Clear of meconium?
- Breathing or crying?
- Good muscle tone?
- Color pink?
- Term gestation?

Assessment

No

- Provide warmth
- Position; clear airway*
  (as necessary)
- Dry, stimulate, reposition
- Give O₂ (as necessary)

A

- Evaluate respirations,
  heart rate, and color

Evaluation

Apnea or *HR <100*

- Provide positive-pressure
  ventilation*

B

HR <60 | *HR >60*

Evaluation

- Provide positive-pressure
  ventilation*
- Administer chest
  compressions

C

HR <60

Evaluation

- Administer
  epinephrine*

D

30 SECONDS / 30 SECONDS / 30 SECONDS

*Endotracheal intubation may be considered at several steps.

FIGURE 4-6 Throughout resuscitation, the infant's respirations, heart rate, and color are evaluated as a basis for decisions and actions. (From Kattwinkel J, ed: *Textbook of neonatal resuscitation,* 4th ed, Elk Grove Village, Ill, 2000, American Academy of Pediatrics and American Heart Association.)

With the ABCs as an overall framework for neonatal resuscitation, the components of the procedure can be examined sequentially:

A—Establish an airway
  Positioning
  Suctioning of mouth, nose, and trachea (in some cases)
  Endotracheal intubation if necessary
B—Initiate breathing
  Tactile stimulation
  Free-flow oxygen, as necessary
  Positive-pressure ventilation

C—Maintain circulation
  Chest compressions
  Medications, volume expansion

At each step of the resuscitation procedure, whether uncomplicated or extended, the cycle of evaluation/decision/action is repeated. Evaluation is based on the infant's respirations, heart rate, and color (Figure 4-6). The importance of the first two elements of resuscitation, establishment of an airway and breathing, cannot be overemphasized with respect to neonatal resuscitation. **Expansion of the lungs with air and adequate ventilation are the**

keys to successful resuscitation. Successful performance of these steps often obviates the need for further intervention, but inadequate lung expansion and ventilation cannot be overcome by performing chest compressions or administering medications.

Apgar Score

The Apgar score, developed by Dr. Virginia Apgar in 1952, provides a comprehensive, objective measure of the infant's condition in the first minutes after birth (Figure 4-7). The Apgar score is not used as an indicator of the need for resuscitation; rather, it may be used to assess an infant's response to resuscitative measures. In term and preterm infants, the Apgar score remains a valuable predictor of infants who will need ongoing support in the immediate postpartum period and those who are at higher mortality risk in the neonatal period.[15]

Although perinatal asphyxia may be associated with low Apgar scores, it is possible for an infant to have a low Apgar score without having asphyxia.[28] For example, an infant born to a mother who received general anesthesia may be flaccid and have depressed reflexes and poor respiratory efforts. These infants usually respond rapidly to bag-and-mask ventilation, and no further intervention is necessary. Conversely, an infant may have an equally low Apgar score as a result of intrauterine asphyxia and require prolonged resuscitative efforts. An infant with a mid-range Apgar score between 6 and 7 may be using homeostatic mechanisms to maintain an adequate central blood pressure and cardiac output. Apgar scores should be assigned at 1 and 5 minutes and every 5 minutes thereafter until the score is 7 or greater. A complete description of resuscitative steps and their timing is vital to interpret a low Apgar score.

Although the Apgar score is not used to guide resuscitation, the experienced clinician performs a rapid visual assessment of an infant at the moment of birth. This rapid assessment incorporates three elements from the Apgar score as well as two key questions that influence the overall conduct of the resuscitation.

Rapid Assessment After Birth

In the first few seconds after birth, a rapid visual assessment of the baby should be performed to answer the following questions[32]:

   Is the amniotic fluid and the skin clear of meconium?
   Is the baby breathing or crying?
   Is there good muscle tone?
   Is the baby's color pink?
   Is the baby term?
If the answer to all of these questions is "yes," the baby can remain with the mother to receive the initial steps of resuscitation (routine care) described below.

   If the answer to any of the questions is "no," the infant should be evaluated under a radiant warmer while the initial steps are carried out. If meconium is present, the vigor of the infant is evaluated first, under the radiant warmer, before the initiation of the initial steps.

   If meconium is present, evaluate the vigor of the infant:

   Does the baby have strong respiratory efforts?
   Is there good muscle tone?
   Is the heart rate above 100 beats/min?
If the answer to all the questions is "yes," the airway may be cleared as described in the airway section below. If the answer to any of the questions is "no," the infant requires endotracheal intubation for suctioning.[32,59] In this circumstance, completion of the initial steps of resuscitation then follows.

Sign	Score		
	0	1	2
A Appearance (color)	Blue, pale	Body pink Extremities blue	Completely pink
P Pulse (heart rate)	Absent	Below 100	Above 100
G Grimace (reflex, irritability to suctioning)	No response	Grimace	Cough or sneeze
A Activity (muscle tone)	Limp	Some flexion	Well flexed
R Respiration (breathing efforts)	Absent	Weak, irregular	Strong cry

FIGURE 4-7   Practical epigram of Apgar score. (From Butterfield J, Covey M: *JAMA* 181:353, 1962.)

Initial Steps of Resuscitation

The initial steps of resuscitation should be performed at every delivery. They include (1) providing warmth, (2) clearing the airway (positioning and suctioning as necessary), (3) initiating breathing by tactile stimulation, and (4) giving oxygen, as indicated.

Many of the initial steps can be performed simultaneously, especially if more than one person is caring for the infant. Positioning and clearing the airway, drying, tactile stimulation, and even oxygen administration may be initiated simultaneously.

Provide Warmth

- Dry the infant and place the baby directly on the mother's chest; cover both with warm linen (routine care).
  or
- Place the infant under a radiant heat source, drying the infant thoroughly and removing the wet linen.

Position and Clear the Airway (as Necessary)

- Ensure that the infant's neck is slightly extended when positioning the baby on the mother's chest; wipe secretions from the mouth and nose or suction with a bulb syringe as necessary (routine care).
  or
- Position the infant supine and flat with the neck slightly extended. A rolled blanket or towel may be used under the shoulders.
- Suction the mouth then the nose to clear the airway. The mouth is suctioned first to clear the largest volume of secretions; when the nasopharynx is suctioned, a reflex cough, sneeze, or cry often results.
- Turn the head (or the head and body) to the side to allow secretions to pool in the cheek, then remove with a bulb syringe or suction catheter. Deep pharyngeal suction in an infant not requiring positive-pressure ventilation or intubation should not be performed during the first few minutes after birth to avoid vagal stimulation, resultant bradycardia, and delay in rise in PaO_2.[11,20]
  or
- If meconium is present, evaluate the vigor of the infant as described above.[59]

Stimulate and Reposition

- Provide tactile stimulation by briefly rubbing the back or gently slapping or flicking the feet.

- Keep the head and neck in a slightly extended position to maintain an open airway.
- Continue gentle rubbing of trunk, extremities, or head to support early respiratory efforts in the newborn.

Provide Free-Flow Oxygen (as Necessary)

- Give free-flow oxygen if the infant is breathing but remains centrally cyanotic. Peripheral cyanosis (acrocyanosis) is not an indication for supplemental oxygen.

Evaluate the Infant

- Evaluation of the infant is a continuous, ongoing process. Evaluation during each step of resuscitation and a decision about whether the response is adequate or not are necessary to guide subsequent action.

Evaluate Respirations

- **Rate and depth of respirations (chest wall movement, air exchange) must be adequate; gasping respirations call for the same intervention as apnea.**

Evaluate Heart Rate

- **The heart rate should be more than 100 beats/ min.** Feel the base of the umbilical cord or listen over the left side of the chest with a stethoscope to count the heart rate. Count the heart rate in 6 seconds and multiply by 10 for the beats per minute. Indicate each beat by tapping the forefinger on the bed or tapping the thumb and index finger together.

Evaluate Color

- **The lips and trunk should be pink.**

Positive-Pressure Ventilation

Indications for positive-pressure ventilation with a bag and mask and 100% oxygen in the newborn infant include:

- **Apnea or gasping respirations, despite a brief period of tactile stimulation**
- **A heart rate below 100 beats/min**
- **Central cyanosis despite 100% free-flow oxygen**

Prolonged tactile stimulation or administration of supplemental oxygen to a baby who is not breathing effectively or who has a heart rate below 100 beats/ min only delays appropriate treatment. If supplemental oxygen is unavailable, positive-pressure ventilation should be initiated with room air.[39]

Chest Compressions

- **If after 30 seconds of effective positive-pressure ventilation with 100% oxygen the heart rate is less than 60 beats/min, begin chest compressions.** Consider intubation and prepare emergency drugs (see Table 4-2).

Administration of Epinephrine and Volume Expansion

- **If the heart rate remains below 60 beats/min despite 30 seconds of positive-pressure ventilation with 100% oxygen and another 30 seconds of ventilation with 100% oxygen and chest compressions, administer epinephrine.**
- **If the baby is not responding to resuscitation, and there is evidence of blood loss, consider administration of a volume expander.**

Each of the major steps in neonatal resuscitation should be accomplished in approximately 30 seconds. The initial rapid assessment can be performed in the first few seconds after birth to determine whether routine care can be provided to the infant, who remains with the mother, or if more extensive evaluation and resuscitation will be necessary during the initial steps. The initial steps of resuscitation can be performed concurrently with more detailed evaluation (heart rate, respirations, and color), especially if more than one person is present to care for the infant. Positive-pressure ventilation with 100% oxygen and chest compressions should both be performed for 30-second intervals before moving to the next level of intervention.

An infant who has received more than the initial steps of resuscitation will require close monitoring for additional or recurrent problems during the postnatal transition and may need supportive care such as oxygen administration. Infants who require more than brief positive-pressure ventilation should be monitored in a nursery setting where they can receive ongoing care.[32]

Skills Required for Neonatal Resuscitation

Initial Steps: Administration of Free-Flow Oxygen

Supplemental oxygen should be administered in a concentration of 100% at a flow rate of 5 L/min. Oxygen may be administered by mask or by holding the oxygen tubing in a cupped hand over the face. 100% oxygen at 5 L/min provides 80% to 100% oxygen to the infant when delivered via a mask or via tubing held adjacent to the nares and surrounded by a cupped hand. The delivered oxygen concentration decreases rapidly as the tubing or mask is withdrawn from the face.

Once the infant becomes pink, gradually withdraw the oxygen tubing or the mask from the infant's face. If cyanosis persists, reevaluate the quality of respirations and the heart rate; perform a brief physical examination; and consider bag-mask ventilation or intubation if there is evidence of respiratory distress.

Initial Steps: Suctioning for Meconium-Stained Amniotic Fluid

Meconium-stained amniotic fluid is seen most often in infants of more than 34 weeks' gestational age, especially in term and postterm neonates. Passage of meconium may be associated with asphyxia. Severe fetal acidosis can result in fetal gasping, leading to in utero aspiration of meconium.[58] Postnatal meconium aspiration often can be avoided by thoroughly suctioning the mouth and hypopharynx at delivery of the head and again after delivery is complete.[12,25]

Tracheal intubation for suctioning is indicated in infants with meconium-stained amniotic fluid who are not vigorous at birth. Vigor is defined by effective spontaneous respirations, a heart rate of more than 100 beats/min, and good muscle tone. A large, multicenter, controlled trial examining management of a vigorous infant with meconium-stained fluid found no difference in the incidence of respiratory distress (meconium aspiration or other respiratory distress) between groups that received routine airway management and endotracheal intubation for suctioning.[59] Nevertheless, any infant born with meconium-stained amniotic fluid who develops signs of airway obstruction or needs positive-pressure ventilation should first have the trachea suctioned and cleared of any meconium present. Controversy still exists over appropriate resuscitation of the infant with thick meconium; this subgroup of infants remains at highest risk for respiratory distress.

If meconium is present in the amniotic fluid, perform the initial steps in the following manner:
- Suction the nose, mouth, and posterior pharynx when the head is delivered.
- If the infant is vigorous, suction the nose, mouth, and posterior pharynx as necessary once the infant is on the radiant warmer and proceed with drying, stimulation, and removal of wet linen.

- If the infant is depressed, clear the oropharynx with a large-bore cathether and suction the trachea under direct visualization using an endotracheal tube, adapter, and mechanical suction or a meconium suction device (Figure 4-8). Dry, stimulate, and remove wet linen after the airway has been cleared.
- Suction the stomach when airway management is complete and vital signs are stable (usually after 5 minutes). Clearing residual meconium from the stomach decreases the risk of postnatal regurgitation and aspiration; however, suctioning too soon after birth can provoke apnea and bradycardia by vagal stimulation and complicate the initial resuscitation.

Bag and Mask Ventilation

The indications for bag and mask ventilation include (1) apnea unresponsive to brief stimulation or gasping respirations, (2) heart rate of less than 100 beats/min and (3) persistent cyanosis despite 100% free-flow oxygen. The equipment for bag and mask ventilation can be either a self-inflating bag with an oxygen reservoir and pressure-release valve or pressure gauge or a flow-inflating bag (anesthesia bag) with a flow-control valve and pressure gauge.

Self-inflating bags more reliably deliver tidal volume in the hands of providers who resuscitate babies infrequently[30]; however, self-inflating bags cannot be used reliably to deliver free-flow oxygen, and they require a special adapter to deliver continuous positive airway pressure (CPAP) (Figure 4-9). Flow-inflating bags require a complete seal between mask and face to deliver a tidal volume. They offer the advantages of ability to achieve high peak pressures, CPAP capability, and delivery of free-flow oxygen. The volume of the bag should generally be between 200 and 750 ml.[32] Smaller bags within this range may not have sufficient volume to deliver a long inspiratory time to a large term baby during opening breaths. Larger bags are more difficult to handle and predispose to overly large tidal volumes, especially for preterm infants.

The face mask should be selected to ensure that it is appropriately sized to cover the chin, mouth, and nose, but not the eyes. Masks are commonly available in term and premature sizes and may be obtained to fit even VLBW infants. Flexible, translucent masks with a cushioned rim generally provide

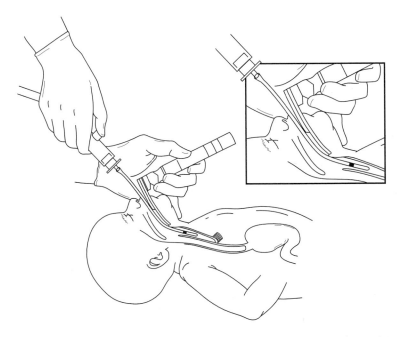

FIGURE 4-8   Equipment for suctioning meconium from the airway. Both meconium aspirator and meconium suction device connect to wall suction. (From Kattwinkel J, ed: *Textbook of neonatal resuscitation,* 4th ed, Elk Grove Village, Ill, 2000, American Academy of Pediatrics and American Heart Association.)

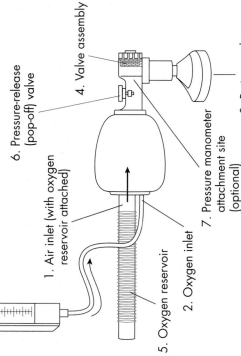

6. Pressure-release (pop-off) valve

4. Valve assembly

3. Patient outlet

1. Air inlet (with oxygen reservoir attached)

7. Pressure manometer attachment site (optional)

5. Oxygen reservoir

2. Oxygen inlet

Parts of a self-inflating bag

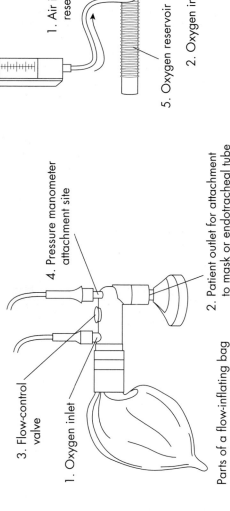

4. Pressure manometer attachment site

2. Patient outlet for attachment to mask or endotracheal tube

3. Flow-control valve

1. Oxygen inlet

Parts of a flow-inflating bag

Flow-inflating bags. Flow-inflating bags contain an inflatable gas reservoir that must be connected to a compressed gas source to refill between breaths.

Advantages:
- Ability to deliver 100% oxygen and any desired inspiratory pressure
- Ability to maintain a positive end-expiratory pressure
- In-line manometer

Disadvantages:
- The bag must be connected to an external oxygen supply to inflate.
- Practice and experience are required to deliver desired tidal volumes and pressures
- Very high inspiratory pressures may cause overinflation or pneumothorax.

Self-inflating bags. Self-inflating bags fill with ambient air and are independent of an external oxygen or compressed air source.

Advantages:
- Simple to use
- Self-inflation (useful backup system in case compressed oxygen source fails)

Disadvantages:
- Maximum pressure-limiting pop-off valve usually set by the manufacturer at 30 to 35 cm H_2O may preclude adequate ventilation in a noncompliant lung. (Some models have a manual override device that will allow increased inspiratory pressures.)
- A reservoir must be attached to deliver 90% to 100% oxygen.
- Free-flow oxygen cannot be delivered reliably through the patient outlet.
- Does not routinely deliver end-expiratory pressure and difficult to retrofit them with an in-line manometer.

FIGURE 4-9 Flow-inflating bag and self-inflating bag. (From Kattwinkel J, ed: *Textbook of neonatal resuscitation,* 4th ed, Elk Grove Village, Ill, 2000, American Academy of Pediatrics and American Heart Association.)

the best seal with minimal trauma and allow monitoring of mouth position and secretions.[42]

Perform the following steps:

- Set the flowmeter to deliver 5 to 10 L/min. Flow rates at the higher end of the range will be necessary to achieve higher pressures and faster ventilation rates with a flow-inflating bag.
- Test equipment before use. Equipment failure can cause resuscitation failure!
- Position the infant with the neck slightly extended and avoid compression of soft tissues of the neck by holding the mask to the face with the thumb and index finger and resting the third, fourth, and fifth fingers along the mandible.
- If the infant has not breathed spontaneously, give an opening breath with pressures of 30 to 40 cm H_2O and an inspiratory time of 1 to 3 seconds.
- **Ventilate at a rate of 40 to 60 breaths/min** with pressures of 15 to 20 cm H_2O for normal lungs or 20 to 40 cm H_2O for diseased or immature lungs.
- Observe chest expansion. If inadequate, (1) reapply the face mask for a better seal, (2) reposition the head, (3) suction secretions, (4) open the infant's mouth slightly, and (5) increase pressure.[32]
- Reevaluate respirations, heart rate, and color.

Insert an orogastric catheter (8 Fr feeding tube) after several minutes of bag and mask ventilation.

- Measure the insertion depth of the catheter by holding the tip at the bridge of the nose and measuring to the earlobe, then to the xiphoid.
- Insert the catheter through the mouth, not the nose.
- Aspirate gastric contents with a 20-ml syringe and leave the catheter open.
- Tape the catheter to the infant's cheek.

The adequacy of bag and mask ventilation must be continuously assessed by auscultation of breath sounds, visualization of chest wall movement, monitoring of heart rate, and observation of skin color. Peak inspiratory pressure should be limited to that necessary to see chest wall movement and hear good air exchange on auscultation of the chest. Infants with collapsed or fluid-filled alveoli may occasionally require inspiratory pressures of 40 to 60 cm H_2O or higher.[55] Inspiratory pressures cannot be judged clinically; bags fitted with in-line pressure manometers are recommended in the delivery room. Data suggest that the neonatal respiratory system responds slowly to mechanical inspiratory pressure[7]; prolonged inspiratory times may be necessary to achieve an adequate inspiratory volume and establish functional residual capacity. Further clinical trials will be necessary to establish the optimal method(s) for achieving lung expansion while minimizing the complications of positive-pressure ventilation.

Potential complications of bag and mask ventilation include trauma to the eyes or face from improper size or position of the mask, air leak (pneumothorax, subcutaneous air), intestinal distention elevating a normal diaphragm, or direct lung compression, in the case of a diaphragmatic hernia (Table 4-3). Complications can be minimized by using gentle technique and equipment of correct size,

Table 4-3	COMPLICATIONS DURING RESUSCITATION AND STABILIZATION		
PROBLEM	**CAUSE**	**DIAGNOSIS**	**REMEDIES**
Persistent cyanosis	Inadequate oxygenation		
	Inadequate FiO_2	Check flowmeter (and blender)	Always administer 100% O_2
	Disconnected O_2 line	Check all connections	Reconnect line
	Empty O_2 cylinder	Check O_2 source	Replace O_2 cylinder
	Inadequate ventilation		
	Inadequate face mask seal	Diminished breath sounds; little chest wall movement; air leak around mask	Readjust face mask; seal tightly against skin
	Compression airway	Diminished breath sounds; little chest wall movement	Apply upward force to mandible to counteract downward force holding face mask in place; extend neck slightly

Continued

Table 4-3	COMPLICATIONS DURING RESUSCITATION AND STABILIZATION—cont'd		
PROBLEM	**CAUSE**	**DIAGNOSIS**	**REMEDIES**
Persistent cyanosis —cont'd	Inadequate ventilation—cont'd Insufficient insufflation pressure	Diminished breath sounds; little chest wall movement	Increase insufflation pressure until breath sounds are audible and chest movement seen
	Compression of lungs by distended stomach	Diminished breath sounds; little chest wall movement; visibly distended stomach	Place orogastric tube
	Malpositioned ET tube	Check tube position with laryngoscope	Reinsert into trachea
		Check breath sounds	Withdraw until breath sounds are bilaterally equal Tape ET tube in place
	Pneumothorax	Check breath sounds Check for chest asymmetry Transillumination Chest x-ray examination	Decompress tension pneumothorax
Bradycardia	Same as cyanosis	Auscultation or palpation of umbilical cord base; pulse oximeter or cardiac monitor	See above for cyanosis External cardiac compression if heart rate <60 beats/min after 30 sec of effective ventilation with 100% oxygen
	Vagal stimulation Perinatal myocardial ischemia	Lack of response to oxygenation, ventilation and chest compressions	Stop oropharyngeal suctioning Emergency medication administration
Hypothermia	Evaporative heat loss; conductive heat loss	Specific symptoms overlap those of asphyxia and shock Low core temperature	Dry infant; remove wet linen Cover wet hair Keep under radiant warmer
Hyperthermia	Excessive warming Maternal fever	Apnea High core temperature	Servo control of warming devices
Hypoglycemia	Using glucose stores before birth or during resuscitation	Specific symptoms overlap those of asphyxia and shock Low blood glucose	Infusion of $D_{10}W$ at 100 ml/kg/24 hr
Hemorrhage	Inadequately secured umbilical arterial or venous line	Pallor Poor capillary filling Leakage of blood	Keep all intravascular tubing connection sites in plain view Tape UAC/UVC in place in addition to suturing lines
	Liver laceration		Perform chest compressions with correct position/depth

careful monitoring of pressures, and insertion of an orogastric tube when indicated.

Endotracheal Intubation

Endotracheal intubation may be performed at several points during neonatal resuscitation.[32] Intubation is indicated when (1) there is a need for tracheal suctioning, as with meconium-stained amniotic fluid in a nonvigorous infant, (2) bag and mask ventilation is ineffective or there is a need for prolonged positive-pressure ventilation, (3) chest compressions are necessary, or (4) epinephrine administration is required. Additional indications for endotracheal intubation include extreme prematurity, surfactant administration, and suspected diaphragmatic hernia.

Equipment for intubation is listed under Airway and Breathing in Box 4-2.

Select a noncuffed, uniform-diameter endotracheal tube of the correct size (Table 4-4). A variety of sizes (2.5 to 4.0 mm) should be available, because estimated weights may be inaccurate or airway anomalies may exist. **Orotracheal intubation is preferable to nasotracheal intubation during acute resuscitation because it can be performed rapidly and without additional equipment.**

Perform the following steps:

- Shorten the selected endotracheal tube to 13 cm and prepare the laryngoscope, tape, suction, oxygen, bag, and mask.
- Position the infant with the neck slightly extended.
- Provide free-flow oxygen.
- Hold the laryngoscope with the left hand; open the mouth with the right index finger and insert the blade.
- Lift the laryngoscope upward and outward so that the blade is nearly parallel to the surface beneath the infant.
- Visualize landmarks; identify the epiglottis, vocal cords, and glottis (Figure 4-10). If the esophagus is seen, withdraw the blade until the epiglottis drops down. If only the tongue is visible, advance the blade further until it enters the vallecula or passes under the epiglottis.
- Apply gentle external pressure over the trachea which may help visualize the vocal cords. This may be applied with the little finger of the hand holding the laryngoscope or by an assistant.
- Insert the endotracheal tube from the right corner of the mouth to the level of the vocal cord guideline at the tip of the tube.
- Limit each intubation attempt to 20 seconds to avoid hypoxia.

Table 4-4	ENDOTRACHEAL TUBE SIZE	
TUBE SIZE (MM) (INSIDE DIAMETER)	**WEIGHT (G)**	**GESTATIONAL AGE (WK)**
2.5	Below 1,000	Below 28
3.0	1,000-2,000	28-34
3.5	2,000-3,000	34-38
3.5-4.0	Above 3,000	Above 38

From Kattwinkel J, ed: *Textbook of neonatal resuscitation,* 4th ed, Elk Grove Village, Ill, 2000, American Academy of Pediatrics and American Heart Association.

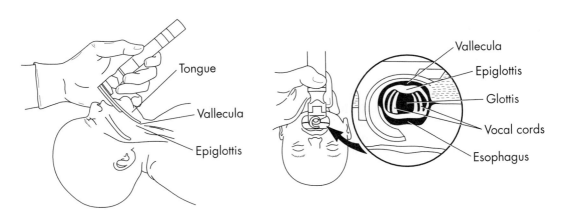

FIGURE 4-10 Anatomic landmarks that relate to intubation. (From Kattwinkel J, ed: *Textbook of neonatal resuscitation,* 4th ed, Elk Grove Village, Ill, 2000, American Academy of Pediatrics and American Heart Association.)

Table 4-5	DEPTH OF ENDOTRACHEAL TUBE INSERTION	
WEIGHT (KG)	DEPTH OF INSERTION (CM FROM UPPER LIP)	
1*	7	
2	8	
3	9	
4	10	

From Kattwinkel J, ed: *Textbook of neonatal resuscitation,* 4th ed, Elk Grove Village, Ill, 2000, American Academy of Pediatrics and American Heart Association.
*Babies weighing less than 750 g may require only 6 cm insertion.

- Confirm endotracheal tube position by auscultation for bilaterally equal breath sounds in the axillae and absence of breath sounds over the stomach. Observe chest wall movement. Note the centimeter marking at the lip (Table 4-5).
- Secure the endotracheal tube with tape and obtain a chest x-ray film.
- Shorten the endotracheal tube to 4 cm beyond the lips, if necessary.

Complications of intubation include hypoxia caused by prolonged intubation attempts or lack of supplemental oxygen; tube malposition; apnea or bradycardia caused by hypoxia or vagal stimulation; and trauma to the oropharynx, trachea, vocal cords, or esophagus (see Table 4-3). Exhaled CO_2 detection devices are commonly used to confirm endotracheal tube position in children; however, a higher rate of false-negative readings with currently available devices limits their usefulness in newborn infants weighing less than 2 kg.[3] Subglottic stenosis may result from prolonged, traumatic, or repeated intubation. To prevent complications, provide free-flow oxygen during intubation, use gentle technique, and limit intubation attempts to 20 seconds.

Chest Compressions

Indications for chest compressions include (1) a heart rate less than 60 beats/min despite effective positive pressure ventilation for 30 seconds with 100% oxygen. It is important to follow the sequence of (A) airway, (B) breathing, and (C) circulation in providing resuscitative support. **Even if the heart rate is below 60 beats/min shortly after delivery, the airway should be cleared and positive-pressure ventilation with 100% oxygen should be given for 30 seconds before beginning chest compressions.** Often, adequate ventilation

alone will result in a rapid increase in heart rate.[44] Beginning chest compressions too early may interfere with the effectiveness of positive-pressure ventilation and actually delay an infant's response to resuscitation.

Perform the following steps:
- Position the infant with the neck slightly extended.
- Provide firm support for the back.
- **Perform compressions using the two-thumb (preferred) or two-finger technique (Figure 4-11):**
  Position: lower third of sternum[23,40]
  Rate: 90 times/min
  Depth: one third the anterior-posterior diameter of the chest
  Support: encircling fingers or hand under back
- **Provide 90 compressions/min and interpose 30 breaths/min with a 3:1 ratio of compressions to breaths (120 events/min)**[9,39]
- Evaluate the heart rate after 30 seconds.
- Continue compressions until the heart rate is above 60 beats/min.
- Administer medications if heart rate remains below 60 beats/min despite at least 30 seconds of adequate ventilation with 100% oxygen and another 30 seconds of coordinated ventilations with 100% oxygen and chest compressions.

When there is poor response to positive-pressure ventilation and chest compressions, reevaluate for technical problems and conditions interfering with ventilation. Confirm that 100% oxygen is connected properly (see Table 4-3). Ensure that the airway is patent, the endotracheal tube is in proper position, the ventilation pressures and rate are optimal, and the chest is expanding with breaths interposed between compressions. Evaluate the infant for pneumothorax, diaphragmatic hernia, or hypovolemia (see Delivery Room Emergencies, p. 65).

Complications of chest compressions include liver laceration, rib fractures, and pneumothorax. To prevent complications, check the position of compressions, maintain contact with the chest during the release portion of the compression cycle, and avoid excessive force during compressions.

Medications

The indications for drugs during newborn resuscitation include the following:

Epinephrine: Heart rate less than 60 beats/min despite at least 30 seconds of adequate ventilation

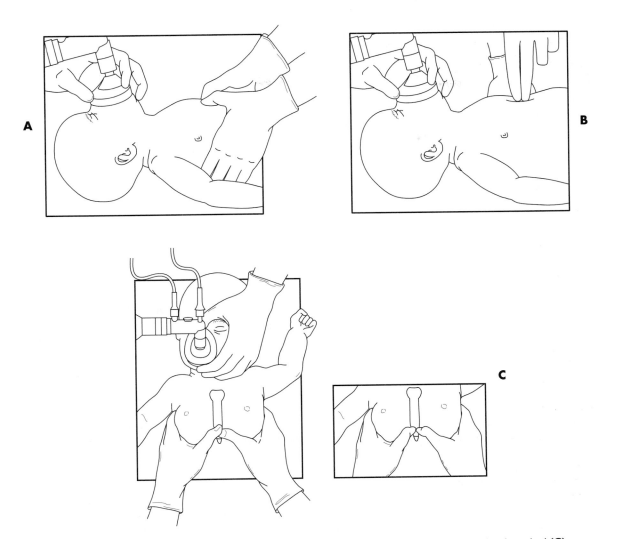

FIGURE 4-11   Two-thumb (**A,** preferred) and two finger (**B**) methods of chest compression. The two-thumb method (**C**) uses two thumbs placed one over the other or side by side (depends on the size of the baby) to compress the sternum and encircle the chest with the hands so that your fingers support the spine. (From Kattwinkel J, ed: *Textbook of neonatal resuscitation,* 4th ed, Elk Grove Village, Ill, 2000, American Academy of Pediatrics and American Heart Association.)

with 100% oxygen and another 30 seconds of coordinated ventilation with 100% oxygen and chest compressions

Volume expanders: Evidence of acute bleeding and signs of hypovolemia; poor response to other resuscitative measures

Sodium bicarbonate: Documented or suspected metabolic acidosis in the presence of adequate ventilation

Perform the following steps (see Table 4-2):
- Calculate the correct dosage of each drug.
- Prepare each drug for administration, draw up

the appropriate concentration and volume, and label.
- Administer each drug by the correct route and at the proper rate.[8]
- Reevaluate for desired effect and take follow-up action.

Epinephrine increases the rate and strength of cardiac contractions; its principal action during resuscitation is that of a peripheral vasoconstrictor; thus it directs cardiac output to the central circulation and increases coronary perfusion pressure.[41,43] Expansion of the plasma and blood volumes may also be required to maintain cardiac output, blood pressure, and peripheral perfusion. Volume expansion should be considered when there is evidence of acute blood loss (e.g., abruptio placentae, fetal-maternal hemorrhage, umbilical cord tear, acute neonatal hemorrhage), or poor response to resuscitation (e.g., pallor, poor capillary filling, bradycardia, or hypotension unresponsive to oxygen therapy, assisted ventilation, and chest compressions). Although acidosis frequently persists after a prolonged resuscitation, many infants will correct an acidosis spontaneously once the asphyxiating circumstances are relieved and adequate ventilation is established. Metabolic correction of pH is a slow process that takes several hours, and treatment with $NaHCO_3$ is not mandatory.

Complications of drug administration include extravasation with intravascular administration, hepatic injury with low umbilical venous catheters, and unpredictable absorption with endotracheal and intramuscular administration. The use of resuscitation drugs may also result in complications from their adverse pharmacologic effects. Epinephrine, administered in high doses, increases the risk of significant hypertension and a hyperadrenergic state which may result in germinal matrix hemorrhage or myocardial damage.[5] Absorption of epinephrine after endotracheal administration is erratic.[38] Sodium bicarbonate results in worsened acidosis in the setting of impaired ventilation; bicarbonate may also worsen intracellular acidosis. Furthermore, bicarbonate adds a high sodium load, which may directly depress myocardial performance.[26,27] Volume overload may result from administration of repeated doses of sodium bicarbonate or volume expanders. Rapid volume expansion, resulting in acute elevation of systolic blood pressure, has been associated with intraventricular hemorrhage.[24]

Distressed newborns have impaired autoregulation of cerebral blood flow, with the blood flow directly related to the systolic blood pressure. Increased cerebral blood flow and elevated systolic pressures may be responsible for intraventricular hemorrhage in the presence of a capillary bed insulted by acidosis and hypoxia.[37] Autopsy studies also suggest that increased cerebral venous capillary pressure can initiate intraventricular hemorrhage (Figure 4-12). Volume expansion should be performed cautiously in preterm or asphyxiated infants, infusing 10 ml/kg aliquots of fluid over a 5- to 10-minute period and evaluating the response before administering repeated aliquots of fluid. The

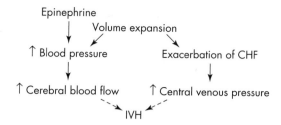

FIGURE 4-12 Potential adverse effects of rapid volume expansion in the setting of asphyxia or prematurity.

exception to this rule is the infant who has experienced acute perinatal hemorrhage with hypovolemia. These infants should have the circulatory fluid volume restored as rapidly as possible. Complications of medication administration can be prevented by choosing the correct dose, rate, and route of administration and positioning umbilical lines carefully. The infant should be evaluated for adverse effects after each medication dose.

Naloxone hydrochloride is indicated during acute resuscitation only in the very specific circumstance of severe neonatal respiratory depression and narcotic administration to the mother in the last 4 hours. **Naloxone is not part of the routine resuscitation of an apneic infant.**[32] Furthermore, naloxone hydrochloride is contraindicated in infants of narcotic-addicted mothers, because administration can result in severe abstinence syndrome, including seizures.

Calcium and atropine have little role in delivery room settings. Calcium is indicated for hypocalcemia or hyperkalemia, which are infrequent problems in the delivery room. Atropine may mask hypoxia-related bradycardia.[35,52]

DELIVERY ROOM EMERGENCIES

Certain conditions can present as emergencies in the delivery room (Table 4-6).[34,47] These conditions may require extensive resuscitation or result in a poor response to resuscitation. Some situations require special intervention immediately; most merit the involvement of a pediatrician or neonatologist for management. Surgical intervention is necessary to complete stabilization of diaphragmatic hernia, abdominal wall defects, and neural tube defects. See Box 4-3 for an outline of emergency procedures in the delivery room.

Table 4-6	DELIVERY ROOM EMERGENCIES		
CONDITION	**SIGNS AND SYMPTOMS**	**ONGOING PROBLEMS**	**INITIAL RESPONSES**
Pneumothorax	Cyanosis, respiratory distress, unequal breath sounds, bradycardia, displaced heart sounds	Continuing asphyxia, shock ($\downarrow$ venous return)	Transilluminate chest, perform needle thoracentesis, evaluate for chest tube placement
Choanal atresia and airway anomalies	Noisy respirations, pink when crying but cyanotic when quiet, inability to pass suction catheter per nares	Respiratory distress, intermittent hypoxemia and bradycardia	Supplemental oxygen, oral/pharyngeal airway, and prone positioning or intubation (lower airway anomalies may require emergency tracheostomy)
Extreme prematurity	Respiratory distress	Continuing hypoxemia, hypothermia, possible sepsis, hypovolemia	Intubate, place umbilical lines, evaluate for use of artificial surfactant, begin antibiotics, consider transport to neonatal center
Sepsis	Respiratory distress, hypotonia, poor perfusion, foul odor	Continuing hypoxemia, shock	Intubate, place umbilical lines, administer antibiotics
Severe asphyxia	Prolonged apnea, bradycardia poor perfusion, pallor, hypotonia, seizures	Hypoxemia, shock, multi-organ system injury	Intubate, place umbilical lines, give volume support and pressors for shock, consider transport to neonatal center
Hydrops fetalis	Body wall edema, ascites, pallor, poor perfusion, respiratory distress, possibly unequal breath sounds (pneumothorax), distant heart sounds (pericardial effusion)	Hypoxemia, anemia, shock, potential for multi-organ system injury	Intubate, perform posterolateral needle thoracentesis bilaterally if unable to ventilate; consider paracentesis if ascites compromises ventilation; place chest tube for pneumothorax, place umbilical lines, evaluate need for partial exchange transfusion, consider transport to neonatal center
Pulmonary hypoplasia and oligohydramnios	Respiratory distress; flattened, deviated nose; infraorbital creases; low-set, crumpled ears; small chin; deformities of the extremities	Hypoxemia, pneumothorax, pulmonary hypertension	Intubate, place umbilical lines, monitor closely for pulmonary air leak, consider transport to neonatal center
Congenital diaphragmatic hernia	Respiratory distress with asymmetrical breath sounds, barrel chest and scaphoid abdomen, point of maximal intensity (PMI) shifted to side opposite hernia	Hypoxemia, pulmonary hypertension, contralateral pneumothorax	Intubate, decompress bowel with orogastric suction to low intermittent suction, place umbilical lines, arrange transport to neonatal center

Continued

Table 4-6   DELIVERY ROOM EMERGENCIES—cont'd

CONDITION	SIGNS AND SYMPTOMS	ONGOING PROBLEMS	INITIAL RESPONSES
Abdominal wall defect	Midline abdominal wall defect at base of umbilical cord (omphalocele) or lateral to cord insertion (gastroschisis) with externalization of abdominal contents	Hypovolemia, respiratory distress, hypothermia, ischemic injury to externalized abdominal contents, infection	Protect exposed tissue with evaporative barrier; begin parenteral fluids at 1.5× maintenance; place an orogastric tube to low intermittent suction, position infant side-lying with support of exposed organs, monitor temperature and urine output, arrange transport to a neonatal center with pediatric surgery
Neural tube defect	Open spinal defect (myelomeningocele), cranial defect with outpouching brain tissue (occipital or frontal encephalocele), failure of formation of skull and brain (anencephaly)	Prolonged apnea, infection, hypothermia	Provide supportive care unless prenatal diagnosis of lethal anomaly has allowed formulation of a plan for limited support; protect exposed tissue with gauze soaked in warmed saline and evaporative barrier; arrange transport to a neonatal center with specialists in spinal defects

Box 4-3   EMERGENCY PROCEDURES IN THE DELIVERY ROOM

A. Umbilical vessel catheterization (see Chapter 7)

B. Thoracentesis and chest tube placement (see Chapter 23)

C. Partial exchange transfusion for anemia (see Chapter 20)
1. Indications
   Profound chronic anemia (Hct <25%), as in the setting of hydrops. Distinct from situations of acute loss of blood volume, chronic anemia results in normal blood volume per kilogram, necessitating partial exchange transfusion to rapidly raise the hematocrit.
2. Procedure
   a. Obtain O-negative packed red blood cells (PRBCs) by emergency release if necessary. PRBCs should be as fresh as possible to minimize risk of hyperkalemia.
   b. Insert a low umbilical venous catheter, and attach a 4-way stopcock (exchange set).
   c. Perform an isovolumetric exchange by alternating withdrawal and infusion of 5 to 10 ml aliquots of patient blood and PRBCs to a total exchange volume of approximately 20 ml/kg. The formula

   $$\text{exchange volume} = \text{est dry wt} \times \text{blood volume/kg} \\ (\text{desired Hct} - \text{current Hct})/\text{Hct of PRBCs}$$

   can be used to estimate the rise in hematocrit for a given exchange volume and a given hematocrit of exchange blood.
   d. Alternatively, place both low UVC and umbilical artery catheter (UAC). Withdraw from the UAC while infusing PRBCs per UVC at the same rate to the total exchange volume.
3. Risks
   a. Thrombotic, embolic events
   b. Infection
   c. Bleeding (from mechanical complications or depletion of clotting factors)
   d. Hyperkalemia (consider use of washed PRBCs for nonemergent partial volume exchanges)

D. Prophylactic administration of exogenous surfactant (see Chapter 23)
1. Indications
   a. Prematurity
   b. Respiratory distress
   c. Presumed surfactant deficiency
2. Procedure
   a. Calculate the appropriate dose of surfactant based on birthweight
   b. Confirm correct endotracheal tube position by centimeter markings at the lip (see Table 4-5) and careful auscultation. Chest x-ray film confirmation is ideal if surfactant is administered during stabilization in the nursery.
   c. Suction the endotracheal tube to clear secretions.
   d. Monitor heart rate and oxygen saturation with pulse oximetry.
   e. Administer surfactant according to manufacturer's directions or experimental protocol. Administration options include rapid bolus or gradual infusion combined with positioning of the infant and hand or mechanical ventilation.
   f. Refrain from suctioning for at least 4 hr after surfactant administration.
   g. Monitor chest wall rise, saturations, and arterial blood gases and adjust ventilator support accordingly.
3. Complications
   a. Hypoxemia
   b. Air leak
   c. Pulmonary hemorrhage

Care During the Transition From the Delivery Room to the Nursery

After the infant is stabilized and vigorous, perform elective procedures, such as clamping and shortening the umbilical cord, footprinting and identification, applying ophthalmic prophylaxis, or weighing. A vigorous, stable infant may breast feed immediately and be held by the parents. The infant may be placed next to mother's skin or wrapped in double blankets. A stocking cap prevents heat loss from the large surface area of the head and wet hair. The stable infant may complete the transition period under appropriate observation in the mother's room.

In the case of the infant who has required more extensive resuscitation in the delivery room, transfer the infant to the nursery when adequate spontaneous or controlled ventilation has been established, the heart rate is greater than 100 beats/min, and the infant has been dried and protected from excessive heat loss. Note the time of the infant's first respiratory effort and sustained, regular respirations. Transfer the infant in a warmed transport incubator with continuation of required support measures (heart rate monitoring by stethoscope, pulse oximeter, or ECG monitor; supplemental oxygen or positive-pressure ventilation). Delay elective procedures until the infant is physiologically stable.[33]

In the intensive care nursery, place the infant on a preheated open warmer with servo control. Avoid overwarming, because hyperthermia may be associated with respiratory depression and worsened neurologic outcome after asphyxial insults.[36,45] Ensure adequate cardiopulmonary monitoring, including ECG, respiratory rate and pattern, and monitoring of oxygen saturation with pulse oximetry. Obtain a serum glucose by heelstick and a blood pressure by a Doppler device and blood pressure cuff. Begin a peripheral intravenous infusion if blood glucose is low or volume expansion is indicated; alternatively, consider rapid placement of a low umbilical vein catheter (UVC) to administer glucose or volume. Evaluate for placement of central umbilical venous and/or arterial lines for maintenance fluid administration, blood sampling, and continuous arterial pressure monitoring. Confirm endotracheal tube and umbilical line placement with an x-ray film.

CARE OF THE FAMILY AND PERINATAL DECISION-MAKING

Encouraging the presence of the father or another mature support person in the delivery room is common obstetric practice and should not interfere with delivery room care. Ideally, members of the obstetric and neonatal resuscitation team should introduce themselves to the parents before the delivery. Parents have a great deal of anxiety concerning procedures performed on their newborn; a few moments spent describing routine procedures will help allay their fears and avoid misinterpretation. When problems are anticipated, a calm, professional explanation of neonatal assessment and life support measures is necessary. Parental awareness that the medical and nursing staff has anticipated and prepared for possible problems can partially relieve their anxieties. Care must be taken, however, to avoid instilling undue alarm. Care providers need to understand ethical principles and the impact of their personal morals and ethical beliefs on the decisions made regarding resuscitation.[57]

If an infant requires resuscitation or prolonged assessment and support, the attending staff's primary obligation is to provide this care and communicate with the parents. Parents should be allowed to have contact with their baby, but the presence of the father or a support person must not be allowed to interfere with or delay the delivery of care. The pediatric staff should tell the parents what is happening at the earliest possible opportunity, because lack of communication prolongs anxiety for the parents. A few brief statements to explain the status of the baby and procedures can relieve the anguish of silence. Especially when a difficult resuscitation is anticipated, it is ideal to designate, in advance, a team member who can keep parents informed.

When severe perinatal problems are anticipated and confirmed, such as extreme prematurity (gestational age less than 23 weeks, birth weight less than 400 g), anencephaly, or trisomy 13 or 18, discussions may be held in advance with obstetric care providers and the family regarding the extent of resuscitative measures.[18,21,39,53] Current data suggest that resuscitation of these infants is very unlikely to result in survival or survival without disability.[22,53] When problems are unanticipated, information is uncertain, or there has been no time for decision-making, intervention in the delivery room is usually warranted.[10,50] This approach allows time for complete information to be gathered and discussed with the family. If appropriate, support measures can be withdrawn later in the nursery[31,48] (see Chapter 32, Perinatal Ethics).

When an infant fails to respond to intensive resuscitative measures in the delivery room, the decision must be made when to stop support. Survival is unlikely if no heart rate has been obtained by 10 minutes.[14,16,29,60] Discontinuation of resuscitation may be appropriate if, after 15 minutes of full resuscitative effort, there has been no return of spontaneous circulation.[39] The data for infants who have an inadequate response to resuscitation remain less clear. The probability of survival diminishes, and the probability of cerebral palsy increases with the length of time Apgar scores remain below 4. If the Apgar score remains below 4 at 20 minutes, the probability of cerebral palsy in surviving infants is greater than 50%. Thus it is important to rapidly rule out remediable causes of poor response to resuscitation and conditions such as congenital heart block. If after 20 minutes of maximal resuscitative efforts the infant does not have a heart rate above 100 beats/min, the team must consider discontinuing supportive measures.[31]

REFERENCES

1. Adamson K, Behrman GS, Dawes GS et al: Resuscitation by positive pressure ventilation and trishydroxymethylaminomethane of rhesus monkeys asphyxiated at birth, *J Pediatr* 65:807, 1964.
2. American Academy of Pediatrics and American College of Obstetricians and Gynecologists: *Guidelines for perinatal care,* ed 5, Elk Grove Village, Ill, 2002, The Academy.
3. Aziz HF, Martin JB, Moore JJ: The pediatric end-tidal carbon dioxide detector role in endotracheal intubation in newborns, *J Perinatol* 19:110, 1999.
4. Bailey C, Kattwinkel J: Establishing a neonatal resuscitation team in community hospitals, *J Perinatol* 10:294, 1990.
5. Berg RA, Otto CW, Kern KB et al: A randomized, blinded trial of high-dose epinephrine versus standard-dose epinephrine in a swine model of pediatric asphyxial cardiac arrest, *Crit Care Med* 24:1695, 1996.
6. Bland RD, Nielson DW: Developmental changes in lung epithelial ion transport and liquid movement, *Ann Rev Physiol* 54:373, 1992.
7. Boon AW, Milner AD, Hopkins IE: Lung expansion, tidal exchange and formation of the functional residual capacity during resuscitation of asphyxiated neonates, *J Pediatr* 95:1031, 1979.
8. Burchfield DJ: Medication use in neonatal resuscitation, *Clin Perinatol* 26:683, 1999.
9. Burchfield DJ, Erenberg A, Mullett MD et al: Why change the compression and ventilation rates during CPR in neonates? Neonatal Resuscitation Steering Committee, American Heart Association and American Academy of Pediatrics, *Pediatrics* 93:1026, 1994 (letter).
10. Byrne PJ, Tyebkhan JM, Laing LM: Ethical decision-making and neonatal resuscitation, *Semin Perinatol* 18:36, 1994.
11. Carrasco M, Martell M, Estol PC: Oronasopharyngeal suction at birth: effects on arterial oxygen saturation, *J Pediatr* 130:832, 1997.
12. Carson BS, Losey RW, Bowes WA et al: Combined obstetric and pediatric approach to prevent meconium aspiration syndrome, *Am J Obstet Gynecol* 126:712, 1976.
13. Carter BS, Haverkamp AD, Merenstein GB: The definition of acute perinatal asphyxia, *Clin Perinatol* 20:287, 1993.
14. Casalaz DM, Marlow N, Speidel BD: Outcome of resuscitation following unexpected apparent stillbirth, *Arch Dis Child Fetal Neonatal Educ* 78:F112, 1998.
15. Casey BM, McIntire DD, Leveno KJ: The continuing value of the Apgar score for the assessment of newborn infants, *N Engl J Med* 344:467, 2001.
16. Davis DJ: How aggressive should delivery room cardiopulmonary resuscitation be for extremely low birth weight neonates? *Pediatrics* 92:447, 1993.
17. Dawes GS: *Foetal and neonatal physiology: a comparative study of the changes at birth,* St Louis, 1968, Mosby.
18. Doron MW, Veness-Meehan KA, Margolis LH et al: Delivery room resuscitation decisions for extremely premature infants, *Pediatrics* 102:3, 574, 1998.
19. Emmanouilides GC, Moss AJ, Duffie ER et al: Pulmonary artery pressure changes in human newborn infants from birth to 3 days of age, *J Pediatr* 65:327, 1964.
20. Estol PC, Piriz H, Basalo S et al: Oro-naso-pharyngeal suction at birth: effects on respiratory adaptation of normal term vaginally born infants, *JPerinat Med* 20:297, 1992.
21. Finer NN, Barrington KJ: Decision-making in delivery room resuscitation: a team sport, *Pediatrics* 102:3, 644, 1998.
22. Finer NN, Horbar JD, Carpenter JH: Cardiopulmonary resuscitation in the very low birth weight infant: the Vermont Oxford Network experience, *Pediatrics* 104:428, 1999.
23. Finholt DA, Kettrick RG, Wagner HR et al: The heart is under the lower third of the sternum: implications for external cardiac massage, *Am J Dis Child* 140:646, 1986.
24. Goldberg RN, Chung D, Goldman SL et al: The association of rapid volume expansion and intraventricular hemorrhage in the preterm infant, *J Pediatr* 96:1060, 1980.
25. Hageman JR, Conley M, Francis K et al: Delivery room management of meconium staining of the amniotic fluid and the development of meconium aspiration syndrome, *J Perinatol* 8:127, 1988.
26. Hein HA: The use of sodium bicarbonate in neonatal resuscitation: help or harm? *Pediatrics* 91:496, 1993.
27. Howell JH: Sodium bicarbonate in the perinatal setting: revisited, *Clin Perinatol* 14:807, 1987.

28. Jain L, Vidyasagar D: Controversies in neonatal resuscitation, *Pediatr Ann* 24:540, 1995.

29. Jain L, Ferre C, Vidyasagar D et al: Cardiopulmonary resuscitation of apparently stillborn infants: survival and long-term outcome, *J Pediatr* 118:778, 1991.

30. Kanter RK: Evaluation of mask-bag ventilation in resuscitation of infants, *Am J Dis Child* 141:761, 1987.

31. Kattwinkel J: Very difficult questions in neonatal resuscitation, *NRP Instructor Update* 5(3 pt, suppl):1S, 1996.

32. Kattwinkel J, ed: *Textbook of neonatal resuscitation,* ed 4, Elk Grove Village, Ill, 2000, American Academy of Pediatrics and American Heart Association.

33. Kattwinkel J, Cook LJ, Hurt H et al: Resuscitating the newborn infant. Perinatal Continuing Education Program, Book I. *Fetal evaluation and immediate newborn care,* Charlottesville, Va, 2001, Division of Neonatal Medicine, Department of Pediatrics, University of Virginia Health Sciences Center.

34. Khan NS, Luten RC: Neonatal resuscitation, *Emerg Med Clin North Am* 12:239, 1994.

35. Leuthner SR, Jansen RD, Hageman JR: Cardiopulmonary resuscitation of the newborn: an update, *Pediatr Clin North Am* 41:893, 1994.

36. Lieberman E, Lang J, Richardson DK et al: Intrapartum maternal fever and neonatal outcome, *Pediatrics* 105:8, 2000.

37. Loe HC, Lassen NA, Friis-Hansen B: Impaired autoregulation of cerebral flow in the distressed newborn infant, *J Pediatr* 94:118, 1979.

38. Lucas VW Jr, Preziosi MP, Burchfield DJ: Epinephrine absorption following endotracheal administration: effects of hypoxia-induced low pulmonary blood flow, *Resuscitation* 27:31, 1994.

39. Niermeyer S, Kattwinkel J, Van Reempts P et al: International Guidelines for Neonatal Resuscitation: an excerpt from the Guidelines 2000 for Cardiopulmonary Resuscitation and Emergency Cardiovascular Care: International Consensus on Science, *Pediatrics* 106:E29, 2000; URL: http://www.pediatrics.org/cgi/content/full/106/3/e29 and *Circulation* 102 (suppl I):I-343, 2000.

40. Orlowski JP: Optimum position for external cardiac compression in infants and young children, *Ann Emerg Med* 15:667, 1986.

41. Otto CW, Yakaitis RW, Blitt CD: Mechanism of action of epinephrine in resuscitation from asphyxiated arrest, *Crit Care Med* 9:321, 1981.

42. Palme C, Nystrom B, Tunell, R: An evaluation of the efficiency of face masks in the resuscitation of newborn infants, *Lancet* 1:207, 1985.

43. Paradis NA, Martin GB, Rivers EP et al: Coronary perfusion pressure and the return of spontaneous circulation in human cardiopulmonary resuscitation, *JAMA* 263:1106, 1990.

44. Perlman JM, Risser R: Cardiopulmonary resuscitation in the delivery room: associated clinical events, *Arch Pediatr Adolesc Med* 149:20, 1995.

45. Perlman JM: Maternal fever and neonatal depression: preliminary observations, *Clin Pediatr* 38:287, 1999.

46. Price WR, Eastlack M, Hall DA et al: Implementing a neonatal resuscitation quality improvement committee, *J Perinat Neonatal Nurs* 7:57, 1993.

47. Ringer SA, Stark AR: Management of neonatal emergencies in the delivery room, *Clin Perinatol* 16:23, 1989.

48. Rivers RP: Decision making in the neonatal intensive care environment, *Br Med Bull* 52:238, 1996.

49. Rudolph AM: High pulmonary vascular resistance after birth. I. Pathophysiologic considerations and etiologic classification, *Clin Pediatr* 19:585, 1980.

50. Sachs BP, Ringer SA: Intrapartum and delivery room management of the very low birthweight infant, *Clin Perinatol* 16:809, 1989.

51. Scarpelli EM: Perinatal lung mechanics and the first breath, *Lung* 162:61, 1984.

52. Sims DG, Heal CA, Bartle SM: Use of adrenaline and atropine in neonatal resuscitation, *Arch Dis Child* 70:F3, 1994.

53. Southgate M, Annibale DJ: Clinical ethics and neonatology: integrating emerging disciplines, *Neonat Intensive Care* 8:42, 1995.

54. Tyson JE, Younes N, Verter J et al: *Viability, morbidity, and resource use among newborn of 501- to 800-g birth weight:* National Institute of Child Health and Human Development Neonatal Research Network, *JAMA* 276:1645, 1996.

55. Vyas H, Field D, Milner AD et al: Determinants of the first inspiratory volume and functional residual capacity at birth, *Pediatr Pulmonol* 2:189, 1986.

56. Wheeler CA, Tudhope AE: Development of a neonatal intensive care nursery resuscitation and triage team: impact on nursing care and infant outcome, *Neonat Net* 13:53, 1994.

57. Wilder MA: Ethical issues in the delivery room: resuscitation of extremely low birth weight infants, *J Perinat Neonatal Nurs* 14:44, 2000.

58. Wiswell TE, Bent RC: Meconium staining and the meconium aspiration syndrome, *Pediatr Clin North Am* 40:955, 1993.

59. Wiswell TE: Meconium in the Delivery Room Trial Group: delivery room management of the apparently vigorous meconium-stained neonate: results of the multicenter collaborative trial, *Pediatrics* 105:1, 2000.

60. Yeo CL, Tudehope DI: Outcome of resuscitated apparently stillborn infants: a ten year review, *J Paediatr Child Health* 30:129, 1994.

5 | Initial Nursery Care

Sandra L. Gardner, Janis L. Johnson, Lula O. Lubchenco

A neonate must demonstrate a condition of well-being before being considered a normal, low-risk infant. Neonatal intensive care professionals must understand the normal neonate to care for the sick neonate. We will discuss the initial assessment, transitional period, and gestational age characteristics to teach health care providers to apply these concepts in initial nursery care.

Physical changes occur so rapidly after birth that the newborn examination can be divided into four time periods. Apgar[12,13] defined the first period in terms of seconds as "exactly 60 seconds after birth" and the next period in minutes. The transition period is considered in hours and the hospital stay in hours or days. Continuing this logarithmic time span for newborns, we use weeks for the first few follow-up visits, then months, and eventually speak of the child's age in years.

Each of these four newborn examinations has a specific purpose. One should consider these examinations in relation to the age of the infant rather than to the location of the mother and infant in the hospital— or to arbitrary nursery routines (delivery room compared with birthing room, transition nursery compared with mother's recovery room, rooming-in compared with low-risk nursery, and so on). The examination at delivery is aimed at detecting life-threatening emergencies. The examination during the next few hours (transition period) is used to evaluate the infant's adjustment to extrauterine life. The complete newborn examination by a qualified health care provider should be performed at about 12 to 24 hours.[9] It is an important examination, because many findings can be treated or complications can be avoided.

The discharge examination is not as detailed as the complete examination. During this examination the professional demonstrates the baby's unique abilities and answers the parents' questions. This is a good time to provide support and encouragement as the parents begin to incorporate the new member into their family.

EXAMINATION AT DELIVERY

Before the delivery occurs, one should obtain pertinent facts about the pregnancy, such as parity, gravidity, fetal losses, estimated birth weight and gestational age of the fetus, and, of course, any problems present in the current pregnancy.[75] Health care providers should note whether the mother was screened for group B *Streptococcus* and whether she received any antibiotic treatment.[9,24]

During labor one can observe the frequency and duration of contractions and the mother's reaction to contractions. Passage of meconium, rupture of membranes, fetal distress, and other signs will alert the attendants to impending problems.

The initial respiratory effort and heart rate, part of the Apgar evaluation (see Chapter 4, Figure 4-7), are noted even before 60 seconds, because one does not wait for the 1-minute Apgar to begin resuscitative procedures if the infant is limp and not breathing.[70] If the baby is vigorous, the care provider may place the baby on the mother's abdomen or in her arms; Apgar assessment can be done there or in a bassinet or warmer. Scoring is repeated at 5 minutes. Under some conditions, such as prolonged resuscitation, it is helpful to have a score at 10 or 15 minutes. Between the 1- and 5-minute Apgar assessments, one systematically evaluates the baby for potential or apparent medical emergencies.

The continued value of the Apgar score as a predictor of neonatal survival was recently reviewed by Casey, McIntire, and Leveno.[23] They noted that for both preterm and term infants, neonatal survival increases with increasing Apgar scores; low 5-minute scores (e.g., 0 to 3) are associated with the highest risk of neonatal death.

With practice and experience the professional will be able to identify approximate gestational age from the physical appearance. One quick and effective way to estimate gestational age is by measuring foot length.[48] Foot length of appropriate-for-gestational-age preterm infants has been correlated

| Table 5-1 | FOOT LENGTH BY GESTATIONAL AGE* |

GESTATIONAL AGE (WK)	FOOT LENGTH (CM)				GESTATIONAL AGE (WK)	FOOT LENGTH (CM)			
	N	MEAN	MEDIAN	SD	RANGE	N	MEAN	MEDIAN	SD	RANGE
24	6	4.22	4.1	.17	3.8-4.4	34	24	6.77	6.8	.20	6.5-7.1
25	12	4.5	4.5	.08	4.4-4.6	35	20	7.1	7.0	.15	6.8-7.3
26	16	4.72	4.7	.07	4.65-4.9	36	22	7.27	7.27	.21	7.0-7.6
27	19	4.99	5.0	.14	4.8-5.2	37	24	7.51	7.5	.24	7.4-8.0
28	18	5.23	5.2	.13	5.0-5.5	38	40	7.92	8.0	.23	7.6-8.3
29	22	5.47	5.4	.129	5.3-5.7	39	42	8.22	8.3	.32	7.9-8.6
30	27	5.75	5.75	.23	5.6-6.2	40	56	8.6	8.7	.37	8.2-8.9
31	24	5.95	6.0	.19	5.7-6.23	41	22	8.75	8.9	.30	8.3-9.1
32	21	6.22	6.2	.13	6.0-6.4	42	12	9.1	9.2	.33	8.7-9.3
33	25	6.5	6.5	.26	6.3-6.9	43	8	9.27	9.3	.25	8.9-9.6

From Hernandez, J et al: Footlength and gestational age in the very-low-birth-weight infant, *The Children's Hospital Pediatric Update*, September 1987, p.4.
SD, Standard deviation.
*Applies to both male and female infants.

with gestational age (Table 5-1 and Figure 5-1). In short gestation (i.e., twenty-fifth to thirty-fourth week) there is a consistent, incremental increase in the mean foot length of 0.5 cm every 2 weeks. Measurement of foot length from the posterior prominence of the heel to the tip of the first (great) toe with a millimeter ruler is a rapid and simple method of assessing maturation of all newborns, even the very ill VLBW infant. With this method, as with other physical measurements of gestational age, one must consider the standard deviation in interpreting the results.

After turning the infant to a prone position, further inspection will reveal congenital abnormalities such as spina bifida, imperforate anus, skeletal abnormalities, or genital defects. Internal abnormalities should be suspected if there is an "empty" or scaphoid abdomen (diaphragmatic hernia) or profuse oral or nasopharyngeal mucus (tracheoesophageal [TE] fistula). Choanal atresia may present as apnea after respirations have been established. If closing the infant's mouth results in cyanosis and/or apnea, this is a positive test result for choanal atresia. Examination of the umbilical cord and vessels may give a clue to other abnormalities. The size and amount of Wharton's jelly, especially if the cord is thin, suggest problems in intrauterine nutrition. A single umbilical artery may be a clue to other anomalies (e.g., genitourinary, gastrointestinal, cardiovascular, CNS, and respiratory).[98,111]

PHYSIOLOGY

Transitional Phases and Significance

With the first breath of life and the cutting of the umbilical cord, all neonates begin the transition from intrauterine to extrauterine life. There are three major changes that take place at birth. First, fluid in the alveoli is reabsorbed, allowing diffusion of air into the surrounding blood vessels. Second, because the umbilical arteries and vein are clamped, the low-resistance placental circuit is gone and systemic blood pressure increases. Third, there is decreased pulmonary vascular resistance as a result of mechanical distention of the alveoli and increased oxygen content in the alveoli. Oxygen is a potent pulmonary vasodilator.

A neonate is a recovering patient, similar to a patient recovering from anesthesia. The transitional phase of the neonate is closely monitored to recognize any abnormalities, initiate appropriate measures for referral, and screen the neonate for common problems in early neonatal life.

Desmond et al[32] described temporal changes occurring in the behavior and physiology of the infant during the first few hours after birth. Figure 5-2 summarizes the physical findings noted during the first 10 hours of extrauterine life in a representative high-Apgar-score infant delivered with the mother under spinal anesthesia without prior medication. Vital signs, including the heart rate, temperature,

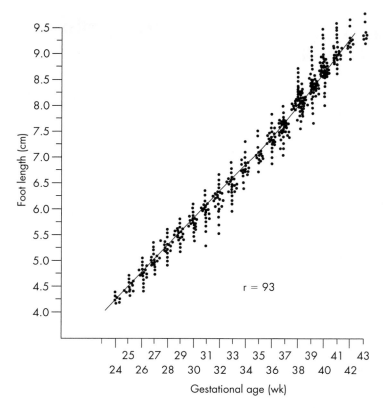

FIGURE 5-1   Foot length and gestational age: a positive linear correlation. (From Hernandez JA, Lazarte R, Pisanos D et al: Foot length and gestational age in the very-low-birth-weight infant, *Child Hosp Pediatr Update* Sept 1987, pp 3-7.)

and blood pressure, are so closely related to age after birth that the examiner can almost estimate the age of the infant from these signs when there are no problems in the transition to extrauterine life. Vital signs thus alert one to problems if the heart rate, respirations, temperature, and blood pressure do not follow the usual time course.

A heart rate of 160 beats/min at any time other than the first hour after birth should alarm the observer. Of course, if this rate persisted, it would indicate some serious problem. In the healthy infant shown on the graph in Figure 5-2, the rate falls to a more usual rate seen in newborns. A persistently elevated heart rate may be caused by a decrease in intravascular volume, so perfusion should also be assessed.

The respiratory rate is also increased after birth. Pulmonary adjustments include (1) alveolar fluid clearance and expansion,[50] (2) a change in pulmonary vascular resistance,[68] (3) an increase in tidal volume and minute ventilation,[45] and (4) a progressive increase in dynamic compliance.[45] When one considers these pulmonary adjustments of the infant, it is not surprising to see tachypnea, but it is disturbing to see barreling of the chest, which usually indicates the presence of extraalveolar air. The spontaneous improvement shown in the figure is just as surprising and gives us even greater respect for the ability of the newborn.

The temperature fall shown in Figure 5-2 may well be iatrogenic. The infant is already stressed by birth and all the adjustments he or she must make. Cold stress requires the infant to use sources of energy that are easily depleted, and if feeding is delayed, hypoglycemia may occur. Hypoglycemia is especially critical in the small-for-gestational-age infant, whose stores of glycogen and fat are limited.

A newborn's activity during the awake and sleep states[56] can help the professional assess the neurologic development and the effect of stimuli on the

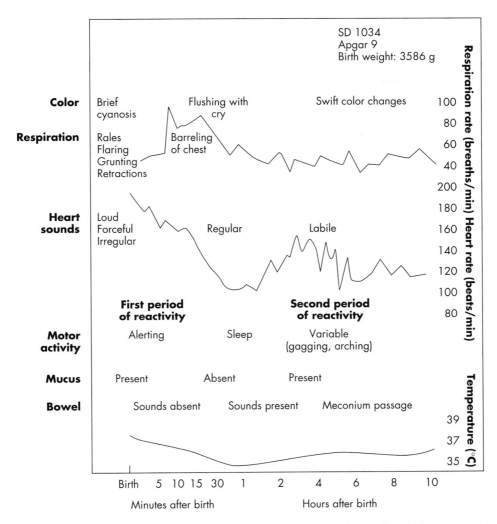

FIGURE 5-2   Neonatal transitional period. (From Desmond MM, Rudolph AJ, Phitaksphraiwan P et al: The transitional care nursery: A mechanism for preventive medicine in the newborn, *Pediatr Clin North Am* 13:651, 1966.)

newborn's ability to recover from the birth process. The infant is usually awake and alert for the first hours after birth and often indicates hunger by mouthing movements or hand-to-mouth contact. A term infant should be fed early in life before it enters its first sleep period. Bowel sounds are present within the first 30 to 60 minutes after birth, and the newborn can successfully feed during this time. After the first feeding the infant falls asleep for several hours and then begins a second stage of activity. The infant awakes from sleep and comes to an alert state if no problems exist. If there are medical problems, the infant will fluctuate between sleeping and crying without an alert period in between. Feeding during a drowsy or fussing state will be unsatisfactory and gives us one of the earliest signs of illness: "poor feeding." More subtle signs of distress in an infant are closed eyes with hands tightly fisted and arms extended rather than kept toward the midline, peripheral or circumoral cyanosis, and regurgitation. The infant attempts to alleviate distress and quiet herself when she brings her hands to her face or mouth.

During these first hours care providers begin to assess the infant's risk for various morbidities. Assessment is aimed at anticipating or preventing problems that interfere with the infant's adjustment to extrauterine life. Of course, warmth and comfort measures are indicated throughout this transition period.

A newborn infant responds to illness or stress by "turning off" reactions, and then the professional has a difficult time recognizing problems. Care providers must learn to suspect illness or problems from very few clues. For instance, illness is suspected when an infant is hypotonic, does not feed well, or is difficult to arouse or bring to an alert state. These signs are the same whether the infant has hypoglycemia[53] or sepsis. Illness may be suspected but requires laboratory documentation to determine the cause. Hence many nurseries have adopted routines that include pulse oximetry, blood glucose determinations, hematocrit counts, x-ray films, and other evaluations for the most common problems. Blood and other cultures, blood typing, screening for congenital infections, and other tests may be indicated, depending on the pregnancy history.

Bowel Activity

Bowel sounds are absent until about 1 hour of age. In some babies bowel sounds will occur earlier, especially if they were stressed during labor or delivery and passage of meconium occurred at this time. Auscultate the abdomen for the presence or absence of bowel sounds.

Temperature

An infant's temperature drops rapidly after delivery and may not begin to stabilize for several hours unless appropriate intervention occurs. **A newborn needs to be dried off immediately after delivery to prevent heat loss caused by evaporation. Until the temperature has stabilized, maternal skin contact, a radiant warmer, or incubator should be used to stabilize the infant's temperature (see Chapter 6). Bathing should be deferred until a normal transition has been achieved.**

Pulse and Respirations

As the cardiopulmonary system changes from fetal to neonatal circulation, the transition from intrauterine to extrauterine life begins (see Chapter 4). **Initially the neonate may exhibit grunting, flaring, retracting, and cyanosis that resolve in the first hour of life (see Figure 5-2). Also, rales may be heard in a normal newborn's chest. As lung fluid is absorbed, the chest sounds clear. Observe, evaluate, and record the infant's respiratory rate and**

effort. A normal respiratory rate is 30 to 60 breaths/min without grunting, flaring, or retracting. Auscultate and record the apical pulse. A normal pulse rate is 120 to 160 beats/min.

Motor Activity

A full-term infant who has not been subjected to medications or stress during labor and birth will be awake and alert immediately after delivery. Observe, evaluate, and record the baby's state and activity.

First Period of Reactivity

The first period of reactivity occurs during the first 1 to 2 hours after birth. This is an excellent time for parents to be with their baby and begin the bonding process. Although the neonate may be physiologically unstable, it is safe to allow the mother and baby to be together under the close observation of the professional staff.

Sleep Period

The baby becomes hungry, will nurse, then falls asleep after an initial awake period and sleeps for several hours. Care providers should avoid disturbing the baby at this time with laboratory work, physical examinations, or feedings so that the infant can recover from the stress of labor and birth. Bathing should be postponed until the baby is awake and the temperature has stabilized.

Second Period of Reactivity

A second period of reactivity occurs between 4 and 6 hours of age. The infant frequently has significant mucoid secretions. The baby will awaken, begin to cry, and demand feeding. Suction secretions as needed.

Awake and Sleep States

Awake and sleep states affect a neonate's behavior and ability to respond to the environment. A newborn may go from one state to another quite frequently in the nursery and at home (see Table 13-3 for newborn states).

ETIOLOGY

Failure to make a normal transition to extrauterine life may result from obstetric anesthesia or analgesia, neonatal illness, or stress such as perinatal asphyxia and its sequelae. **If the infant's pulse, respirations, color, and activity have not stabilized** within the normal ranges after 1 hour of life, a problem should be suspected and investigated.

Prevention

Determination of the infant's gestational age provides a reference point for individualizing care. Whether the infant is term and admitted to the normal newborn nursery or preterm and admitted to the intensive care nursery, attention to care practices that support development and neurologic integrity is essential in preventing iatrogenic disruptions or injury.

In utero the fetus depends on the mother's physiologic systems to automatically regulate its own. At birth the neonate's basic physiologic needs (feeding, elimination, heat balance, communication) are met in new and different ways. Emerging from physiologic dependence into a physiologically independent neonatal state introduces new variables for both mother and baby in the development of their extrauterine relationship. **For both term and preterm newborns, the primary developmental task is to reestablish biorhythmic balance by (1) establishing homeostasis through self-regulation of states (e.g., arousal and sleep/wake cycles), (2) processing, storing, and organizing internal and external stimuli, and (3) establishing a reciprocal relationship with primary care providers and the environment.**

Although biorhythmic balance is internally determined, caretaking interaction between newborn and parent or caretaker either facilitates or disturbs this transition. After birth, balance is facilitated by contact with familiar surroundings (the mother's body). The mother's sensorimotor (auditory, tactile, visual), thermal, and nutrient stimuli provide regulatory effects on the infant's behavior (activity level, sucking, sleep and wake cycles, and circadian rhythms) and physiology (endocrine secretion, oxygen consumption, and cardiovascular status).[49] **Full-term newborns placed on the mother's chest immediately after delivery display a stereotypic innate sequence of prefeeding behavior:** no sucking activity in the first 15 minutes, rooting and sucking activity begins and reaches maximum intensity at 45 minutes, first hand-to-mouth movement at 35 minutes, spontaneous and unassisted finding of nipple and initiation of breastfeeding.[114,115] Within the first 90 minutes after birth, neonates cared for in close body contact with the mother are quiet.[28,29] However, **infants separated from their mothers during this period** and cared for in a crib cry and exhibit a "separation distress call" (also seen in several other mammalian species) that ceases at reunion.[28,29]

Care practices (e.g., separation of the mother and infant, gastric suction, supine positioning, noise levels in the newborn nursery) **that have become "routine" in maternal child care are (1) based on few scientific foundations,[57,62,79] (2) disrupt maternal and infant regulation and establishment of innate behaviors,* (3) may have hidden consequences that surpass human adaptability,[57,62,79,92] and (4) may contribute to behavioral deviations that result from violations of an innate agenda.†** For example, gastric suction after birth evokes aversive reflexes (e.g., retching, combative movements, increased mean arterial blood pressure, and varied heart rate, including bradycardia), disrupts development of early feeding behaviors, is unpleasant, and has no advantages in a healthy term infant after normal pregnancy, vaginal delivery, and clear amniotic fluid.[115] Use of maternal analgesia may interfere with the newborn's spontaneous breast-seeking and breastfeeding behavior and may increase neonatal temperature and crying.[92]

During transition of a term neonate, prone position has been shown to improve oxygenation, decrease heart and respiratory rates, and encourage more favorable behavioral states.[99] In the newborn nursery the lack of diurnal rhythm in noise levels and care-providing activities disrupts reestablishment of biorhythmic balance, sleep and wake cycles, and state lability.[41] **Significant differences in nighttime sleep and wake patterns exist between newborns cared for in the nursery (exposed to more light, noise, crying, and noncontingent care) than for newborns rooming with the mother (more quiet sleep and less crying).**[55] In another study, 20 white, term infants exposed to soothing music in the newborn nursery spent less time in high arousal states (i.e., nonalert waking and crying) and had fewer behavioral state changes.[52] Studies of outcomes of early discharge have not evaluated behavioral states, sleep and wake cycles, and state lability of infants at home versus infants hospitalized after birth.[16]

For full-term babies who must have heelstick bloodwork, presentation of heartbeat sounds and white noise (at 85 dB) have been shown to have a

---

*References 49, 57, 79, 92, 95, 101, 113-116.
†References 57, 62, 79, 92, 96, 97, 102, 114.

calming effect, as measured by less-pronounced behavioral responses and reduced adrenocortical release.[54] **Placing full-term babies skin-to-skin in whole-body contact with their mothers during heelstick procedures reduces heart rate, crying (by 82%), and grimacing (by 65%).**[46]

If adaptation to extrauterine life of full-term neonates is influenced either positively or negatively by nursery care practices, **adaptation of preterm or sick neonates may be even more influenced by early care and handling.** Use of stress-reduction techniques to prevent fluctuations in blood pressure, vital signs, and oxygenation are often not initiated until after the preterm infant has been admitted and stabilized in the NICU.[71,105] **Individualized developmental care (e.g., dimmed lights, decreased noise, gentle handling, contingent stimuli) (see Chapter 13) may be delayed in the urgency of expeditious assessment, diagnosis, and life-supporting interventions by care providers in the delivery room and on admission to the nursery.** However, the physiologic, anatomic, and psychologic transition to extrauterine life makes neonates, especially preterm or sick neonates, extremely vulnerable to the stress of resuscitation and initial nursery care.

Minimizing stress and conserving energy should accompany establishing and maintaining an airway, adequate oxygenation and ventilation, and circulatory support.[71,105] An immature preterm infant (under 32 weeks' gestation) (see Chapter 13) who is physiologically unstable may deteriorate if not handled gently and protected from overstimulation. **Rapid fluctuations in oxygenation and blood pressure, overwhelming stimuli, too-rapid volume expansion, suction, unrelieved pain, and hypothermia contribute to the incidence of intraventricular hemorrhage that most commonly occurs in the first 24 hours after birth (see Chapters 4, 6, 7, 12, 23, and 26). In preterm infants, "routine" procedures such as bathing result in increased heart rate and blood pressure, motor stress behaviors, changes in stability and reorganizational behavior, hypoxia, and increased intracranial pressure.**[30,85,86,89,101] Overwhelmed by external stimuli, a neonate's global response to stress may be apnea and bradycardia.

Based on the infant's ability to tolerate an intervention and the benefits of early assessment and intervention, **the admission process should be prioritized to (1) provide life-supportive care, (2) conserve energy, and (3) collect data and com-** **plete the health care record.**[105] **Table 5-2 outlines developmental interventions for neonatal admissions and initial nursery care that decrease stress, reduce energy consumption, improve oxygenation and respiratory and heart rates, and prevent iatrogenic stress and injury. Developmentally supportive care should begin immediately following birth.**[21]

Kangaroo Care

Very early skin-to-skin "kangaroo" care (KC), beginning in the delivery room and continuing for 6 hours after birth, in six 34- to 36-week preterm infants resulted in (1) neutral thermal temperature, (2) vital signs and oxygen saturation within normal limits, (3) disappearance of grunting respirations in two neonates with warmed, humidified oxygen, (4) a predominance of sleep state, and (5) discharge at 48 hours with full breastfeeding.[78] These researchers concluded that KC was conducive to recovery from birth-related fatigue. Other studies of KC immediately after birth show either no significant difference or higher temperature, more optimal glucose levels and less crying than babies placed in cribs[26,29,110] (Table 5-2).

Kangaroo care not only prevents hypothermia but also is effective in treating hypothermia. KC warms healthy, low-risk, hypothermic preterm infants better (90%) than does incubator care (60%).[27] In a study of fathers providing KC after cesarean section, they were able to significantly increase the axillary temperature and blood glucose levels of their full-term newborns, compared with these parameters when the infants received incubator or crib care.[26] During KC preterm infants remain clinically stable, with improved gaseous exchange and temperature stability.[40] **The benefits of KC were especially significant (e.g., smallest increase in heart rate; highest decrease in respiratory rate; a doubling of oxygen saturation) in infants under 1000 g.**[40] Kangaroo care promotes stable cardiorespiratory functions, minimizes unnecessary movement, improves behavioral state, and facilitates maternal-infant and paternal-infant interaction.[77]

Knowledge of the normal vital processes of an infant's first 24 hours of life assists the care provider in early recognition of deviations from normal extrauterine life and in early initiation of corrective interventions.[42,73] **Delay in recognizing and initiating therapy increases morbidity and mortality.**[108]

Table 5-2	DEVELOPMENTAL INTERVENTIONS DURING ADMISSION AND INITIAL NURSERY CARE
Oxygenation	Apply noninvasive monitor (see Chapter 7)
	Titrate FiO$_2$ to maintain saturation at 92% to 94% (see Chapters 7, 11)
	Handle gently, minimally (see Chapters 13, 23)
	Kangaroo care improves gaseous exchange, especially in preterms <1000 g[40]
	Position prone to maximize oxygenation (see Chapter 13 and below)
	Delay or defer bathing[85,86,89] (see Chapter 18)
Thermoregulation	Maintain temperature: axillary (>36.5° to 37.5° C in term infants); skin (36° to 36.5° C in preterm infants) (see Chapter 6)
	Skin-to-skin (kangaroo care) provided by mothers or fathers to preterm/term newborns warms better than incubator care[26,27,29,110]
	Prewarm linen, scales, radiant warmer, incubator (see Chapter 6)
	Decrease heat loss with position (i.e., prone, flexion) (see Chapters 6, 13)
	Use warm water on skin before applying probe, electrodes (see Chapter 18)
	Delay or defer bathing[85,86,89] (see Chapter 18)—healthy term infants with axillary temperature >36.8° C can be bathed after 1 hour of age when appropriate care is taken to support thermal stability[109] (see Chapters 6, 13)
Nutrition	Screen at-risk and symptomatic infants for hypoglycemia (see Chapter 15)
	Provide fluids and/or calories (orally or intravenously) (see Chapters 14-17)
	Decrease energy expenditures by decreasing internal (i.e., hypothermia, hypoxia) and external (i.e., noise, light) stressors (see Chapters 13, 15)
Pain	Minimize painful stimuli (see Chapters 12, 13)
	Relieve pain with pharmacologic management (see Chapter 12)
	Provide comfort measures (e.g., pacifier, containment, grasping) (see Chapters 12, 13)
Environmental stimuli	Tactile: (see Chapter 13)
	Handle gently and minimally
	Support and contain in flexion
	Rest periods between procedures, handling
	Visual: (see Chapter 13)
	Shield from bright, direct light
	Dim lights as soon as possible
	Cover oxygen hood, face with wash cloth
	Cover incubator with blanket or cover
	Auditory: (see Chapter 13)
	Talk quietly
	Respond quickly to alarms
	Parents to softly talk to infant
	Keep ill neonates away from crying babies[55]
Position	Promote flexion in side-lying position with blankets, rolls (see Chapter 13)
	Prone (oxygenation better; quiet; more restful sleep; decreased caloric expenditure; decreased reflux)[99] (see Chapter 13)
	Swaddle (see Chapter 13)
	Avoid supine (see Chapter 13)
Assess and interpret infant cries	Assess avoidance and approach behaviors so that care is individualized (see Chapter 13)
	Support infant strengths, adaptive and coping behaviors (see Chapter 13)
	Modulate environmental and caregiver stimuli based on infant cues (contingent on cues rather than noncontingent stimuli and interaction) (see Chapter 13)
	Teach parents infant cues (see Chapter 13)

DATA COLLECTION

History

Good perinatal care requires the identification of social, demographic, and medical-obstetric risk factors that correlate with fetal outcome. This must be an ongoing process, because high-risk patients may be identified on the first prenatal visit, during follow-up prenatal visits, or not until the intrapartum and postpartum periods. **Review of the perinatal history is important in determining significant factors for neonatal health management.** Identification of an at-risk maternal situation is essential to plan and organize care for an at-risk neonate. Review of the perinatal history includes antepartum and intrapartum events (see Chapter 2) and events of the neonatal course, such as normal or abnormal transition, timing and onset of symptoms, and the ability to feed.

Signs and Symptoms

Unlike the verbalizing adult patient, the nonverbal neonate communicates needs primarily by behavior. **Through objective observations and evaluations the neonatal care provider interprets this behavior into information about the individual infant's condition. Assessment of the neonate includes the following:**
- **Estimation of gestational age**
- **Physical examination**
- **Neurologic examination**
- **Brazelton examination**

All care providers must not only be familiar with these tools but also be proficient in performing and interpreting them.

Estimation of Gestational Age

An assessment of gestational age should be done on all newborns to assign a newborn classification, determine neonatal mortality risk, generate a problem list of potential morbidities, and quickly initiate appropriate screening procedures and/or interventions for recognized morbidities.[14,33,76,107] Gestational age can be assessed by obstetric methods and by pediatric methods.

The obstetric methods for determining maturity will have already been performed by the time the newborn reaches the nursery. However, the newborn's care providers should be familiar with dating a pregnancy. Dating the last menstrual period (LMP) could be the most accurate method if the mother is sure of the dates of her last menstrual period. Some women will have spotting or even a light period after becoming pregnant, making them unsure of the time of conception. The use of birth control pills may also make the time of ovulation and conception unknown; therefore pregnancy tests are useful in confirming the pregnancy and not the timing of conception.

The most accurate assessment is the ultrasonographic examination during the first trimester.[25] Ultrasonography is preferred because it confirms conception, assesses gestation, and evaluates fetal growth.

Pediatric methods of determining gestational age are based on physical characteristics and neurologic examination. Within two hours of birth,[9] **every newborn should have an assessment of gestational age by physical characteristics. Numerous tables, charts, and graphs are available for determining gestation. Some tables are more subjective than others, but at least one form should be used by all nurseries.**

Three of the available charts for determining gestational age by physical characteristics are shown in Figures 5-3, 5-4, and 5-5. Figure 5-3 does not place much emphasis on the neurologic assessment, which may not be valid in the first 24 hours because of birth recovery.[3] To use this chart, an X or ditto marks (" ") are placed in each appropriate slot. Then an age is assigned according to a line drawn through the point where most of the marks have been placed. The disadvantage of this system is the subjectivity of the chart; the advantage is that items relate to gestational age, not a score. The examiner must therefore be experienced to offset the possibility of error in the chart.

Figures 5-5 incorporates physical maturity and neuromuscular maturity on an equal basis. An X is placed in the appropriate box for each category. The score for the neuromuscular and physical maturity is added and noted under the maturity rating column. Weeks of gestation are assigned according to the maturity rating score.

Accuracy in estimation of gestational age is important, because for VLBW infants, small differences in gestational age result in large differences in outcome and may be a criteria in decision-making by parents and professionals, whether comfort care or intensive care is utilized.* Research has shown that estimation of gestational age in very immature preterm

---

*References 4, 34, 48, 59, 88, 103, 106.

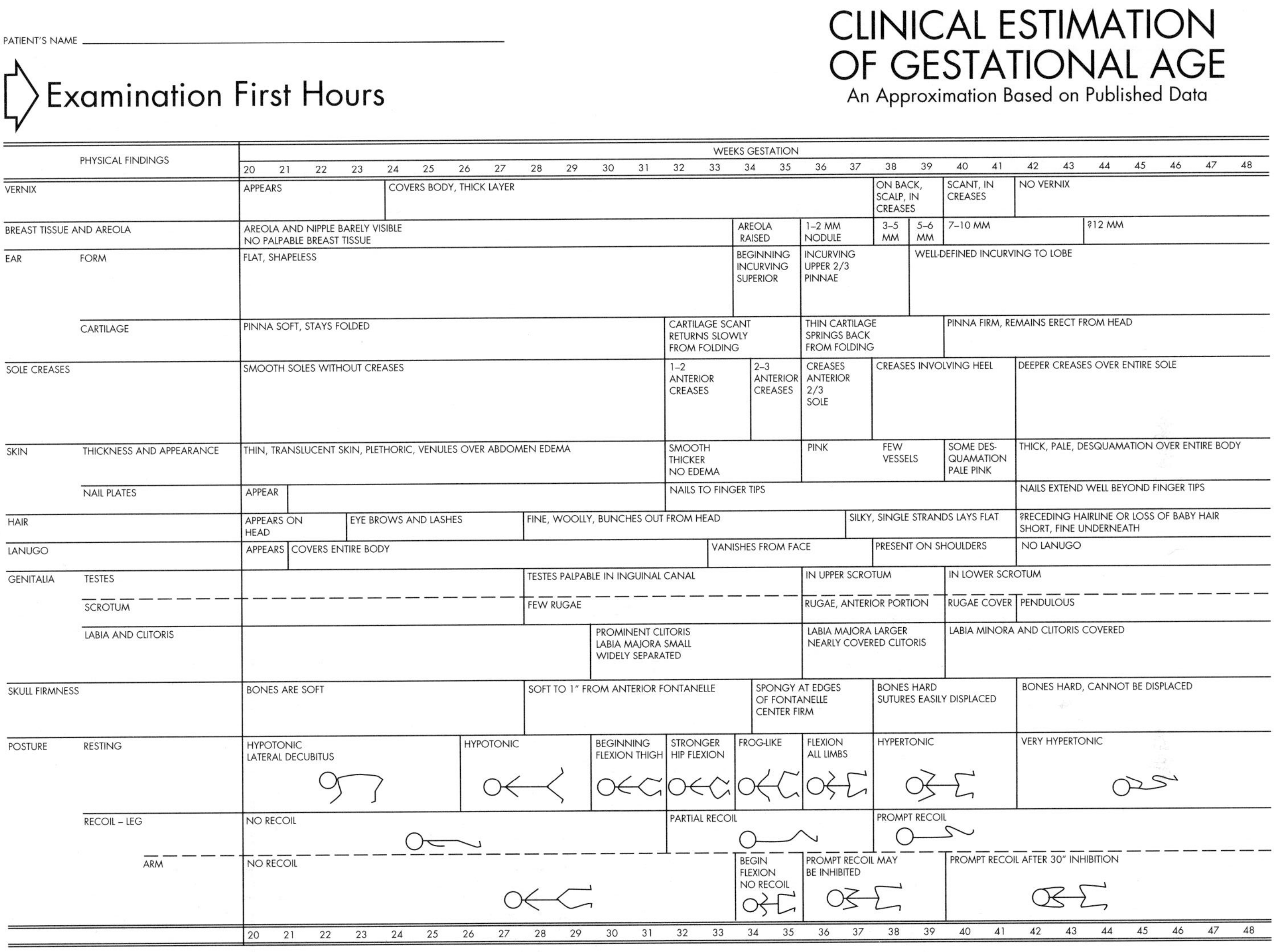

PATIENT'S NAME

Examination First Hours

CLINICAL ESTIMATION OF GESTATIONAL AGE
An Approximation Based on Published Data

WEEKS GESTATION (20–48)

Physical Findings	Findings (with approximate weeks gestation)
VERNIX	APPEARS (21); COVERS BODY, THICK LAYER; ON BACK, SCALP IN CREASES (38); SCANT, IN CREASES (40); NO VERNIX (42)
BREAST TISSUE AND AREOLA	AREOLA AND NIPPLE BARELY VISIBLE, NO PALPABLE BREAST TISSUE; AREOLA RAISED (34); 1–2 MM NODULE (36); 3–5 MM (38); 5–6 MM (39); 7–10 MM (40); ≥12 MM (44)
EAR — FORM	FLAT, SHAPELESS (20); BEGINNING INCURVING SUPERIOR (34); INCURVING UPPER 2/3 PINNAE (36); WELL-DEFINED INCURVING TO LOBE (39)
EAR — CARTILAGE	PINNA SOFT, STAYS FOLDED (24); CARTILAGE SCANT, RETURNS SLOWLY FROM FOLDING (32); THIN CARTILAGE SPRINGS BACK FROM FOLDING (36); PINNA FIRM, REMAINS ERECT FROM HEAD (39)
SOLE CREASES	SMOOTH SOLES WITHOUT CREASES (22); 1–2 ANTERIOR CREASES (32); 2–3 ANTERIOR CREASES (34); CREASES ANTERIOR 2/3 SOLE (36); CREASES INVOLVING HEEL (38); DEEPER CREASES OVER ENTIRE SOLE (42)
SKIN — THICKNESS AND APPEARANCE	THIN, TRANSLUCENT SKIN, PLETHORIC, VENULES OVER ABDOMEN EDEMA (23); SMOOTH THICKER, NO EDEMA (32); PINK (36); FEW VESSELS (38); SOME DESQUAMATION PALE PINK (40); THICK, PALE, DESQUAMATION OVER ENTIRE BODY (42)
SKIN — NAIL PLATES	APPEAR (20); NAILS TO FINGER TIPS (34); NAILS EXTEND WELL BEYOND FINGER TIPS (43)
HAIR	APPEARS ON HEAD (20); EYE BROWS AND LASHES (25); FINE, WOOLLY, BUNCHES OUT FROM HEAD (28); SILKY, SINGLE STRANDS LAYS FLAT (37); RECEDING HAIRLINE OR LOSS OF BABY HAIR, SHORT, FINE UNDERNEATH (43)
LANUGO	APPEARS (20); COVERS ENTIRE BODY (24); VANISHES FROM FACE (33); PRESENT ON SHOULDERS (38); NO LANUGO (42)
GENITALIA — TESTES	TESTES PALPABLE IN INGUINAL CANAL (28); IN UPPER SCROTUM (37); IN LOWER SCROTUM (40)
GENITALIA — SCROTUM	FEW RUGAE (29); RUGAE, ANTERIOR PORTION (37); RUGAE COVER (40); PENDULOUS (42)
GENITALIA — LABIA AND CLITORIS	PROMINENT CLITORIS, LABIA MAJORA SMALL, WIDELY SEPARATED (30); LABIA MAJORA LARGER, NEARLY COVERED CLITORIS (36); LABIA MINORA AND CLITORIS COVERED (40)
SKULL FIRMNESS	BONES ARE SOFT (24); SOFT TO 1″ FROM ANTERIOR FONTANELLE (29); SPONGY AT EDGES OF FONTANELLE, CENTER FIRM (35); BONES HARD, SUTURES EASILY DISPLACED (38); BONES HARD, CANNOT BE DISPLACED (43)
POSTURE — RESTING	HYPOTONIC, LATERAL DECUBITUS (21); HYPOTONIC (26); BEGINNING FLEXION THIGH (30); STRONGER HIP FLEXION (32); FROG-LIKE (34); FLEXION ALL LIMBS (36); HYPERTONIC (38); VERY HYPERTONIC (44)
RECOIL — LEG	NO RECOIL (21); PARTIAL RECOIL (32); PROMPT RECOIL (39)
RECOIL — ARM	NO RECOIL (21); BEGIN FLEXION NO RECOIL (34); PROMPT RECOIL MAY BE INHIBITED (36); PROMPT RECOIL AFTER 30″ INHIBITION (41)

FIGURE 5-3   Clinical estimation of gestational age: examination in the first hour. (From Kempe CH, Silver HK, O'Brien D: *Current pediatric diagnosis and treatment*, ed 3, Los Altos, Calif, 1974, Lange Medical.)

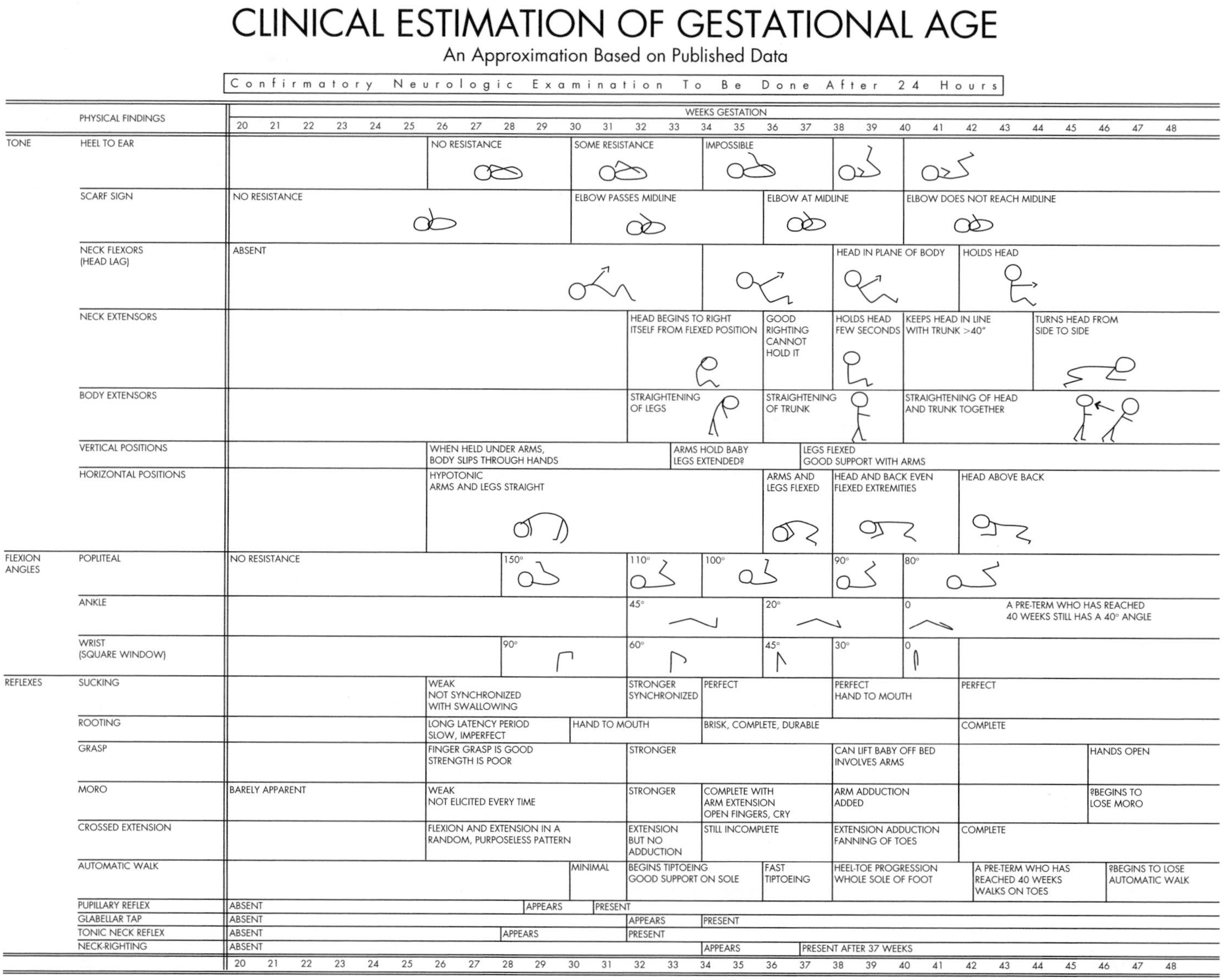
CLINICAL ESTIMATION OF GESTATIONAL AGE
An Approximation Based on Published Data
Confirmatory Neurologic Examination To Be Done After 24 Hours
PHYSICAL FINDINGS
WEEKS GESTATION
20 21 22 23 24 25 26 27 28 29 30 31 32 33 34 35 36 37 38 39 40 41 42 43 44 45 46 47 48
TONE
HEEL TO EAR
NO RESISTANCE
SOME RESISTANCE
IMPOSSIBLE
SCARF SIGN
NO RESISTANCE
ELBOW PASSES MIDLINE
ELBOW AT MIDLINE
ELBOW DOES NOT REACH MIDLINE
NECK FLEXORS (HEAD LAG)
ABSENT
HEAD IN PLANE OF BODY
HOLDS HEAD
NECK EXTENSORS
HEAD BEGINS TO RIGHT ITSELF FROM FLEXED POSITION
GOOD RIGHTING CANNOT HOLD IT
HOLDS HEAD FEW SECONDS
KEEPS HEAD IN LINE WITH TRUNK >40°
TURNS HEAD FROM SIDE TO SIDE
BODY EXTENSORS
STRAIGHTENING OF LEGS
STRAIGHTENING OF TRUNK
STRAIGHTENING OF HEAD AND TRUNK TOGETHER
VERTICAL POSITIONS
WHEN HELD UNDER ARMS, BODY SLIPS THROUGH HANDS
ARMS HOLD BABY LEGS EXTENDED?
LEGS FLEXED GOOD SUPPORT WITH ARMS
HORIZONTAL POSITIONS
HYPOTONIC ARMS AND LEGS STRAIGHT
ARMS AND LEGS FLEXED
HEAD AND BACK EVEN FLEXED EXTREMITIES
HEAD ABOVE BACK
FLEXION ANGLES
POPLITEAL
NO RESISTANCE
150°
110°
100°
90°
80°
ANKLE
45°
20°
0
A PRE-TERM WHO HAS REACHED 40 WEEKS STILL HAS A 40° ANGLE
WRIST (SQUARE WINDOW)
90°
60°
45°
30°
0
REFLEXES
SUCKING
WEAK NOT SYNCHRONIZED WITH SWALLOWING
STRONGER SYNCHRONIZED
PERFECT
PERFECT HAND TO MOUTH
PERFECT
ROOTING
LONG LATENCY PERIOD SLOW, IMPERFECT
HAND TO MOUTH
BRISK, COMPLETE, DURABLE
COMPLETE
GRASP
FINGER GRASP IS GOOD STRENGTH IS POOR
STRONGER
CAN LIFT BABY OFF BED INVOLVES ARMS
HANDS OPEN
MORO
BARELY APPARENT
WEAK NOT ELICITED EVERY TIME
STRONGER
COMPLETE WITH ARM EXTENSION OPEN FINGERS, CRY
ARM ADDUCTION ADDED
?BEGINS TO LOSE MORO
CROSSED EXTENSION
FLEXION AND EXTENSION IN A RANDOM, PURPOSELESS PATTERN
EXTENSION BUT NO ADDUCTION
STILL INCOMPLETE
EXTENSION ADDUCTION FANNING OF TOES
COMPLETE
AUTOMATIC WALK
MINIMAL
BEGINS TIPTOEING GOOD SUPPORT ON SOLE
FAST TIPTOEING
HEEL-TOE PROGRESSION WHOLE SOLE OF FOOT
A PRE-TERM WHO HAS REACHED 40 WEEKS WALKS ON TOES
?BEGINS TO LOSE AUTOMATIC WALK
PUPILLARY REFLEX
ABSENT
APPEARS
PRESENT
GLABELLAR TAP
ABSENT
APPEARS
PRESENT
TONIC NECK REFLEX
ABSENT
APPEARS
PRESENT
NECK-RIGHTING
ABSENT
APPEARS
PRESENT AFTER 37 WEEKS
20 21 22 23 24 25 26 27 28 29 30 31 32 33 34 35 36 37 38 39 40 41 42 43 44 45 46 47 48

FIGURE 5-4 Clinical estimation of gestational age: examination after the first 24 hours. (From Kempe CH, Silver HK, O'Brien D: *Current pediatric diagnosis and treatment,* ed 3, Los Altos, Calif, 1974, Lange Medical.)

Neuromuscular maturity

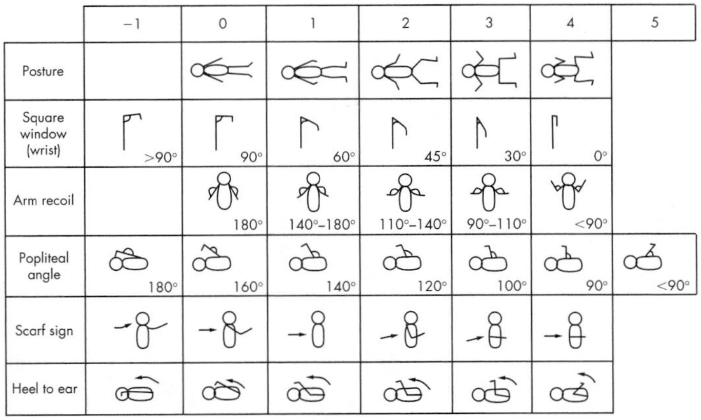

	−1	0	1	2	3	4	5
Posture							
Square window (wrist)	>90°	90°	60°	45°	30°	0°	
Arm recoil		180°	140°–180°	110°–140°	90°–110°	<90°	
Popliteal angle	180°	160°	140°	120°	100°	90°	<90°
Scarf sign							
Heel to ear							

Physical maturity

	−1	0	1	2	3	4	5
Skin	Sticky friable transparent	Gelatinous red, translucent	Smooth pink, visible veins	Superficial peeling and/or rash, few veins	Cracking pale areas rare veins	Parchment deep cracking no vessels	Leathery cracked wrinkled
Lanugo	None	Sparse	Abundant	Thinning	Bald areas	Mostly bald	
Plantar surface	Heel-toe 40–50 mm: −1 <40 mm: −2	>50 mm no crease	Faint red marks	Anterior transverse crease only	Creases ant. 2/3	Creases over entire sole	
Breast	Imperceptible	Barely perceptible	Flat areola no bud	Stippled areola 1–2 mm bud	Raised areola 3–4 mm bud	Full areola 5–10 mm bud	
Eye/ear	Lids fused loosely: −1 tightly: −2	Lids open pinna flat stays folded	Sl. curved pinna, soft, slow recoil	Well-curved pinna; soft but ready recoil	Formed and firm instant recoil	Thick cartilage ear stiff	
Genitals male	Scrotum flat, smooth	Scrotum empty faint rugae	Testes in upper canal rare rugae	Testes descending few rugae	Testes down good rugae	Testes pendulous deep rugae	
Genitals female	Clitoris prominent labia flat	Prominent clitoris small labia minora	Prominent clitoris enlarging minora	Majora and minora equally prominent	Majora large minora small	Majora cover clitoris and minora	

Maturity rating

Score	Weeks
−10	20
−5	22
0	24
5	26
10	28
15	30
20	32
25	34
30	36
35	38
40	40
45	42
50	44

FIGURE 5-5 Clinical estimation of gestational age (revised to include extremely premature infants). (From Ballard JL, Khoury JC, Wedig K et al: New Ballard score, expanded to include extremely premature infants, *J Pediatr* 119:417, 1991.)

infants is inaccurate.[34,112] For preterm infants of 22 to 28 weeks' gestation, estimates of gestational age (by the scoring system shown in Figure 5-5) exceeded the gestational age (by dates) by 1.3 to 3.3 weeks.[34] These inaccuracies must be considered in decision-making, and better scoring systems are needed.[34,103]

To use these charts accurately the examiner must assess the following physical characteristics.[76,107]

Vernix. At 20 to 24 weeks, vernix is produced by sebaceous glands. **Note the amount and distribution of vernix on the baby's skin (best done in the delivery room).** Vernix is high in fat content and protects the skin from the aqueous amniotic fluid and

bacteria. At 36 weeks, the white, cheeselike material begins to decrease and disappears by 41 weeks.

Skin. **In early gestation the skin of the fetus is very transparent, and veins are easily seen. As gestation progresses, the skin becomes tougher, thicker, and less transparent.**

By 37 weeks, very few vessels are visible. From 36 weeks to delivery, fat deposits begin to form and grow. In a postterm infant, desquamation will be prominent at the ankles, wrists, and possibly palms and soles. As gestation progresses, the loss of vernix and subcutaneous tissue causes wrinkling. **Note skin turgor, color, texture, and the prominence of vessels, especially on the abdomen.**

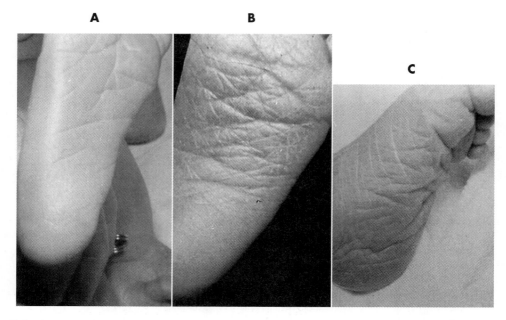

A   **B**   **C**

FIGURE 5-6   Sole creases at different gestational ages. **A,** Age 31 to 33 weeks' gestation. **B,** Age 34 to 38 weeks' gestation. **C,** Term.

Lanugo. At 20 weeks, fine downy hair (lanugo) appears over the entire body of the fetus. At 28 weeks, it begins to disappear around the face and anterior trunk. At term, a few patches of lanugo may still be present over the shoulders. **Note the distribution of lanugo, first on the face and anterior trunk, then on the rest of the body.**

Hair on the Head. Hair appears on the head at 20 weeks. At 20 to 23 weeks, the eyelashes and eyebrows develop. From 28 to 34 or 36 weeks the hair is fine and woolly and sticks together. It appears disheveled and sticks out in bunches from the head. At term the hair lies flat on the head, it feels silky, and single strands are identifiable. **Note the quality and distribution of the hair and feel its texture.**

Sole Creases. Sole creases develop from toe to heel, progressing with gestational age. An infant with IUGR and early loss of vernix may have more sole creases than expected. **By 12 hours after birth, the skin has dried to a point that sole creases are no longer a valid indicator of gestational age. Note the development of sole creases as they progress from the superior to inferior aspects of the foot (Figure 5-6).**

Eyes. **In the third month of fetal life, the eyelids fuse and reopen between 26 and 30 weeks.**

In neonates of 27 to 34 weeks' gestation, examination of the anterior vascular capsule of the lens is useful in assessing gestational age. Gestational age is determined by assessing the level of remaining embryonic vessels on the lens (Figure 5-7). Before 27 weeks, the hazy cornea prevents visualization of the vascular system. After 34 weeks, only remnants of the vascular system are visible. Because rapid atrophy occurs in the vascular system, an ophthalmoscopic examination should be performed during the first physical examination or within 24 to 48 hours after birth.

Ears. Before 34 weeks, the pinna of the ear is a slightly formed, cartilage-free double thickness of skin. When it is folded, it remains folded. **As gestation progresses, the pinnas develop more cartilage, resulting in better form, so that they recoil when folded (Figure 5-8).** Check ear recoil by folding the ear in half or into a three-corner-hat shape. Consistently folding it the same way helps the care provider develop a baseline for judging maturity. **Note the form and cartilage development of the ear. Examine both ears to be sure they are the same and without defects.**

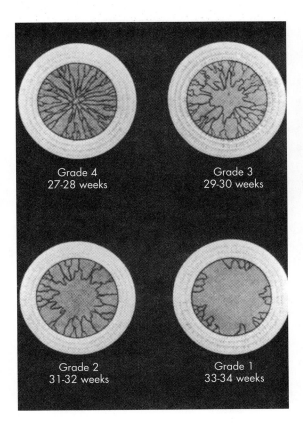

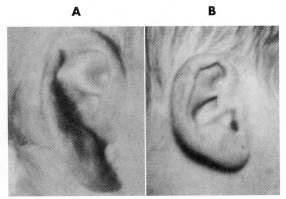

A   **B**

FIGURE 5-8   Ear form and gestational age. **A,** Age 34 to 38 weeks' gestation. **B,** Term.

FIGURE 5-7   Anterior vascular capsule and gestational age. (From Hittner H, Hirsch NJ, Rudolph AJ: Assessment of gestational age by examination of the anterior vascular capsule of the lens, *J Pediatr* 91:455, 1977.)

Breast Development. **Breast development is the result of the growth of glandular tissue related to high maternal estrogen levels and fat deposition.** The areola is raised in an infant of 34 weeks' gestation. **Note the size, shape, and placement of both breasts.** Palpate the breast nodule and determine its size. If the infant is growth retarded, breast size may be less than expected at term.

Genitalia

Male Genitalia. At 28 weeks, the testes begin to descend from the abdomen. By 37 weeks, they are high in the scrotum. By 40 weeks, the testes are completely descended, and the scrotum is covered with rugae. As gestation progresses, the scrotum becomes more pendulous (Figure 5-9). **Note the presence of rugae on the scrotum and its size in relation to the position of the testes.** When examining the baby for descended testes, put the fingers of one hand over the inguinal canal to prevent the testes from ascending into the abdominal cavity and palpate the scrotal sac with the other hand.

Female Genitalia. Early in the female's gestation the clitoris is prominent with small and widely separated labia. By 40 weeks the fat deposits have increased in size so that the labia majora completely cover the labia minora (Figure 5-10). **Note the labial development in relation to the prominence of the clitoris.**

Newborn Classifications. **The clinical estimate of gestation is defined by weeks of gestation into the following categories (Figures 5-11 and 5-12):**
- **Preterm (PR)—through 37 completed weeks**
- **Full-term (F)—38 through 41 completed weeks**
- **Postterm (PO)—42 weeks or more**

Intrauterine growth curves for the 10th and 90th percentiles are represented in Figure 5-11. Small-for-gestational-age (SGA) infants are those below the 10th percentile. Appropriate-for-gestational-age (AGA) infants are those between the 10th and 90th percentiles. Large-for-gestational-age (LGA) infants are above the 90th percentile. Based on birth weight, the infant's intrauterine growth will be SGA, AGA, or LGA.

Using the clinical estimate of gestational age (in weeks) and the birth weight (in grams), one determines the newborn's classification. The combined gestational age and weight criteria shown in

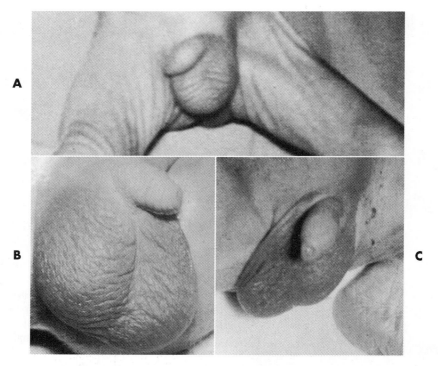

FIGURE 5-9 Male genitalia and gestational age. **A,** Age 28 to 35 weeks' gestation. **B,** Term. **C,** Age 42 or more weeks' gestation.

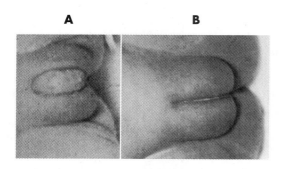

FIGURE 5-10 Female genitalia and gestational age. **A,** Age 30 to 36 weeks' gestation. **B,** Term.

Figure 5-11 form nine possible newborn classifications: preterm, full-term, and postterm large-for-gestational-age (PRLGA, FLGA, and POLGA); preterm, full-term, and postterm appropriate-for-gestational-age (PRAGA, FAGA, and POAGA); and preterm, full-term, and postterm small-for-gestational-age (PRSGA, FSGA, and POSGA).

Using Figure 5-11, it is possible to plot the newborn weight in grams against the clinical gestational age (marking an X on the chart) by determining to which of the nine categories the baby belongs, then classifying and noting the newborn's classification on the record.

Neonatal Mortality Risk. Neonatal mortality risk (NMR), the chance of dying in the neonatal period, can be determined from graphs such as that shown in Figure 5-11 and is based on birth weight and gestational age. This figure is based on the Lubchenco Perinatal Database, University of Colorado Hospital, 1980 to 1992. On the chart the area of least risk is the full-term appropriate-for-gestational-age (FAGA) infant. Deviations from this area of least risk in relation to either weight or gestational age increase the newborn's mortality risk.

Over time there has been a change in mortality because an increasingly physiologic basis of care has been used, coupled with sophisticated professional care, technology, transport systems, and aggressive management to handle increasingly at-risk populations. For example, before recent years, LGA

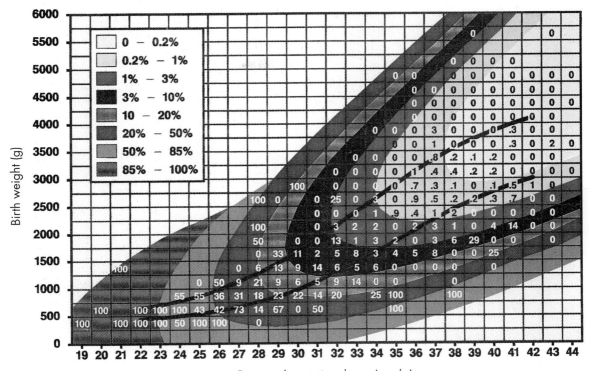

FIGURE 5-11   Neonatal mortality risk by birth weight and gestational age. (From Johnson JL, Merenstein G, Coll J et al: Colorado intrauterine growth curve 1980-1992: the new Lubchenco growth curve, *Pediatr Res* 35:274A, 1994.)

infants were at increased risk for mortality; this is no longer true because of earlier recognition and better obstetric management (see Chapter 2). Babies with greater than 10% risk of neonatal mortality usually require level II or III care. Note the infant's NMR on the chart (see Figure 5-11) and insert an entry in the newborn record. NOTE: To determine the appropriate NMR, read to the right of the vertical lines and above the horizontal line.

Examination of NMR in Figure 5-11 also reveals that two infants with the same birth weight but with different gestational ages may have very different risks of death. For example, infant A may have a birth weight of 2000 g and a gestational age of 33 weeks. Plotting these values on Figure 5-11, one determines the NMR for this infant at 2%. Infant B, on the other hand, may also weigh 2000 g but have a gestational age of 39 weeks. The infant's risk is 0%. Infant A thus has a mortality risk 10 times

greater than that of infant B, even though they have the same birth weight.

Neonatal Morbidity Risk. **Neonatal morbidity risk (see Figure 5-12) is determined by deviations of intrauterine growth and newborn classification. Classification of the newborn assists in identification, observation, screening, and treatment of the most commonly occurring problems. For every newborn, formulate a problem list based on the morbidities common to the newborn classification. Observe, screen, intervene, and refer as necessary to prevent complications.**

Physical Examination
The purpose of the physical examination is (1) to discover common variations of normal or obvious defects, (2) to quickly initiate intervention or referral for deviations from normal, and (3) to

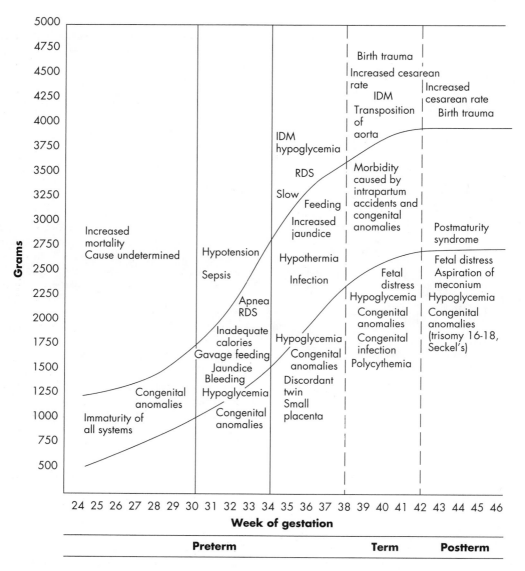

FIGURE 5-12 Specific neonatal morbidity by birth weight and gestational age based on statistics from Newborn and Premature Center at the University of Colorado Medical Center. (From Lubchenco LO: *The high-risk infant,* Philadelphia, 1976, WB Saunders.)

establish a database for serial observations and comparisons. **The best data are obtained from the neonate when the physical examination is organized to limit stress, maximize interaction with the examiner, and not overwhelm the newborn. To maximize data and minimize stress, the physical examination should entail observation, quiet examination, and head-to-toe examination.**

The order of the first, thorough examination is determined by using the least stressful items first to obtain optimal information on organ systems. However, the examination is usually recorded in an orderly manner from head to toe.

When one appreciates how stressful it is to the newborn to be undressed, it becomes obvious that as much as possible should be done without exposing the infant. Warm hands and instruments are essential, and a warm environment helps. Before touching the infant or removing any covers, observe the face, head, and hands as they appear.

Observation. **Observation of the neonate provides pertinent data without touching the newborn. General condition, anomalies, resting posture, and respirations of the infant should be observed.**

General Condition. The general condition of the infant should be assessed by noting the color, activity, and neonatal state.

Color. **The color of the newborn is normally pink. Acrocyanosis, or peripheral cyanosis of the hands and feet, is commonly present in the first 24 hours of life and may be the result of immature circulation or cold stress.** Ecchymotic areas, especially on the presenting part, are common; however, they may be confused with cyanosis. To differentiate the two, apply pressure to the area. An ecchymotic area remains blue with pressure, whereas a cyanotic area will blanch.

General cyanosis and central cyanosis of the lips, mouth, and mucous membranes may indicate CNS, heart, or lung disease. Jaundice appearing at birth or within the first 12 hours of life is abnormal. Physiologic jaundice appears after 24 hours, but jaundice may indicate other abnormalities. **Pallor at or directly after birth is a sign of circulatory failure, anoxia, edema, or shock.** Pallor of anoxia is associated with bradycardia, and the pallor of anemia with tachycardia. **Plethora, a beef-red color, may indicate polycythemia and is confirmed by hemoglobin and hematocrit determinations.** However, lack of plethora does not rule out polycythemia or hyperviscosity.

Activity and Neonatal State. **Activity and the neonatal state at the beginning of the examination and appropriate changes throughout the examination should be observed.** If the infant is asleep, is it quiet or rapid-eye-movement (REM) sleep? Spontaneous, symmetric movements are normal. Tremors and twitching movements of short duration are normal in relation to states of coldness or startling. Good muscle tone is established with adequate oxygenation soon after birth.

Flaccidity, floppiness, or poor muscle tone should be noted. Spasticity, hyperactivity, opisthotonos, twitching, hypertonicity, tremors, or seizures may be indicative of CNS damage. Asymmetry may result from intrauterine pressure or birth trauma rather than a CNS insult. **A lack of crying or evasive behavior in response to the manipulations of a physical examination is abnormal.**[89]

Crying. **Attempts to calm and console a crying infant during this part of the examination assist in better data collection during the quiet examination.** Acoustic qualities (e.g., melody, pitch, duration, latency, and so on)[89] reflect the newborn's neurophysiologic status and are general assessors of risk.[69,89] Crying is beneficial in (1) ductal closure and transition from fetal to neonatal cardiorespiratory status, (2) improving pulmonary capacity, (3) maintaining homeostasis, (4) facilitating vocal tract development, and (5) cueing and care-eliciting behavior.[89] Negative effects include (1) changes in cardiovascular (e.g., tachycardia, hypoxia, changes in cerebral blood flow) and endocrine systems, (2) stress production and energy drainage,[93] (3) strong, sometimes negative feelings in care providers.[89]

Although uniquely individual, types of cries that reflect the infant's state and contextual basis have been identified as birth, distress call, hunger, pain, spontaneous, and pleasure.[28,105,115,117] At birth, the term neonate has a loud, lusty cry (a signal of robustness and wellness),[15] whereas the preterm's cry may be weak or absent. Observe the infant's ability to quiet himself or herself when crying.

A **high-pitched cry** suggests CNS irritation from increased intracranial pressure, injury, infection, or abnormality. **Weak crying,** no crying, or constant, irritable crying may indicate brain injury, infection, or abnormality. **Hoarse cries or crowing inspirations** result from laryngeal inflammation, injury, vocal cord dysfunction (e.g., paresis/paralysis) or anomalies. **A weak, groaning cry or expiratory grunt** is indicative of respiratory disease.

Anomalies. **Obvious bodily malformations such as omphalocele, cleft lip and palate, imperforate anus, syndactyly, polydactyly, spina bifida, or myelomeningocele should be observed and recorded as anomalies. Odd facies or body appearances that are often associated with specific syndromes should also be noted.**

Resting Posture. **Resting posture should be observed while the infant is quiet and not disturbed.** The infant's posture systematically develops according to gestational age[3]: (1) from extension to flexion of the lower extremities, and (2) to flexion of the upper extremities. Asymmetry may result from intrauterine pressure or birth trauma. The infant may take a position of comfort assumed in utero.

Respirations. **Respirations should be evaluated while the infant is at rest and before any** manipulation. **The normal rate is 30 to 60 breaths/min. Count the respiratory rate and rhythm, noticing the infant's use of accessory muscles. Respiration is normally abdominal or diaphragmatic.**

After the first hour of life a respiratory rate of more than 60 breaths/min indicates tachypnea. Tachypnea is the earliest sign of many neonatal respiratory, cardiac, metabolic, and infectious illnesses. Tachypnea, apnea, dyspnea, or cyanosis may indicate cardiorespiratory distress. Labored respirations include retractions, flaring nares, and expiratory grunt.[39]

If the infant is swaddled, the observation examination will not be as extensive as is possible when the infant is unclothed in an incubator or under a radiant warmer. If the infant is swaddled, unwrap gently so that observations of the thorax, abdomen, genitalia, and extremities may also be done during this phase of the examination.

Without touching the infant, one can rule out a multitude of conditions. In fact, more than 80% of the newborn examination is made through observation.

Quiet Examination. **Quiet examination is defined as any part of the examination in which data are best collected from the quiet, cooperative newborn. The heart, lungs, head and neck, scalp and skull, abdomen, eyes, and blood pressure are areas that should be checked during the quiet examination.** Using pacifiers, warming hands and stethoscopes, and holding and gently manipulating the infant are ways to avoid overwhelming the baby and to prevent crying.

Auscultation

Heart. Auscultation of the heart, lungs, and abdomen is most effective when the infant is quiet. When the infant is quiet and at rest, auscultate the heart rate, rhythm, and regularity at the apex. The normal rate is 120 to 160 beats/min at a regular rhythm. Sinus dysrhythmia is normal and may be heard. The point of maximal intensity (PMI) of the neonatal heart is lateral to the midclavicular line at the third to fourth interspace. Note the PMI.

A rate of less than 80 beats/min is bradycardia. A rate greater than 160 beats/min is tachycardia that may be associated with respiratory problems, anemia, or congestive heart failure when accompanied by cardiomegaly, hepatomegaly, and generalized edema.

Murmurs are noted for loudness, quality, location, and timing. They are best auscultated at the base of the third or fourth interspace. Heart murmurs in the newborn period are very common, perhaps as frequent as 10% of the population (see Chapter 24). Note dextrocardia—heart sounds audible on the right side of the chest. Pneumothorax, pneumomediastinum, dextrocardia, or diaphragmatic hernia result in muffled heart sounds or a shift in PMI. To complete the cardiac assessment careful attention to the femoral pulses is necessary and diminished femoral pulses suggest coarctation of the aorta (see Chapter 24).

Lungs. Normally the lungs and chest are resonant after birth, and fine rales may be present for the first few hours. Auscultation reveals bronchial breath sounds bilaterally. Air entry should be good, particularly in the midaxilla. A normal respiratory rate is 30 to 60 breaths/min.

Hyperresonance suggests pneumomediastinum, pneumothorax, or diaphragmatic hernia. **Decreased resonance** is a result of decreased aeration—atelectasis, pneumonia, or respiratory distress syndrome. **Expiratory grunt** suggests difficulty in aeration and oxygenation. Peristaltic sounds heard in the chest may be caused by a diaphragmatic hernia.

Abdomen. Bowel sounds are normally heard shortly after birth.

Palpation. **Palpation of the fontanels and abdomen is best accomplished before the infant begins crying, because guarded muscles and the normally tense fontanels of the crying infant give little useful data.**

Head and Neck. **The head and neck of a newborn make up 25% of the total body surface.** The head is usually 2 cm larger than a newborn's chest. Normal head circumference ranges between 32 and 38 cm for an FAGA infant. Note the size, shape, symmetry, and general appearance.

Microcephaly is characterized by a small head size in proportion to body size. **Craniosynostosis** is a small head size caused by early closure of sutures. **Hydrocephalus** is a condition in which an increase in cerebrospinal fluid creates an abnormally large and growing head.

Scalp and Skull. **Temporary deformation of the head is caused by pressures during labor and de-**

livery. The head circumference measurements may be altered so that the occipitofrontal circumference (OFC) on the first day of life may be smaller than on the second or third. **Caput succedaneum** is an edematous area over the presenting part of the scalp that extends across suture lines and resolves in 24 to 48 hours. A **cephalhematoma** is a soft mass of blood in the subperiosteal space on the surface of the skull bone. The blood mass does not extend across suture lines and resolves in 6 to 8 weeks.

Deviating from the normal, **skull fractures may be linear or depressed, palpable or nonpalpable.**

The **anterior fontanel,** a diamond-shaped space normally measuring from 1 to 4 cm, may be gently palpated at the junction of the sagittal suture and coronal suture and between the two parietal bones. Normally the anterior fontanel softly pulsates with the infant's pulse, becomes slightly depressed when the infant sits upright and is quiet, and may bulge when the infant cries. Within 24 to 48 hours after birth, the initial molding of the head and overlap of the sutures resolve, resulting in a larger fontanel and in suture lines that should be palpated as depressions.

The **posterior fontanel,** formed at the juncture of the sagittal suture and the lambdoidal suture, is palpated between the occipital and parietal bones. Normally it is triangular shaped and barely admits a fingertip.

A **bulging, tense, or full fontanel** may be associated with increased intracranial pressure caused by birth injury, bleeding, infection, or hydrocephalus. A **depressed fontanel,** a very late sign in the newborn, may indicate dehydration. A **third fontanel,** located along the sagittal suture between the anterior and posterior fontanels, may be a sign of congenital infection, Down syndrome, or a normal variant.

Sutures are palpable ridges between skull bones. The coronal suture is located between the frontal and two parietal bones. The sagittal suture intersects the two parietal bones, and the lambdoidal suture lies between the occipital and the two parietal bones. With increasing gestational age, the suture edges become firmer and with gentle palpation are felt as hard ridges. Sutures may be open to a varying degree or may be overlapped because of molding. Lack of normal expansion may indicate microcephaly or craniosynostosis. Abnormally rapid expansion indicates hydrocephalus or increased intracranial pressure.

Abdomen. **The abdomen will appear slightly scaphoid at birth but will become distended as the bowel fills with air. Gentle palpation of the abdomen for organs or masses reveals that the spleen tip can be felt from the infant's left side and is sometimes 2 to 3 cm below the left costal margin. The liver is palpable 1 to 2 cm below the right costal margin. Superficial veins over the abdominal wall may be prominent.**

A markedly scaphoid abdomen coupled with respiratory difficulty may indicate a diaphragmatic hernia. **Abdominal distention and lack of bowel sounds** may occur because of intestinal obstruction, paralytic ileus, ascites, imperforate anus, meconium plug, peritonitis, omphalocele, Hirschsprung's disease, or necrotizing enterocolitis. The infant should be observed for **abdominal wall defects,** such as umbilical hernia; omphalocele, a herniation into the base of the umbilical cord; and gastroschisis, a defect of the abdominal wall.

The **umbilical cord** may also be observed and inspected while the abdomen is being palpated. The diameter of the cord varies, depending on the amount of Wharton's jelly present. **Two arteries and one vein are normally present in the umbilical cord.** The umbilical cord begins to dry soon after birth, becomes loose from the skin by 4 to 5 days, and falls off by 7 to 10 days. Redness, foul odor, or wetness of the cord may indicate omphalitis. Persistent drainage may indicate a patent urachus.

Inspection

Eyes. Inspection of an infant's eyes is best accomplished when the infant is found in the quiet alert state or when the infant has been aroused to wakefulness during the examination. The eyes cannot be observed while the baby is crying. Tipping the baby backward and raising him or her slowly or shading the infant's eyes from bright light often causes the eyes to open.

The newborn's eyes open spontaneously, look toward a light source, fix, focus, and follow. Uncoordinated eye movements are common. Subconjunctival or scleral hemorrhages are a common result of the pressures of labor and birth. The size, shape, and structure of the eye should be noted.

The **pupils** of the normal newborn respond to light by constricting. **Red reflex** is normally present and indicates an intact lens. Tears are not normally produced until 2 months of age. The iris is usually dark blue until 3 to 6 months of age. Doll's eye maneuvers are normally associated with eyes that follow movement of the head, often with a lag and/or nystagmus.

Discharge from the eyes may represent irritation or infection. A lateral upward slope of the eyes with an epicanthal fold may indicate syndromes of mental, physical, or chromosomal aberrations. The **absence of red reflex** may indicate tumors or congenital cataracts accompanying rubella, galactosemia, or disorders of calcium metabolism. **Chorioretinitis** is often found in congenital viral diseases such as cytomegalovirus and toxoplasmosis. White speckles on the iris known as **Brushfield's spots** are associated with Down syndrome and mental retardation or are a normal variant. **Scleral blueness** is associated with osteogenesis imperfecta and scleral yellowness with jaundice. Brain injury may be indicated by a constricted pupil, unilaterally dilated fixed pupil, nystagmus, or strabismus.

Blood Pressure. **Blood pressure with noninvasive Doppler devices is best determined before the infant is upset. Although blood pressure screening is not specifically recommended by the AAP,[9] we recommend it. The blood pressure should be checked in all four extremities to screen for coarctation of the aorta. Because the blood pressure proximal to the area of obstruction is higher than the blood pressure distal to the area of obstruction, blood pressure in the upper extremities is higher (above 15 mm Hg) than in the lower extremities (Figures 5-13 and 5-14).**

Head-to-Toe Examination. **The infant's crying will not affect the data to be gathered in the head-to-toe examination.**

Skin. **As each body part is examined, the skin is also inspected. Vernix,** a white, cheeselike material, containing quantities of α-tocopherol and surfactant proteins that provide significant protection from infection,[80,87] normally covers the body of the fetus and decreases with increased gestational age. Discoloration of the vernix occurs with intrauterine distress, postmaturity, hemolytic disease, and breech presentations.

The color of the skin is normally pink. Mongolian spots caused by the presence of pigmented cells may cover the sacral-gluteal areas of infants of color (e.g., black, Hispanic, Asian). The degree of generalized pigmentation varies and is less intense in the newborn period than later in life. **Nevus flameus** may be present at the nape of the neck or on the eyelids.

Note the size, shape, color, and degree of ec-

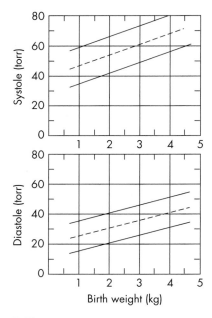

FIGURE 5-13 Aortic blood pressure during first 12 hours after birth. Linear regression (broken lines) and 95% confidence limits (solid lines) of systolic and diastolic blood pressures on birth weight in healthy newborn infants. (From Versmold HT, Kitterman JA, Phibbs RH et al: Aortic blood pressure during the first 12 hours of life in infants with birth weight 610 to 4,220 grams. *Pediatrics* 67:607, 1981.)

chymosis, erythema, petechiae, or hemangiomas. **Meconium staining, which occurs in 10% to 20% of newborns, is indicative of prior fetal distress. Erythema toxicum** appears as a generalized red rash in the first 3 days of life. **Milia** caused by retained sebum are pinpoint white spots on the cheeks, chin, and bridge of the nose.

The normal texture of a neonate's skin is soft. A preterm infant's skin is more translucent than a term infant's skin. **Slight desquamation** may occur as skin becomes dry. **Moderate to severe esquamation** occurs in postterm infants with IUGR. **Puffy, shiny skin is symptomatic of edema.** Localized edema of a presenting part is caused by trauma and is only temporary. Edema should be distinguished from increased subcutaneous fat. **Lanugo** coverage decreases with increasing gestational age.

Tissue turgor is the sensation of fullness derived from the presence of hydrated subcutaneous tissue and intrauterine nutrition. Test the elasticity of the skin by grasping a fold of skin between the thumb and forefinger. When released, the skin should promptly spring back to the surface of the body. A

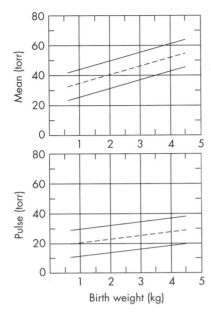

FIGURE 5-14 Mean aortic and pulse pressures during first 12 hours after birth. Linear regression *(broken lines)* and 95% confidence limits *(solid lines)* on birth weight in healthy newborn infants. (From Versmold HT, Kitterman JA, Phibbs RH et al: Aortic blood pressure during the first 12 hours of life in infants with birth weight 610 to 4,220 grams. *Pediatrics* 67:607, 1981.)

loss of normal skin turgor resulting in peaking of the skin is a late sign of dehydration. A generalized hardness of the skin is a sign of sclerema that occurs in debilitated, stressed infants. A recent study of AGA infants found a correlation between smaller skinfold thickness (tricipital, bicipital and subscapular) and hypoglycemia.[72]

Ears. Cartilage development and ear form progress according to gestational age. Observe the external ears for size, shape, and position. **The angle of placement** of the ears is almost vertical. If the angle of placement is greater than 10 degrees from vertical, it is abnormal. The level of placement is determined by drawing an imaginary line from the outer canthus of the eye to the occiput. If the ear intersects the line, it is placed normally. Slapping hands or other sharp noises will normally elicit a twitching in the eyelid or a complete Moro reflex.

Malformed or malpositioned (lowset or rotated) ears are often associated with renal and chromosomal abnormalities and other congenital anomalies. **Abnormalities such as skin tags or sinuses may be associated with renal problems or hearing loss.** A recent study found a significant prevalence of urinary tract abnormalities in infants with preauricular tags.[64] Forceps or difficult deliveries may injure the outer ear. Congenital deafness is suspected if the infant does not respond to noise. It is confirmed by standardized hearing screening tests and follow-up.

Nose. Note the shape and size of the nose. Deformities caused by intrauterine pressure may be temporary. **Neonates are obligatory nasal breathers and must have patent nasal passages. Check the patency of the alae nasi by (1) obstructing one nostril, closing the mouth, and observing breathing from the open nostril, (2) placing a stethoscope under the nostrils that will "fog" the diaphragm and auscultate breathing, or (3) passing a soft catheter (if necessary).**

Abnormal configuration may be associated with congenital syndromes. Obstructions can be caused by drugs, infections, tumors, nasal discharge, and mucus. **Choanal atresia,** a membranous or bony obstruction in the nasal passage, may be unilateral or bilateral. Choanal atresia is characterized by the noisy breathing, cyanosis, and apnea of the quiet infant (mouth closed) as opposed to the pink color of the same crying infant (mouth open).

Mouth. Examination of the mouth may be done here or at the end of the examination when the infant is crying loudly with a wide, open mouth. **At birth a normal infant is able to suck and swallow (this ability develops at 32 to 34 weeks' gestation) and root and gag (this ability develops at 36 weeks' gestation). Elicit each.**

Lips and mucous membranes are normally pink. Observe the lips and mucous membranes for pallor and cyanosis. If the infant is well hydrated, the membranes should be moist. Open the mouth to look for anomalies. **Palpate the hard and soft palates for a membranous cleft or submucous cleft. Epithelial pearls** are common along the gum margins and the palate.

Natal teeth may be present and may require removal to prevent aspiration.[60] **A large tongue (macroglossia), cleft lip or palate (including submucous cleft), or high-arched palate may be associated with abnormal facies or be an isolated finding. Esophageal atresia and tracheoesophageal fistula** are often present with copious secretions or distress in feeding.

Thorax. Conformation of the newborn chest is cylindric with an anteroposterior ratio of 1:1.

Note the shape, symmetry, position, and development of the thorax. **Asymmetry of the chest** may be caused by diaphragmatic hernia, paralysis of the diaphragm, pneumothorax, emphysema, pulmonary agenesis, or pneumonia. **Fullness of the thorax** caused by increased anteroposterior diameter occurs with an overexpansion of the lung. **Retractions,** an inward pull of the soft parts of the chest while inhaling, indicate air-entry interference or pulmonary disease.

Breasts. Breast tissue systematically develops according to gestational age. Enlargement of breasts because of maternal hormones occurs in either sex on the second or third day. Milky secretions may be present. Unilateral redness or firmness indicates infection.

Clavicles. Observe and palpate the area above each clavicle. A fracture of the clavicle is evidenced by a palpable mass, crepitation, tenderness at the fracture site, and limited arm movements on the affected side.

Genitalia. Male and female genitalia systematically develop according to gestational age.

MALE. Inspect the genitalia for the presence and position of the urethral opening. Palpate the testes either in the inguinal canal or scrotum. The scrotum appears large and pendulous with the presence of descended testes. A tight prepuce may be found. In dark-skinned races, darker pigmentation of the genitalia is normal. **Hypospadias exists** if the urethral opening is on the ventral surface of the penis. **Epispadias** exists if the opening is on the dorsal surface. **Hydroceles** are a common finding.

FEMALE. Inspect the genitalia for the presence and position of the urethral opening. The introitus is posterior to the clitoris. A **vaginal skin tag** is a visible hymenal ring.

Edema of the genitalia in both sexes is common in breech deliveries. Note the presence of a hydrocele or hernia. Fecal urethral discharge may indicate **rectourethral fistulas.**

Rectum. Visualize and check the patency of the anal opening by gently inserting a soft rubber catheter (do not use rigid objects such as glass rectal thermometers). Observe the anatomy and feel the

muscle tone. **Meconium** is normally present during the first days of life.

Imperforate anus, irritation, or fissures may be present. Meconium passage before birth suggests fetal intrauterine distress. Failure to pass meconium within 48 hours suggests obstruction. **Meconium ileus** is associated with cystic fibrosis.

Back. Place the infant in a prone position and observe for a flat and straight **vertebral column.** Separate the buttocks to observe the coccygeal area. To check incurving reflex, stroke one side of the vertebral column. The baby will turn the buttocks toward the side stroked. **Deviations from normal include curvature of the vertebral column, pilonidal dimple, pilonidal sinus, spina bifida, or myelomeningocele.**

Extremities
UPPER EXTREMITIES. **Note the size, shape, and symmetry of the arms and hands.** Observe and feel for fractures, paralysis, and dislocations. Count and inspect the fingers. The hands are normally clenched into fists. The infant is capable of adduction, flexion, internal rotation, extension, and symmetry of movement. Note the tone of the muscles. Flexion develops with increasing gestational age.

Simian creases may indicate chromosomal abnormalities that are frequent causes of deformity. **Polydactyly and syndactyly** of the fingers may be found. **Osteogenesis imperfecta** is characterized by multiple fractures and deformities. **Palsies** caused by fractures, dislocations, or injury to the brachial plexus are recognized by limited movement of the extremity. **Fractures** may also be present with edema, palpable crepitus, or the "palpable spongy mass sign" over the clavicle.[94]

LOWER EXTREMITIES. **Note the size, shape, and symmetry of the feet and legs.** Note the normal position of flexion (develops according to gestational age) and abduction. Note symmetry of movement, thigh folds, and gluteal folds. A full range of motion is possible, including the "frog position"—a rotation of the thighs with the knees flexed. Observe and feel for fractures, paralysis, and dislocations. Palpate femoral pulses.

Polydactyly and syndactyly of the toes may exist. **Osteogenesis imperfecta** results in multiple fractures and deformities. Paralysis of both legs is caused by severe trauma or congenital anomaly of the spinal cord. A unilaterally or bilaterally **dislocated hip** (more common in females) causes a hip click when the baby's legs are abducted into the frog position. Although soft clicks are common, a sharp click indicates dislocation. Fractures may be present and are characterized by limited movement and edematous, crepitant areas. Chromosomal abnormalities are frequent causes of deformity.

Recoil is a test of flexion development and muscle tone. Recoil systematically develops as flexion develops in the lower extremities first and then in the upper extremities. Extend the legs and then release. Both legs should return promptly to the flexed position in accordance with the gestational age of the infant. Extend the arms alongside the body. On release, prompt flexion should occur at the elbows.

Hypotonia causes the infant to become limp and "floppy," with little control. The extremities fall without resistance when the infant is raised off the bed. Recoil may be partial or absent. **Hypertonia** causes the infant to tremble and startle easily. The fists are tightly clenched, arms flexed, and legs stiffly extended.

Neurologic Examination

Clinical, electric, and anatomic studies of the nervous systems of premature and full-term neonates have confirmed the belief that the CNS of the human fetus matures at a fairly constant rate. Neurologic findings, clinical signs, and electroencephalogram (EEG) findings specifically correlating to gestational age have been established.[35,63,73] However, there are recognized limitations in clinical applications of the neurologic evaluation. **The evaluation is of little value in the first 24 hours of life unless there is an obvious palsy or seizure.** Because a newborn is recovering from the stress of birth, the neurologic examination is not valid until after the infant has successfully completed the transition to extrauterine life. Therefore the neurologic examination should be performed after the first 24 hours of life (see Figure 5-4). If the infant is ill or has obstetric anesthesia or analgesia, the neurologic examination may not be valid even after 24 hours.

Brazelton Examination

The Neonatal Behavioral Assessment Scale[17,90] assesses the interactive behavior of the newborn. This psychologic scale for the neonate enables assessment of the infant's individual capabilities for social relationships. Clinical application of the Brazelton scale includes neonatal research and evaluation of infant capabilities after illness, prematurity, or maternal medications. **A modified version of the Brazelton examination is useful in teaching parents about their individual infant's patterns of behavior, temperament, and states.**[22,43,44,81]

By understanding the uniqueness of their infant, parents may more intelligently assess and interpret their baby's cues for interaction and distance. If the parents know their infant's individual strengths and weaknesses, they will be more capable of realistically reacting to their infant. It is important for the care provider to elicit the parents' assessment of their infant's behavior and responsiveness. Unrealistic expectations or incorrect parental perceptions may exist. The care provider therefore uses this opportunity for parent teaching, counseling, and possibly referral.[28,44]

The Brazelton examination is usually performed at 2 to 3 days of life, at discharge, or on the follow-up visit at 1 to 2 weeks. This examination assesses the infant's best performance in response to stimulation and handling by the examiner. For research purposes, the scoring technique by a certified examiner is required. For clinical use, knowledge of the specific techniques and interpretation of results is all that is required. Because the state of consciousness influences a newborn's reactions, the most important variable in the examiner's observation is knowledge of the infant's state (see Table 13-3 for neonatal states). **Performing the examination with the parents present provides the opportunity for parental participation and observation of their infant's response.**

Interventions

After the newborn has been examined and assessed, certain admission procedures should be performed. Vital signs should include pulse, respirations, and skin or axillary temperature (never rectal). **During the transitional period, vital signs should be recorded frequently enough to monitor the infant's condition and provide appropriate care:**

- **If the infant is distressed (elevated heart rate or respiratory rate, retracting and/or nasal flaring), vital signs may be required every ½ to 1 hour.**
- **If the baby's vital signs are normal on admission (heart rate 120 to 160 beats/min, respiratory rate 30 to 60 breaths/min, and temperature 36° to 36.5° C [97.8° F to 98.6° F]), he or**

she should be monitored and the data charted every 30 minutes until the infant's condition has remained stable for 2 hours.[9]

- **Vital signs should be recorded at least once every 8 hours.**
- **Measuring the temperature rectally is contraindicated in newborn infants because of the risk of rectal perforation (see Chapter 6).**

Weight, length, and head circumference should be graphed on the appropriate intrauterine growth chart to show at which percentile the baby falls. The parameters should be set at less than 10%, between 10% and 90%, and greater than 90%. **Determine the weight/length ratio (Figure 5-15), which normally increases with fetal age because baby becomes heavier for length as term approaches.** In intrauterine growth retardation the weight/length ratio decreases because the rate of growth in weight is

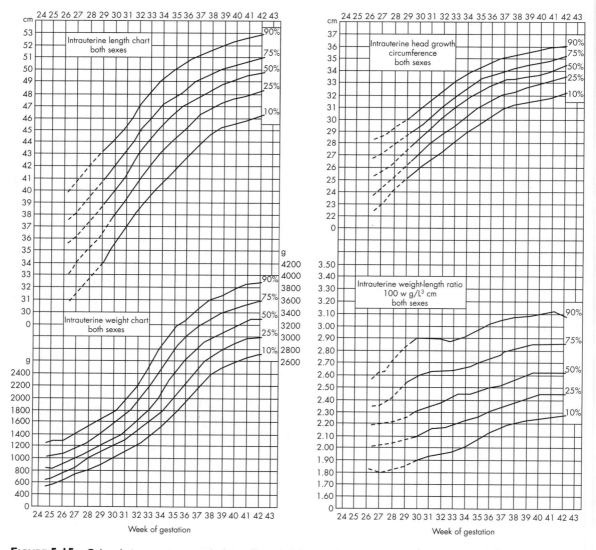

FIGURE 5-15 Colorado intrauterine growth charts. (From Lubchenco LO, Hansman C, Boyd E et al: Intrauterine growth in length and head circumference as estimated from live births at gestational ages from 26-43 weeks, *Pediatrics* 37:403, 1966. Courtesy Ross Laboratories, Columbus Ohio.)

affected more than length. Severe and prolonged intrauterine malnutrition may affect head, weight, and length ratios.

Complications

Complications of common morbidities (see Figure 5-12) are prevented by classification, assessment, and screening of all newborns at birth. Preterm SGA/IUGR infants have more gross motor and neurologic dysfunction, but less cerebral palsy (CP) than AGA infants do. SGA infants are at increased risk of mortality and cognitive disorders needing special education when compared with AGA infants.[65] Complications of the morbidities listed in Figure 5-12 are thoroughly discussed in the appropriate chapters.

Parent Teaching

Transitional care, neonatal assessment, and initial care need not take place in a nursery where the newborn and family are isolated from each other. Alternative settings for initial care include birthing rooms, recovery rooms in which family and baby are kept together, the mother's postpartum room, or at a home visit. **In fact, keeping the family together not only facilitates bonding but also provides unique opportunities for teaching parents about the uniqueness and individuality of their newborn.** At this time parents are most receptive to information about the baby, who is the center of attention.

The assessments of gestational age and physical condition are best performed with the mother and father in attendance so that deviations from normal such as caput, cleft lip, cleft palate, or clubfoot can be explained. Eliciting parental cooperation is important. For example, when the major

concern is "Will the procedure hurt?" a response such as "It is routine" will not comfort and reassure well-informed, noninterventionist consumers. Rather, a more physiologically oriented explanation about the condition being screened, why their particular infant is at increased risk, and what interventions are available encourages parental cooperation.

Professional care providers are only temporary caretakers. It is the care providers' responsibility to help parents become confident, primary caretakers of their own infants. **Actively involving parents in the treatment of their newborn further solidifies their position as primary caretakers.** Encouraging active parental involvement enhances the parents' self-esteem and confidence in their abilities[43]; thus the care providers' actions must tell the parents, "You are able to care for this baby."

At discharge, performing the physical examination in the room with the parents offers a final opportunity to teach, counsel, and advise them before they take their new baby home. Information about feeding, cord care, bathing, elimination patterns, safety, signs of illness, medications, and the importance of follow-up care is essential for parents of a full-term, healthy newborn as well as for parents taking home an infant after prolonged hospitalization. In addition, a modified version of Brazelton's examination on all neonates enables parents to become familiar with a newborn's competencies for reacting to and shaping his or her environment and with strategies for parental intervention. Developing written materials for parents about normal newborn care and documenting teaching sessions and return demonstrations ensure that no important information is forgotten.[82,91,95]

Both term and preterm neonates are being discharged earlier (Table 5-3). Although evidence

Table 5-3	AVERAGE HOSPITAL LENGTH OF STAY		
	1982*	1992†	1994-1995‡
Term	3.7 days	1.7 days	1.6 days
Preterm	>40 days	18 days	1750-2499 g = 1.6-2.4 days
			1500-1749 g = 13-24.3 days
			1000-1499 g = 40.6-42.8 days
			500-999 g = 70.9-72.2 days

*From Commission on Professional and Hospital Activities: *Length of stay by operation, United States, 1982,* Ann Arbor, Mich, Commission on Professional Hospital Activities, 1983.
†From HCIA Inc: *Length of Stay by Diagnosis and Operation, United States, 1994,* Baltimore, Md.
‡From HCIA Inc: *Length of Stay by Diagnosis and Operation, United States, 1996,* Baltimore, Md.

Box 5-1	CRITERIA FOR DISCHARGE WITHIN 24 HOURS OF DELIVERY

Maternal

- Uncomplicated vaginal delivery
- Stable condition after delivery: normal vital signs, able to urinate and ambulate
- Laboratory data obtained: Hgb/Hct; ABO blood group; Rh typing; RhIg administered
- Support system available first few days after delivery
- Demonstrates knowledge, ability, and skill in self and newborn care, recognizing complications and how to access care

Neonatal

- Term (38 to 42 weeks' gestation), appropriate for gestational age newborn (2500 to 4500 g)
- Examined by qualified health care provider and found to be normal
- Newborn course: (1) normal and without complications, (2) normal thermoregulation, and (3) able to successfully feed, void, and stool
- Follow-up for mother and newborn within 48 hours of discharge

Modified from American Academy of Pediatrics and American College of Obstetricians and Gynecologists: *Guidelines for perinatal care,* ed 5, Washington, DC, 2002, The Academy.[9]

of the safety, efficacy, and effectiveness of traditional hospital practices and procedures is lacking and has been questioned,* **early discharge has been generalized from a birth alternative by a self-selected population to virtually all low-risk mothers and babies.**[16] Concerns about the mother include (1) rest, (2) readiness to learn and assume self and newborn care, (3) readiness to parent, and (4) availability of support systems. Concerns about the newborn include (1) transition from intrauterine to extrauterine life, (2) ability to feed and hydrate adequately, and (3) the early development and recognition of complications. **Until scientific evidence is available, individualized discharge plans requiring strict predischarge screening and postdischarge follow-up are recommended**[9,10,11,58,82] **(Box 5-1). Because in the first 24 hours after delivery women have transient deficits in cognitive function, particularly memory,**[38] **verbal instruc-**

tions may be poorly remembered and should be augmented with written information.[6,9,11,38,82] In a recent study of early discharge (within 36 hours) of full-term babies, no association with alterations in breastfeeding at 3 months, mother-infant interaction at 3 to 9 months, or attachment at 12 months of age was found.[18]

For preterm infants, the attainment of a weight of 5 pounds is no longer the criterion for discharge. **Rather, the ability of a preterm or recovering neonate to maintain physiologic stability and the ability of the family to care for the infant's physiologic and developmental needs are the criteria for discharge (Box 5-2).** There are significant variations in inter-NICU discharge criteria, with assessment of apnea and feeding behavior significantly influencing duration of hospitalization in a healthy preterm infant.[37]

Recent studies document the positive effects of home visitation programs.[36,61,67,83] After meeting specific criteria, early discharge of preterm infants using advanced practice nurses who provide a comprehensive program of transitional home follow-up has been shown in a randomized clinical trial to (1) decrease hospital stay by 11 days, (2) not increase rehospitalization or emergency room visits, and (3) reduce hospital charges by 27%.[20] In lieu of continued hospitalization, chronically ill VLBW infants were provided with 8 to 24 hours/day of home nursing care and were retrospectively found to have fewer rehospitalizations, emergency department and specialty clinic visits, and no doctor's office visits for illness in the first year of life.[20]

A randomized controlled trial (RCT) of early discharge for preterm SGA infants weighing 1300 to 1350 g found no difference in weight gain or incidence of infection when compared to hospitalized infants.[31] Behavioral criteria for discharge included that the infant (1) maintain temperature in the crib, (2) be able to nipple at least 120 cal/kg/day, (3) gain weight consistently for at least 3 days, and (4) be symptom free and without medications for 3 days. Family cooperation for early discharge included (1) learning CPR and orogastric feeding methods, (2) the parent actively feeding the baby for 5 days, and (3) a home environment that included a single family in the home, basic utilities, phone, and transportation. **Benefits of early discharge of infants meeting these behavioral and environmental criteria included (1) improved parental bonding, (2) less exposure to nosoco-**

*References 2, 26, 49, 62, 95, 96, 102, 115

Box 5-2	CRITERIA FOR DISCHARGE OF PRETERM OR NEONATE WITH SPECIAL NEEDS

Infant

- Maintain temperature between 36° and 37° C per axilla in an open crib
- Maintain fluid and nutrition status—take in adequate calories to grow and maintain adequate weight gain (20 to 30 g/day)
- Maintain oxygenation status
  In room air, without oxygen
  In nasal cannula oxygen to maintain saturation ≥92% to 95%
  Pass room air challenge*—able to maintain saturation ≥92% after 40 min in room air
  Free of apnea and bradycardia for at least 5 days
- Maintain oxygenation and ventilation status on home ventilator

Parents/Family

- Demonstrate knowledge, ability, and skill to
  Provide infant care: bathing, diapering, dressing, cord and circumcision care
  Maintain infant's thermal state—able to take temperature and dress appropriately
  Feed infant adequate calories to gain weight by breast, bottle, or alternative methods (e.g., nasogastric tube, gastrostomy)

Parents/Family—cont'd

  Manage oxygen and oxygen equipment
  Manage monitoring equipment (e.g., cardiorespiratory, apnea, or pulse oximetry)
  Manage home ventilator equipment, suction and retrach procedure
  Maintain safe environment—car seat adapted for infants with special needs†
  Administer medications in proper doses, at proper times, and know side effects
  Recognize signs of illness, know when to call primary care provider
  Administer CPR
- Availability of support system to assist in infant's care (e.g., family, friends, or community resources)
- Demonstrate emotional and relationship stability
- Financial resources (e.g., insurance, Medicaid) available for equipment, medications, and ongoing care and services
- Understand importance of follow-up care and know when and whom to call for problems or questions
- Able to read and respond to infant cues for hunger, pain, more or less stimuli, increasing distress, sleep and wake cycles

Modified from American Academy of Pediatrics: Guidelines for home care of infants, children and adolescents with chronic disease, *Pediatrics* 96:161, 1995; and American Academy of Pediatrics: Hospital discharge of the high-risk neonate: proposed guidelines, *Pediatrics* 102:411, 1998.
*Modified from Simoes E, Rosenberg A, King S et al: Room air challenge: prediction for successful weaning of oxygen-dependent infants, *J Perinatal* 17:125, 1997.[100]
†Modified from American Academy of Pediatrics: Transporting children with special health care needs, *Pediatrics* 104:988, 1999.[8]

mial infection, **(3) shortened length of stay (by about 3 weeks), and (4) cost effectiveness.**[31] As in other aspects of health care delivery, care of high-risk infants from hospital to home is happening sooner with more technology and is more common. Although this reduces direct health care costs, earlier home care of these infants increases family burdens of care, expenses, and stressors and without collaborative follow-up, complications and problems may go undetected.[19]

REFERENCES

1. Abman S, Wolfe RR, Accurso FJ et al: Pulmonary vascular response to oxygen in infants with severe bronchopulmonary dysplasia, *Pediatrics* 75:80, 1985.
2. Alberts J: Learning as adaptation of the infant, *Acta Paediatr Suppl* 397:77, 1994.
3. Allen MC, Capute A: Tone and reflex development before term, *Pediatrics* 85(suppl):393, 1990.
4. Allen M, Donohue P, Dusman A: The limit of viability: neonatal outcome of infants born 22-25 weeks' gestation, *N Engl J Med* 329:1597, 1993.
5. American Academy of Pediatrics: Guidelines for home care of infants, children and adolescents with chronic disease, *Pediatrics* 96:161, 1995.
6. American Academy of Pediatrics: Hospital stay for healthy term newborns, *Pediatrics* 96:788, 1995.
7. American Academy of Pediatrics: Hospital discharge of the high-risk neonate: proposed guidelines, *Pediatrics* 102:411, 1998.
8. American Academy of Pediatrics: Transporting children with special health care needs, *Pediatrics* 104:988, 1999.
9. American Academy of Pediatrics and American College of Obstetricians and Gynecologists: *Guidelines for perinatal care*, ed 5, Washington, DC, 2002, The Academy.

10. American College of Obstetricians and Gynecologists: *Statement on decreasing length of hospital stay following delivery,* Washington, DC, 1995, The College.

11. American Nurses Association: *Home care for mother, infant, family following birth,* Washington, DC, 1996, The Association.

12. Apgar V: A proposal for a new method of evaluation of the newborn infant, *Anesth Analg* 32:260, 1953.

13. Apgar V: The newborn (Apgar) scoring system, reflections and advice, *Pediatr Clin North Am* 13:645, 1966.

14. Attico N, Meyer DJ, Bodin HJ et al: Gestational age assessment, *Am Fam Physician* 41:535, 1990.

15. Barr R: Reflections on measuring pain in infants: dissociation in responsive systems and "honest signaling," *Arch Dis Child Fetal Neonatal Educ* 79:152, 1998.

16. Braverman P, Egerter S, Pearl M et al: Early discharge of newborns and mothers: a critical review of the literature, *Pediatrics* 96:716, 1995.

17. Brazelton TB: *Neonatal behavioral assessment scale,* ed 2, Philadelphia, 1984, JB Lippincott/Spastics International Medical Publishers.

18. Britton J, Britton H, Gronwaldt V: Early perinatal hospital discharge and parenting during infancy, *Pediatrics* 104:1070, 1999.

19. Brooten D: Perinatal care across the continuum; early discharge and nursing home follow-up, *J Perinat Neonatal Nurs* 9:38, 1995.

20. Brooten D, Kumar S, Brown LP et al: A randomized clinical trial of early hospital discharge and home follow-up of very low-birth-weight infants, *N Engl J Med* 315:934, 1986.

21. Brown L, Heerman J: The effect of developmental care on preterm infant outcome, *Appl Nurs Res* 10:190, 1997.

22. Buckner E: Use of Brazelton neonatal behavioral assessment in planning care for parents newborns, *J Obstet Gynecol Neonatal Nurs* 12:26, 1983.

23. Casey B, McIntire D, Leveno K: The continuing value of the Apgar score for assessment of newborn infants, *N Engl J Med* 344:467, 2001.

24. Centers for Disease Control and Prevention (CDC): Prevention of perinatal group B streptococcal disease: a public health perspective, *MMWR* 45(RR-7):1, 1996.

25. Chervenak F, Skupski DW, Romero R et al: How accurate is fetal biometry in the assessment of fetal age? *Am J Obstet Gynecol* 178:678, 1998.

26. Christensson K: Fathers can effectively achieve heat conservation in healthy newborn infants, *Acta Paediatr* 85:1354, 1996.

27. Christensson K, Bhat GJ, Amadi BC et al: Randomized study of skin-to-skin versus incubator care for rewarming low-risk hypothermic neonates, *Lancet* 352:1115, 1998.

28. Christensson K, Cabrera T, Christensson E et al: Separation distress call in the human neonate in the absence of maternal contact, *Acta Paediatr* 84:468, 1995.

29. Christensson K, Siles C, Moreno R et al: Temperature, metabolic adaptation and crying in healthy full-term newborn infants cared for skin-to-skin or in a cot, *Acta Paediatr* 81:488, 1992.

30. Conway A: The effects of routine nursing procedures on the behavior of preterm infants in the NICU. In *Proceedings of the NAAN Clinical Update and Research Conference,* Washington, DC, 1992, NAAN.

31. Cruz H, Guzman N, Rosales M et al: Early hospital discharge of preterm VLBW infants, *J Perinatol* 17:29, 1997.

32. Desmond MM, Rudolph AJ, Phitaksphraiwan P et al: The transitional care nursery: a mechanism for preventive medicine in the newborn, *Pediatr Clin North Am* 13:65, 1966.

33. Dodd V: Gestational age assessment, *Neonatal Netw* 15:27, 1996.

34. Donovan EF, Tyson JE, Ehrenkranz RA et al: Inaccuracy of Ballard scores before 28 weeks' gestation, *J Pediatr* 135:147, 1999.

35. Dubowitz L, Dubowitz V, Goldberg C: Clinical assessment of gestational age in newborn infant, *J Pediatr* 77:1, 1970.

36. Eckenrode J: Preventing child abuse and neglect with a program of nurse home visitation, *JAMA* 284:1385, 2000.

37. Eichenwald E, Lloyd J, Tran T et al: Inter-NICU variation in discharge timing: effects of relationship between apnea and feeding management, *Pediatr Res* 45:195A, 1999.

38. Eidelman A, Hoffman N, Kaitz M: Cognitive deficits in women after childbirth, *Obstet Gynecol* 81:764, 1993.

39. Estol P, Piriz H, Pintos L et al: Assessment of pulmonary dynamics in normal newborn: a pneumotachographic method, *J Perinat Med* 16:183, 1988.

40. Fohe K, Kropf S, Avenarius S: Skin-to-skin contact improves gas exchange in premature infants, *J Perinatol* 5:311, 2000.

41. Freudigman K, Thoman E: Ultradian and diurnal cyclicity in the sleep states of newborn infants during the first two postnatal days, *Early Hum Dev* 38:67, 1994.

42. Galloway K: Early detection of congenital anomalies, *J Obstet Gynecol Neonatal Nurs* 2:37, 1973.

43. Gardner SL: Mothering the unconscious conflict between nurses and new mothers, *Keep Abreast J* 3:192, 1978.

44. Gibes RM: Clinical uses of the Brazelton neonatal behavioral assessment scale in nursing practice, *Pediatr Nurs* 7:23, 1981.

45. Goyal M, Suresh BR, Reinersman G et al: Evolution and variability of pulmonary mechanics during postnatal transition in term infants, *J Perinatol* 15:441, 1995.
46. Gray L, Watt L, Blass E: Skin-to-skin contact is analgesic in healthy newborns, *Pediatrics* 105:110, 2000.
47. Hernandez JA, Hall DM, Goldson EJ et al: Impact of infants born at the threshold of viability on the neonatal mortality rate in Colorado, *J Perinatol* 20:21, 2000.
48. Hernandez JA, Lazarte R, Pisanos D et al: Foot length and gestational age in the very-low-birth-weight infant, *Child Hosp Pediatr Update* Sept 1987, pp 3-7.
49. Hofer M: Early relationships as regulators of infant physiology and behavior, *Acta Paediatr Suppl* 397:9, 1994.
50. Jain L: Alveolar fluid clearance in developing lungs and its role in neonatal transition, *Clin Perinatol* 26:585, 1999.
51. Johnson JL, Merenstein G, Coll J et al: Colorado intrauterine growth curve 1980-1992: the new Lubchenco growth curve, *Pediatr Res* 35:274A, 1994.
52. Kaminski J, Hall W: The effect of soothing music on neonatal behavioral states in the hospital newborn nursery, *Neonatal Netw* 15:45, 1996.
53. Karp TB, Scardino C, Butler LA et al: Glucose metabolism in the neonate: the short and sweet of it, *Neonatal Netw* 14:17, 1995.
54. Kawakami K, Takai-Kawakami K, Kurihara H et al: The effect of sounds on newborn infants under stress, *Infant Behav Dev* 19:375, 1996.
55. Keefe M: Comparison of neonatal nighttime sleep-wake patterns in nursery vs. rooming-in environments, *Nurs Res* 36:114, 1987.
56. Keefe MR, Kotzer AM, Reuss JL et al: Development of a system for monitoring infant state behavior, *Nurs Res* 38:344, 1989.
57. Kennell J, McGrath S: Commentary: what babies teach us: the essential link between baby's behavior and mother's biology, *Birth* 28:20, 2001.
58. Kessel W, Kiely M, Nora AH et al: Early discharge: in the end, it is judgment, *Pediatrics* 96:739, 1995.
59. Kilpatrick SJ, Schlueter MA, Piecuch R et al: Outcome of infants born at 24-26 weeks' gestation. I. Survival and cost, *Obstet Gynecol* 90:803, 1997.
60. King MM: Prematurely erupted teeth in newborn infants, *J Pediatr* 114:807, 1989.
61. Kitzman H, Olds DL, Sidora K et al: Enduring effects of nurse home visitation on maternal life course: a 3-year follow-up of a randomized trial, *JAMA* 283:1983, 2000.
62. Kjellmer I, Winberg J: The neurobiology of infant-parent interaction in the newborn: an introduction, *Acta Paediatr Suppl* 397:1, 1994.
63. Koeingsberger R: Judgment of fetal age. I. Neurologic evaluation, *Pediatr Clin North Am* 13:823, 1966.
64. Kohelet D, Arbel E: A prospective search for urinary tract abnormalities in infants with isolated preauricular tags, *Pediatrics* 105:1148, 2000.
65. Kok J, den Ouden L, Verloove-Vanhorick P et al: Outcome of very preterm SGA infants: the first nine years of life, *Br J Obstet Gynaecol* 105:162, 1998.
66. Koops BL, Morgan LJ, Battaglia FC et al: Neonatal mortality risk in relation to birthweight and gestational age: update, *J Pediatr* 101:969, 1982.
67. Korfmacher J, O'Brien R, Hiatt S: Differences in program implementation between nurses and paraprofessionals providing home visits during pregnancy and infancy: a randomized trial, *Am J Publ Health* 89:1847, 1999.
68. Lakshminrusimha S, Steinhorn R: Pulmonary vascular biology during neonatal transition, *Clin Perinatol* 26:601, 1999.
69. Lester BM, Anderson LT, Boukydis CF et al: Early detection of infants at risk for later handicap through acoustic cry analysis, *Birth Defects Orig Artic Ser* 25:99, 1989.
70. Letko MD: Understanding the Apgar score, *J Obstet Gynecol Neonat Nurs* 25:299, 1996.
71. Little D, Riddle B, Saule C: The power in our hands: integrating developmental care into neonatal transport, *Neonatal Netw* 13:19, 1994.
72. Lizo C, Azevedo-Lizo Z, Segre C et al: Neonatal skinfold thickness in Brazilian newborns: correlation with maternal and neonatal anthropometrical data, *Neonatal Intensive Care* 13:60, 2000.
73. Lubchenco L: Watching the newborn for disease, *Pediatr Clin North Am* 8:471, 1961.
74. Lubchenco L: *The high-risk infant,* Philadelphia, 1976, WB Saunders.
75. Lubchenco LO, Hansman C, Boyd E et al: Intrauterine growth in length and head circumference as estimated from live births at gestational ages from 26-43 weeks, *Pediatrics* 37:403, 1966.
76. Lubchenco LO, Searls DT, Brazie JV et al: Neonatal mortality risk: relationship to birthweight and gestational age, *J Pediatr* 81:814, 1972.
77. Ludington-Hoe S: Developmental aspects of kangaroo care, *J Obstet Gynecol Neonatal Nurs* 25:691, 1996.
78. Ludington-Hoe SM, Anderson GC, Simpson S et al: Birth-related fatigue in 34-36 week preterm neonates: rapid recovery with very early kangaroo (skin-to-skin) care, *J Obstet Gynecol Neonatal Nurs* 28:94, 1999.
79. MacMullen N, Dulski L: Factors related to sucking ability in healthy newborns, *J Obstet Gynecol Neonatal Nurs* 29:390, 2000.

80. Narendran V, Wickett RR, Pickens WL et al: Vernix caseosa contains surfactant proteins: potential role in innate immune function in the fetus, *Pediatr Res* 47:420A, 2000.

81. Nugent J: The Brazelton neonatal behavior assessment scale: implications for interventions, *Pediatr Nurs* 7:18, 1981.

82. Nurses Association of the American College of Obstetricians and Gynecologists: *Standards for the nursing care of women and newborns,* ed 4, Washington, DC, 1991, The Association.

83. Olds D, Hill P, Robinson J et al: Update on home visiting for pregnant workers and parents of young children, *Curr Probl Pediatr* 30:109, 2000.

84. Parker S, Zuckerman B, Bauchner H et al: Jitteriness in full-term neonates; prevalence and correlates, *Pediatrics* 85:17, 1990.

85. Peters K: Does routine nursing care complicate the physiologic status of the premature infant with RDS? *J Perinat Neonatal Nurs* 6:67, 1992.

86. Peters K: Dinosaurs in the bath, *Neonatal Netw* 15:71, 1996.

87. Pickens W, Zhou Y, Wickett R et al: Antioxidant defense mechanisms in veinix caseosa: potential role of endogenous vitamin E, *Pediatr Res* 47:425A, 2000.

88. Piecuch RE, Leonard CH, Cooper BA et al: Outcome of infants born at 24-26 weeks' gestation. II. Neurodevelopmental outcome, *Obstet Gynecol* 90:809, 1997.

89. Pineyard B: Infant cries: physiology and assessment, *Neonatal Netw* 13:15, 1994.

90. Pressler J, Hepworth J: Newborn neurologic screening using NBAS reflexes, *Neonatal Netw* 16:33, 1997.

91. Pridham KF, Lytton D, Chang AS et al: Early postpartum transition: progress in maternal identity and role attainment, *Res Nurs Health* 14:21, 1991.

92. Ransjo-Arvidson AB, Mathiesen AS, Lilja G et al: Maternal analgesia during labor disrupts newborn behavior: effects on breastfeeding, temperature and crying, *Birth* 28:5, 2001.

93. Rao M, Blass E, Brignol M et al: Effect of crying on energy metabolism in human neonates, *Pediatr Res* 33:309A, 1993.

94. Reiners C, Souid A, Oliphant M, Newman N: Palpable spongy mass over the clavicle, an underutilized sign of clavicular fracture in the newborn, *Pediatr Res* 47:429a, 2000.

95. Robinson T: Discharge teaching: sending babies home safely, *Neonatal Netw* 13:77, 1994.

96. Rosenblatt J: Psychobiology of maternal behavior: contribution to the clinical understanding of maternal behavior among humans, *Acta Paediatr Suppl* 397:3, 1994.

97. Rosenblum L, Andrews M: Influences of environmental demand on maternal behavior and infant development, *Acta Paediatr Suppl* 397:57, 1994.

98. Schuman A: The single umbilical artery: what work up is needed? *Contemp Pediatr,* Dec 1991, p 65.

99. Schwartz R: Effect of position on oxygenation, heart rate, and behavioral state in the transitional newborn infant, *Neonatal Netw* 12:73, 1993.

100. Simoes E, Rosenberg A, King S et al: Room air challenge: prediction for successful weaning of oxygen-dependent infants, *J Perinatol* 17:125, 1997.

101. Smail K: *The effects of routine bathing on the behavior of preterm infant in an NICU,* NANN annual meeting procedure, Sept 1992, p 158.

102. Smotherman W, Robinson S: Milk as the proximal mechanism for behavioral changes in the newborn, *Acta Paediatr Suppl* 397:64, 1994.

103. Sola A, Chow L: The coming of (gestational) age for preterm infants, *J Pediatr* 135:137, 1999.

104. Thoden C, Koivisto M: Acoustic analysis of the normal pain cry. In Murry M, Murry J, eds: *Infant communication: crying and early speech,* Houston, 1980, College Hill Press.

105. Tribotti S: Admission to the NICU: reducing the risk, *Neonatal Netw* 8:17, 1990.

106. Tyson J, Younes N, Verter J et al: Viability, morbidity and resource use among newborns of 501-800 gm birth weight, National Institute of Child Health and Human Development Neonatal Research Network, *JAMA* 276:1645, 1996.

107. Usher R, McLean F, Scott KE et al: Judgment of fetal age. II. Clinical significance of gestational age and an objective method for its assessment, *Pediatr Clin North Am* 13:835, 1966.

108. Van Leewan G: The nurse in prevention and intervention in the neonatal period, *Nurs Clin North Am* 8:5089, 1973.

109. Varda K, Behnke R: The effect of timing of initial bath on newborns temperature, *J Obstet Gynecol Neonatal Nurs* 29:27, 2000.

110. Vaughn B: Early maternal-infant contact and neonatal thermo-regulation, *Neonatal Netw* 8:19, 1990.

111. Vlietinck R, Thiery M, Orye E et al: Significance of the single umbilical artery. A clinical, radiological, chromosomal and dermatoglyphic study, *Arch Dis Child* 47:639, 1972.

112. Wariyar U, Tin W, Hey E: Gestational assessment assessed, *Arch Dis Child Fetal Neonatal Educ* 77:216, 1997.

113. Wasz-Hockert O, Lind J, Vuorenkoski V et al: The infant cry: a spectographic and auditory analysis. In *Clinics in developmental medicine 29,* Lavenham, Suffolk, England, 1968, Spastics International Medical Publications.

114. Widstrom A, Thingstrom-Paulsson J: The position of the tongue during rooting reflexes elicited in newborn infants before the first suckle, *Acta Paediatr* 82:281, 1993.

115. Widstrom A, Ransjo-Arvidson AB, Christensson K et al: Gastric suction in healthy newborn infants. Effects on circulation and developing feeding behavior, *Acta Paediatr Scand* 76:566, 1987.

116. Widstrom A, Wahlberg V, Werner S et al: Short-term effects of early suckling and touch of the nipple on maternal behavior, *Early Hum Dev* 21:153, 1990.

117. Wolff P: The natural history of crying and other vocalizations in early infancy. In Foss B, ed: *Determinants of infant behavior IV,* London, 1969, Metheum.

118. Zahr L, Montijo J: The benefits of home care for sick premature infants, *Neonatal Netw* 12:33, 1993.

6

Heat Balance

W. Woods Blake, Judith A. Murray

Optimal care of sick newborn and premature infants requires meticulous attention to detail. The consequences of overlooking some details may not as yet be clinically apparent, whereas other details may affect the very survival of the neonate. Such was the case early in the twentieth century when the beginning of the science of neonatology was marked by the discovery of the importance of maintaining adequate warmth in the newborn. Tarnier, an obstetrician in Paris and Lion in Nice during the late nineteenth century, reported improving the survival of premature infants using crude incubators to warm them. These were impressive first steps in attempting to control the fragile heat balance of weak preterm infants. Manual adjustment of the oil or gas flames that warmed these incubators (undoubtedly resulting in both hypothermia and hyperthermia) dramatically improved the survival rate of these infants.[12,35,56]

Building on these early findings, researchers have gained insight into the physiology of thermoregulation and developed the technology to maintain thermal neutrality in the tiniest and sickest neonates. Although the staff of modern NICUs have the expertise and equipment to avoid the consequences of inadequate thermoregulation, determining the most appropriate ways of attaining the best temperature balance is the subject of ongoing investigation.[5] This chapter discusses the current knowledge of the physiology and pathophysiology of neonatal thermoregulation and approaches not only to prevent heat loss but to manage heat balance.

PHYSIOLOGY

Animals that maintain their body temperature within a narrow range through a wide range of environmental temperatures are known as *homeotherms*. Humans, as homeotherms, maintain a "normal" body temperature by balancing the amount of heat lost from the body with the amount of heat generated from within the body. Our ability to cope with changing thermal environments improves physically

and physiologically with age. Eventually we are physically able to move to a different place with a more suitable environment or dress more appropriately when the temperature is uncomfortable. Babies, especially preterm or SGA babies, of course cannot physically respond as older children would, and even their physiologic responses are different and limited. Adults lose some thermoregulatory control during REM sleep. Because newborns spend a great deal of time in active sleep, loss of their ability to compensate for changes in environmental temperatures may be detrimental to their well-being. Recent evidence suggests that thermoregulation is not impaired during active sleep, which indicates the developmental importance of both thermoregulation and active sleep in the maturation of newborn infants.[4]

Physiologic responses to a cold environment involve metabolic reactions that consume substrate and oxygen and result in the production of heat. A neutral thermal temperature is the body temperature at which an individual baby's oxygen consumption is minimized. Thus a minimal amount of the baby's energy is expended for heat maintenance, and energy is conserved for other basic functions and growth. Minimal metabolic activity is possible within a narrow range of temperatures, so temperatures that are too high or too low add stress and increase metabolic rate. Extreme deviations from this range will overwhelm the thermoregulatory mechanisms, leading to body temperature changes and eventually death.

CAUTION: **All studies used to develop Figures 6-1 and 6-2 were conducted under specific, controlled environments that may not exist in the clinical setting. The ideal temperature varies with the particular baby and environmental variables, such as relative humidity, type of incubator used, and clothing used.**

The goal in controlling a neonate's environment is to minimize energy expended to maintain a "normal" temperature, thus eliminating thermal stress. This neutral thermal environ-

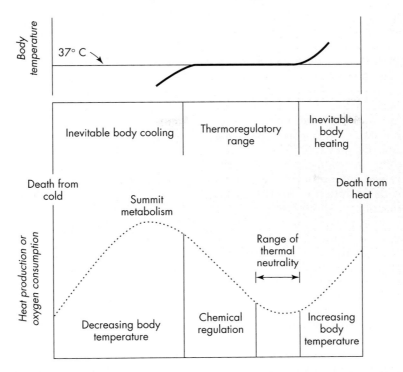

FIGURE 6-1 Temperature versus oxygen consumption. Effect of environmental oxygen consumption and body temperature. (From Klaus M, Fanaroff A: *Care of the high-risk neonate,* ed 2, Phildelphia, 1979, WB Saunders.)

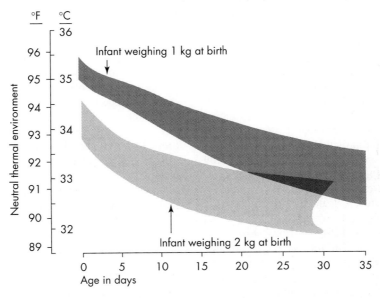

FIGURE 6-2 Thermal neutral environments. Range of temperature to provide neutral environmental conditions for infant lying naked on warm mattress in draft-free surroundings of moderate humidity (50% saturation) when mean radiant temperature is same as air temperature. Shaded areas show average neutral temperature range for healthy infant weighing 1 kg *(dark)* or 2 kg *(light)* at birth. Optimal temperature probably approximates to lower limit of neutral range as defined here. Approximately 1° C (1.8° F) should be added to these operative temperatures to derive appropriate neutral air temperature for single-walled incubator when room temperature is less than 27° C (80° F) and more if room temperature is much less. (From Hey EN, Katz G: The optimum thermal environment for naked babies, *Arch Dis Child* 45:328, 1970.)

ment is the sum total of factors at which a baby with a normal body temperature has a minimal metabolic rate and therefore minimal oxygen consumption. Both traditional indirect calorimetry and the more accurate and sensitive direct calorimetry are used to study the production and expenditure of heat in newborns. **Factors such as ambient air temperature, air flow velocity, relative humidity, and temperature and composition of objects in direct contact with the infant or to which heat may be radiated compose the infant's thermal environment.**

When exposed to a cold environment, a neonate senses the reduced skin surface temperature (using sensors in the skin, primarily the face) and reduces core body temperature (using sensors along the spinal cord and in the hypothalamus). Information from these various sensors is processed (probably in the posterior hypothalamus), including average temperature, rate of temperature change, and size of the stimulated area. Cold stress results in the initiation of a series of reactions to increase heat production and decrease heat loss. In adults the most significant involuntary method of heat production is shivering. **Neonates rarely shiver and must rely on nonshivering, or chemical, thermogenesis to produce the needed heat.** This process is initiated in the hypothalamus and transmitted through the sympathetic nervous system, leading to the release of norepinephrine at the site of brown fat. Brown fat, found mostly in the nape of the neck, axillas, and between the scapulas of newborns, is a specialized type of fat. It is unique in that it contains thermogenin, which is the key enzyme regulating nonshivering thermogenesis. Norepinephrine causes the release of free fatty acids, which with thermogenin undergo combustion in the mitochondria of brown fat cells, releasing heat. Lipoprotein lipase also provides further triglyceride substrate for heat production.

When servocontrol is used, the thermistor must not be placed over an area of brown fat, which may directly heat the overlying skin, causing a decrease in the amount of servocontroller heat output. Oxygen and glucose are also consumed during nonshivering thermogenesis. Thus an infant who already has low oxygen or glucose levels may become hypoxemic or hypoglycemic if added thermal stress occurs. The tiniest premies may not have developed sufficient brown fat stores to mount a significant heat production response to compensate for even minimal cold stress.[49]

Heat generated within the body is transferred by conduction through tissues along a gradient to cooler areas such as the skin surface. An initial response to a cold environment is to constrict superficial blood vessels to minimize the transfer of heat from the core to the surface of the body. Superficial vasoconstriction in response to cold stimulus gives a lower skin temperature reading to the thermocontroller and consequently causes an increase in the incubator temperature. The smaller the body size, the less effective vasoconstriction is in conserving heat. Compared with adults, newborns have a very large surface area/body mass ratio and therefore have a relatively large area exposed to the environment from which heat can be lost. More mature infants may try to minimize their surface area by changing positions when faced with cold stimulus, but immature infants are unable to flex the trunk and extremities effectively. They also have little subcutaneous fat tissue that could act as insulation to help prevent heat conduction to the body's surface, where it is lost.[33]

Heat is transferred from the infant's body to the environment (i.e., everything in close proximity to the baby) along a temperature gradient from warmest to coolest. This transfer of heat occurs by four principal mechanisms: radiation, conduction, evaporation, and convection. Figure 6-3 illustrates these four mechanisms and identifies interventions to minimize their effects.

Much less frequently, a newborn calls on physiologic responses to an environment that is too warm, and these responses are somewhat limited. As skin temperature rises, superficial blood vessels dilate, increasing the transfer of core body temperature to the surface. Increasing the temperature gradient between the skin and the environment increases heat loss from the body. When exposed to elevated environmental temperatures, babies of less than 36 weeks' gestation are generally unable to generate sweat to eliminate heat by evaporation. Maturing babies develop this eccrine gland function first on the forehead, followed by the chest, upper arms, and more caudal areas.[31]

Temperature Measurement

A neonate's temperature can be determined by various methods. Deep body (core) temperature may be measured in the rectum, in the esophagus, and on the tympanic membrane. Rectal thermistors are thin, flexible probes that must be inserted at least 5 cm to obtain an accurate reading. Insertion to this depth runs the risk of perforation, because the sig-

RADIATION **EVAPORATION**

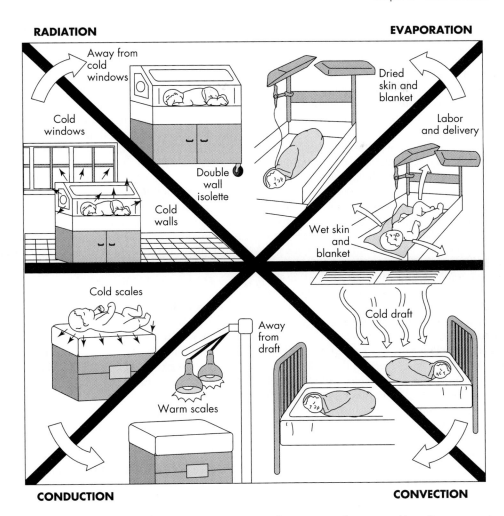

CONDUCTION **CONVECTION**

FIGURE 6-3 *Radiation,* or heat loss in the form of electromagnetic photons, occurs from warm skin surfaces to a cooler object not in contact with the newborn (e.g., inside the incubator wall, nursery wall, or window). Radiant heat loss is independent of ambient air temperature and is the main source of heat loss because of the infant's large surface area. *Conduction* is the loss of heat to a cooler object in direct contact with the newborn (e.g., cold scale, unwarmed bed, stethoscope, or examiner's hand). *Convection* is the loss of heat to moving air at the skin surface and depends on the air's velocity and temperature. *Evaporation* of water from the skin and mucous membranes also causes heat loss, especially in the delivery room. The thinner stratum corneum layer of skin of VLBW infants makes evaporative heat and water loss and fluid management ongoing problems. (Courtesy Lynn Jones, RN.)

moid colon makes a right-angle turn approximately 3 cm from the anal opening.[46] Esophageal and tympanic readings are difficult to obtain and usually impractical. Noninvasive infrared thermometry, a rapid and painless method of determining tympanic membrane or axillary temperature in children, is not recommended for use in newborns at this time. Studies have failed to demonstrate an accurate correlation between infrared thermometer readings and axillary or rectal temperature readings in newborn infants.[54,65,66] Continuous monitoring of abdominal skin temperature when lying supine is a noninvasive method that has been reported to show good correlation with rectal temperatures.[19] It is impractical to keep babies in a supine position constantly, so research to find the best practice to monitor and servocontrol infants' temperatures continues.[12] Correlation with this method and core temperature requires further study, and whether its use with servocontrol is appropriate is yet to be determined, because incubators are programmed to respond to insulated skin temperature, not core temperature.

Rectal temperature can be obtained using a glass or electronic thermometer, but there are risks of vagal stimulation and rectal perforation,[23,46] and, as previously noted, one must be cautious about insertion depth. Care must be taken that the thermometer is inserted less than 3 cm to avoid perforation at the site where the sigmoid colon turns. Rectal glass thermometers should be held in place at least 3 minutes to obtain an accurate reading. Electronic thermometers may provide a reading in less time. **Because of the risks involved, rectal temperatures should not be taken on a routine basis in neonates.** Some nurseries routinely obtain rectal temperatures when the neonate is admitted to check patency of the anus. However, a soft, flexible catheter can easily maneuver the turns in the colon and would be a safer method for determining patency while reducing the risk of perforation.

Axillary temperatures are safe and easy to obtain and may be measured using glass, electronic, or disposable thermometers. The tip of the thermometer should be held firmly in the midaxillary area for at least 3 minutes in preterm infants and 5 minutes in term infants. **When taken properly, axillary temperatures provide readings as accurate as rectal and core temperature methods. By consensus axillary temperatures should be maintained at 36.5° to 37.5° C (97.7° to 99.5° F) in term infants. For preterm infants the normal axillary temperature ranges between 36.3° and 36.9° C (97.3° to 98.6° F).**[2] Infants nursed under radiant warmers may have higher axillary readings compared with rectal measurements and compared with infants cared for in incubators.

In critically ill infants the skin temperature is usually routinely monitored in addition to regular axillary temperature readings. A skin probe is secured to the right upper quadrant of the abdomen. Because an infant responds to cold stress by vasoconstriction, a drop in skin temperature may be the first sign of hypothermia. The core temperature may not fall until the infant is no longer able to compensate. The axillary temperature may remain normal because of close proximity to brown fat stores.

ETIOLOGY

The ambient temperature range in which a healthy full-term infant maintains a stable core temperature is narrower than the temperature range in which an adult maintains a normal temperature. When measures are taken to provide a neutral thermal environment for the neonate, thus avoiding excessive heat loss or gain, heat balance is maintained. Recognition of infants at risk for heat imbalance is essential in the prevention of thermal stress.

Premature infants have a limited ability to control body temperature and are extremely susceptible to hypothermia. Factors that contribute to temperature instability include very thin skin, large surface area relative to body mass, limited substrate for heat production, decreased subcutaneous tissue, and an immature nervous system. These infants often have multiple health problems that necessitate frequent interventions by health care providers with consequent disruption of the infant's neutral thermal environment.

A premature infant's very thin skin and larger surface area/body mass ratio allow for increased evaporative heat loss. Term infants can reduce surface area by flexing their extremities onto their trunk, a skill that increases with gestational age. Unable to maintain flexion, a preterm infant lies primarily with extremities extended. Care providers may reduce the surface area by positioning infants in flexion and supporting them with blankets and rolls. The shortened gestation limits lipid supplies, brown fat, and the accumulation of subcutaneous tissue. The immature nervous system delays or mutes the infant's response to thermal stress. The premature infant is likely to experience other complications (e.g., respiratory distress, sepsis, intraventricular hemorrhage, and hypoglycemia) that may increase basal metabolic rate and oxygen consumption, thus interfering with the ability to maintain thermal stability. Numerous procedures and interventions (e.g., medication administration, starting intravenous fluids, and obtaining vital signs) may impede efforts to maintain a neutral thermal environment. Care providers should routinely check the infant's temperature before initiating treatments. If the temperature is low, treatment should be delayed until a more normal temperature is obtained. If interventions are prolonged, temperature should be monitored frequently, an external heat source provided, and the intervention stopped if hypothermia occurs.

SGA infants, as with preterm infants, have a large surface area relative to body mass and decreased subcutaneous tissue, brown fat, and glycogen stores, all of which contribute to heat imbalance.[57] Decreased placental blood flow frequently contributes to the small size and possible intrauterine hypoxia.

The relatively large surface area of an SGA infant increases evaporative and radiant heat loss, whereas limited subcutaneous tissue and brown fat stores contribute to a decreased ability to produce heat. Some flexion of the extremities may be present because flexion depends on gestational age and not weight. SGAs have a higher metabolic rate compared with infants at similar weights but appropriate for gestational age. This is believed to be caused by the larger brain size compared with body weight.[57] Hypoxia in utero may depress the infant's CNS and alter the ability to regulate temperature. Increased energy requirements coupled with limited glycogen stores may result in hypoglycemia and limited ability to produce heat. SGAs may require numerous interventions that disrupt the neutral thermal environment. Care providers should ensure that the infant has a stable temperature before initiation of treatments. Should treatments be prolonged, temperature should be monitored frequently, an external heat source provided, and treatments stopped if hypothermia occurs.

Infants with neurologic damage or depression may experience difficulty maintaining a stable temperature. Hypoxia before, during, or after delivery, neurologic defects, and exposure to drugs such as analgesics and anesthetics may depress the infant's neurologic response to thermal stress.

Hypoxia decreases the effect of norepinephrine on nonshivering thermogenesis, the main route of thermal regulation in the newborn infant. Hypoxia may also reduce the oxidative capacity of the mitochondria in brown fat and skeletal muscles, which are involved in thermogenesis. Infants who have experienced hypoxia in utero may have increased norepinephrine concentrations, which result in peripheral vasoconstriction. This may cause a delayed metabolic response to cold stress and delayed vasodilation to heat stress.[13]

Neurologic defects that affect the hypothalamus may also interfere with heat balance. The hypothalamus coordinates temperature input from various sensors. Such drugs as analgesics and anesthetics cause CNS depression and reduce the infant's ability to respond to thermal stress. Neuromuscular blocking agents inhibit the infant's ability to maintain a flexed position, increasing exposed body surface and heat loss. **Care providers must be alert to the effect of drugs on the CNS and the infant's ability to regulate temperature.**

Infants with sepsis may have hypothermia or hyperthermia. In a newborn infant an elevated temperature may begin as a response to cold stress, with peripheral vasoconstriction and thermogenesis. Heat production continues as the infant attempts to achieve a higher core body temperature. Exogenous and endogenous pyrogens may enhance thermogenesis.[13]

Initially an infant with sepsis may feel cool to the touch and may have a low body temperature. As fever progresses temperature may rise, and the infant feels warm to the touch. Infants nursed in servocontrolled incubators may not have an elevated temperature. The lower heater output in response to increasing skin temperature (by manual or servo-control adjustment) may mask a fever by keeping the baby's temperature within normal limits. The care provider should be alert to a sudden decreased need for incubator heat support in a previously stable infant.

Many times hyperthermia is iatrogenic, caused by inappropriate control of the neonate's environmental temperature. The most common cause is the use of external heat sources. Dehydration may also contribute to hyperthermia. **Infants nursed with the use of external heat sources should have their temperatures monitored frequently. Phototherapy, sunlight, and the use of excessive clothing and blankets contribute to overheating.** Dehydration may be avoided by early recognition of infants at risk for increased fluid loss. Increased insensible water loss occurs in preterm infants because of increased skin permeability and the use of phototherapy and radiant warmers. Vomiting, diarrhea, gastric suction, and ostomy drainage also increase fluid loss. These infants should receive additional fluids to replace the increased losses (see Chapter 14).

PREVENTION

Heat balance is determined by the amount of heat lost to the baby's environment offset by the amount of heat generated by the body plus the amount of heat supplied from outside sources. Because a smaller, more immature, and sicker baby is less able to regulate body temperature, it is crucial that care providers understand the physical and physiologic principles of heat balance and be able to maintain a neutral thermal environment. **Two broad categories of interventions foster thermal neutrality: (1) blocking avenues of heat loss and (2) providing external heat and environmental support to**

maintain temperature within the normal range of 36.5° to 37.5° C (97.7° to 99.5° F). The theoretically neutral thermal environment required for neonates of 1 and 2 kg at a given age is listed in Figure 6-2. Newborns of less than 800 g are not adequately addressed in currently available tables but should have a starting environmental temperature setting of 36.5° C (97.7° F).

Attention to the details of these interventions begins in the delivery room, where the first step is to adjust the ambient delivery room temperature to a minimum of 22° C (71° F), with a relative humidity of 60% to 65%. Warming the room and placing the resuscitation table away from doors or drafts minimizes convective heat loss. The newborn's skin temperature may drop by as much as 0.3° C/min, with core temperature dropping more slowly after delivery.[2] At birth, most heat loss results from evaporation of amniotic fluid from the baby's skin surface. Drying the infant with prewarmed towels and immediately replacing used ones with dry warm towels minimizes evaporative heat loss. Dry towels conduct heat poorly when contacting the neonate's skin. However, cold examiner hands, stethoscopes, scales, and bare mattresses are good heat conductors and can add significant cold stress if not warmed before coming in contact with the newborn.

Skin-to-skin contact between mother and infant may reduce conductive and radiant heat loss and is an excellent way to maintain a neutral thermal condition for the healthy newborn.[16] If the infant remains with the parents for an extended time, temperature should be monitored. In the case of a preterm infant in stable condition, the use of an additional heat source (e.g., a radiant warmer) enables parents to spend more time with their infant before transfer to the NICU.[61] Skin-to-skin contact should be delayed at least until week 2 of life in extremely premature infants, because they have been shown to lose heat during skin-to-skin contact during the first week of life.[6]

Resuscitation should take place on a preheated radiant warmer so that the adverse consequences of hypothermia are avoided. Because a significant amount of heat is lost through the surface area of the head, with its abundant blood supply and the brain's high heat production, covering the infant's head with some insulating material conserves heat during transfer to the nursery or NICU and afterward. Stockinette material is relatively ineffective for this purpose and provides poor insulation. The best material is thick, maintains its shape with use, and has a high percentage of air volume trapped in the fibers. Knitted wool caps or Thinsulate material may provide the best results.[17,25]

There are a variety of ways to maintain thermal neutrality. Accessibility, insensible water loss, servocontrol versus manual control of temperature, and safety are major considerations when determining the method to use for an individual neonate.

Incubators

Incubators provide a controlled, enclosed environment, heated convectively with warm air. The temperature in an incubator may be servocontrolled to maintain a desired skin temperature or air temperature.[9] As the temperature varies from the desired "set point," proportional control units gradually increase or decrease heat output to maintain a constant temperature (without the wider temperature fluctuations seen with simple on-off controllers). **When servocontrolling the incubator to the desired skin temperature, the sensor should be attached to the right upper quadrant of the abdomen with insulated temperature patches. The sensor should not be placed over areas of brown fat deposits, because the higher-than-expected temperature information to the controlling unit will result in a lower-than-desired heat output.** Inadvertent cooling may take place if the sensor is covered with clothes or a blanket or if the baby lies on it. If the sensor becomes disconnected from the skin, unwanted heating may occur because an erroneously low temperature reading will cause an unwanted increase in heat output. One must also consider that when an insulated patch is used to cover the thermistor, skin temperature is sensed as being higher than if tape covers the thermistor, resulting in decreased heat output by the warming device.[20] The desired skin temperature used for skin servocontrol is generally 36.0° to 36.5° C (96.8° to 97.7° F).[40] Modern incubators can also be servocontrolled to a desired air temperature. This mode has been shown to provide a more stable thermal environment and less temperature variation when compared with skin servocontrol.[21,35] Air servocontrol maintains a constant ambient air temperature when other factors such as phototherapy, external radiant heat, unstable room temperature, or direct sunlight are not confounding variables.[18] **Recently it has been shown that infants who had been skin servocontrolled had greater variability but higher** air temperatures and spent more time in a neutral thermal environment. Babies air servocontrolled had less variability in air temperatures but more variability in infant body temperature.[60] A review of published trials concluded that VLBW babies who were skin servocontrolled at 36° C had a lower mortality rate than those air servocontrolled at 31.8° C.[58] The question of air versus skin servocontrol or manual control is still debatable for any given situation, and probably neither is the perfect solution for all babies.[18]

Radiant heat loss to cooler incubator walls, especially in single-walled incubators, is a significant source of heat loss. The use of double-walled incubators (with the inner wall warmed to the ambient air temperature inside the incubator) results in less radiant heat loss from the baby.[8,42] With a skin-set servocontrol temperature, the decreased radiant heat loss (because of warmer incubator walls) is offset by increased convective heat loss (because the ambient air temperature required for the desired skin temperature is lower[9]); consequently there is no net change in the mean environmental temperature. Double-walled incubators provide less temperature fluctuation when doors are open, thus providing a more stable caretaking environment. Evaporative heat loss is not appreciably different with single- and double-walled incubators. One may increase the humidity in incubators to decrease the infant's metabolic rate only if a neutral thermal environment cannot be achieved by increasing the ambient temperature.

The tiniest neonate has a large evaporative heat loss, and maximum air temperature is limited by the incubator controls, thus making it difficult to reach an air temperature high enough for thermal support. In such cases hypothermia can be avoided by increasing the ambient humidity within the incubator by (1) using the water reservoir or (2) supplying warmed humidified air into the incubator with respiratory humidifiers. Careful attention should be given to preventing bacterial growth in the humidification system[27] (see Chapter 23). Incubator temperatures may also be controlled manually by estimating the appropriate temperature for the baby's age and weight from Table 6-1 and setting the incubator to that temperature.

Regardless of whether one is using skin or air servocontrol or manual temperature adjustments, the baby's temperature and the air temperature must be monitored and recorded regularly. The incubator should be kept away from air conditioning ducts, direct sunlight, and cool windows that may cool or warm the incubator. Room temperature should be kept between 22.2° and 24.4° C (72° and 76° F). Alarms for both high and low temperature levels should always be turned on.

The principal disadvantage of maintaining sick newborns in incubators is the limited access to the infant when extensive procedures are required. Incubators may also be perceived by mothers as a barrier between them and their infants and prolong feelings of fear and insecurity, compared with heating methods that provide easier access to the baby.[53] Holding their baby for short periods of time outside the incubator may help to promote bonding and relieve some of their fears. Stable preterm infants dressed in a diaper, shirt, and cap and wrapped in two blankets can maintain a normal temperature when held close to their parent's body. Keeping the skin probe attached to the infant and plugged into the incubator allows for frequent monitoring of the infant's temperature.[45] We also now have an increasing awareness of and concern regarding the high noise levels within incubators. Such noise poses a potential deleterious effect on the hearing development of preterm infants (see Chapter 13). Improved alarm technology minimizes the risk of inappropriate heating, but malfunctions still occur occasionally. When experienced nurses provide care, infants can be appropriately managed in incubators using any of the three modes of temperature control.

Weaning an infant from an incubator to an open crib is an important step in preparing for discharge. Indicators that an infant may be successfully weaned include weight of at least 1500 g, 5 days of consistent weight gain, an absence of medical complications, and the baby's tolerating enteral feeds. Weaning may occur over several days and involves dressing the infant in a shirt, hat, and diaper and swaddling with a blanket. The incubator temperature is manually lowered while monitoring the infant's temperature. Abdominal skin temperature should be 36° to 37° C (96.8° to 98.6° F). After weaning has been successful, the crib should be placed in a draft-free environment.[37,44]

Radiant Warmers

Radiant warmers provide infrared energy to heat the baby's skin while he or she lies naked on an open bed. The radiant warmer must generate enough energy to offset the tremendous amount of radiant heat

Table 6-1	NEUTRAL THERMAL ENVIRONMENTAL TEMPERATURES					
AGE AND WEIGHT	STARTING TEMPERATURE (° C)	RANGE OF TEMPERATURE (° C)		AGE AND WEIGHT	STARTING TEMPERATURE (° C)	RANGE OF TEMPERATURE (° C)
0-6 hr				72-96 hr		
Under 1200 g	35.0	34.0-35.4		Under 1200 g	34.0	34.0-35.0
1200-1500 g	34.1	33.9-34.4		1200-1500 g	33.5	33.0-34.0
1501-2500 g	33.4	32.8-33.8		1501-2500 g	32.2	31.1-33.2
Over 2500 g	33.9	32.0-33.8		Over 2500 g	31.3	29.8-32.8
(and >36 wk)				(and >36 wk)		
6-12 hr				4-12 days		
Under 1200 g	35.0	34.0-35.4		Under 1500 g	33.5	33.0-34.0
1200-1500 g	34.0	33.5-34.4		1501-2500 g	32.1	31.0-33.2
1501-2500 g	33.1	32.2-33.8		Over 2500 g		
Over 2500 g	32.8	31.4-33.8		(and >36 wk)		
(and >36 wk)				4-5 days	31.0	29.5-32.6
12-24 hr				5-6 days	30.9	29.4-32.3
Under 1200 g	34.0	34.0-35.4		6-8 days	30.6	29.0-32.2
1200-1500 g	33.8	33.3-34.3		8-10 days	30.3	29.0-31.8
1501-2500 g	32.8	31.8-33.8		10-12 days	30.1	29.0-31.4
Over 2500 g	32.4	31.0-33.7		12-14 days		
(and >36 wk)				Under 1500 g	33.5	32.6-34.0
24-36 hr				1501-2500 g	32.1	31.0-33.2
Under 1200 g	34.0	34.0-35.0		2-3 wk		
1200-1500 g	33.6	33.1-34.2		Under 1500 g	33.1	32.2-34.0
1501-2500 g	32.6	31.6-33.6		1501-2500 g	31.7	30.5-33.0
Over 2500 g	32.1	30.7-33.5		3-4 wk		
(and >36 wk)				Under 1500 g	32.6	31.6-33.6
36-48 hr				1501-2500 g	31.4	30.0-32.7
Under 1200 g	34.0	34.0-35.0		4-5 wk		
1200-1500 g	33.5	33.0-34.1		Under 1500 g	32.0	31.2-33.0
1501-2500 g	32.5	31.4-33.5		1501-2500 g	30.9	29.5-32.2
Over 2500 g	31.9	30.5-33.3		5-6 wk		
(and >36 wk)				Under 1500 g	31.4	30.6-32.3
48-72 hr				1501-2500 g	30.4	29.0-31.8
Under 1200 g	34.0	34.0-35.0				
1200-1500 g	33.5	33.0-34.0				
1501-2500 g	32.3	31.2-33.4				
Over 2500 g	31.7	30.1-33.2				
(and >36 wk)						

From American Academy of Pediatrics and American College of Obstetricians and Gynecologists: *Guidelines for perinatal care,* ed 2, Evanston, Ill, 1988, American Academy of Pediatrics and American College of Obstetricians and Gynecologists. Data from Scopes JW, Ahmed I: Minimal rates of oxygen consumption in sick and premature infants, *Arch Dis Child* 41:407, 1966; and Scopes JW, Ahmed I: Range of critical temperatures in sick and premature newborn babies, *Arch Dis Child* 41:417, 1966.

NOTE: For their table, Scopes and Ahmed had the walls of the incubator 1° to 2° C warmer than the ambient air temperatures. Generally speaking, the smaller infants in each weight group require a temperature in the higher portion of the temperature range. Within each time range, the younger the infant, the higher the temperature required.

lost to the room by a naked baby lying in an open environment. Heat output can be servocontrolled or manually controlled. With manual control no feedback from the infant is used; this poses a greater risk of overheating or overcooling. **Therefore manual control should not be used routinely except for short periods (e.g., while initiating resuscitation).** The servocontrol sensor measuring skin temperature must be protected from the infrared heat source, or the probe will sense a temperature higher than the skin temperature and decrease radiant heat output, leading to cold stress. Conversely, insulating the sensor with an aluminum reflective patch protects the underlying skin from the radiant heat and keeps the protected skin cooler than the surrounding skin. When the skin under the patch is warmed to the desired temperature, the rest of the skin may be overheated. Vasodilation may then increase convective heat loss, resulting in an effective, though precarious, heat balance. **Caregivers must use caution to ensure that the sensor does not become detached from the skin, or the baby could be exposed to excess heat and become hyperthermic.**

Insensible water loss (IWL) under radiant warmers is increased by 40% to 50% compared with losses in incubators. Directly related to the amount of heat required from the warmer, this loss is also influenced by other factors (e.g., relative humidity and convective air currents) on an open bed. With very premature infants, severe dehydration may occur if water intake is not increased to replace the inordinate IWL (see Chapter 14). Plexiglas heat shields and polyethylene blankets (plastic wrap) have been used in an attempt to prevent large IWLs; studies have shown these to be somewhat effective for this purpose.[7,11,22] However, the microenvironment created by these blankets undergoes drastic change every time the blanket is removed. Even without such blankets the baby will experience wide swings in heat balance when the infrared heat is blocked from reaching the newborn by hands, heads, or drapes during a procedure.

Incubators and radiant warmers are both effective in maintaining an appropriate thermal balance in sick and preterm infants. The method chosen should be individualized to the infant and to the situation. Experience, skill, and nurse preference often influence the choice of heating methods. These factors also influence the extent to which incubators are perceived to interfere with the performance of care providers' tasks. Basic principles of care (e.g., keeping bed linens dry to prevent evaporative heat loss) apply to use of both heating methods. Radiant warmers provide easy access for performing procedures, a definite advantage over incubators, in which procedures must be done through portholes. Advances in equipment technology now make it possible to convert a single unit between radiant mode and convection mode without moving the baby from one platform to another. This seems to be an efficient way to provide the improved access needed when a baby's condition changes while maintaining appropriate warming without the potential risks of moving the baby.[24] Fluid management is easier for infants in incubators because humidity is easily added to the enclosed environment. The large flux of heat exchange between radiant heat source, the baby, and the environment make wide fluctuations in heat balance more likely when compared with the more easily controlled temperature within an incubator. Oxygen consumption using these two heating methods has many variables, but the metabolic rate and oxygen consumption of infants under radiant warmers is slightly higher than in incubators. However, the clinical significance of this finding is uncertain. Infection rates are comparable between the two methods.[33,43,62] Regardless of the type of heat supplied, care must be taken to minimize thermal instability during nursing interventions. Radiant warmers may be able to rewarm a baby faster than an incubator with convective heating after a procedure. Organizing interventions so their frequency and duration limit as much as possible the exposure to a thermally unstable environment can minimize this instability.[47,55]

Other Methods

In the tiniest preterm infants, a conductive heat source (e.g., a heating pad) may also be needed to raise and maintain body temperature. Heated water mattresses provide a neutral thermal environment for less critically ill babies lying in open cribs (making access easier than in closed incubators).[52] This may also provide a feasible and effective means of rewarming hypothermic infants. Heated, water-filled mattresses are most useful in the newborn units of developing countries.[51]

Swaddling materials include various types of infant wrappings (e.g., blanket, clothing, foil, or bubble wrap). The use of swaddling materials makes observation of the infant more difficult and blocks heat from overhead radiant warmers. Before one wraps the infant in insulating materials, the infant must be warm, because these merely retain body warmth and do not generate heat.

Oxygen and air delivered to the neonate should be warmed and humidified to minimize convective and evaporative heat loss (see Chapter 23).

Skin-to-skin (kangaroo) care provides a safe and effective alternative method of caring for premature infants.[3] The infant, dressed only in a diaper and hat, is held upright against the mother's or father's bare chest and covered with the parent's shirt or a blanket. Both AGA and SGA infants experience a beneficial warming effect and a stable skin and core temperature when held skin to skin.[1,38,39,63,64] Mothers exhibit thermal synchrony with the infants, so that their body temperature increases or decreases to maintain the infant's thermal neutrality.[3,38,39] In one study each mother's skin temperature met the neutral thermal environmental zone of her particular infant.[38] Mothers also preferred this method for holding their infant, compared with the traditional method of wrapping the infant in a blanket and the infant being cradled in the parent's arms.[37]

Transport

The same principles of heat balance that apply to infants in an NICU apply to infants during transport. Infants should have a stable temperature before transport. The infant should be transferred from nursery to transport incubator rapidly to prevent prolonged exposure to an uncontrolled thermal environment. Transport incubators that can provide thermal stability inside the transport vehicle must be used. Oxygen provided during transport should also be warmed and humidified. Monitor temperature continuously or at least every 30 minutes.[29] Thin plastic wrap may be useful in decreasing IWL or convective and radiant heat loss. Chemically heated mattresses can also be used to provide a short-term heat source.[34]

DATA COLLECTION

Anticipation and early recognition of the infant at risk for temperature instability is important in the management and prevention of complications associated with both hypothermia and hyperthermia. The perinatal history and ongoing neonatal evaluation identify events and early risk factors of temperature instability.

HISTORY

Events during pregnancy and the early neonatal period may increase an infant's risk for thermal instability. Review of the maternal history should include estimated date of confinement because preterm infants at delivery are at increased risk for hypothermia. Exposure to viral agents (e.g., herpes) as well as vaginal and cervical colonization increases the risk of acquiring an infection before or during delivery (see Chapter 22). Intrapartal use of analgesics and anesthetics may depress the infant's CNS and mute the thermoregulatory ability.

Fetal stress manifested as fetal decelerations, meconium-stained fluid, or low Apgar scores may suggest an impaired thermoregulatory response.

Neonatal interventions that may depress the CNS and thermal response include resuscitation and administration of analgesics, anesthetics, or neuromuscular blocking agents. Invasive procedures (e.g., endotracheal intubation and umbilical catheterization) increase the infant's chance for infection and need for prolonged use of antibiotics. Poor handwashing by care providers may also contribute to infectious nursery outbreaks, such as outbreaks of necrotizing enterocolitis (see Chapters 22 and 28).

Physical Examination/Signs and Symptoms

Physical assessment of the infant should include not only gestational age but also appropriateness of size. Evaluation of the infant's neurologic status (tone, activity, alertness, etc.) may give the caretaker an indication of the extent of neurologic impairment. Hypotonia results in decreased flexion, with an increased exposed surface area and resultant heat loss.

Temperature Determinations

Temperature determinations may need to be made as often as every 30 minutes until stable. After that, temperatures should be recorded every 1 to 3 hours in LBW and preterm infants and every 4 hours in the healthy term infant. Critically ill infants should have continuous monitoring of skin temperature, with axillary determinations every 1 to 2 hours.[2] Documentation should include environmental temperature (e.g., air temperature in the incubator or radiant warmer settings). Measuring the skin and core temperatures simultaneously may help to differentiate fever as a result of disease versus environmental overheating. Noting that the baby's servocontrolled skin temperature is relatively stable but that the environmental temperature has dropped may also be indicative of fever as the incubator responds to the high probe reading by cooling the infant's environment.

Hypothermia

As the infant attempts to conserve heat by vasoconstriction, he or she may be pale and feel cool to touch, particularly on the extremities. Acrocyanosis and respiratory distress may occur as the infant increases oxygen consumption in an attempt to increase heat production. If hypothermia continues, apnea, bradycardia, and central cyanosis may occur. The hypothermic infant may initially be irritable but may become lethar-

gic as cold stress continues. Other behavioral changes that may occur include hypotonia, apnea, weak cry, weak suck, increased gastric residuals, abdominal distention, or emesis. Infants generally do not shiver in response to cold stress, but shivering may occur in more mature babies in the presence of severe hypothermia. Chronic hypothermia may result in poor weight gain.

Hyperthermia

The hyperthermic infant may feel warm to touch, and skin color may be red as the infant attempts to increase heat loss by vasodilation. Sweating may occur in a term infant but generally is not present in infants of less than 36 weeks' gestation. Sweating may first appear on the forehead followed by the chest, upper arms, and lower body.[31]

The hyperthermic infant may be irritable, lethargic, hypotonic, apneic, have a weak or absent cry, and feed poorly. Tachypnea may be seen as the infant attempts to increase heat loss.

Infants with thermal instability should be closely watched for changes in behavior, feeding patterns, and respiratory status. Temperatures should be monitored frequently in any infant exhibiting these symptoms or who feels cool or warm to touch. Early recognition of thermal instability may prevent further consequences and possibly permanent injury or death.

Laboratory Data

The following laboratory data should be used to evaluate metabolic derangements associated with thermal instability:

- Arterial blood gas (to assess for hypoxemia and metabolic acidosis)
- Complete blood count (to assess for sepsis)
- Blood glucose level (to assess for hypoglycemia)
- Electrolytes (to assess for hyperkalemia)
- Blood urea nitrogen (BUN) (elevated with dehydration)
- Serum and urine osmolality (to assess hydration)

TREATMENT AND INTERVENTION

Hypothermia

To avoid the complications of hypothermia, rewarming of cold infants should begin immediately by providing external heat. Rewarming too rapidly, however, may further compromise the already cold-stressed infant and result in apnea. Oxy-gen consumption is minimal when the difference between the skin and the ambient air temperature is less than 1.5° C (35° F).[30] **Avenues of heat loss should be blocked, temperatures should be monitored, and iatrogenic or pathologic causes should be investigated.**

If hypothermia is mild, slow rewarming is preferred. External heat sources should be slightly warmer than the skin temperature and gradually increased until the neutral thermal environmental temperature range is attained. Efforts to block heat loss by convection, radiation, evaporation, and conduction should be initiated. Skin, axillary, and environmental temperatures should be measured and recorded every 30 minutes during the rewarming period. **For more extreme hypothermia (i.e., core temperatures less than 35° C) more rapid rewarming with radiant heaters (servocontrol 37° C) and/or heated water mattresses prevents prolonged metabolic acidosis or asymptomatic hypoglycemia and decreases mortality.**[29,48,59]

Hyperthermia

The usual approach to treating the hyperthermic infant is to cool by removing external heat sources and by removing anything that blocks heat loss. The most common causes of hyperthermia in intensive care nurseries are iatrogenic. Check the heating controls for proper function and thermistors for proper position. Consider sources of heat (e.g., direct sunlight, heaters, and lights) as possible causes of hyperthermia. Excessive bundling with blankets and a hat and elevated environmental temperature can cause a newborn's body temperature to rise into the febrile range. When evaluating the treatment options in the hyperthermic infant, one should consider removing extra blankets or swaddling materials.[15] Nonenvironmental causes of hyperthermia (e.g., infection, dehydration, and/or CNS disorders) should be considered. During the cooling process, skin, axillary, and environmental temperatures should be monitored and recorded every 30 minutes.

COMPLICATIONS

Hypothermia

Acute cold stress results in the release of norepinephrine, which causes vasoconstriction to reduce heat loss and initiate thermogenesis. As glycogen stores are depleted and oxygen consumption increases, the infant uses anaerobic metabolism to increase heat production, resulting in lactic acid production (metabolic acidosis). Pulmonary vasoconstriction, accentuated by metabolic acidosis, is associated with hypoxia, decreased surfactant production, and further acidosis (see Chapter 23). Blood flow to vital organs is diminished, and pulmonary hemorrhage and death may occur if hypothermia continues.[41]

Hyperbilirubinemia and kernicterus may occur as nonesterified free fatty acids from brown fat metabolism compete with bilirubin for albumin-binding sites. Acidosis not only decreases the affinity of albumin for bilirubin but also increases the permeability of the blood-brain barrier, allowing bilirubin to enter brain tissue. If hypothermia continues, carbohydrate, protein, and fat supplies will be used for heat production instead of growth.[28]

Close monitoring of the hypothermic infant is essential for early identification and prevention of complications. Evaluation of vital signs, arterial blood gas, and oxygen saturation may give early indication of hypoxia and metabolic acidosis. The infant may be dusky or bright red because failure of dissociation of oxyhemoglobin occurs at low body temperatures. Respirations may be rapid, shallow, and grunty, accompanied by bradycardia. Oxygen and ventilation should be initiated as needed to reduce hypoxia. Sodium bicarbonate may be given to correct metabolic acidosis. Seizures may occur as a result of hypoxia, requiring the administration of anticonvulsants.

IV glucose may be necessary to prevent or correct hypoglycemia. Blood glucose levels should be monitored hourly until stable (see Chapter 15).

Blood pressure and urine output should be measured to evaluate hydration and kidney function. An elevated BUN and hyperkalemia may be indicators of decreased renal perfusion and impaired renal function. As fluid is retained, edema of the extremities and face may occur.

Bilirubin should be monitored on a regular basis, and phototherapy may be initiated at a lower than usual level to prevent kernicterus. Adequate nutrition to promote growth should be given either intravenously or enterally. While the infant is hypothermic, nipple feedings should be avoided to conserve calories and energy for heat production and growth and to avoid aspiration.

During the rewarming process the hypothermic infant should be observed for hypotension as vasodilation occurs. Volume expanders may be needed to maintain an adequate blood pressure. Apnea and seizures may occur as a result of hypoxia or decreased cerebral blood flow after vasodilation.

Currently the usefulness of selective head cooling in asphyxiated newborns to reduce the damage done to their brain cells is being investigated. There is preliminary evidence that this may be an effective and safe procedure, but further multicenter investigation to evaluate this technique is required.[26]

Hyperthermia

Vasodilation to increase heat loss may also cause hypotension and dehydration as a result of increased IWL. Seizures and apnea may also occur as a result of high core temperature.

Fluid status should be monitored by assessing intake, output, electrolytes, serum and urine osmolality, skin turgor, and mucous membranes. Fluids should be adjusted to include IWL. Blood pressure should be assessed for hypotension, and volume expanders should be administered as needed.

Cardiorespiratory monitoring to detect apnea should be used. Ventilation may be needed if apnea persists or is unresponsive to stimulation. Subtle signs of seizures may include facial grimacing, nystagmus, tremors, apnea, opisthotonic posturing, tongue thrusting, or staring (see Chapter 26).

PARENT TEACHING

Parents should be taught the importance of maintaining a normal temperature. Temperature should be taken before parents touch the infant through the portholes of the incubator or hold the infant. While the infant is outside the incubator, monitor the skin temperature continuously with a telethermometer. Unwrapping the infant to check the temperature exposes the baby to cold stress. Additional heat sources (e.g., a radiant warmer, a hat, and extra blankets) may be needed while parents hold the infant. Teach parents to monitor their infant's temperature and notify the nurse if it rises or falls.

Before discharge, teach parents to take an accurate axillary temperature and to notify their physician if it drops below 36° C (96.8° F) or rises above 37.8° C (100° F). A parent should not routinely take a rectal temperature. The temperature should be taken whenever the infant feels cool or warm to the touch. The nurse should observe the parents taking the infant's axillary temperature before discharge.

The home environment should be kept at a temperature that prevents heat and cold stress. A room temperature that is comfortable for the parent is usually suitable for the infant. The infant should be in clothing appropriate for the room temperature. For example, if the parent requires a sweater to be comfortable, then the infant probably also requires a sweater. Parents often overdress the infant or overheat the home, and this may cause hyperthermia. Parents should be given written instructions before discharge on how and when to take an axillary temperature, when to call the physician, and how to maintain a comfortable environment for their infant.

REFERENCES

1. Acolet D, Sleath K, Whitelaw A: Oxygenation, heart rate and temperature in very low birthweight infants during skin-to-skin contact with their mothers, *Acta Paediatr Scand* 78:189, 1989.
2. American Academy of Pediatrics and American College of Obstetricians and Gynecologists: *Guidelines for perinatal care,* ed 4, Evanston, Ill, 1997, The Academy.
3. Anderson GC: Current knowledge about skin-to-skin (kangaroo) care for preterm infants, *J Perinatol* 21:216, 1991.
4. Bach V, Bouferrache B, Kremp O et al: Regulation of sleep and body temperature in response to exposure to cool and warm environments in neonates, *Pediatrics* 93:789, 1994.
5. Baker JP: The incubator controversy: pediatricians and the origins of premature infant technology in the United States, 1890 to 1910, *Pediatrics* 87:654, 1991.
6. Bauer K, Pyper A, Sperling P et al: Effects of gestational and postnatal age on body temperature, oxygen consumption, and activity during early skin-to-skin contact between preterm infants of 25-30 week gestation and their mothers, *Pediatr Res* 44:247, 1998.
7. Baumgart S: Reduction of oxygen consumption, insensible water loss, and radiant heat demand with use of a plastic blanket for low-birth-weight infants under radiant warmers, *Pediatrics* 74:1022, 1984.
8. Baumgart S, Engle WD, Fox WW et al: Effect of heat shielding on convective and evaporative heat losses and on radiant heat transfer in the premature infant, *J Pediatr* 99:948, 1981.
9. Bell EF, Rios GR: Air versus skin temperature servocontrol of infant incubators, *J Pediatr* 103:954, 1983.
10. Bell EF, Rios GR: A double-walled incubator alters the partition of body heat loss of premature infants, *Pediatr Res* 17:135, 1983.
11. Bell EF, Weinstein MR, Oh W et al: Heat balance in premature infants: comparative effects of convectively heated incubator and radiant warmer, with and without plastic heat shield, *J Pediatr* 96:460, 1980.
12. Blackburn S, DePaul D, Loan LA et al: Neonatal thermal care. Part III: the effect of infant position and temperature probe placement, *Neonatal Netw* 20:25, 2001.
13. Bruck K: Neonatal thermal regulation. In Polin R, Fox W, eds: *Fetal and neonatal physiology,* Philadelphia, 1991, WB Saunders.
14. Butterfield LS: Martin Couney's story revisited. The AAP Perinatal Section Ad Hoc Committee on Perinatal History, *Pediatrics* 100:159a, 1997.
15. Cheng T, Partridge J: Effect of bundling and high environmental temperature on neonatal body temperature, *Pediatrics* 92:238, 1993.
16. Christensson K, Siles C, Moreno L et al: Temperature, metabolic adaptation and crying in healthy newborns, *Acta Paediatr Scand* 81:488, 1992.
17. D'Apolito K: Hats used to maintain body temperature, *Neonatal Netw* 13:93, 1994.
18. D'Apolito K: Temperature control: servo versus nonservo: which is best? *Neonatal Netw* 15:75, 1996.
19. Dollberg S, Atherton HD, Heath SB et al: A trancutaneous alternative to rectal thermometry for continuous measurement of core temperature in preterm infants, *Pediatr Res* 35:222A, 1994.
20. Dollberg S, Atherton HD, Sigda M et al: Effect of insulated skin probes to increase skin-to-environment temperature gradients of preterm infants cared for in convective incubators, *J Pediatr* 124:799, 1994.
21. Ducker DA, Lyon AJ, Ross Russell R et al: Incubator temperature control: effects on the very low birthweight infant, *Arch Dis Child* 60:902, 1985.
22. Fitch CW, Korones SB: Heat shield reduces water loss, *Arch Dis Child* 59:886, 1984.
23. Frank J, Brown S: Thermometers and rectal perforation of the neonate, *Arch Dis Child* 53:824, 1978.
24. Greenspan JS, Cullen AB, Touch SM et al: Thermal stability and transition studies with a hybrid warming device in neonates. *J Perinatol* 21:167, 2001.
25. Greer P: Head coverings for newborns under radiant warmers, *J Obstet Gynecol Neonatal Nurs* 17:265, 1988.
26. Gunn AJ, Gluckman PD, Gunn TR et al: Selective head cooling in newborn infants after perinatal asphyxia: a safety study, *Pediatrics* 102:885, 1998.
27. Harpin VA, Rutter N: Humidification of incubators, *Arch Dis Child* 60:219, 1985.
28. Kanto WP, Calvert LJ: Thermoregulation of the newborn, *Am Fam Phys* 16:157, 1977.
29. Kaplan M, Eidelman AI: Improved prognosis in severely hypothermic newborn infants treated by rapid rewarming, *J Pediatr* 105:470, 1984.
30. Klaus MH, Fanaroff AA: *Care of the high-risk neonate,* ed 3, Philadelphia, 1986, WB Saunders.
31. Lane A: Sweating in the neonate. In Polin R, Fox W, eds: *Fetal and neonatal physiology,* Philadelphia, 1991, WB Saunders.
32. LeBlanc MH: Evaluation of two devices for improving thermal control of premature infants in transport, *Crit Care Med* 12:593, 1984.

33. LeBlanc MH: Neonatal heat transfer. In Polin R, Fox W, eds: *Fetal and neonatal physiology,* Philadelphia, 1991, WB Saunders.

34. LeBlanc MH: Relative efficacy of radiant and convective heat in incubators in producing thermoneutrality for the premature, *Pediatr Res* 18:425, 1984.

35. LeBlanc MH: Skin, rectal, or air temperature control in the neonate: which is the preferred method? *J Perinatol* 5:2, 1985.

36. LeBlanc MH: Thermoregulation: incubators, radiant warmers, artificial skins, and body hoods, *Clin Perinatol* 18:403, 1991.

37. Legault M, Goulet C: Comparison of kangaroo and traditional methods of removing preterm infants from incubators, *J Obstet Neonatal Nurs* 24:501, 1995.

38. Ludington-Hoe SM, Anderson GC et al: Synchrony in maternal and premature infant temperature during skin-to-skin contact. Poster presented at the American Nurses Association Council of Nurse Researchers Conference, Chicago, Ill, September 1989.

39. Ludington-Hoe SM, Hadeed A, Anderson GC: Physiologic response to skin-to-skin contact in hospitalized premature infants, *J Perinatol* 11:19, 1991.

40. Malin SW, Baumgart S: Optimal thermal management for low birth weight infants nursed under high-powered radiant warmers, *Pediatrics* 79:47, 1987.

41. Mann TP, Elliott RIK: Neonatal cold injury due to accidental exposure to cold, *Lancet* 1:299, 1957.

42. Marks KH, Lee CA, Bolan CD Jr et al: Oxygen consumption and temperature control of premature infants in a double-wall incubator, *Pediatrics* 68:93, 1981.

43. Marks KH, Nardis EE, Momin MN et al: Energy metabolism and substrate utilization in low birth weight neonates under radiant warmers, *Pediatrics* 78:465, 1986.

44. Medoff-Cooper B: Transition of the preterm infant to an open crib, *J Obstet Gynecol Neonatal Nurs* 23:329, 1994.

45. Mellien A: Incubators versus mothers' arms: body temperature conservation in very-low-birth-weight premature infants, *J Obstet Gynecol Neonatal Nurs* 30:157, 2001.

46. Merenstein G: Rectal perforation by thermometer, *Lancet* 1:1007, 1970.

47. Mok Q, Bass CA, Ducker DA et al: Temperature instability during nursing procedures in preterm neonates, *Arch Dis Child* 66:783, 1991.

48. Motil KJ, Blackburn MG, Pleasure JR et al: The effects of four different radiant warmer temperature set-points used for rewarming neonates, *J Pediatr* 84:546, 1974.

49. Nedergaard J, Cannon B: Brown adipose tissue: development and function. In Polin R, Fox W, eds: *Fetal and neonatal physiology,* Philadelphia, 1991, WB Saunders.

50. Rao M, Koenig E, Li S et al: Direct calorimetry for the measurement of heat release in preterm infants: methods and applications, *J Perinatol* 15:375, 1995.

51. Sarman I, Tunell R: Providing warmth for preterm babies by a heated, water filled mattress, *Arch Dis Child* 64:29, 1989.

52. Sarman I, Can G, Tunell R et al: Rewarming preterm infants on a heated, water filled mattress, *Arch Dis Child* 64:687, 1989.

53. Sarman I, Tunell R, Vastberg L et al: Mothers' perception of their preterm infants treated in an incubator or on a heated water filled mattress: a pilot study, *Acta Pediatr* 82:930, 1993.

54. Seguin J, Terry K: Neonatal infrared axillary thermometry. *Neonatal Intens Care* 12:40, 1999.

55. Sequin J, Vieth R: Thermal stability of premature infants during routine care under radiant warmers, *Arch Dis Child* 74:F137, 1996.

56. Silverman WA: Incubator-baby side shows, *Pediatrics* 64:127, 1979.

57. Sinclair J: Heat production and thermoregulation in the smaller-for-date infant, *Pediatr Clin North Am* 17:147, 1970.

58. Sinclair JC: Servo-control for maintaining abdominal skin temperature at 36C in low birth weight infants (Cochrane Review). In *The Cochrane library,* Issue 3, 2001.

59. Sofer S, Yagupsky P, Hershkowits J et al: Improved outcome of hypothermic infants, *Pediatr Emerg Care* 2:211, 1986.

60. Thomas KA, Burr R: Preterm infant thermal care: differing thermal environments produced by air versus skin servo-control incubators, *J Perinatol* 19:264, 1999.

61. Vaughans B: Early maternal-infant contact and neonatal thermoregulation, *Neonatal Netw* 8:19, 1990.

62. Walther FJ, Wu PY, Siassi B et al: Cardiovascular changes in preterm infants nursed under radiant warmers, *Pediatrics* 80:235, 1987.

63. Whitelaw A: Skin-to-skin contact in the care of very low birthweight babies, *Matern Child Health* 7:242, 1986.

64. Whitelaw A, Heisterkamp G, Sleath K et al: Skin-to-skin contact for very low birthweight infants and their mothers: a randomized trial of "kangaroo care," *Arch Dis Child* 63:1377, 1988.

65. Weiss ME, Pue AF, Smith J III et al: Infrared tympanic thermometry for neonatal temperature assessment, *J Obstet Gynecol Neonatal Nurs* 23:798, 1994.

66. Yetman RJ, Coody DK, West MS et al: Comparison of temperature measurements by an aural infrared thermometer with measurements by traditional rectal and axillary techniques, *J Pediatr* 122:769, 1993.

7 Physiologic Monitoring

John R. Pierce, Barbara S. Turner

Since the clinical usefulness of the umbilical vessels was first demonstrated by Diamond in 1947 when exchange transfusions were being performed to prevent kernicterus, there have been many advances. In most nurseries it is a matter of routine to use the umbilical artery for monitoring blood gas status and arterial blood pressure. Because of the frequency and clinical significance of complications, alternatives to indwelling arterial catheters have been vigorously sought. The development of noninvasive physiologic monitoring devices has been a major step toward this goal.

The purpose of this chapter is to review the procedures and advances in physiologic monitoring.

PHYSIOLOGY

Pulmonary

Gas exchange takes place in the alveoli of the lung. Ventilation is the movement of air in and out of these air spaces. Diffusion is the movement of oxygen from the alveolar space into the pulmonary capillary and the movement of carbon dioxide from the pulmonary capillary into the alveolar space for eventual exhalation. Pulmonary perfusion is the flow of blood through the pulmonary capillaries that surround the alveolar spaces. Once oxygen diffuses through the alveolar lining cells and into the capillaries, it is bound to hemoglobin within the red blood cell.

Oxygen content in the arterial blood is the sum of the amount of oxygen dissolved in the plasma and the amount bound to hemoglobin. Approximately 3% of the oxygen content is dissolved in the plasma, with the remaining 97% bound to hemoglobin. PaO_2 is the partial pressure of the oxygen dissolved in the plasma. Fetal hemoglobin has a higher affinity for oxygen than does adult hemoglobin; therefore at any given PaO_2 more oxygen is bound to adult hemoglobin (Figure 7-1). Oxygen saturation (SaO_2) is the percentage of oxygen bound to hemoglobin.

Noninvasive Blood Gas Monitoring

Oxygen

Noninvasive monitoring of oxygenation can be accomplished by using two monitoring technologies. Oxygen saturation monitoring is the most common and widely used method for assessing oxygenation status. This technology relies on a pulsating arterial vascular bed between a dual light source and a photoreceptor.[1] As blood passes between the light source and the photoreceptor, different amounts of red and infrared light are absorbed, depending on the percentage of oxygen saturation. This difference in light absorption is electronically processed and displayed by the monitor as arterial hemoglobin oxygen saturation.[19]

The second method of noninvasive monitoring of oxygenation is transcutaneous oxygen tension, which relies on the principle of oxygen diffusing from the skin capillaries through the dermis to the surface of the skin. To measure the oxygen, it is necessary to heat the skin, which then dilates the local capillaries and arterializes the capillary bed as well as promotes faster diffusion of the oxygen from the skin.[19]

Carbon Dioxide

As with noninvasive monitoring of oxygen, carbon dioxide can also be assessed using two types of monitors. Transcutaneous carbon dioxide works under similar principles as transcutaneous oxygen monitoring. Although heating of the skin is not required for carbon dioxide, the values are more reliable and valid if a heated probe is used.[3] A second method used to measure the content of the carbon dioxide in the respiratory gases during the respiratory cycle is end-tidal carbon dioxide ($PetCO_2$) monitoring. The carbon dioxide content varies widely with the phase of the respiratory cycle. During inspiration there are minimal amounts of carbon dioxide, whereas at the end of expiration the carbon dioxide values are at their maximum level (Figure 7-2). Until recently the relatively fast respiratory

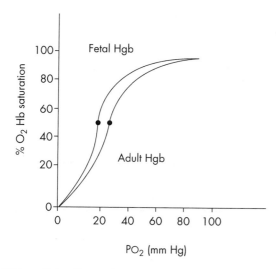

FIGURE 7-1   Oxygen dissociation curve for fetal hemoglobin (Hgb) *(left)* and adult hemoglobin *(right).*

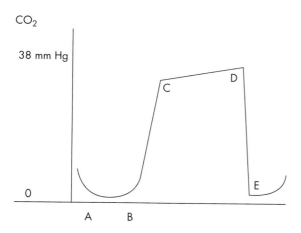

FIGURE 7-2   Variations in the content of carbon dioxide during phases of the respiratory cycle. *A,* End of inspiration. *B,* beginning of exhalation; *C,* end of mixed gases washout (deadspace and alveolar gases); *D,* end of expiration of alveolar gases; *E,* inspiration.

rate of newborns, combined with the small tidal volumes, resulted in inaccurate values when measured by end-tidal carbon monoxide monitors. Advances in technology have improved the reliability of this monitoring technique for newborn infants.

Cardiorespiratory Monitoring

The electrical activity of an infant's heart is picked up by chest leads (usually three) placed on the in-

fant and recorded by a cardiorespiratory monitor. The recording is displayed on a visual screen as the infant's electrocardiographic pattern. The infant's respiratory pattern is also recorded, because the chest leads electronically detect movement of the infant's chest with each respiration.

Blood Pressure Monitoring

Systolic blood pressure (measured in millimeters of mercury) is the pressure at the height of the arterial pulse and coincides with left ventricular systole. Diastolic blood pressure (measured in millimeters of mercury) is the lowest point of the arterial pulse and coincides with left ventricular diastole. Mean arterial pressure is the diastolic pressure plus one third the pulse pressure. Central venous pressure is the pressure in the right atrium and may be approximated by the blood pressure in any of the large central veins.

DATA COLLECTION

The indications for using the various techniques for physiologic data collection depend on the infant's clinical situation.

Umbilical Artery Catheters

An umbilical artery catheter (UAC) is placed in those infants requiring frequent blood gas determinations, continuous monitoring of arterial blood pressure and infusion of fluids and medications. Infants who are candidates for indwelling catheters are those with congenital heart disease or disorders that cause respiratory insufficiency, such as surfactant deficiency, meconium aspiration syndrome, persistent pulmonary hypertension, and diaphragmatic hernia.[11] Although use of an indwelling umbilical artery catheter allows arterial pressure monitoring and accessibility for parenteral infusions, it is not acceptable to place a UAC for these indications alone.

Umbilical Vein Catheters

Umbilical vein catheter (UVC) use is reserved for exchange transfusions, central venous pressure monitoring, and emergency administration of fluids or chemicals in delivery room resuscitation. There are more complications associated with umbilical venous lines than with umbilical arterial lines, but the complications are less severe.[3,11,27] UVCs are being used with increasing frequency for initial management of ELBW infants. There is a continued need for research into the efficacy and safety of UVCs.

Noninvasive Oxygen/Carbon Dioxide Monitoring

Oxygen monitoring is indicated in an infant receiving oxygen for any reason. Acute monitoring is used as a part of the management of acute respiratory disorders. Long-term monitoring is used to wean infants with chronic lung disease from oxygen therapy. During transportation of infants, noninvasive oxygen monitoring is helpful. Carbon dioxide monitoring is useful for verifying that the endotracheal tube is in the trachea (end-tidal CO_2 monitoring) and for the infant with a respiratory disease in which retention of carbon dioxide may become clinically significant (end-tidal CO_2 and transcutaneous CO_2 monitoring). There is a report of end-tidal CO_2 monitoring used for the diagnosis of an H-type tracheoesophageal fistula.[10]

Cardiorespiratory Monitoring

Cardiorespiratory monitoring should be used in any infant who requires intensive or intermediate care and in any infant at risk for apnea or rhythm disturbances.

Blood Pressure Monitoring

Blood pressure monitoring should be used in the infant requiring surgery and in the infant acutely ill with cardiorespiratory distress or with any other illness in which hypotension may be a significant contributor to the pathologic state. Central venous pressure should be monitored in infants who may experience an excess or loss of blood volume.

INTERVENTIONS

Umbilical Artery Catheters

Determine the size and length of the catheter to be inserted. For infants weighing more than 1250 g, use a 5 Fr catheter, and for infants weighing less than 1250 g, use a 3.5 Fr catheter. (Figures 7-3 and 7-4 correlate total body length to the length of the catheter to be inserted.) Place the infant in a supine position on a radiant heater or in an incubator. Skin temperature should remain between 36° and 37° C (96.8° and 98.6° F). Provide appropriate oxygenation and ventilation. Restrain the infant's hands and feet to prevent the infant's contaminating the sterile field and interfering with the placement procedure. Wash hands before and after the procedure. Put on a gown and gloves. Open the catheterization tray;

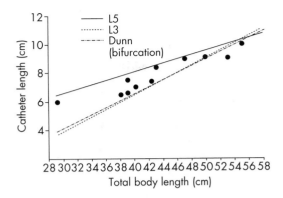

FIGURE 7-3 Graph for distance of catheter insertion from umbilical ring for low placement.(From Rosenfeld W, Biagtan J, Schaeffer H et al:A new graph for insertion of umbilical artery catheters, *J Pediatr* 96:735, 1980.)

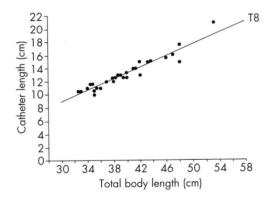

FIGURE 7-4 Graph for distance of catheter insertion from umbilical ring for high placement (T8). (From Rosenfeld W, Estrada R, Jhaveri R et al: Evaluation of graphs for insertion of umbilical artery catheters below the diaphragm, *J Pediatr* 98:627, 1981.)

most units now use commercially available disposable trays. Catheterization tray contents are shown in Figure 7-5. Connect the catheter to the stopcock and flush and fill the entire system with flush solution. Turn off the stopcock to the catheter to prevent fluid from draining out of the catheter during insertion and securing of the catheter. Prepare the catheter by flushing it with a flush solution. Prepare the cord and base of the umbilicus with povidone-iodine (Betadine) solution and then alcohol. Infants weighing less than 1000 g may experience iodophor skin burns. Therefore avoid using an excess of povidone-iodine solution so the infant is not lying in

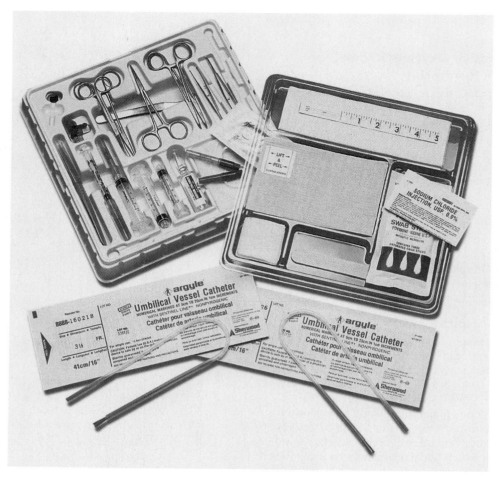

FIGURE 7-5   Argyle Umbilical Vessel Catheter Insertion Tray. (Courtesy Tyco/Healthcare Kendall-LTP.)

the solution during the procedure. Any residual iodophor should be carefully washed off the infant after the procedure is completed. Drape the infant by placing an eye sheet over the umbilicus (alternatively, use sterile drapes). Hold the diagonal corners of one drape and allow the top half to fold over the bottom half. The result will be a V shape. Place the tips of the V on either side of the umbilicus. Repeat with another drape and place on the other side of the umbilicus. The umbilical stump is now visible, yet surrounded by drapes. After the UAC is inserted, the drapes can be easily removed without the need to pass the stopcock and catheter through an eyehole of a drape. Ensure that the infant's head and feet remain visible during the procedure to assess the infant's color. A small eye drape with adhesive

backing (Steri-Drape) has the advantage of being transparent, so that the infant's color can be seen and temperature can be maintained. Towel drapes may interfere with a radiant heat source used for temperature regulation.

Because the tie will be left in place, tie umbilical tape around the base of the cord to ensure that the tape is not around skin. The tape is used to control bleeding. A single overhand knot is preferred, because it allows tightening as needed. Using tissue forceps, pick up the cord and cut it with a scalpel about 1 to 1.5 cm above the base. Arterial spasm allows only minimal bleeding. **Identify the vessels. There are usually two arteries and one vein. The arteries are small, thick walled, and constricted. The vein is larger, thin walled, and usually gap-**

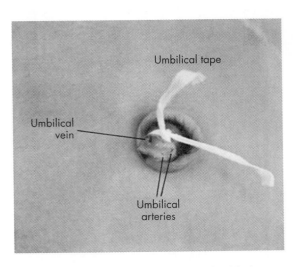

FIGURE 7-6 Umbilical tape and position of umbilical vessels.

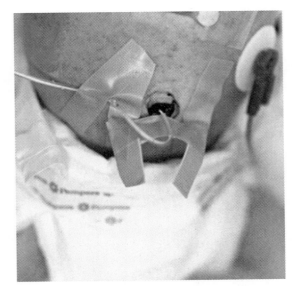

FIGURE 7-7 Umbilical artery catheter secured in "goalpost" design.

ing open. If the vein is at the 12 o'clock position, the arteries are usually at the 4 and 8 o'clock positions (Figure 7-6). Stabilize the umbilical stump by grasping the cord between the thumb and index finger or grasping the edge of the stump with a mosquito hemostat. Ensure that the hemostat does not crush the umbilical vessels. With iris forceps, dilate one of the arteries by placing the tips of the forceps in the artery and gently allowing them to spring open. You may need to repeat this procedure several times. While grasping one side of the wall of the dilated artery, gently insert the catheter or insert the catheter between the open prongs of the forceps, dilating the artery. Instructional aids such as Baby Umb* and the Umbilical Artery Catheterization Slide-Tape Neonatal Educational Program† are helpful. As the catheter passes into the artery, you may meet resistance at several different points:

- At the umbilical tape: The tape may be tied too tightly. Loosen slightly.
- At the point at which the umbilical artery turns downward (caudal) into the abdomen: Steady,

gentle pressure is important, because forceful pressure may cause the catheter to perforate the artery wall and create a false channel.
- At the point at which the umbilical artery joins the external iliac artery: Once again, steady gentle pressure is important.

Insert the catheter to the predetermined length. Aspiration on the syringe should provide immediate blood return. Lack of blood return may indicate the following:

- The catheter is not inserted far enough. Insert farther.
- The vessel wall has been perforated, or a false channel has been created. If the catheter has pierced the vessel wall, repeat the procedure using the other artery.
- The catheter is kinked. Pull back slightly and then advance.
- The stopcock is turned off. Correct the stopcock position. Return aspirated blood to the infant and flush until the catheter clears.

Observe the infant's feet, legs, and buttocks for signs of vascular compromise. If any blanching or blueness occurs, follow the steps outlined under Complications on p. 129-130. Secure the catheter by making a "goalpost," using skin prep on the skin (Figure 7-7). Properly secured by the goalpost taping method, the catheter is secure, and foreign

---

*Medical Plastics Laboratory, Inc., P.O. Box 38, Gatesville, TX 76528.
†Charles R. Drew Postgraduate Medical School, 1621 E. 120th St., Los Angeles, CA 90059.

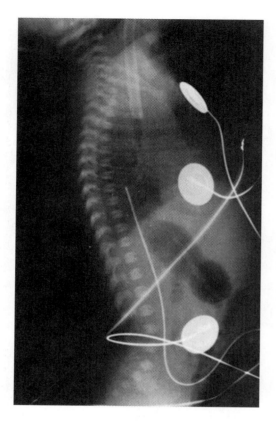

FIGURE 7-8 High catheter demonstrating "leg loop."

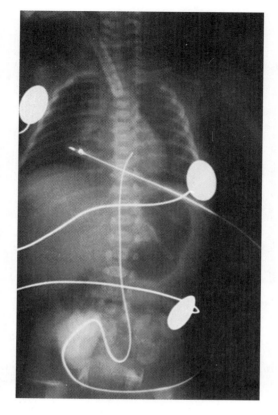

FIGURE 7-9 Umbilical artery catheter in high position (T8).

bodies such as sutures are avoided. (However, many centers use sutures to secure the catheter.) Connect the stopcock to the intravenous (IV) solution and set an appropriate infusion rate. Ensure that no air is in the tubing, stopcock, or catheter. All connections must be secure. Automatic infusion pumps must be used for UACs. Determine catheter placement by an abdominal x-ray examination. Figure 7-8 shows how the UAC will appear on a lateral x-ray film. **Note that the catheter enters the umbilicus and travels inferiorly before turning superiorly. This "leg loop" is characteristic of an arterial catheter. Optimal placement is at L3 to L4 for a low catheter and T8 for a high catheter.**[11,27] A large study found that more than 56% of practitioners preferred high placement for UACs.[11] Figure 7-9 shows high catheter placement, and Figure 7-10 shows low catheter placement. If the catheter is too high, measure on the x-ray film the distance from the tip of the catheter to the desired level and pull the catheter back the appropriate distance. Some

clinicians multiply this length by 0.8 to account for the magnifying effect of the x-ray film. If the catheter is placed too low, the catheter cannot be advanced but must be removed because the external portion of the catheter is no longer sterile.

Teaching Model
The umbilical cord can be used for teaching the procedure of both arterial and venous catheterization. Many of the steps can be effectively carried out using a fresh placenta.

Special UACs and monitors are available for continuous PaO_2 and/or oxygen saturation monitoring.

Nursing Care and Use of Umbilical Artery Catheters
Infants can be positioned on their sides or their backs. The abdominal position is avoided, because accidental slipping, kinking, and removal of the catheter may occur without being immediately apparent. Care needs to be taken so that the infant is positioned to

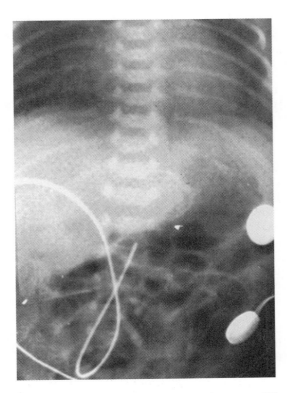

FIGURE 7-10 Umbilical artery catheter in low position (L3).

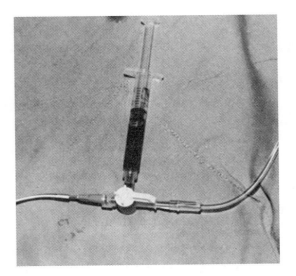

FIGURE 7-11 Stopcock off to IV solution; 1 to 2 ml aspirated into syringe.

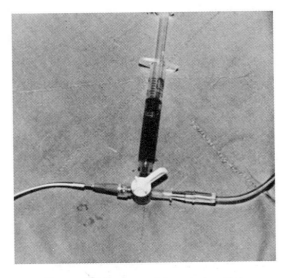

FIGURE 7-12 Stopcock in neutral position.

prevent dislodgement of the catheter. Diapers are effective for preventing the feet and toes from becoming entangled in the catheter. The diaper is folded below the umbilicus. If the infant is receiving phototherapy and thus is not diapered, leg restraints may be indicated. A dressing over the umbilicus is unnecessary; dressings inhibit inspection of the umbilicus and evaluation of the catheter. The IV tubing, connecting tubing, and stopcock should be changed daily. Clots form in the stopcock, so changing it daily prevents the likelihood of emboli formation. Blood backing into the catheter can be caused by the following:

- Increased intraabdominal pressure commonly caused by the infant crying vigorously
- Disconnection of tubing
- Stopcock turned in wrong direction
- Infusion pump malfunction
- A leak in the filter or tubing

The procedure for drawing blood gases from an umbilical catheter must be kept sterile. It requires one syringe flushed with heparin, and one filled with flush solution. Syringes are used for aspirating fluid and blood from the line, collecting blood gas samples, and flushing the line.

Procedure for Drawing Arterial Blood Gas

Turn the stopcock so that the IV solution stops flowing. Aspirate 1 to 2 ml from the catheter into the dry syringe (Figure 7-11). The IV fluid is prevented from infusing, and aspiration clears the catheter of its IV fluid. Turn the stopcock to the neutral position (Figure 7-12), remove the syringe, and replace it with the heparinized syringe. The neutral position of the stopcock prevents contaminating the sample with IV fluid and prevents blood loss from the infant.

CAUTION: Never allow blood to drip from an open stopcock. Using steady, even pressure, aspirate blood into the heparinized syringe. Turn the stopcock to the neutral position and remove the syringe (Figure 7-13). Remove the air from the syringe, cap the end, and chill it to preserve values. Usually 0.2 to 1 ml of blood is needed, depending on the laboratory requirements. Replace the syringe that has the aspirated blood in it with the syringe filled with flush solution. Turn off the stopcock to the IV line. Slightly aspirate to remove any air in the stopcock and slowly insert the syringe. After infusing the flush solution, return the stopcock to the neutral position. Record the amount of blood removed from the infant. Replace the syringe filled with flush solution with a clean, dry syringe. Turn the stopcock so that the IV line can be infused.

To ensure the integrity of all connections, the stopcock and other connections must be visible at all times. Do not place the stopcock and other connections under linen, because this would hamper the immediate detection of an accidental disconnection that would cause severe blood loss in the infant. Immediately remove any air in

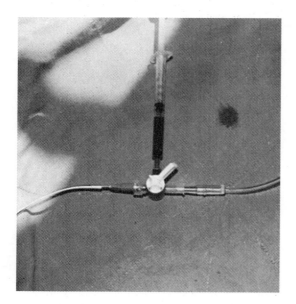

FIGURE 7-13 After blood is aspirated into heparinized 1-ml syringe, stopcock is placed in neutral position before syringe is removed.

the tubing or catheter, because air is a potential embolus. It is best removed through the stopcock. If the air has passed the stopcock, it can easily be aspirated back into a syringe.

Umbilical Vein Catheter Placement Procedure

A 5 Fr catheter is normally used in the umbilical vein catheter (UVC) placement procedure. To determine the length of the catheter to be inserted, the distance from the umbilicus to the sternal notch should be measured and multiplied by 0.6. Complete steps for the placement procedure are found in this chapter's section on UACs. The only difference is that the vein is used instead of the artery up to the point of stabilizing the cord. The vein is usually gaping open and does not require dilation. The catheter can be easily advanced to the desired position. The catheter should lie in the inferior vena cava with the UVC above the diaphragm but below the heart, as demonstrated on x-ray film. UVCs do not have the "leg loop" found on the lateral x-ray film of UACs. The catheter should be taped in the same manner as for a UAC.

Percutaneously Inserted Central Catheter

Percutaneously inserted central catheter (PICC) lines are inserted in neonates for intravenous access that is expected to last for an extended period of time, for those infants with limited access, as a transition from umbilical catheters in infants weighing less than 1000 g, as a first line catheter for infants weighing 1000 to 1500 g, or for infants with gastrointestinal anomalies, gastrointestinal diseases that will require surgical correction, or necrotizing enterocolitis.[22] The catheters are most often made of Silastic, but some units use polyurethane catheters.[9] The insertion sites for PICC lines include the brachial cephalic veins; the axillary subclavian junction when the line is inserted through the arm or hand; the saphenous veins; or the jugular veins when the line is inserted through scalp vessels.

This sterile procedure can be performed when the neonate is on a radiant warmer or in an incubator.

Supplies

PICC insertion tray (Figure 7-14)
PIC catheter and introducer: 24-gauge 8-, 10-, or 30-cm catheter (Figure 7-15)
Sterile gloves (two sets)

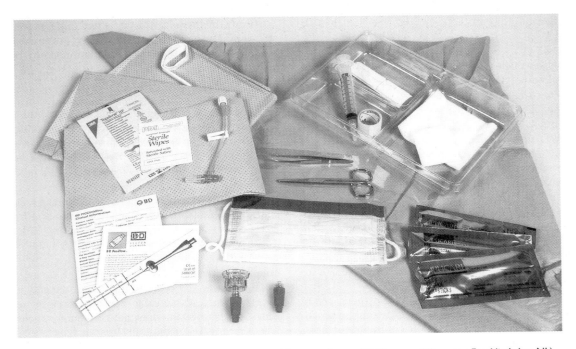

FIGURE 7-14 Disposable tray used for PICC insertion. (Courtesy Becton, Dickinson and Company, Franklin Lakes, NJ.)

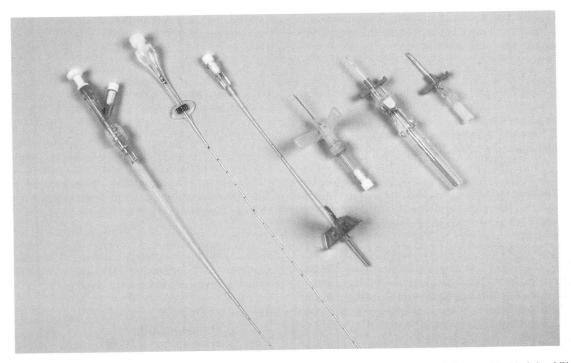

FIGURE 7-15 Peripherally inserted central catheters and introducers. (Courtesy Becton, Dickinson and Company, Franklin Lakes, NJ.)

Gown
Hat
Mask
Heparin flush
Lipid-compatabile T-connector extension tubing
Steri-strips or sterile tape
Transparent film dressing
Normal saline
Sterile drapes

Procedure

For an arm or hand insertion measure the distance from the insertion site to the axilla, then to 1 cm above the nipple line. If the catheter is to be inserted in the scalp, measure from the insertion site to 1 cm above the nipple line, and for a leg insertion measure from the insertion site to 1 cm above the umbilicus or to the site of the superior vena cava or inferior vena cava.

Lidocaine-prilocaine (EMLA) anesthetic cream or a local anesthetic can be used before the procedure is begun. The individual inserting the catheter wears a sterile gown, hat, mask, and gloves. Swaddle the infant, with the site to be used exposed. Grasp the extremity to be used with sterile gauze so that an occlusive dressing can be applied to the distal part of the extremity, thus allowing manipulation of the extremity and precluding contamination of the insertion site by bacteria from distal sites. Prepare the site with a povidone-iodine swab three times and allow the site to air dry. Clean the area with alcohol. For infants weighting less than 750 g or those with fragile skin, prepare the area with povidone-iodine solution, permit the site to dry, and then rinse with sterile water. Place sterile drapes under the exposed site. Prime the extension tubing with heparinized flush solution. Keeping the catheter sterile, remove it from the protective wrapper with sterile forceps. **Measure the catheter and withdraw the stylet just past the desired length, then trim the catheter without cutting the stylet. Some units do not cut the catheter because it removes the tapered tip, which is easier to insert than a blunt-cut tip. Reglove and place the catheter, introducer, needle, syringe, and sterile forceps on the sterile field near the planned insertion site. For hand or arm insertion sites, turning the infant's head toward the insertion site will cause a slight occlusion of the jugular vein so that as the catheter is passed into the subclavian vein, the risk of the catheter advancing upward into the jugular is diminished.**

Insert the introducer tip at a flat angle to access the vein. The needle is *not* advanced into the vein; rather, it is used only as an introducer. At this point there will most likely be no blood return. Once the introducer is in the vein, gently advance the catheter with forceps; blood should fill the catheter. If the catheter is not advancing, pull the catheter back beyond the point of the introducer and reattempt to cannulate the vein. Rastogi et al[22] reported that gentle surface massaging of the vein 1 cm distal to the tip of the catheter was useful in successfully advancing the catheter. Once the vein has been cannulated, advance the catheter to the premeasured length, then remove the stylet entirely. Blood should be easily aspirated with a syringe. Flush the catheter with 0.5 to 1.0 ml of NS with 1 U heparin/ml. Secure the catheter using sterile tape or nonfiber steri-strips. A lipid-compatible T-connector should be Luer-locked into the hub of the catheter. Dress the area with a clear, occlusive dressing; ensure that the dressing does not completely encircle the extremity. Wrap long catheters that have not been precut into a coil above or below the joint to prevent occlusion. Label the dressing with the gauge and length of the catheter, the line type (PICC), and your initials. The occlusive dressing should be changed only when the integrity of the dressing has been lost. Confirm the placement of the catheter with an x-ray assessment. PICC lines that are placed in central veins have complication rates lower than those that reside in noncentral veins.[20]

PICC Line Dressing Change

The dressing is changed under sterile conditions. Changing is indicated when the current dressing is no longer occlusive. If the infant is on a radiant warmer rather than in an incubator, the person performing the dressing change wears a hat, mask, and sterile gloves. Changing the dressing entails removing the transparent film covering the area, cleaning the insertion site with povidone-iodine solution, allowing this to dry, and then cleaning the site with sterile water to remove the preparation agent from the skin. If the Steri-strips are no longer adhesive, they are replaced and the area is once again dressed with transparent film.

Removing Umbilical Arterial, Venous, and Percutaneous Catheters

When there is no longer a need for the UAC, UVC, or PICC, the catheter is removed. For UAC catheter removal, make certain the cord tie is snug. Turn off the stopcock to the patient and the infusate. Sterile gauze is needed, and a suture removal kit should be available if the catheter was sutured in place. For umbilical arterial catheters, withdraw the catheter to 3 cm and leave it in place for 30 minutes before withdrawing it completely. Alternatively, withdraw the catheter slowly over several minutes, allowing for the artery to spasm. Pinch the umbilical stump with the sterile gauze for approximately 5 minutes until hemostasis is achieved. Observe the umbilicus for active bleeding or oozing. The procedure is similar for umbilical venous catheters, with the exception that the catheter can be slowly withdrawn in one step, followed by pinching of the umbilical stump for 5 minutes with a sterile gauze pad. For PICC lines clamp the catheter, turn off the infusion, and withdraw the catheter, applying pressure over the insertion site for 5 minutes with a sterile gauze pad. As with the UAC and UVC, observe the site for bleeding.

Noninvasive Oxygen/Carbon Dioxide Monitoring

End-Tidal Carbon Dioxide Monitoring*

End-tidal CO_2 monitors use either sidestream or mainstream analysis.[15,16,18] For sidestream analysis the endotracheal tube has a second narrow lumen that opens at the end of the endotracheal tube. Gases are analyzed from samples taken from the end of the tube. The advantages of this system are that there is no increased deadspace in the ventilator circuit and less chance of inspiratory gases contaminating the sample. The disadvantage to this method is that secretions may pool at the tip of the endotracheal tube and occlude the sampling port. The response time to changes in carbon dioxide content is slower than that used with mainstream analysis.

Mainstream analysis of carbon dioxide samples gases in the ventilator circuit. These gases are thought to be reflective of gases at the tip of the endotracheal tube. This method requires a separate chamber attached to the end of the endotracheal tube adapter, thus adding increased dead space and additional weight at the endotracheal tube adapter.

When sidestream and mainstream analysis of end-tidal CO_2 were compared, it was found that distal values were higher than proximal values and that distal values correlated more closely with $PaCO_2$ values.[15] This discrepancy was thought to result from the mixing of end-tidal gases with fresh gases in the ventilator circuit. In an infant with a large A-a gradient, $PetCO_2$ monitoring cannot be relied on for accuracy. In premature infants, it may be useful if the lung disease is mild to moderate; in infants with normal lung function this method is reliable.

The waveform output of the end-tidal CO_2 monitor can be used clinically if the clinician understands how the waveform corresponds to the exchange of gases in the lung. The waveform has a sharp rise on expiration that reflects the carbon dioxide content of the alveolar gases. This expiration is followed by a plateau that reflects the cessation of dead space gases and the measurement of alveolar gas. At the end of the plateau is a sharp drop that reflects the inspiration of fresh gases with minimal carbon dioxide content.

When using the monitor, the clinician should recognize that a sharp rise indicates compromised exhalation. Partial plugged endotracheal tubes and dislodged tubes will change the angle of rise on the capnogram.[6] **The plateau phase of the capnogram can be altered by severe hypotension or decreased cardiac output, whereas a leak around the endotracheal tube will alter the slope of the drop of the waveform caused by entrainment of tracheal carbon dioxide.[6]**

Transcutaneaous Oxygen/Carbon Dioxide Monitoring

Skin oxygen tension ($TcPO_2$) and carbon dioxide tension ($TcPCO_2$) are measured by using one or two electrodes, depending on the model and brand of the monitor. The electrodes, once positioned on the skin, heat the area under the probe and cause certain physiologic changes as previously discussed. Oxygen and carbon dioxide that diffuse through the heated skin are measured by the electrode, and the value is digitally displayed on the monitor. If intervals between calibration are longer than 4 hours, the readings are subject to drift. The calibration procedures vary with the instruments used. Inherent in the calibration process is the necessity to change the position of the skin electrode on the infant. In the clinical setting the correlation of the $TcPO_2$ and PaO_2 has been reported to vary from $r = 0.84$ to as low as $r = 0.16$.[24] Better correlations are found when the instrument is calibrated every 4 hours, the temperature is set correctly, and the infant is well perfused and normothermic. If the temperature of the probe cannot be maintained at 43° to 44° C (109° to 111° F), a lower temperature should be selected to avoid possible burns. At a lower temperature the $TcPO_2$

---

*References 28, 29.

monitor can be used to monitor trends but should not be interpreted as actual arterial PaO$_2$ values. The range of accuracy of TcPO$_2$ monitors is limited; hypoxia (less than 40 mm Hg) and hyperoxia (more than 120 mm Hg) may not be accurately reflected.[26]

In an infant with suspected significant right-to-left shunting through a patent ductus arteriosus such as in persistent pulmonary hypertension, two transcutaneous oxygen electrodes can be placed on the infant: one preductally (right shoulder) and the other postductally (lower abdomen or legs). Significant right-to-left shunting through the patent ductus arteriosus is present when the preductal oxygen tension is significantly higher than the postductal oxygen tension.

The disadvantages of the use of transcutaneous monitoring are that the instrument requires frequent calibration, requires the use of a heated electrode, requires a 15-minute period after calibration to heat the skin to the correct temperature, and has a 15- to 20-second delay in the readings as compared with the patient's real-time values. The advantages are that it is not invasive, does not require the removal of blood for analysis, and displays a continuous readout of skin oxygen/carbon dioxide tensions.

Nursing Care of Infants With Noninvasive Transcutaneous Oxygen and Carbon Dioxide Monitors

The electrode can be placed on any portion of the infant's body as long as good contact between the electrode and the skin is maintained. **Uneven areas of skin such as skin over bones should be avoided because of poor contact between the membrane and the skin surface. The infant should not lie on the electrode. Placing the infant on top of the electrode increases the pressure on the underlying capillaries, thus affecting the flow of blood under the probe and resulting in a drop in TcPO$_2$ values. Because of the heat generated by the electrode (43° to 44° C), small red areas are produced on the infant's skin. To minimize trauma to the infant's skin, the electrode should be repositioned every 2 to 4 hours, depending on the infant's skin sensitivity.** Grouping of nursing interventions has resulted in minimizing the time that the infant receives less than optimal oxygenation.

Oxygen Saturation Monitoring by Pulse Oximetry

Oxygen saturation monitoring by pulse oximetry involves placing a small sensor on the infant in such a manner that the infant's finger, toe, foot, or wrist comes between the light source and the photoreceptor. The light source emits two wavelengths of light: red (660 nm) and infrared (940 nm). The difference between the absorption of the light is picked up by the receptor that is placed directly opposite the light source. The calculation of the ratio of oxyhemoglobin and deoxyhemoglobin is displayed as the percent of oxygen saturation. Key to accuracy of the monitor is the placement of the light source and the receptor must be directly opposite each other over an area in which a pulse can be detected.

The monitor does not require any heat source or warm-up period; nor does it require calibration or changing of the probe position. Oxygen saturation monitoring provides the care provider with continuous and instantaneous readout of the oxygen saturation in the infant. In comparison with a blood gas analyzer, which calculates the relative oxygen saturation based on established nomograms, the oxygen saturation monitor measures the actual saturation of the hemoglobin. **Calculated values using standard nomograms do not reflect shifts in the affinity of oxygen for hemoglobin based on changes in the patient's temperature, pH, PCO$_2$, or 2,3-DPG.**

The oxygen saturation monitor relies on adequate perfusion to the site and the ability to detect arterial pulsations; thus, if it is placed distal to a blood pressure cuff, there will be an inaccurate reading while the cuff is inflated. Newer models of pulse oximetry are in development that reduce the artifact that results from motion and low perfusion.[12] There may be incorrect readings when the probe is placed under or near infrared heat lamps and under phototherapy lamps.[2] The light from these external sources interferes with the light receptor on the infant's extremity. Newer neonatal probes have built-in external light source protectors that are not found on adult probes.

Oxygen saturation is more indicative of the total oxygen content of the blood than is PaO$_2$ and is the most sensitive to hypoxemia when it is on the steep part of the oxygen dissociation curve (see Figure 7-1). Keeping the SaO$_2$ at 90% to 92% will keep the infant in a normoxemic state under most conditions.

There are no complications associated with the use of oxygen saturation monitoring other than the potential for skin trauma caused by adhesive on the probe. Newer probes held in position by gentle elastic pressure have no adhesive touching the infant's skin.

Oxygen saturation monitoring by pulse oximetry is reliable and practical for use in infants over a wide range of birth weights and postnatal ages.[1,2,8,17,21] There is one report in recent literature of an infant with meconium-stained skin in whom pulse oximetry produced a false low reading because the meconium staining absorbed more red, thereby filtering the infrared light.[14] Poets et al[19] make a compelling argument for the use of both transcutaneous oxygen monitoring and pulse oximetry monitoring in critically ill neonates, because each monitor has its own shortcomings.

Cardiorespiratory Monitoring

The chest leads are applied in a triangular pattern on the infant's chest. Integrity of the leads must be ensured. Allowing the contact gel to dry or inadvertently dislodging the lead during procedures such as x-ray examination, echocardiography, and lumbar puncture may account for inaccurate tracings. Various components of the electrocardiogram (ECG) pattern may be diagnostically helpful. The QRS complex should be monitored for baseline height. A sudden decrease in QRS complex height that is not caused by artifact may be an indication of pneumothorax. The QT interval is helpful in diagnosing hypocalcemia in some infants. Other portions of the strip may be evaluated for electrolyte imbalance and possible cardiac ischemia. Changes registered on the visual display or strip recorder should be verified by a 12-lead ECG.

Blood Pressure Monitoring

Arterial pressure monitoring may be accomplished via the UAC attached to a transducer and monitor. Newer transducers require calibration only once daily. Central venous pressure monitoring may be carried out in the same manner. The same type of transducer may be used for either arterial or venous pressure recording.

Event Monitoring

The advancement of physiologic monitors with memory capability has enhanced the ability of the practitioner to review the physiologic status of the infant on multiple physiologic parameters for the past 24 to 48 hours. In many NICUs the monitor output is integrated into the electronic or computerized chart. This integration allows the care provider to "pull" the data from the monitors into the chart at preselected times either prospectively or retrospectively. When the monitors are programmed with critical value ranges, any deviation outside these ranges is noted as an "event," which can then be reviewed, tallied, or otherwise annotated. For care

providers at the bedside, the challenge is to keep iatrogenic events (such as lead removal, excessive activity of the infant, a stopcock turned the wrong direction) minimized such that the infant's record is as valid a reflection of its actual physiologic status as possible. Any circumstances noted at the time of the event that may produce false readings should be recorded so that when the infant's record is reviewed, these events can be placed in context of the circumstances at the time.

COMPLICATIONS*

UACs act as foreign bodies, causing fibrin deposition and thrombus formation around the catheter. Although most catheters are associated with thrombus formation, it is of clinical significance in less than 10% of patients. **The most common problem associated with major complications of UACs is ischemic disease resulting from emboli or spasms.[13] In such cases the catheter should be removed immediately, and heparin therapy should be considered. Although vasospasm is quite common, usually it does not require immediate removal of the catheter. Blue discoloration is seen rather than blanching. Obviously a hemorrhage may occur when the catheter slips out or when any of the various connections loosen. For reasons such as these, UACs require constant attention.**

If the extremities or buttocks blanch, the catheter should be removed immediately, and heparin therapy should be considered. To prevent bleeding once the catheter is removed, pressure should be applied immediately below the umbilicus. When the color has returned to the affected area and the infant is stable, replacement of the catheter can be considered. If vasospasm occurs in one leg or foot, apply warm wraps (diapers wet with warm water) to the opposite leg or apply wraps to the upper extremities, thereby producing a reflex vasodilation to the legs. Inherent in this action, however, is the hazard of obscuring recognition of compromise in that extremity. The wraps need to be reheated every 10 to 15 minutes until the spasm has resolved. The skin temperature of the infant must be greater than 36° C (96.8° F) for wraps to be effective. For infants with UACs, blood must be available for immediate transfusion.

UVCs may cause thrombi. Clots may form in the portal vessels, resulting in portal hypertension.

*References 11, 27.

Hepatic necrosis, gut ischemia, and hemorrhage have been associated with UVCs.[15]

PICC lines are associated with sepsis, occlusion, breakage, clotting, leaking, phlebitis, and peripheral edema.[4,9,22,25]

Transcutaneous blood gas monitoring may cause burns to the skin.

CONTROVERSIES

Complications involving high UAC placement (T8) are fewer but more severe than the complications involving low UAC placement (L3 to L4).[27] Prophylactic administration of antibiotic agents is not indicated. Use of the UAC for infusion of antibiotic agents, calcium, hyperalimentation solutions, or blood varies, and no definitive studies are available. Blood cultures can be drawn from the UAC for up to 6 hours after insertion. The use of heparin in the infusate is controversial. Practices vary widely, and definitive studies are lacking; however, it appears safe to feed infants enterally with a UAC in place.[7] Routine monitoring of all infants is the standard of care. Indwelling catheters for blood pressure monitoring have the advantage of continuous readout, but external cuffs are less invasive.

PARENT TEACHING

As for the many other invasive procedures in neonatology, the clinician obtains permission from the parents for umbilical vessel catheterization. This may be the clinician's first contact with the family and thus sets the atmosphere for future contacts. Although parents are initially hesitant about umbilical catheter placement, they are generally comforted to learn that it will result in a painless way of drawing blood. Before visiting the infant, parents need to be told what the umbilical catheter, transcutaneous monitors, cardiorespiratory monitors, and blood pressure monitors look like in place and what they are registering. Often parents are confused as to where the catheter goes once it enters the umbilicus and what the purpose of other monitoring devices is. Some parents are uncomfortable with the arm and leg restraints on their infant. It may be unwise for parents to hold their infant while an umbilical catheter is in place, because manipulating the infant may accidentally dislodge the catheter, and subsequently the infant may lose blood. Also, when the infant is being held out of the incubator and is wrapped in blankets, the integrity of the catheter and connections cannot be evaluated.

ACKNOWLEDGMENT

The authors appreciate the careful review of this chapter by Wanda Bradshaw, RN, MSN, PNP, NNP.

REFERENCES

1. Anderson JV: The accuracy of pulse oximetry in neonates: effects of fetal hemoglobin and bilirubin, *J Perinatol* 7:309, 1987.
2. Barrington JK, Finer NN, Ryan CA: Evaluation of pulse oximetry as a continuous monitoring technique in the critical care unit, *Crit Care Med* 16:1147, 1988.
3. Cassady G: Transcutaneous monitoring in the newborn infant, *J Pediatr* 103:837, 1987.
4. Chathas MK: Percutaneous central venous catheters in neonates, *J Obstet Gynecol Neonatal Nurs* 15:324, 1986
5. Comer DM: Pulse oximetry implications for practice, *Obstet Gynecol Neonatal Nurs* 21:35, 1992.
6. Cote CJ, Ryan JF: *A practice of anesthesia for infants and children,* Philadelphia, 1993, WB Saunders.
7. Davey AM, Wagner CL, Cox C et al: Feeding premature infants while low umbilical catheters are in place: a prospective, randomized trial, *J Pediatr* 124:795, 1994.
8. Emery JR: Skin pigmentation as an influence on the accuracy of pulse oximetry, *J Perinatol* 7:329, 1987.
9. Evans M, Lentsch D: Percutaneously inserted polyurethane central catheters in the NICU: one unit's experience, *Neonatal Netw* 18:37, 1999.
10. Fazlollah TM: End-tidal carbon dioxide monitoring may help diagnosis of H-type tracheoesophageal fistula, *Anesthesiology* 83:878, 1995.
11. Fletcher MA, Brown DR, Landers S et al: Umbilical arterial catheter use: report of an audit conducted by the Study Group For Complications of Perinatal Care, *Am J Perinatol* 11:94, 1994.
12. Goldstein MR, Martin GI, Sindel BD et al: Novel pulse oximetry technology resistant to noise artifact and low perfusion: "the neonatal model," *Am J Respir Crit Care Med* 155:A717, 1997.
13. Hogan MJ: Neonatal vascular catheters and their complications, *Radiol Clin North Am* 37:1109 1999.
14. Johnson N, Johnson VA, Bannister J et al: The effect of meconium on neonatal and fetal reflectance pulse oximetry, *J Perinat Med* 18:351, 1990.
15. McEvedy BA, McCloud ME, Kirpilani H et al: End-tidal CO_2 measurements in critically ill neonates: a comparison of side-stream and mainstream capnometers, *Can J Anaesth* 37:322, 1990.
16. Meredith KS, Monaco FJ: Evaluation of a mainstream capnometer and end-tidal carbon dioxide monitoring in mechanically ventilated infants, *Pediatr Pulmonol* 9:254, 1990.

17. Mower WR, Sachs C, Nicklin EL et al: Pulse oximetry as a fifth pediatric vital sign, *Pediatrics* 99:681, 1997.
18. Paige PL: Noninvasive monitoring of the neonatal respiratory system, *Clin Issues Crit Care Nurs* 1:416, 1990.
19. Poets CF, Southall DP: Noninvasive monitoring of oxygenation in infants and children: practical consideration and areas of concern, *Pediatrics* 93:737, 1994.
20. Racadio JM, Doellman DA, Johnson ND et al: Pediatric peripherally inserted central catheters: complication rates related to catheter tip location, *Pediatrics* 107:28, 2001.
21. Ramanathan R, Durand M, Larrazabal C: Pulse oximetry in very low birth weight infants with acute and chronic lung disease, *Pediatrics* 79:612, 1987.
22. Rastogi S, Bhutada A, Sahni R et al: Spontaneous correction of the malpositioned percutaneous central venous catheter, *Pediatr Radiol* 28:694, 1998.
23. Rejjal AR, Galal MO, Nazer HM et al: Complications of parenteral nutrition via umbilical vein catheter, *Eur J Pediatr* 152:624, 1993.
24. Rooth G, Huch A, Huch R: Transcutaneous oxygen monitors are reliable indicators of arterial oxygen tension (if used correctly), *Pediatrics* 79:283, 1987.
25. Trotter CW: Percutaneous central venous catheters in neonates: A descriptive analysis and evaluation of predictors of sepsis, *J Perinat Neonatal Nurs* 10:56, 1996.
26. Turner BS: Nursing procedures. In Askin DF, ed: *Acute respiratory care of the neonate,* Petaluma, Calif, 1997, NICU.
27. Umbilical Artery Catheter Trial Study Group: Relationship of intraventricular hemorrhage or death with the level of umbilical artery catheter placement: a multicenter randomized clinical trial, *Pediatrics* 90:881, 1992.
28. Watkins AMC, Weindling AM: Monitoring of end-tidal CO_2 in neonatal intensive care, *Arch Dis Child* 62:837, 1987.
29. Weingarten M: Respiratory monitoring of carbon dioxide and oxygen: a ten year perspective, *J Clin Monit* 6(3):217, 1990.

8

Diagnostic Imaging in the Neonate

John D. Strain, Rita T. Keuten

Imaging has become an important part of the diagnosis and work-up of medical problems of newborns. The ability to use a noninvasive means to diagnose disease, screen for potential pathologic conditions, monitor the effects of therapy, and assist in defining the prognosis for counseling has made imaging an essential part of health care. With refinements in diagnostic equipment and capabilities, the role of imaging has expanded significantly in recent years. There are many ways to assess any problem, and the vast potential of the new imaging modalities makes appropriate imaging a constant challenge (Table 8-1). The boom in technology has meant the introduction of new modalities as well as added sophistication to established modalities. Nearly 60% of diagnostic imaging involves modalities that weren't even available 20 years ago.

There are many excellent reference books and textbooks on neonatal imaging, and specific questions can be most adequately addressed through these resources. Our goal is to acquaint readers with the various imaging modalities available for diagnosis and intervention. A short summary of each imaging modality includes background information, a discussion of image acquisition, and the risks and benefits of each. We have provided a thumbnail description of each modality; however, for clarity we have taken significant liberty and license in discussing the physics of image acquisition. Each section addresses the most common usage of the modality in neonates, followed by a focused discussion of one or two aspects of image interpretation.

Because there may be more than one appropriate way to evaluate any given problem, it is essential to understand the inherent advantages and limitations of each modality to decide which might be most effective. We have pointed out some of the challenges associated with diagnostic imaging. A focused problem-solving approach with appropriate collaboration and consultation can yield positive results.

X-RAY

Background

The 1896 introduction of the roentgenogram was met with great enthusiasm and quickly became an indispensable diagnostic tool in clinical settings throughout the world. Until 25 years ago the field of radiology was based almost exclusively on use of the x-ray.

A beam of ionizing radiation from a source (x-ray tube) passes through the patient, and various structures within the body interact to attenuate the x-ray before it is received on the other side. The x-rays pass through the patient, then expose a film, just as light exposes a negative in black and white film photography. The film is developed, and the resultant image (radiograph) is a map that corresponds to the transmitted x-ray (that portion of the x-ray not attenuated by absorption or scattered as it passes through the patient). Somewhat analogous to the shadows that result from objects in the sun, the images from x-ray are a reflection of the object being x-rayed. (Hence the slang term "Shadow Doctor" came into use in reference to early radiologists.) Bone attenuates a greater amount of the x-ray (or allows for the penetration of fewer x-rays) than lung tissue does; this results in a film on which the rib is white and the lung black. In some ways this can be compared with the different shadows cast by the trunk of a tree from that of its leaves. With x-ray the spatial resolution is exquisite, although the contrast resolution is lacking. One can capture between 10 and 20 line pairs per millimeter with film radiography, although **only five different densities can be routinely distinguished: air, fat, water (which includes all solid viscera—liver, spleen, kidney, pancreas, and heart), bone, and metal.**

The most recent development in x-ray technology is computed radiography (CR) and direct radiography (DR). Although the physics of x-ray generation

Table 8-1	COMPARATIVE ANALYSIS OF IMAGING MODALITIES					
	IONIZING RADIATION	SPATIAL RESOLUTION	CONTRAST RESOLUTION	COST	SEDATION	MISCELLANEOUS
X-ray	Very low	Excellent	Fair	Low	Never	Very fast acquisition eliminates motion
Fluoroscopy	Low	Excellent	Fair	Moderate	Never	Evaluate motion real-time
Ultrasonography	None	Good	Fair	Moderate	Never	Portable; evaluate motion real-time
CT	Low	Good	Good	Moderate to high	Sometimes	Cross-sectional imaging
MRI	None	Good	Excellent	High	Frequent	Multi-planar (i.e., in multiple planes) imaging, flowing blood without contrast
Nuclear medicine	Very low	Poor	Excellent	Moderate to high	Sometimes	Physiologic imaging

is essentially the same, the receiver has changed. With CR a phosphorescent plate replaces film, and the latent image can be either exposed to film or captured digitally. With DR the image is directly captured in a digital mode. The introduction of these products was driven by the desire to capture, archive, distribute, and display digital images.

Clinical Utility in the Neonatal Setting

Chest x-rays are most commonly used to evaluate the heart and lungs. Abdominal imaging allows one to assess the solid viscera (the liver, spleen, and kidneys) as well as the bowel gas pattern, useful in evaluating a neonate with a feeding intolerance (Figure 8-1). Bones of the trunk and extremities are easily assessed with plain film radiology.

In addition to helping to determine a specific diagnosis, imaging is frequently a valuable means for assessing patient response to therapy. For instance, lung compliance and volume, as assessed by x-ray film, helps determine the patient's response to various ventilator rates and pressures. The x-ray findings can therefore be very useful in the selection of the most appropriate ventilator settings. X-rays also make it possible to visualize the appropriate locations of lines and tubes. Many endotracheal, feeding, and thoracostomy tubes as well as PICC lines and other devices are marked with radiopaque stripes that make it possible to localize them in the patient.

Focused Discussion: Chest Radiographs

The most common use of x-ray imaging in the neonatal unit is for evaluation of the chest, to help define abnormalities that might contribute

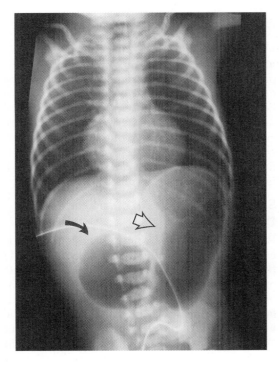

FIGURE 8-1 Frontal chest and abdomen show gaseous distention of the stomach *(open arrow)* and duodenal bulb *(curved arrow)*, the classic double bubble seen in duodenal atresia. Incidental note is made of thirteen pairs of ribs in this patient with Down syndrome.

to respiratory distress. Respiratory distress in newborns can be divided into three categories: conditions that are managed medically, those that are managed surgically, and iatrogenic respiratory distress.

Table 8-2	MEDICALLY MANAGED CAUSES OF RESPIRATORY DISTRESS IN THE NEWBORN (CHIMP DIFFERENTIAL)					
		GESTATIONAL AGE	HEART SIZE	LUNG VOLUME	NATURE OF INFILTRATE	PROGRESSION	ANCILLARY FINDINGS
C	Congenital heart disease		Increased	Normal or increased	Increased pulmonary vascularity or edema	Stable or progressive	Abnormal situs, aortic discordance
H	Hyaline membrane disease	Less than 36 weeks		Decreased	Diffuse granular with air bronchograms	Progressive over first 24 hours	No pleural effusions or body wall edema
I	Immature lung	Less than 26 weeks	Normal	Decreased	Diffuse granular	Progressive	Absent thymus from stress
M	Meconium aspiration	39 weeks or greater	Normal	Increased	Streaky and patchy	Stable	Air leak (i.e., pneumothorax)
P	Neonatal pneumonia		Normal or increased		Either diffuse or focal		Pleural effusions and body wall edema

Medically Managed Respiratory Distress

Table 8-2 summarizes plain film diagnosis of respiratory distress in newborns. Use of this approach takes advantage of the fact that there are only a limited number of changes that can be identified radiographically, and a constellation of findings can define a specific group of etiologic factors. A systematic analysis of these various characteristics helps to determine a specific group that has a fairly limited differential diagnosis (Box 8-1).

Surgically Managed Respiratory Distress

Respiratory conditions that are managed surgically can be subdivided into three groups: (1) those associated with aspiration, such as cleft palate, laryngeal cleft, or tracheoesophageal fistula; (2) those that compromise functional lung volume including congenital diaphragmatic hernia (CDH), congenital lobar emphysema (Figure 8-2), and congenital cystic adenomatoid malformation (CCAM); and (3) structures associated with tracheal or bronchial narrowing, such as a double aortic arch, congenital tracheal stenosis, and bronchogenic cyst.

Iatrogenic Respiratory Distress

Most iatrogenic respiratory distress results from either a misplaced catheter or tube or from barotrauma. An endotracheal tube (ETT) can be placed too deep and will preferentially ventilate only a single lung. An ETT may even be inadvertently placed into the esophagus, resulting in inadequate ventila-

Box 8-1	CHIMP DIFFERENTIAL

Congenital heart disease
    Transient tachypnea of the newborn (resolves over first 24 hours)
    Extracardiac shunts
Hyaline membrane disease*
    Diffuse atelectasis
Immature lung
    Represents anectasis rather than atelectasis
Meconium aspiration
    Amniotic fluid aspiration
Pneumonia
    Diffuse
        Birth asphyxia
    Focal
        Pulmonary hemorrhage
Bronchopulmonary dysplasia (BPD) represents the chronic lung disease that may result from any of the causes of respiratory distress.

*The use of exogenous surfactant modifies the picture of HMD significantly. The irregular distribution after endotracheal administration causes a much less uniform infiltrate, and the patchy pattern that results has a look that is similar to meconium aspiration, which might be seen in a term or postterm infant.

tion (Figure 8-3), which is further compromised by distention of the esophagus and small bowel limiting lung expansion.

Air leaks are considered to result from barotrauma (Figure 8-4). Although barotrauma occurs much less frequently since the introduction of exogenous surfactant and high-frequency ventilation, air leaks continue to be a problem that causes significant

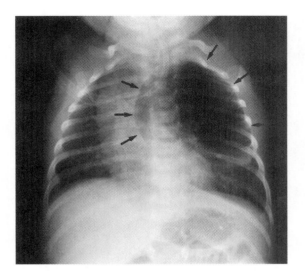

FIGURE 8-2   Frontal view of the chest shows a hyperaerated lucent left upper lobe *(small arrows)* associated with mediastinal shift from left to right and is characteristic of congenital lobar emphysema.

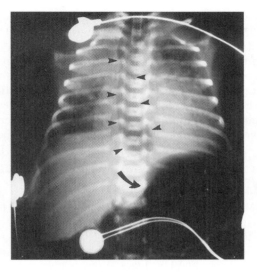

FIGURE 8-3   Frontal chest. Although the endotracheal tube projects over the midline mediastinum near the thoracic inlet, the dilated esophagus *(arrowheads)* and distended stomach *(arrow)* associated with right upper lobe and left lower lobe atelectasis suggested esophageal intubation, which was diagnosed in this patient.

A

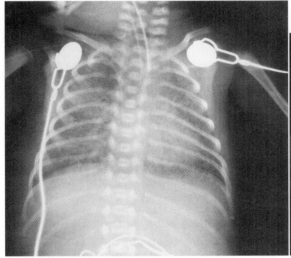

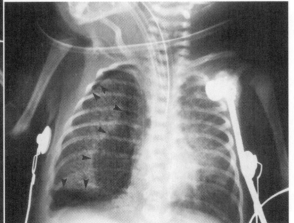

B

FIGURE 8-4   **A,** Frontal chest. Hyaline membrane disease in this patient is defined by the diffuse symmetric granular infiltrates with small lung volumes. This patient required intubation, and the endotracheal tube tip projects in satisfactory position. **B,** Follow-up examination in the same patient demonstrates linear lucencies within the right lung resulting from pulmonary interstitial emphysema. A tension pneumothorax *(arrowheads)* is identified on the right with mild mediastinal shift from right to left. The lack of atelectasis on the right is the result of extremely poor lung compliance that accompanies pulmonary interstitial emphysema. The endotracheal tube tip projects in satisfactory position, but the nasogastric tube is in the mid esophagus.

concern. Appropriate ventilation management requires timely and accurate diagnosis. One goal in review of a chest x-ray film is to define the location of the extrapulmonary gas. **Abnormal extrapulmonary gas can include any one or a combination of the following: pulmonary interstitial emphysema, subcutaneous emphysema, pneumomediastinum, pneumothorax, pneumopericardium, pneumocardia, and portal venous gas.**

FLUOROSCOPY

Background

In fluoroscopy an x-ray tube similar to that used for plain film radiography is used. The x-ray is generated in the same manner as in plain film, but it is received in most cases by a camera that is similar to a TV camera or VCR. Fluoroscopy allows real-time evaluation of a patient and can be performed with or without contrast material. Spatial resolution in fluoroscopy is not as good as that of plain film radiography, but it is still excellent. Contrast resolution is about the same: air, fat, water, and bone are about the only densities that can be separated. A contrast medium given orally, per rectum, instilled into the urinary bladder, or given intravenously provides various compounds that attenuate the radiation beam to a variable extent related to physical properties and thickness of the attenuator. Most contrast agents are compounds that use either inert barium or iodine as the attenuator of the radiation beam. **The most important characteristic of fluoroscopic imaging is the ability to evaluate motion in real-time. This is an essential in the evaluation of swallowing function, gastrointestinal (GI) peristalsis, and diaphragmatic motion.**

Clinical Utility in the Neonatal Setting

The most common fluoroscopic examinations requested for neonates include the upper gastrointestinal series (upper GI, or UGI), the contrast enema, and voiding cystourethrography. The upper GI is useful in the evaluation of swallowing, aspiration, feeding intolerance, vomiting, and abdominal distention with possible bowel obstruction.

A contrast enema can be diagnostic in Hirschsprung's disease (Figure 8-5). It can be both diagnostic and therapeutic in meconium plug syndrome and meconium ileus.

A voiding cystourethrogram is used to evaluate the urinary bladder and the urethra and to look for vesicoureteral reflux (Figure 8-6), which is associ-

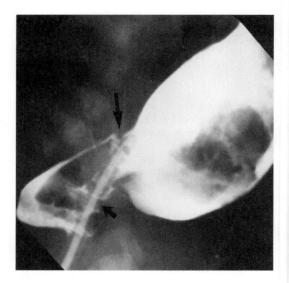

FIGURE 8-5 A lateral film from the early filling phase of a barium enema demonstrates spasm of the distal rectal segment *(small arrow)* with a transition zone to dilated colon *(long arrow)*. These findings are characteristic of colonic Hirschsprung's disease.

ated with urinary tract infection. Vesicoureteral reflux is a common cause of hydronephrosis, which is now frequently identified during prenatal ultrasonography. Ureteroceles, periureteral diverticulae, and posterior urethral valves can all be associated with hydronephrosis in the neonatal period and all can be demonstrated with cystourethrography.

Air works as a fine contrast agent, and fluoroscopic evaluation of the nasal and oral airway as well as the trachea and proximal bronchus can be easily performed fluoroscopically. Because the diaphragm is immediately adjacent to aerated lung, diaphragmatic motion and its relationship to inspiratory effort help in the evaluation of phrenic nerve injury and diaphragmatic paralysis. Eventration of the diaphragm can also be evaluated fluoroscopically.

Focused Discussion: Upper GI Series

Indications for performing a UGI include swallowing dysfunction, aspiration, vomiting, choking, and apnea. An appropriately performed UGI offers a systematic approach to the upper gastrointestinal tract. Starting with the patient in a left-side-down recumbent position, deglutition is evaluated. Tongue action, transport, nasopharyngeal regurgitation, aspiration, and laryngeal penetration can all

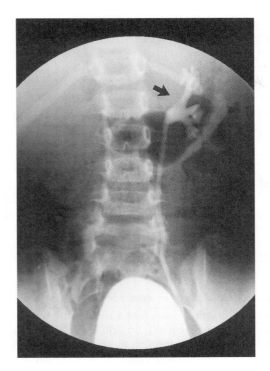

FIGURE 8-6 Frontal view from a voiding cystourethrogram demonstrates grade II vesicoureter on the left *(arrow)*.

be assessed. The right-side-down position better separates the esophagus and the tracheal air column; however, if this position is used routinely for the patient, the stomach may empty, filling the proximal small bowel and obscuring the location of the ligament of Treitz. The left-side-down position allows one to evaluate swallowing without concern that the stomach may empty prematurely. Once deglutition is satisfactorily evaluated, one can concentrate on the esophagus. Vascular rings and slings are evaluated in both the frontal and lateral positions.

Esophageal atresia is usually diagnosed clinically; plain film observation of intraluminal bowel gas defines the most common form, which is associated with a distal tracheal esophageal fistula. The benefit of a proximal pouch study in esophageal atresia is controversial. There is a small incidence of fistula from the proximal pouch to the trachea; this incidence is independent of the presence or absence of a distal fistula. If the surgical approach to esophageal atresia repair includes direct visualization of the proximal pouch, the pouch contrast study

is superfluous. If on the other hand esophagoscopy is not routinely performed, there is some value in evaluating the proximal pouch before surgery. In the absence of esophageal atresia, the location of the fistula (H type) is at the thoracic inlet. This is higher than the fistula that occurs in the most common form of esophageal atresia, in which the fistula is at the level of the carina.

The caliber of the esophagus is informative, because it is usually dilated in association with significant gastroesophageal reflux. Esophageal contour, mucosal detail, and peristalsis are assessed. The configuration of the gastroesophageal junction can indicate gastroesophageal reflux, and rare hiatal hernias can be diagnosed. Gastric emptying is evaluated and gastric peristalsis examined. Because the rotation and fixation of the bowel have important consequences in the newborn period, this is an important part of a complete exam. The duodenal bulb, C-loop, and ligament of Treitz are defined. The lateral film is essential in localizing the ligament of Treitz. For proximal bowel rotation and fixation to be considered normal, the duodenal jejunal junction (ligament of Treitz) must be retroperitoneal and therefore posterior, to the left of the spine, and at the level of the retroperitoneal portion of the second portion of the duodenum (just distal to the duodenal bulb).

Because the rotation of the proximal bowel may be independent of the rotation of the hindgut, and therefore if the clinical question is malrotation and possible volvulus, the UGI is the examination of choice. The caliber, contour, and fold pattern of the proximal bowel are evaluated and the transit time observed. This simple, systematic, yet comprehensive approach to an upper GI series yields a tremendous amount of information.

ULTRASONOGRAPHY

Background

One of the first applications of ultrasound (US) was in the 1912 search for the Titanic. Although that initial search was unsuccessful, the basic imaging principles of diagnostic US are the same as those used by Bouchard in finding the Titanic and later in his search for Noah's ark. Medical US found its roots in *so*und *na*vigation and *r*anging (SONAR) developed during World War II.

In medical US a transducer (essentially a piezoelectric crystal) converts electrons into mechanical vibration that create high frequency sound waves within the body. The same transducer serves as both the transmitter of the sound wave and the receiver of the reflected sound. Within the body these high-frequency sound waves propagate through the soft tissues until they meet a reflective surface that reflects some of those fluid waves back to the transducer. The percent of the sound beam reflected relates to the difference in the acoustic impedance of the material being evaluated. When the acoustic impedance of material is similar, as is the case with the abdominal wall musculature—the liver and the kidney, for example—most of the sound is transmitted and a small percent reflected at each interface. As the sound beam travels through the abdominal wall to the liver, the abdominal wall–liver interface reflects the beam and transmits it through the liver to the liver-kidney interface. The small difference in acoustic impedance between the liver and kidney causes the reflection of some of the beam and transmission of most to the posterior abdominal wall. This allows the visualization of multiple interfaces that are deep to the first structure encountered. If the velocity of the sound beam in tissue is known, the distance to the reflective surface can be estimated by measuring the time it takes for the pulse to travel the distance to and back from the object imaged.

Most of the tissues in the body have similar acoustic impedance; however, air has extremely low impedance and bone extremely high impedance. This means that there is a big difference in the acoustic impedance between these substances and the organs most commonly imaged. **For this reason both bone and air reflect nearly all of the sound that reaches them. This is why a coupling gel is used on the skin surface to eliminate the air gap between the transducer and the skin.** This is also why imaging through the liver gives a good acoustic window to deeper structures, but bowel gas obscures imaging lower in the abdomen. For ultrasonographic imaging of the brain in a neonate, the anterior fontanel serves as the acoustic window because the bone of the skull acts as a reflective surface that severely limits thorough transmission of US to deeper structures. Bulk fluid within the body, such as urine in the urinary bladder, bile in the gall bladder, or CSF in the ventricles, has no internal interfaces and therefore is seen as solid black on conventional US. Cysts have a sharp posterior wall and have increased through transmission, because the sound wave penetrates the fluid without any reflections to block transmission of the sound.

Doppler ultrasonography takes advantage of the physical principle that the US reflection from a moving object distorts the wavelength and the distortion is related to the velocity of the object being measured. This is the principle that causes the pitch of a train whistle to change from high to low as a train passes an observer. It is the same principle used by police in monitoring the speed of cars and baseball teams use with the Judd gun to measure the velocity of a pitcher's fastball.

One of the major advantages of US is the lack of ionizing radiation. Although most diagnostic imaging, which requires ionizing radiation, is of low dose, any radiation exposure is a concern and should be avoided when possible. The portability of ultrasonographic equipment has made it a valuable adjuvant to the diagnostic imaging in the neonatal intensive care setting.

Clinical Utility in the Neonatal Setting

Ultrasonography has had a major impact in the evaluation of the neonatal brain. Most of the early work focused on intracranial hemorrhage, which was a common occurrence in preterm neonates. Even though the incidence has decreased, intracranial hemorrhage remains an issue for which US is extremely well suited. Ultrasonographic instrumentation has improved tremendously, and with the addition of color and pulse Doppler technology, great strides have been made in the refinement and sophistication of intracranial imaging. Numerous complex structural abnormalities can be recognized, and screening for developmental abnormalities can largely be accommodated with intracranial ultrasonography. Because bone reflects most of the sound-limiting through-transmission, the open fontanel is the window to the brain. As the fontanel closes over time, ultrasonography becomes less and less useful for intracranial imaging. This same limitation affects the utility of ultrasonographic evaluation of the spine as the patient ages.

Renal imaging offers another major role for ultrasonography in the neonatal unit. The kidneys are well visualized ultrasonographically, either through a posterior approach or more commonly using the liver or spleen as soft tissue acoustic windows to the kidneys. Ultrasonography is an excellent way to evaluate hydronephrosis, which is now frequently picked up on routine prenatal evaluations. Ultrasonography has a role in the evaluation of a jaundiced patient, because it is ideal for evaluating cystic structures, such as the gallbladder, and can readily define dilated biliary ducts. Jaundice caused by biliary obstruction from a choledochal cyst, for instance, can be readily defined ultrasonographically. Because of the reflectivity related to bone and bowel gas, US is much more effective in the upper abdomen, where the liver and spleen serve as the acoustic windows, or in the pelvis, where the urinary bladder can function as the window.

Even though US is reflected by bone, it has a significant role in the evaluation of the hips in the neonate. Because the capital femoral epiphysis is cartilage in the newborn, the hip can be well imaged in a neonate. Maternal estrogen causes ligamentous laxity. This changes significantly during the first weeks of life; therefore the accuracy of hip ultrasonographic examinations improves after the first 3 to 4 weeks. Ultrasonography is very good for the detection of developmental dysplasia of the hip and can be used to evaluate the degree of femoral head coverage, the acetabular angle, and any instability of the hip.

Focused Discussion: Cranial Ultrasonography

Ultrasonography is an ideal tool for evaluating the brain in a newborn. **In general, an ultrasonographic examination is the first step in the imaging evaluation for any neurologic question. Structural abnormalities, intracranial hemorrhage, sequelae of anoxia or ischemia events and infection are all well assessed via US.** The most common approach is through the anterior fontanel but additional information can be gained with axial imaging through the squamosa of the temporal bone. The posterior fossa can be evaluated through the posterior lateral fontanel. Familiarity with the normal anatomy is essential. Coronal and parasagittal views are generally obtained. Normal structures can be easily recognized; their absence or deformity is key to defining developmental abnormalities of the brain. The ventricular size and configuration are assessed. Characteristic ventricular configurations can define lobar or semilobar holoprosencephaly. In addition, the ventricular configuration can suggest septooptic dysplasia, or agenesis of the corpus callosum. The corpus callosum can be readily visualized; abnormalities of the corpus callosum are commonly associated with Chiari malformation and other structural abnormalities of the brain, such as Dandy-Walker malformation. **Dilatation of one or**

more of the ventricles can be an indication of a pathologic condition. An obstruction of CSF flow in the region of the aqueduct of Sylvius would manifest with disparity in ventricular size. The third and lateral ventricles might be enlarged, whereas the fourth ventricle remains normal in size. **Dilatation of one of the lateral ventricles especially when associated with an area of porencephaly is indicative of an in utero destructive event.**

Seizures or apnea may indicate an anoxic or ischemic event in a neonate. Certain structural abnormalities can suggest a specific diagnosis. Periventricular nodules and cortical tubers, for instance, define tuberous sclerosis. US is less sensitive than CT and MRI in defining subtle areas of gray matter heterotopia or focal pachygyria, examples of developmental abnormalities associated with seizures. **US is very sensitive to intracranial hemorrhage and areas of increased echogenicity can be demonstrated in areas of edema.** Increased sulcal echogenicity is suggestive of meningitis, and encephalitis results in increased parenchymal echogenicity which is a manifestation of localized brain swelling.

Intracranial hemorrhage is generally a concern in a premature neonate (Figure 8-7). It is classified into four grades, with each grade generally associated with a prognosis. Grade I hemorrhage usually has a good outcome, whereas the prognosis with grade IV hemorrhage is usually poor. Grade I hemorrhage is confined to germinal matrix in the caudothalamic groove. This is the last fetal germinal matrix to mature and is prone to hemorrhage in preterm babies. Grade II intraventricular hemorrhage (IVH) has intraventricular blood. Grade III hemorrhage is associated with ventricular dilatation as the intraventricular clot enlarges the lateral ventricles. Grade IV hemorrhage must demonstrate parenchymal extension. It has been hypothesized that grade IV hemorrhage may be the result of venous infarction that occurs from obstruction of the septal veins by the swollen germinal matrix hemorrhage. **Periventricular leukomalacia is a consequence of anoxic or ischemic injury to the brain that manifests as increased echogenicity in the deep periventricular white matter of the centrum semiovale. This may progress to cavitation and is then called *cystic leukoencephalomalacia*.** Ultrasonographic examination is a very sensitive way to detect this change, which is usually apparent within about 2 weeks of birth.

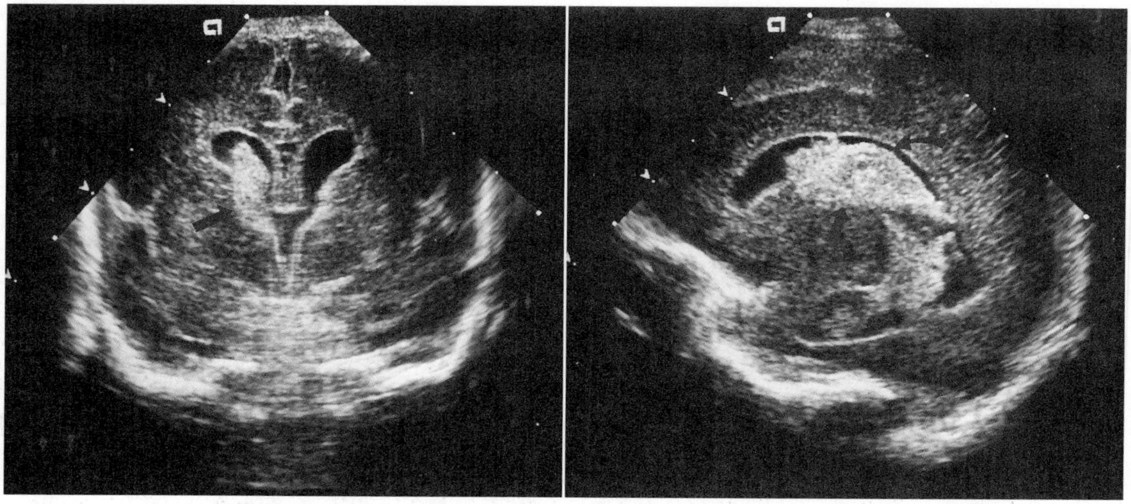

FIGURE 8-7 Coronal **(A)** and parasagittal **(B)** ultrasound images from a cranial ultrasound demonstrate an echogenic clot *(arrows)* within the dilated right ventricle. The intraventricular clot with ventricular dilatation defines a grade III hemorrhage.

COMPUTED TOMOGRAPHY

Computed axial tomography (CAT, or more frequently, CT) was initially developed in 1972 in Middlesex, England. Image acquisition takes place with a fairly sophisticated algorithm that interprets projections made by x-rays taken from multiple different positions around a single axial plane. These multiple projections are analyzed and composite image developed. **In essence a series of multiple x-rays from various angles are obtained in a single imaging plane. This renders a cross-sectional slice that can show all of the structures within that slice.** For instance, a slice through the upper abdomen may show the liver, spleen, pancreas, both kidneys, and the spine, each separated by a plane of fat and each with a subtly different density.

Spiral CT imaging, which is most commonly used today, allows a gantry to continuously rotate while the table translates through the scanning plane, generating a data set resembling a coil spring around the body. Multidetector arrays are now available by which four and even more image planes can be acquired simultaneously, significantly reducing the time required to obtain a complete image. Eliminating the mechanical movement of the tube and detectors allows the fastest image acquisition. In this system, the x-ray beam is focused through all of the various angles of the slice by electromagnetic manipulation of the beam to a circular array of detectors. A single slice can be acquired in less than 0.2 seconds, in essence stopping motion from interfering with image acquisition.

The radiation dose with CT is significantly higher than that of plain film imaging. The sophistication, utility, and availability of CT have raised concern related to the possible consequences to a population of increased radiation exposure. CT now accounts for more that 40% of the radiation exposure from medical imaging in the United States. When CT is used appropriately, there should be little concern about the low-dose radiation exposure used in medical imaging. However, it is prudent to be aware of the potential adverse effects of unnecessary radiation exposure to a vulnerable population (e.g., neonates). Unnecessary risk can be minimized if one limits the use of ionizing radiation to instances in which imaging is appropriate. The possibilities of noninvasive diagnosis are tremendous, and it would be inappropriate to allow the fear of radiation exposure to dissuade or discourage appropriate use of imaging. Scan times now are so short that imaging can be acquired in almost any age-group. **Radiation dose can be decreased significantly in the neonatal setting because the low tissue density of the neonate allows acceptable imaging at low radiation exposure.**

Common Utility in the Neonatal Intensive Care Setting

Cranial imaging is the most common use of CT in most neonatal intensive care settings. CT adds significant specificity to the abnormalities recognized with ultrasonography. Concern about ionizing radiation and the fact that CT equipment is generally not portable make obtaining a CT film more difficult than obtaining a sonogram. **CT is more accurate in assessing extraaxial fluid collections and is very helpful in further defining structural abnormalities of the brain, particularly those associated with abnormal distribution of gray or white matter. It is also very good for evaluating intracranial hemorrhage and infection.** Exquisite bone detail defines craniofacial anomalies, choanal atresia and stenosis, and abnormalities of the petrous bone associated with hearing loss. Chest imaging is becoming much more frequent in the NICU. It is used to evaluate abnormalities detected during intrauterine ultrasonographic examination and for potential surgical lesions identified on chest x-ray films. **Ultrasonography remains the first diagnostic tool for the evaluation of kidneys, liver, and spleen, but when a pathologic condition of the abdomen is a concern and a good acoustic window for US is not available, CT is frequently the examination of choice. CT can be performed with significantly less sedation than that required for MRI. CT eliminates many of the artifacts, including those of vascular flow, respiratory motion, and even bowel peristalsis, that limit the utility of MRI.** Skeletal lesions are well visualized with CT. Ultrasonography is the first method of choice in the evaluation of congenital hip dysplasia, but CT can be very helpful in evaluating the position of the femoral heads following reduction and treatment of congenital hip dysplasia when the patient is immobilized in a plaster cast.

CT can be very helpful in identifying the organ of origin of a specific pathologic condition. This of course is the first step in narrowing a differential diagnosis. The addition of intravenous contrast is very useful in defining tumor thrombus in renal arteries and inferior vena cava, which may affect surgical approach to renal and hepatic neoplasm. The nature of abnormalities seen on CT can frequently lead to a specific diagnosis. **Although the spatial resolution of CT is inferior to plain film radiography, the contrast resolution is significantly better and CT has taken advantage of this trade-off. Acquisition time for CT is much slower than that of radiogra-**

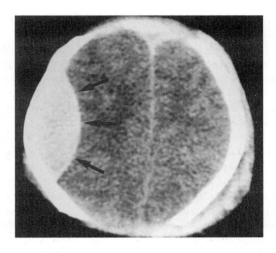

FIGURE 8-8   A single axial image near the vertex demonstrates a high-density lenticular mass *(arrows)* in the extraaxial space over the right cerebral cortex. The lenticular configuration is that of an epidural fluid collection and the high-density characteristic of acute hemorrhage.

phy and therefore motion artifact is more of a problem. The cross-sectional rendition of anatomy, which allows deep structures to be distinguished from one another, is the most significant advantage that CT has over radiography.

Focused Discussion: Intracranial Blood

CT is extremely sensitive and specific for the detection and localization of intracranial blood (Figure 8-8). Acute blood has a density (measured in Hounsfield numbers) higher than any normal structure except bone. The increased contrast resolution that is available through CT allows for the separation of gray matter from white matter, which affords detailed structural evaluation of the brain. The ventricles are low in density (0 Hounsfield units of water), the white matter more dense, and the gray matter more dense still, followed by acute blood and finally calcium of bone. Acute blood is visualized as white as soon as a clot is formed, and this high density will slowly decrease in density over time. By 2 to 3 weeks, for instance, the acute blood in a subdural hematoma will become lower and lower density until it assumes a density indistinguishable from water, which is equal to CSF in the ventricular system. MRI has the ability to differentiate blood from a chronic subdural hematoma for a longer time interval than CT because the protein within a chronic subdural hematoma modifies the signal on MRI for a long period of time.

Although all intracranial blood does change density over time, the compartment in which the blood is found affects the rate of change to some extent. Therefore the timing of an event responsible for the blood cannot be precisely determined based on the density alone. The location of the blood is the next issue. **CT is the most accurate imaging method for detection of subarachnoid blood.** The presence of subarachnoid blood is common even after a relatively nontraumatic birth. Unfortunately, on rare occasions subarachnoid blood can cause vasospasm of vessels near the skull base, which can result in relative ischemia or hypoperfusion of the peripheral cortex. Areas of edema can be detected by looking for loss of the normal gray-white differentiation or by finding a focal area of brain edema characterized by an area of relatively low density caused by the addition of the low-density water to an otherwise normal area of brain.

The shape of a collection of blood is an important variable used in evaluating intracranial hemorrhage. Subarachnoid blood assumes a configuration that follows the arachnoid space. Therefore it is most frequently seen in the suprasellar cistern, the ambient cistern, the sylvian fissure, the interhemispheric fissure, or layering on the tentorium. The most sensitive locations for identifying subarachnoid blood are in the region of the quadragerminal plate cistern, the posterior aspect of the third ventricle, and the interpeduncular cistern. **Subdural hematomas occur most frequently over the convexities or along the interhemispheric fissure.** Those over the convexity can be differentiated from epidural hematomas by their crescentic configuration. This is opposed to the lenticular configuration of an epidural hematoma. The dura is the periosteum of the inner table of the skull; therefore an epidural hematoma is limited by the adhesion of the periosteum to the skull and hence the lenticular configuration. This is also why epidural hematomas are most often associated with the higher-pressure arterial bleeding and subdural hematomas are frequently associated with venous bleeding. **Another key to differentiating the compartment is the relationship to cranial sutures.** An epidural hematoma will not cross a suture line because of the anatomic limitation of the dura by the suture. A similar limitation by dural attachment at suture lines helps distinguish a cephalohematoma from a caput succedaneum.

MAGNETIC RESONANCE IMAGING

Background

Magnetic resonance imaging (MRI) is a modality that images protons or hydrogen ions within the body. Rapid development of magnetic resonance was in part because of the transfer of some of the sophistocated reconstruction algorithms used in CT and the computer power developed in other fields, such as 3-D graphics used in cartoon animation, cartology, and seismology. These technologic advances allow tremendous amounts of information to be manipulated quickly enough to make image reconstruction a reality. MRI is essentially hydrogen imaging, and because the human body is 98% water, there is a lot of hydrogen available to image.

MRI is performed by placing a patient in a strong magnetic field, which varies slightly from the head to the foot. Each proton acts as a small magnet, and just as the needle on a compass orients itself in one direction when placed next to a magnet, the protons in the body align when placed into the magnetic field of the imaging magnet. This alignment of protons is essential to create an environment that can have a net electromagnetic field effect which can induce the movement of electrons. Without the alignment of protons by the magnetic field, the random orientation of protons would have no measurable net field effect when stimulated and therefore would create no signal to image.

Once the patient is in the magnet, a radiofrequency pulse is delivered. In current imaging systems the pulse wave has a frequency of an FM radiowave. Less than 1 in 1 million hydrogen ions will absorb any energy, and only certain radiofrequencies will allow the transfer of energy from the radiofrequence (RF) pulse to a hydrogen ion.

An analogy of this energy transfer can be seen on a schoolyard playground. Visualize a child on a swing. If you push the swing in rhythm or resonance with the natural frequency of the motion of that swing, the swing will absorb the energy and the child will swing higher and higher with each push. This natural rate of harmonic motion depends on the length of the rope on the swing and the mass of the swing and the child. If you were to push at a rate that was not syncrynous with the swing's natural rhythm, pushing would not allow the energy to assist in propelling the swing higher and higher, and in fact, you would disrupt the normal rhythm of the swing.

In the memorable TV commercial in which Aretha Franklin was recorded by Memorex and the playback of her voice caused a goblet to break, the phenomenon being demonstrated was resonance frequency being absorbed by the crystal in the goblet. That absorbed energy caused the goblet to shatter. In MRI, FM radiofrequency energy is used to stimulate hydrogen ions or protons in the body.

Because the field strength of the magnet used for imaging varies slightly from one end of the patient to the other, and the resonance frequency is dependent on the field strength of the magnet, one can selectively stimulate various locations within the patient. By changing the radiofrequency slightly, a different specific group of protons is stimulated. Protons stimulated by a radiofrequency pulse absorb that energy and move to an unstable higher energy state. They give up that energy as a radiofrequency pulse or "echo" of the pulse they received. The echo is received by an antenna just like a radio receiver and converted to an image. The signals or echos received are the result of T1 and T2 relaxation times, which are simply physical parameters that describe the environmental interactions that influence the signal released from a proton. Spin-echo pulse sequences are the most frequently used sequences in routine MR imaging.

A spinning top analogy can help to explain the T1 and T2 relaxation times that result in spin-echo imaging. Each hydrogen ion has a dipole moment (a positive pole and a negative pole) and therefore acts like a small magnet within the powerful magnetic field of the imaging magnet. These protons spin or *precess* with a precessional frequency that is related to the field strength of the magnet. Electromagnetic energy can be transferred to these protons if the energy is delivered at the resonance frequency. Once an RF pulse of resonance frequency is delivered, a certain number of protons (less than 1 in 1 million) will absorb this energy and move to a higher energy state. The T1 relaxation time reflects the time it takes for these excited protons to give up their higher energy and return to baseline.

T2 relaxation times relate to a second parameter of physical interactions. Although the protons are rotating at a frequency proportionate to the magnetic field in which they exist, they are not in phase. In other words, there is no net direction of polarity from all of these spinning magnets. Once the RF pulse perturbs or stimulates these protons, they begin to spin synchronously and therefore create a net

magnetic field. This spinning net magnetic field generates an electromagnetic wave that can be picked up by the RF antenna of the imaging system as an "echo" of the original RF pulse delivered. (The principle of a spinning magnet inducing an electromagnetic pulse is the basis for the turbines of hydroelectric generators.)

Because its immediate electromagnetic environment affects each proton differently, these protons will only remain synchronous in their precession for a very short period of time. As they move out of phase or synchrony, the net magnetic field that was created dissipates, and therefore the signal received by the RF antenna diminishes. The T2 relaxation time indicates the time it takes the protons to go from a state of synchronous rotation, at which maximal signal is created, to random, out-of-phase precession, with zero net magnetic field and hence no signal.

This is a rather simplified explanation of the physics required for image acquisition, but it is important to recognize that the images are acquired without the use of ionizing radiation. **There is therefore no risk from ionizing radiation with MRI, and this is particularly attractive in pediatrics. No known harmful effect of either magnetic exposure or radiofrequency exposure at the levels used in MRI has been observed.** However, MRI is still relatively new, and one should be cautious in using fetal and newborn imaging. Energy deposition is a concern, and protocols have been established that limit patient exposure.

Another concern is the effect a magnetic field might have on electronic instrumentation, such as pacing devices and metalic surgical clips. The torque on metallic implants can be quite high, but this is rarely of clinical significance. However, the artifact caused by the disturbance of the magnetic field can be significant. **The most important and real safety concern is that of the magnetic field attraction of ferromagnetic material. Pens, stethoscopes, or even oxygen cannisters can act as a projectile when inadvertently brought too close to a magnetic field.** One should also be cautious about the effect that a magnetic field might have on magnetic strips of credit cards and identification badges, but this is more of a nuisance than a safety concern.

There are two very significant advantages of MRI: (1) the ability to accurately acquire and reconstruct images in any plane and (2) the ability

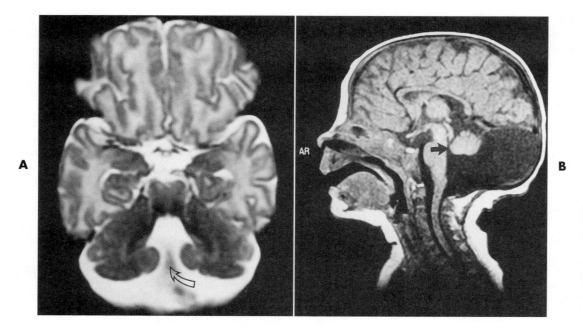

FIGURE 8-9 **A,** Axial T2 weighted image through the posterior fossa demonstrates the high-signal CSF fluid in the posterior fossa cyst, which communicates with the fourth ventricle more anteriorly *(open arrow)*. **B,** Midsagittal T1 weighted image demonstrates a Dandy-Walker variant in this patient. The partial formation of the vermis seen best on the sagittal image defines a Dandy-Walker variant *(arrow)*.

to image flowing blood without the need for an intravenous contrast medium. The main drawback of current MRI technology is the time it takes to acquire an image. **Motion-free imaging is necessary for optimal image quality, and because image acquisition in MRI takes minutes to obtain, sedation is frequently required.** Respiratory and cardiac gating can help for physiologic motion, but even physiologic motion can be problematic.

Focused Discussion: Practical Consideration (Figure 8-9)

The physics of MRI is complex, and variables that influence the signal received are protean. These influences variably affect the T1 and T2 relaxation times in spin-echo imaging. Imaging sequences tend to be referred to as *T1* or *T2 sequences,* depending on which physical parameter has the most influence upon the appearance of the image. **A simplified approximation of spin-echo imaging that can be helpful for the novice is that in T1-weighted spin-echo sequences fluid is black and in T2 imaging fluid is white.** Most pathologic conditions are characterized either by the distortion of the normal anatomy or by edema, which is manifested by in-

creased fluid in an otherwise normal structure or within the particular lesion. Therefore if one looks for a fluid collection, CSF in the ventricles of the brain, CSF in the subdural space around the cord, orbital fluid of the aqueous humor, fluid in the heart or urinary bladder, one can easily determine whether the imaging sequence is T1 weighted where the fluid is black or T2 weighted where the fluid is white. **On T1-weighted sequences, a pathologic condition would be seen as a black or lower signal, because a pathologic state is associated with increased water in the area of abnormality. In T2-weighted sequences, the pathologic lesion would tend to be white.**

NUCLEAR SCINTIGRAPHY

Nuclear scintigraphy is the most physiologic of the tools commonly used in neonatal imaging. A pharmaceutical is tagged with a *radiotracer,* which is a radioactive isotope that can be detected by a nuclear medicine camera. The pharmaceutical may be injected intravenously, be given orally, or be delivered directly into the urinary bladder. The pharmaceutical is distributed in the body based on the parent compound, to which the radioisotope is chelated or bound. The patient is then imaged using a detector that maps the distribution of the tagged isotope in the body.

The radiation dose in scintigraphy is small. With the doses used for diagnostic purposes, there is no risk to the individual or anyone who is in immediate contact with the patient. The pharmaceutical agents have both a biologic half-life, which is related to the natural elimination of the parent compound from the body and a radioactive half-life, which is determined by the isotope used to label the pharmaceutical. The spatial resolution is poor, but contrast resolution is exquisite, because the radiopharmaceutical is distributed so specifically within the body.

Common Utility and the Neonatal Intensive Care Setting

Three common investigations for which nuclear medicine is well suited include renal scintigraphy, hepatobiliary imaging, and splenic imaging. In patients with vertebral, anal, cardiac, tracheal, esophageal, renal, or limb (VACTERL) anomalies, renal scans can be helpful in determining the number and location of the kidneys. Renal scintigraphy can be used to quantify relative renal function. Scintigraphy is a functional way to evaluate the degree of obstruction in hydronephrosis. Nuclear cystography has a very low radiation dose and therefore a good method for following vesicoureteral reflux. Fluoroscopic cystography is usually performed for the initial evaluation, because the excellent spatial resolution can assist in defining anatomic abnormalities that may be responsible for reflux, for example, that might be missed with the poor spatial resolution of nuclear imaging.

Hepatobiliary imaging can assist in the evaluation of the jaundice patient. The radiopharmaceutical is extracted from the blood pool by the liver and excreted like bile, allowing one to determine transit time and flow of the bile from the liver into the gallbladder, through the common bile duct and into the duodenum. Hepatobiliary imaging can help diagnose neonatal hepatitis, in which there is limited clearance of the pharmaceutical agent from the blood by the liver; therefore the liver shows little activity compared with the background. In biliary atresia, the clearance or extraction of the radiopharmaceutical agent from the blood is closer to normal, but activity never leaves the liver and therefore no activity is seen in the duodenum and small bowel,

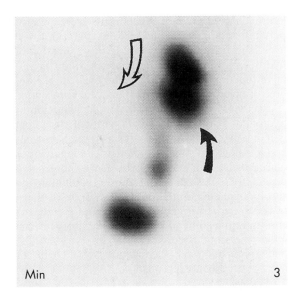

Min   3

FIGURE 8-10 This posterior image from a DTPA renal scan demonstrates the collecting system, ureter and urinary bladder associated with the functioning right kidney *(black arrow)*. The multicystic dysplastic kidney on the left shows no functional renal tissue *(open arrow)*.

even on delayed images. A choledochal cyst will accumulate radiotracer and is diagnosed by an intense area of focal activity and a dilated biliary system more proximally.

Splenic imaging can be performed either with technetium sulfur colloid, which is taken up both in the Kupfer cells in the liver and spleen. Alternatively, radiolabeled damaged red blood cells can be used for splenic images, because they are sequestered in the spleen. Splenic imaging is frequently helpful in patients with complex congenital heart disease and situs abnormalities to diagnose asplenia or polysplenia.

Focused Discussion: Renal Scintigraphy

The radiopharmaceutical choices for renal imaging are either cortical agents which bind in the renal cortex, filtered agents which transit the cortex and then are excreted into the collecting system, or a combination both cortical and filtered agents. Cortical agents are useful in defining size, number, location, and relative function of the kidneys when there are two. The US characteristics of multicystic dysplastic kidney (MDK) are usually diagnostic (Figure 8-10); however, occasionally renal scintigraphy can help differentiate the hydronephrotic form of MDK from severe uretero-pelvic junction (UPJ) obstruction. A combination agent such as MAG3 is useful in the evaluation of hydronephrosis, because one can determine the relative function of each kidney and evaluate the degree of obstruction. The addition of the furosemide (Lasix) washout study augments the evaluation of hydronephrosis by rendering a washout curve that is indicative of the severity of obstruction. In general it is helpful when evaluating hydronephrosis to place a catheter in the urinary bladder to prevent the possibility of vesicoureteral reflux confounding the results of the examination. Although all of these tests can be performed in the newborn period, the concentrating ability of the newborn kidney is marginal. Therefore the tests are often reserved until the patient is 3 to 6 months of age to improve their accuracy and prognostic capability.

INTERVENTION

Intervention is one of the newest but most rapidly growing subspeciality areas in medical imaging. Interventional radiology has assumed an important role as a minimally invasive way to treat disease. Imaging is used to direct the surgical approach. From a practical standpoint, **there are four major areas of radiology intervention: (1) vascular access, (2) tissue sampling for minimally invasive diagnosis of neoplasm or infection, (3) catheter or needle drainage of fluid collections or abscesses, and (4) directed delivery of cells, chemotherapy, or embolic material, which may be used to diminish flow in a vascular lesion.**

Any of the imaging modalities may be used to guide the intervention, but the most commonly used are fluoroscopy, ultrasonography, and CT.

Common Utility in the Neonatal Intensive Care Setting

Vascular access is the most commonly requested radiologic intervention in most pediatric institutions. Ultrasonography or fluoroscopy can be used to visualize veins for venous access.

Most tissue sampling is performed for the diagnosis of neoplasm. In general, a needle can be placed into an area of abnormal tissue and either a fine-needle aspirate obtained, or, in solid tumors, a core needle biopsy may be performed. The advantage of a core needle biopsy is that adequate tissue is obtained, frequently a volume sufficient to complete many of the biologic studies necessary in the preoperative evaluation of the neoplasm. This can be particularly helpful in patients in whom a neoplasm, once defined, can be pretreated before definitive surgical resection is performed.

Cysts or abscesses can be drained, obviating the need for an open surgical procedure and thus minimizing morbidity and shortening recovery time.

A gastrostomy or gastrojejunostomy tube can also be placed in a minimally invasive manner, rather than a more invasive standard surgical procedure. This can be an ideal approach for a temporary feeding method.

Directed delivery of chemotherapy has been used in neonatal units for the treatment of hepatoblastoma, in which chemotherapy can be directed through the hepatic artery into the specific lobe involving the hepatoblastoma and the tumor reduced in size before excision. This reduces the size in some patients, allowing a tumor that would previously been deemed nonresectible to be resected.

Another example of directed delivery is the embolization of hepatic hemangioendothelioma. Hemangioendothelioma is an infrequent cause of congestive failure as a result of an extracardiac shunt in the neonatal period. It is possible to embolize the benign neoplasm, thereby diminishing the shunt and correcting the patient's failure. Vein of Galen aneurysm is another extracardiac vascular shunt that frequently predisposes the patient to high-flow cardiac failure. There is a significant spectrum of disease related to vein of Galen aneurysms, and the success of embolization is highly dependent on the degree of vascular insufficiency related to the steal associated with a high-flow lesion. In patients who present early and in florid heart failure, the outcomes are predictably less positive than in patients who present later with an abnormality discovered during a routine physical examination, where an intracranial bruit might be identified.

Finally, directed delivery in cell implantation and genetic engineering shows great promise. These areas are early in their development, but the ability to direct a catheter to a specific organ for cell implantation or genetic engineering will clearly have a role in future applications of interventional radiology.

Focused Discussion: Vascular Access

The availability of ultrasonographic equipment can allow placement of PICC lines or central venous catheters in vessels as small as 2 mm. With US the vessel is visualized directly. Fluoroscopic guidance requires limited venography through a peripheral IV line. Indirect visualization of the venous system is possible because intravascular contrast defines the vascular lumen. After visualization with either ultrasonography or fluoroscopy, a 21-gauge needle is placed into the vessel selected. Once good blood return confirms the intraluminal position of the needle tip, an 18-gauge wire is passed through the needle. The needle is removed and the tract is dilated. Next a peel-away sheath is placed over the wire. The catheter is sized and then passed through the peel-away sheath. The location of the catheter tip is confirmed fluoroscopically.

INFORMATICS

Picture Archive and Communications System (PACS) is radiology's entrant in the age of medical informatics. PACS allows images to be stored or archived in digital format for distribution throughout an entire health care system. The implementation of a PACS network requires digital acquisition of images. Except for x-ray equipment, most modern imaging equipment acquires the image in a digital format. Some older systems may require an analog to digital conversion. Computed radiology (CR) and direct radiology (DR) are the most recent methods of acquiring x-rays without the need for a separate step required to translate the plain film by some digitizing process. X-rays recorded on film in a conventional manner can be converted to a digital format through a laser scanner. Once acquired, the image is interpreted and the image with report stored in a digital archive. The images and interpretations are then available for general distribution. PACS facilitates simultaneous and distributed viewing of imaging and reports. PACS is a powerful tool that helps clinicians improve medical decision-making by translating bits of data into clinically relevant information. It is the imaging component of the electronic medical record.

SUMMARY

There are numerous alternatives available for the evaluation of any patient condition. The best imaging choice may vary, depending on local expertise or availability. It should also be obvious that a clear understanding of the differential diagnosis, along with a thoughtful and specific analysis of the clinical question, is essential for optimal imaging consultation. The pros and cons of each modality should be considered by the clinician, and if there is any uncertainty as to the best method of imaging, consultation with a radiologist is advisable.

BIBLIOGRAPHY

Amplatz K, Moller JH: *Radiology of congenital heart disease,* St. Louis, 1993, Mosby.

Barkovich AJ: *Pediatric neuroimaging,* ed 3, Philadelphia, 2000, Lippincott Williams & Wilkins.

Cohen M, Edwards M: *Magnetic resonance imaging of children,* Philadelphia, 1990, Decker.

Kirks DR: *Practical pediatric imaging: diagnostic radiology of infants and children,* ed 2, Boston, 1991, Little, Brown.

Osborn AG: *Diagnostic neuroradiology,* St. Louis, 1994, Mosby.

Rumack CM, Wilson SR, Charbonneau JW: *Diagnostic ultrasound,* ed 2, St Louis, 1998, Mosby.

Siegel M: *Pediatric sonography,* Philadelphia, 1996, Lippincott-Raven.

Silverman FN, Kuhn JP: *Caffey's pediatric x-ray diagnosis: an integrated imaging approach,* ed 9, St. Louis, 1993, Mosby.

Stark D, Bradley W Jr: *Magnetic resonance imaging,* ed 2, St. Louis, 1992, Mosby.

Swaiman KF: *Pediatric neurology: principles and practice,* St. Louis, 1989, Mosby.

Swischuk LE: *Imaging of the newborn, infant, and young child,* ed 4, Baltimore, 1997, Williams & Wilkins.

Volpe JJ: *Neurology of the newborn,* ed 3, Philadelphia, 1995, WB Saunders.

9 Pharmacology in Neonatal Care

C. Michael Cotton, Barbara S. Turner, Mary Miller-Bell

Optimal pharmacotherapy delivers maximal beneficial effect with minimal toxicity. Determining the optimal pharmacotherapy for neonates is problematic in that much of the data have been extrapolated from research in adults, children, and laboratory animals. Neonates show dramatic differences in the way they respond to drugs compared with older children and adults and within the neonatal population.[25] Gestational age, chronologic age, and disease state alter a neonate's ability to metabolize medications and affect the infant's response to the drug.

We will discuss pharmacology as it relates to the neonate and illustrate how rational medication decisions can be made for NICU patients. We will also discuss strategies to avoid medication errors and strategies for drug delivery.

PHYSIOLOGY

Pharmacodynamics and Pharmacokinetics

The drug-receptor theory states that the amount and duration of a drug's availability to a receptor determine its effectiveness. *Pharmacodynamics* describes what the drug does to the body, whereas *pharmacokinetics* describes what the body does to the drug, how much drug will be available to the receptors, and for how long (Figure 9-1).[25] A drug's *disposition* can be described by four processes: drug entry (absorption), distribution, biotransformation, and elimination. *Pharmacogenomics,* not covered in this chapter, is a relatively new science that attempts to explain the variability of drug effects by the genetic makeup of an individual.[23]

Pharmacodynamics relates the amount of available drug (or active metabolite) to the effect, and is dependent on receptor availability, affinity of the drug to the receptor, and cellular function.

Antagonist drugs block a receptor's cellular and physiologic activity (e.g., naloxone), whereas agonist drugs elicit the receptor's action (e.g., cardiovascular agents such as dopamine and ep-inephrine). **Some drugs act with receptors to increase or decrease gene expression (e.g., antenatal steroids), whereas others affect cell membrane permeability.** Some drugs, such as methylxanthines, increase or decrease the amount or activity of "second messenger" molecules within cells. Antibiotics and antiviral agents act through some of these mechanisms to reduce the viability of pathogenic organisms by changing vital characteristics and functions. Readers should note that most drugs have more than one effect, so although the desired therapeutic effect may occur, the drug's other effects can limit its usefulness. Side effects, which can vary from the minor to the prohibitive, occur within the therapeutic range of concentration. Toxic effects result from drug overdose or serum concentrations higher than the recommended therapeutic range.

Individual infants may have idiosyncratic as well as expected responses to medications. Infants who are low sensitivity responders exhibit a drug response less than that expected for a usual dose, whereas infants who are extreme sensitivity responders exceed the expected response for a given dose and drug level. Unpredictable adverse reactions differ from expected responses. Patients may become tolerant to a given drug dosage, as is commonly seen with opiates. Tachyphylaxis, a rapid decrease in drug response without a dosage change, may be related to limited receptors or other intracellular mechanisms.[21]

Developmental differences in number and function of receptors and intracellular mechanisms are critical to estimating drug actions. An example of developmental effect on pharmacodynamics is the diminished sensitivity of the cardiovascular system to digitalis in the youngest patients; the receptor number increases with age. Changes in alpha- and beta-adrenergic receptors also occur with gestational and chronologic age and must be considered when determining dosage with pressors and inotropes.[5]

To elicit the desired therapeutic effect the drug must be delivered to the receptor and remain avail-

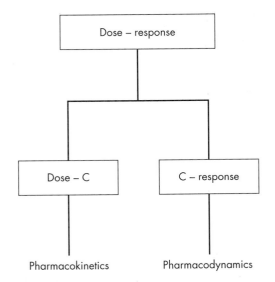

FIGURE 9-1 Variability in dose-response relationship can be the result of differences in pharmacokinetics or pharmacodynamics. *C*, Drug concentration (plasma or serum).

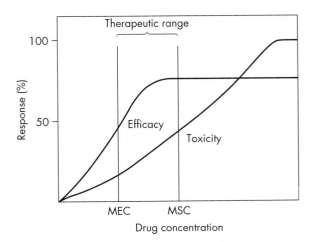

FIGURE 9-2 Percentage of patients with desired and toxic responses as a function of drug concentration. Therapeutic range is bounded by minimum effective and maximum safe concentrations. *MEC*, Minimum effective concentration; *MSC*, maximum safe concentration.

able for an appropriate amount of time.[25] ***Pharmacokinetics*** **describes the delivery and removal of the drug to and from the body. Doses and dose intervals are expressed mathematically by pharmacokinetic disposition parameters related to distribution, biotransformation, and elimination, such as clearance, volume of distribution, and half-life.**

A clinician bases drug choice and dose regimen largely on the desired therapeutic response and toxic effect in "average" patients. Plasma concentration provides a surrogate for effect when the relationship between concentration (C) and effect has been demonstrated in similar patients. The minimum effective concentration (MEC) is that at which 50% of patients exhibit the desired response (Box 9-1). The maximum safe concentration (MSC) is that at which 50% of patients exhibit a toxic response (Figure 9-2). To continue the desired effect, the clinician aims to obtain a target plasma concentration at "steady state" (Css), somewhere between the MEC and the MSC, where most patients would exhibit the desired effect and few suffer toxic effects. With ideal maintenance therapy, drug input equals drug elimination. The variability around the Css depends on dose, dose interval, and drug disposition.

Box 9-1	ABBREVIATIONS	
C	Drug concentration (plasma or serum)	mg/L
Css	Steady state concentration (average)	mg/L
MEC	Minimum effective concentration	mg/L
MSC	Maximum safe concentration	mg/L
F	Extent of drug availability (0 to 1); how much active drug gets to the systemic circulation	unitless
V	Volume of distribution; relates to loading dose	L/kg
Cl	Clearance: relates to maintenance dose	L/kg/hr
$t_{1/2}$	Drug elimination half-life; relates to the time course of changes in drug concentration	hours

L = liter = 1000 milliliters
mg = milligram = 1000 micrograms

The target Css is influenced by the amount of drug bound to plasma protein. In a newborn, free unconjugated bilirubin can displace numerous medicines of lower protein affinity, and numerous medicines can displace unconjugated bilirubin, increasing unconjugated bilirubin's serum concentration and its potential for toxicity. Intravenous lipid infusions can also affect protein binding of both bilirubin and some medicines. The drug concentration measured is usually the total, both protein-bound and free; therefore the available concentration at the receptor is usually somewhat less than the total serum concentration.

Dose-Concentration Considerations Related to Age

The reported therapeutic range for theophylline in adults is 10 to 20 μg/ml. In neonates the reported range is 4 to 12 μg/ml.[25] Theophylline is reported to be 36% bound to plasma protein at a total concentration of 8 μg/ml in newborns, compared with 70% bound in adults. A total theophylline concentration of 10 μg/ml in an adult would represent 3 μg/ml free theophylline available to receptors, whereas in a neonate a total of 4.7 μg/ml equals 3 μg/ml of free theophylline (not to mention the metabolism of theophylline in neonates leads to measurable free caffeine, which will be discussed below). Decreased bound theophylline in neonates could explain why therapeutic effect is achieved with lower total serum concentration in neonates.

In the NICU doses and intervals must be adjusted based on changes in the dose-concentration and the concentration-response relationships. We can be more predictive and respond more precisely to changes in dose-concentration effects, especially total concentrations, but as with the theophylline case, we must watch for clinical effects and estimate other factors' influences to estimate the free concentration's effectiveness and the receptor and cellular responsiveness. Potential causes of changes in dose-concentration relationships unique to newborns are described for the pharmacokinetic processes that follow.

Absorption

The process of absorption defines the rate and amount of drug that enters the blood stream. The parameter F indicates the percentage of dosed drug available in the systemic circulation, with F = 1 indicating the drug is 100% available. We lack systematic studies of absorption in sick newborns, and differences in absorptive processes are expected but remain generally unmeasured. Some differences in newborns that potentially affect bioavailability include developmental changes in surface area and permeability of gastrointestinal (GI) mucosa, age-dependent changes in acid secretion in the stomach (higher pH than older children and adults), changes in gastric emptying time and total gastrointestinal transit time, and the characteristics of GI flora. Drugs such as ranitidine and metaclopramide will also affect absorption of other medications by means of the same mechanisms.

"First pass" pharmacokinetics means the drug is absorbed through the GI mucosa, travels directly to the liver where it is metabolized and excreted in significant amounts, limiting bioavailability. Different drugs are absorbed at different rates, and different formulations of the same medication may be protected from "first pass" metabolism. Drugs may also be given by inhalation, intranasally, intrarectally, topically, intramuscularly, subcutaneously, and intravenously.[21]

Distribution

Medications rely on blood flow and drug solubility for distribution to their sites of therapeutic effect. The *volume of distribution* for a drug is a parameter that relates total amount of drug distributed throughout the body to the serum or plasma concentration.[13,25] It is an attempt to quantify the space where the drug can go. Strictly defined, it is the hypothetical volume of body fluid required to dissolve the total amount of drug as found in the serum. Volume of distribution must be used to estimate the amount of a loading dose or a change in plasma concentration with any bolus dose:

Loading dose $\times$ F (the absorption parameter) = Change in concentration (ΔC) $\times$ V (volume of distribution)

Or, put another way:

$$\Delta C = F \times \text{loading dose}/V$$

Volume of distribution is usually expressed as a function of body weight, with units of volume per kilogram. Major factors that affect distribution volume are plasma protein binding and body composition.[5,14] Changes in body composition happen throughout fetal and newborn life. Total body water decreases with increasing age: 85% in the smallest, most preterm infants; 70% in term infants; and 55% in most adults. Total body water may increase with such conditions as the syndrome of inappropriate antidiuretic hormone excretion (SIADH), which increase total body water. Extracellular water composes about half this amount in a healthy term neonate. Large water-soluble molecules reach this compartment. Intravascular water composes about 10% of the body weight; protein-bound medications stay in this small compartment. Water-soluble drugs such as penicillins, aminoglycosides, and cephalosporins are distributed in a greater volume in smaller, more preterm infants, therefore requiring a higher loading dose per kilogram, if total body water were the only determinant of volume of distribution.

Plasma protein amounts and binding capacities also differ with gestational and chronologic age. Protein binding is decreased in newborns, because lower amounts of albumin are available than later in life, and fetal albumin has less capacity to bind some drugs. Acidic drugs such as ampicillin, phenytoin, phenobarbital bind less well, thus increasing the free (available to receptor) fraction of the drug, with resultant increase in effect. Changes in pH also can affect a drug's affinity for albumin. Fat content will vary with gestational age and degree of illness; increased fat content increases the volume of distribution. Lipid-soluble molecules are also distributed in this space.

Of particular concern in newborns is the interaction of circulating unconjugated bilirubin and protein-bound drugs. Several anionic compounds bind to albumin and can displace bilirubin, increasing free bilirubin, thus increasing its potential of toxicity. Bilirubin has a higher affinity for albumin than some other medications; it may displace them from albumin, increasing the medication's availability and potential to reach toxic levels.

Biotransformation

Biotransformation, or drug metabolism, occurs most commonly in the liver. Phase I metabolism describes the nonsynthetic metabolism of medications. Phase II, usually conjugation, or the addition of a substance to a medication, is synthetic metabolism. Oxidation, conjugation, glucuronidation, and hepatic blood flow change with gestational and chronologic age, disease, states and use of certain medications. For example, oxidation and glucuronidation are decreased in newborns. Drugs such as acetaminophen, phenobarbital, and phenytoin, which require oxidation for elimination, remain available longer and may be transformed to other active metabolites (the neonatal liver metabolizes theophylline to caffeine), or the drug may remain at significant free concentrations for a prolonged period. The possibility of prolonged peak concentrations of available drug or active metabolites for many pharmaceuticals mandates careful monitoring of drug levels and clinical conditions to titrate dose intervals. To further the potential for confusion and trouble, and further the argument for careful assessment of levels and clinical signs of ef-

fectiveness and toxicity, a decrease in plasma protein binding (or any other change in volume of distribution) may increase the hepatic clearance of a drug.

Clearance (Elimination)

Drug clearance or elimination occurs by excretion of unaltered drug or biotransformation to an inactive metabolite. Most drug elimination pathways can become saturated if the dose is high enough and dose intervals too frequent. Most drugs in use in the NICU have therapeutic doses less than those necessary to saturate the elimination system. When clearance mechanisms are not saturated, the steady-state concentration (Css) in plasma is proportional to the dose rate. Clearance equals the rate of drug elimination divided by the drug concentration.[13] Just as volume of distribution relates to loading dose and initial concentration, clearance relates to a maintenance dose that keeps a drug's concentration at steady state. So for an ideal drug maintained at steady-state concentration:

$$(\text{Dose/dose interval}) \times F = Cl \,(\text{clearance}) \times Css$$

Stated another way:

$$Cl = F \times \text{Dose}/(\text{dose interval} \times Css)$$

Or, to tailor the dose for a desired steady state concentration:

$$\text{Dose rate} = (Cl \times Css)/F$$

If the clinician can specify the desired steady-state plasma concentration and knows the clearance and bioavailability of a drug (from peak and trough levels in a particular patient), the appropriate dosing rate can be calculated.

For example, clearance of theophylline in preterm infants is reported to be 0.017 L/kg/hr. If the desired Css = 8 mg/L, assuming F = 1, particularly if the dose is to be given intravenously:

$$\text{Dose rate} = (Cl \times Css)/F = (0.017 \times 8)/1 =$$
$$0.136 \text{ mg/kg/hr or } 1.1 \text{ mg/kg q 8 hr}$$

Renal Excretion

The kidney is the primary route of excretion for many drugs commonly used in the NICU. The kidney clears drugs through glomerular filtration and tubular secretion. Examples of medications eliminated through the kidney include aminoglycosides, digoxin, diuretics, and penicillins. Doses and dose intervals of drugs that have renal excretion must change with age and disease state.

The glomerular filtration rate (GFR), that is, the amount of blood filtered by the kidney in a unit of time, is low at birth and gradually increases over the first weeks. In preterm infants GFR starts even lower than term infants with a somewhat significant increase occurring at 34 weeks postconception. Tubular secretion also matures with increasing gestational age and depends on tubular function. In adults, aminoglycosides may be dosed based on creatinine clearance, but in neonates less than 1 week old, serum creatinine may reflect maternal levels as well as renal impairment. Acidosis and a history of hypoxia or ischemia may also modify an infant's renal function, slowing excretion and altering pharmacokinetics. Again, measuring levels in cases of suspected renal impairment, whether from suspicious history or lab values, is important to determining an appropriate dosing strategy.

Half-Life

A drug's "half-life"($t_{1/2}$) is the time required for the drug level to decline by 50%. Half-life is re-lated to both volume of distribution (V) and clearance (Cl), so that:

$$t_{1/2} = 0.7 \times V/Cl$$

The $t_{1/2}$ is used to predict and interpret the time course of changes in plasma drug concentrations. For example, the time to steady state is 4 to 5 half-lives. The half-life is useful in selecting dose intervals. This concept is illustrated in Figure 9-3.

Loading doses help expedite reaching desired therapeutic concentrations, especially for drugs with long half-lives, where a desired effect is needed immediately. For drugs with one-compartment distribution that stay in the circulation and are not stored in cells or tissue, the loading dose may be given as a simple single dose. Drugs that are fat soluble or stored intracellularly are more difficult to assess, and therapeutic levels must be included in the loading dose assessment.

LD (loading dose) = (Vd × Concentration)/F

If the volume of distribution for theophylline in preterm infants is 0.7 L/kg, and 8 mg/L is the desired

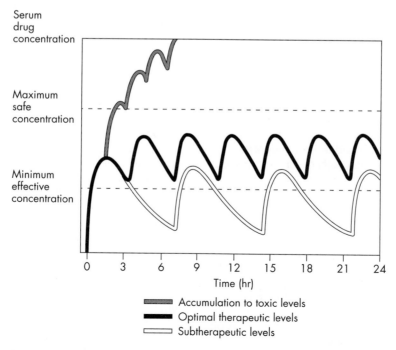

FIGURE 9-3   Effect on serum drug concentration of multiple dosing along with different time intervals between doses. (From Roberts RJ: *Drug therapy in infants*, Philadelphia, 1984, WB Saunders.)

concentration, and F, for an intravenous dose, is assumed to be 1.0, a loading dose can be calculated.

$$LD = (Vd \times C)/F = 0.7 \text{ L/kg} \times 8 \text{ mg/L} =$$
$$5.6 \text{ mg of theophylline/kg}$$

DATA COLLECTION

Clinicians should be aware of a medication's desired effects, side effects, and toxicities, know when they are expected to occur, and monitor for these effects. Whether a dose effect occurs or not should be noted. Dose-plasma concentration results should be recorded when therapeutic drug monitoring is done. If the drug's serum concentration relates to clinical response, the blood concentration should be followed in addition to clinical signs. To optimally use drug serum levels, the expected blood concentration is calculated from the dosing history, and patient variables that may affect pharmacokinetics with the timing of blood samples are considered. A comparison of expected values with measured values allows rational adjustment of future dosing.[15] Potential explanations for differences between measured and expected concentrations are listed in Box 9-2.

Even if predictable pharmacokinetic and pharmacodynamic changes are taken into account, other factors may influence a drug's effect. Clinical endpoints must be followed and recorded and dose regimens adjusted accordingly. One example is the monitoring of renal function with indomethacin dosing; if clinical signs of renal dysfunction are noted, the drug is not administered. A pharmacist should be included in the caregiving team to clarify dose and disposition parameters for individual patients with their various conditions.

If a suboptimal clinical response is noted in conjunction with a subtherapeutic plasma concentration, revised estimates of clearance should be adjusted with one or two available plasma concentrations. If a single level is drawn after absorption and distribution is complete or near steady state, then the maintenance dose formula can be rearranged to calculate the revised clearance. The common-sense approach suggests that if a patient has half the expected concentration of a drug, then perhaps the clearance is twice the initial estimate. If the patient has twice the expected concentration, the clearance likely is half the initial estimate. However, this technique is misleading if steady state has not been reached. If a drug's level is higher than expected and higher than what is considered safe, or if toxicity is noted, the drug should be discontinued until the concentration decays to the appropriate target. If two concentrations are available after absorption and distribution, half-life is determined by plotting the concentrations on semilog paper. The revised clearance is calculated by rearranging the half-life formula:

$$\text{Clearance} = 0.7 \times Vd/t_{1/2}$$

Once the clearance and desired steady state is known, a new dose rate can be calculated:

$$\text{Dose rate} = (Cl \times Css_{desired})/F$$

EXAMPLES

The following example illustrates the need to pay close attention to issues of drug delivery and clinical effects.

EXAMPLE 1: A 15-day-old 1-kg preterm infant receives oral theophylline for apnea of prematurity. He has received 1 mg every 8 hours for 5 days. At 0800 on the fifth day, 4 hours after the last dose, the baby's heart rate is more than 180 beats/min, but apnea has not been a problem. Clinical and laboratory evaluation of tachycardia includes consideration of theophylline toxicity. Blood samples for caffeine (a pharmacologically active metabolite of theophylline) and theophylline are sent to the laboratory. Estimate what the concentration will be.

Necessary data:
Total body weight: 1 kg
Vd = 0.7 L/kg = 0.7 L in this patient
Cl = 0.017 L/kg/hr = 0.017 L/hr in this patient
$t_{1/2} = 0.7 \times Vd/Cl = 0.7 \times 0.7$ L/(0.017 L/hr) = 28.8 hr
Time to steady state (Tss) = $4 \times t_{1/2}$ = 115.3 hr
Assume F = 1, MSC = 12 mg/L, MEC = 4 mg/L

Box 9-2	POTENTIAL EXPLANATIONS FOR DISCREPANCIES BETWEEN MEASURED AND EXPECTED DRUG CONCENTRATION

Inadequate compliance
Inadequte medication delivery
Inappropriate timing of samples
Laboratory error
Revision in initial estimates of pK required

Therefore:

$$Css = F \times dose/(dose\ interval \times Cl) =$$
$$1 \times 1.0\ mg/(8\ hr \times 0.017\ L/hr) =$$
$$7.38\ mg/L$$

The Css was estimated based on average Vd and Cl values reported in similar infants, adjusted for this infant's weight. If this infant has diminished clearance relative to "average," toxicity may result from the standard dose. Toxicity may not have been noted until day 5 because of the estimated Tss of 115 hours.

EXAMPLE 2: At 1600 hours, when the next dose is due, 8 hours after the last dose, theophylline concentration of 15 mg/L is reported. This is higher than the expected level and is most likely the result of decreased clearance. Using this concentration, estimate the time when the concentration will decline to 8 mg/L and determine a 12-hour dose schedule to maintain that concentration. The 1600 dose is held, and the tachycardia resolves 8 hours later.

$$Clearance\ revised = F \times dose/(interval \times Css) =$$
$$1 \times 1\ mg/(8\ hr \times 15\ mg/L) = 0.008\ L/hr$$

$$Revised\ t_{1/2} = 0.7 \times Vd\ /\ Cl_{revised} =$$
$$0.7 \times 0.7\ L/0.008\ L/hr = 61.25$$

Therefore the concentration 40 hours later should be one half of the measured 15 mg/L, or about 8 mg/L. To maintain a concentration of 8 mg/L:

$$Dose = (interval \times Cl_{revised} \times Css)/F =$$
$$12\ hr \times 0.008\ L/hr \times 8\ mg/L)/1 =$$
$$0.8\ mg\ theophylline\ PO\ q\ 12\ hr$$

EXAMPLE 3: Before the new oral regimen is initiated, another level is drawn 60 hours after the first and is 7.5 mg/L. Because apnea has resolved, an oral regimen based on the last two levels is begun to maintain a theophylline concentration of 7 mg/L. Estimate the necessary maintenance dose.

The concentration fell 50%, from 15 to 7.5 mg/L in 60 hours, which confirmed our original estimate of half-life. It should be noted that monitoring and dosing for theophylline can be complicated by measurable levels of caffeine.

DRUG CATEGORIES

Antimicrobial Agents

Antimicrobial agents inhibit growth or kill microorganisms; they include antibacterial, antiviral, and antifungal agents. Bacteriostatic agents limit growth, allowing host defenses to control spread; this will not reliably eliminate a pathogen. Bactericidal agents kill the pathogen. Bactericidal agents at low concentrations may be bacteriostatic. Minimum inhibitory concentration (MIC) is the lowest concentration of an antimicrobial that stops the spread of an organism in laboratory culture media. This cannot be directly measured in an infected neonate and depends on tissue concentration and numbers of bacteria present. Minimum bactericidal concentration (MBC) is the lowest concentration of antimicrobial that reduces microbial number in laboratory media by 99.9%. Pathogens can develop resistance to antimicrobials by changing their cellular structures or producing enzymes that reduce antimicrobial activity.

For effective antimicrobial action, the drug must reach an adequate concentration in the infected tissue. The ideal concentration elicits maximal effect on the pathogen with minimal effects on the patient. Selection criteria for antimicrobials include the microorganism's sensitivity, the availability of the drug to the target tissue (some antibiotics do not cross the blood-brain barrier), bioactivity of the antimicrobial in the target tissue, the known MIC and MBC relative to side and toxic effect levels for the medication, and the individual infant's biologic state—that is, whether the systems of absorbance and elimination are working adequately for effective and safe drug delivery and removal. When the use of antimicrobial agents is planned in a seriously ill infant, as with other drugs, greater consideration must be made for clinical status than the gestational or chronologic age.

Diuretics

Diuretics are used in the NICU to remove excessive extracellular fluid. Diuretics commonly cause a loss of electrolytes along with water. Response to any diuretic depends on renal function and the drug's ability to reach its target in adequate amounts. Most diuretics work within the tubule, but any drug that increases glomerular filtration rate can increase water loss. Drugs that increase cardiac output without decreasing renal perfusion, or others that specifically increase renal blood flow, also cause diuresis.

In infants renal tubular function improves with increasing chronologic and gestational age. Because of its poor absorption and poor response to aldosterone (especially in extremely preterm infants), electrolyte losses can be clinically significant with the addition of a loop diuretic such as furosemide or bumetadine. The ongoing losses may lead to hypochloremic metabolic alkalosis and less response to the diuretic.

Delivery of diuretics to the kidney loop will increase with increasing chronologic and gestational age. Most diuretics rely on secretion from the proximal tubule and filtration through the glomerulus to reach their site of action. Both these functions improve with age. Enteral absorption of some diuretics is limited, so clinical effectiveness and electrolyte stability must be monitored closely to help determine safe and effective dosage regimens. The kidney is also responsible for diuretic excretion, again through tubular secretion and glomerular filtration. Because these functions are age dependent, the clinician must take care that clearance time is adequate to avoid toxic levels.

Cardiovascular Drugs

Medicines used to improve cardiovascular function include digitalis and the sympathomimetic amines, which include drugs such as dopamine, dobutamine, and epinephrine. Antiarrhythmics, including digoxin, act to control the electrical conduction within the myocardium.

The sympathomimetic amines bind to β and Γ receptors; the number and availability of receptors determine response. $β_1$ Receptor response leads to constriction of vascular smooth muscle. $β_2$ Receptors cause decrease in GI motility. $Γ_1$ Receptor stimulation stimulates cardiac contractility, and $Γ_2$ response includes vascular and bronchial smooth muscle relaxation. The response in any individual, and in any individual's specific organ system, depends on the relative amount of these receptors. Receptor numbers and their linked response elements within cells vary with gestation and clinical condition, and response must be monitored to aid in dosing decisions. Prolonged administration of sympathomimetic amines can lead to decreased response, an example of tachyphylaxis.

Antihypertensive agents are occasionally used in neonates for essential hypertension and occasionally to decrease afterload in neonatal patients with heart failure. These include volume reducers like diuretics, inhibitors of physiologic regulators of blood pressure like enalapril, and drugs that decrease vascular resistance through β and Γ receptors.

The pathophysiology of neonatal disease should direct choice of cardiovascular agent. Extremely close monitoring of physiologic effects helps to determine safety and efficacy of therapy. Monitoring must include very frequent, if not continuous monitoring of blood pressure, heart rate, perfusion, oxygen saturation (preductal and postductal in some cases). Because other drugs are often given as a neonate receives cardiovascular medicines, thorough knowledge of possible drug interactions is mandatory.

Absorption of cardiovascular drugs is unpredictable. The sympathomimetic amines must be given intravenously, unless used in an emergency situation when endotracheal administration of epinephrine is indicated. Once dosed, the drug must be delivered to the target organ system. Infants in shock may not have the circulatory wherewithal to deliver the medication to elicit the desired therapeutic response. Because of the variability in β and Γ receptor development and distribution, undesired side effects in various organ systems may accompany desired responses. Rapid metabolism of the sympathomimetic amines demands continuous IV infusion, and infiltration of IV fluids may lead to significant tissue damage. Along with the physiologic effects, these IV lines must be carefully monitored.[19]

Central and Peripheral Nervous System Drugs

Nervous system drugs include analgesics, which decrease pain sensations; anesthetics, which control pain peripherally or in the CNS (central nervous system); sedative/hypnotics including barbiturates (phenobarbital) and nonbarbiturates (chloral hydrate, lorazepam), which do not control pain and can control some seizures; and antiepileptic agents, which are designed to control seizures (phenytoin, fos-phenytoin). These drugs are associated with problems of addiction, tolerance, dependence, and withdrawal.

Addiction is a complex lifestyle change that involves drug-seeking behavior that is not applicable to neonates. Tolerance occurs with many drug types. Tolerance exists when increasing doses and serum concentrations of a medicine are necessary to achieve a desired effect. A patient is dependent on a medication when regular drug administration is required for physical well-being. Withdrawal is a collection of physiologic and behavioral signs attributed to the absence of a medication in a dependent individual. Withdrawal has been identified for many medications, but classified and described, along with weaning protocols, for opiate analgesics.[8]

The mechanism of action of most CNS medications is not clearly known. Again, careful monitoring of therapeutic effects relative to dose, duration, and serum concentrations is extremely important. Significant respiratory depression can occur with most CNS medications, so appropriate resuscitation equipment must be available. Variations in hepatic metabolism and volume of distribution are important in the ongoing assessment of dose-response. Some medications are highly fat bound and are slowly released into the circulatory system, causing prolonged effects, both therapeutic and undesired (such as respiratory depression, poor gastric motility, and abnormal neurologic function, such as feeding difficulties).

PREVENTION OF THERAPEUTIC MISHAPS

More individuals die each year in the United States from medical error than from traffic accidents. A large portion of medical errors is from medication errors.[10] Even after making a correct choice of medication, one must pay attention to the appropriate dose and interval based on factors that affect a drug's pharmacokinetics and pharmacodynamics. Drug delivery must be ensured: this includes appropriate dose calculations, appropriately written and read orders, appropriate mixing with diluents, attention to drug interactions, incompatabilities, and contraindications and drug delivery systems. In addition, effects of therapy at the chosen dose, and systematic monitoring for therapeutic and toxic effects must be included in NICU care when medications are used.

Human error may occur, and it is in hospital areas of highest acuity, such as intensive care units and emergency departments, that the majority of medication errors have been described. In a review of medication errors in a large general hospital, pediatric medication errors occurred at a higher rate than patients in the emergency department and medicine, surgery, and OB-GYN units (5.89 errors per 1000 patients), with dosage calculation errors being the most common problem.[17] The authors suggested initiatives designed to prevent, detect, and avert problems associated with the major factors leading to errors. In addition to calculation errors, problems included availability and information on drug therapy such as pharmacokinetic and drug interaction information, appreciation of patient characteristics that alter drug therapy, and confusing drug nomenclature.[17] In another review of hospital errors involving dosage equations,[18] antibiotics were the principal drug class involved. Errors in the equa-

Box 9-3	THE "FIVE RIGHTS" OF DRUG ADMINISTRATION
Right drug	Right dose
Right patient	Right time
Right route	

tions used to calculate doses for all drug classes accounted for 29.5% of the errors.

Completing the "five rights" of medication administration (Box 9-3) is complicated by the small doses and dosage adjustments based on infant weight or surface area. It has been estimated that 8% of drug doses calculated and administered by competent NICU nurses are at least 10 times greater or less than the ordered dose.[22] Another risk with neonatal pharmacotherapy is that many drugs must be diluted, because they are ordered in amounts that are not commercially available. The rate of drug entry, or absorption, also varies, depending on route of administration. Calculations can be difficult and must be at least double-checked. Examples should be readily available to those responsible for calculating doses. Other suggestions include the use of standardized drug preparations and dosing and standardized nomenclature or computer/digital order entry, with alerts for unusual doses. To avoid errors with emergency "code" medications, the doses of emergency medications should be calculated on admission, along with appropriate infusion rates (Figure 9-4). The calculated doses for the most commonly administered medications should be posted at the bedside; these need to be updated routinely with the passage of days and weight changes (as the pharmacokinetics and pharmacodynamics change).

Including a pharmacist in more direct patient care and consultation than the traditional role of drug preparation and dispensing can reduce medication errors. In addition, designing the ordering system to reduce complexity and provide rule-based order screening and double-checking of calculations and developing effective information delivery may be more effective than traditional education or process-improvement efforts that target interventions after an error occurs.[10,17]

The AAP has published recommendations for reducing medication errors for pediatric patients.[1] These include some hospital-wide actions, including the establishment of a clearly defined system for

NEONATAL RESUSCITATION MEDICATIONS

Name: _____   Weight: _____   Suction depth: _____

Date of birth: _____   ET tube size: _____

Drug	Strength	Dose	Route	Amount to administer
NaHCO$_3$	0.5 mEq/ml	1-2 mEq/kg	IV	_____
Epinephrine	1:10000	0.1 ml/kg	IV, ET	_____
Atropine	0.1 mg/ml	0.1 ml/kg	IV	_____

Other drugs and dosages could be added (see Table 4-2).

_____
Signature of preparer

FIGURE 9-4   Calculations for neonatal resuscitation medications.

drug ordering, dispensing, and administration, with review of the original drug order before dispensing and administration. Confirmation of patient weight and drug dosage and strength are also recommended. Avoiding the use of the terminal zero to the right of the decimal point (e.g., writing 5 instead of 5.0), and using a zero to the left of a dose less than 1 (e.g., using 0.1 rather than .1) will help reduce medication errors. For pediatric nurses, recommendations include:

- **Familiarity with the medication ordering and use system**
- **Verification of drug orders before administration**
- **Confirmation of patient identity before each dose**
- **Verification of calculations with a second individual**
- **Verification of any unusually large volumes or dosage units for a single patient dose**
- **Listening to the patient or parent or other caregiver**
- **Asking questions as to whether a drug should be administered**
- **Maintain familiarity with the operation of administration devices and the potential for errors with such devices**

METHODS OF ADMINISTRATION

Once a clinician orders a medication and the drug and dose are found to be appropriate for that particular infant, the nurse's challenge is to administer the medication correctly. The following section addresses some of the means of delivery that help improve accuracy of drug delivery.

Oral Administration

Variations in oral bioavailability and unanticipated and immeasurable loss of drug complicates administering oral medications to newborns. Loss of medication occurs when infants regurgitate or require gastric suctioning and lose residual fluid that may include medication. If an infant is receiving orogastric (OG) or nasogastric (NG) feedings, medication should be placed into the center of the barrel of a syringe containing a small portion of the feeding. Medication may adhere to the plastic and decrease the amount of medicine delivered. The nurse must document drug administration attempts and any possible loss of drug, with an estimate of the amount lost. For infants receiving oral medications, documenting the color of the emesis or residual material helps determine presence of medications that have distinctive color.

If an infant is bottle fed, the nurse may put the medication in the full bottle. If the infant fails to take the whole volume, however, he or she has not received the full dose. One option is to finish the volume with gavage feeding. Another option is to gently introduce very small portions of a dose into the cheek pouch and wait for the infant to swallow. Another method is to put 5 to 10 ml of a feeding in a small bottle and let the infant take that amount, then continue with the remainder of the feeding. Medication may also be placed into a nipple with a small volume of formula and offered to an infant. For breastfeeding infants, medication may be administered into the mouth as above, with or without a small volume of expressed breast milk. As with all dosing of medicines, it is imperative to record doses and volume and characteristics of any residual material or emesis.

Intramuscular Injection

A newborn infant has relatively little muscle mass to receive injections. When IM injections are required, as with vitamin K, the anterior thigh is the site of choice. Comfort measures should be given before and after injection. Clean the site with alcohol, insert a 22- to 25-gauge needle into the muscle, and for most medications, draw back on the syringe to ensure safe needle placement (unless specifically contraindicated), then inject the medication. After injection the area is massaged. For an infant weighing less than 1500 g, the volume injected into one leg should not exceed 0.5 ml. Document the administration.

Intravenous Administration

IV medication can be given by push or antegrade injection, pump infusion, and retrograde injection.[3,9] Although drugs directly enter the bloodstream, the time required to complete drug delivery to receptors is a function of dosage volume, IV flow rate, and injection site (depending on particular IV methods).[24] Failure to recognize these potential time lags could result in inappropriate expectations of the timing of physiologic responses and peak and trough concentrations. The use of microbore IV tubing will facilitate rapid drug delivery because the volume of the fluid in the tubing is reduced. An example of a pediatric syringe infusion preparation and delivery chart for common neonatal drugs may be useful to the reader.[20] Some drugs should never be administered into the umbilical vein or artery, and drug incompatabilities should be recognized before setting up multiple drug dosing through the same IV line.

Careful monitoring for infiltrates and knowledge of drug-specific treatment for this complication are essential to safe IV drug administration. Continuous IV infusion of pressors is a common event in the NICU, and because of their rapid clearance and physiologic importance, these infusions should never be interrupted without orders. Because of the sudden influx of potent medication, flushes to clear lines with continuous infusions of sympathomimetic amines should be avoided.

Push Injection

IV push medications must be mixed in appropriate volumes, delivered through appropriately sized syringes, and followed with an appropriate flush: heparin with normal saline solution (NS), 10% or 5% dextrose and water (D_5W or $D_{10}W$). If numerous flushes are given, care must be taken with the osmolality of the flush solution. D_5W is hypoosmolar and can lead to dangerous intracellular fluid shifts and hemolysis.

To administer an IV push injection, prepare the IV port closest to the patient. Administer a small volume of appropriate flush, then administer the medication over 1 to 2 minutes. Slow pushes are sometimes ordered, but the rate should be specified by the ordering medical caregiver. A postmedication flush is given at the same rate as the medication to clear the line of remaining medication. IV push administration of many medications used in the NICU is contraindicated because of the possibility of immediate adverse reactions associated with rapid bolus injections. Opiates and sedatives should be given with great care and constant attention to respiratory and cardiovascular parameters. Check a pharmacology reference if there is any uncertainty.

Antegrade Injection

Antegrade injection is the introduction of medication into an entry port along the course of the IV tubing. The flow of maintenance fluid carries the medication to the patient at its rate. Because infusion rates in neonates are characteristically low, significant delays in drug delivery result. If rapid infusion is required, as with emergency resuscitation medications, more rapid infusion rates are necessary. This can lead to a significant medication error if, after drug delivery, the IV rate is not returned to baseline.

Pump Infusion

To avoid delay of drug delivery, two methods of pump infusion using a mechanical infusion device allow control of drug amount and delivery rate. Pumps vary by manufacturer, and consist of a pump that can be set to deliver a specific volume over a specific time, a syringe or other container that holds the medication or fluid to be delivered, and connecting tubing to connect the pump to a port for drug delivery. Because pumps vary by manufacturer and some may be used in a variety of ways, each NICU should have a policy to ensure that each staff member carries out pump infusions in the same manner. If different care providers start and end an infusion, the method used must be communicated.

Method 1. An exact ordered amount of medication is drawn into a syringe and diluted if necessary to provide the volume necessary for pump operation. This drug plus diluent fluid is flushed through the tubing, and the syringe is placed in the pump. After the pump finishes the infusion, some medication remains in the tubing and syringe hub. This medication needs to be flushed into the IV with a flush solution to deliver the entire ordered dose.

Method 2. Medication is drawn into the syringe through the connecting tubing until the desired volume is in the syringe. The syringe is then placed on the pump and a volume carrying the ordered amount of drug is infused. The tubing and syringe hub need not be flushed, because the infant has already received the entire ordered dose.

Retrograde Injection
Injection of medication in the opposite direction of IV fluid flow is *retrograde injection*. This requires injection of medication into the IV tubing, resulting in displacement of a portion of the IV fluid. The excess fluid moves into an upstream syringe. An alternative is to use specifically developed retrograde tubing for administration of the medication or retrograde sets containing a collection bag for displaced fluid.

Retrograde injection as currently available is not recommended for premature infants. Reported disadvantages include limitations in fluid amount because of the size of the tubing, syringe, or collection bag. Microbial contamination risk increases and, because medication is usually calorie-poor, calories are lost.

Other Considerations
Health-care providers must remain attuned to additional concerns when administering IV medications.

Medications may require filters, protection from light sources, or have significant specific gravity osmolarity. A 0.22-μm filter may provide "cold sterilization" (i.e., remove particulate matter and bacterial contamination). Some medications cannot be administered through a filter, because the filter removes the active ingredient. Medications with a specific gravity less than IV fluid have a tendency to accumulate at high points in the IV tubing, whereas those with a higher specific gravity settle into low tubing loops, both resulting in delayed and inaccurate drug delivery.

How to Get IV Access: Inserting Peripheral IV Lines
Common sites for IV placement in neonates include the hands, feet, arms, legs, or scalp veins. A transilluminator may help outline vessels in extremities. (When using a transilluminator, be mindful of potential burns from the high-intensity light source.)
Equipment
Catheters with needles appropriate for vessel size
Tape
Alcohol
Gauze
Syringe with flush solution
Tourniquet
Arm or leg board
Restraints (as necessary)
Gloves
Comfort measures

Procedure. Always consider comfort measures with any potentially painful procedure. Local anesthetic or other analgesia should also be considered. Assemble equipment at the bedside. Provide adequate temperature support. Tear tape into two pieces, about 2 inches × ½ inch wide, and three 6-inch pieces. Select a vessel after confirming it is not an artery. Determine the direction of flow; veins fill toward the heart, arteries away from the heart.

Restrain the infant enough to prevent movement that prevents line placement. Some care providers place a leg or arm board before the catheter is placed; others secure the limb after the catheter is in position. Flush the needle/catheter and remove the syringe. Place a tourniquet around the extremity, taking care to not pinch the skin. (Some caregivers prefer not to use a tourniquet and with practice may achieve success equal to those using one.) Clean the site with alcohol and allow it to dry. After gloving, insert the needle catheter into the vessel using hand

and fingers to anchor the skin surrounding the vessel. Insert at an acute angle and *in the direction of blood flow.* Observe for blood return or flashback into the tubing or cannula of the catheter. Some vessels will not provide blood return; babies in hemodynamic shock may also not have blood return. If you feel the needle is in the vessel but note no blood return, a small amount of flushing solution may be injected. If the needle is not in the vessel, the tissue will swell. If it blanches, the vessel is most likely an artery. If blood return is seen, inject flushing solution to clear the needle; remove the needle and gently advance the catheter.

Place a short piece of tape across the catheter to secure it. Cross a longer piece around the back of the catheter and cross the ends across the front of the catheter. Check for proper position by disconnecting the IV from the syringe to note blood return or infuse a small amount of flushing solution. If necessary use gauze behind the needle for support. Secure the IV in place by using another long piece of tape. Cover the IV site to protect it. Leave adequate access to skin close to the IV site to allow monitoring for infiltrates.

If the medication is to be administered intermittently and the line is not otherwise used, it may be "heparin-locked" and flushed every shift with heparin solution (0.2 U of heparin per milliliter of solution). Heparin solutions are available in several concentrations. It is good unit practice to standardize the volume and container type for each concentration and to individualize how each concentration-specific container looks and where they are kept. Controversy exists over the use of heparin versus normal saline solution for flushing lines. Two recent articles may be of interest: in one a rabbit model was used to determine the length of time for patency of catheters "locked" with heparin compared with those with normal saline solution; the second article examined the same issue in newborns and included a useful table comparing and contrasting the literature on the topic. Both studies found no significant difference in length of time for catheter patency based solely on the infusate.[12,16]

Teaching Model. Models for teaching IV insertion with various needles and catheters vary from the highly sophisticated (and expensive) computerized human patient simulator to the "low-tech" and inexpensive human placenta. The computerized Human Patient Simulator is currently available in two models, adult and pediatric, but there are plans to develop a neonatal model. The simulator allows lines to be inserted in vessels, then bar-coded syringes of "drugs" can be administered through the lines, and the simulator will respond with the appropriate physiologic response, which may include changes in blood pressure, heart rhythms, respiratory effort, and changes in pupil dilation. Less-advanced techniques include various models of neonatal-sized manikins with visible "vessels" in the scalp, arms, legs, and feet.

The fetal side of a human placenta is an inexpensive and easy-to-use model. The needed supplies and procedure follow.

Supplies

Placenta
Assorted needles and catheters
Syringes with flush solution
Gloves
Tape

Procedure. Place the placenta fetal side up on drapes. Remove the fetal membranes, exposing the rich network of vessels. After gloving, insert IV needles with catheters into the larger vessels first, then smaller vessels with improving technique. Tortuous or branching vessels can be used for various methods. Once catheters are in position, practice securing with various taping methods.

Complications of IV Therapy

Complications include phlebitis, infiltration, hematomas, chemical burns, compartment syndrome, and emboli.[19] Long-term complications include disfigurement, contractions, and the need for surgical repair or amputation. Frequent (at least hourly) assessment of IV sites helps reduce, but does not absolutely prevent, IV complications. Swelling or discoloration of the extremity or skin at the needle tip are signs of trouble, and the line should be removed. In the scalp, infiltration may be difficult to assess, because swelling is not only at the IV site, but also on the dependent side of the head. Scalp edema on the dependent side or a swollen eye is an indicator of scalp vein infiltration.

Footdrop[7] and compartment syndrome, in which nerves and vessels are damaged by swelling of tissue within a limited space, have been associated with positioning a footboard along the lateral aspect of the fibula, with or without an IV infiltration. The use of rolled washcloths as footboards or extensive padding of IV boards with cotton or gauze may prevent excessive pressure. Unnoticed infiltrations may result in significant tissue loss. Warm soaks are contraindicated, because when warmed, extravasated

Table 9-1	TREATMENT OPTIONS FOR EXTRAVASATION	
DRUG SUPPLIED	DOSAGE/ADMINISTRATION	COMMENTS
Hyaluronidase* 150 U/1 ml vial	1 ml (15 units) given as 4-5 subcutaneous or intradermal 0.2 ml injections with a 25-gauge needle around the periphery of the IV extravasation site.	• Prepare a 1:10 dilution • Use with extravasation of hyperosmolar or extreme pH drugs • Administer within 1 hr of event • Not for use with vasoconstrictive drugs
Phentolamine 5 mg/ml in 1-ml vial	0.5 mg/ml given as 4 or 5 subcutaneous or intradermal 0.2-ml injections with a 25-gauge needle around the periphery of the IV extravasation site.	• Prepare a dilution • Used for extravasation of vasoconstrictive drugs • May be given up to 12 hr after an event

Modified from Roberts RJ: Intravenous administration of medication in pediatric patients: problems and solutions, *Pediatr Clin North Am* 28:23, 1981.
*Wyeth has recently discontinued manufacturing this product.

fluid may exacerbate the burn, maceration, and necrosis. In addition, heat increases oxygen demand in already compromised tissues.

Elevating the infiltrated area increases venous and lymphatic drainage helping to decrease the edema. Hyaluronidase[6] destroys extracellular barriers, allowing rapid diffusion and absorption of the extravasated fluid. For vasoconstrictive substances that extravasate, local use of vasodilators like phentolamine can aid in reperfusion.

Table 9-1 lists treatment approaches for extravasation.

PARENT TEACHING

IV lines in newborns may frighten the child's parents, especially scalp vein lines. Without information, parents may mistakenly believe the fluid or a needle is going directly into their baby's brain. It is helpful to reassure the parents that a needle, the fluid, and possibly medications are going into large veins. Also, reminding parents that although their infant has an IV line in place, they may still touch, hold, and feed their child may help parents to cope with interventions.

Parents should be made aware that pain assessment and control are part of the caregiver's ongoing efforts, and both are addressed during IV placement and maintenance. They should be told that a newborn's venous fragility, combined with the types of solutions used, make restarting IV lines and multiple sticks per line relatively commonplace. The potential for infiltration should also be addressed,

and parents need to be included in the effort to monitor the appearance of IV sites.

As for an infant's medications, the parents should be made aware of treatment choices in the NICU. They need not know the details of medication dosing but should be made aware of significant medications in their child's treatment regimen. At discharge parents *must* know the names of their child's medications and the dosage, frequency of administration, and side effects as well as where to obtain refills for each drug. Caregivers must teach parents to administer prescribed medicines, and the parents must demonstrate their ability to safely and reliably give their child the recommended doses. The parents should receive written drug information instructions that may be developed by the unit for their families or may be commercially available from such companies as MICROMEDEX Thomson Healthcare (www.micromedex.com). Instructions must include dosing amounts, routes of administration, dosing schedule, and potential side effects.

REFERENCES

1. American Academy of Pediatrics Committee on Drugs and Committee on Hospital Care: Prevention of medication errors in the pediatric inpatient setting, *Pediatrics* 102:428, 1998.
2. American Academy of Pediatrics: *Red Book 2000, Report of the Committee on Infectious Diseases,* ed 25, Elk Grove Village, Ill, 2000, The Academy.
3. Burch SM, Chadwick JV: Use of a retroset in the delivery of intravenous medications in the neonate, *Neonatal Netw* 6:51, 1987.

4. Cloherty, JP, Stark AR, *Manual of neonatal care,* ed 4, Philadelphia, 1988, Lippincott-Raven.

5. Evans ME, Bhat R, Vidyasagar D: Factors modulating drug therapy and pharmacokinetics. In Yeh TF, ed: *Drug therapy in the neonate and small infant,* St. Louis, 1985, Mosby.

6. Few BJ: Hyaluronidase for treating intravenous extravasations, *Am J Matern Child Nurs* 12:23, 1987.

7. Fischer AQ, Strasburger J: Footdrop in the neonate secondary to the use of footboards, *J Pediatr* 101:1003, 1982.

8. Franck L, Vilardi J: Assessment and management of opioid withdrawal in ill neonates, *Neonatal Netw* 14:39, 1998.

9. Glass SM, Giacoia GP: Intravenous drug therapy in premature infants: practical aspects, *J Obstet Gynecol Neonatal Nurs* 16:310, 1987.

10. Glauber J, Goldmann DA, Homer CJ et al: Reducing medical error through systems improvement: the management of febrile infants, *Pediatrics* 105:1330, 2000.

11. Gomella TL, ed: *Neonatology, management, procedures, on-call problems, diseases, drugs,* Stamford, Conn, 1999, Appleton & Lange.

12. Hanrahan KS, Kleiber C, Berends S: Saline for peripheral intravenous locks in neonates: evaluating a change in practice, *Neonatal Netw* 19:19, 2000.

13. Heimann G: Basic pharmacokinetic principles. In Polin R, Fox W, eds: *Fetal and neonatal physiology,* Philadelphia, 1998, WB Saunders.

14. Hilligoss D: Neonatal pharmacokinetics. In Evans W, ed: *Applied pharmokinetics,* San Francisco, 1986, Applied Therapeutics.

15. Holford NHG: Clinical interpretation of drug concentrations. In Katzung BG, ed: *Basic and clinical pharmacology,* East Norwalk, Conn, 1987, Appleton & Lange.

16. Kyle LA, Turner BS: Efficacy of saline vs. heparin in maintaining 24-gauge intermittent intravenous catheters in a rabbit model, *Neonatal Netw* 18:49, 1999.

17. Lesar T, Briceland L, Stein DS: Factors related to errors in medication prescribing, *JAMA* 277:312, 1997.

18. Lesar TS: Errors in the use of medication and dosage equations, *Arch Pediatr Adolesc Med* 152:340, 1998.

19. MacCara ME: Extravasation: a hazard of intravenous therapy, *Drug Intell Clin Pharm* 17:71, 1983.

20. McCurdy DE, Arnold MT: Development and implementation of a pediatric/neonatal IV syringe pump delivery system, *J Neonatal Nurs* 16:9, 1995.

21. Martin, RG: Pharmacology in neonatal care. In Beach P, Deacon J, eds: *Core curriculum for neonatal intensive care nursing,* Philadelphia, 1993, WB Saunders.

22. Perlstein PH, Callison C, White M et al: Errors in drug computation during newborn intensive care, *Am J Dis Child* 133:376, 1979.

23. Rioux PP: Clinical trials in pharmacogenetics and pharmacogenomics: methods and applications, *Am J Health Syst Pharm* 57:887, 2000

24. Roberts RJ: Intravenous administration of medication in pediatric patients: problems and solutions, *Pediatr Clin North Am* 28:23, 1981.

25. Roberts RJ: *Drug therapy in infants,* Philadelphia, 1984, WB Saunders.

26. Taketomo CK, Hodding JH, Kraus DM: *Pediatric dosage handbook,* ed 7, Cleveland, 2000, Lexi-Comp.

27. Young TE, Mangum OB: *Neofax: a manual of drugs used in neonatal care,* ed 12, Raleigh, NC, 1999, Acorn Publishing.

28. Zenk KE: *Neonatal medication and nutrition,* Santa Rosa, Calif, 1999, NICU.

10 Drug Withdrawal in the Neonate

Susan M. Weiner, Loretta P. Finnegan

The epidemic of maternal substance abuse over the last 30 years has continued to escalate at an alarming rate. The extent of drug use during pregnancy is often underestimated, as are the effects on the fetus and neonate. Brown et al[6] reported that the estimated possible prevalence of opiate use among pregnant women ranges from under 1% to 2% to as high as 21%. This lack of awareness is related in part to a tendency of human nature to minimize the existence of socially undesirable problems, especially among those of higher socioeconomic standing. Nevertheless, the sequelae of both licit and illicit substance abuse by the mother during pregnancy must be recognized and addressed to provide optimal medical care of the neonate. Stereotypic biases should not interfere with the diagnosis or treatment. Drug dependence in pregnancy crosses all socioeconomic and racial barriers. Therefore health care providers should not rule out drug exposure in any neonate who is exhibiting symptoms at birth related to withdrawal or exposure to drugs.

Opioid addiction of the mother during pregnancy has been studied in detail for nearly four decades in terms of its effects on the woman, the fetus, and the developing child.* However, as time, circumstances, and knowledge change, other factors need to be considered when treating neonates. Diagnostic data can no longer be gathered on the assumption that one drug or substance was used. Polydrug use and the combination of illicit substances with those that are legal are more the norm. The impact on the fetus and neonate is not necessarily minimized by the legality of the substance.[5] Patterns of abuse, purity of the illicit drug, and sometimes potent or poisonous additions to them may also cause catastrophic sequelae in newborns.

A recent phenomenon studied by Franck and Vilardi[25] concerned iatrogenic neonatal abstinence syndrome (NAS), a condition caused by the abrupt withdrawal of analgesics and sedatives administered during the neonatal period. Recent advances in neonatology have continued to broaden the period of viability as many more premature infants are being kept alive. What appears to be decreased severity of abstinence in preterm infants may be related to developmental immaturity of the CNS or to differences in total drug exposure. This proves to be a problem in evaluating the severity of abstinence signs in a preterm infant, because scoring tools were largely developed for use with term or near-term infants.[1,56] In addition to prematurity, a myriad of procedures are performed on these infants, requiring the use of narcotic sedation and causing narcotic dependence (see Chapter 12).

This chapter presents current information about treatment issues surrounding drug-exposed neonates, with the main focus on opioid withdrawal. The effects of other substances such as stimulants, hallucinogens, nonopioid CNS depressants, tobacco, and alcohol will be addressed when symptoms deviate from those of NAS.

PHYSIOLOGY

Because of their low molecular weight and lipid solubility, all drugs of abuse reach the fetal circulation by crossing the placenta, causing direct toxic effects on the fetus.* Although certain drugs may produce specific effects, many abused drugs produce similar manifestations of fetal and neonatal disease. In addition, the effects of legal drugs such as tobacco, caffeine, and alcohol may confound simple drug-effect relationships.[1] A hostile intrauterine environment may also be caused by adverse effects of the mother's drug addiction and must be considered when diagnosing the neonate's problems. **Examples of factors that could have an impact on neonatal outcome include lifestyle, homelessness, physical and/or sexual abuse, prostitution, poverty, poor or no prenatal care, polydrug abuse, intravenous**

---

*References 20, 23, 32, 34, 37, 38, 52, 54, 58, 60.

*References 1, 12, 23, 34, 58, 60.

drug abuse, binge and withdrawal cycles, anorexia, poor maternal nutrition, pica, dehydration, alcoholism, sexually transmitted diseases, dental abscesses, preexisting medical conditions requiring pharmacologic therapy, HIV-positive status or AIDS infection, and hepatitis B and C.[1,20]

Opioid Substances

When the major opioid drugs such as heroin, methadone, morphine, and meperidine cross the placenta, the fetus may become passively addicted. Morphine, the major metabolite of heroin, and methadone have been identified and measured in amniotic fluid, cord blood, breast milk,[28,42] neonatal urine, and meconium.* Stimulants (amphetamines and cocaine) have been found in breast milk in extremely high levels.[28] Nonopioid CNS depressants (benzodiazepines and barbiturates) and the minor opioids (codeine and propoxyphene) have all been identified in neonatal urine and meconium.† Ethanol and its primary metabolite, acetalehyde, have been identified in placental tissue and amniotic fluid.‡

Human and animal studies have shown that use of opioids during pregnancy directly affects fetal growth. Heroin is associated with IUGR, with only a slight reduction in gestational length. However, the mechanism by which heroin inhibits growth is not known.[17,30] Studies comparing methadone-exposed infants with nonexposed infants have found that methadone-exposed infants had lower birth weights.[30] But infants born to methadone-maintained women have been reported to have higher birth weights than those born to women using heroin.[30] Decreased head circumference has been an inconsistent finding with theses babies. Hulse et al[30] conducted a metaanalysis comparing birth weights of newborns of mothers using heroin to that of newborns whose mothers used methadone alone and that of newborns whose mothers used both heroin and methadone during their pregnancy. A mean reduction of 489 g in birth weight was associated with heroin use, compared with a reduction of 279 g with methadone use. The use of both heroin and methadone produced a mean reduction of 557 g, suggesting that the use of both drugs may counteract the birth weight advantage seen with women on methadone alone.

Neither heroin nor methadone has been associated with congenital malformations or a specific dysmorphic syndrome in offspring.[5]

Recent research has found that when compared with a control group, fetuses who are heroin and methadone exposed do not demonstrate a higher incidence of meconium staining.[34,54,58,60] Heroin exposure during pregnancy has also been reported to accelerate fetal lung maturity.[27] However, it is not known whether this occurs from the direct heroin exposure or from the growth restriction and chronic stress.[54]

Neonatal withdrawal from all the substances that the fetus is exposed to occurs in varying degrees. Several studies have shown that symptoms of NAS in heroin-exposed infants occur earlier than in infants of methadone-maintained mothers. This is a result of heroin's shorter half-life.[5,14,18-22] NAS resulting from in utero exposure to opioids may be severe and may necessitate pharmacologic intervention.

Nonopioid Substances

Cocaine crosses the placenta by simple diffusion. This occurs because of its high lipid solubility, low molecular weight, and low ionization at physiologic pH.[26,47] Cocaine has a significant vasoconstrictive property, which decreases blood flow to the placenta and fetus, contributing to fetal growth retardation and hypoxia.[4,11,41,47,58] These infants have an increased risk of prematurity, perinatal cerebral infarctions, abnormal EEGs at birth, nonduodenal intestinal and anal atresias, necrotizing enterocolitis, terminal limb defects, cardiovascular effects, and genitourinary anomalies.* Maternal cocaine abuse has also been shown to produce neuromotor deficits, which include impaired muscle tone leading to abnormal movement patterns and tremors.[29,47]

Alcohol has been shown to cause diminished deoxyribonucleic acid (DNA) synthesis, disruption of protein synthesis, and impaired cellular growth, differentiation, and migration. These cellular effects can be seen with both ethanol and acetaldehyde and are instrumental in inducing fetal malformations. Alcohol interferes with the transport of amino acids across the placenta to the fetus. Thus embryonic or-

---

* References 7, 17, 33, 38, 45, 63.
†References 7, 17, 26, 33, 38, 44, 45, 63.
‡References 9, 10, 12, 47, 53-55.

*References 1-5, 11, 29, 41, 47, 57.

ganization is altered, with IUGR and chronic fetal hypoxia as the result.[4,53-55] Alcohol causes many of the same anomalies that are observed in cocaine-exposed neonates. When marijuana is added, the incidence of delivering an infant with the features of fetal alcohol syndrome (FAS) are increased nearly fivefold.[2,39,44,47]

When cocaine and alcohol are used together, as is often the case, a unique metabolite, cocaethylene, is formed.[47] Cocaethylene is reported to be 10 times more potent than cocaine alone, which also suggests that it is more toxic in its effects on the growing fetus.[4] In light of this, Bauer stated that the expression of fetal cocaine effects or nonspecific anomalies could be expected to increase when the parturient is combining cocaine with the teratogen ethanol, because the toxicity is augmented.[4]

Amphetamines and methamphetamines known as *crystal, ice,* or *crank* are abused by pregnant women in many geographic areas in the United States with the same frequency as cocaine. Like cocaine and "crack," the amphetamines are potent stimulants, and effects on the fetus and neonate are similar.[5,33,46] In their 1995 article "Perinatal and neonatal issues of substance abuse," Bell and Lau[5] discussed how in utero amphetamine exposure can lead to congenital brain lesions, including hemorrhage, infarction, or cavitary lesions. They also described the sites of these lesions as frontal lobes, basal ganglia, posterior fossa, or general atrophy; the effects of the lesions are not exhibited until the child is older. Plessinger[46] reported on structural and adverse outcomes that are also associated with amphetamine use during pregnancy. These include cleft lip, cardiac defects, low birth weight, growth reduction, reduced head circumference, biliary atresia, prematurity, stillbirth, hyperbilirubinemia requiring exchange transfusion, low body fat, mongolian spots, systolic murmur, and undescended testes.

A review of the most recent literature documents lack of prenatal care as the hallmark of maternal cocaine and amphetamine use with an increase in maternal morbidity and mortality as its consequence.* The use of these stimulants is toxic to the fetal brain, and there is an increase in sudden infant death syndrome (SIDS) and neonatal seizure activity.† These infants also demonstrate poor state control,

difficulty with habituation, and impairment of some neonatal reflexes.*

ETIOLOGY OF NEONATAL ABSTINENCE SYNDROME

NAS is presently occurring in two ways: (1) by the passive exposure to opioids in utero as a consequence of maternal addiction to heroin, methadone, and other narcotic analgesics; and (2) iatrogenically, by the administration of opiates such as fentanyl, morphine, and methadone to the neonate for analgesia and sedation.[25] Infants born to heroin- or methadone-dependent mothers have a high incidence of NAS. Less-potent opioids or opioidlike agents also have been implicated in the development of NAS (Box 10-1 gives a complete list). **Neonatal abstinence is described as a generalized disorder characterized by CNS hyperirritability, gastrointestinal dysfunction, respiratory distress, and autonomic dysfunction manifesting vague**

---

* References 1, 2, 4, 5, 29, 47.

Box 10-1	DRUGS ASSOCIATED WITH NAS

Opioids

Heroin
Fentanyl
Methadone
Morphine
Meperidine (Demerol)

Less Potent Opioids and Opioidlike Agents

Propoxyphene hydrochloride
Codeine
Pentazocine (Talwin)

Nonopioid Central Nervous System Depressants

Tranquilizers and sedatives
Bromides
Chlordiazepoxide (Librium)
Desipramine (Pertofrane; Norpramin)
Diazepam (Valium)
Ethchlorvynol (Placidyl)
Glutethimide (Doriden)
Hydroxyzine HCl (Atarax)
Oxazepam (Serax)
Alcohol

---

*References 1, 2, 5, 33, 46, 53.
†References 2, 4, 5, 11, 12, 33, 41, 44, 46, 47, 57, 61.

symptoms such as yawning, hiccups, sneezing, mottled color, and fever.[18,19,32,33]

When narcotics cross the placenta, an equilibrium is established between maternal and fetal circulations. Before birth, the drug is cleared from the infant's circulation primarily by the mother's excretory and metabolic mechanisms.[22]

The onset of withdrawal symptoms varies from minutes or hours after birth to 2 weeks of age, but the majority of symptoms appear within 72 hours. Many factors influence the onset of NAS (Boxes 10-2 and 10-3).

Once the umbilical cord has been cut, the neonate is no longer exposed to the drug, and symptoms of withdrawal can be expected. Because heroin is not stored in appreciable amounts by the fetus, signs of heroin withdrawal usually are apparent shortly after delivery and generally within 48 hours. However, methadone is stored in the fetal lung, liver, and spleen, facilitating the slow decline of methadone levels, but the rate of metabolic disposition varies for each infant, making the age of onset of NAS unpredictable.[17,24,33,48] Withdrawal may be mild and transient and delayed in onset, or it may increase stepwise in severity. Symptoms may be intermittently present or follow a biphasic course characterized by acute NAS signs, followed by improvement and then the onset of a subacute withdrawal reaction.* Withdrawal seems to be more severe in infants whose mothers have taken large amounts of drugs for an extended period. **In general, the closer to delivery a mother takes the drug, the more severe the symptoms and the greater the delay in onset.**[14]

Usually the origin of NAS lies in the abnormal intrauterine environment. A series of steps appears to be necessary for the onset of NAS and thus the recovery of the infant. The growth and ongoing survival of the fetus is threatened by the continuing or episodic transfer of addictive substances from the maternal to fetal circulation. During this time the fetus goes through a biochemical adaptation to the abnormal element. At delivery abrupt removal of the drug is the catalyst needed to start the onset of symptoms. The newborn continues to metabolize and excrete the substance, so that withdrawal signs occur when critically low tissue levels have been reached. Recovery from NAS is gradual and occurs as the infant's metabolism is reorganized to adjust to the absence of the offending drug.[14,20,33] In another instance, Malpas and Darlow[42] reported two infants who appeared to develop NAS after an abrupt discontinuation of breast feeding. The women's methadone doses were 70 mg and 130 mg, respectively. The data available on the relationship between maternal methadone dose and the drug's concentration in breast milk are sparse and limited to women receiving relatively small doses of methadone.

PREVENTION

Neonatal drug withdrawal is preventable if women do not use dependence-producing substances, licit or illicit, during pregnancy. Through intense educational efforts the desirability and availability of drugs may be thwarted. Unfortunately, the psychosocial and socioeconomic milieu of modern society continues to propagate dysfunctional families, victimization of women, and an intergenerational cycle of substance abuse.

Therefore our goals must be to provide prenatal care for the pregnant drug-dependent woman and her fetus to diminish or eliminate the sequelae of passive addiction. The medical community is challenged to become more astute in its assessment and intervention regarding the problems of drug-dependent parturients. More treatment is required for these women

Box 10-2	FACTORS INFLUENCING THE ONSET OF PASSIVELY ACQUIRED NAS

Drugs used by the mother
Both the timing and the dose of the drugs before delivery
Character of labor
Type of analgesia and/or anesthesia given during labor
Maturity, nutritional status, and the presence of intrinsic disease in the neonate

NAS, Neonatal abstinence syndrome.

Box 10-3	FACTORS INFLUENCING THE ONSET OF IATROGENIC ACQUIRED NAS

Prolonged opiate sedation for mechanical ventilation
Duration of opioid analgesia use during extracorporeal membrane oxygenation (ECMO)
Type of opiate used
Maturity and presence of intrinsic disease in the neonate

NAS, Neonatal abstinence syndrome.

---

*References 1, 14, 17, 21, 22, 32, 33.

and their neonates through inpatient and residential care and outpatient interdisciplinary clinics that focus on the elimination, as well as the consequences, of addiction.

Franck and Vilardi,[25] in addressing iatrogenic NAS, stated that guidelines for effective weaning of neonates from opiate analgesics and sedatives are not yet well established. Researchers encourage dose reductions of 10% to 20% per day (see Chapter 12). Further suggestions for the prevention of iatrogenic NAS include limiting total doses of fentanyl during extracorporeal membrane oxygenation (ECMO) therapy by administering morphine boluses or using continuous morphine infusions to replace fentanyl.[25]

DIAGNOSIS

History

A comprehensive prenatal medical and drug history, especially with respect to polydrug abuse, is of prime importance. All pregnant patients who are substance abusers, regardless of the drug used, are considered to be high risk because of the effects of the drug as well as complications arising from concomitant infections and lifestyle.[5,23,34,37,60] Fear of referral to child welfare agencies or the legal system has, in recent years, prompted women to conceal their drug abuse and/or pregnancy. This fear and denial may prevent the parturient from seeking prenatal care. Thus she may appear at the emergency room of the hospital either in crisis or ready to deliver. In this instance, a prenatal history is absent, making neonatal assessment more difficult.

Signs and Symptoms of NAS

At birth most infants exposed to narcotics appear physically and behaviorally normal. Symptoms of withdrawal begin shortly after birth to 2 weeks of age, but the majority are exhibited within 72 hours.* Acute symptoms may persist for several weeks, whereas subacute symptoms (**irritability, sleep problems, hyperactivity, feeding problems, and hypertonia) may persist for 4 to 6 months.**[12,13,25,33,43] Mayes and Carroll[43] reported that infants of mothers who used cocaine in conjunction with their methadone had significantly higher first withdrawal scores on the NAS score sheet. However, these infants did not require more

pharmacologic intervention, nor did it lengthen their number of days treated.

The most common signs and symptoms of neonatal withdrawal are those of CNS hyperirritability, gastrointestinal dysfunction, respiratory distress, and autonomic instability. The NAS scoring system that is used in monitoring abstinence will be discussed later in the chapter. However, for the convenience of referencing, the signs and symptoms will be discussed here in the order in which they appear on an assessment sheet entitled "Neonatal Abstinence Scoring System."

Initially, the infants appear only to be restless. Tremors develop, which are mild and occur only when the infants are disturbed, but these progress to the point at which they occur spontaneously without any external stimulation of the infant. A high-pitched cry, increased muscle tone, and further irritability develop to the point of inconsolability. When examined, the infant tends to have increased deep tendon reflexes and an exaggerated Moro reflex.*

Infants undergoing narcotic withdrawal have seriously disturbed sleep patterns. Sisson et al[51] studied electroencephalographic tracings and simultaneous electromyographic recordings of eye and mouth movements before, during, and after treatment of withdrawal in 10 infants. REM and non-REM sleep patterns were correlated with muscular and respiratory activity. This study concluded that narcotics obliterate REM sleep in neonates; withdrawal prevents normal adequate periods of deep sleep; proper therapy will cause the return of REM and sleep cycles; and maintenance of therapy can be best regulated by use of polygraphic recordings rather than observed absence of gross signs and symptoms of withdrawal. Schulman[50] reported the absence of quiet sleep in eight full-term infants whose mothers used heroin until delivery. Recent studies by Pinto et al[45a] substantiated the findings of previous sleep studies.[50]

One of the most serious consequences of neonatal abstinence is the development of seizures. **Seizures occur in about 1% to 2% of heroin-exposed neonates and approximately 7% of methadone-exposed neonates.**[1,5,33] The relationship between maternal methadone dosage and the frequency or severity of the seizures has not been established. In addition, no significant differences were found

---

*References 1, 17, 18-22, 32, 33.

*References 5, 18-20, 22, 23, 33.

between neonates with seizures and those without seizures in birth weight, gestational age, occurrence of their withdrawal symptoms, day of onset of withdrawal symptoms, or the need for specific pharmacologic treatment.[20,24] **The mean age of seizure onset was 10 days. Generalized motor seizures, or myoclonic jerks, are the principal seizure manifestation, although in some infants, the seizure manifestation can be complex.** Seizures may occur even while the infant is being treated for NAS. Abnormal EEG tracings tend to occur only during the active seizure, with normal interictal tracings.* The short-term prognosis for abstinence-associated seizures is favorable when compared with the prognosis after seizures associated with other causes. Finnegan and Kaltenbach[20,21] suggested that this observed improvement in neurologic function may be based on the replenishment of neurotransmitters after transient depletion in the neonatal period.

Infants with NAS frequently exhibit respiratory distress symptoms such as rhinorrhea, a stuffy nose, tachypnea, nasal flaring, chest retractions, intermittent cyanosis, and apnea. Increased severity of these symptoms may occur when the infant regurgitates, aspirates, or develops aspiration pneumonia.

There is some evidence of transient abnormality of lung compliance and tidal volume in infants born to methadone- or heroin-abusing mothers and tachypnea in the NAS, suggesting that opioids may alter the fetal development of the respiratory system.[23] Infants with acute heroin withdrawal have shown increased respiratory rates associated with hypocapnia and an increase in blood pH during the first week of life. The observed respiratory alkalosis was thought to have a beneficial role in the binding of indirect serum bilirubin to albumin and possibly in the prevention of RDS, which is rarely observed in infants of opioid-abusing mothers. However, alkalosis can decrease the levels of ionized calcium and lead to tetany.[21]

The risk of sudden infant death syndrome (SIDS) should be considered when the neonate has an especially difficult course of NAS, when the mother supplemented her methadone with other substances (stimulants, nicotine), and when a combination of therapeutic agents is used for treatment, because an increase in SIDS in these infants has been demonstrated to be 5 to 10 times over the general population. Bell and Lau[5] re-

ported that the risk of SIDS is increased in opiate-exposed infants and varies from 2.5% to 4%.[33] Wingkun et al[61] and other researchers studied carbon dioxide sensitivity in infants of substance-abusing mothers and found that these infants have abnormal sleep ventilatory patterns and "an impaired repertoire" of protective responses to hypoxia and hypercapnia during sleep cycles.

Infants undergoing withdrawal from narcotics have disturbed sleep patterns and exhibit excessive spontaneous generalized sweating, which may result from the predominantly central-neurogenic stimulation of sweat glands induced by heroin withdrawal.[20] **Other autonomic nervous system signs include yawning, elevation of temperature, sneezing, and mottling. The rooting reflex is exaggerated. It is not surprising then that these infants frequently suck their fists or thumbs; yet when fed, their suck and swallow reflexes are uncoordinated and ineffectual. Therefore they tend to regurgitate or vomit in a projectile manner. The infant may also develop loose stools and is susceptible to dehydration and electrolyte imbalance.**[17,20,22,33]

These symptoms are exhibited as a result of exposure to opioids as well as nonopioid CNS depressants. However, with nonopioid CNS depressant exposure, symptoms tend to begin at a later age, with malnourishment at birth not a usual feature. Because barbiturate withdrawal may not develop until an infant has been discharged from the nursery, it may not be treated unless suspicion has been aroused by the mother's symptoms or actions. **Furthermore, there is a greater risk of seizure activity in neonates withdrawing from barbiturates than those withdrawing from opioids.**[1,17,18,20,33]

Symptoms exhibited by stimulant-exposed newborns differ significantly from those associated with maternal opioid use, unless the mother was using cocaine or amphetamines along with the opioids. **Recent literature describes cocaine-exposed infants as tremulous, irritable, lethargic, unable to respond appropriately to stimuli, and having abnormal state control and abnormal cry patterns.**[1,5,13,29] **Also described are abnormalities in orientation, motor ability, state regulation, muscular hypertonia, and abnormal reflexes. Infants may show symptoms of lethargy intermittently with irritability, poor sucking patterns, and sleep disturbances.** When cocaine has been the primary drug of abuse, most clinicians have not seen symptoms severe enough to treat the infant pharmacologically.[13,20,47,57] Most would not refer to the symp-

---

* References 15, 17, 20-22, 33, 35.

toms associated with cocaine as withdrawal, but instead as a manifestation of toxicity.[47,57]

Laboratory Data

Before initiating medication for treatment of NAS, one must rule out common neonatal metabolic alterations that can mimic or compound withdrawal, such as hypocalcemia, hypomagnesemia, hypoglycemia, and hypothermia. Serum glucose and calcium tests may be indicated. If the mother has had no prenatal care, it would be prudent to thoroughly assess the infant at birth, including testing for occult disease, sepsis, and intracranial bleeding. **A urine test for toxicology should also be obtained. Meconium testing, although expensive and not readily available in all institutions, appears to be more accurate and can detect a longer period of drug exposure.**[1,58] Recent articles by Zenewicz and Kuhn[63] and Ostrea[45] support meconium drug analysis, because the test is noninvasive, highly accurate, and able to detect prior drug use over a 20-week period. Although hair analysis of the mother and infant shows some promise, this approach is still in the investigative stages, and problems exist with regard to hair color, texture, and acceptability to postpartum women. Drugs of abuse are retained in hair for prolonged periods, and, unlike urine, hair samples cannot be adulterated. Unfortunately, hair sampling is invasive, and the sample may be insufficient in newborns.[45] However, depending on the confidentiality laws of the state and whether members of the medical team are responsible by law for reporting the results of any drug testing to child protection agencies, informed consent may be needed from the mother. Health care professionals caring for infants of mothers who have received no prenatal care will need to check their own state laws and institutional policies for clarification regarding this procedure.[11]

Treatment and Intervention

To determine whether an infant will need pharmacologic treatment for withdrawal, appropriate assessment of symptoms is essential. **Because only 50% to 60% of exposed infants have symptoms significant enough to require medication, an assessment tool is helpful.**

We have used a scoring system to monitor the neonate in a comprehensive and objective way. With this score one can assess the onset, progression, and resolution of symptoms. The score is also used to monitor the infant's clinical response to pharmacotherapy for the control of NAS symptoms. Titration of therapeutic agents is thus based on the degree of withdrawal symptomatology that corresponds to a specific score (Figure 10-1). The nurse is vital in the assessment of withdrawal symptoms, because he or she will administer and record

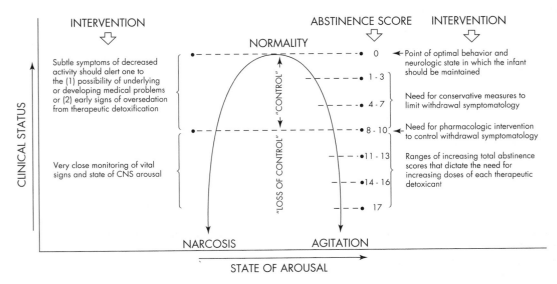

FIGURE 10-1   Management of the neonatal abstinence syndrome (NAS). (From Finnegan LP: Neonatal abstinence syndrome. In Nelson N, ed: *Current therapy in neonatal-perinatal medicine*, ed 2, Ontario, 1990, BC Decker.)

the score and any other activities that may affect the infant's progress. Therefore it is essential that inter-rater reliability be developed between all nurses responsible for the infant.

The Abstinence Scoring Sheet uses a weighted scoring of 31 items most commonly observed in an opioid-exposed neonate.[1] Signs are recorded as single entities or in several categories if they occur in varying degrees of severity. Each symptom, with its associated degree of severity, has been assigned a score. Higher scores are assigned to symptoms found in infants with more severe withdrawal. The total score is determined by adding the score assigned to each symptom observed throughout the entire scoring interval. The scoring system is dynamic rather than static; all of the signs and symptoms observed during the 4-hour intervals at which infant symptoms are monitored are point-totaled for that interval. **Infants are assessed 2 hours after birth and every 4 hours afterward. If at any time the infant's score is 8 or higher, scoring every 2 hours is instituted and continued for 24 hours from the last total score of 8 or higher. If subsequent 2-hour scores continue to be 7 or less for 24 hours, 4-hour scoring intervals may be resumed.**

If medication is not warranted, the infant is scored for the first 4 days of life at the prescribed intervals. **If the symptoms are severe enough to require medication, the infant is scored at 2- or 4-hour intervals, depending on whether the score is less than or greater than or equal to 8, as described previously, throughout the duration of the therapy. Once medication is discontinued, if there is no resurgence of the total score to 8 or higher after 3 days, scoring may be discontinued. However, if there is a resurgence of symptoms with scores consistently equaling 8 or higher, scoring should be continued for a minimum of 4 days after discontinuation of medication to ensure that the infant is not discharged prematurely, with the consequent development of symptoms at home.**

Figure 10-2 shows the Neonatal Abstinence Scoring System. Symptoms are listed on the left, scores to the right. Times of each evaluation are listed at the top, and the total score is listed for each evaluation. A new sheet should be started at the beginning of each day. A "Comments" column has been provided for nursing and medical staff to record important notes about the infant's progress.

Salient points to consider when using the scoring system are as follows:

- **The first score should be recorded approximately 2 hours after the neonate's admission to the nursery.** This score reflects all infant behaviors from admission to that first point in time when the scoring interval is complete. The times designating the end of the scoring intervals (whether every 2 or 4 hours) have been left blank to permit the nursing staff to choose the most appropriate times for scoring intervals in relation to effective planning and implementation of nursing care.
- **All infants should be scored at 4-hour intervals unless high scores indicate a need for more frequent scoring.**
- **All symptoms exhibited during the entire scoring interval, not just a single point in time, should be included.**
- **The infant should be awakened to elicit reflexes and specified behavior, but if the infant is awakened to be scored, one should not score him or her for diminished sleep after feeding.** Sleeping should never be recorded for a scoring interval except when the infant has been unable to sleep for an extended period of time: more than 12 to 18 hours. If the infant is crying, he or she must be quieted before assessing muscle tone, respiratory rate, and the Moro reflex.
- **Respirations are counted for 1 full minute.**
- **The infant is scored if prolonged crying is exhibited, even though it may not be high pitched in quality.**
- **Temperatures should be taken (mild pyrexia is an early sign indicating heat production by increased muscle tone and tremors).**
- If the infant is sweating solely because of conservative nursing measures (e.g., swaddling), a point should not be given. **Medication is not indicated if consecutive total scores or the average of any three consecutive scores continues to be 7 or less during the first 4 days of life.**

The total scores dictate the specific dose of medication, such as paregoric, morphine, or phenobarbital, and all subsequent doses are determined by and titrated against the total score. In the phenobarbital loading dose approach, an initial dose of 20 mg/kg is administered in an attempt to achieve an expected therapeutic serum level with a single dose.

NEONATAL ABSTINENCE SCORING SYSTEM

SYSTEM	SIGNS AND SYMPTOMS	SCORE	AM						PM						COMMENTS
CENTRAL NERVOUS SYSTEM DISTURBANCES	Excessive high pitched (or other) cry	2													Daily weight:
	Continuous high pitched (or other) cry	3													
	Sleeps <1 hour after feeding	3													
	Sleeps <2 hours after feeding	2													
	Sleeps <3 hours after feeding	1													
	Hyperactive Moro reflex	2													
	Markedly hyperactive Moro reflex	3													
	Mild tremors disturbed	1													
	Moderate-severe tremors disturbed	2													
	Mild tremors undisturbed	3													
	Moderate-severe tremors undisturbed	4													
	Increased muscle tone	2													
	Excoriation (specific area)	1													
	Myoclonic jerks	3													
	Generalized convulsions	5													
METABOLIC/VASOMOTOR/RESPIRATORY DISTURBANCES	Sweating	1													
	Fever <101 (99-100.8° F/37.2-38.2° C)	1													
	Fever >101 (38.4° C and higher)	2													
	Frequent yawning (>3-4 times/interval)	1													
	Mottling	1													
	Nasal stuffiness	1													
	Sneezing (>3-4 times/interval)	1													
	Nasal flaring	2													
	Respiratory rate >60/min	1													
	Respiratory rate >60/min with retractions	2													
GASTROINTESTINAL DISTURBANCES	Excessive sucking	1													
	Poor feeding	2													
	Regurgitation	2													
	Projectile vomiting	3													
	Loose stools	2													
	Watery stools	3													
	TOTAL SCORE														
	INITIALS OF SCORER														

FIGURE 10-2   Neonatal Abstinence Score Sheet. (From Finnegan LP: Neonatal abstinence syndrome. In Nelson N, ed: *Current therapy in neonatal-perinatal medicine,* ed 2, Ontario, 1990, BC Decker.)

The need for medication is indicated when the total score is 8 or higher for three consecutive scorings (e.g., 9-8-10) or when the average of any three consecutive scores is 8 or higher (e.g., 9-7-9). Once an infant's score is 8 or higher, the scoring in- terval automatically becomes 2 hours, so that the in- fant exhibits symptoms that are out of control for no longer than 4 to 6 hours before therapy is initiated.

If the infant's total score is 12 or higher for two consecutive intervals or the average of any

two consecutive scores is 12 or higher, therapy should be initiated at the appropriate dosage for that score before more than 4 hours elapse.

The longer the delay in initiating an appropriate medication dose, the greater the risk of increased infant morbidity. **Comfort measures employed for the infant should include the following**[5,13,44]:

- **Swaddling**
- **Offering a pacifier** for nonnutritive, excessive sucking
- **Aspirating nasal secretions** when needed
- **Changing the diaper frequently;** exposing hyperemic buttock in severe cases for air drying
- **Providing soft sheets or sheepskin** to decrease excoriations

- **Positioning prone or right side–lying** to reduce aspiration if vomiting or regurgitation is a problem
- **Protecting the infant from face scratching** by using mitten cuffs on the undershirt or tying a rubber band to the end of the shirt sleeves
- **Considering demand feedings** if weight change patterns are an issue
- **Modifying the infant's environment (noise and light control);** for severe cases, Oro and Dixon[44] recommend self-activated nonoscillating waterbeds as a useful adjunct to supportive care of narcotic-exposed neonates.

Table 10-1 describes the symptoms of withdrawal and appropriate nursing interventions.

Table 10-1	CREATING A SUPPORTIVE ENVIRONMENT FOR THE DRUG-EXPOSED NEONATE	
INFANT BEHAVIOR	**OBSERVATIONS**	**INTERVENTION**
High-pitched cry	Note onset Note length of time the cry persists—is it continuous? Is it high pitched and piercing as though infant were in pain? Observe infant for other causes of abnormal crying patterns (meningitis, intracranial bleeding, pain, etc.) • Is anterior fontanel full or bulging? • Are cranial sutures widely separated? • Is head circumference increased? • Does infant stare without blinking and exhibit adder's tongue? • Is cry aggravated or alleviated when infant is picked up?	Soothe infant by swaddling, holding firmly and close to your body; soft-pack baby carrier; smooth, slow rocking Nonnutritive sucking Decrease feeding intervals and/or implement a demand-feeding schedule Reduce environmental stimuli (noise, light) Waterbeds, lambskin
Inability to sleep	Note how long infant sleeps after feeding Note general sleep and wake patterns If drug therapy has been initiated, note changes in sleep patterns, ability to rest, and whether there is decreased activity indicative of drug overdose	Decrease environmental stimuli (noise, light) Swaddle or use soft-pack baby carrier Feed small amounts at frequent intervals Waterbeds, lambskin Organize care to minimize handling
Frantic sucking of fists	Note onset and amount of fist sucking Observe for blisters on fingertips and knuckles If blistering occurs, observe sites for signs of infection	Use infant shirts with sewn-in sleeves for mitts to prevent skin trauma Offer pacifier for nonnutritive sucking Keep skin area clean; use aseptic technique
Yawning	Note onset and frequency	None
Sneezing	Observe onset and frequency	Aspirate nasopharynx as needed
Nasal stuffiness	Note severity of nasal stuffiness and determine whether it hinders breathing and feeding; if mucus is excessive, consider possibility of other underlying problems, such as esophageal atresia, tracheoesophageal fistula, and congenital syphilis	Allow more time for feeding with rest between sucking Aspirate trachea if tracheal mucus is increased Check rate and character of respirations frequently Cardiorespiratory monitor with alarms set

Modified from Finnegan LP, MacNew BA: *Am J Nurs* 74:685, 1974.

Table 10-1	CREATING A SUPPORTIVE ENVIRONMENT FOR THE DRUG-EXPOSED NEONATE—cont'd	
INFANT BEHAVIOR	**OBSERVATIONS**	**INTERVENTION**
Poor feeding	Note sucking pattern—is infant uncoordinated in attempt to suck/swallow/breathe? Observe for other possible causes of poor feeding (sepsis, hypoglycemia, immaturity, bowel obstruction, pyloric stenosis)	Daily weights Decrease environmental stimuli Feed small amounts at close intervals Wrap securely Maintain fluid and caloric intake required for infant's weight Consider demand feedings Use alternative feeding methods (e.g., gavage) Avoid rocking; may be helpful for some babies Avoid talking or eye contact during feeding
Regurgitation	Note when regurgitation or vomiting occurs—is there a precipitating factor (medication, handling, manipulation, position, etc.)? Observe for signs of dehydration • Specific gravity >1.015 • Urinary output <1 ml/kg/hr • Dry mucous membranes • Marked loss of weight • Poor skin turgor • Sunken anterior fontanel Note time, color, consistency, and quantity of vomitus and/or stool When stools are loose, estimate amount of water loss with stools Note whether vomiting is nonforceful or projectile Observe for electrolyte imbalance	Measure intake and output closely and correlate with infant's general condition, progress, and therapy Offer supplementary fluids if signs of dehydration appear Weigh frequently if weight loss, vomiting, and diarrhea persist Maintain IV at prescribed rate Maintain infant in prone or side-lying position to prevent aspiration of vomitus Head of bed may be elevated Give skin care to prevent excoriation of neck folds, buttocks, and perineum Frequent diaper changes, exposure of hyperemic buttocks for air drying Consider barrier dressings on knees, elbows, etc.
Hyperactive Moro reflex	Is reflex moderately or markedly exaggerated? If drug therapy has been started, note a diminished or absent Moro reflex Is there asymmetry of the reflex? Asymmetry may indicate underlying pathophysiology—Erb's palsy, fractured clavicle, intracranial hemorrhage	None
Hypertonicity	Note degree (mild, moderate, or severe) of increased muscle tone by • Attempting to straighten arms and legs and recording degree of resistance • Picking infant up by hands and noting body rigidity with degree of head lag (a withdrawing infant often exhibits trunk rigidity and holds the head on a plane with the body for a prolonged time) • Raising infant by arms and letting him or her stand (a withdrawing neonate exhibits marked leg rigidity and can support body weight for considerable periods) Correlate mother's obstetric history and delivery with infant's condition and observe baby for other pathophysiology—hypocalcemia, hypoglycemia, meningitis, asphyxia, and intracranial hemorrhage	Change infant's position often since prolonged or marked rigidity predisposes the infant to develop pressure areas Use sheepskin to reduce pressure, plus for relaxation and comfort Decrease environmental temperature if infant's temperature is >37.6° C (99° F)

Continued

Table 10-1	CREATING A SUPPORTIVE ENVIRONMENT FOR THE DRUG-EXPOSED NEONATE—cont'd	
INFANT BEHAVIOR	**OBSERVATIONS**	**INTERVENTION**
Hypertonicity—cont'd	Observe for reddened areas over heels, occiput, sacrum, and knees Observe temperature frequently; increased activity may cause hyperthermia	
Tremors, convulsions	Note whether tremors occur when infant is disturbed and/or undisturbed Note location of tremors • Upper extremities • Lower extremities • Generalized Note whether degree of tremors is mild, moderate, or severe Observe skin over nose, elbows, fingers, toes, knees, heels for excoriation Observe face for scratches Observe for underlying pathology mentioned under "Hypertonicity" Check temperature often for hyperthermia Observe for seizures; if they occur, note onset, length, origin, body involvement, whether tonic, clonic, or both, eye deviation, and infant's color	Change position frequently to prevent excoriation Give frequent skin care (cleansing, ointment, and exposure to air and/or a heat lamp) Use sheepskin Observe excoriations for healing, worsening, infection Decrease environmental temperature if infant exhibits hyperthermia If infant convulses, maintain patent airway and prevent self-trauma If infant is apneic after seizure, stimulate appropriately and be prepared to resuscitate Decrease environmental stimuli Organize nursing care to decrease handling Support movements during caregiving Swaddle as much as possible during caregiving

Modified from Finnegan LP, MacNew BA: *Am J Nurs* 74:685, 1974.

The pharmacologic agents most commonly used in the treatment of withdrawal include paregoric (camphorated tincture of opium) and tincture of opium (10 mg/ml) with the latter preferred. The AAP supports the use of a 25-fold dilution of tincture of opium, which contains the same concentration of morphine equivalent as paregoric (0.4 mg/ml morphine equivalent) without the additives or high alcohol content found in paregoric.[1] A review of recent literature finds that some NICUs treating NAS have switched from the use of paregoric to an oral morphine solution because of concerns about the contents of the paregoric mixture: morphine or opioid alkaloids, camphor, alcohol (46%), anise oil, and benzoic acid. Oral morphine solution contains only 10% alcohol.[25,56]

Table 10-2 outlines drug treatment for NAS. Any infant who exhibits a precipitous drop in a total score of 8 points or higher should be monitored for vital signs immediately. It is important to determine whether any underlying medical problems are developing, such as sepsis, meningitis, hypocalcemia, or hypoglycemia. Detection of underlying medical problems may be difficult, because poorly controlled abstinence may mimic and/or disguise many common neonatal conditions.

An infant may become increasingly depressed by a medication that is not specific for withdrawal. This situation may be reflected in the gradual development of depression, with concomitant poorly controlled withdrawal, requiring reevaluation for appropriateness of the medication (Box 10-4).

The efficacy of the medication must always be assessed. Two common situations indicate the need for reassessment: (1) CNS depression and (2) failure to achieve "control" despite aggressive pharmacologic intervention and/or near-toxic serum levels of the agents. In these situations, the following measures are indicated:

• **Evaluate the infant for metabolic derangements, sepsis, and CNS disturbances to detect an occult problem compounding the clinical picture.** Evaluate laboratory data in-

Table 10-2	DRUGS USED FOR NAS	
DRUG	**DOSAGE**	**COMMENTS**
Morphine	0.08-0.2 mg/dose PO q3-4 hr Use a 0.4 mg/ml dilution: 1 ml of the 4 mg/ml injectable solution added to 9 ml preservative-free normal saline solution. Protect from light; stable for 7 days, refrigerated.	Advantages: Diminishes bowel motility and loose stools; 20%-40% bioavailability when administered orally. Disadvantages: Respiratory depressant, hypotension, delayed gastric emptying, ileus, urine retention.
Paregoric	Starting dose: 0.8 ml/kg/ day in six divided doses. If score is ≥8, increase in increments of 0.4 ml/kg/day until control is achieved or signs of overtreatment occur. Maintain dose for 72 hours. Decrease dose: lower total daily dose by 10%. Adjust dose by weight gain or loss of ≥50 g. Discontinue: when dose is 0.5 ml/kg/day. Observe (depending on symptom severity) for 2-4 days after medication is discontinued.	Signs of control: scores are ≤8, infant is easily consoled, rhythmic sleep and feeding cycle, steady weight gain. Signs of overtreatment: lethargy, hypotonia, irregular respirations, and/or bradycardia. Advantages: diminishes bowel motility and loose stools; increases sucking coordination; controls symptoms in 90% of infants; reduces incidence of seizures. Disadvantages: large doses often necessary; duration of therapy longer than with other drugs; contains 45% alcohol, numerous additives with potential for toxic effects.
Phenobarbital	Loading dose: 20 mg/kg to achieve an expected therapeutic level in a single dose. If score ≥8, give 10 mg/kg every 12 hours until control or signs of toxicity appear. Maintenance dose (once under control): 2-6 mg/kg/day for 3-4 days. Decrease dose to 3 mg/kg/day. Discontinue: serum levels <15 μg/ml.	Daily serum levels can be obtained. Advantages: drug of choice for polydrug use; especially effective in controlling irritability and insomnia; controls symptoms in 50% of infants. Disadvantages: does not prevent loose stools. Infant should be in a nursery where he or she can be monitored closely.

NAS, Neonatal abstinence syndrome.

Box 10-4	COMPLICATIONS OF EXCESSIVE PHARMACOLOGIC TREATMENT

- Diminished or absent reflexes: Moro, sucking, swallowing, Galant, Perez, tonic neck, corneal, grasp (palmar or plantar)
- Truncal (central) or circumoral cyanosis or persistent mottling not associated with ambient temperature decreases
- Decreased muscle tone with passive resistance to extension of extremities or decreased neck or trunk tone
- Altered state of arousal (e.g., obtunded or comatose)
- Diminished response to painful stimuli
- Failure of visual following
- Hypothermia
- Altered respirations: irregular (periodic breathing in full-term infants), shallow (decreased air entry), decreased respiratory rate (<20/min), apnea
- Cardiac alterations: irregular rate, distant heart sounds with weak peripheral pulses, heart rate of 80 to 100 beats/min, poor peripheral perfusion (pale, gray, mottled), cardiac arrest

cluding serum calcium, electrolytes, glucose determinations, and blood cultures.
- **Review maternal drug history along with both maternal and infant urine toxicology results to ensure appropriate medication.**
- **If a single medication is ineffective, consider a combination of therapeutic agents.**

PARENT TEACHING

It is important for primary caretakers to understand that infants exposed to narcotics through maternal addiction have been found to be more irritable and less cuddly, exhibit more tremors, and have increased tone. These infants are also less responsive to visual stimulation and are less likely to maintain an alert state. **Some symptoms of withdrawal may persist for 2 to 6 months, and the nurse should discuss this possibility with the caretakers well before discharge so that they may begin building the skills they will need under the watchful eye of supportive staff.** The infant may continue to feed poorly and regurgitate, yet vigorously suck fists and hands. Mothers frequently misread this continued, exaggerated rooting reflex as hunger and therefore may overfeed the infant. Loose stools may continue.

These infants are easily disturbed by normal household sounds and do not sleep well. They sweat more than the other infants and, when crying, continue to have a high-pitched cry. Hypertonia may continue, and the mother may interpret this as a sign of rejection. Nursing support, including thorough descriptions of the potential symptoms and their management and the fact that they are time limited, is vital if maternal-infant attachment is to occur and potential neglect and abuse are to be avoided.

In recent studies drug-dependent mothers and their infants were assessed for patterns of interaction. Both drug-dependent mothers and their newborns demonstrated poor performance on a measure of social engagement. The drug-dependent mothers demonstrated significantly less positive affect and greater detachment, and the drug-exposed infants presented fewer behaviors promoting social involvement. **Drug-exposed infants and their mothers experience a difficult early period during which both are less available, less likely to initiate, and less responsive to social involvement.**[52,58] Therefore parents of the drug-exposed infant may need assistance in recognizing important symptoms that signal problems and cues necessary for caretaking.

All drugs of abuse pass through the breast milk. However, breastfeeding in the methadone-maintained mother need not be discouraged, because it does not appear to shorten or worsen the course of withdrawal.[28,42,60] On the other hand, women using stimulants and other drugs as well as those who are infected with the HIV virus should not be encouraged to breastfeed because of the potential toxic and negative effects on the neonate (see Chapter 19). **Finally, secondary crack smoke, crystal methamphetamine smoke, marijuana smoke, and tobacco smoke can be detrimental to the health of the newborn; therefore parents should be warned of the consequences of using these substances around their infant.**

REFERENCES

1. American Academy of Pediatrics, Committee on Substance Abuse: Neonatal drug withdrawal, *Pediatrics* 101:1079, 1998.
2. Bandstra ES: Assessing acute and long-term physical effects of in utero drug exposure on the perinate, infant, and child. In Kibley MM, Asghar K, eds: *Methodological issues in epidemiological, prevention, and treatment and research on drug-exposed women and their children,* NIDA Research Monograph 117, Washington, DC, 1992.
3. Battin M, Albersheim S, Newman D: Congenital genitourinary tract abnormalities following cocaine exposure in utero, *Am J Perinatol* 12:425, 1995.
4. Bauer CR: Perinatal effects of prenatal drug exposure: neonatal apects, *Clin Perinatol* 26:87, 1999.
5. Bell GL, Lau K: Perinatal and neonatal issues of substance abuse, *Pediatr Clin North Am* 42:261, 1995.
6. Brown HL, Britton KA, Mahaffey D et al: Methadone maintenance in pregnancy: a reappraisal, *Am J Obstet Gynecol* 179:459, 1998.
7. Buchi KF: The drug-exposed infant in the well-baby nursery, *Clin Perinatol* 25:335, 1998.
8. Chumley Jones H: Shorter dosing interval of opium solution shortens hospital stay for methadone babies, *Fam Med* 31:327, 1999.
9. Church MW, Abel EL: Fetal alcohol syndrome: hearing, speech, language, and vestibular disorders, *Obstet Gynecol Clin North Am* 25:85, 1998.
10. Coleman FS, Kay J: Biology of addiction, *Obstet Gynecol Clin North Am* 25:1, 1998.
11. Collier DN: Protecting the fetus from in-utero cocaine exposure, *N C Med J* 60:40, 1999.
12. D'Apolito K: Substance abuse: infant and childhood outcomes, *J Pediatr Nurs* 13:307, 1998.
13. D'Apolito K: Comparison of a rocking bed and standard bed for decreasing withdrawal symptoms in drug-exposed infants, *Am J Mat Child Nurs* 24:138, 1999.
14. Desmond MM, Wilson GS: Neonatal abstinence syndrome: recognition and diagnosis, *Addict Dis* 2:113, 1975.
15. Doberczak TM, Shanzer S, Cutler R et al: One-year follow-up of infants with abstinence-associated seizures, *Arch Neurol* 45:649, 1988.
16. Ehrlich S, Finnegan LP: Trends and changes in a treatment program for drug-dependent pregnant women: an 8-year study [abstract], *Pediatr Res* 21:1324, 1987.
17. Finnegan LP: Clinical perinatal and developmental effects of methadone. In Cooper JR et al, eds: *Research on the treatment of narcotic addiction, state of the art,* Washington, DC, 1983, US Department of Health and Human Services, National Institute of Drug Abuse.
18. Finnegan LP: Neonatal abstinence syndrome: assessment and pharmacology. In Rubaltelli FF, Granati B, eds: *Neonatal therapy: an update,* New York, 1986, Elsevier.

19. Finnegan LP: Influence of maternal drug dependence on the newborn. In Kacew S, Lock S, eds: *Toxicologic and pharmacologic principles in pediatrics,* Washington, DC, 1988, Hemisphere.

20. Finnegan LP, Kaltenbach K: Neonatal abstinence syndrome. In Hoekelman RA, Nelson N: *Primary pediatric care,* ed 2, St Louis, 1992, Mosby.

21. Finnegan LP, Kaltenbach K: The assessment and management of neonatal abstinence syndrome. In Hoekelman RA, Friedman SB, Nelson NM et al, eds: *Primary pediatric care,* ed 3, St Louis, 1997, Mosby.

22. Finnegan LP, Macnew B: Care of the addicted infant, *Am J Nurs* 74:685, 1974.

23. Finnegan L, Wapner RJ: Drug use in pregnancy. In Neibyl JR, ed: *Narcotic addiction in pregnancy,* Philadelphia, 1987, Lea & Febiger.

24. Finnegan LP, Kron RE, Connaughton JF et al: Assessment and treatment of abstinence in the infant of the drug-dependent mother, *Int J Clin Pharmacol Biopharmacol* 12:19, 1975.

25. Franck L, Vilardi J: Assessment and management of opioid withdrawal in ill neonates, *Neonatal Netw* 14:39, 1995.

26. Garland M: Pharmacology of drug transfer across the placenta, *Obstet Gynecol Clin North Am* 25:21,1998.

27. Hanlon-Lundberg KM, Williams M, Lund T et al: Accelerated fetal lung maturity profiles and maternal cocaine exposure, *Obstet Gynecol* 87:128, 1996.

28. Howard CR, Lawrence RA: Breast-feeding and drug exposure, *Obstet Gynecol Clin North Am* 25:195, 1998.

29. Huffman DM, Price BK, Langel L: Therapeutic handling techniques for the infant affected by cocaine, *Neonatal Netw* 13:9, 1994.

30. Hulse GK, Milne E, English DR et al: The relationship between maternal use of methadone and infant withdrawal, *Addiction* 92:1571, 1998.

31. Jones HE, Balster RL: Inhalant abuse in pregnancy, *Obstet Gynecol Clin North Am* 25:153, 1998.

32. Kaltenbach K, Finnegan LP: Prenatal opiate exposure: physical, neurobehavioral, and developmental effects. In Miller M, ed: *Development of the central nervous system: effects of alcohol and opiates,* New York, 1992, Wiley-Liss.

33. Kandall S: Treatment strategies for drug-exposed neonates, *Clin Perinatol* 26:231, 1999.

34. Kandall S, Doberczak, TM, Jantunen M et al: The methadone-maintained pregnancy, *Clin Perinatol* 26:173, 1999.

35. Kandall S, Gartner LM: Late presentation of drug withdrawal symptoms in newborns, *Am J Dis Child* 127:58, 1974.

36. Kandall SR et al: Differential effects of maternal heroin and methadone use on birth weight, *Pediatrics* 58:681, 1976.

37. Kandall SR et al: The narcotic-dependent mother: fetal and neonatal consequences, *Early Hum Dev* 1:159, 1977.

38. Kreek MJ: Opioid disposition and effects during chronic exposure in the perinatal period in man. In Stimmel B, ed: *Advances in alcohol and substance abuse,* New York, 1982, Haworth.

39. Lee MJ: Marihuana and tobacco use in pregnancy, *Obstet Gynecol Clin North Am* 25(1):65, 1998.

40. Maichuk GT, Zahorodny W, Marshall R: Use of positioning to reduce the severity of neonatal narcotic withdrawal syndrome, *J Perinatol* 19:510, 1999.

41. Malanga CJ, Kotofsky BE: Mechanisms of action of drugs of abuse on the developing fetal brain, *Clin Perinatol* 26:17, 1999.

42. Malpas TJ, Darlow BA: Neonatal abstinence syndrome following abrupt cessation of breastfeeding, *N Z Med J* 112:12, 1999.

43. Mayes LC, Carroll KM: Neonatal withdrawal syndrome in infants exposed to cocaine and methadone, *Subst Use Misuse* 31:241, 1996.

44. Oro AS, Dixon SD: Perinatal cocaine and methamphetamine exposure: maternal and neonatal correlates, *Pediatrics* 111:571, 1987.

45. Ostrea EM: Testing for exposure to illicit drugs and other agents in the neonate: a review of laboratory methods and the role of meconium analysis, *Curr Prob Pediatr* 29:37, 1999.

45a. Pinto F, Torrilli M, Casella G et al: Sleep in babies born to clinically heroin-addicted mothers: a follow-up study, *Drug Alcohol Dep* 1:43, 1998.

46. Plessinger, MA: Prenatal exposure to amphetamines: risks and adverse outcomes in pregnancy, *Obstet Gynecol Clin North Am* 25:199, 1998.

47. Plessinger MA, Woods, JR: Cocaine in pregnancy: recent data on maternal and fetal risks, *Obstet Gynecol Clin North Am* 25:99, 1998.

48. Rosen TS, Johnson HL: Children of methadone-maintained mothers: follow-up to 18 months of age, *J Pediatr* 101:192, 1982.

49. Rosen TS, Pippenger CE: Pharmacologic observations on the neonatal withdrawal syndrome, *J Pediatr* 88:1044, 1974.

50. Schulman L: Alteration of the sleep cycle in heroin addicted and "suspect" newborns, *Neuropaediatrie* 1:89, 1969.

51. Sisson TRC, Wickler M, Tsai P et al: Effect of narcotic withdrawal on neonatal sleep patterns, *Pediatr Res* 8:451, 1974.

52. Smeriglio VL, Wilcox HC: Prenatal drug exposure and child outcome, *Clin Perinatol* 26:1, 1999.

53. Streissguth AP: Alcohol and motherhood: physiological findings and the fetal alcohol syndrome. In Research Monograph No. 16, *Women and alcohol: health related issues,* Washington, DC, 1986, US Department of Health and Human Services.

54. Streissguth AP, Finnegan LP: Effects of prenatal alcohol and drugs. In Kinney, J, ed: *Clinical manual of substance abuse,* ed 2, St Louis, 1996, Mosby.

55. Streissguth AP, LaDue RA: Fetal alcohol syndrome: teratogenic causes of developmental disabilities. In Schroeder S, ed: *Toxic substances and mental retardation,* Washington, DC, 1987, American Association on Mental Deficiency.

56. Tran JH: Treatment of neonatal abstinence syndrome, *J Pediatr Health Care* 13:295, 1999.

57. Tronick EZ, Beeghly M: Prenatal cocaine exposure, child development, and the compromising effects of cumulative risk, *Clin Perinatol* 26:151, 1999.

58. Wagner CL, Katikaneni LD, Cox TH et al: The impact of prenatal drug exposure on the neonate, *Obstet Gynecol Clin North Am* 25:169, 1998.

59. Wallach RC, Jerez ME, Blinick G: Pregnancy and menstrual function in narcotic addicts treated with methadone, *Am J Obstet Gynecol* 105:1226, 1969.

60. Wang EC: Methadone treatment during pregnancy, *J Obstet Gynecol Neonatal Nurs* 28:615, 1999.

61. Wingkun JG, Knisely JS, Schnoll SH et al: Decreased carbon dioxide sensitivity in infants of substance-abusing mothers, *Pediatrics* 95:864, 1995.

62. Zacharia Boukydis CF, Lester BM: The NICU network neurobehavioral scale, *Clin Perinatol* 26:213, 1999.

63. Zenewicz D, Kuhn PJ: Routine meconium screening versus drug screening per physician order: detecting the true incidence of drug-exposed infants, *Pediatr Nurs* 24:543, 1998.

Acid-Base Homeostasis and Oxygenation

William H. Parry, Jan Zimmer

Examination of arterial blood gases and interpretation of acid-base balance are essential to proper diagnosis, management, and outcome in an ill neonate. The measurement of arterial blood gases allows analysis of two interrelated but separate processes: acid-base homeostasis and oxygenation. This chapter describes the parameters that designate oxygenation and acid-base balance, their measurements, and the effects of proposed treatment to maintain homeostasis.[7] Common abbreviations and their meanings are listed in Box 11-1.

Measurement of arterial blood gases involves (1) actual values (PaO_2, $PaCO_2$, and pH) and (2) calculations from these values (oxygen saturation, base excess, and bicarbonate concentration). Some analyzer systems also estimate hemoglobin concentration. To assess acid-base homeostasis, one examines the pH, PCO_2, base excess, and bicarbonate components. The parameters used to assess the adequacy of oxygenation are PaO_2, saturation (SaO_2), and hemoglobin[4,11] (Table 11-1).

PHYSIOLOGY

Acid-Base Homeostasis

An acid is a hydrogen ion donor, and a base is a hydrogen ion receptor. The puissance hydrogen (pH), which refers to the concentration of the hydrogen ion [H^+] in the blood, specifies the acid-base balance in the blood. The quantity of hydrogen ions is minute, amounting to approximately 0.0000001 moles/L. In logarithmic units this is 1×10^{-7} moles/L. The pH is the negative log of the hydrogen ion concentration (pH = 7) (equation 1). A pH of 7 represents a neutral solution, a pH of less than 7 represents increasing acidity, and a pH greater than 7 shows increasing alkalinity:

(1)

$$pH = -\log[H^+]$$
$$pH = -\log[0.0000001]$$

$$pH = -[-7]$$
$$pH = 7$$

The Henderson-Hasselbalch equation describes the pH as a constant (pK) plus the logarithm of the ratio of the base-to-acid concentration (equation 2). Thus, if there is too much acid (an increase in the hydrogen ion reflected in the denominator), the blood pH value decreases. This condition is acidemia. Conversely, if there is less acid or more base, the pH value increases. This is alkalemia.

(2)

$$pH = pK + \log \frac{base}{acid}$$

The pK is the pH at which a substance is half dissociated (cations and anions) and half undissociated (conjugate pair). The pK of whole blood is 6.1; therefore the pH of blood is:

(3)

$$pH = 6.1 + \log \frac{base}{acid}$$

Considering pH is the first step in determining acid-base homeostasis.

The suffix *-osis* denotes physiologic and pathophysiologic processes that tend to change the pH. Thus a process that tends to lower the pH is acidosis, and the process that tends to raise the pH is alkalosis. The normal human pH is between 7.35 and 7.45; therefore a pH of less than 7.35 is acidemia, and the process that caused it is acidosis.

Acid-base homeostasis refers to the physiologic mechanisms that maintain the pH in normal range. Pathophysiologic mechanisms result in pH changes that lead to acidemia or alkalemia. A *tendency* to change the pH, not the actual resultant change, connotes a pathophysiologic mechanism.

Arterial carbon dioxide and bicarbonate values in the blood gas analysis evaluate the processes of acidosis and alkalosis that affect the acid status of

Box 11-1	ABBREVIATIONS
A	Alveolar
a	Arterial
c	Capillary
C	Content
D	Difference
E	Expiration, expired
ET	End tidal
F	Fraction
I	Inhalation, inspired
P	Partial pressure (tension, driving force)
pH	Negative log of hydrogen ion concentration
Q	Flow per unit time
Q̇	Perfusion (flow)
tc	Transcutaneous
v	Venous
V̇	Volume
V	Volume per unit time
VD	Volume of the dead space
VT	Tidal volume

Combined Abbreviations

PaO_2	Partial pressure of arterial oxygen
FiO_2	Fraction of inspired oxygen
$Petco_2$	Partial pressure of carbon dioxide at the end of a tidal volume breath
PIO_2	Partial pressure of inspired oxygen

Table 11-1	NORMAL (ARTERIAL) BLOOD GAS VALUES
BLOOD GASES	**VALUES**
pH	7.35-7.45
$Paco_2$	35-45 mm Hg
HCO_3^-	22-26 mEq/L
Base excess	$(-4) - (+4)$
PaO_2	60-80 mm Hg
O_2 saturation	92%-94%

the body. These parameters assess separate components of the acid-base homeostasis: (1) respiratory contribution ($Paco_2$) controlled by alveolar ventilation and (2) nonrespiratory or metabolic contribution (HCO_3^-) controlled primarily by renal excretion, retention, or manufacture of HCO_3^-.[3,10]

Respiratory Contribution

Carbon dioxide, produced by each cell as a waste product of metabolism, is a gas and follows the laws of gas transport. As carbon dioxide is produced, it dissolves in the intracellular fluid and can be measured as the partial pressure (P) of the dissolved gas (CO_2). As the pressure of the dissolved gas increases in the cell, a pressure gradient develops between this pressure and the extracellular fluid. Accordingly, the dissolved carbon dioxide gas moves out of the cell and into the bloodstream (i.e., from the area of greater pressure to the area of less pressure). Blood transports the dissolved carbon dioxide gas (some combined with hemoglobin as carboxyhemoglobin, most as bicarbonate) to the lung, where the partial pressure in the pulmonary capillary is greater than that in the alveoli.[5] The alveoli receive carbon dioxide according to the direction of the pressure gradient. **Ventilation is the only method of excreting carbon dioxide. The amount of carbon dioxide in the blood is a consequence of the body's metabolism (production) and the alveolar ventilation (excretion). Because metabolism does not change greatly, the measurement of $Paco_2$ accurately reflects the alveolar ventilation.**

Dissolved carbon dioxide is an acidic substance. The plasma ratio of the dissolved carbon dioxide to carbonic acid is 1000:1. In the erythrocyte, carbonic anhydrase combines dissolved carbon dioxide gas with water to form carbonic acid, which dissociates into a hydrogen ion and a bicarbonate ion:

(4)
$$H_2O + CO_2 \leftrightarrows H_2CO_3 \leftrightarrows H^+ + HCO_3^-$$

Elevated $Paco_2$, resulting in too much "acid" in the blood, causes the pH to fall ($\uparrow Pco_2$, $\downarrow$ pH). Hypoventilation causes an increase in carbon dioxide. This process is an acidosis because the acid in the body increases. Because only the lung regulates the amount of carbon dioxide in the body, the process is respiratory acidosis.

Depressed $Paco_2$, resulting in less acid in the blood, causes the pH to rise ($\downarrow Pco_2$, $\uparrow$ pH). A pathophysiologic process that causes hyperventilation reduces the dissolved carbon dioxide. The result is a decreased amount of acid, with a subsequent increase in the pH value. This process is alkalosis. Because only the lung controls the parameter that is changing, the process is respiratory alkalosis.

Nonrespiratory (Metabolic) Contribution

Nonrespiratory (metabolic) factors involved in acid-base homeostasis are regulated mainly by generating fixed acid in the kidney but are also influenced by pathologic conditions of the gastrointestinal system and other organ systems.[3,10] The bicarbonate ion is a base (i.e., a hydrogen ion receptor). The calculated bicarbonate ion concentration, or its corollary, the *base excess,* evaluates the nonrespiratory contribution to acid-base homeostasis.

The base excess primarily represents the actual excess or deficit of bicarbonate, but it also incorporates the buffering action of red blood cells. Multiplying the calculated bicarbonate by 1.2 and subtracting the normal bicarbonate value (24 mEq) from the product estimates the base excess. A positive value suggests a deficit of fixed acid or an excess of base; a negative value indicates an excess of fixed acid or a deficit of base.

Thus when there is a base excess or the bicarbonate ion increases above normal (normal = 21 to 24 mEq/L), too much base is in the blood, and the pH increases. Any process that raises the pH is an alkalosis. Because the bicarbonate ion or base excess is involved (and not carbon dioxide, the respiratory parameter), the process will be a nonrespiratory (metabolic) alkalosis. Conversely, when the bicarbonate ion is below normal, a base deficit or negative base excess is present, and because there is less base (or more acid) than normal, the pH decreases, reflecting an acidosis. Because bicarbonate is a nonrespiratory parameter, this represents a nonrespiratory (metabolic) acidosis.

In the Henderson-Hasselbalch equation discussed previously, the pH was equal to a constant, pK, plus the log of the base/acid ratio. We can substitute the bicarbonate ion concentration for the base, and substitute the dissolved carbon dioxide concentration for the acid. The Henderson-Hasselbalch equation is as follows:

$$pH = pK + \log \frac{base}{acid}$$

Substituting:

(5)

$$pH = pK + \log \frac{[HCO_3^-]}{[Paco_2]}$$

The normal bicarbonate concentration is 24 mEq/L. $Paco_2$ is 40 mm Hg.
Substituting:

(6)

$$pH = pK + \log \frac{24 mEq/L}{40 \ mm \ Hg}$$

However, HCO_3^- units are in milliequivalents per liter, and $Paco_2$ is measured in millimeters of mercury. Multiplying $Paco_2$ by its solubility coefficient (0.03 mEq/L) converts $Paco_2$ to milliequivalents per liter:

(7)

$$pH = pK + \log \frac{24 mEq/L}{40 \ mm \ Hg \times 0.03}$$

Converting to common units: 40 mm Hg × 0.03 mEq/L = 1.2 mEq/L.
Solving:

(8)

$$pH = pK + \log \frac{24 \ mEq/L = 20}{1.2 \ mEq/L = 1}$$

The ratio of base (bicarbonate) to acid (carbon dioxide) is 20:1. The pK of blood is 6.1. The log of 20 is 1.3. Therefore:

$$pH = 6.1 + 1.3 = 7.4$$

Changes in the 20:1 ratio accordingly have profound effects on the pH. For example, should some process occur causing hypoventilation (respiratory acidosis) of sufficient degree that the $Paco_2$ is doubled from 40 to 80, the mEq/L of carbon dioxide gas would be 2.4, and the ratio of bicarbonate to carbon dioxide gas becomes 24:2.4, or 10. The logarithm of 10 is 1, and the pH would be 6.1 + 1, or 7.1. Conversely, if respiratory alkalosis, which results from hyperventilation, occurred, lowering the Pco_2 to 20 mm Hg, the resulting ratio would be (24 mEq/L):(0.6 mEq/L) or 40:1. The log of 40 is 1.6, and the subsequent pH would be 7.70. Similarly, if metabolic acidosis reduced the bicarbonate ion from 24 mEq/L to 12 mEq/L, the ratio would be 12:1.2 or 10:1, and the pH value would be 7.1. If a metabolic alkalosis acutely raised the bicarbonate ion concentration from 24 mEq/L to 36 mEq/L, the ratio of bicarbonate to carbon dioxide gas would be 30:1, and the subsequent pH would be log 30 = 1.47 + 6.1 = pH 7.57.

Thus far these derangements (Figure 11-1) have been discussed as if they happened in isolation, but combined respiratory and nonrespiratory problems often occur, depending on pathologic processes in the body.[1] Besides the four single acid-base derangements, there are combined acid-base derangements: (1) respiratory acidosis and metabolic acidosis, (2) respiratory acidosis and metabolic alkalosis, (3) respiratory alkalosis and metabolic acidosis, and (4) respiratory alkalosis and metabolic alkalosis. The combined acidoses or combined

	Respiratory parameter pCO_2	Metabolic parameter HCO_3^-	Cause
Respiratory acidosis	⬆	↑	Hypoventilation
Respiratory alkalosis	⬇	↓	Hyperventilation
Metabolic acidosis	↓	⬇	Add acid or lose base
Metabolic alkalosis	↑	⬆	Add base or lose acid

FIGURE 11-1 Acid-base derangements. *Large arrow* indicates primary process that produces change in pH. *Small arrow* indicates compensatory process.

alkaloses have a cumulative effect on the pH, whereas an acidosis and alkalosis combination tends to negate the effects of each on the pH value.

Compensation

Acid-base homeostasis maintains the pH value near the normal range. Thus if either the respiratory or nonrespiratory acid-base system is "deranged," the other system will become "unbalanced" in the opposite direction in an attempt to counterbalance the primary process. Compensation occurs when the body attempts to maintain equilibrium by balancing one pathophysiologic process with a second pathophysiologic process that opposes the pH effect of the primary process.

For example, any respiratory process that leads to retention of carbon dioxide (respiratory acidosis) stimulates a nonrespiratory system (i.e., the kidney retains bicarbonate) to return the pH to normal range. The nonrespiratory compensation is actually a second pathophysiologic process, and the retention of bicarbonate (metabolic alkalosis) counteracts the primary defect (respiratory acidosis). Thus a neonate with an increased $Paco_2$ and a compensating elevated bicarbonate is both acidotic and alkalotic but has a pH near the normal range.

Metabolic compensations to respiratory processes can go to remarkable extremes, but respiratory compensations to metabolic processes are limited. For example, hyperventilation cannot lower the $Paco_2$ much below 8 to 10 mm Hg. Similarly, **hypoventilation (in the presence of an intact CNS) in compensation for a metabolic alkalosis is severely limited by the onset of hypoxemia. Hypoxemia, of course, stimulates the respiratory drive, overriding the compensatory hypoventilation, resulting in the alkalemia continuing unabated.**

Correction

Correction of an acid-base disturbance occurs when the health care provider detects the pathophysiologic process and directs therapy at the primary pathologic process, rather than counterbalancing it with a second pathologic process.

For example, if a respiratory acidosis is present, the clinician assesses the patient to discover the cause of the carbon dioxide retention and directs therapy at improving the ventilatory capacity of the lung, rather than attempting to increase the retention of bicarbonate.

Oxygenation

The remaining components of the blood gas analysis are the PO_2, hemoglobin, and oxygen saturation. Oxygenation is distinct from, although related to, ventilation. As previously stated, the $Paco_2$ correlates inversely to ventilation, whereas other factors besides ventilation influence oxygenation. **What is important is the degree of oxygenation at the tissue level.[8,9]**

Many factors cause tissue hypoxia, including the inability of the lung to oxygenate the blood

(arterial hypoxemia). **Another cause of tissue hypoxia is interference with oxygen delivery to the tissue, such as that seen in congestive heart failure (venous hypoxemia).** In this situation the PaO_2 may be normal, but because of heart (pump) failure, oxygen is not delivered to the tissue. Treatment should be directed toward improving delivery by the pump (Chapter 24).

A third cause of tissue hypoxia may result from a decrease in oxygen content (which occurs with anemia). In this instance the heart and lungs work adequately, so the PaO_2 is normal, but there is insufficient hemoglobin to provide an adequate amount of oxygen to the tissues.

Finally, tissue hypoxia may result from an abnormal affinity of oxygen to the hemoglobin molecule.[5] In this situation, the heart and lungs are performing properly, but the red blood cell releases inadequate oxygen amounts at the tissue level because of the abnormal affinity. Fetal hemoglobin has a greater affinity for oxygen than adult hemoglobin and thus requires a lower tissue PO_2 to release comparable amounts of oxygen molecules from the hemoglobin. On the other hand, the greater affinity of fetal hemoglobin enhances oxygen uptake from the hypoxemic maternal placenta blood (see Figure 7-1).

Interestingly, nitric oxide is a compound that has a high affinity for hemoglobin oxygen–binding sites (8000 times that of oxygen). (Compare that affinity with carbon monoxide that has 200 times the affinity of oxygen.) However, a globin chain–binding site tends to protect the heme-binding site and has the benefit of carrying nitric oxide to the tissues, where it acts to reduce vascular resistance.[5] Nevertheless, the effect of therapeutic levels of inhaled nitric oxide on reducing the pulmonary artery resistance and improving the ventilation/perfusion ratio and oxygenation outweighs the risk of reducing oxygen content through nitric oxide–bound hemoglobin.[6]

Because PaO_2 measures only partial pressure of oxygen in the arterial blood (i.e., measures the amount of dissolved oxygen gas in the blood), it reflects how the lung is working but does not measure tissue oxygenation. **Despite oxygenation complexities at the tissue level, the PaO_2 taken with the clinical assessment of tissue perfusion is probably an adequate and accurate reflection of tissue oxygenation.**[8] In a few instances hemoglobin determination may be needed for assessing the cause of tissue hypoxia.

Because respiratory disease is an important aspect of neonatal care, the PaO_2 or the SaO_2 is frequently measured. **Most tissue oxygenation problems are directly related to a respiratory problem rather than to oxygen delivery, oxygen content, or hemoglobin affinity problems. A high PaO_2 can be as dangerous as a low PaO_2. Retinopathy of prematurity has been related to arterial oxygen tensions greater than 100 mm Hg and is directly related to PaO_2 but not to the FiO_2 (see Chapter 23).**

In cyanotic congenital heart disease there is a fixed shunt that does not allow the PaO_2 to rise when supplemental oxygen is given; thus a low PaO_2 is not related to lung disease. In respiratory distress, hypoxemia because of intrapulmonary shunting or ventilation and perfusion inequality can be overcome by increasing the inspired oxygen tension.

Theoretically, in a normal lung with matched ventilation and perfusion, the alveolar (PAO_2) and the arterial oxygen tension (PaO_2) should be equal. The body never obtains this ideal situation, and a difference (gradient) in gas tension exists between the PAO_2 and the PaO_2. An inequality in ventilation and perfusion creates the gradient, the functional intrapulmonary shunt, and the anatomic shunt. **The alveolar-arterial oxygen gradient $D(A\text{-}a)O_2$ is useful in estimating the degree of pulmonary involvement in hypoxemia. The difference between the value of the alveolar oxygen and arterial oxygen tensions should be less than 20. The $D(A\text{-}a)O_2$ will be greater than 20 in pulmonary disease.**

To calculate the alveolar-arterial oxygen difference:

(9)

$$D(A\text{-}a)O_2 = PAO_2 - PaO_2$$

Substitute the calculation of alveolar oxygen tension:

(10)

$$D(A\text{-}a)O_2 = \left(FiO_2 - \frac{PaCO_2}{RQ} \right) - PaO_2$$

Substitute the calculation of inspired oxygen tension:

(11)

$$D(A\text{-}a)O_2 = \left[(PB - 47)\, FiO_2 - \frac{PaCO_2}{RQ} \right] - PaO_2$$

Blood gas analysis measures the arterial PO_2. The alveolar (PAO_2) is calculated as follows. First determine the inspiratory PO_2, which is the barometric pressure minus the water vapor pressure multiplied by the fraction of the inspired oxygen.

To calculate the inspired oxygen tension:

(12)

$$PI_{O_2} = (P_B - P_{H_2O})Fi_{O_2}$$

BUT

$$P_{H_2O} = 47$$

THUS

$$PI_{O_2} = (P_B - 47)Fi_{O_2}$$

Thus the inspired oxygen pressure when one is breathing room air at sea level is $(760 - 47)(0.21) = 150$ mm Hg.

The alveolar oxygen is equal to the inspired oxygen minus the alveolar carbon dioxide divided by the respiratory quotient (RQ). Clinically, the alveolar carbon dioxide is equal to the arterial carbon dioxide, and RQ is 0.8.

To calculate the alveolar oxygen tension:

(13)

$$PA_{O_2} = PI_{O_2} - \frac{PA_{CO_2}}{RQ}$$

BUT

$$PA_{CO_2} = Pa_{CO_2}$$

AND

$$RQ = 0.8$$

THUS

$$PA_{O_2} = PI_{O_2} - \frac{PA_{CO_2}}{0.8}$$

Therefore when one is breathing room air at sea level with a Pa_{CO_2} of 40 mm Hg, the alveolar oxygen pressure is equal to the PI_{O_2} (150 mm Hg) minus 40 divided by 0.8 (which is 50), or 100 mm Hg. The alveolar-arterial oxygen gradient in an infant with a Pa_{O_2} of 160 mm Hg and a Pa_{CO_2} of 40 mm Hg in an atmosphere of 40% oxygen at sea level is 75 mm Hg.

(14)

$$D(A\text{-}a)_{O_2} = \left[(760 - 47)\,0.4 - \frac{40}{0.8}\right] - 160 = 75$$

The alveolar-arterial oxygen gradient is useful in predicting the Fi_{O_2} necessary for a desired Pa_{O_2}. Working from a known $D(A\text{-}a)_{O_2}$ and rearranging equation 11:

(15)

$$Fi_{O_2} = \frac{D(A\text{-}a)_{O_2} + \dfrac{Pa_{CO_2}}{RQ} + Pa_{O_2}}{(P_B - 47)}$$

For example, to obtain a Pa_{O_2} of 90 mm Hg in an infant with an alveolar-arterial gradient of 75 mm Hg

and a Pa_{CO_2} of 40 mm Hg at sea level, the infant requires an atmosphere of 30% oxygen ($Fi_{O_2} = 0.3$).

(16)

$$Fi_{O_2} = \frac{75 + \dfrac{40}{0.8} + 90}{(760 - 47)} = 0.3$$

Knowledge of the $D(A\text{-}a)_{O_2}$ can help the clinician adjust the arterial oxygen concentration by working the equation backward (equation 15). Thus if the alveolar-arterial gradient is known, we can set an Fi_{O_2} on the ventilator that will predict a desired Pa_{O_2}.

Equation 15 can be simplified. The rule of seven states that the estimated percentage change in inspired oxygen is equal to the desired change in Pa_{O_2} divided by 7.

(17)

$$\%O_2 \text{ change} = \frac{\text{New } Pa_{O_2} - \text{Old } Pa_{O_2}}{7}$$

For example, to obtain a Pa_{O_2} of 90 mm Hg in an infant with a Pa_{O_2} of 160 mm Hg, a reduction of 10% inspired oxygen is required.

(18)

$$\%O_2 \text{ change} = \frac{90 - 160}{7} = \frac{-70}{7} = -10\%$$

Saturation

Saturation is the percentage of hemoglobin that is combined with oxygen. Oxygen binding with hemoglobin increases as the partial pressure of oxygen increases, but not linearly.[5] The oxygen dissociation curve is a measure of the affinity that hemoglobin has for oxygen (Figure 11-2).

The "30-60-90 rule" is useful in remembering percent saturation and reconstructing the hemoglobin dissociation curve if required (see Figure 11-2). At Pa_{O_2} of 30 mm Hg, the oxygen saturation is 60%; at a Pa_{O_2} of 60 mm Hg, saturation is 90%; and at 90 mm Hg Pa_{O_2} the hemoglobin is 95% saturated. At the normal venous oxygen tension of 40 mm Hg, the oxygen saturation is 75%.

Factors that affect this affinity include temperature, pH, and hemoglobin structure. Hypothermia, alkalemia, hypocapnia, and fetal hemoglobin increase the affinity of hemoglobin for oxygen (shift the curve to the left), whereas fever, acidemia, and hypercapnia decrease the affinity of hemoglobin for oxygen (shift the curve to the

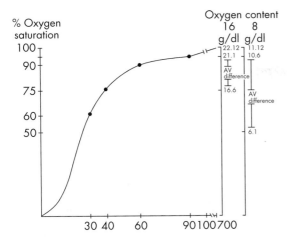

FIGURE 11-2   Oxygen hemoglobin dissociation curve; the 30-60-90 rule is demonstrated. *Right,* the oxygen content for a hemoglobin concentration of 16 g/dl and 8 g/dl is given, demonstrating the effect of anemia on venous saturation and tissue.

right). At a given tissue Po_2 an increased affinity for oxygen releases less oxygen at the tissue level, whereas a decreased affinity releases more oxygen to the tissue. Alternately, the Po_2 at which the oxygen-binding sites of hemoglobin are 50% saturated (the P_{50}) is low when the hemoglobin affinity is great and higher when the hemoglobin affinity is low.[5]

Content

Oxygen content is calculated from the hemoglobin saturation and hemoglobin concentration. One gram of hemoglobin binds 1.39 ml of oxygen. The oxygen content in milliliters per deciliter is the product of the saturation percentage and the hemoglobin in grams per deciliter plus the amount of dissolved oxygen. For clinical purposes we can neglect the amount of dissolved oxygen in plasma, because it is only 0.003 ml/dl/mm Hg.

Oxygen content becomes critical in anemia, which can cause a significant derangement in tissue oxygenation. An infant with a hemoglobin of 8 g/dl will have half the oxygen content of an infant with a hemoglobin of 16 g/dl at an equivalent percentage saturation. In Figure 11-2, an infant with 16 g hemoglobin that is 95% saturated ($Pao_2 = 90$ mm Hg) carries 21.1 ml/dl oxygen, whereas the infant with 8 g hemoglobin carries 10.6 ml/dl oxygen. The tissues require approximately 4 to 5 ml/dl oxygen

for metabolism. Therefore venous blood contains 4 to 5 ml/dl oxygen less than the arterial blood. The venous oxygen content in an infant with 16 g hemoglobin would be between 16 and 17 ml/dl ($21.1 - 4.5 = 16.6$), which corresponds to approximately 75% saturation ($16.6/22.4 = 74.6\%$), or a Pvo_2 of 40 mm Hg. However, the venous oxygen content in an infant with 8 g hemoglobin would be 6.1 ml/dl oxygen ($10.6 - 4.5 = 6.1$). The saturation is 55% ($6.1/11.12$), which corresponds to a Po_2 of less than 30, suggests tissue hypoxia, as compared with an infant with 16 g/dl hemoglobin.

Blood Flow

The product of oxygen content (Cao_2) and the pulmonary blood flow determines the total amount of oxygen in arterial blood. The total blood flow (t) can be divided into the amount of blood in the pulmonary capillaries (c) and in the shunt (s). Knowing the venous oxygen content, arterial oxygen content, and oxygen content in the pulmonary capillaries exposed to ventilated alveoli permits calculation of shunting.

(19)

$$\frac{\dot{Q}s}{\dot{Q}t} = \frac{Cco_2 - Cao_2}{Cco_2 - Cvo_2}$$

A shunt occurs when blood passes from the systemic venous to the systemic arterial circulation without receiving oxygen, because of anatomic defects in the heart (such as cyanotic congenital heart disease) or because of blood perfusing alveoli that are not ventilated (such as intrapulmonary shunts). Shunts lower the final arterial oxygen saturation. The usual degree of shunt in a newborn is 15% to 20% of the cardiac output.

The degree of oxygen saturation in the components estimates the percentage of shunt. (The equation is derived in terms of oxygen content, but in the absence of significant anemia, hemoglobin saturation is adequate for clinical purposes.)

(20)

$$\frac{\dot{Q}s}{\dot{Q}t} = \frac{Sco_2 - Sao_2}{Sco_2 - Svo_2} \times 100$$

Venous and arterial saturation can be calculated from venous and arterial blood gases, and the pulmonary capillary saturation can be estimated from the calculated alveolar oxygen tension (see equation 13). Calculation of the shunt helps distinguish lung disease from congenital heart disease or helps document changes in the severity of lung disease.

ETIOLOGY FACTORS

Acid-Base Homeostasis

Ventilation is usually defined as the amount of gas leaving the mouth per units of time (e.g., minute ventilation, $\dot{V}E$). Minute ventilation is equal to the product of the tidal volume (VT) and the respiratory frequency in breaths per minute:

(21)

$$\dot{V}E = VT \times f$$

The tidal volume can be divided into (1) the gas in the airway plus the gas in nonperfused alveoli (physiologic dead space, VD) and (2) the gas in the alveolar space, which is involved in gas exchange (alveolar volume, VA). Therefore:

(22)

$$\dot{V}E = (VD + VA)f$$

or

(23)

$$\dot{V}E = \dot{V}D + \dot{V}A$$

Alveolar ventilation ($\dot{V}A = \dot{V}E - \dot{V}D$) is measured by collecting the volume of expired gas ($\dot{V}E$) and measuring the concentration of carbon dioxide gas in the expired volume ($FEco_2$) and the arterial carbon dioxide tension ($Paco_2$) and a constant:

(24)

$$\dot{V}A = \frac{\dot{V}E\ (FEco_2)}{Paco_2} \times K = \frac{Vco_2(K)}{Paco_2}$$

Thus the $Paco_2$ is inversely related to alveolar ventilation.

A disturbance in alveolar ventilation (a change in Pco_2) causes an acid-base derangement. In a respiratory acidosis when carbon dioxide excretion is below normal, several conditions must be considered. The most common cause of carbon dioxide retention is obstructive lung disease. Meconium aspiration is a common cause of obstructive lung disease in the neonate, and transient tachypnea of the newborn is an obstructive lung disease. Obstructive lung disease is found in the recovery phase of uncomplicated respiratory distress syndrome and in bronchopulmonary dysplasia. Alveolar ventilation is decreased in these conditions from the increased physiologic dead space that occurs with (1) debris in the large and small airways, (2) inflammation in the large and small airways, and (3) ventilation and perfusion mismatch. An increase in dead space leads to carbon dioxide retention.

Another major cause of carbon dioxide retention is poor respiratory effort from (1) narcosis because of maternal anesthesia before delivery, (2) depressed respiratory drive because of sepsis, (3) severe intracranial hemorrhage, including intraventricular hemorrhage, or (4) metabolic disturbances, such as hypoglycemia, affecting the respiratory center.

The third cause involves injuries or changes in the thoracic cage, such as diaphragmatic hernia, phrenic nerve paralysis, or pneumothorax. These result in a decline in tidal volume or respiratory rate, or a combination of these.

In respiratory alkalosis the carbon dioxide excretion is greater than normal. The mechanism for this increased excretion is hyperventilation. Respiratory alkalosis because of hyperventilation may be (1) iatrogenic, resulting from vigorous ventilator therapy in a neonate with respiratory disease; (2) a result of restrictive lung disease, such as early respiratory distress syndrome (RDS); (3) caused by CNS stimulation of the respiratory drive (e.g., high altitude and encephalitis); and (4) present in hypoxemia, which stimulates the respiratory centers through chemoreceptors.

In nonrespiratory (metabolic) acidosis the metabolic component results from either adding nonvolatile acid (an acid other than carbon dioxide) or losing base bicarbonate.[3] Abnormal acids that are associated with diseases are lactic acid in hypoxia, organic acids in renal failure, and ketoacids in diabetic acidosis. Loss of base occurs in renal tubular acidosis (a defect in the ability of the renal tubules to reabsorb bicarbonate), diarrhea with loss of bicarbonate in the feces, or through urinary excretion resulting from the effects of certain drugs, such as acetazolamide (Diamox).

Measurement of the *anion gap* may distinguish the nature of the metabolic acidosis.[2,3] The anion gap is variably calculated: taking value of the serum sodium minus the serum chloride minus the serum bicarbonate,[2] or alternately, the sodium plus the serum potassium minus the chloride.[3] Acidosis with an increased anion gap probably results from the addition of nonvolatile acids. In the presence of a normal anion gap, loss of base is the likely source of the acidosis.

Nonrespiratory (metabolic) alkalosis is caused either by a loss of acid or an addition of base, principally bicarbonate.[3] A bicarbonate addition is most likely iatrogenic. Loss of acid occurs with nasogastric suctioning or severe vomiting, which may occur in pyloric stenosis. Acid loss also occurs from the kidney through the influence of certain drugs such as diuretics, digitalis therapy, and corticosteroids, which preferentially excrete sodium and potassium, causing depletion. A hydrogen ion is therefore substituted in the urine to conserve sodium or potassium. Acid is lost because the hydrogen ion is excreted, the base remains, and the body fluids become alkaline.

Oxygenation

Although delivery system failure (heart failure), anemia, abnormal hemoglobin affinity for oxygen, and a decreased PaO_2 may cause tissue hypoxia, hypoxemia results from only lung disease or cyanotic congenital heart disease. The most common abnormality of the lung leading to hypoxemia is mismatched ventilation and perfusion. Perfect matching of ventilation and perfusion takes place when an adequate amount of blood flows past oxygenated and ventilated alveoli, but this ideal situation rarely occurs. There is always some degree of ventilation and perfusion mismatch. Two extreme examples of mismatch are (1) ventilated and oxygenated alveoli without perfusion (e.g., pulmonary emboli or persistent pulmonary hypertension of the newborn) and (2) the well-perfused but nonventilated alveoli (atelectasis). The former is an example of wasted ventilation ($\dot{V}\dot{Q}$ = infinity), and the latter is an example of an intrapulmonary shunt ($\dot{V}\dot{Q}$ = O). Either extreme of ventilation and perfusion abnormality is incompatible with life, and thus the degree of ventilation and perfusion mismatch is somewhere between the ends of the spectrum.

Hypoxemia because of ventilation and perfusion mismatch can be overcome by administering supplemental inspired oxygen. Despite poorly ventilated alveoli, raising the inspired oxygen tension will wash nitrogen from the alveoli, resulting in a higher alveolar oxygen tension, which increases artery oxygen tension. However, in an extrapulmonary shunt, no oxygen is exposed to any of the shunted blood, and the PaO_2 cannot increase.

To perform the "shunt test," place a neonate with hypoxemia in 100% oxygen; if the PaO_2 rises to more than 150 mm Hg pressure, cyanotic congenital heart disease is unlikely.

Central hypoventilation from narcosis may cause hypoxemia. As the alveolar carbon dioxide rises, the PaO_2 falls, and subsequently PaO_2 decreases. However, this condition should be clinically evident and should not be confused with lung or congenital heart disease. Other causes of hypoxemia are sufficiently rare in the infant that we need only mention them: decreased inspired oxygen tension, which may occur at high altitude, and oxygen diffusion limitations.

Most conditions that were thought to be diffusion limited are caused by ventilation and perfusion mismatch. The oxygen molecule must diffuse from the alveolus across the alveolar cell, interstitial space, the capillary endothelial cell, and the plasma to the red blood cell. A pathologic condition may occur that interferes with the diffusion process (e.g., thickening of the interstitial space). These processes, however, do not affect oxygen diffusion as much as they alter ventilation and perfusion relationships. Consequently the abnormal ventilation and perfusion relationship causes the hypoxemia rather than diffusion limitation.

PREVENTION

Perinatal asphyxia has profound effects on neonatal oxygenation, involving the following factors: (1) decreased inspired oxygen tension, (2) an aggravated ventilation and perfusion mismatch (increased intrapulmonary shunt) and anatomic shunt through the ductus arteriosus and foramen ovale, (3) decreased cardiac output through asphyxic cardiomyopathy, and (4) decreased oxygen affinity by shifting the oxygen dissociation curve to the right during asphyxic acidemia that resulted from combined metabolic and respiratory acidosis.[1]

Prevention of acid-base and oxygenation disturbances and maintenance of acid-base homeostasis require attention to detail. Prevention of premature births or transport of pregnant women who may deliver a high-risk infant to tertiary care centers for treatment can minimize perinatal asphyxia. Prompt and efficient resuscitation measures can also significantly improve the survival rate of premature infants with acid-base and oxygenation problems.

With respiratory disturbances, immediate assessment and prompt therapy, including supplemental inspired oxygen and assisted ventilation when indicated, minimize the respiratory component of acid-base and oxygenation disturbances (see Chapter 23). Careful monitoring of fluid intake and output, minimizing blood loss, observing for sepsis, and monitoring urine electrolytes for potential abnormalities will enable the clinician to control the continuous nonrespiratory conditions and ideally prevent development of nonrespiratory acid-base disturbances.

Monitoring inspired oxygen tensions and arterial oxygen tensions and supplying appropriate concentrations of additional inspired oxygen will prevent low arterial oxygen tensions (see Chapter 23). Monitoring may be accomplished intermittently through indwelling arterial catheters or continuously through transcutaneous oxygen monitors and pulse oxygen saturation devices (see Chapter 7). Monitoring hemoglobin concentration and blood loss, with replacement to an adequate hemoglobin concentration, potentially ensures adequate oxygen content. Careful attention to fluids, electrolytes, and acid-base homeostasis minimizes adverse effects of asphyxic cardiomyopathy by reducing the strain on the heart.

DATA COLLECTION

Reviewing the patient's history, performing a physical examination, and evaluating laboratory data augment each other in the assessment of disturbances in acid-base homeostasis and oxygenation (Box 11-2).[4]

History

An adequate obstetric and perinatal history may warn of potential acid-base and oxygenation disturbances:
- Premature delivery predisposes the infant to shock and respiratory distress.
- Meconium staining may portend respiratory difficulties.

Box 11-2	EVALUATION OF ACID-BASE DISTURBANCES AND OXYGENATION PROBLEMS IN NEONATES

1. History
   a. Obstetric and perinatal
   b. Neonatal
   c. Family
2. Physical examination
   a. Vital signs
   b. General appearance
   c. Respiratory effort
   d. Pulmonary examination
   e. Cardiac examination
   f. Abdominal examination
   g. Neurologic examination
3. Laboratory
   a. Chest x-ray film
   b. Arterial blood gases
   c. Urinalysis
   d. In selected cases: sepsis evaluation, urine electrolytes, and serum electrolytes

---

- Prolonged rupture of membranes, infants of diabetic mothers, or abnormal maternal bleeding may be associated with either metabolic or respiratory acid-base disturbances and hypoxemia.
- A neonatal history of vomiting, diarrhea, or other gastrointestinal disturbances can cause acid-base disturbances.
- The infant's general appearance, feeding habits, and activity level may indicate sepsis or CNS injury, both of which promote acid-base disturbances and hypoxemia.
- Nosocomial infections and pneumonia may significantly influence acid-base and oxygenation disturbances.
- A family history of inherited renal problems such as tubular acidosis may suggest an acid-base disturbance.
- A family history of salt-losing endocrinopathies may produce an acid-base disturbance.

Physical Examination: Signs and Symptoms

Signs of acid-base disturbance vary widely and often go undetected.[1] Vital signs that show hypothermia and low blood pressure imply metabolic derangements in acid-base homeostasis. Respiratory rate and pattern, grunting, flaring, and retractions indicate respiratory derangements of acid-base homeostasis and oxygenation. Abnormal auscultation of the chest or heart may suggest present or future acid-base or oxygenation disturbances, including possible congenital heart disease. Examining the abdomen, particularly for the proper number and size of kidneys, is important in assessing potential acid-base disturbances. Lethargy, seizures, generalized neurologic signs, or focal neurologic signs increase concern about either potential respiratory or metabolic acid-base disturbances or hypoxemia.

Laboratory Data

Chest X-ray

A chest x-ray examination may identify a respiratory cause for acid-base disturbance and hypoxemia.

Urinalysis

The routine urinalysis records urine specific gravity and demonstrates that urine is being produced.

Arterial Blood Gases

Interpretation of the arterial blood gases will point to the primary acid-base derangement and may reveal a secondary compensation and define the degree of hypoxemia.[2,4,11] Presently, methods for monitoring of the components of acid-base analysis comprise both invasive and noninvasive techniques. Intermittent arterial punctures or indwelling catheters in various vessels (often the umbilical arteries or veins) supply the requisite data. However, we can continuously measure transcutaneous PO_2 or O_2 saturation. Monitors can continuously measure expired end-tidal CO_2, which corresponds to the alveolar CO_2. (We have seen earlier that alveolar and arterial CO_2 are equivalent.) Additionally, skin electrodes are available that measure PaO_2 and $PaCO_2$.

Although the pathophysiologic condition of the acid-base disturbance is determined through the analysis of arterial blood gases, further assessment of the infant is required[1,2]:

- Respiratory alkalosis or acidosis should be evident from the physical examination, arterial blood gas analysis, and chest x-ray examination.
- Consider shock and sepsis in metabolic acidosis. The anion gap and urine electrolytes may provide additional information to delineate causes. Blood pressure measurement, a complete blood cell count, serum and urine electrolyte and glucose determinations, and assessment of intake and output of fluids are necessary to assess a metabolic disturbance.
- Oxygenation disturbances may be analyzed from the preceding laboratory tests, and when indicated, electrocardiogram and arterial blood gas response to increased inspired oxygen concentrations are used to evaluate the possibility of cyanotic congenital heart disease.

Another calculation, the oxygenation index (OI), has come into favor for assessing and following the course of critically ill neonates receiving ventilator therapy. The OI is $(FiO_2 \times 100 \times$ Mean airway pressure$)/PaO_2$. An OI of 25 or greater has been considered an indication for extraordinary ventilatory support, such as inhaled nitric oxide or extracorporeal membrane oxygenation.[6]

TREATMENT

In respiratory acidosis the pathophysiologic condition is hypoventilation, which is associated with hypoxemia. Treatment is directed at the underlying cause.[1,2] Where primary lung disease exists, we must provide ventilatory assistance. Hypoxemia, because of ventilation and perfusion mismatch in respiratory disease, is treated with increased inspired oxygen concentration or ventilatory support. Ventilatory techniques that may be of benefit include continuous positive airway pressure (CPAP), standard ventilation, high-frequency ventilation, extracorporeal membrane oxygenation (ECMO), inhaled nitric oxide, and others (see Chapter 23).

Asphyxia often leads to combined respiratory and metabolic acidosis. Ventilation will resolve the respiratory acidosis, and the improved oxygenation may allow the lactic acidosis to resolve without bicarbonate therapy. In narcosis, temporary ventilatory support may be required. The narcosis may be reversed with administration of naloxone (Narcan) at a dose of 0.1 mg/kg. (Repeated doses may be required; see Chapter 4.)

With the other acidoses and alkaloses a careful search must be instituted for the causes, with therapy directed toward them. This may require drug therapy, replacement of losses, or surgical correction of abnormalities.[1,2]

COMPLICATIONS

The outcome of unrecognized and untreated acid-base or oxygenation disturbances may be an increased mortality or an increased morbidity in the survivors.[1] Complications of the correction of the acid-base and oxygenation disturbance vary according to the disturbance and treatment provided.

The major effect of acidosis on the body is CNS depression. In metabolic acidosis the rate and depth of respiration are increased, whereas in respiratory acidosis respiration is depressed. The major effect of alkalosis on the body is increased excitability of the CNS and tetany (often of the respiratory muscles).

Respiratory acidosis with treatment by assisted ventilation can produce all of the complications of assisted ventilation, including infection, trauma, oxygen toxicity, sepsis, air leak, subglottic stenosis, and others (see Chapter 23).

Complications of oxygen therapy include the risks of hypoxemia and hyperoxemia. Immediate effects of hypoxia include pulmonary vasoconstriction, a change from aerobic to anaerobic metabolism (with eventual metabolic acidosis), cyanosis, bradycardia, hypotonia, and decreases in CNS and cardiac functions. Prolonged high inspired oxygen concentrations increase pulmonary morbidity through pulmonary oxygen toxicity and contribute to retinopathy of prematurity. If ventilatory support is required to attain adequate oxygenation, the complications are those of ventilator therapy (see Chapter 23).

PARENT TEACHING

Obtaining blood for blood gas analysis by invasive techniques (arterial punctures and heel sticks) is stressful for parents and their infant. Explaining the rationale for the test, eliciting parental assistance (if they are present), and encouraging them to comfort their crying baby involves parents as primary caregivers. Explaining the results of the analysis and needed changes in therapy keeps parents apprised of their baby's progress. Many parents become quite adept at blood gas interpretation and are able to anticipate therapeutic alterations: "Did you change the Fio_2? The ventilator rate?" This helps parents master a difficult situation. Beyond sharing technical information, the care provider should also personalize the infant to his or her parents (see Chapter 28).

REFERENCES

1. Androgue HJ, Madias NE: Management of life-threatening acid-base disorders, *N Engl J Med* 338(1): 26, 1998; 338(2):107, 1998.
2. Fall PJ: A stepwise approach to acid-base disorders: practical patient evaluation for metabolic acidosis and other conditions, *Postgrad Med* 107:249, 2000.
3. Gluck SL: Acid-base, *Lancet* 352:474, 1998.
4. Horne C, Derrico D: Mastering ABGs: the art of arterial blood gas measurement, *Am J Nurs* 99:26, 1999.
5. Hsia CC: Respiratory function of hemoglobin, *N Engl J Med* 338:239, 1998.
6. Kinsella JP, Abman SH: Recent developments in the pathophysiolgy and treatment of persistent pulmonary hypertension of the newborn, *J Pediatr* 126: 853, 1995.
7. Lowenstein J: *Acid and basics: a guide to understanding acid-base disorders,* New York, 1993, Oxford University Press.
8. Richard C: Tissue hypoxia: how to detect, how to correct, how to prevent? *Intensive Care Med* 22: 1250, 1996.
9. Siegemund M, van Brommel J, Ince C: Assessment of regional tissue oxygenation, *Intensive Care Med* 25:1044, 1999.
10. Williamson JC: Acid-base disorders: classification and management strategies, *Am Fam Physician* 52: 584, 1995.
11. Wong FWH: A new approach to ABG interpretation, *Am J Nurs* 99:34, 1999.

12 Pain and Pain Relief

Rita Agarwal, Mary I. Enzman Hagedorn, Sandra L. Gardner

Pain is a complex phenomenon that is at best elusive in the neonate. Rationalization for inadequate treatment of pain has resulted in unnecessary suffering for these fragile infants. Research has shown that the "unchecked release of stress hormones by untreated pain may exacerbate injury, prevent wound healing, lead to infection, prolong hospitalization, and even [lead] to death."[160] These fragile neonates are simply too sick to not have their pain treated. Health care professionals are responsible for influencing positive change in clinical practice regarding neonatal pain.[140]

In the past neonates have not been given analgesia and/or anesthesia for surgery because of the controversy as to whether they feel pain and whether they are physiologically stable enough to tolerate the effects of these drugs. The rationale for withholding analgesia and/or anesthesia included the following beliefs:

- Neonates have an immature CNS with nonmyelinated pain fibers and are thus incapable of perceiving pain. Neonates have no memory of pain.
- Pain is a highly subjective experience that is difficult to objectively assess in nonverbal neonates.
- Anesthetics and analgesics are dangerous when administered to neonates, and neonates are safer being unmedicated.

There is increasing evidence from recent research that neonates, including preterm infants, have a CNS that is much more mature than previously thought.[6,15,54,55] Pain pathways are myelinated in the fetus during the second and third trimesters, and are completely myelinated by 30 to 37 weeks' gestation. Even thinly myelinated or nonmyelinated fibers carry pain stimuli. Incomplete myelination implies only a slower transmission, which is offset in the neonate by the shorter distance the impulse must travel.[15]

Even though pain is not expressed verbally in semiconscious patients, nonverbal adults (intubated, mute), or infants, this does not negate their experience of pain. In response to the question of whether the neonate's responses are reflexive or a perception of pain, research has focused on measuring the infant's pain experience. The infant's capacity for memory is far greater than previously thought,[6,85,154] and a neuropsychologic complex of altered pain threshold and pain-related behavior has been identified.[73,74,78,175]

Concern has been expressed that giving potent medications to an already critically ill infant might be dangerous. Local and systemic drugs now available, as well as new techniques and devices for monitoring, enable neonates (including preterm infants) to be safely anesthetized and provide safe and effective analgesia while maintaining a stable condition.[15]

Neonates, including premature infants, exhibit (1) physiologic, (2) hormonal, (3) metabolic, and (4) behavioral responses to invasive procedures that are similar to, but more intense than, adult responses.* Exposure to multiple pain procedures may increase the vulnerability of preterm infants to gross neurologic damage (IVH, PVL).[10,11,114,125,189] Pain relief benefits the neonate by decreasing physiologic instability, hormonal and metabolic stress, and the behavioral reactions accompanying painful procedures.† The Committee on Fetus and Newborn of the American Academy of Pediatrics has recommended the administration of local and/or systemic drugs for anesthesia or analgesia to neonates undergoing surgical procedures.[6] The committee further states that any decision to withhold these drugs should not be based solely on the infant's age or perceived degree of cortical maturity but should be based on the same criteria used in older patients.[6] The AAP, in an updated version of the guidelines, cites that prolonged exposure to untreated pain increases morbidity and alters subsequent behavioral and physiologic responses to pain.[7] National associ-

---

*References 8, 10, 13, 15, 71, 93, 107.
†References 8, 13, 15, 16, 123, 135, 176, 187.

ations have promulgated standard of care guidelines and/or position statements regarding neonatal pain management.[2,12,133] The focus of these documents is on the proactive assessment and management of pain in the neonate. NANN's guidelines outline the following recommendations[133]:

- Parents should be informed of pain relief as an important part of the neonates health care plan and should be encouraged to actively participate in their neonate's assessment and management of pain.
- Every institution must mandate clinical practice guidelines that ensure access and safe administration of pain control to the neonate. Institutions should also develop guidelines for assessing and monitoring pain management practices that include parental input with the goal of measuring the adequacy of pain relief/control in the neonate.
- Institutional support of interdisciplinary research and ongoing education that includes a description of neonatal pain, accurate pain assessment, interventions to improve patient care and reduce morbidity as well as guidelines ensuring adequate administration of analgesia/sedation for the neonate.

PHYSIOLOGY AND PATHOPHYSIOLOGY

"Pain is an unpleasant sensory and emotional experience associated with actual or potential tissue damage, or described in terms of such damage."[126] The neonate's expression of pain does not fit the self-report aspect of this definition that often results in the health care provider's failure to recognize and treat pain.[27,44] Because self-report is absent in the preverbal neonate, nonverbal behavioral information needs to be assessed and used to determine the treatment options for neonates.[14] Although we are unable to assess the emotional experience associated with pain in these babies, the sensory pathways required are now better understood. Neonates have a developing, incompletely myelinated nervous system at birth; however, all the components of the nociceptive (pain) pathways are present.[54,55] To better understand neonatal responses and their differences from adults, the basic mechanisms of adult pain transmission are presented in Figure 12-1.

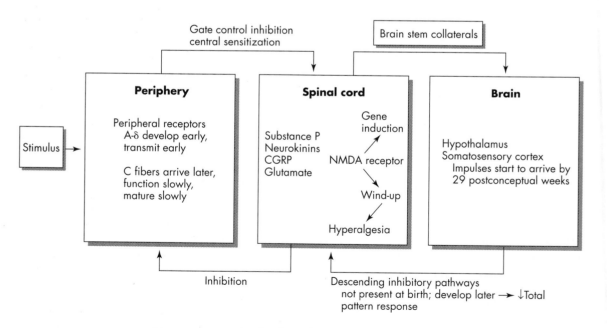

Neonates react to localized pain by moving the whole body.
Maturation results in more individual response.

FIGURE 12-1 Schematic representation of transmission of noxious stimuli from the periphery to the brain.

Neuroanatomy

Peripheral Nervous System

Peripheral nerves can be classified into three broad categories based on fiber diameter and velocity (Table 12-1). Pain receptors (nociceptors) are the A-delta fibers (A-δ) and C fibers that are widely spread in the superficial layers of the skin, periosteum, fascia, peritoneum, joints, muscle, pleura, dura, and tooth pulp. Most visceral tissues have fewer nociceptors, and these transmit to the spinal cord through the sympathetic, parasympathetic, and splanchnic nerves. Tissue damage and inflammation cause the release of arachidonic acid and other chemicals that can sensitize nerve endings and cause vasodilatation and plasma extravasation. This causes pain, swelling, and hyperalgesia.[47,48]

A-δ fibers are myelinated and therefore capable of fast impulse conduction. These nerves are responsible for "fast" or "first" pain. They are also known as high threshold mechanoreceptors (HTMs), because they respond to strong pressure or tissue injury. The C fibers (polymodal nociceptors) are unmyelinated, conduct impulses more slowly, and are the main nociceptors for transmitting chemical, thermal, and mechanical noxious stimuli to the spinal cord.[127] The A-δ fibers develop ahead of the C fibers in the skin and the spinal cord. A-δ fibers are involved in the cutaneous flexion reflex. This reflex is exaggerated in the preterm. Thresholds to mechanical skin stimulation (that may or may not be perceived as pain in a newborn) are both lower and responses last longer. Complete myelination occurs during the second and third trimesters. Lack of myelination had been thought to indicate the inability of a neonate to perceive pain; however, incomplete myelination leads only to slower conduction, which is offset by the shorter distances traversed in the infant.[15]

Reflex responses to somatic stimuli begin at 7½ weeks postconceptual age (PCA) in the perioral skin and continue to develop in the palms of the hands before finally reaching the hindlimbs by 13 to 14 weeks.[55] It is likely that both A-δ fibers (touching) and A-δ fibers (pinching) transmit painful stimuli in the human fetus. In rat pups the C fibers reach the spinal cord but do not start to stimulate dorsal horn cells until the end of the first postnatal week. They subsequently continue to mature for several weeks. This slow maturation in rats may be due to low levels of neuropeptides such as substance P (SP), neurotransmitters, or immature receptor sites. These changes in rat pups appear to correlate with the third trimester and the early neonatal period in humans.[54,55]

Spinal Cord

Once a noxious stimulus is detected by the nociceptors, the signal is transmitted via the primary afferents to the dorsal root ganglia and from there to the dorsal horn of the spinal cord.[47] Neurotransmitters and their receptors amplify or attenuate the signal in the dorsal horn before sending the signal to the brain.[48]

Excitatory neurotransmitters such as SP and other neurokinins are increased after acute inflammation and may be required for the transmission of painful stimuli to the brain.[92] Glutamate and aspartame are amino acids that appear to be involved in central hypersensitivity and *wind-up*.[47] **Wind-up is**

Table 12-1	CLASSIFICATION AND CHARACTERISTICS OF PERIPHERAL NERVES	
NAME/CHARACTERISTIC	**FUNCTION**
A-alpha (A-α) d: 10-20 μ v: 70-120 m/sec myelinated	Innervate skeletal muscle
A-beta (A-β) d: 12-20 μ v: 30-70 m/sec myelinated	Light touch or pressure may be involved in peripheral sensitization and allodynia; in the premature and newborn infant, may be involved in the transmission of noxious stimuli
A-gamma (A-γ) d: 3-6 μ v: 15-30 m/sec myelinated	Muscle tone
A-delta (A-δ) d: 2-5 μ v: 12-30 m/sec myelinated	Fast, well-localized pain; high threshold mechanoreceptors
B d: 3 μ v: 3-15 m/sec myelinated	Preganglionic autonomic fibers may be involved in sensory or sympathetic coupling
C d: 0.4-1.2 μ v: 0.5-2 m/sec unmyelinated	Slow pain, touch, temperature, postganglionic sympathetic fibers, polymodal nociceptors

d, Nerve diameter; *v*, nerve velocity.

Box 12-1   NEONATAL PAIN RESPONSE*

Physiologic

Increase in
  Heart rate
  Blood pressure
  Intracranial pressure, *which leads to higher risk for intraventricular hemorrhage*
  Respiratory rate
  Mean airway pressure
  Muscle tension
  Carbon dioxide ($\uparrow$ $TcPCO_2$; PCO_2)
Decrease in
  Depth of respirations (shallow)
  Oxygenation ($\downarrow$ $TcPO_2$; PO_2; SaO_2) *which leads to apnea/bradycardia*
Pallor or flushing
Diaphoresis or palmar sweating
Dilated pupils

Behavioral

Vocalizations
  Crying (higher-pitched, tense, and harsh)
  Whimpering
  Moaning
Facial expressions
  Grimacing
  Furrowing or bulging of the brow
  Quivering chin
  Eye squeeze
Bodily movements
  General diffuse body activity
  Limb withdrawal, swiping, thrashing

Behavioral—cont'd

  Changes in tone
    Hypertonicity, rigidity, fist clenching
    Hypotonicity, flaccidity
  Touch aversion
States
  Sleep-wake cycle changes—wakefulness
  Activity level changes: increased fussiness, irritability, listlessness, lethargy
  Feeding difficulties
  More difficult to comfort, soothe, quiet
  Disrupts interactive ability with parents

Hormonal/Catabolic Stress Response

Increase in
  Plasma renin activity
  Catecholamine levels (epinephrine and norepinephrine)
  Cortisol levels
  Nitrogen excretion
  Release of
    Growth hormone
    Glucagon
    Aldosterone
  Serum levels of
    Glucose
    Lactate
    Pyruvate
    Ketones
    Nonesterified fatty acids
Decrease in
  Insulin secretion

*References 8, 9, 13, 15, 45, 62, 66, 71, 72, 74, 81, 96, 97, 119, 141, 142, 146, 149, 164, 167, 169, 174, 181, 190.

---

a phenomenon whereby repetition of the same noxious stimulus leads to an exaggerated response. This response continues even after the noxious stimulus ceases. Wind-up may also be responsible for converting a low-level, pain-related activity to a high-level, pain-related activity.[47,125] The preterm experiences increased stress and activity in the nociceptive pathways after prolonged periods of exposure to painful stimuli. After prolonged exposure, the preterm exhibits similar pain responses when exposed to other caretaking activities (e.g., handling, suctioning the ETT, positioning).[125]

An additional factor in the development of hypersensitivity and hyperalgesia is the presence of nociceptive specific receptors, which respond only to pain. In the presence of peripheral inflammation, the threshold of these receptors is decreased so that they are capable of responding to other nonnoxious stimuli.[47,125] **For example, an infant whose heel has been repeatedly stuck for blood samples may demonstrate pain behavior, even when the heel is merely touched. Many of these responses can be blocked by low doses of opioids. However, once these responses are established, a tenfold increased dose of opioids may be required to reverse them.**[56,123,187]

The spinal cord also contains inhibitory neurotransmitters (γ-aminobutyric acid [GABA], glycine), which are activated by descending neural pathways (from the brain to the spinal cord) and decrease the intensity of pain transmission.[54] Descending inhibition is necessary to modulate the pain response and yet to allow for specific pain responses (i.e., withdrawal from a needle stick). Lack of inhibition produces exaggerated, generalized, but definite responses to pain such as body wriggling, facial grimacing, and excessive crying. These pathways, in contrast to the excitatory ones, are not fully developed at birth in rat pups and probably in humans; therefore the neonatal spinal cord is more excitable.[54]

Neurotransmitters in the developing nervous system may be expressed early but are not necessarily located in areas normally found in an adult.[54] This is particularly true of SP and glutamate, which may contribute to the unorganized responses noted with pain stimuli in the newborn (i.e., the whole body moves when an IV is started).

Brain
Much less is known about the development of the pathways to the higher brain centers, such as the hypothalamus and cortex. Once again there is evidence of immaturity of the inhibitory pathways.[54,55] Development in the human cortex continues for many years after birth. Contrary to prior beliefs that newborns do not feel pain, it appears that in fact cutaneous responses are exaggerated, occur at much lower thresholds, and reflex muscle contractions last longer in newborns when compared with mature individuals.[55] In summary, the newborn's nervous system, though still developing, is fully capable of transmitting, perceiving, responding to, and probably remembering noxious stimuli.

Physiologic Responses
Acute pain in adults is associated with increased sympathetic stimulation, heart rate, respiratory rate, blood pressure, cardiac output, myocardial oxygen consumption, peripheral resistance, anxiety, emotional distress, hormonal imbalance, and greater morbidity and mortality.[43] Rao et al[152] reported that infant energy expenditure increased by at least 7.5% with crying when compared with a resting state. **Numerous studies have shown that both premature and full term infants express the same physiologic responses to pain and noxious stimuli (e.g., intubation) as adults (Box 12-1).**[4,6,13,15,17,19] **Infants undergoing circumcision without the use of pain medication demonstrated increased irritability after the procedure, an altered sleep-wake state, and abnormal feeding patterns for up to 22 hours.**

These responses can be attenuated or blocked with the appropriate use of analgesics.[30,57,166]

Grunau et al[76,77] examined pain reactivity in VLBW infants at 32 weeks' PCA and found that younger gestational ages at birth and increased numbers of invasive procedures at birth resulted in a "dampening" of normal pain reactions. In this study infants had higher baseline heart rates that may have indicated these infants were in a perpetual state of stress/pain. Previous exposure to morphine was associated with a "normalization" of responses to painful stimuli.

ETIOLOGY

Invasive Procedures
Pain is produced with any invasive procedure[146] (Table 12-2). One study found that the number of invasive procedures in 54 neonates during admission to the NICU was 3283.[25] The most common (56%) was heelstick, followed by endotracheal suctioning (26%) and intravenous cannula insertion (8%). The most premature infants underwent the highest number of procedures, with one infant undergoing 488 procedures!

Another study examining the use of analgesics for "minor" procedures in NICUs and pediatric intensive care units (PICUs), found that analgesics were rarely used for the placement of intravenous catheters, suprapubic bladder aspiration, urinary bladder catheterization, venipuncture, arterial line placement, lumbar puncture, and paracentesis in NICUs. **Analgesics were used approximately 60% of the time in the NICU for the placement of chest tubes, central lines, and bone marrow aspiration.**[29] By contrast, analgesics were used in the majority of patients in the PICU undergoing arterial line placement, lumbar puncture, and paracentesis and in greater than 90% of chest tube insertions, central line placements, and bone marrow aspirations. Possible reasons for these differences were that (1) neonates were more often critically ill and the use of analgesics may have prolonged the procedure or exacerbated the infants' medical problems, (2) the use of neuromuscular blocking agents prevented the physical response to pain, and (3) not all infants respond to pain by crying loudly, withdrawing, or otherwise "protesting." This study indicates that considerable work needs to be done to educate practitioners about the benefits of appropriate pain management in neonates.

Table 12-2	SELECTED COMMON CAUSES OF PAIN IN NEONATES	
INVASIVE PROCEDURES	**SURGICAL PROCEDURES**	**OTHERS**
Intravenous cannulation	Central line placement	Clavicle, rib fracture
Venipuncture	PDA ligation	Extremity fracture
Heelstick	TEF repair	Chest pain
Intramuscular injection	Gastroschisis repair	Central pain syndrome (i.e., pain derived from
Arterial line, blood gas	Omphalocele repair	CNS damage)
Umbilical catheterization	CDH repair	Spasticity
Cutdown for vascular access	Inguinal hernia repair	Abdominal pain resulting from shortgut
Chest tube insertion or removal	Cardiac surgery	syndrome, multiple abdominal surgeries
Bone marrow aspiration	Circumcision	Necrotizing enterocolitis
Lumbar puncture	Broviac catheter insertion or removal	Bowel obstruction
Paracentesis	ECMO catheter insertion or removal	Prolonged and/or improper positioning
Endotracheal intubation		Position changes
Endotracheal suction		NG tube placement
Mechanical ventilation		Flushing lines
Nasal CPAP		Dressing changes
Bladder catheterization		Eye examination for ROP
Suprapubic aspiration		IV administration of medications
		Addition/withdrawal of fluid from umbilical
		catheter

Data from Barker D, Rutter N: Exposure to invasive procedures in neonatal intensive care unit admissions, *Arch Dis Child Fetal Neonat Educ* 72:F47, 1995; Bauchner H, May A, Coates E: Use of analgesic agents for invasive medical procedures in pediatric and neonatal intensive care units, *J Pediatr* 4:647, 1992; and Evans JC, Vogelpohl DG, Bourguignon CM et al: Pain behaviors in LBW infants accompany some "nonpainful" caregiving procedures, *Neonat Netw* 16:33, 1997.

CDH, Congenital diaphragmatic hernia; *ECMO,* extracorporeal membrane oxygenation; *PDA,* patent ductus arteriosus; *ROP,* retinopathy of prematurity; *TEF,* tracheoesophageal fistula.

Endotracheal intubation has been associated with hypoxia, catabolism, increased ICP, increased IVH/PVL, increased blood pressure and increased stress hormones.* Researchers have shown that even a single dose of fentanyl during mechanical ventilation decreases pain scores, heart rate, blood pressure, and serum cortisol levels and increases clinical stability of the infant.[81] **Other researchers have documented the possible protective role of continuous low-dose analgesia on the neurologic outcome in certain infants.**[18,114,159,189] Furthermore, studies have compared fentanyl with morphine for analgesia during mechanical ventilation in neonates and found that fentanyl was equianalgesic with fewer side effects, thus leading to decreased plasma adrenaline and noradrenaline concentrations.[79,157]

Surgery

Painful stimuli, surgery, and traumatic injuries have been shown in adults to trigger the "stress response," which causes the release of a variety of hormones, including epinephrine, norepinephrine, corticosteroids, glucagon, and growth hormones.[43] These hormones prepare the body for a fight-or-flight response and cause, among other things, an increase in heart rate, respiratory rate, glucose production, muscle, and fat breakdown. This response in the short term allows the body to deal with an insult. If the insult continues or is untreated, the ongoing catabolic stress response may become deleterious to the body's well-being by promoting more tissue breakdown while preventing growth and tissue repair.[43] **Both premature and full-term infants have a decreased stress response with the use of appropriate analgesia both during and immediately after surgery.**[8,9,13,15-17,19] A special example of untreated operative pain is newborn circumcision. In addition to the previously mentioned short-term effects of not treating the pain associated with circumcision, male infants who have undergone circumcision without analgesia have an increased pain response to vaccination at 4 to 6 months of age.[175,176] It is possible, therefore, that newborns have a much greater capacity for memory than previously thought!

Other Causes

Rib, clavicular, and extremity fractures are not uncommon and should be considered in the presence of prolonged crying and failure to move the affected extremity.[60] Bronchopulmonary dysplasia is a common problem in infants who were premature and may cause chest pain, a syndrome known to occur in some older patients with chronic lung disease. Neurologic dysfunction can leave patients with ongoing pain from central pain syndrome or excessive spasticity. A recent study showed that 27% of former extremely-low-birth-weight (ELBW) infants who were now teenagers had neurosensory impairment, and 9% reported moderate or severe pain.[158]

PREVENTION

Prevention of pain in the neonate and preterm infant begins with a proactive plan of care aimed at preventing the pain cycle.[161] The key approaches in this plan include (1) anticipation, (2) comprehensive and ongoing assessment of the variables, (3) distinguishing agitation and irritability from pain expressions and responses of the preterm infant, (4) ongoing communication among health care providers, using input from the parents, (5) advocating and implementing timely and effective treatment for irritability, agitation, and pain (e.g., pharmacologic and comfort measures), and (6) ongoing reevaluation of this proactive plan of care.[2] **Individualized behavioral and developmental care is another important area in preventing stress and sensory overload that often contribute to an ongoing pain cycle.**[61] These approaches help prevent disorganization in the neonate. To facilitate stability and self-regulation before and during an invasive, painful procedure, (1) assess the infant's state and facilitate a change to an alert state, (2) contain extremities (see Chapter 13), (3) provide a pacifier and an opportunity to grasp (a finger, hand, or blanket), and (4) utilize another person (e.g., parent or caregiver) to support, contain, and observe for stress. After the procedure, provide support,

comfort, and slow withdrawal so that the infant remains calm.[181]

The suffering of neonates can be avoided. Needless suffering is prevented by an established plan of care for assessment, management, and evaluation of pain and attempts to relieve pain. Neonates depend on the skilled observations, assessments, and interventions of care providers for prompt, safe, and effective relief. **A cooperative effort among health care providers and the parents in the form of pain management teams**[31] **and well-established pain protocols prevents unnecessary suffering of both neonates and their families.** Controlling environmental stimuli (e.g., dimming lights, controlling noise level, turning radios off, speaking softly when near the incubator or warmer, and performing rounds outside of the unit), although often difficult in the NICU, is crucial for decreasing stress and preventing unnecessary agitation. Use of an individualized, developmentally appropriate plan of care reduces the need for sedation in severely ill, very-low-birth-weight neonates.[84] Quieting techniques are also a useful way to help control pain response in the neonate; these include nonnutritive sucking, containment interventions, and rocking[140] (see Chapter 13).

DATA COLLECTION

History

Neonates experiencing procedural, surgical, and/or chronic pain must be provided measures to alleviate pain. Neonatal irritability and agitation (Box 12-2) secondary to chronic conditions (e.g., BPD, necrotizing enterocolitis [NEC], short bowel syndrome, neurologic deficits) **and/or environmental overstimulation may also require a combination of environmental interventions and sedation.**[7]

SIGNS AND SYMPTOMS

Assessment of pain in neonates is often challenging because they cannot verbalize their subjective experience. However, "pain assessment must be designed to conform to the communication capabilities of the suffering person."[14] There are four objectives in the assessment of pain: (1) detection of the presence of pain, (2) impact of pain, (3) pain-relieving interventions, and (4) effectiveness of interventions.[111,144] **Expression of pain through**

Box 12-2	INDICATORS OF IRRITABILITY AND AGITATION

Physiologic

Increase in
    Heart rate and blood pressure only with activity
    Oxygenation ($\uparrow$ $TCPO_2$; PO_2; SaO_2)
    Respiratory rate and effort
Decrease in
    Oxygenation ($\downarrow$ $TCPO_2$; PO_2; SaO_2) after prolonged
      agitation
    Heart rate (bradycardia)
    Respirations (apnea)
Alterations in color: cyanosis, mottling, duskiness, pallor
Diaphoresis
Vomiting
Poor pattern of weight gain

Behavioral

Vocalizations
    Whining cry
    Intense, urgent cry
    High-pitched cry
    Resumes fussiness when consolation ceases
Facial expressions
    Frowning
    Worried facies

Behavioral—cont'd

    Gaze aversion
    Closes eyes to tune out
Bodily movements
    Random movements of head and body
    Hypertonic, rigid posturing; arching; hyperextended neck
    Flailing, thrashing, frantic activity of extremities during fuss
      or cry
    Decreased activity
    Tremulousness
States
    Hyperalert—easily aroused from sleep; startles easily
    Rapid and frequent state changes to fuss or cry
    Sleep-wake cycles unpredictable
    Feeding difficulties
    Difficult to console, soothe
    High level of persistence
    Needs environmental structure to fall asleep; takes a long
      time to fall asleep
    Ineffective in self-consoling; requires vestibular stimulation
      or body containment to console; responds
      inconsistently to consolation
    Noncuddly

Modified from Broome ME, Tanzillo H: Differentiating between pain and agitation in premature neonates, *J Perinat Neonat Nurs* 4:53, 1990; Burdeau G, Kleiber C: Clinical indicators of infant irritability, *Neonat Netw* 9:23, 1991; and Franck LS: A national survey of the assessment and treatment of pain and agitation in the NICU, *J Obstet Gynecol Neonat Nurs* 16:387, 1987.

behavior is one of the neonate's only means of communicating about pain. Behavioral cues may include diffuse or localized motor activity (e.g., pulling extremity away, hypotonia), facial grimacing, crying, agitation, and level of activity (see Box 12-1). In both preterm and term neonates gender differences in pain expression may exist—female infants express more facial expressions of pain when compared to male infants.[80] **Assessment of pain in the neonate is further complicated by the infant's state and level of neural development.**[71] The younger the gestational age, the more immature the CNS and more limited the autonomic and self-regulatory abilities to deal with pain and stress and disorganized ineffective responses that make it more difficult to communicate pain.[4,45,181] A more immature, fragile neonate may manifest alterations in sleep-wake cycles and habituate to the overwhelming stimuli of the NICU (see Chapter 13) and thus be unable to exhibit any response to pain.

Behavioral expressions of pain by the neonate are further hampered by intubation, use of restraints, and neuromuscular blockers. Similarly, chronically ill infants who have developed what has been described as learned helplessness (see Chapter 13) have difficulty generating a pain response.[140] Preterm infants who have experienced: (1) more invasive procedures, (2) are lower gestational age at birth, (3) have spent more days on ventilators have a diminished behavioral and cardiac autonomic pain response (i.e., a blunted response) to acute pain at 32 weeks' PCA.[76,77] Another study indicates that neonates (both preterm and term) who undergo handling and immobilization may exhibit exaggerated behavioral and physiologic response to later painful procedures.[145] VLBW infants with parenchymal brain injury exhibit a bio-behavioral response to pain that is unaltered from VLBW infants without brain injury.[134]

Physiologic parameters may also indicate pain (e.g., increased heart and respiratory rates, elevated blood pressure, desaturation, apnea, palmar sweat-

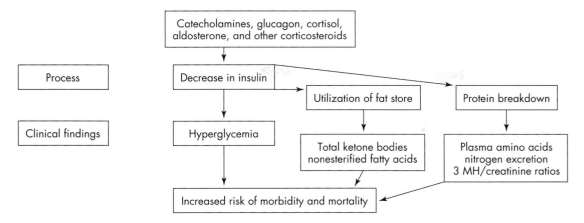

FIGURE 12-2   Hormonal response to pain in infants. (From Johnston C, Stevens B: Pain in infants. In Watt-Watson J, Donovan M, eds: *Pain management: nursing perspective,* St. Louis, 1992, Mosby.)

ing). These symptoms are the result of sympathetic nervous system activation (see Box 12-1). A recent study found that some physiologic responses to pain (e.g., facial activity and state) moderately correlated to heart rate changes while other behavioral expressions (e.g. finger splay) did not correlate with any autonomic changes.[130] However, in the same study specific measures of cardiac autonomic modulation did not correlate with behavioral change suggesting that cardiac alterations may be independent measures of pain in the preterm.[130] Some preterm infants respond to pain with more behavioral changes, while others respond with more physiologic changes.[168,170]

When pain is repetitive or persists for hours or days, there is a decompensatory response, resulting in hormonal and metabolic alterations (Figure 12-2 and Box 12-1). The fight-or-flight mechanism of the sympathetic nervous system is no longer able to compensate, so an adaptation syndrome begins with a return to baseline physiologic parameters. The return of the heart rate, respirations, and blood pressure to baseline parameters makes assessment of the infant's pain more difficult and does not mean that the infant has "adjusted" to or no longer is experiencing pain.[164]

The lack of an expression of pain through physiologic and behavioral responses does not mean that the neonate is not experiencing pain.[77] Pain responses may be delayed, cumulative, or absent. In the preterm infant sustained elevations in vital signs and decreased oxygenation confirm the persistence of physiologic alterations after painful stimuli.[45,169] Very critically ill neonates and immature preterm infants may be so weak and overwhelmed that they have completely exhausted their energy and are unable to respond.[59,75,168,185] **The incidence of crying in response to painful or noxious stimuli is less than 50% in the preterm infant.**[98,169] Depending on gestational age, a preterm infant's behavioral responses (e.g., facial changes and bodily movements) to pain are similar to the term infant. The responses of the very preterm infant are highly variable (a reflection of continuous maturation of the CNS) and less robust.[45,77,98,169] Preterm infants exhibit significant variability in behavioral and physiologic responses to preparatory procedures and handling, making it unclear if these responses are related to stress, behavioral disorganization, or a conditioned response and/or pain perception.[75,95,168,169]

Pain responses of the neonate are also influenced by the number and timing of painful procedures, the technique used, and the degree of professional expertise.[7,61,77] Lack of a response to a painful stimuli occurs more frequently in younger newborns (both gestational and postconception age [PCA]) who are asleep and who have recently undergone another painful procedure.[77,95,99] Use of mechanical lancets rather than manual lancets results in less behavioral and physiologic distress, fewer repeat punctures, and less bruising.[37,83,124,182] Venipuncture has been shown to be associated with less pain in the neonate than heelstick.[106,132,162,163]

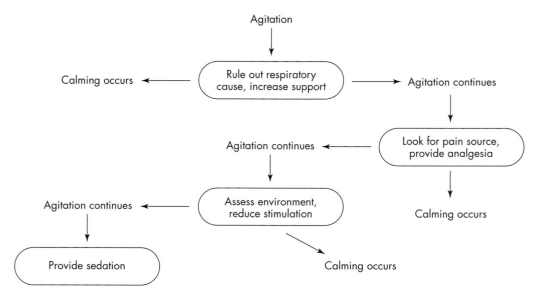

FIGURE 12-3 Decision tree for assessing and managing pain and/or agitation. (From Gordin P: Assessing and managing agitation in the critically ill infant, *Matern Child Nurs* 15:26, 1990.)

Differentiation between pain and agitation is a challenge (Figure 12-3). **Agitation is a behavioral symptom of many problems, including environmental overstimulation, respiratory insufficiency, neurologic irritability, and pain.**[140] Causes of agitation other than pain should first be eliminated before pain management is initiated. Assessment of environmental stimuli should be a routine part of the neonate's care. The neonate may associate certain stimuli with unpleasant events over time, and repeated exposure (e.g., ventilator alarms, placement of heel warmer, the odor of an alcohol wipe) may trigger agitation. Although these stimuli are inevitable, identifying, avoiding, or limiting them will help prevent anticipatory decompensation in these fragile infants.[140]

**Assessment of neonatal pain is influenced by the attitudes and beliefs of care providers, amount of time spent observing for and having knowledge of pain responses, discrepancy between attitudes and practice, and prioritization of pain recognition and relief in the NICU.*

Researchers have examined the beliefs and management techniques of 374 clinicians (both physicians and nurses) regarding procedural pain in newborn infants. Although the majority of clinicians believe that infants experience pain in the same or greater degree than adults, 9 of 12 commonly performed bedside procedures (e.g., intubation, chest tube insertion, arterial or venous catheter insertion, heelsticks) were rated as "moderately to very painful." Neither pharmacologic nor comfort measures were frequently used.[146]

To quantify and objectify a neonate's pain experience and to facilitate health care professionals' recognition of the presence and severity of pain in neonates, ongoing research is aimed at tool development.

Although pain tools have been developed for research purposes, limited reliability and validity have been established for clinical practice.[1,168] **The two most commonly used pain assessment tools in clinical practice are CRIES and PIPP.**

The CRIES assessment tool (Table 12-3), developed to measure physiologic and behavioral pain responses postoperatively, is utilized hourly with vital sign assessment. CRIES uses a scoring system similar to the Apgar score: a score of 4 or above indicates pain and requires intervention.[31] Validity and reliability to measure postoperative pain has been established,[103] whereas use of CRIES to measure procedural pain has not been validated.[31]

The Premature Infant Pain Profile (PIPP) (Table 12-4) is a multidimensional (physiologic and

---

*References 23, 46, 63, 79, 82, 96, 100, 120, 136, 160, 164, 183, 184.

Table 12-3   CRIES: NEONATAL POSTOPERATIVE PAIN ASSESSMENT SCORE

	SCORING CRITERIA FOR EACH ASSESSMENT			INFANT'S SCORE
	0	1	2	
Crying	No	High-pitched	Inconsolable	_____
Requires O₂ for saturation >95%	No	<30%	>30%	_____
Increased vital signs*	HR and BP within 10% of preoperative value	HR or BP 11%-20% higher than preoperative value	HR or BP 21% or more above preoperative value	_____
Expression	None	Grimace	Grimace/grunt	_____
Sleepless	No	Wakes at frequent intervals	Constantly awake	_____
			Total score†	_____

From Krechel S, Bildner J: Neonatal pain assessment tool developed at the University of Missouri–Columbia.
*BP should be done last.
†Add scores for all assessments to calculate total score.

Table 12-4   PREMATURE INFANT PAIN PROFILE (PIPP)

Infant Study Number: _____

Date/time: _____

Event: _____

PROCESS	INDICATOR	0	1	2	3	SCORE
Chart	Gestational age	36 weeks and more	32-35 wk, 6 days	28-31 wk, 6 days	Less than 28 wk	
Observe infant 15 sec	Behavioral state	Active/awake; eyes open; facial movements	Quiet/awake; eyes open; no facial movements	Active/asleep; eyes closed; facial movements	Quiet/asleep; eyes closed; no facial movements	
Observe baseline Heart rate Oxygen saturation						
Observe infant 30 sec	Heart rate Max	0-4 beats/min increase	5-14 beats/min increase	5-24 beats/min increase	25 beats/min or more increase	
	Oxygen saturation Min	0%-2.4% decrease	2.5%-4.9% decrease	5.0%-7.4% decrease	7.5% or more decrease	
	Brow bulge	None 0%-9% of time	Minimum 10%-39% of time	Moderate 40%-69% of time	Maximum 70% of time or more	
	Eye squeeze	None 0%-9% of time	Minimum 10%-39% of time	Moderate 40%-69% of time	Maximum 70% of time or more	
	Nasolabial furrow	None 0%-9% of time	Minimum 10%-39% of time	Moderate 40%-69% of time	Maximum 70% of time or more	
					Total Score	_____

From Stevens B, Johnston C, Petroshen P et al: Premature Infant Pain Profile: development and initial validation, *Clin J Pain* 12:13, 1996.
Scoring method for the PIPP
1. Familiarize yourself with each indicator and how it is to be scored by looking at the measure.
2. Score gestational age (from the chart) before you begin.
3. Score behavioral state by observing the infant for 15 seconds immediately before the event.
4. Record baseline heart rate and oxygen saturation.
5. Observe the infant for 30 seconds immediately after the event. You will have to look back and forth from the monitor to the infant's face. Score physiologic and facial action changes seen during that time and record immediately after the observation period.
6. Calculate the final score.

Table 12-5	POSTOPERATIVE PAIN SCORE*		
BEHAVIOR	**0 (POOR)**	**1 (MEDIOCRE)**	**2 (SATISFACTORY)**
1. Sleep during preceding hour	None	Short naps between 5 and 10 min	Longer naps ≥10 min
2. Facial expression of pain	Marked, constant	Less marked, intermittent	Calm, relaxed
3. Quality of cry	Screaming, painful, high-pitched	Modulated (can be distracted by normal sound)	No cry
4. Spontaneous motor activity	Thrashing around, incessant agitation	Moderate agitation	Normal
5. Spontaneous excitability and responsiveness to ambient stimulation	Tremulous, clonic movements; spontaneous Moro reflexes	Excessive reactivity (to any stimulation)	Quiet
6. Flexion of fingers and toes	Very pronounced, marked, constant	Less marked, intermittent	Absent
7. Sucking	Absent or disorganized sucking	Intermittent (three or four) and stops with crying	Strong, rhythmic with pacifying effect
8. Global evaluation of tone	Strong hypertonicity	Moderate hypertonicity	Normal for age
9. Consolability	None after 2 minutes	Quiet after 1 minute of effort	Calm before 1 minute
10. Sociability (eye contact) response to voice, smile, real interest in face	Absent	Difficult to obtain	Easy and prolonged

Modified from Attia J, Barrier G, Ahia J et al: Measurement of postoperative pain and narcotic administration in infants using a new clinical scoring system, *Intensive Care Med* 15:1537, 1989.

*Infants with a total score of 15 to 20 have arbitrarily been considered to have adequate postoperative pain management.

behavioral) assessment tool intended for use within clinical practice.[170] The PIPP is a seven-item, four-point scale whose maximum score is dependent on the infant's gestational age. The PIPP has been validated with both full-term and preterm neonates and is able to distinguish between pain and nonpain events.[24]

The Postoperative Pain Score (Table 12-5) is an assessment tool developed to measure postoperative pain after minor surgical procedures in 1- to 7-month-old infants. This scale has not been standardized or validated in full-term or preterm neonates. The Neonatal Facial Coding System (Table 12-6) is an assessment tool based on nine facial expressions of term newborns in four sleep-wake states while experiencing the discomfort of heel rub and the pain of heel lance. Quiet, awake neonates demonstrate the most facial activity, whereas those in quiet sleep demonstrate the least.[71,72] Facial activity also increases with gestational age, so that both infant state and gestational age must be considered when using this scale.[45,168] Because this tool is sensitive to changes in pain intensity, it is also

useful for evaluating the effectiveness of interventions. There is recent evidence of reliable clinical use of this tool, although it is time consuming and requires experienced coders.[1,75,156]

The Neonatal Infant Pain Scale (NIPS) (Table 12-7) is a behavioral assessment tool for preterm and term neonates responding to a needle puncture. NIPS scores reveal an increase in behavioral response during the procedures and a decline in response scores after the procedure (Figure 12-4). Thus NIPS provides a measurement of intensity of infant responses to painful procedure during and after the event.[109] NIPS scores have been correlated with gestational age (e.g., maturity and level of behavior) and Apgar scores. NIPS provides an objective measure of pain-relieving interventions and their effectiveness.[109] The NIPS scale is objective, nonintrusive, and assesses only behavioral response to pain; it has been used as a research tool and has not been used in clinical practice.[1] Flow sheets have also been designed to facilitate the documentation of pain scores and behaviors.[109]

Table 12-6	NEONATAL FACIAL CODING SYSTEM
ACTION	**DESCRIPTION**
Brow bulge	Bulging, creasing, and vertical furrows above and between brows occurring as a result of the lowering and drawing together of the eyebrows
Eye squeeze	Identified by the squeezing or bulging of the eyelids; bulging of the fatty pads about the infant's eyes is pronounced
Nasolabial furrow	Primarily manifested by the pulling upwards and deepening of the nasolabial furrow (a line or wrinkle that begins adjacent to the nostril wings and runs downward and outward beyond the lip corners)
Open lips	Any separation of the lips
Stretch mouth (vertical)	Characterized by a tautness of the lip corners coupled with a pronounced downward pull on the jaw; seen when an already wide open mouth is opened a fraction further by an extra pull at the jaw
Stretch mouth (horizontal)	Appears as a distinct horizontal pull at the corners of the mouth
Lip purse	Lips appear as if an "oo" sound is being pronounced
Taut tongue	Characterized by a raised, cupped tongue with sharp tense edges; the first occurrence of taut tongue is usually easy to see, often occurring with a wide open mouth; after this first occurrence, the mouth may close slightly; taut tongue is still scorable on the basis of the still visible tongue edges
Chin quiver	An obvious high-frequency up-down motion of the lower jaw

From Grunau RVE, Craig KD: Pain expression in neonates: facial action and cry, *Pain* 28:399, 1987; and Grunau R, Craig K: Facial activity as a measure of neonatal pain expression. In Tyler DC, Krane EJ, eds, *Advances in pain, research and therapy,* vol 15, New York, 1990, Raven.

Table 12-7	NEONATAL INFANT PAIN SCALE (NIPS) OPERATIONAL DEFINITIONS
Facial Expression	
0-Relaxed muscles	Restful face, neutral expression
1-Grimace	Tight facial muscles; furrowed brow, chin, jaw (negative facial expression—nose, mouth, and brow)
Cry	
0-No cry	Quiet, not crying
1-Whimper	Mild moaning, intermittent
2-Vigorous cry	Loud scream; rising, shrill, continuous (Note: Silent cry may be scored if baby is intubated as evidenced by obvious mouth and facial movement.)
Breathing Patterns	
0-Relaxed	Usual pattern for this infant
1-Change in breathing	Indrawing, irregular, faster than usual; gagging; breath holding
Arms	
0-Relaxed/restrained	No muscular rigidity; occasional random movements of arms
1-Flexed/extended	Tense, straight arms; rigid and/or rapid extension, flexion
Legs	
0-Relaxed/restrained	No muscular rigidity; occasional random leg movement
1-Flexed/extended	Tense, straight legs; rigid and/or rapid extension, flexion
State of Arousal	
0-Sleeping/awake	Quiet, peaceful sleeping or alert and settled
1-Fussy	Alert, restless, and thrashing

From Children's Hospital of Eastern Ontario, 1989.

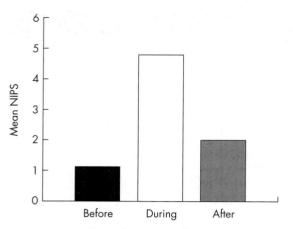

FIGURE 12-4   Mean NIPS scores over time in 22 infants. (From Lawrence J, Alcock D, McGrath P et al: The development of a tool to assess neonatal pain, *Neonatal Netw* 12:62, 1993.)

Box 12-3	CRITICAL QUESTIONS TO ASK ABOUT PAIN MANAGEMENT IN NEONATES

Is the infant being adequately assessed at appropriate intervals?

Are analgesics ordered for prevention and relief of pain?

Is the analgesic strong enough for the pain expected or the pain being experienced?

Is the timing of the drug administration appropriate for the pain expected or being experienced?

Is the route of administration appropriate (preferably PO or IV) for the infant?

Is the infant adequately monitored for side effects?

Are side effects appropriately managed?

Has the analgesic regimen provided adequate comfort and satisfaction from the family's perspective?

Questions to Consider Regarding Nonpharmacologic Strategies

Is the strategy appropriate for the infant's developmental level, condition, and type of pain?

Is the timing of the strategy sufficient to optimize its effects?

Is the strategy adequately effective in preventing or alleviating the infant's pain?

Is the family satisfied with the strategy for prevention or relief of pain?

From Acute Pain Management Guideline Panel: *Acute pain management: operative or medical procedures and trauma: clinical practice guideline,* AHCPR Pub No 92-0032, Rockville, Md, 1992, Agency for Health Care Policy and Research, Public Health Service, US Dept of HHS.

The National Practice Guidelines provides a list of assessment questions to ask when assessing pain management in the neonate (Box 12-3). Lack of validated assessment tools may leave health care providers wondering if behaviors are indicators or responses to pain. The Acute Pain Management Guideline suggests that "if care providers are unsure whether a behavior indicates pain, and if there is reason to suspect pain, an analgesic trial can be diagnostic as well as therapeutic."[2] Assessment of pain and delivery of effective pain relieving interventions in daily clinical practice must not be delayed while adequate, objective assessment tools are developed.[169] All health care providers must utilize their highly developed assessment skills, along with input from the parents, to gather information about infant behavioral, physiologic, and hormonal or catabolic stress responses before, during, and after painful stimuli. These same assessment skills enable care providers and parents to evaluate the effectiveness of pharmacologic and comfort interventions and institute more and/or different interventions as necessary to relieve pain and suffering.

Laboratory Data

Hormonal and metabolic changes are listed in Box 12-1. Serum glucose levels and reagent test strips monitor for hyperglycemia, which may result in increased serum osmolality and increase the risk of intraventricular hemorrhage (IVH). Glucosuria, ketonuria, and proteinuria result in elevated specific gravity. Metabolic acidosis may result from increased serum levels of lactate, pyruvate, ketones, and nonesterified fatty acids. This data may also be indicative of other serious neonatal problems (e.g., sepsis, acute tubular necrosis).

TREATMENT

The neonate relies on the skilled observations, assessment, and interventions of care providers for prompt, safe, and effective relief. Limiting factors in providing adequate analgesia in these patients has been an unfamiliarity with medication doses, regional techniques, and concern over increased drug sensitivity in neonates. Since routine care can be irritating to newborns, differentiating between agitation, which may respond well to comfort measures, and pain, which won't, is mandatory. **Opioids are**

Table 12-8	PHARMACOLOGIC DIFFERENCES BETWEEN NEWBORNS AND ADULTS	
DIFFERENCES	**CAUSE**	**EFFECT**
Altered gastric acidity	Presence of alkaline amniotic fluids at birth Immature gastric mucosa Consumption of alkaline milk	Variable drug absorption
Decreased gastric emptying time		Increased absorption of some drugs
Decreased protein binding	Lower levels of albumin, a-acid glycoprotein Increased competition for binding sites by endogenous substances (bilirubin)	Increased levels of free drug (opioids, local anesthetics)
Increased volume of distribution	Larger volume of body water in the newborn	Larger initial dose may be needed for effect (neuromuscular blocking agents, local anesthetics)
Decreased drug metabolism	Immature liver enzyme systems	Prolonged effect of some medications (morphine, fentanyl, neuromuscular blockers)
Decreased drug clearance	Immature renal system and decreased glomerular filtration rate	Prolonged effect of some medications (morphine)

From Rovee-Collier C, Hayne H: Reactuation of infant memory: implications for cognitive development, *Adv Child Dev* 10:185, 1987.

the mainstay of pharmacologic treatment; however, there are other useful medications and techniques that may be used for pain relief.[7]

Pharmacologic

Absorption, metabolism, distribution, and clearance of drugs in the neonate differs from the older child and adult (see Chapter 9). These differences are summarized in Table 12-8.

Opioids

Opioids have their primary effect on the μ-receptor in the brain and spinal cord. High-affinity μ-receptors are associated with analgesia, and low-affinity μ-receptors are associated with respiratory depression. There may be fewer high-affinity μ-receptors in the newborn that are less sensitive to the analgesic effects of opioids. Higher initial doses of opioids may therefore be required for effect, which may in turn increase the risk of respiratory depression. Decreased protein binding, drug metabolism, and drug clearance may contribute to higher plasma and CNS concentrations and prolonged drug effect.[60]

All the opioids have similar mechanisms of action; however, there are a few important differences in side effects[192] (Table 12-9). Morphine commonly causes hypotension in dehydrated patients or when used in high doses. **Fentanyl is the preferred drug in many NICUs because of its cardiovascular stability and its ability to decrease pulmonary**

vascular resistance. It can, however, cause chest wall rigidity and decreased lung compliance if administered too quickly. Neuromuscular blocking agents or slow administration of the drug will prevent this problem.[60,121,192] Fentanyl is also commonly used in patients on ECMO to provide sedation and analgesia and to prevent increases in pulmonary vascular resistance and pressure.[112] Sufentanil is 10 times more potent than fentanyl and significantly more expensive. It is shorter acting and can have even greater effects on lung and chest wall compliance.

Dosing by PRN schedule may result in peaks and valleys of pain relief and increases in side effects. Because analgesia is most effective if given before the peak of pain (wind-up), continuous infusions or regular dosing can help prevent undue neonatal suffering.[7,164] Figure 12-5 illustrates the variability in serum levels of analgesia with PRN and continuous dose, loading dose, and breakthrough pain.

Local Anesthetics

Local anesthetics have a variety of uses and provide analgesia by preventing the transmission of noxious stimuli either at the peripheral receptor site or the spinal cord. Bupivacaine and lidocaine are the two most commonly used local anesthetics (see Table 12-9).

Bupivacaine is longer acting but more cardiotoxic than lidocaine. Both are more toxic in neonates than

Table 12-9	ANALGESICS, SEDATIVES, AND REVERSAL AGENTS FOR THE NEONATE	
DRUG	**DOSAGE**	**COMMENTS**
Analgesics		
Narcotic		
Morphine	0.05-0.2 mg/kg/dose q 2-4 hr PRN IV, IM, or SC Continuous IV infusion: 10-15 μg/kg/hr	CNS and respiratory depressant; bronchospasms; peripheral vasodilation with hypovolemic infants; hypotension; decreases intestinal motility; increases intracranial pressure; easily reversed with naloxone; slower onset but longer duration than fentanyl; withdrawal symptoms may occur.
Fentanyl (Sublimaze)	1-5 μg/kg/dose q 1-2 hr PRN IV or SC Continuous IV infusion: 1-5 μg/kg/hr	Same as morphine. Rapid onset of action; decreases motor activity; does not increase intracranial pressure in the absence of respiratory depression; easily reversed with naloxone; short duration of action; may cause bradycardia, hypotension, apnea, seizures, or rigidity if given too rapidly; withdrawal symptoms occur with prolonged use.
Sufentanil citrate (Sufenta)	0.5-1 μg/kg/dose q 30 min to 1 hr	Ten times more potent than fentanyl; has a quicker onset and shorter duration of action than fentanyl. Use with caution in neonates with IVH, hepatic or renal impairment, or pulmonary disease. Same side effects as in fentanyl, above.
Meperidine (Demerol)		Not recommended in preterm or term infants. The active metabolite, normeperidine, accumulates in tissues and causes CNS stimulation (e.g., tremors, muscle twitching, hyperactive reflexes, and dilated pupils) and also lowers the seizure threshold level.[7,22]
Nonnarcotic		
Acetaminophen (Tylenol)	10-15 mg/kg/dose q 4-6 hr PO or PR	May cause hepatotoxicity in overdose. Potentiates effects of narcotics but alone does *not* relieve surgical pain or heel lance pain.[7] Do not use in patients with G6PD deficiency.
Ibuprofen (Advil, Motrin)	4-10 mg/kg/dose q 6-8 hr PO	Gastric irritant—administer with or after feeding; use with caution in neonates with necrotizing enterocolitis, impaired renal function, hypertension, or compromised cardiac function.
Local Anesthetics		
Lidocaine	0.5%-1% solution (to avoid systemic toxicity, volume should be <0.5 ml/kg of 1% lidocaine solution—5 mg/kg)	Local infiltration anesthesia for invasive procedures; use solution *without epinephrine* to avoid vasoconstriction.
Bupivacaine Levobupivacaine Ropivacaine	2.5 mg/kg one-time epidural dose Continuous IV infusion: 0.2 mg/kg/hr (maximum dose)	Monitor for CNS (i.e., seizures, irritability) and cardiotoxic (i.e., ventricular dysrhythmias) side effects. Monitor catheter site integrity. Epidural infusion is titrated to effect but *must not* exceed maximum dose. Levobupivacaine and ropivacaine have decreased cardiotoxicity more than bupivacaine.
EMLA (Lidocaine and Prilocaine)	2.5-5 g to site for at least 60 min	Vasoconstriction at the site. Site must be covered with water-impermeable dressing (i.e., Tegaderm). Single doses have not been shown to cause methemoglobinemia in preterm or term neonates.[177] Does not relieve pain of heel lance.[7]

CNS, Central nervous system; *G6PD,* glucose-6-phosphate dehydrogenase; *IM,* intramuscularly; *IV,* intravenously; *IVH,* intraventricular hemorrhage; *PO,* per os; *PR,* per rectum; *PRN,* as needed; *SC,* subcutaneously.

Table 12-9	ANALGESICS, SEDATIVES, AND REVERSAL AGENTS FOR THE NEONATE—cont'd	
DRUG	**DOSAGE**	**COMMENTS**
Local Anesthetics—cont'd		
Amethocaine gel* (4%) (liposome-encapsulated tetracaine) (Ametrop)	1.5 g to site for 30 min-1 hr	Site must be covered with water-impermeable dressing (i.e., Tegaderm). Vasodilation at the site—mild transient (~20 min) erythema.[26,90,91]
Sedatives/Hypnotics **Barbiturates**		Do *not* provide pain relief; help reduce agitation precipitated by painful events. Frequently produce hyperalgesia and increased reaction to painful stimuli; contraindicated for neonates who have pain and also require sedation.
Phenobarbital	Loading: 10-20 mg/kg IV to maximum 40 mg/kg Maintenance: 5-7 mg/kg in 2 divided doses beginning 12 hr after last loading dose	Prolonged sedation possible once therapeutic levels achieved (20-25 mg/ml); depresses CNS—motor and respiratory; slow onset of action; little or no pain relief; not easily reversed; withdrawal symptoms may occur; incompatible with other drugs in solution.
Nonbarbiturates		
Chloral hydrate	10-30 mg/kg/dose q 6 hr PRN PO to maximum daily dose of 50 mg/kg/day; PR	Gastric irritant—administer with or after feeding; paradoxic excitement; prolonged use associated with direct hyperbilirubinemia[104]; not to be used for analgesia; respiratory depressant; in repeated doses to premature infants—adverse effects—CNS depression, arrhythmias, and renal failure.[65]
Diazepam (Valium)	0.02-0.3 mg/kg IV, IM, or PO q 6-8 hr	Do not dilute injection; venous sclerosing; may displace bilirubin and result in kernicterus; respiratory depression; hypotension; may cause agitation; induces sleep; relaxes muscles; withdrawal symptoms may occur; no analgesic effect; this drug should be used with caution in the neonate because of its long half-life, long-acting metabolites, and its preservative (benzyl alcohol).[7]
Lorazepam (Ativan)	0.05-0.1 mg/kg/dose IV (give over ≥3 min) q 4-8 hr	Respiratory depressant, partial airway obstruction, drowsiness; respiratory depression potentiated when narcotics or barbiturates also being given; infuse slowly to avoid apnea, bradycardia, and hypotension.
Midazolam (Versed)	0.05-0.2 mg/kg/dose IV (give over ≥3 min) q 4-8 hr PRN Continuous IV infusion: 0.2-6 μg/kg/min	Same as for lorazepam; continuous IV infusion enables precise titration until sedative effect is obtained; calms agitated infant on ventilator. Rapid bolus delivery and/or use with fentanyl is associated with (1) myoclonus—rhythmic twitching of all extremities that ceases with discontinuation of drug and does not return and (2) respiratory depression and hypotension—caution use in hypotensive and hypovolemic neonates.[89,115]
Reversal Agents		
Naloxone (Narcan)	1-10 μg/kg	Reverses effects of opioids (both side effects and analgesia).
Flumazenil (Mazicon)	10 μg/kg	Reverses the effects of benzodiazepines (midazolam, diazepam, lorazepam).

*Not yet approved by the FDA for use in the United States.

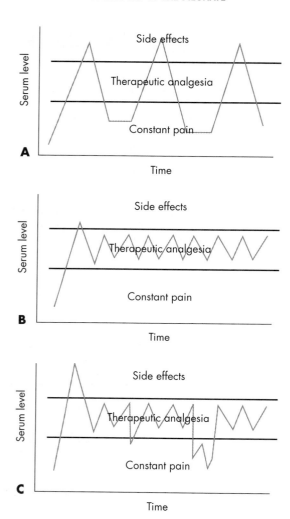

FIGURE 12-5   Administration of analgesic medication. **A,** PRN administration results in peaks and troughs in serum levels of analgesia. **B,** Continuous or around-the-clock administration produces effective pain relief with lower doses of analgesia and fewer side effects. **C,** Loading dose represented in first elevated serum level. Breakthrough pain (i.e., situational pain that "breaks through" baseline analgesia) requires additional analgesia and/or nonpharmacologic interventions. (From Hester N, Foster R: Integrating pediatric postoperative pain management into clinical practice, *Parmaceu Care Pain Symptom Control* 1:5, 1993.)

in adults because of increased organ sensitivity and free fraction of drug. The cardiovascular toxicity may be enhanced if epinephrine containing local anesthetics is used.[51] The new long-acting local anesthetics levobupivacaine and ropivicaine are as effective as bupivicaine, but are less cardiotoxic.[58,68,188,191]

Regional Technique. **Regional techniques provide adequate analgesia thus reducing the need for higher doses of opioids** (Table 12-10). Advantages include (1) stress responses are significantly decreased, (2) normal respiratory patterns return more quickly, (3) the need for postoperative ventilation may be avoided or shortened, (4) intestinal motility recovers more quickly, and (5) morbidity decreases with the use of regional techniques,[43] particularly epidural blocks.[43,131]

Dorsal Penile Nerve/Ring Block. **Dorsal penile nerve block is extremely easy to perform with a high degree of success that can provide surgical anesthesia for circumcision.** The block is performed by injecting 1% lidocaine 3 to 5 mm below the skin at the 2 o'clock and 10 o'clock positions on the dorsum of the penis (Figure 12-6).[121] In a full-term neonate, 0.5 ml/side is used, and 0.2 ml/kg/side is used in premature infants. An alternative technique less likely to cause hematoma is to inject a subcutaneous ring of 0.5% or 1.0% lidocaine around the base of the penis. **All solutions should be without epinephrine.**

Epidural Block. The epidural space is an area surrounding the dura of the spinal cord. This space can be accessed from the caudal, lumbar, or thoracic region. An epidural block is performed by a skilled pediatric anesthesiologist, often under general anesthesia.[49,122,131] A small catheter can be left in the space or a one-time dose of medication can be given. Local anesthetics act by anesthetizing either the local nerve roots or the spinal tracts at the level of the spinal cord where they are placed. The most commonly used medications are the local anesthetics lidocaine or bupivacaine. They are often used in combination with low doses of opioids, which have both a local and systemic action. **The major advantages of these techniques are the ability to provide continuous pain relief and the potential to minimize respiratory depression, facilitate extubation, and hasten recovery.**

EMLA and Infiltration. **Eutectic mixture of local anesthetic (EMLA) is a local anesthetic cream that anesthetizes the skin. It can be used for a variety of procedures (lumbar puncture, venipuncture).**[102] EMLA has been used for analgesia with circumcisions in newborns and has been shown to be efficacious.[3,30] However its analgesic properties are not as effective as those of dorsal penile

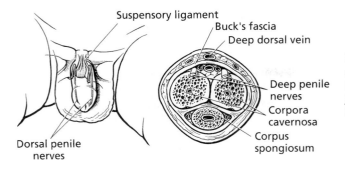

FIGURE 12-6 Anatomic landmarks for placement of a dorsal penile nerve block. (From McClain B, Anand KS: Neonatal pain management. In Deshpande J, Tobias J, eds: *The pediatric pain handbook*, St Louis, 1996, Mosby.)

Table 12-10	TYPES OF REGIONAL BLOCKADE: POTENTIAL USES	
BLOCK	**POTENTIAL USES**	**COMPLICATIONS**
Spinal	In place of general anesthesia for surgery below the umbilicus; decreased incidence of postoperative apnea	Inability to access space; incomplete block or inadequate duration of anesthesia
Caudal/epidural	Intraoperative and postoperative analgesia for thoracic, abdominal, perineal, and lower extremity surgery	Inadequate block; local or opioid-related toxicity: nerve damage, paralysis
Dorsal penile nerve/ring block	Circumcision, analgesia for any penile surgery	Hematoma formation; end-organ damage if epinephrine-containing solutions are used
Intercostal nerve block	Rib fractures, thoracic surgery	Pneumothorax; local anesthetic toxicity (highest rate of absorption)

blocks.[86] **Use of combined modalities (e.g., EMLA, penile block, and a sucrose pacifier) has been shown to provide the greatest analgesia and comfort during invasive procedures.**[178] A meta-analysis of the efficacy of EMLA for a variety of procedures in neonates found that EMLA diminishes pain during circumcision, venipuncture, arterial puncture, and placement of a peripheral/central IV.[64,155,177] **For maximum effectiveness, EMLA should be applied and left on for at least 1 to 2 hours before starting an invasive procedure. Unfortunately, EMLA does not appear to alleviate pain resulting from heelsticks.**[105,124] Infiltration of local anesthetic can also help decrease pain for such procedures as placement of percutaneous central lines, removal of Broviac catheters, and circumcision.[21] Methemoglobinemia does not appear to be a problem in premature neonates, but studies are ongoing to address this issue.[105] Amethocaine gel (lysosome-encapsulated tetracaine) is a topical local anesthetic preparation that provides more effective superficial analgesia than EMLA in adults.[53] Studies have documented its effectiveness in neonates: (1) relieves pain during venipuncture[26,90] and (2) does not relieve pain from heelsticks.[91]

Other Medications
Acetaminophen and nonsteroidal antiinflammatory drugs (NSAIDs) can be helpful in providing mild to moderate analgesia (see Table 12-9). These medications are more effective when administered on a regular schedule and can augment the effects of narcotics. Sedatives can help decrease agitation and improve comfort but do not by themselves provide analgesia.[21,60]

Comfort Measures
Comfort measures alone do not relieve pain; however, their use reduces agitation, which indirectly reduces pain by promoting behavioral organization, relaxation, general comfort, and sleep.[7,70,164] Nonnutritive sucking (e.g., on his or her own fingers, hands, or a pacifier) soothes by reducing the infant's level of arousal and duration of cry while increasing the quiet alert state.[38,40,52,108,129] Nonnutritive sucking is effective in reducing pain in preterm infants during heelstick.[173]

Distressed infants offered oral sucrose calmed quickly, stayed calm longer, and spent more time in a quiet alert state than infants offered only a pacifier.[33,150,165] Sucking soothes, reduces heart and metabolic rates, induces hand-to-mouth behavior, and elevates the pain threshold through opioid and nonopioid systems.[32] **Administration of sucrose (into the mouth)[149] within 2 minutes before an invasive procedure (e.g., heelstick) has been shown to decrease crying duration, heart rate, and facial activity associated with pain in full-term and postterm infants.[88,171-173]** In these studies the amount (0.05 to 2 ml) and concentrations (12% to 24%) of sucrose varied but even the smallest dose administered once to preterm infants of 26 to 34 weeks' gestation reduced pain behaviors.[94] Other studies have found no significant pain-relieving effects of sucrose with heelsticks, venipuncture, or eye examinations.[132,138] When sucrose is paired with developmental interventions such as rocking[94] and prone positioning,[173] sucrose is more effective in decreasing behavioral pain responses. However, giving sucrose to preterm infants (less than 32 weeks' gestational age) for all painful procedures in the NICU in the first week of life does not significantly improve neurodevelopmental outcomes.[98]

Body containment of extremities in a flexed position (e.g., holding, swaddling, nesting; providing an opportunity to grasp a finger or pacifier) decreases gross motor movements that contribute to the infant's increased level of arousal, reduces physiologic and behavioral stress, and facilitates energy conservation in the preterm.[40,94,108,139,179] Improper body position contributes to discomfort and pain. **Facilitated tucking—gentle containment of flexed extremities in the midline on the trunk while sidelying or supine—during a painful procedure (e.g., heelstick) results in lower heart rate, shorter crying time, less sleep disruption, and fewer sleep-state changes.[42]** Motoric boundaries (e.g., containment of extremities) assist a preterm infant to maintain a more secure, controlled response and facilitate self-regulation. **Therapeutic interventions include the use of positions that support flexion and restraint in physiologic position, periodic release of restraint and exercise of extremities, gentle change in body position, and positioning to guard operative sites.** Along with comfort measures, minimizing stimulation in the NICU environment enables a neonate who is agitated and/or in pain to use internal and external resources in organizing his or her behavior and developing self-soothing strategies (see Chapter 13).[7,61,139] Individualizing these techniques to the infant's likes and dislikes and listing these at the bedside helps to maintain consistency of care and builds trust in these developing neonates.[69,140]

Picking up, holding, and rocking provide tactile soothing, vestibular stimulation, and the soothing of rhythmic, repetitive movement. Use of massage, rocking, and water mattresses provides tactile, vestibular, and kinesthetic stimuli that modify and accelerate behavioral, state control, and decreased stress behaviors (see Chapter 13). Skin-to-skin contact (kangaroo care) between mothers and healthy newborns during heelstick is a potent analgesic intervention that reduces cry (by 82%), grimace (by 65%), and heart rate.[67]

Complementary healing modalities (e.g., therapeutic touch, acupressure, reiki) are gaining increasing interest among neonatal health care providers. Little research exists, but clinical reports have depicted the benefits of pain relief with integration of these modalities. Research in this area is desperately needed to validate the use of these modalities for pain management.

Activation of cutaneous sensory nerves with a transcutaneous electrical nerve stimulation (TENS) unit and application of thermal (topical skin refrigerant) blocks inhibit transmission of peripheral pain impulses from procedural pain.[113,117] Low-frequency, monotonous sounds (e.g., heartbeat, vacuums) quiet and increase behavioral organization.[113] Use of music (see Chapter 13) and tape recordings of family voices soothe term and preterm infants, resulting in fewer state changes, less time in the arousal state, and increased behavioral organization.[41,101,110] However, during circumcision, music (with or without a pacifier) is not an effective distraction or soothing strategy for relief of the pain of the procedure.[118]

Although comfort measures may prevent the intensification of pain (e.g., guarding an abdominal incision by positioning is less painful than four-point restraint), they may not relieve moderate to severe pain. Comfort measures are helpful but inadequate by themselves, considering the intensity of the noxious stimuli causing moderate to severe pain.[7,42,118]

END-OF-LIFE CARE

When the decision is made to terminate or not begin aggressive medical intervention, the neonate receives end-of-life care, also known as *comfort care* or *palliative care* (see Chapter 31). Neonates who receive end-of-life care are at the threshold of viability, have multiple congenital anomalies that are incompatable with life, or are not responding to NICU interventions (e.g., deterioration in condition despite medical efforts).

End-of-life care should combine comfort measures, pharmacologic management, and psychosocial support for the neonate and family. The family are provided a quiet, private, homelike area in which to touch, hold, and interact with their terminal neonate. Parents, siblings, and extended family members remain with their infant during and after death. Clergy are present for family support and may perform a religious service, such as baptism or blessing.

For comfort care, all invasive procedures, including measurement of vital signs, monitors, machines, and artificial feeding, are discontinued. The infant, cleaned and wrapped in a warm blanket, is held by the family. Intravenous access may remain in place for administration of pain medications or sedatives. **Medication is administered in sufficient doses to provide comfort, relieve pain, and ensure that the infant does not suffer at the end of his or her life.**

In the only study that documents use of analgesia for dying infants whose life support is withdrawn or withheld, 165 deaths in a university-based NICU were reviewed.[137] Opioid analgesia was administered to 84% of infants when life support was withdrawn or withheld. Infants with major congenital anomalies (93%) and necrotizing enterocolitis (100%) were more likely to receive opioids than were ELBW infants (66% to 83%). Overall opioid analgesia was administered to at least 65% of infants. Reasons for life support discontinuation also influenced administration of opioids: (1) futility of treatment (84% medicated), (2) severe lifelong impairment (85% medicated), and (3) suffering caused by treatment (100% medicated). The median dose of opioids was within the usual pharmacologic range (64%) and greater (36%). Ninety-four percent of the infants receiving a higher dose had previously been receiving analgesia and may have required a higher dose as a result of tolerance. The median time until death from the discontinuation of life support was 18 minutes for those who received the standard dose and 20 minutes for those who received the higher dose.

COMPLICATIONS

A neonate's complex behavioral response to pain has both short-term and long-term ramifications. These behavioral changes may disrupt parent-infant interaction and attachment, adaptation to the postnatal environment, and feeding behaviors.[15] An alteration in brain development and maldevelopment of sensory systems can occur when distorted or inappropriate sensory input occurs during a critical period in development.[4,5,20] Because of a neonate's memory, painful experiences increase his or her sensitivity to subsequent medical encounters.[56,155,176,177] These initial experiences may affect the development of attitudes, fears, anxiety, conflicts, wishes, expectations, and patterns of interactions with others.[180]

As previously mentioned, unanesthetized surgery and/or unrelieved pain causes suffering that might itself be a risk to life.[15,44] Maintaining metabolic homeostasis by the appropriate use of anesthetics and analgesics improves postoperative outcome by preventing (1) protein wasting, (2) electrolyte imbalance, (3) impaired immune function, (4) sepsis, (5) metabolic acidosis, (6) pulmonary and cardiac insufficiency, (7) hypermetabolic state, and (8) death.[8,16,96] Increasing evidence confirms that exposure to prolonged, severe or untreated pain increases morbidity, and alters subsequent behavioral and physiologic responses to pain.[7]

Narcotic analgesics may produce respiratory depression severe enough to require mechanical ventilation. Naloxone (0.1 mg/kg IV or IM) is the specific antidote for narcotic overdose (see Table 12-9). Lower doses of naloxone (0.001 to 0.01 mg/kg IV or IM) can be used for moderate respiratory depression. Complete opioid reversal with 0.1 mg/kg naloxone increases agitation and stress response in neonates with ongoing pain. Subsequently it is more difficult to manage the neonate's pain until the effects of the naloxone wear off. Lower doses of naloxone should be used and the dose titrated to prevent this outcome. **An ampule of neonatal naloxone should always be immediately available with the appropriate dose precalculated on the infant's emergency card.** Flumazenil is a specific antagonist for the benzodiazepines and should be used to treat respiratory depression (see Table 12-9). **Respiratory depression may produce hypoxemia so that a pulse oximeter should be standard equipment along with cardiorespiratory monitoring.**[7] **If available, TcPCO$_2$ monitors should also be used to watch for hypercapnia. All equipment for assisted ventilation should be at the bedside.**[7]

An overdose of local anesthetics can cause seizures, ventricular tachycardia, bradycardia, and cardiovascular collapse. Toxic doses for neonates should be carefully calculated, and lower doses should be administered. Benzodiazepines or phenobarbital can be used to treat refractory seizures;

cardiopulmonary resuscitation (CPR) and defibrillation may be necessary to treat the cardiovascular complications.[51] **Patients who are receiving epidural analgesia for postoperative pain control need to be monitored for signs of potential CNS toxicity** (e.g., irritability, jitteriness, twitching, myoclonic jerking). If an opioid is being administered with the local anesthetic infusion, then respiratory depression is also a possibility and patients should be monitored as described above. Other extremely rare complications of epidurals are nerve injury or paralysis.

Hematoma formation can occur (1.2%) with the placement of a dorsal penile nerve block.[57] Using a ring block usually avoids this problem. **Epinephrine-containing solutions must never be used, because this can lead to compromise of the blood supply to the penis and severe tissue damage.**

Tolerance and Withdrawal

Tolerance is the need for escalating doses of drug to achieve the same effect. Physical dependence is the state wherein continued drug is needed to prevent the signs of withdrawal.[60,192,193] **Withdrawal arises when discontinuing the drug causes symptoms such as irritability, diarrhea, tachycardia, hypertension, insomnia, restlessness, diaphoresis, or palmar sweating and muscle twitches.** Addiction occurs when there is psychological as well as physical dependence, and is associated with active drug-seeking behavior and use (abuse) of the drugs for nonmedical conditions. Tolerance, dependence, and withdrawal can occur with opioids and benzodiazepines; however, addiction is exceedingly rare when these medications are used for medical purposes. **Medications should not be restricted because of fear of addiction. Critically ill infants sometimes need long-term infusions of opioids and/or benzodiazepines to provide analgesia and sedation.** ECMO and prolonged mechanical ventilation are two examples of this situation. Use of fentanyl for more than 5 to 7 days can lead to tolerance and withdrawal (also known as opioid abstinence syndrome). Opioid use should be decreased by no more than 10% to 20% every 1 to 3 days, depending on the duration of the medication's use and the infant's response to the changes. Shorter-acting medications such as fentanyl and midazolam can be switched to methadone and lorazepam, which have the advantage of being longer acting as well as being available in an oral form. **Addition of oral clonidine 1.5-3.0 μg/kg bid can help alleviate withdrawal symptoms. The dose of**

clonidine can be titrated up to 5 to 10 μg/kg bid as tolerated. The side effects of clonidine include bradycardia, hypotension, and sedation. In addition, minimal handling and a quiet, darkened environment help decrease external stimuli. A pacifier, swaddling, and holding are effective comfort measures. Positioning the withdrawing infant prone rather than supine, decreases the level of distress, lowers withdrawal scores, and facilitates sleep.[116]

PARENT TEACHING

Parents are excellent observers of their infant and often recognize when the infant is experiencing pain even before the care provider does.[140] The health care provider loses credibility when he or she does not acknowledge the infant's pain. Listening to parents' concerns about their infant's pain, including the parent's report of their assessment, communication of the plan of care regarding analgesia and/or sedation, and offering the rationale behind the medication decision-making help the parents become active participants in the management of their infant's pain. Parents of medically fragile infants have identified specific sources of stress in the NICU: (1) parental role alterations, especially inability to comfort the infant, and (2) infant appearance and behavior, especially pain and difficulty breathing.[35] The most common fear expressed by parents is that their infant will experience undue pain while being cared for in the NICU.[140] Three years after their infant's NICU experience mothers are still able to recall the pain and procedures that their infants endured.[186] The care provider's sensitivity to the neonate's pain and advocating for pain relief are comforting for parents.[153] Teaching parents to report their assessments and encouraging parents to comfort their infants will help them in the attachment process and foster a trusting relationship with the health care team. **Comfort measures are ideally provided by parents who may then actively participate in their infant's pain relief.**

REFERENCES

1. Abu-Saad H, Bours G, Stevens B: Assessment of pain in the neonate, *Semin Perinatol* 22:402, 1998.
2. Acute Pain Management Guideline Panel: Acute pain management: operative or medical procedures and trauma, clinical practice guideline, AHCPR Pub No 92-0032, Rockville, Md, 1992, Agency for Health Care Policy and Research, Public Health Service, US Dept of HHS.

3. Alkalay A, Sola A: Analgesia and local anesthesia for non-ritual circumcision in stable healthy newborns, *Neonat Intensive Care* 13:19, 2000.

4. Als H: Toward a synactive theory of development: promise for the assessment and support of infant individuality, *Infant Mental Health J* 3:299, 1982.

5. Als H, Lawhon G, Duffy FH et al: Individualized developmental care for the very low-birth-weight preterm infant, *JAMA* 272:853, 1994.

6. American Academy of Pediatrics, Committee on Fetus and Newborn, Committee on Drugs, Section on Anesthesiology and Section on Surgery: Neonatal anesthesia, *Pediatrics* 80:446, 1987.

7. American Academy of Pediatrics and Canadian Paediatric Society: Prevention and management of pain and stress in the neonate, *Pediatrics* 105:454, 2000.

8. Anand KJ: Neonatal stress responses to anesthesia and surgery, *Clin Perinatol* 17(1):207, 1990.

9. Anand KJ: Relationship between stress responses and clinical outcomes in newborns, infants and children, *Crit Care Med* 21(suppl):358, 1993.

10. Anand KJ: Clinical importance of pain and stress in preterm neonates, *Biol Neonate* 73:1, 1998.

11. Anand KJ: Effects of perinatal pain and stress. In Mayer E, Saper C, eds: *Progress in brain research,* Amsterdam, 2000, Elsevier.

12. Anand KJ: Consensus statement for the prevention and management of pain in the newborn, *Arch Pediatr Adolesc Med* 155:173, 2001.

13. Anand KJ, Carr DB: The neuroanatomy, neurophysiology and neurochemistry of pain, stress and analgesia in newborns and children, *Pediatr Clin North Am* 36:795, 1989.

14. Anand KJ, Craig KD: New perspectives on the definition of pain, *Pain* 67:3, 1996.

15. Anand KJ, Hickey PR: Pain and its effect in the human neonate and fetus, *N Engl J Med* 317:1321, 1987.

16. Anand KJ, Hickey PR: Halothane-morphine compared with high-dose sufentanil for anesthesia and postoperative analgesia in neonatal cardiac surgery, *N Engl J Med* 326:1, 1992.

17. Anand KJ, Sippel WG, Aynsley-Green A: Randomised trial of fentanyl anesthesia in preterm neonates undergoing surgery: effects on the stress response, *Lancet* 1:62, 1987.

18. Anand KJ, Barton BA, McIntosh N et al: Analgesia and sedation in preterm neonates who require ventilatory support, *Arch Pediatr Adolesc Med* 153:331, 1999.

19. Anand KJ, Sippell WG, Schofield NM, et al: Does halothane anesthesia decrease the metabolic and endocrine stress responses of newborn infants undergoing operation? *Br Med J* 296:668, 1988.

20. Anders T, Zeanah C: Early infant development from a biological point of view. In Call J, Galenson E, Tyson R, eds: *Frontiers of infant psychiatry,* New York, 1984, Basic Books.

21. Anderson C, Zeltzer L, Fanurik D: Procedural pain. In Schecter N, Berde C, Yaster M, eds: *Pain in infants, children and adolescents,* Baltimore, 1993, Williams & Wilkins.

22. Armstrong P, Bersten A: Normeperidine toxicity, *Anesth Analog* 65:536, 1986.

23. Balda R, Guinsburg R, Fernanda M et al: Are adults capable of recognizing facial expression of pain in full term newborn infants? *Pediatr Res* 47:387A, 2000.

24. Ballantyne M, Stevens B, McAllister M et al: Validation of the premature infant pain profile in the clinical setting, *Crit J Pain* 15:297, 1999.

25. Barker D, Rutter N: Exposure to invasive procedures in neonatal intensive care unit admissions, *Arch Dis Child Fetal Neonat Educ* 72:F47, 1995.

26. Barker D, Rutter N: Skin blood flow and topical local anaesthesia in preterm infants, *Early Human Dev* 45:163, 1996.

27. Barr R: Reflections on measuring pain in infants: dissociation in responsive systems and "honest signalling," *Arch Dis Child Fetal Neonat Educ* 79: F152, 1998.

28. Barrington K, Finer N, Ryan C: Evaluation of pulse oximetry as a continuous monitoring technique in the NICU, *Crit Care Med* 16:1147, 1988.

29. Bauchner H, May A, Coates E: Use of analgesic agents for invasive medical procedures in pediatric and neonatal intensive care units, *J Pediatr* 4:647, 1992.

30. Benini F, Johnston CC, Faucher D et al: Topical anesthesia during circumcision in newborn infants, *JAMA* 270:850, 1993.

31. Bildner J, Krechel S: Increasing staff nurse awareness of post operative pain management in the NICU, *Neonat Netw* 15:11, 1996.

32. Blass E: Behavioral and physiological consequences of suckling in rat and human newborns, *Acta Paediatr Suppl* 397:71, 1994.

33. Blass EM, Hoffmeyer LB: Sucrose as an analgesic for newborn infants, *Pediatrics* 87:215, 1991.

34. Broome ME, Tanzillo H: Differentiating between pain and agitation in premature neonates, *J Perinat Neonat Nurs* 4:53, 1990.

35. Brunssen S, Miles M: Sources of environmental stress experienced by mothers of hospitalized medically fragile infants, *Neonat Netw* 15:88, 1996.

36. Burdeau G, Kleiber C: Clinical indicators of infant irritability, *Neonat Netw* 9:23, 1991.

37. Burns ER: Development and evaluation of a new instrument for safe heelstick sampling of neonates, *Lab Med* 29:481, 1989.

38. Campos R: Soothing neonate's response to a stressful procedure, *Neonat Netw* 12:93, 1993.
39. Campos RG: Rocking and pacifiers: two comfort interventions for heelstick pain, *Res Nurs Health* 17:321, 1994.
40. Campos RG: Soothing pain-elicited distress in infants with swaddling and pacifiers, *Child Dev* 60:781, 1989.
41. Collins S, Kuch K: Music therapy in the NICU, *Neonat Netw* 9:23, 1991.
42. Corff K, Seideman R, Venkataraman PS et al: Facilitated tucking: a nonpharmacologic comfort measure for pain in preterm neonates, *J Obstet Gynecol Neonat Nurs* 24:143, 1995.
43. Cousins M: Acute and postoperative pain. In Wall P, Melzack R, eds: *Textbook of pain,* Edinburgh, 1994, Churchill Livingstone.
44. Craig K, Badali M: On knowing an infant's pain, *Pain Forum* 8:74, 1999.
45. Craig K, Whitfield MF, Grunau RV et al: Pain in the preterm neonate: behavioural and physiological indices, *Pain* 52:287, 1993.
46. Cunningham N: Ethical perspectives on the perception and treatment of neonatal pain, *J Perinat Neonat Nurs* 4:75, 1990.
47. Devor M: Pain mechanism and pain syndromes. In Campbell J, ed: *Pain 1996: an updated review,* Seattle, 1996, IASP Press.
48. Dickenson A: Pharmacology of pain transmission and control. In Campbell J, ed: *Pain 1996: an updated review,* Seattle, 1996, IASP Press.
49. Ecoffey C, Dubousset A, Samii K: Lumbar and thoracic epidural anesthesia for urologic and upper abdominal surgery in infants and children, *Anesthesiology* 65:87, 1986.
50. Evans JC, Vogelpohl DG, Bourguignon CM et al: Pain behaviors in LBW infants accompany some "nonpainful" caregiving procedures, *Neonat Netw* 16:33, 1997.
51. Eyres R: Local anesthetic agents in infancy, *Paediatr Anaesth* 5:213, 1995.
52. Field T, Goldson E: Pacifying effects of nonnutritive sucking on term and preterm neonates during heelstick procedures, *Pediatrics* 74:1012, 1984.
53. Fischer R, Hung O, Mezei M: Topical anaesthesia of intact skin: liposome encapsulated tetracaine vs. EMLA, *Br J Anaesth* 81:972, 1998.
54. Fitzgerald M: Neurobiology of fetal and neonatal pain. In Wall P, Melzad R, eds: *Textbook of pain,* Edinburgh, 1994, Churchhill Livingstone.
55. Fitzgerald M, Anand KJ: Developmental neuroanatomy and neurophysiology of pain. In Schector N, Berde C, Yastor M, eds: *Pain in infants, children and adolescents,* Baltimore, 1993, Williams & Wilkins.
56. Fitzgerald M, Millard C, Macintosh N: Hyperalgesia in premature infants, *Lancet* 1:292, 1988.
57. Fontaine P, Dittberner D, Scheltema K: The safety of dorsal penile nerve block for neonatal circumcision, *J Fam Pract* 39:243, 1994.
58. Foster R, Markham A: Levobupivacaine, *Drugs* 59:551, 2000.
59. Franck L: Identification, management, and prevention of pain in the neonate. In Kenner C, Brueggemeyer A, Gunderson L, eds: *Comprehensive neonatal nursing: a physiologic perspective,* Philadelphia, 1998, WB Saunders.
60. Franck L, Gregory G: Clinical evaluation and treatment of infant pain in the neonatal intensive care unit. In Schecter N, Berde C, Yastor M, eds: *Pain in infants, children and adolescents,* Baltimore, 1993, Williams & Wilkins.
61. Franck L, Lawhon G: Environmental and behavioral strategies to prevent and manage neonatal pain, *Semin Perinatol* 22(5):434, 1998.
62. Franck L, Miaskowski C: Measurement of neonatal responses to painful stimuli: a research review, *J Pain Symptom Manage* 14:343, 1997.
63. Franck LS: A national survey of the assessment and treatment of pain and agitation in the NICU, *J Obstet Gynecol Neonat Nurs* 16:387, 1987.
64. Garcia O, Reichberg S, Brion L, Schulman M: Topical anesthesia for line insertion in very low birth weight infants, *J Perinatol* 17:477, 1997.
65. Goldsmith J: Ventilation management casebook: chloral hydrate intoxication, *J Perinatol* 14:74, 1994.
66. Goldstein R, Brazy J: Narcotic sedation stabilizes arterial blood pressure fluctuations in sick premature infants, *J Perinatol* 11:365, 1991.
67. Gray L, Watt L, Blass E: Skin-to-skin contact is analgesia in healthy newborns, *Pediatrics* 105(1):110, 2000.
68. Groban L, Deal DD, Vernon JC et al: Cardiac resuscitation after incremental overdosage with lidocaine, bupivacaine, levobupivacaine and ropivacaine in anesthetized dogs, *Anesth Analog* 92:37, 2001.
69. Grossman R, Lawhon G: Individualized supportive care to reduce pain and stress. In Anand KJ, McGrath P, eds: *Pain in neonates,* Amsterdam, 1995, Elsevier.
70. Gruenwald P, Becker P: Developmental enhancement: implementing a program for the NICU, *Neonat Netw* 9:29, 1991.
71. Grunau RVE, Craig KD: Pain expression in neonates: facial action and cry, *Pain* 28:395, 1987.
72. Grunau R, Johnston C, Craig K: Neonatal facial and cry responses to invasive and non invasive procedures, *Pain* 42:295, 1990.
73. Grunau RV, Whitfield MF, Petrie JH: Pain sensitivity and temperament in extremely low-birth weight premature toddlers and preterm and full term controls, *Pain* 58:341, 1994.

74. Grunau R et al: Extremely low birth weight (ELBW) toddlers are relatively unresponsive to pain at 18 months corrected age compared to larger birth weight children, Abstract 18, *Proc Neonat Soc* 1993.

75. Grunau RE, Oberlander T, Holsti L et al: Bedside application of the neonatal facial coding system in pain assessment of premature neonates, *Pain* 76: 277, 1998.

76. Grunau R, Oberlander T, Whitfield M et al: Stressful early NICU experience dampens subsequent pain reactivity in preterm infants at 32 weeks PCA, *Pediatr Res* 47:400a, 2000.

77. Grunau RE, Oberlander TF, Whitfield MF et al: Demographic and therapeutic determinants of pain reactivity in VLBW infants at 32 weeks gestational age, *Pediatrics* 107:105, 2001.

78. Grunau RV, Whitfield MF, Petrie JH et al: Early pain experience, child and family factors, as precursors of somatization: a prospective study of extremely premature and full term children, *Pain* 56:353, 1994.

79. Guinsburg R, Fernanda M, Almeida B et al: Contributing factors to analgesic prescription in mechanically ventilated newborn infants, *Pediatr Res* 45:200A, 1999.

80. Guinsburg R, Fernanda M, Almeida B et al: Differences in pain expression between male and female newborn infants, *Pediatr Res* 45:200A, 1999.

81. Guinsburg R, Kopelman BI, Anand KJ et al: Physiological, hormonal and behavioral responses to a single fentanyl dose in intubated and ventilated preterm neonates, *J Pediatr* 132:954, 1998.

82. Hancock S, Newell S, Brierley J et al: Premedication for neonatal intubation: current practice in Australia and the United Kingdom, *Arch Dis Child Fetal Neonat Educ* 82:A29, 2000.

83. Harpin VA, Rutter N: Making heel pricks less painful, *Arch Dis Child* 58:226, 1983.

84. Heller S, Constantinou J, Vandenberg K et al: Sedation administration to VLBW premature infants, *J Perinatol* 17:107, 1997.

85. Herzog JM: A neonatal intensive care syndrome: a pain complex involving neuroplasticity and psychic trauma. In Galenson E, Tyson RL, eds: *Frontiers in infant psychiatry,* New York, 1983, Basic Books.

86. Hester N, Foster R: Integrating pediatric postoperative pain management into clinical practice, *J Pharmaceut Care Symptom Control* 1:5, 1993.

87. Howard C, Howard FM, Fortune K et al: A randomized controlled study of a eutectic mixture of local anesthetic cream versus penile nemeblock for pain relief during circumcision, *Am J Obstet Gynecol* 181:1506, 1999.

88. Isik U, Ozek E, Bilgen H et al: Comparison of oral dextrose and sucrose solutions on pain response in neonates, *Pediatr Res* 47:403A, 2000.

89. Jacqz-Aigrain E, Daoud P, Burton P et al: Placebo-controlled trial of midazolam sedation in mechanically ventilated newborn babies, *Lancet* 344:646, 1994.

90. Jain A, Rutter N: Local anaesthetic effect of topical amethocaine gel in neonates: randomised controlled trial, *Arch Dis Child Fetal Neonat Educ* 82:F42, 2000.

91. Jain A, Rutter N, Ratnayaka M: Topical amethocaine gel for pain relief of heel prick blood sampling: a randomised double blind controlled trial, *Arch Dis Child Fetal Neonat Educ* 84:F56, 2001.

92. Ji R, Hiroshi B, Brenner G et al: Nociceptive-specific activation of ERK in spinal neurons contributes to pain hypersensitivity, *Nature Neurosci* 2:1114, 1999.

93. Johnston CC, O'Shaughnessy D: Acoustical attributes of pain cries: distinguishing features. In Dubner R, Gebbart GF, Bond MR, eds: *Advances in pain research,* New York, 1988, Raven.

94. Johnston CC, Stemler RL, Stevens BJ et al: The effect of simulated carrying and sucrose on pain response to heel stick in preterm neonates, *Pain* 72:193, 1997.

95. Johnston CC, Stevens B: Experience in a neonatal intensive care unit affects pain response, *Pediatrics* 98:925, 1996.

96. Johnston CC, Stevens B: Pain assessment in newborns, *J Perinat Neonatl Nurs* 4:41, 1990.

97. Johnston CC, Filion F, Majnemer A et al: The efficacy of sucrose analgesia for procedural pain in preterm infants <32 week in the first week of life, *Pediatr Res* 47:405A, 2000.

98. Johnston CC, Stevens B, Craig KD et al: Developmental changes in pain expression in premature, full term, two and four month old infants, *Pain* 52:201, 1993.

99. Johnston CC, Stevens B, Franck L et al: Factors explaining lack of responses to heel stick in preterm newborns, *J Obstet Gynecol Neonat Nurs* 28:587, 1999.

100. Kahn DJ, Richardson DK, Gray JE et al: Variation among neonatal intensive care units in narcotic administration, *Arch Pediatr Adoles Med* 152:844, 1998.

101. Kaminski J, Hall W: The effect of soothing music on neonatal behavioral states in the hospital newborn nursery, *Neonat Netw* 15:45, 1996.

102. Koren G: Use of eutectic mixture of local anesthetics in young children for procedure-related pain, *J Pediatr* 122:530, 1993.

103. Krechel SW, Bildner J: CRIES: a new neonatal postoperative pain measurement score: initial testing of validity and reliability, *Paediatr Anaesth* 5:53, 1995.

104. Lambert GH, Muraskas J, Anderson CL et al: Direct hyperbilirubinemia associated with chloral hydrate administration in the newborn, *Pediatrics* 86:277, 1990.

105. Larsson B: Pain management in neonates, *Acta Paediatr* 88:1301, 1999.
106. Larsson BA, Jylli L, Lagercrantz H et al: Does a local anaesthetic cream (EMLA) alleviate pain from heel lancing in neonates? *Acta Anaesthesiol Scand* 39:1028, 1995.
107. Larsson BA, Tannfeldt G, Lagercrantz H et al: Venipuncture is more effective and less painful than heel lancing for blood tests in neonates, *Pediatrics* 101:882, 1998.
108. Lawhon G: Providing developmentally supportive care in the newborn intensive care unit: an evolving challenge, *J Perinat Neonat Nurs* 10:48, 1997.
109. Lawrence J, Alcock D, McGrath P et al: The development of a tool to assess neonatal pain, *Neonat Netw* 12:59, 1993.
110. Leonard J: Music therapy: fertile ground for application of research in practice, *Neonat Netw* 12:47, 1993.
111. Lepley M, Gardner S, Hagdorn M et al: High-risk obstetrical care. In Gardner S, Hagedorn M, eds: *Legal aspects of maternal child nursing practice,* Menlo Park, Calif, 1997, Addison-Wesley.
112. Leuschen MP, Willard LD, Hoie EB et al: Plasma fentanyl levels in infants undergoing extracorporeal membrane oxygenation, *J Thorac Cardiovasc Surg* 105:885, 1993.
113. Lynam L: Research utilization: nonpharmacological management of pain in neonates, *Neonatal Netw* 14:59, 1995.
114. MacGregor R, Evans D, Sugden D et al: Outcome at 5-6 years of prematurely born children who received morphine as neonates, *Arch Dis Child Fetal Neonat Educ* 79:F40, 1998.
115. Magny JF, d'Allest AM, Nedelcoux H et al: Midazolam and myoclonus in neonate, *Eur J Pediatr* 153:389, 1994.
116. Maichuk GT, Zahorodny W, Marshall R: Use of positioning to reduce the severity of neonatal narcotic withdrawal syndrome, *J Perinatol* 19:510, 1999.
117. Maikler V: Effects of a skin refrigerant/anesthetic and age on the pain response of infants requiring immunizations, *Res Nurs Health* 14:397, 1991.
118. Marchette L, Main R, Redick E et al: Pain reduction interventions during neonatal circumcision, *Nurs Res* 40:241, 1991.
119. Marlow N, Weindling M, Shaw B: Opiates, catecholamine concentrations and ventilated preterm babies, *Lancet* 342:997, 1993.
120. May KA, Britt R, Newman MM et al: Pediatric registered nurse usage and perception of EMLA, *J Soc Pediatr Nurs* 4:105, 1999.
121. McClain B, Anand KJ: Neonatal pain management. In Deshpande J, Tobias J, eds: *The pediatric pain handbook,* St Louis, 1996, Mosby.
122. McGown R: Caudal analgesia in children: 500 cases for procedures below the diaphragm, *Anaesthesia* 37:806, 1982.
123. McIntosh N: Pain in the newborn: a possible new starting point, *Eur J Paediatr* 156:173, 1997.
124. McIntosh N, Van Veen L, Brameyer H: Alleviation of the pain of heel prick in preterm infants, *Arch Dis Child* 70:F177, 1994.
125. Menon G, Anand KJ, McIntosh N: Practical approach to analgesia and sedation in the neonatal intensive care unit, *Semin Perinatol* 22:417, 1998.
126. Mersky, H: The definition of pain, *Euro J Psychiatr* 6:153, 1991.
127. Meyer R, Campbell J, Raja S: Peripheral neural mechanisms of nociception. In Wall P, Melzack R, eds: *Textbook of pain,* Edinburgh, 1994, Churchill Livingstone.
128. Millar C, Bissonnetter B: Awake intubation increases intracranial pressure without affecting cerebral blood flow velocity in infants, *Can J Anaesth* 41:281, 1994.
129. Miller H, Anderson G: Nonnutritive sucking: effects on crying and heart rate in intubated infants requiring assisted mechanical ventilation, *Nurs Res* 42:305, 1993.
130. Morison S, Grunau R, Oberlander T et al: Is there a correlation between behavioral and autonomic reactivity to pain in preterm infants at 32 wks PCA? *Pediatr Res* 47:418A, 2000.
131. Murrell D, Gibson P, Cohen R: Continuous epidural analgesia in newborn infants undergoing major surgery, *J Pediatr* Surg 28:548, 1993.
132. Mutti D, Mariani GL, Lequizamon E: Randomized trial of different methods to reduce the pain response associated with blood extraction in term neonates, *Pediatr Res* 45:213A, 1999.
133. National Association of Neonatal Nurses: *Pain assessment and management: guideline for practice,* Glenview, Ill, 2000, The Association.
134. Oberlander T, Grunau R, Whitfield M et al: Does parenchymal brain injury affect biobehavioral pain responses in VLBW infants at 32 wks P.C.A.? *Pediatr Res* 47:421A, 2000.
135. Oberlander TF, Grunau RE, Whitfield MF et al: Biobehavioral pain responses in former extremely low birth weight infants at 4 months' corrected age, *Pediatrics* 105:e6, 2000.
136. Ohlsson A, McMillan D, Schmidt B et al: Variations in use of narcotics, benzodiazepines and pancuronium in newborn babies with assisted ventilation, *Pediatr Res* 45:313A, 1999.
137. Partridge JC, Wall SN: Analgesia for dying infants whose life support is withdrawn or withheld, *Pediatrics* 99:76, 1997.

138. Pearson C, Jorgenson K, Blocker R et al: Reducing the pain of neonatal eye examination: a randomized trial of plain and sugar dipped pacifier, *Pediatr Res* 45:218A, 1999.

139. Peters K: Infant handling in the NICU: does developmental care make a difference? An evaluative review of the literature, *J Perinat Neonat Nurs* 13:83, 1999.

140. Phillips P: Neonatal pain management: a call to action, *Pediatr Nurs* 21:195, 1995.

141. Pokela M: Effect of opioid-induced analgesia on beta-endorphin, cortisol and glucose responses in neonates with cardiorespiratory problems, *Biol Neonate* 64:360, 1993.

142. Pokela M: Pain relief can reduce hypoxemia in distressed neonates during routine treatment procedures, *Pediatrics* 93:379, 1994.

143. Pokela M, Koivisto M: Physiological changes, plasma beta-endorphin and cortisol responses to tracheal intubation in neonates, *Acta Paediatr* 83:151, 1994.

144. Porter F: Pain assessment in children and infants. In Schecter N, Bende C, Yaster M, eds: *Pain in infants, children and adolescents,* Baltimore, 1993, Williams & Wilkins.

145. Porter F, Wolf C, Miller J: The effect of handling and immobilization on the response to acute pain in newborn infants, *Pediatrics* 102:1383, 1998.

146. Porter FL, Wolf CM, Miller JP et al: Procedural pain in newborn infants: the influence of intensity and development, *Pediatrics* 104:105, 1999.

147. Quinn MW, deBoer RC, Ansari N et al: Stress responses and mode of ventilation in preterm infants, *Arch Dis Child Fetal Neonat Educ* 78:F195, 1998.

148. Quinn MW, Wild J, Dean HG et al: Randomised double-blind controlled trial of effect of morphine on catecholamine concentrations in ventilated preterm babies, *Lancet* 342:324, 1993.

149. Ramenghi L, Evans D, Levene M: "Sucrose analgesia": absorptive mechanism or taste perception? *Arch Dis Child Fetal Neonat Educ* 80:F146, 1999.

150. Ramenghi LA, Wood CM, Griffith GC et al: Reduction of pain response in premature infants using intraoral sucrose, *Arch Dis Child Fetal Neonat Educ* 74:F126, 1996.

151. Raju TN, Vidyasagar D, Papazafiratou C et al: Intracranial pressure during intubation and anesthesia in infants, *J Pediatr* 96:860, 1980.

152. Rao M, Blass E, Brignol M et al: Effect of crying on energy metabolism in human neonates, *Pediatr Res* 33:309A, 1993.

153. Reed M: Principles of drug therapy. In Behrman R, Kliegman R, Aruon A, eds: *Textbook of pediatrics,* ed 15, Philadelphia, 1996, WB Saunders.

154. Rovee-Collier C, Hayne H: Reactuation of infant memory: implications for cognitive development, *Adv Child Dev* 10:185, 1987.

155. Rubio D, Soto A, Oliveria F et al: EMLA cream for percutaneous venous central line placement in preterm infants: a randomized controlled trial, *Pediatr Res* 47:415A, 2000.

156. Rushforth J, Levere M: Behavioural response to pain in healthy neonates, *Arch Dis Child Fetal Neonat Educ* 70:F174, 1994.

157. Saarenmaa E, Huttenun P, Leppaluoto J et al: Advantages of fentanyl over morphine in analgesia for ventilated newborn infants after birth: a randomized trial, *J Pediatr* 134:144, 1999.

158. Saigals S, Feeny D, Rosenbaum P et al: Self-perceived health status and health related quality of life of extremely low-birth-weight infants at adolescence, *JAMA* 276:453, 1996.

159. Santiero ML, Christy J, Stromquist C et al: Pharmacokinetics of continuous infusion fentanyl in newborns, *J Perinatol* 17:135, 1997.

160. Schecter N, Berde C, Yaster M: *Pain in infants, children and adolescents,* Baltimore, 1993, Williams & Wilkins.

161. Schechter NL, Blankson V, Pachter LM et al: The ouchless place: no pain, children's gain, *Pediatrics* 99:890, 1997.

162. Shah V, Ohlsson A: Venipuncture should replace heel lance to obtain blood samples for neonatal screening: a systematic review, *Pediatr Res* 45:224A, 1999.

163. Shah VS, Taddio A, Bennett S et al: Neonatal pain response to heelstick vs. venipuncture for blood sampling: a randomized controlled trial, *Pediatr Res* 41:177A, 1997.

164. Shapiro C: Pain in the neonate, *Neonat Netw* 8:7, 1989.

165. Smith BA, Fillion RJ, Blass EM: Orally-mediated sources of calming in 1-3 day old human infants, *Dev Psychol* 26:731, 1990.

166. Snellman L, Stang H: Prospective evaluation of complications of dorsal penile block for neonatal circumcision, *Pediatrics* 95:705, 1995.

167. Stevens B, Johnston C: Physiological responses of premature infants to a painful stimulus, *Nurs Res* 43:226, 1994.

168. Stevens B, Johnston C, Gruanau R: Issues of assessment of pain and discomfort in neonates, *J Obstet Gynecol Neonat Nurs* 24:849, 1995.

169. Stevens B, Johnston C, Hurton L: Factors that influence the behavioral pain responses of premature infants, *Pain* 59:101, 1994.

170. Stevens B, Johnston C, Petroshen P et al: Premature Infant Pain Profile: development and initial validation, *Clin J Pain* 12:13, 1996.

171. Stevens B, Taddio A, Ohlsson A: The efficacy of sucrose for relieving procedural pain in neonates: a systematic review and meta-analysis, *Acta Paediatr* 86:837, 1997.

172. Stevens B, Ohlsson A: Sucrose in neonates undergoing painful procedures. In Sinclair JC, Bracken MB, Soll RS et al, eds: *Neonatal module of the Cochrane data base of systematic reviews,* Cochrane Library (database on disk and CD ROM). The Cochrane Collection: Issue 2, Oxford, 1998, Update Software.

173. Stevens B, Johnston C, Franck L: The efficacy of developmentally sensitive interventions and sucrose for relieving procedural pain in VLBW infants, *Nurs Res* 48: 35, 1999.

174. Storm H: Development of emotional sweating in preterms measured by skin conductance changes, *Early Hum Dev* 62:149, 2001.

175. Taddio A, Goldbach M, Ipp M: Effect of neonatal circumcision on pain responses during vacation in male infants, *Lancet* 345:291, 1995.

176. Taddio A, Katz J, Ilersich AL: Effects of neonatal circumcision on pain response during subsequent vaccination, *Lancet* 349:599, 1997.

177. Taddio A, Ohlsson A, Einarson TR: A systematic review of lidocaine-prilocaine cream (EMLA) in the treatment of acute pain in neonates, *Pediatrics* 101:El, 1998.

178. Taddio A, Pollock N, Gilbert-MacLeod C: Analgesia and local anesthesia to minimize pain during circumcision, *Arch Pediatr Adolesc Med* 154:620, 2000.

179. Taquino L, Blackburn S: The effects of containment during suction and heelstick on physiological and behavioral responses of preterm infants, *Neonat Netw* 13:55, 1994,

180. Tyson P: Developmental lines and infant assessment. In Call JD, GalensonE, Tyson RL, eds: *Frontiers of infant psychiatry,* New York, 1984, Basic Books.

181. Van Cleve L, Johnson L, Andrews S: Pain responses of hospitalized neonates to venipuncture, *Neonat Net* 14:31, 1995.

182. Vertanen H, Fellman V, Brommels M et al: An automatic incision device for obtaining blood samples from the heels of preterm infants causes less damage than a conventional lancet, *Arch Dis Child Fetal Neonat Educ* 84:F53, 2001.

183. Vogel S, Gibbins S, Simmons B et al: Pharmacological management of pain and stress during mechanical ventilation in neonates: a Canadian perspective, *Pediatr Res* 47:43A, 2000.

184. Vogel S, Gibbins S, Simmons B et al: Premedication for ET intubation in neonates: a Canadian perspective, *Pediatr Res* 47:438a, 2000.

185. Vogelpohl D, Evans J, Cedargren D: Behavioral pain response of the LBW premature neonate in the NICU, *Neonat Intensive Care* Sept/Oct 1995, 1996, p 28.

186. Wereszczak J, Miles M, Holditch-Davis D: Maternal recall of the neonatal intensive care unit, *Neonat Netw* 16:33, 1997.

187. Whitfield M, Grunau R: Behavior, pain perception and the extremely LBW survivor, *Clin Perinatol* 27:363, 2000.

188. Wilder R: Local anesthetics for the pediatric patient, *Pediatr Clin North Am* 47:545, 2000.

189. Winberg J: Do neonatal pain and stress program the brain's response to future stimuli? *Acta Paediatr* 87:723, 1998.

190. Wood CM, Rushforth JA, Hartley R: Randomized double blind trial of morphine vs. diamorphine for sedation of perterm neonates, *Arch Dis Fetal Neonat Educ* 79:F34, 1998.

191. Wulf H, Peters C, Behnke H: The pharmacokinetics of caudal ropivacaine 0.2% in children, *Anesthesia* 55:757, 2000.

192. Yaster M, Maxwell L: Opioid agonists and antagonists. In Schecter N, Berde C, Yaster M, eds: *Pain in infants, children and adolescents,* Baltimore, 1993, Williams & Wilkins.

193. Yaster M, Kost-Byerly S, Berde C et al: The management of opioid and benzodiazepine dependence in infants, children and adolescents, *Pediatrics* 98:135, 1996.

13 The Neonate and the Environment: Impact on Development

Sandra L. Gardner, Edward Goldson

For centuries the newborn baby has been considered a *tabula rasa*—a blank slate on which parents and the world "write" to create the individual. In the first half of the twentieth century, research emphasized the contributions of the environment in shaping the infant and child. Only recently has the individuality of the infant been recognized as a powerful shaper of the caregiver, the care given, and thus the environment.

In this chapter we will explore the psychosocioemotional development of term and preterm neonates. Infant development is a reflection of the dynamic relationship between endowment and environment. Along the continuum of development, development of the infant is the beginning of the child and, ultimately, of adult competence in the world. Understanding the dynamic relationship between endowment and environment is enhanced by a review of the principles of development in Box 13-1. First, the developmental tasks of infancy are presented, along with the influences of endowment and environment on mastery. Home and family life, in which most infants are raised, is then contrasted with the experiences of babies in the NICU. Intervention strategies to normalize the NICU environment are then presented, along with strategies for parent teaching. The developmental and social outcomes of infants exposed to the NICU are then presented.

DEVELOPMENTAL TASKS OF THE NEONATE AND INFANT

Neonates begin extrauterine life able to attend with their sensory capabilities and communicate with their environment through a complex repertoire of behaviors. They are able to accumulate experience in memory. Infancy (birth to 12 months) is the time of further development and maturation of these capabilities through self-mastery and adaptation to the extrauterine environment.

Biorhythmic Balance: The Primary Developmental Task of Newborns

In utero the fetus depends on the mother's physiologic systems to regulate its own systems. At birth the neonate's basic physiologic needs (feeding, elimination, cleaning, heat balance, stroking, and communicating) are met in new and different ways. The process of emerging from a physiologically dependent state as a fetus into a physiologically independent as a neonate introduces new variables for both mother and infant in the development of their extrauterine relationship.

The primary task of newborns is to reestablish biorhythmic balance by stabilizing the function of sleep-wake cycles, respiratory and heart rates, blood chemistry levels, metabolic processes, and eating patterns.

Although biorhythmic balance is internally determined, caregiving interaction between newborn and parent/caregiver either facilitates or disturbs this transition.[402] After birth this balance is facilitated by contact with familiar surroundings (the mother's body) (see Chapter 5).

When immediate recontact between the neonate and the mother is not possible, such as when the mother refuses or is ill, or the neonate is preterm or sick and requires immediate emergency medical intervention or transport, the primary "mothering" role is temporarily transferred to professional (medical and nursing) care providers. Interactional dynamics necessary for reestablishing biorhythmic balance and fostering the psychosocioemotional development of the newborn are also transferred into the NICU.

Just as in a home or family setting, the infant's personality and behavioral development are affected by the nature and dynamics of the stimuli and relationships encountered with the staff in a nursery or NICU setting.[195] The level of function or dysfunction in the biorhythmic balance affects the neonate's long-range outcomes and is interwoven with the development of a sense of self and a basic trust.

Sense of Self

In utero the fetus has continuous tactile-kinesthetic stimulation that develops and matures the CNS and establishes kinesthesis as the most natural pathway for growth and development. The interaction between infants and the extrauterine environment is also kinesthetic. Tactile contact and vestibular stimulation are essential for (1) the development of a physical identity (body image), (2) organization and sorting of stimuli, (3) coordination of sensorimotor

skills, (4) a psychologic and social sense of self, (5) normal neurophysiologic development (mental and cognitive abilities), and (6) emotional stability and temperament.[67,292,420,435]

Daily caregiving and interactions, such as feeding, diapering, holding, and playing with the parent or caregiver, provide infants with reciprocal stimuli for further developing their identity. Through the manner in which the infant is handled, he or she receives messages about how the caregiver feels about him or her. Response cues given by an infant affect the caregiver's response to and interaction with the infant.[18,67,176] As the infant quiets in response to caregiving, the parent is positively reinforced to continue nurturing and soothing behaviors. Withdrawal, irritability, or continuous crying is perceived by the caregiver as rejection and may result in parental frustration, withdrawal, and decreased interaction. Repeated exposure to the caregiver's style and nonverbal messages thus enables the infant to adapt to these patterns of caregiving. **The self of the infant is formed through interaction with people and objects within the environment.**

Because the nature (amount and kind) of the kinesthetic interaction between infants and caregivers influences how infants develop and mature, a lack of appropriate stimulation can have long-term consequences. **Stimulus deprivation results in impairment, retardation, or deviancy in skill development for productive living.** The degree or extent of impairment depends on the severity of the restrictions and limitations encountered. Studies have demonstrated that infants who were well cared for physically (fed, diapered, and cleaned) but who did not receive tactile or kinesthetic stimulation either died or were seriously impaired mentally, emotionally, and socially.[67,176,486] Institutionally reared infants who had minimal contact and no social interaction with their caregivers displayed significant developmental delays.[425] The effect of kinesthetic deprivation was seen in the minimal expression of social skills (cooing, babbling, and crying), minimal interest in objects in the environment, increased self-stimulation (rocking), touch aversion, flat or withdrawn affect, and retarded mental and motor development. **Environmental deprivation may also affect the physical growth of the infant.**[176] Montagu[370] stated that infants are able to overcome mental and nutritional deprivation as long as they are not deprived of tactile stimulation.

The Psychosocial Task:
Trust Versus Mistrust

Trust versus mistrust in oneself and the environment is solidified during infancy.[18] The response of the environment from the moment of birth is the means by which neonates continue to develop trust in themselves and decide on the reliability of their new environment. **Two major factors influence the development of trust versus mistrust: (1) the infant's ability to communicate needs to the environment and (2) the reliability and constancy of the responding environment.**

In the course of routine caregiving, an infant associates the caregiver with either comfort and trust or with lack of need satisfaction and mistrust. The infant cries to communicate a need (e.g., "I'm hungry"; "I'm wet"). The caregiver responds to the infant and meets the need—the infant is fed; the infant is changed. Thus the newborn learns to communicate when the need arises again, because the environment or caregiver has responded and will respond. This **contingent response** of the caregiver to the infant's need is the necessary reinforcement for the development of trust in self, in others, and ultimately in humankind. The infant develops a sense of mastery over his or her world and a sense that it is okay to have needs and to have them met.

Caregiving that ignores or delays needs gratification is **noncontingent** to the infant's cues for care. Need meeting that is externally defined by the caregiver's agenda (e.g., feeding schedule, rigid or inflexible routines, medical or nursing procedures in the NICU) discourages the infant from being aware of and experiencing needs and communicating them. Such infants will eventually detach themselves (emotionally and kinesthetically) from the sensation of their needs, thus no longer experiencing or communicating them.[69,176]

As a result, these infants conclude that they and their needs (which they perceive as one and the same) are not important and that they have no effect on their environment. They do not cultivate their sense of self or of their own existence, physically (where their boundaries end and another's begin) or psychologically (their identity that exists independent of another). Some people with severe mistrust in themselves and their environment do not experience the sensation of hunger when hungry or express appropriate emotional responses to situations. They also do not kinesthetically feel where their body ends and another's begins when they are

hugging—they totally merge and experience the two as one and the same person. Low self-concept and self-esteem and a sense of helplessness about succeeding in life are a result of lack of trust. Behaviorally this is manifested in touch aversion; avoidance of eye contact; flat, withdrawn, or depressed affect; or hyperactivity, restlessness, low frustration level, demanding behavior and perpetual dissatisfaction, and poor social relationships.[68,292,425,486]

Survival depends on the caregiver's meeting the newborn's needs. Need meeting is either contingent on the infant's cues or noncontingent on an external agenda. The degree of the mother's emotional investment and connectedness with the newborn will determine the nature and quality of the caregiving. Likewise, the temperament and responsiveness of the infant will affect the mother's feelings of competency, success, and emotional connectedness to her infant.[69,176] Parents who relate to the newborn as an individual (i.e., a person with feelings, wants, and needs; a person who knows what these are) will be sensitive and responsive to the infant's needs and interact with the baby during caregiving. This relationship facilitates the ongoing development of a good sense of self (esteem, confidence, and emotional security) and mastery of the world. Caregivers who do not perceive infants as individuals do not respond to their "need cry" or interact with the child during caregiving. This style fosters the development of mistrusting, suspicious, helpless, emotionally insecure, and isolated children and adults.

ENDOWMENT

Infants possess innateness and individuality. **Primitive reflex behaviors, higher cognitive abilities, temperament, and sensorimotor competencies are the endowment of the individual infant.** Individual variation and utilization of these endowments are influenced by the environment of the newborn.

Even before conception, the genetic endowment of the parents and preceding generations affects the fetus or newborn. Everything that the individual will inherit from his or her parents is determined at the moment of conception. Of the vast number of possible combinations of chromosomes, chance determines which characteristics the individual receives. Thus each individual, except monozygotic twins, is genetically and biologically different from every other person. Either a faulty gene (e.g., sickle cell anemia) or an altered number of chromosomes (e.g., Down syndrome) is responsible for inherited defects (see Chapter 27).

Although after the moment of conception hereditary endowment can never be changed, it is influenced by the intrauterine environment. Some birth defects are caused by teratogens—any environmental agent (drugs, virus, chemical, or pollutant) that interferes with normal fetal development. An individual's potential for growth and development is limited by his or her genetic endowment. As Montagu[369] stated, "Genetic endowment determines what we can do—environment what we do do."

The exception to individual genetic endowment is identical twins, who share the same heredity. Identical twins have been extensively studied, because it is hypothesized that any differences between them are the result of environmental effects. Identical twins raised apart have been found to be more similar in intelligence, temperament, and personality characteristics than are fraternal twins raised together.

Genetic endowment imposes limits on a child's potential. Studies show that children resemble their parents both physically and mentally more than they differ from them. Parental expectations that are unrealistic or beyond the child's capacity may set the child up for disappointment when he or she fails to meet these expectations. All too often abilities and potential are stifled within this environment, so that the child is unable to achieve what is within his or her capability.

The exact influence of genetics for most psychologic traits is unknown. Introverted (timid, shy, and withdrawn) and extroverted (active, friendly, and outgoing) personality types may be partially genetically controlled. The degree to which intelligence is inherited is currently unknown, although the intelligence of children is most often similar to parental intelligence (i.e., intelligence is more similar between child and biologic mother than child and adopted mother).

Freedman[169] studied newborns of many ethnic groups to see if there were any similarities in disposition within the group or differences from other ethnic groups. He found that Chinese-American newborns were more adaptable, less irritable, and easier to console than Caucasian-American newborns. Maneuvers such as the Moro and covering the face with a cloth elicited very different responses, depending on the newborn's ethnic origin.

The same environmental stimuli elicit very different behavioral responses, which are individual and genetically influenced. These genetically influenced behaviors are also influenced by environment—both

internal and external. Thus an individual may be more vulnerable to or more resilient in a specific environment. Therefore we are totally endowment and totally environment (100% endowment + 100% environment = an individual).[169]

Temperament

Parents often notice behavioral differences in their children from the first day. These differences are obvious in motor activity, irritability, and passivity. Some infants are quiet and placid, others are irritable and easily upset, and others are somewhere in between. **Nine categories of behavior that describe individual temperament are outlined in Table 13-1.** These temperamental qualities enable three basic types of infants to be identified:

- The "easy" child who is seen as regular, pleasant, and easy to care for and love
- The "difficult" child who is difficult to rear and reacts with protest and withdrawal to strange events or people
- The "slow to warm" child who reacts with withdrawal or passivity to new events

Neurologic Development

Brain growth of the fetus and newborn occurs in two stages.[123]

Stage I

Stage I occurs from 10 to 18 weeks of pregnancy. The number of nerve cells that the individual has develops during this period. Any environmental perturbation (e.g., maternal malnutrition, medications, and infections) that affects brain growth during this stage may also affect neonatal behavioral responses.

Stage II

Stage II occurs from 20 weeks' gestation to 2 years of age. This period marks a brain growth spurt and the most vulnerable period of growth of the dendrites of the human cortex.

The maturity of an infant is reflected in his or her behavior. Infants of a younger gestational age have less-mature responses than infants of an older gestational age. A neurologic assessment of the newborn includes evaluation of (1) newborn reflexes, (2) neonatal states, (3) psychosocial interaction, and (4) sensory capabilities. The neonate is born with behaviors that are unlearned, instinctual, and of an adaptive and survival nature. They reflect the state of the nervous system and the level of neonatal maturation (see Figure 5-4). **Table 13-2 summarizes neonatal reflex behaviors, their**

Table 13-1	BEHAVIORAL CATEGORIES DESCRIPTIVE OF INDIVIDUAL TEMPERAMENT
TEMPERAMENTAL QUALITY	**RATING**
Activity level	*Low*—Decreased movement when dressed or during sleep
	High—Increased movement when asleep; increased wiggling and activity when diaper changed
Rhythmicity	*Regular*—Establishes own feeding; sleep and bowel movement pattern is fairly predictable
	Irregular—Amounts of sleep, feeding variable; "no two days are alike"; no pattern established
Approach and withdrawal	*Positive*—Eagerly tries new foods; interested in new surroundings and people
	Negative—Rejects new foods, new toys, and new environments; apprehensive, cries with new people
Adaptability	*Adaptive*—Little resistance to first bath; may enjoy bath
	Nonadaptive—Startles easily; resists diapering, bathing, and other manipulating
Quality of mood	*Positive*—Pleasant, easygoing disposition; easy to comfort; smiles
	Negative—Fussy; cries easily and is not easily comforted by external stimuli; unable to comfort self easily
Intensity of mood	*Mild*—No crying when wet; frets instead of crying when hungry
	Intense—Vigorously cries; rejects food
Sensory threshold (intensity of stimulus necessary to elicit a response)	*High*—Not startled or interrupted by noise or other stimuli
	Low—Noise, activity, or other stimuli enough to interrupt infant's behavior
Distractibility	*Distractible*—Rocking, pacifier, toy, voice, music will decrease fussing
	Nondistractible—No stimulus will decrease distress until need is met—food; stop changing diaper; bath over
Attention span and persistence	*Short*—Cries when awakened but stops immediately; mild objection if needs are not immediately met
	Long—Repeatedly rejects substitutions for perceived needs (no pacifier until diaper is changed; no water if milk is wanted)

Modified from Thomas A. Chess S: *The dynamics of personality development,* New York, 1980, Brunner/Mazel.

Table 13-2	NEONATAL REFLEX BEHAVIORS	
BEHAVIOR	**BEGINS (IN UTERO) (WK)**	**INTEGRATES**
Protection		
Moro	28	At 6-8 mo to allow sitting and protective extension of the hands
Palmar grasp	28	At 5-6 mo to allow voluntary grasping of objects
Plantar grasp	28	At 7-8 mo with foot rubbing on objects; complete at 8-9 mo for standing and walking
Babinski	28	(Same as plantar grasp)
Tonic neck	35	At 4 mo, so rolling over and reaching or grasping may occur
Gag*	36	Protects against aspiration—does *not* disappear
Blink	25	Does *not* disappear
Crossed extension	28	Disappears around 2 mo of age
Survival		
Rooting*	28	At 3 mo; decreased response if baby is sleepy or with satiety
Sucking*	26-28	Not yet synchronized with swallowing
Swallowing*	12	32-34 wk, stronger synchronization with sucking; perfect by 34-37 wk

*Although isolated components of feeding behaviors are all present before 28 weeks' gestational age, they are not effectively coordinated for oral feedings before 32-34 weeks' gestational age.[187,208,347] Coordination of respiration with sucking and swallowing during bottle feeding is consistently achieved by infants >37 weeks postconceptual age.[38,81]

significance, and the time of their integration into voluntary movement. Serial testing of reflex behavior gives more reliable data than one observation. Observations indicative of major deviations include asymmetry—total absence or no response on one side or in upper or lower extremities.

Psychologic Interaction and Neonatal States

For years newborn behavior was thought to occur only on a reflexive, instinctual level. **Through the work of Brazelton[73] and others, newborns have been shown to have the ability to interact with and shape their environment. With the the Neonatal Behavioral Assessment Scale (NBAS),[73] care providers can observe and score the interactive behavior of newborns.** The NBAS enables assessment of the infant's individual capabilities for social relationships rated on the infant's best performance. Interest in the best performance is based on the belief that newborns may briefly respond to external stimuli from higher centers of the nervous system (i.e., the cerebrum). Six categories of abilities are considered in evaluating an infant's performance: habituation, orientation to auditory and visual stimuli, motor maturity, state changes, self-quieting ability, and social behaviors.

Response decrement (i.e., habituation) is the protective mechanism by which an infant decreases responsivity to external stimuli.[406] Habituation represents the cerebral behavior of memory—the infant stores the memory of the stimulus and with repeated presentation learns not to respond. Infants who are able to habituate are able to "tune out" mild to moderate stimuli in the environment and protect themselves from overstimulation.

Infants who become "bored" with their toys have habituated to them—infants like variety. **Dishabituation represents increasing attention to a new stimulus (new mobile, toy, face) after habituation to an old stimulus.** The infant thus "recognizes" the novelty of the new stimulus and chooses to respond.

An infant who is unable to habituate will continue to react vigorously to repeated stimuli. Compared with term infants, preterm infants are more reactive (e.g., less able to control their level of excitation) and less able to self-regulate (e.g., modulate reactivity, reflected in habituation rate and self-soothing abilities).[135] **VLBW infants are less able to (1) modulate attention, (2) take brief breaks from processing information, and (3) habituate to stimuli.**[135,372] **Thus the preterm is easily over-**

stimulated and less able to deal with multiple sources of stimuli.[17]

Neonates are able to imitate the facial and manual gestures of adults.[353] Infants as young as 12 days old imitate gestures such as mouth opening and tongue protrusion. Because a neonate has never seen his or her own face, this innate ability to match behaviors to those of another is a remarkable utilization of the cerebral cortex. Imitation may operate as a positive feedback mechanism to caregivers; thus it is important in parent-infant reciprocity and represents early learning behaviors.

Learning, a function of the cerebral cortex, occurs with habituation and imitation. Early cognitive development is important to later learning and future cognitive function. Knowledge of the cognitive ability of the neonate enables care providers to provide opportunities for learning. Learning occurs in the context of experience[12,406] and influences structural development; there is increased CNS development during the first 2 years of life.[73,123]

The state of consciousness influences the reactions of a newborn to internal and external stimuli. The infant's state at the time of observation must be considered in interpretation of the findings. **Table 13-3 shows the six states of the newborn and specific considerations for caregiving in each state.**

Clinical application of the NBAS includes evaluation of infant capabilities after illness, prematurity, or maternal medications. The most important application of the NBAS is in anticipatory guidance for parents. Demonstration of parts of the examination for parents enables them to become familiar with their infant's individual patterns of behavior, temperament, and states. Thus parents are able to more accurately assess and interpret their infant's cues for interaction and for distance.

Circadian Rhythms

Circadian rhythms are cyclic variations in function that occur daily at about the same time. Humans cycle their bodily functions (e.g., temperature, hormonal changes, blood pressure, urine volume, sleep-wake cycles) in a 24-hour period.[436,467] These daily fluctuations are innately controlled by the individual's "biologic clock" in the suprachiasmatic nuclei (SCN) in the anterior hypothalamus. The SCN are located at the base of the third ventricle, above the optic chiasm.[436] The circadian pacemaker must be reset daily by the relay of photic information from the retina to the SCN, along the direct pathway from

Table 13-3	NEWBORN STATES AND CONSIDERATIONS FOR CAREGIVING
NEWBORN STATE	**COMMENTS**

Sleep States

Newborn State	Comments

Deep sleep (non-REM or quiet sleep)
  Slow state changes
  Regular breathing
  Eyes closed; no eye movements
  No spontaneous activity except startles
    and jerky movements
  Startles with some delay and
    suppresses rapidly
  Lowest oxygen consumption
	Infant is very difficult if not impossible to arouse. Infant will not breastfeed or bottle-feed in this state, even after vigorous stimulation. Infant is unable to respond to environment; frustrating for caregivers.
	Term infants may exhibit a "slow" heart rate (80-90 beats/min), which may trigger heart rate alarms and result in unnecessary stimulation by NICU staff.
	At birth, preterm infants have altered states of consciousness:
	Early dominant states are light sleep, quiet, and active alert. "Protective apathy" enables the preterm to remain inactive, unresponsive, and in a sleep state to conserve energy, grow, and maintain physiologic homeostasis.[523]
	As maturation occurs, there is an increase in quiet alert.

Light sleep (REM or active sleep)
  Low activity level
  Random movements and startles
  Respirations irregular and abdominal
  Intermittent sucking movements
  Eyes closed, REM
  Higher oxygen consumption
	Full-term infants begin and end sleep in active sleep; preterm infants are more responsive (than term infants) to stimuli in active sleep.
	Infant may cry or fuss briefly in this state and be awakened to feed before they are truly awake and ready to eat.
	Lower and more variable oxygenation states.

Awake States

Newborn State	Comments

Drowsy or semidosing
  Eyelids fluttering
  Eyes open or closed (dazed)
  Mild startles (intermittent)
  Delayed response to sensory stimuli
  Smooth state change after stimulation
  Fussing may or may not be present
  Respirations—more rapid and shallow
	Infant may awaken further or return to sleep (if left alone).
	Quietly talking and looking at the infant, or offering a pacifier or an inanimate object to see and listen to may arouse the infant to the quiet alert state.
	Less mature infants (30 weeks) demonstrate a more drowsy than quiet alert state than older infants (36 weeks).

Quiet alert, with bright look
  Focuses attention on source of
    stimulation
  Impinging stimuli may break through;
    may have some delay in response
  Minimal motor activity
	Immediately after birth, term newborns exhibit a period of quiet alert, their first opportunity to "take in" their parents and the extrauterine environment. Dimmed lights, quiet talking, and stroking optimize this time for parents.
	Best state for learning to occur, because infant focuses all of attention on visual, auditory, tactile, and sucking stimuli; best state for interaction with parents—infant is maximally able to attend and reciprocally respond to parents.

Active alert—eyes open
  Considerable motor activity—thrusting
    movements of extremities; sponta-
    neous startles
  Reacts to external stimuli with increase
    in movements and startles (discrete
    reactions difficult to differentiate
    because of general higher activity level)
  Respirations irregular
  May or may not be fussy
	Infant has decreased threshold (increased sensitivity) to internal (hunger, fatigue) and external (wet, noise, handling) stimuli. Infant may quiet self, may escalate to crying, or with consolation by caregiver may become quiet alert or go to sleep.
	Infant is unable to maximally attend to caregiver or environment because of increased motor activity and increased sensitivity to stimuli.

Crying—intense and difficult to
    disrupt with external stimuli
  Respirations rapid, shallow, and
    irregular
	Crying is infant's response to unpleasant internal or external stimulation—infant's tolerance limits have been reached (and exceeded). Infant may be able to quiet self with hand-to-mouth behaviors; talking may quiet a crying infant; holding, rocking, or putting infant upright on caregiver's shoulder may quiet infant.

Modified from Brazelton TB: *Neonatal behavioral assessment scale*, ed 2, Philadelphia, 1984, Spastics International Medical Publishers JB Lippincott; and Blackburn S: *J Obstet Gynecol Neonatal Nurs* (Suppl) 805, 1983.

the retinohypothalamic tract (RHT) to the SCN.[164,436] During the eighteenth week of prenatal life[431] the SCN form and continue maturation after birth.[500] In utero the fetus expresses endogenous circadian rhythms (in heart/respiratory rates and steroid secretion) that are influenced by the mother.[364,464] The RHT has been identified in human newborns of 36 weeks' gestation.[183] Although the limitations of human study have made it impossible to determine whether the circadian clock of the human infant is functionally responsive to light at birth, animal data show that the SCN is functionally innervated by the retina at stages equivalent to 25 weeks after conception in human infants.[213]

In infants the development of circadian rhythm is influenced by genetic factors, brain maturation, and the environment.[158,337,436,513] Although there are individual differences in the development of circadian rhythms, both in preterm and full-term infants,[170,264,365,366,444] the influences of prenatal rhythms and/or postnatal environmental influences are being studied.[364] Research and experimental outcomes in the development of circadian rhythms in the neonate are influenced by the environment: (1) feeding, (2) environmental lighting, and (3) chronologic/postconceptual age.[364] Intrauterine growth influences the development of circadian rhythms—in one study more AGA than SGA infants developed body temperature and heart rate rhythms.[182] More mature infants (i.e., greater postconceptual age) of 35 to 37 weeks' gestation have a higher amplitude on body temperature rhythm when compared with infants of 32 to 34 weeks' gestation.[182] Infant biorhythms have been studied in the areas of temperature, heart and respiratory rates, blood pressure, sleep-wake cycles, endocrine secretion, and feeding frequency.*

At birth and for the first few weeks of life, term newborns generally distribute sleep over a 24-hour period and sleep from 16 to 19 hours a day. As sleep begins, a term infant enters active, rather than quiet, sleep and spends more time in active sleep than does an adult.[129] Active sleep durations vary from 10 to 45 minutes, whereas quiet sleep lasts about 20 minutes.[129] An infant's sleep cycle is 50 to 60 minutes, as compared with an adult's 90- to 100-minute cycle.[32] Although day-night rhythms are difficult to detect in the neonatal period, some infants exhibit such rhythms as early as a week of age.[436,437] **Mat-**

uration of infant sleep is characterized by: (1) increased organization of sleep states, (2) decrease in total sleep time, (3) increase in quiet sleep, (4) decrease in active sleep, and (5) increase in active and quiet waking.* Arousability from sleep is altered by gestational and postnatal age.[243] In term infants, arousal thresholds are significantly elevated in quiet sleep compared with active sleep (at 2 to 3 weeks and 2 to 3 months of age), so that spontaneous arousal is greater in active than in quiet sleep.[243]

Infants have their own "clock" for sleep-wake, hunger, and feeding or fussy times. This clock often does not coincide with the family's rhythms and may cause disruption and conflict.[540] Sleep-wake states reflect the underlying status of the neurologic system. The infant's maturity at birth greatly affects his or her rhythms and development of normal circadian rhythm. Rhythmicity of sleep-wake cycles is influenced more by brain maturation than environmental influences.[103,363,473] Early relationships with caregivers provide the organization and stabilization necessary for sleep regulation as well as other biologic functions. At 6 weeks infants are awake more during the day than at night; by 12 weeks more sleep occurs at night as daytime sleep duration continues to decrease. A term newborn has innate rhythms and over a period of time (about 16 to 18 weeks) develops adult regularity (e.g., more sleep at night than in the daytime).[32]

In preterm infants, active and quiet sleep cycles are less well organized and of shorter duration (a sleep cycle is about 30 to 40 minutes) than in term infants.[128] Active sleep is "lighter" than quiet sleep—there is more response to stimuli in active sleep.[128] Quiet sleep is a more controlled state and occurs more frequently in term infants than in premature infants. Quiet sleep does not become significant in the preterm until approximately 36 weeks' gestation. Hence a third sleep state, *transitional sleep,* has been identified for premature infants.[393] This state is characterized by quiet sleep with periods of closed eyes, regular or periodic respirations, no body movements, and no REM. Before 36 weeks' gestation a preterm infant's predominant sleep state is transitional sleep. As the preterm infant matures, he or she spends progressively less time in transitional sleep, has more quiet than active sleep, and has more awake, alert time. How-

---

*References 32, 63, 182, 264, 320, 342, 364, 473, 513.

*References 32, 129, 236, 237, 243, 511, 540.

ever, a preterm of 40 weeks' postconceptional age does not have sleep patterns that are as well organized as those of a term newborn.[393,540] Spontaneous arousal from sleep is greater in active sleep compared with quiet sleep (at 2 to 3 weeks' and 2 to 3 months' postterm age).[243] During quiet sleep, spontaneous arousals at 2 to 3 weeks do not differ in preterm infants compared with term infants; however, at 2 to 3 months of age preterm infants have significantly fewer spontaneous arousals compared with term infants.[243] Long-term follow-up studies fail to show a difference in sleep distribution between preterm and term infants when corrected for age.[32,473,474] Both preterm and full-term infants who are exposed to an appropriate light intensity at home develop day-night rhythmicity by 44 and 48 weeks of postconceptual age.[364,473,474]

As day and night rhythms in sleep-wake cycles develop, so diurnal rhythm in hormone production also develops: (1) melatonin production is detectable at 12 weeks of age and (2) variations in cortisol levels appear between 3 to 6 months of age.[436] Sleep disruption may interfere with growth and development by altering neuronal maturation and growth hormone secretion. **Human growth hormone has a rhythmic pattern associated with sleep-wake cycles.** The highest peaks of growth hormone in infants occur during REM (active) sleep. A fetus (29 to 32 weeks' gestation) spends 80% of the time in utero in REM sleep; a term newborn's sleep is 50% REM sleep.[128,129] **Because growth hormone secretion depends on the regular recurrence of sleep, any disturbance of the sleep-wake cycle results in irregular spikes of growth hormone during a 24-hour period.**

Although infant circadian rhythms are synchronous with those of the mother, desynchronous rhythms at birth may occur.[393,436,437] An infant whose cycles are discrepant from his or her family's may be perceived as "difficult." Because this behavior does not fit parental expectations of regular eating, sleeping or eliminating, the parent-child interaction is off to a rocky start.[540] Gradually, through caregiving, parents teach the infant synchronization with family rhythms. By 9 months of age a term infant has developed day-night fluctuations that are similar to adult patterns.

Sensory Capabilities

At birth a neonate's senses are developed and functioning. Sensory development proceeds in a specific order: tactile/vestibular, olfactory/ gustatory, and auditory/visual.[294] Stimuli (e.g., type, timing) to one sense affects the development of other senses.[294] Sensory enhancement or deprivation of a later developing sensory system (e.g., vision) could either accelerate or decelerate the development of behavior mediated by earlier developing sensory systems (e.g., tactile and olfactory).[294]

A newborn is able to communicate—react to and initiate a reaction from those in the environment. Through the neonate's sensory perception learning occurs by (1) habituating to some stimuli while attending to other stimuli, (2) discriminating between related and unrelated sensory events, and (3) integrating multisensory stimuli.[406] As the neonate takes in the sensory information, he or she associates features of the environment that occur together (e.g., sound, smell, sight, and touch of "mother" or "father"), demonstrating complex and intermodal abilities for handling the sensory input from the environment.[66]

Tactile/Kinesthetic

Touch is the major method of communication for neonates and infants. Touch is the first sense to develop (at about 7.5 weeks' gestational age) and the last sense to fade. In utero a fetus's existence has been primarily one of movement—floating within the amniotic fluid and rhythmic maternal movements. The sense of touch, temperature, and pressure are all well developed, and receptors lie in the newborn's skin. **The sensitivity to touch is especially well developed in the face, around the lips (root reflex), and in the hands (grasp reflex).** Because newborns are nonverbal, they pick up messages through the manner in which they are held and handled—by the adult's "body language." Infants are often barometers for adult feelings—if the adult is tired and irritable, the infant knows and may respond with irritability and crying.

Infants love to be held, rocked, and carried—note the soothing effects on a crying infant. Adults do *not* spoil infants by providing these important stimuli. Increased carrying of infants contributes to less crying at 6 weeks of age.[52] In response to being held, infants adjust their body posture to the body of the caregiver. Adults describe infants as "cuddly" (comfortable, relaxed curl; snuggles to adult body and attempts to root or suck) or "noncuddly" (sprawls, tenses or stiffens, and "pushes away"). The most comforting position for a crying infant is upright on an adult's shoulder.[272] Responsiveness to tactile stimulation has been found to be greater in female than in male neonates.[272]

Hearing

The fetus in utero has heard the voices of mother, father, and siblings from the twenty-second to the twenty-fourth week of intrauterine life.[3,179,211,545] **These voices are "familiar" to newborns, so they "know" their family and are able to differentiate them from the voices of strangers.**[117,118] Neonates prefer their mother's voice and the maternal language that they heard in utero.[179,371] Studies have suggested that fetuses and neonates exhibit memory.[117,118,371] Newborns who had been read a particular story while in utero responded to the story reread to them after birth with a recognition and attentiveness that was not exhibited in response to unfamiliar stories.[117,118,371] The ability to hear the outside world, particularly the spoken word, is a prerequisite to further verbal language development.

Fetal responses to sound include increases in breathing, body movements, fetal heart rate, cerebral blood flow and glucose utilization and changes in behavior states.[3,179] Neonates with an intact CNS are able to orient and respond to the auditory environment.[372,406] In response to a sound, the neonate will:

- Change motor activity (eye blink, decrease in activity, limb movements, head turn)
- Change heart rate and/or respiration—if the infant is quiet, the heart rate increases with stimuli; if the infant is crying, the heart rate decreases with stimuli; increase in respiratory rate, decrease in amplitude, or decrease in respiratory cycle rate
- Smile
- Startle or grimace
- Alert or arouse
- Cry or cease to cry
- Stop sucking

The response to sound depends on the sound's quality. The intensity of intrauterine noise is approximately 85 dB. When frequency and pitch are low, the infant is soothed and distress is decreased; high frequency and pitch alert, distress the infant, and disturb sleep. Therefore monotonous low-frequency sounds are an auditory soother and induce sleep.[406]

Frequencies below 4000 Hz (the range of human speech is 500 to 3000 Hz) produce the most newborn response.[384] Infants are maximally reactive to the human voice in typical speech patterns (rather than disconnected syllables). Infants prefer the high-pitched (such as female) voice over the low-pitched (such as male) voice. Note how adults and children instinctively pitch their voices higher when talking to an infant. The higher pitched voice elicits sustained attention from newborns.[104] Presented with a female and a male voice, the infant always turns toward the female voice. Parents who talk with their infants elicit increasing eye contact with the infant.

Experience with sound improves an infant's behavioral responses to sound.[406] Stimuli presented for 5 to 15 seconds elicit the best reaction. Stimuli lasting longer than several minutes are less effective, because the term infant habituates to the sound and ceases responding. **The ability to habituate to sound is indicative of an intact CNS. Full-term newborns habituate to sound better and faster than do preterm infants.** Infants will exhibit startle behavior if the stimulus rapidly reaches maximal loudness. A slower time to reach maximal loudness is associated with infant alerting and searching for the stimulus. Infant state is important in evaluation of response to auditory stimuli—light sleep is the optimal state. Infants quiet and soothe in response to rhythmic sounds (rather than dysrhythmic ones). Neonates move their bodies in rhythmic synchrony (*entrainment*) with the spoken word.

Vision

Eye development begins 22 days after conception. The eyelids fuse at about 10 weeks' gestation and remain fused until about 26 weeks' gestation. Eyelid opening is a function of maturity—more mature neonates open their eyes more than younger gestation neonates.[442] At birth photoreceptors are already developed, but maturation is not complete for several months. The fetus is able to distinguish light from dark and recoils from a bright light shone at the mother's abdomen. Even at term birth the visual system is immature, and significant development occurs over the next 6 months to a year. **The ability to fix, follow, and alert is indicative of an intact CNS.**[362]

At birth infants are able to see an object within 8 to 10 inches of the face (visual acuity of 20/140).[150] **Within seconds after birth the neonate is able to recognize his or her mother's face.**[66] **The cradled-in-the-arms position of feeding is the exact distance from the adult's face that the newborn can see.** In response to an interesting visual stimulus, neonates stop sucking to look, alert, and attend to the object, horizontally scan the object, and fix and follow a moving object in a 90-degree arc.

Infants prefer the human face as a visual stimulus, prefer a patterned over a nonpatterned stimulus, and attend longer to larger patterns with more complex patterns and angles.[150] Infants prefer black and white because of the greater contrast and will focus on the outside of a figure where the contrast is greatest.[362] Newborns are sensitive to bright light and will tightly close their eyes in its presence. They prefer moderate, diffuse lighting. Newborns exposed to cycled light (e.g., day/night changes) open their eyes more than those exposed to continuous bright light.[442] Presentation of visual stimuli enables development of the neural pattern for vision. During the infant's first year of life, visual investigation of the environment is a primary mode of learning.

Smell and Taste[452]

The fetus increases its amniotic fluid consumption when saccharine is added to the fluid and decreases consumption with the injection of distasteful substances.[72] Taste may be a way the fetus monitors the intrauterine environment.[72] **Olfaction is well developed at birth. Olfactory cues guide the full-term newborn to the maternal nipple.**[534] At 5 days of age a neonate is able to differentiate his or her mother's breast pad and demonstrates a preference for the smell over that of a "stranger." The infant's response to pleasant odors is to arouse and suck. After several presentations of the stimuli, the infant will habituate to the odor. Infants withdraw from unpleasant odors such as vinegar and ammonia. They are also able to differentiate tastes, preferring sweet solutions and refusing bitter, acid, and sour substances. Asphyxiated infants demonstrate a loss of olfaction that parallels the suppression of brainstem reflexes and activities.

Communication Skills

A neonate's ability to communicate is a naturally endowed survival skill. Crying is an infant's language to communicate needs. Crying may also be a response to the environment—noisy, cold, overstimulating, multiple caregiving, or lack of synchrony. Because the cry brings someone to meet the need, the infant soon learns that the caregiver gives attention and the world is a trustworthy place. The more responsive the caregiver is to the infant's crying, thus the infant's needs, the less crying behavior is necessary.[52] Learning occurs as the infant associates comfort with the caregiver. The temperament of the individual infant and his or her ability to habituate to disturbing stimuli influence the amount of crying behavior. Tension in the caregiver or the environment is communicated nonverbally to the infant and may potentiate or contribute to the infant's crying.

The amount and tone of the newborn's cry are influenced by birth weight, gestational age, and the events of birth. **Types of cries include birth cry, hunger cry, pain cry, and pleasure cry.**[93,94,510,558] **Infants separated from their mothers in the first**

90 minutes after birth exhibit a "separation distress call" (also seen in other mammal species) that ceases at reunion.[93,94] The newborn's cry physiologically affects the mother—her breasts change and prepare to nurse. Neonates possess a repertoire of self-quieting behaviors when in a fussy state: (1) hand-to-mouth efforts, (2) sucking on fist or tongue, and (3) use of visual and/or auditory stimuli from the environment.[73]

After birth, crying develops a diurnal pattern—term infants cry more during the day than at night.[487] Persistent crying (more than 3 hours a day) is more likely to be done by breastfed babies, whereas early evening crying is more likely from formula-fed infants.[487] Postnatal age is a significant predictor of crying—crying decreases with increasing chronologic age.[514] The neonatal cry may be a signal of robustness or wellness,[46] a signal of pain or diagnostic of existing conditions or trauma. CNS insult often results in a high-pitched, shrill cry. The pain cry of asphyxiated newborns differs significantly from that of healthy term infants[357] (see Chapter 5).

A smiling infant is a joy to the caregiver. Smiling may be either spontaneous (from birth) or a response to the social human face (at 4 to 12 weeks of life). A smile is most easily elicited by the stimulus of a moving, smiling human face. The ability to smile begins before 40 weeks in a preterm infant, as observed during REM sleep. The social implications of the smile include positive feedback to the caregiver that the infant is happy and contented, which results in parental feelings of adequacy and competence.

ENVIRONMENT

Prenatal Environment

In utero the fetus depends totally on its mother's emotional and physical health and well-being for their own. It is through her that he or she receives the nurturance, housing, and stimulation to develop the body, the sensory organs, and the rudiments of his or her personality and temperament.

Intrapartal Environment

Birth is a major transition from physiologic dependence to physiologic independence. At term a neonate's physiologic systems are developed, sensory organs function, and the foundation of personality and temperament are established. Birth is disorienting and disruptive. The amount of disruption depends on the degree of trauma incurred during the labor and birth process. Not having a social support system compounds the stress, often escalating it beyond the mother's tolerance and coping skills. Anxious and fearful women have longer labors and more delivery complications than women who are confident about themselves and their infants. The recent shift toward family-centered birth enables mothers to receive support from their families, to be an active participant in the birth process, and to have immediate contact with their newborns.

A neonate is also influenced by medications and the events of labor and birth (see Chapter 2). Maternal medications for analgesia and anesthesia affect neonatal behaviors, resulting in decreased sucking ability, lethargy, and decreased habituation. Medicated infants are less able to evoke caregiver behaviors such as smiling, touching, and vocalization. They also give less feedback to their parents than unmedicated infants. The parents may feel rejected, tend to stimulate the infant less, and thus begin a pattern of aberrant interaction.

Postnatal Environment

Home and family are the primary media through which newborns (1) reestablish their biorhythmic balance, (2) stabilize themselves in the extrauterine world, (3) develop a sense of self and mastery in the world, and (4) become socialized as human beings. Socialization teaches the adaptive psychosocial skills necessary for survival and functioning in society. Cultural and family values, behavioral expression, and ways of meeting social-emotional needs are learned within the family. Thus the home and family environment is considered to be a "normalized" environment for human development.

Caregiver Factors

The dyadic relationship continues postpartally between the caregiver and the infant—the behavior of one reinforces the behavior of the other. The infant's physical and emotional needs are satisfied by caregivers. The infant's response to the caregiver depends on how he or she perceives and receives ministrations; this response affects the level of emotional satisfaction the caregiver receives from the interaction. Parental expectations have a major effect on their perceptions and their behavior and ultimately affect the child's development. Parents must work out the discrepancy between the wished-for and the actual child, especially if the infant is preterm, ill, or has an anomaly. How attached the parents are to the infant influences their relationship to and ability to care for their infant (see Chapter 29). If the pregnancy has failed to produce a normal, healthy infant, the parents must grieve the loss of their expectations. Parents are unable to attach to and care for the infant until they have completed their grief work (see Chapter 30).

A caregiver and infant have a reciprocal interaction when their cycles and signals are synchronized with each other. The biorhythmic cycle of the newborn has been in synchrony with one person (mother) in utero, and the infant is accustomed to her cycles and rhythms for developing adaptive behavior. Consistent maternal caregiving enables a newborn to regulate his or her rhythms to those of the mother and begin adapting to the postnatal environment.[235,270] From her they expand their adaptation to the family and to the larger world of society.[156]

Experience in relating to infants does influence the caregiver's efficiency in interpretation of and sensitivity to infant cues. Multiparous women have more sensitivity to infant cues than do primiparous mothers. Mothers with little or no experience exhibit more difficulty in quieting a crying infant. The competence of parents may be improved through acquisition of knowledge about infants, so that the quality of interaction between parent and infant is enhanced. In one study, prenatally, first time mothers received videotaped education about infant behavior, states, and communication cues which resulted in significant differences in sensitivity to infant cues and social-emotional growth fostering behaviors in early (first 24 hours) mother-infant interaction.[286]

Consistency in maternal responses is especially important as the infant continues to learn the accepted patterns of cues from the caregiver. Cared for by one or two people, an infant is able to develop synchrony with and expectations of the parents. Single caregiving improves establishment of biorhythms for sleep-wake cycles, feeding, and visual attentiveness. Consistent cues soon elicit a consistency of response from the infant. Consistency and promptness of maternal response result in less infant crying during the first year of life. A predictable and responsive environment enables the infant to progress to varied types of communication (not just crying). Care by parents provides for mutual cueing and mastery of the environment through interaction. Inconsistent cues distress and confuse the infant. Multiple caregiving confuses the infant, increases distress with feeding, causes irritability, and upsets visual attention.

Regardless of how stable or unstable, consistent or inconsistent it is, family life has a rhythm, synchronicity, and predictability of its own. Through interaction with parents and siblings, infants further develop their ability to form relationships. From these primary relationships, the foundation and format for other relationships are established. The quality of subsequent relationships depends on the quality of the relationship experienced within the primary family from birth throughout infancy.[192]

Neonatal Factors

The neonate is not a passive recipient of the environment of the family but is an active participant in shaping that environment. Infants send cues about their ability and readiness for interpersonal interactions. Infants in the first 4 months of life interact differently with persons than with inanimate objects (Figure 13-1). The excitement generated by interpersonal interaction is seen in an infant's arm and leg movements, bodily movement toward the other person, smiling, vocalizing, and increased visual attention. Because of the infant's immaturity, he or she is unable to maintain a continuous interaction. The infant attends for short periods and then turns away to decrease excitement, to protect himself or herself from bombardment by overwhelming stimuli, and to process the experience. **Maternal or care provider sensitivity to the attention-withdrawal cycle of interaction enables the adult to modulate her behavior in synchrony with the infant's cues.** Successful interaction with an infant includes reading the infant's cues, responding appropriately, and not overwhelming the infant with too much stimulation (thus overstepping the infant's tolerance for interaction). Overwhelming the infant results in withdrawal for progressively

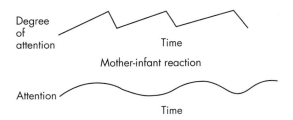

FIGURE 13-1   Interaction pattern with object and with mother. Object interaction is characterized by abrupt attention and excitement phases followed by sudden and abrupt looking away. Interaction with person is cyclical and involves initiation of interaction, orientation to person, acceleration of excitement, peak of excitement, deceleration of excitement, and withdrawal or turning away. (From Brazelton TB, Koslowski B, Main M: The origins of reciprocity: the early infant-mother interaction. In Lewis M, Rosenblum LA, eds: *The effect of the infant on its caregiver,* New York, 1974, John Wiley & Sons.)

longer periods of time to protect himself or herself from overstimulating and insensitive others.

Just as the parent has expectations, the infant also has expectations of the relationship. The infant expects relief or protection from painful experiences, maintenance of comfort, and homeostasis. Relief from the discomforts of hunger, cold, sleeplessness, and boredom enables the infant to respond positively to the care provider.

Care-eliciting behaviors are those neonatal cues used to signal the caregiver that attention is needed. Crying, visual following, and smiling are care-eliciting behaviors. Newborn responses to care include quieting, suckling, clinging and cuddling, looking, smiling, and vocalizing. These social interactions positively reward the care provider and encourage and promote continued care. Infant characteristics that modify maternal attitudes include (1) a healthy or sickly infant, (2) an attractive, pretty infant or an infant with obvious congenital anomaly, (3) a premature infant, (4) a calm and contented or a fussy and irritable infant, and (5) an infant responsive to or rejecting of maternal care. A maternal or care provider ability to soothe the infant reinforces a feeling of success (or failure) in her feelings of competence.

The infant's sex also affects the cues and the caregiver's response. Male infants exhibit more startles, more muscle activity, and more physical strength. In response, they receive more holding from caregivers as a means of soothing.[272] Females exhibit more tactile and oral sensitivity, more smiling, and more responsivity to sweet taste. As a result, girls are more often soothed by talking, eye-to-eye contact, and a pacifier.[272]

The infant's level of neurophysiologic development influences the appropriateness of maternal and caregiving behaviors. The neurologically mature term infant who has already mastered autonomic, motoric, and state regulation is able to actively elicit and respond to caregiving behaviors.[73,156] **Because of the immaturity of the CNS, a preterm infant lags behind a term infant in care eliciting and responsivity to the care provider.**[42,186,340] **Stages and characteristics of behavioral organization in preterm infants are described in Table 13-4.** Because a young preterm infant's priority is mere survival, interaction with the environment and care providers is at the expense of physiologic stability.[523] Because a preterm infant sends cues different from those of a term infant, knowledge of these stages enables caregivers to modulate their behavior and the environment. Although overwhelming the term infant results in

Table 13-4	STAGES AND CHARACTERISTICS OF BEHAVIORAL ORGANIZATION IN PRETERM INFANTS
ALS ET AL*	**GORSKI†**
Physiologic homeostasis—stabilizing and integrating temperature control, cardiorespiratory function, digestion, and elimination. Characteristics: becomes pale, dusky, cyanotic; heart and respiratory rates change—all symptoms of disorganization of autonomic nervous system.	"In turning"—physiologic stage of mere survival characterized by autonomic nervous system responses to stimuli (rapid color changes caused by swings in heart and respiratory rates); no or limited direct response; inability to arouse self spontaneously; jerky movements; asleep (and protecting the CNS from sensory overload) 97% of the time. Preterms (<32 weeks) are easily physiologically overwhelmed by stimuli.
Motor development may infringe on physiologic homeostasis, resulting in defensive strategies (vomiting, color change, apnea, and bradycardia).	"Coming out"—first active response to environment may be seen as early as 34-35 weeks (provided some physiologic stability has been achieved). Characteristics: remains pink with stimuli; has directed response for short periods; arouses spontaneously and maintains arousal after stimuli ceases; if interaction begins in alert state: maintains quiet alert for 5-10 min, tracks animate or inanimate stimuli; spends 10%-15% of time in alert state with predictable interaction patterns.
State development becomes less diffuse and encompasses full range: sleep, awake, crying. States and state changes may affect physiologic or motor stability.	
Alert state is well differentiated from other states; may interfere with physiologic or motor stability	"Reciprocity"—active interaction and reciprocity with environment from 36-40 weeks. Characteristics: directs response; arouses and consoles self; maintains alertness; interacts with animate/inanimate objects; copes with external stress.

*Modified from Als H et al: A new model of assessing the behavioral organization in preterm and fullterm infants: two case studies, *J Am Acad Child Psychiatry* 20:239, 1981.

†Modified from Gorski PA: Stages of behavioral organization in the high-risk neonate: theoretical and clinical considerations, *Semin Perinatol* 3:61, 1979.

withdrawal from interaction, overwhelming the preterm infant first results in a real threat to physiologic survival, then to withdrawal from interaction.

The ability of an infant to be a social partner and to respond in a social interaction is developmentally determined and influenced by the infant's physical condition. The response of preterm infants (weight less than 1500 g) to social stimulation (e.g., talking and talking combined with touching) evolves developmentally: (1) at 29 to 32 weeks' gestation, respond with distress (e.g., eye closing) to all forms of social stimuli, (2) at approximately 33 weeks' gestational age, begin to respond with increased attention to talking; they remain distressed with combined stimuli, and (3) at approximately 35 to 36 weeks' gestational age, pay more attention to talking; more distress at combined stimuli is seen in high-risk infants and better habituation seen in healthier infants.[134] Sicker preterm infants have a more difficult time in attending to and modulating their response to social interactions than do healthier preterm infants.[134,135] Although VLBW preterm infants respond to talking with increased attention and eye opening, the addition of touch results in increased eye closing and facial grimacing.[135] Sicker infants demonstrate the

same pattern of response but in a more exaggerated way that reflects their increased reactivity (e.g., level of excitation) and decreased ability for self-regulation (e.g., modulate reactivity).[135,523]

Because preterm infants are not as neurologically mature as term infants, the NBAS has little value with this population. **A behavioral assessment scale for preterm infants, Assessment of Preterm Infant's Behavior (APIB), has been developed that evaluates the preterm infant's behavioral organization along five subsystems of functioning: autonomic, motor, state, attentional-interactive, and self-regulatory.**[20] Although subsystems are observed independently, they are interdependent because disorganization in one system affects other systems. This examination delineates the quality and duration of the preterm infant's response, the difficulty in eliciting the response, and the effort and cost to the preterm infant of achieving and maintaining a response. Because it, too, is an interactive test, the nature and amount of organization provided by the care provider is an indication of the preterm infant's lack of integrative skill. As the preterm infant matures and advances in development of organization, he or she is more able to interact with the environment (animate

Table 13-5	OUTCOMES OF INDIVIDUALIZED DEVELOPMENTAL INTERVENTION IN THE NICU*		
PHYSIOLOGIC BENEFITS	**DEVELOPMENTAL BENEFITS**		**COST SAVINGS**

Decreases in
  Incidences of IVH or pneumothorax, and
    severity of BPD, ROP
  Ventilator/CPAP use
  Need for supplemental oxygen
  Need for gavage feedings
  Number of apneic episodes
  Need for less sedation/analgesia
Increase in
  Daily weight gain; head growth
  Stability of cardiorespiratory function
  Sleep states
  Significant electrophysiologic differences
    in frontal, temporal, central, occipital,
    and parietal lobes of the brain
	Improvement in
	  Behavioral organization of autonomic, motor,
	    attention modulation, and self-regulatory
	    abilities
	  Interactive capability of infant with staff and
	    parents
	  Quality of parent-infant interaction
	  Cognitive function/IQ
	  Development of feeding skills (earlier full oral
	    feedings)
	  Fewer behavioral problems and attentional
	    difficulties
	  Continuation of maternal ability to read and
	    respond to infant behavioral cues
			Shorter length of stay
			Earlier discharge at
			  younger age
			Decrease in hospital
			  charges

*References 16, 21-23, 50, 51, 77, 80, 161, 166, 231, 269, 305, 374, 404, 429, 430, 432, 490, 491, 530, 547, 548.
BPD, Bronchopulmonary dysplasia; *CPAP*, continuous positive airway pressure; *IVH*, intraventricular hemorrhage; *ROP*, retinopathy of prematurity.

and inanimate). However, it must be remembered that this maturation process is "uneven"—as the preterm infant advances in one area of development, he or she may become, at least temporarily, more vulnerable (i.e., experience difficulties) in other areas such as physiologic stability.[192]

INTERVENTIONS

Life in a special care nursery is characterized by sensory deprivation of normal stimuli that the preterm infant would have experienced in the womb and that term infants would experience at home with their families. However, the NICU is also an environment of sensory bombardment—constant noise, light, and tactile stimulation; intrusive, invasive procedures; upset of sleep-wake cycles; and multiple caregivers; etc. **Rather than too much or too little stimulation, infants in the NICU receive an inappropriate pattern of stimulation**[192,195,294] **(e.g., noncontingent, nonreciprocal, painful [rather than pleasant], and multiple stimuli).** Because the immature CNS of the premature infant is unable to tolerate these stimuli, the easily overstimulated preterm infant protects himself or herself by physiologic and interactional defensive maneuvers that threaten survival and social ability and may lead to lifelong maladaptations. Long-term physiologic instability is linked with poor outcomes in preterm infants.[332] Exposure to acute and chronic stress may lead to enduring alterations in the individual's threshold for activation and arousal, alter thresholds for hyperarousal and increase the risk for stress-related diseases.[333]

Research has shown medical, developmental, and cost benefits to low-birth-weight infants from individualized behavioral and environmental care in the NICU (Table 13-5). The most effective interventions (1) are contingent on the infant's responses, (2) balance protection from sensory overload with provision of enough stimulation to promote emerging capabilities, and (3) involve parents.*

Preterm infants are not the only infants at risk from the stress of overstimulation in the NICU. **Acutely ill infants and chronically ill infants with prolonged hospitalization also experience stress.**[206] A term infant with persistent pulmonary hypertension (see Chapter 23) is particularly vulnerable to repeated handling, procedures, and interventions that decrease PaO_2. Thus these infants are managed on a minimal intervention regimen—care is organized, coordinated, and individualized to decrease noxious stimuli and physical manipulations. Even when a "minimal handling" (i.e., parents and staff are discouraged from providing any unnecessary tactile stimulation) protocol[280,360] is encouraged for the sickest neonates, one study documented no difference in the amount of handling the infant

---

*References 23, 80, 161, 191, 195, 202, 341, 379, 429, 431, 432.

endured.[546] The chronically ill infant with BPD has been shown to improve when behavioral or environmental changes were initiated.[21,22] The term SGA infant is sleepy and not alert in the first few weeks of life, which may result in the infant's being left alone or overstimulated to awaken for interaction.[19] After a few weeks these infants become very irritable, fussy, and disorganized in spontaneous and social behaviors. Anticipatory guidance, reassurance that the disorganization is in the infant rather than a result of parental care, and practical intervention strategies enable the parents to shape the environment and the infant's response.[19,192]

The ultimate goal of intervention strategies in the NICU is to facilitate and promote infant growth and development and thus task mastery.[274,402,532] **In the NICU, this goal is achieved by (1) altering the environmental and caregiving stressors that interfere with physiologic stability, (2) promoting individual neurobehavioral organization and maturation by identifying and facilitating stable behaviors and reducing stressful behaviors, (3) conserving energy, (4) teaching parents to interpret infant behavior, and (5) promoting infant-parent interaction and caregiving.** Establishing biorhythmic balance and physiologic homeostasis is necessary for survival and is enhanced by a sensitive, responsive NICU environment. **An unresponsive environment may so stress the preterm infant that apnea, bradycardia, and other physiologic instabilities severely compromise and prolong recovery.*** For the hospitalized infant, development of the sense of self and trust is undermined by noncontingent stimulation that prevents a sense of competence and control of the environment from being established.[195] When the ventilated infant experiences hunger or is wet, he or she is unable to signal the care provider with a cry because of the tube. Thus the infant experiences a need, but is unable to signal and bring care and relief. The infant soon learns that he or she is not in control of the situation. Another intubated infant may be quietly asleep and not experiencing a need; yet it is "care time," so the nurse moves, wakes, changes, and generally disturbs the infant. This infant also soon learns about not being in control of the situation.

Hospitalized infants, especially those with prolonged stays, may exhibit the classic signs of in-stitutionalized infants or infants suffering from maternal deprivation[176,486] (Box 13-2). **It is the goal of "environmental neonatology"**[195] **to prevent this maladaptive behavior by altering the NICU to be more developmentally appropriate and responsive for infants.** Normalizing the environment begins with an assessment of the stimulation to which the individual infant is exposed. The type (i.e., noxious versus pleasant; contingent versus noncontingent), amount, and timing of stimulation should be noted. To decrease noxious stimuli, no infant should have "routine" care (e.g., all infants are suctioned every 2 hours; all infants have a Dextrostix test every 4 hours).[21,192] Care should be individualized by asking the questions: "Why are we doing this procedure?" and "Is this procedure necessary for this infant's care?" Overstimulation in the

---

Box 13-2	CLASSIC SIGNS OF "HOSPITALITIS"

Asocial Behavior

Gaze aversion—fleeting glances at caregiver with inability to maintain eye contact

Flat affect—social unresponsiveness (little fixing and following; little smiling) to caregiver

Little or no quiet alert state—infant abruptly changes state and often is described as "either asleep or awake and crying" (crying is only "awake" state); out-of-control crying

Touch Aversion*

Becomes hypotonic or hypertonic with caregiving or attempts at socialization

Fights, flails, and resists being cared for or held

Aversive responses (see Table 13-8) to caregiving or holding persist

Feeding Difficulties[181,249]

Have multiple origins, including delayed onset of oral feedings; touch aversion around mouth secondary to invasive procedures; multiple caregivers; feeding on schedule, rather than demand

Rumination syndrome—voluntary regurgitation, a form of self-comfort and gratification when environment is not nurturing or gratifying[469]

Failure to Thrive

Poor or no weight gain despite adequate caloric intake
Develops mental delays (language, motor, social, emotional)

From Gardner LI: *Sci Am* 227:76, 1982; Spitz R: *Psychoanal Study Child* 1:53, 1945.
*Infant associates human touch with pain.

NICU occurs when procedures (81% to 94% of all contacts are medical or nursing procedures, an average of 40 to 132 times per day) are performed.[143,546] The frequency, pattern, and trends of caregiver encounters and disturbance has not changed over the last 20 years,[37,402] although caregivers grossly underestimate the amount of handling to which NICU infants are exposed.[37] Nurses, who are best able to control overstimulation, provide the majority of handling, excessive disturbance, and noncontingent interaction to these fragile infants (ranging in number of contacts from 79 to 164 times, evenly distributed over a 24-hour period).[37] Painful, invasive procedures that are not vital to the individual infant are stress-producing events that should be eliminated.

Rest may be the most important environmental change.* Although rest periods are necessary for normal growth and development, care continues to be evenly distributed over 24 hours without adequate periods of undisturbed rest.[402] **Rest periods of less than 60 minutes' duration are ineffective and insufficient for the preterm to complete a normal sleep cycle.**[402] The length of rest periods in most NICUs have not changed (Table 13-6), and institution of a rest period (even of only 1 hour in length) does not necessarily decrease the amount of disturbance.[244]

A fetus in utero and a term infant at home relate to a minimum of caregivers and thus need to learn one or only a few sets of cues. **Consistency of caregivers is essential for an infant's developmental agenda.**[79] Multiple caregivers in the NICU confuse the infant by providing many care-related cues for the infant to learn—many techniques of handling and many emotional, nonverbal messages to decode. Primary nursing minimizes the number of care providers, because the primary nurse and one or two associates always (or as much as possible) care for the infant; assess, revise, and write the care plan; and coordinate care. Primary nursing also adds consistency and continuity for parents.[21,51,206]

The infant's state or level of arousal provides an appropriate context for caregiving.[175] Some infants exhibit a low threshold for stimuli—they are easily overwhelmed and fatigued. Others with a higher threshold are quieter, more difficult to arouse, initiate less, and thus receive less interaction.[20] **Organizing care to be reciprocal to the infant's state reinforces the infant's competence in signaling a need (sense of self) and having it met (sense of**

Table 13-6	REST PERIODS FOR **NICU** INFANTS: RESEARCH BASIS	
AUTHOR/YEAR	**LENGTH OF REST PERIOD**	
Korones, 1976[271]	Range of mean rest period 5.6-19.2 min	
Duxbury, 1984[132]	Average of 30.2 min	
Evans, 1994[143]	Time between handling:	
	1-38.45 min in first nursery	
	1-60 min in second nursery	
Appleton, 1997[37]	2-59 min	

trust and mastery). As the infant matures, feeding on demand rather than on a schedule not only teaches this valuable lesson but also increases absorption and utilization of caloric intake.[192,453] If the infant is asleep, ask: "Do we need to do this now? Would another time be better?" In some centers physicians make an appointment with the nurse to examine the infant—at a time that is optimal for the infant.

Because preterm infants exhibit short duration of state cycles until around 38 weeks, they have decreased tolerance for stimuli. **The smaller, sicker, and less mature the infant, the less he or she is able to handle stimuli.** Some preterm infants tolerate all care done at once and long periods of rest; others do not and need care spread out to decrease overstimulation and decompensation. Clustering of care—performance of several procedures together in a short period of time—may result in more physiologic alterations (changes in cardiorespiratory stability and blood pressure) than a single caretaking event or the actual length of the handling episode.[146,397] Clustering care may not ensure long rest periods, because 50% of all rest periods in several NICUs were less than 10 minutes in length[143] (see Table 13-6). If the practice of clustering care, with its prolonged disturbance of the preterm infant, results in alterations of vital signs and oxygen saturation, care should be individualized and provided to minimize physiologic and behavioral disturbances.[401,402] Even "premie growers" may be unable to tolerate more than one stimulus at a time—they feed best if visual, auditory, and social stimuli are not provided until after the feeding. As the infant matures and is able to tolerate integrated experience, multimodal stimuli are provided.[290]

Alterations in the individual infant's daily schedule are made to accommodate a more flexible or structured schedule—whichever is better for the infant.[195] **Assessing the infant before, during, and**

---

*References 205, 240, 241, 290, 402, 497, 520.

Table 13-7	PARAMETERS FOR ASSESSING INTERACTION AND INTERVENTION WITH NEONATES
TIME FRAME	**ASSESSMENT**
Before	
Gather baseline data *before* touching the infant	Gestational age and postconceptual age
	Diagnosis
	Level of physiologic homeostasis
	Previous vital signs
	Oxygenation state—(continuous pulse oximetry or transcutaneous monitor)
	Neonatal state
	Sleep—deep, light, drowsy
	Awake—quiet, active alert, crying
	Self-regulatory vs stress behaviors (Table 13-8)
During	
Gently and as nonintrusively as possible assess physiologic and behavioral signs *during* intervention	Level of (current) physiologic homeostasis: vital signs and changes
	Observation (without touching infant)—color, posture, general appearance, respiratory rate, temperature (skin, incubator), blood pressure (transducer), oxygenation (from continuous monitor)
	Quiet (with minimal disturbance)—ausculate heart, lungs, and abdomen; axillary temperature, blood pressure (cuff); head-to-toe assessment; oxygenation (saturation decreases with stressful, disturbing stimuli)
	Neonatal state change
	Sleep—deep, light, drowsy
	Awake—quiet alert, active alert, crying
	Self-regulatory vs stress behaviors (Table 13-8)
After	
Assess physiologic and behavioral signs *after* intervention (delayed reactions may occur minutes after care)	Level of physiologic homeostasis
	Vital signs—returned to baseline values? More or less stable than baseline values?
	Neonatal state change—return to baseline state? To a higher state? Unable to be consoled? More consolable left alone?

after an interaction or intervention guides the care provider in adapting care and the environment to the individual infant (Table 13-7). An organized infant is able to interact with the environment without disrupting his or her physiologic and behavioral functioning.[20] **When a disorganized preterm interacts with the environment, signs of physiologic and behavioral stress may occur (Table 13-8), in which case the interaction should cease.**[272,290] An intubated preterm infant cared for in a NICU with a strict suction "routine" every 2 hours responds with profound cyanosis, lowered $TcPO_2$ and pulse oximetery, and bradycardia, and requires bagging after every suction (with no secretions obtained)—an obviously unnecessary and stressful intervention. In a less rigid, more individualized care setting, that same infant may signal the need for suction by becoming restless, by a decrease in oxy-

genation, and/or by heart rate changes (tachycardia or bradycardia). Suctioning improves the infant's condition—the infant lies quietly and has improved oxygenation, and the heart pattern stabilizes. This infant has signaled his or her need, and the care providers have read the cues and responded with a stabilizing intervention—the infant has not been stressed by an unnecessary procedure.

Knowledgeable professionals are able to role model for and teach parents how to relate to their premature infant.[429] Parents are taught to recognize and use infant states to maximize appropriate interaction.[16,199,286,290,429] The drowsy premature infant may be unable to engage in eye-to-eye contact with the parents or be able to sustain it for too short (for the parents) a period. Waiting until the infant is more awake to initiate eye contact will be more rewarding to the parent and less stressful to

Table 13-8	SELF-REGULATORY VERSUS STRESS BEHAVIORS	
ORGANIZATION	**DISORGANIZATION**
Physiologic	**Physiologic**
Cardiorespiratory: stable heart and/or respiratory rate; regular, slow respirations	Cardiorespiratory: increase or decrease in respiratory rate; irregular respirations; apnea; gasping; bradycardia; blood pressure instability; sneezing, hiccoughs, coughing, sighing
Color: pink, stable	Color: mottling, duskiness; cyanosis—central or generalized; pallor or plethora
Gastrointestinal: tolerates feedings	Gastrointestinal: abdominal distention; spitting up; vomiting; gagging; stooling
Behavioral	
Body movements smooth and synchronous: consistent tone of all body parts; arms and legs flexed with smooth movements	Tremors, jittery and jerking movements; hypotonia or hypertonia (flaccid trunk, extremities; arching, flailing, extended extremities; finger splays, fisting)
States; well-defined sleep-wake	Unable to modulate states: sudden state changes; more active than quiet sleep; awake states with gaze aversion, frowning, grimacing, staring, irritability, wide-eyed "help me" look
Self-quieting behaviors: hand-to-mouth, hand or foot clasping, finger folding or grasping, sucking, foot or leg bracing	Limited use of self-quieting behaviors (may need assistance from caregiver)
Attentive behaviors: alert gaze; fixes and follows visual stimuli; ceases to suck or slows suck rate, turns toward auditory stimuli, smiles; imitates: mouth opening, tongue extension; vocalizes: cooing, babbling, habituates to stimuli	May demonstrate any of above stress signals when attempting to interact with one or more modes of stimuli (e.g., rocking and talking) simultaneously in environment (either animate or inanimate)

Modified from Als H et al: A new model of assessing the behavioral organization in preterm and fullterm infants: two case studies, *J Am Acad Child Psychiatry* 20:239, 1981; Gorski PA: Stages of behavioral organization in the high-risk neonate: theoretical and clinical considerations, *Semin Perinatol* 3:61, 1979.

the infant. Role model for parents that this infant is an individual and even though premature, is able to signal for more or less stimulation (see Table 13-8).

A preterm infant who is lightly touched may startle, jerk, or withdraw from parental touch. In response, the parent suddenly and sadly pulls his or her hand away and is reticent to touch the infant again. Intervention includes helping parents read cues and learn appropriate responses to their infant. The infant may be interpreted to the parents: "Jamie likes firm touch . . . like this." Teach parents how to recognize a stressed infant and how to intervene. The prime rule of relating to infants is: the infant leads; the adult follows.

Feeding a premature infant may be difficult, because the infant "goes to sleep" or "gets lazy" during feedings. The usual parental ministrations of talking to the infant, soothing with touch, or holding upright on the shoulder may not work with a fussy, irritable preterm infant. The preterm infant's behavior may be so disorganized, unpredictable, or misunderstood by

the parents that an appropriate response is not possible.[17,192] Thus parents often become exhausted, bewildered, and frustrated in their encounters with their preterm infant's behavioral response to their care as rejecting and unloving: "My baby doesn't like me."[156] Teach parents that their infant's disorganization with stimuli is related to prematurity (i.e., an immature CNS) and not to parent ministrations. Reassure them that as the premature infant grows and evidences maturational changes, he or she will be able to tolerate more stimulation and will be more responsive to their care.

Just as parent-infant interaction is responsible for normal development of the term infant, parent-infant interaction is crucial in the development of at-risk infants.[429,432] Many parents of premature infants have been observed making heroic efforts, over long periods of time, to interact with their less alert, active, and responsive infants.[42,186,190,192,340] Parenting the preterm has been described as "more work and less fun."[186] **"Setting parents up to succeed"** involves placing parents in situations where they will experience positive feedback from their infants. Suggesting and role modeling intervention strategies shows parents what and how to play and interact with their infants. Parent participation in intervention strategies is ensured by stressing how important it is to infant development, that professionals are too busy to provide all necessary interventions, and that parents are in a unique position to provide developmental care in the hospital and at home after discharge. **Parents, with help from professionals, are the ideal planners and providers of developmentally appropriate intervention strategies.** Beneficial effects of parent involvement in developmental care of VLBW infants include better interaction with and perception of the infant and improved cognitive development (see Table 13-5).

A rooming-in setting for parents and their at-risk newborns is the best environment for cues to be learned and care given according to these cues. **Unlimited and unrestricted contact of parents and newborns should be the policy in every normal, medium-risk, and high-risk nursery (see Box 29-2).** Providing a "family room," "bonding room," or "apartment" where parents and their soon-to-be discharged newborn can room-in helps the transition from hospital to home care. Rooming-in before discharge gives mothers and fathers an opportunity to assume full responsibility for their infant's care, tests the reality of caregiving, helps them to learn caregiving activities and their infant's behavior patterns, and confirms their readiness for independent parenting and the infant's readiness for discharge.[107,238,531]

Intervention Strategies

Because infants experience their environment through sensory capabilities, intervention strategies are based on tactile/kinesthetic, auditory, visual, olfactory/gustatory, and communication skills. Interventions must be individualized according to the infant's state, sensory threshold, physiologic homeostasis, and stability or stress cues.[16,143,523]

Circadian Rhythms

In utero the states of the fetus are regulated by the sleep-wake cycles of the mother. **In the NICU multiple intrusions disrupt regulation. How this affects an infant is not fully known, although limited energy may be drained, the infant subjected to further stress,[21,195,206] and outcomes of therapeutic interventions may not be optimized.[467]** To minimize interruptions and excessive handling,

infants should not be awakened when asleep; if they must be awakened for care, it should be during active sleep by talking softly and gentle stroking.[98,128,525] Appointments for examinations should be made before feeding to decrease unnecessary disturbance of sleep, but with enough rest time (if needed) before actual feeding.

Adequate numbers of caregiving encounters—physical assessment, vital signs, diaper or linen change, and procedures—must be balanced against constant manipulations.[21,192] **Because essentially all NICU (level II and III) infants are continuously monitored, "laying on of hands" every 1 to 2 hours is often unnecessary. Thorough physical assessment and vital sign recording every 4 hours is easily alternated with recordings from the monitors every 4 hours. Thus the infant is evaluated every 2 hours but not disturbed that often.** An acutely ill infant may need closer observation, but alternating "hands-on" with monitor readings accomplishes the goal without overwhelming an infant with few reserves.

Sleep-wake patterns are influenced by feeding method,[426,514] temperature,[503,515] position,[307,311] central nervous system maturation,[236,364] birth weight,[237] caregiving practices,[366,415] and environmental effects (e.g., ambient light, noise).[130,343,364] Sleep-wake patterns in breastfed and bottlefed infants differ. Full-term breastfed infants awaken more and sleep less during the night.[426] In one study preterm breastfed infants cried approximately 1 hour more during the day than preterm infants being bottlefed with formula.[514] Although being held in skin-to-skin contact, babies sleep 50% to 75% of the time with no change in the amount of quiet sleep.[63,307,311]

Day-night cycles are facilitated by afternoon nap time and nighttime in which the dimming of lights or covering of incubators and cribs with blankets and quieting of NICU noise enables infants to sleep.[55,56,319,497] Deep, quiet sleep is facilitated by quiet and dark, soft (classical) music, gentle stroking of the head, and self-regulated tasks (self-sought proximity of infant to breathing bear).[512] Maintaining daily nap time and nighttime hours helps infants reset their diurnal rhythms and become accustomed to sleeping in dim light and a quiet environment[56] (something that babies discharged from the hospital for even short stays have difficulty doing). Among convalescing preterm infants (less than 34 weeks' gestational age), four standard rest periods per day resulted in (1) increased daily weight gain, (2) increased sleep, (3) less-active states during nap time, (4) decreased occurrences of apnea, and (5) by 3 weeks, less quiet waking time and longer uninterrupted sleep episodes.[240,241,518] Uninterrupted sleep and diurnal rhythmicity is also associated with improved state organization in VLBW infants.[149]

Tactile/Kinesthetic Intervention

Because the sense of touch is highly developed in utero, even a very immature preterm has acute tactile sensitivity. **For newborns, human touch is the most important tactile stimulation.** Not all touch is equal, however, nor is it responded to equally by term or preterm infants who are well, critically ill, or recovering from illness. Any type of tactile stimulation is composed of six factors: duration, location, action, intensity, frequency, and sensation.[293] **Tactile sensation both arouses and quiets—gentle but firm handling quiets infants, because they feel more secure; light, uncertain touch often results in agitation and withdrawal.**[274,298] **Handling for routine care (i.e., vital signs, changing the diaper or position, venipuncture for blood draws or placement of IVs, feeding, heelsticks, suction, and physical or neurologic examinations) results in physiologic alterations of hypoxia, increased intracranial pressure, and increased/decreased heart rate and blood pressure.***

How a neonate is handled during care affects his or her physiologic and behavioral response. Use of body containment during suction decreases the physiologic and behavioral responses to this stressful procedure.[141,504,527] Comparing preterm responses to swaddled and unswaddled weighing, unswaddled infants exhibit more physiologic distress, more motor disorganization, poorer self-regulation, and more need for caregiver facilitation than when they were swaddled for weighing.[381] Transferring preterm infants from the incubator to the parent for holding or kangaroo care may be stressful. In one study, with preterm infants of 28 weeks' gestation receiving ventilatory therapy, it was found that keeping the infant connected to the ventilator during transfer resulted in adequate oxygenation and heart rate stability.[309] Another study documented physiologic disorganization in nurse-to-parent or parent transfer from the incubator for kangaroo care.[382] Both transfer methods resulted in increased physiologic and motor disorganization

(i.e., oxygen desaturation, tachycardia, cyanosis/pallor, hypotonia, decreased self-regulation, and increased need for caregiver facilitation to maintain physiologic stability during transfer). In both methods of transfer (which lasted 6 to 9 minutes) the ventilator was disconnected (for a duration of 5 seconds). Both the infant's desaturation readings and tachycardia recovered to baseline levels faster with the parent transfer; during and after kangaroo care oxygen saturation and heart rate returned to baseline values.[382]

Excessive handling of preterm or sick neonates results in significant physiologic consequences, such as (1) blood pressure changes, (2) alterations in cerebral blood flow, and (3) hypoxia and other stress behaviors.[301] A total body position change is not considered a painful procedure, but in LBW preterm infants with endotracheal tubes and umbilical artery catheters the handling necessary to change the infant's position elicits pain behaviors.[147]

In the NICU, infants who are repeatedly subjected to painful, intrusive procedures develop touch aversion—the association of human touch with pain. These infants cry uncontrollably, squirm away, flail arms and legs, and recoil when touched, knowing that pain will soon follow. An infant who has received ventilatory therapy may have touch aversion around the mouth: the infant is averse to facial stroking and rooting, has a hypersensitive gag reflex, and refuses to nipple feed. **Painful procedures should be minimized to those absolutely (medically) indicated—*no* infant should be subjected to "routine" painful procedures. During those necessary procedures it is essential to provide body containment, comfort measures (such as a pacifier), and adequate pain relief (see Chapter 12).**

Touch that is not related to caregiving (i.e., social contact) should be provided by parents and professionals when the preterm infant is aware, alert, and receptive.[88,290] When parents touch their babies they provide a wide variety of amounts and types of touch—most frequently holding, stroking, rubbing, or making physical contact (placing a finger in the infant's hand).[218] Preterm infants respond individually and physiologically to their parents' touch—there is more variation in heart rate and oxygen saturation levels compared to baseline values. These variations depend on gestational age, infant state, and the amount of handling before parent handling.[219,220] Less touching by the nurse within the 2 hours before parental holding results in less mean

---

*References 88, 114, 115, 141, 301, 346, 383, 397-399.

decrease in heart rate during parental holding.[219] Parents provide more positive touch (kissing and stroking); preterm infants are more likely to smile and sleep for their parents when compared with the increase in sleep-wake transitions, larger body movements, and jitters exhibited after a nurse's touch.[360] In animal studies increased parental touching in infancy results in changes in brain structure, decreased levels of stress hormones, and better ability to survive a stressful environment.[299] Perhaps parental touch of preterm humans enables them to withstand the stress of illness and the NICU environment.

Kangaroo care, skin-to-skin contact between parents and infant by placing the infant in a vertical position between the maternal or paternal breasts, benefits both parents and neonates (Box 13-3). Kangaroo care for the healthy preterm has been used in the delivery room and the transitional period (see Chapter 5). Kangaroo care is well tolerated in the first week of life by preterm infants with current or resolving neonatal illness.[463] Kangaroo care improves gas exchange in preterm infants of less than 1800 g. The smallest infants (less than 1000 g) remained more clinically stable (i.e., smallest increase in heart rate, highest decrease in respiratory rate and increase in oxygen saturation, and no hypothermia) when compared with infants larger than 1000 g.[162] Parental perceptions of kangaroo care while their infant requires ventilation are characterized by three themes: (1) ambivalence toward kangaroo care: yearning to hold the infant yet apprehensive about it, (2) the necessity of a supportive environment, and (3) the special quality of parent-infant interaction: intense connectedness and active parenting.[380] When kangaroo care was compared with conventional cuddling care (i.e., mother holding her swaddled, clothed infant) there was no difference in maintenance of temperature, weight gain, length of stay, and duration of breastfeeding between the two groups.[438]

Nonpainful touch such as stroking (the head, trunk, or hands) during care may calm, soothe, and prevent touch aversion. **Stroking of physiologically stable preterm infants has been associated with increased activity and alertness, a faster regaining of birth weight, more rapid weight gain, less crying and apnea, enhanced developmental status, and better social scores.** * In a recent study

---

*References 6, 44, 260, 455, 456, 484, 485.

Box 13-3	BENEFITS OF KANGAROO CARE/SKIN-TO-SKIN CONTACT*

Parental

Activates maternal processes of search for meaning and mastery of the experience of premature birth
Increases maternal self-confidence, competence, and self-esteem
Enhances parent-infant attachment
Initiates and maintains maternal behavior
Positive and personally beneficial experience
Positively impacts parental identity and knowledge of infant
Increases confidence in meeting infant's needs
More frequent visiting
Parental eagerness for infant's discharge

Neonatal

Thermal synchrony—mother's body temperature rises and falls to maintain infant in neutral state (see Chapter 6)
Cardiopulmonary
    Adequate or improved oxygenation
    Fewer episodes of periodic breathing, apnea, and bradycardia
Breastfeeding
    Increased incidence and length
    Increased milk supply

Neonatal—cont'd

Behavioral
    Increased alert activity
    Increased deep sleep
    Decreased or no crying[93,94]
    Increased enface positioning
Earlier discharge
    Increased weight gain
    No increased infection; decreased severity of infection and mortality
    Out of incubator earlier
Regulatory interaction[235]

Behavioral	Cardiovascular
Sucking	Endocrine
Neurochemical	Immune
Metabolic	Circadian

Sleep-wake cycles
Long term
    Increased length and head circumference at 9 mo/1 year of age
    More consistent/contingent maternal responses at 15 mo of age
    Less crying at 6 mo of age

---

*Data compiled from references 8, 9, 33, 34, 49, 58, 63, 90, 91, 92, 119, 162, 173, 175, 308, 310, 311, 352, 380, 438, 507, 551.

12 strokes of controlled pressure were applied to preterm infants in an intermediate care setting; no difference was found in weight/length/head circumference or oxygen saturation levels between the experimental and control groups.[57] **However, in preterm infants (26 to 30 weeks' gestation) who are *not* physiologically stable, stroking results in decreased oxygen saturation and signs of behavioral stress (e.g., grasping, grunting, and gaze aversion).**[386] Other behavioral and physiologic effects include heart rate and blood pressure changes, changes in respiratory rate and rhythm, increase in avoidance signals (increased startle reflex, agitation, and crying), increase in activity and movement, and decreased visual responsivity.*

If the preterm infant becomes agitated with stroking, a hand firmly placed on the head and lower back, buttocks, or abdomen often quiets.[105,222] Hand placement without stroking does not decrease oxygen saturation or alter heart rate and has a soothing effect (i.e., decreases active sleep, increases quiet sleep, and decreases motor activity and behavioral distress) in small preterm infants.[221,222,368,522] Handle gently to avoid stressful reactions (e.g., flailing, arching, and oxygen desaturation) and enable the infant to become calm and rest between caregiving. Gentle touch causes no skin discoloration because of applied pressure.[227] Parents should be taught and encouraged to provide their preterm with "gentle human touch"[222,368,522,552] in the form of supportive containment with their hands,[222] use of gradual and rhythmic action,[227] observation of infant responses (see Table 13-8), and modification, alteration or cessation of touch when necessary.[79,217,293]

The touching and stroking of massage stimulates nerve pathways and aids myelinization by increasing hypothalamic activity and production of the growth hormone somatotrophin. In animal studies touch deprivation decreases growth hormone secretion, which results in undergrowth of all organ systems; a return to normal secretion occurs with tactile stimulation.[458] More recently a growth gene that responds to tactile stimulation has been discovered; this suggests a genetic origin for the touch/growth relationship.[154] Because touch stimulation of the inside of a neonate's mouth increases the release of gastrointestinal food absorption hormones (i.e., gastrin and insulin),[526] it is postulated that the tactile stimulation of massage leads to a similar hormone release.[157] Current assay

of glucose and insulin levels in heelstick samples of preterm infants suggest that massaged infants show increased levels of insulin.[154]

Research on massage therapy with preterm infants has been conducted on medically stable growing infants (i.e., premie growers) (Table 13-9). Massage therapy provides social touch, rather than painful touch, prevents or treats touch aversion, and should be taught to and provided by parents in the hospital and at home. Confidence in parenting skills and tactile communication between parents and infant are encouraged when parents massage their infant. **Because massage has not been studied in acutely ill preterm infants, its use should be confined to premie growers.**[79,154] Chronically ill infants (i.e., babies with bronchopulmonary dysplasia [BPD] or congenital heart disease) may exhibit physiologic and behavioral disorganization with massage so that the risk-benefit ratio must be carefully assessed.[79,346,542,543]

There is a lack of evidence of the safety and efficacy of sponge bathing preterm babies in the NICU on a daily or every-other-day schedule.[167,376,478] **Sponge bathing critically ill preterm infants (28 to 34 weeks' gestational age) results in significant increases in behavior state and activity levels (i.e., motor stress behavior, stability, and reorganization), stress cue frequency, increase or decrease in heart rate, and decrease in oxygen saturation.**[398,399] These detrimental effects caused by handling were exhibited most frequently by neonates of the younger gestational ages. Because sponge bathing of critically ill preterm infants clearly increases physiologic risk and provides no clear benefits, the procedure of routine bathing of these infants is unnecessary and not recommended.[29,400] Frequency of sponge bathing can be reduced to every 4 days without increasing skin flora colony counts or colonization with pathogens.[167] **Waiting to bathe these infants until they are physiologically stable and introducing the bath as a "recovery milestone" for parents to complete is a more developmentally and physiologically appropriate practice.**[259,400] Parents may tub bathe the premature grower, which provides a soothing, relaxing, tension-relieving experience of multiple textures (water, water temperature, soap, and washcloth).[21,259] (See Chapter 18 for skin care practices.)

Varying sensation and touch pattern keeps infants interested in stroking and massaging. As a preterm infant matures and is able to tolerate variety, he or she should be introduced to different textures (e.g., lambskins, stuffed toys, cotton, satin). Baby clothes

---

*References 114, 141, 217, 301, 383, 386, 397.

Table 13-9 BENEFITS OF MASSAGE WITH NICU INFANTS: RESEARCH BASIS	
STUDY	RESULTS
Forty preterm "growers" (31 wk ga; 1280 g BW; 20 days of NICU care) massaged for 15 min, three times/day for 10 days[157]	• Gained 47% more weight (no difference in caloric intake) • More awake/active time • Better performance on habituation, orientation, and motor activity; regulation of state behavior • Hospitalized 6 days less (cost saving $3000/infant) • Infant preferred some degree of pressure (rather than light stroking) • 1 year later—weight advantage, better performance on developmental scales—higher mental and motor scores[155]
Metaanalysis of 19 studies[391]	• 72% of infants receiving some form of tactile stimulation were positively affected • Increased weight gain • Better performance of developmental tasks
Three times/day massage of cocaine-exposed infants[549]	• Fewer postnatal complications • Fewer stress behaviors • 28% greater daily weight gain • More mature motor behavior
Three times/day massage by mothers to HIV-exposed infants[454]	• 100% compliance by mothers • Greater weight gain • Better performance on habituation, motor, range of state and autonomic stability clusters • Better performance on stress behavior scale, including alert responsiveness, cost of attention, examiner persistence, state regulation, motor tone, and excitability
Three times/day massage of pre-terms with physiologic and biochemical measurements[455,457]	• 21% increase in daily weight gain • Discharged 5 days earlier • Superior performance on habituation • Fewer stress behaviors (mouthing, grimacing, clenched fists) • Increase in catecholamine secretion in neonatal period (analogous to the normal developmental increase following birth)[278] • Increase in vagal activity

From Field T: Infant massage therapy. In Goldson E, ed: *Nurturing the premature infant,* New York, 1999, Oxford University Press.
BW, Birth weight; *ga,* gestational age.

provide various textures, decrease heat loss (especially hats), and make the infant more attractive ("He looks like a real baby!"; "She looks like a girl, since her shaved head is covered!").

Consoling hand-to-mouth behaviors are observed more frequently during caregiving (by nurses, rather than parents) and before and after feeding (especially in gavage-fed infants).[55] Hand-to-midline behaviors are encouraged by cradling the infant for feedings (for both bottle and gavage feedings if the infant tolerates it) with both arms in the midline. If a premature infant needs an oxygen hood, using one large enough so that the infant's whole upper body will fit inside encourages hand-to-mouth quieting (Figure 13-2). VLBW preterm infants whose whole body was not inside the oxygen hood have been videotaped expending energy in persistent attempts (30 to 40 minutes) to self-console and reduce stress by trying to get their hands to their mouths.[55]

Use arm restraints only when necessary and immobilize the extremity in a physiologic position. Release and exercise the restrained extremity with each caregiving encounter. Avoid restraining both arms so that one is free for hand-to-mouth behaviors. If both must be restrained (e.g., the infant pulls out the orogastric tube), give the infant a pacifier.

Positioning. **Preterm infants display different motor development from that of term infants.**[109,451] A continuous assessment of muscle tone, response to positioning and handling, oral-motor function, and response to sensory stimuli provide data for individualizing intervention.[109,157] The goal of intervention is to provide opportunities for normal development and organization of the sensory systems, to detect early developmental problems, and to educate parents about stimulation, handling, and positioning. Although some studies have shown that

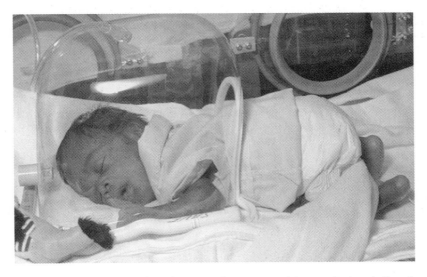

FIGURE 13-2   Preterm infant in oxygen hood that is large enough to accommodate upper body to facilitate hand-to-mouth behavior. Note sling that helps maintain flexion without frog-leg position.

specific positioning for premature infants does not significantly affect development,[7] others have shown that a developmental approach to care of VLBW infants greatly reduces the long-term effects of prematurity.[51,127,374] VLBW and full-term infants achieve the same fine and gross motor milestones although the developmental pathways of milestone achievement is different—early (in the first 8 months of life of the VLBW infant), fine motor control develops almost to the exclusion of gross motor development.[481]

Preterm infants usually have less developed physiologic flexion in the limbs, trunk, and pelvis than term newborns (Table 13-10). Even at term conceptual age, preterm infants have less flexion than their full-term counterparts do.[214,374] For preterm infants long periods of immobilization without a positioning device on a firm mattress with the influences of gravity result in a number of abnormal characteristics: (1) increased neck extension[181] with a right-sided head preference, (2) shoulder retraction and abduction (reduces forward rotation and ability to reach midline), (3) increased trunk extension with "arching" of the neck and back,[181] (4) frog-leg position: hips abducted and externally rotated, and (5) ankle and feet eversion[523] (Figure 13-3). These characteristics interfere with development of eye-hand coordination, cognitive development, and equilibrium.[62,205,451] **Box 13-4 lists the reasons for proper positioning in the NICU.**

To prevent overstretching of the joints and to fa-

Table 13-10	DEVELOPMENT OF TONE*
GESTATIONAL AGE (WK)	**DEVELOPMENT**
28	Completely hypotonic and lacks all physiologic flexion
32	Hips and knees begin to show some flexion while arms remain extended
34	Flexor tone apparent in legs
36	Loose flexion of arms and legs evident and grasp reflex present
40	Develops tone in utero and develops flexed position in intrauterine space; after birth, reflex activity and CNS maturity help term infant to unfold and extend; term infant holds all four limbs in flexed position

From Anderson J, Auster-Liebhaber J: *Phys Occup Ther Pediatr* 4(1):89, 1984; Dubowitz L et al: *J Pediatr* 77:1, 1970; Palisano R, Short M: *Phys Occup Ther Pediatr* 4(4):43, 1984.
*Muscle tone develops in caudocephalic and centripetal (distal to proximal) directions and interacts with simultaneous cephalocaudal development of movement to help affect posture. Although knowledge of normal development before term helps detect signs of abnormality, variability of ±2 weeks' gestational age must be taken into consideration.[13]

cilitate development of flexor tone, the infant should be provided with a variety of positions. **Side-lying (Figure 13-4) is used to improve visual awareness of hands, to encourage hands-to-midline movement, and to discourage the frog-leg position. In**

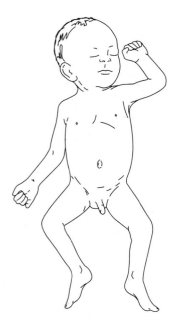

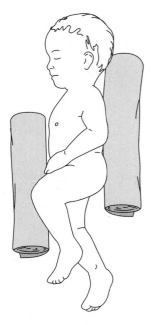

FIGURE 13-3   Premature infant resting posture exhibiting shoulder retraction and abduction and frog-leg position: hips abducted and externally rotated and ankles and feet everted. (From Pelletier-Sehnar JM, Palmeri A: High-risk infants. In Pratt PN, Allen AS, eds: *Occupational therapy for children,* ed 2, St. Louis, 1989, Mosby.)

FIGURE 13-4   Side-lying is facilitated by using a rolled blanket behind infant's head and trunk. Additional support is added by placing another roll in front of infant's chest and abdomen with infant's top leg over it. Placing a blanket over the infant and tucking it under the mattress helps hold this position. Placing the rolled blanket in a stockinette helps provide a firm boundary for the roll. To avoid neck flexion of hyperextension, the infant's head should be monitored and the position of the neck changed as necessary. Blanket roll at the feet gives the infant a boundary on which to brace the feet.

Box 13-4 **REASONS FOR PROPER POSITIONING**	
1. Inhibits or shortens dystonic phase while infant remains in fetal position during postnatal period 2. Facilitates hand-to-midline and midline orientation 3. Stimulates visual exploration of environment (through head to midline) 4. Facilitates development of head control (making feeding easier and helping respiratory problems)[181] 5. Helps balance flexors and extensors to facilitate symmetric posture[127,374,451]	6. Helps develop antigravity movement 7. Enhances comfort and decreases stress 8. Has an organizing effect that facilitates development of flexor tone 9. Promotes normal and prevents abnormal development[127,451] 10. Helps enhance development of motor skills, reflexes, and postural tone[127,374,451]

From Pelletier-Sehnar JM, Palmeri A: High-risk infants. In Pratt PN, Allen AS, eds: *Occupational therapy for children,* ed 2, St. Louis, 1989, Mosby.

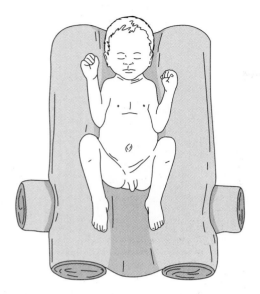

FIGURE 13-5 Supine positioning with rolled blankets or pads on either side. *NOTE:* Supine positioning should be used with caution. Preterm infants who have not developed gag reflex (<36 weeks gestation) are at particularly high risk for aspiration. Supine position should not be used until most of the feeding has been absorbed (at least 1 to 1½ hours after feeding). (From Pelletier-Sehnar JM, Palmeri A: High-risk infants. In Pratt PN, Allen AS, eds: *Occupational therapy for children,* ed 2, St. Louis, 1989, Mosby.)

this position the infant is able to bring the hands to the mouth for sucking and self-comforting.

Acutely ill preterm infants are often positioned supine with the head to the side or in the midline to accommodate their ventilators, umbilical catheters, and other devices. **Supine positioning does not promote flexion and may be stressful to acutely ill infants.**[16,70] A recent study of 22 preterm infants with apnea and bradycardia found no significant difference in the incidence of clinically significant events between supine and prone positioning.[262] Placed supine, infants exhibit more startle behaviors and sleep disturbance from environmental stimuli. Prolonged supine positioning is associated with the hypertonic "arched" position (hyperextension of head, neck, and shoulder girdle) of many chronically ventilated infants. Supine positioning should promote as much flexion as possible (Figure 13-5). Use of a positioning device of foam with the middle cut out and sloping under the scapulae is another method of obtaining supine flexion. Use of hip support results in less lower extremity abduction and external rotation

than in infants without such hip support.[127] Pillows filled with polystyrene beads (i.e., premie bean bags) require skill for optimal positioning and close infant monitoring[263] but are useful in providing positioning for very small premature infants (1000 to 1500 g).

Body containment increases the infant's feeling of security, promotes quieting and self-control, enhances physiologic stability, promotes energy conservation, reduces physiologic and behavioral stress, and enables stress to be better endured.[504] Many premature infants "travel" (no matter how many times they are moved) to the sides or bottom of their incubator. Just as premature infants are able to seek proximity to a breathing bear,[512] they are able to seek out security. Parents and professionals are inclined to move the uncomfortable-looking infant back to the middle of a "boundaryless" world. Infants should be left where they feel safe and comfortable; if they become uncomfortable they will let you know. Providing boundaries (e.g., blanket rolls) often stops this migration.

Small, acutely ill premature infants who are positioned supine are often extremely agitated, thrashing arms and legs, tachycardic, and expending precious energy and calories. Instead of medications, these infants are often calmed by providing a nest of blankets on either side and at the head and feet. The infant's limbs are then flexed inside this artificial womb, and the infant quietly rests (Figure 13-6). If agitation recurs, a limb (usually a leg) has extended outside the infant's secure boundary; flexing and returning it to the "womb" quiets the infant.[16,20,525]

Body containment maneuvers such as swaddling, holding onto a finger or hand, and crossing the infant's arms in the midline and holding them securely help with self-regulation during feeding, procedures, or other stressful manipulations.* Because being wrapped in a blanket with extremities flexed simulates in utero position, swaddling (1) improves flexed posture and flexor muscle tone, (2) facilitates behavioral responses, and (3) improves the development of primitive reflexes.[477] Picking the preterm infant up from a supine position often produces startles, apnea, or head hyperextension.[151] A better technique is to roll the infant prone, which flexes the head, and then flex the limbs onto the trunk and pick the infant up.[525] If the infant has difficulty breathing in prone position, swaddle or contain the extremities before picking the infant up.

---

*References 85, 105, 142, 153, 504, 527.

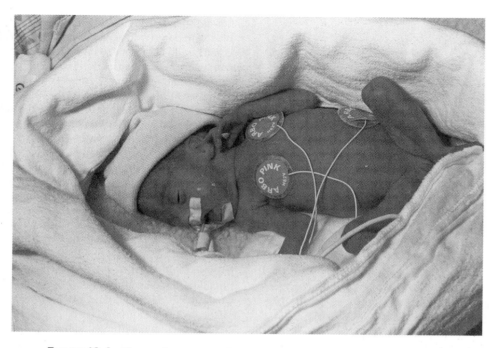

FIGURE 13-6 Very small premature infant resting quietly in a "nest" of pads and blankets.

Prone positioning encourages the infant to work on using neck extension and promotes flexion of the extremities. This position does not require the use of any device—it merely encourages knee and arm flexion; a small hiproll or sling (see Figure 13-2) assists in maintaining flexion.[151] **Prone (versus supine) positioning has numerous benefits and is the position of choice for many NICU infants (Box 13-5).** Although in one study prone position did not decrease pain,[490] prone positioning of highly agitated fretful narcotic-withdrawing neonates experienced less distress (i.e., lower withdrawal scores and lower caloric intake) than supine-lying infants.[316] Use of a sheepskin or lambskin helps to further facilitate flexion and prevents skin abrasion, especially on the knees.

Many of the beneficial effects of prone positioning listed in Box 13-5 become detrimental in increasing the risk of sudden infant death syndrome (SIDS) (Table 13-11). In 1996 the American Academy of Pediatrics updated its position paper on infant sleep and recommends placing healthy infants only supine for sleep.[31] In this updated statement, side-lying is no longer endorsed because the infant may spontaneously roll from side-lying to prone.[230] Use of side-lying and prone positioning as well as containment with soft bedding for physiologically compromised term and preterm infants is

Box 13-5	EFFECTS OF PRONE POSITIONING

1. Decreases heart rate variability[71,168]
2. Enhances respiratory control[59,326]
3. Improves oxygenation by 15% to 25%[306,325,459,539]
   a. Increased $TcPO_2$ values
   b. Increased PaO_2 values
4. Improves lung mechanics and lung volumes[247,539]
   a. Increased lung compliance
   b. Increased tidal volume
5. Decreases energy expenditure[194,256,284,331,459]
   a. Increased quiet sleep; higher arousal threshold[25,71,168,256,482]
   b. Decreased awake time; more sleep time
   c. Decreased caloric expenditure (median difference supine versus prone: +3.1 kcal/kg/day)
   d. (?) Decreased heat loss
   e. Less crying[71]
   f. Lower levels of activity[87,224]
6. Decrease in gastric reflux in prone position with head of bed elevated 30 degrees[390]

safe and appropriate in a NICU setting.[300] Parents may question these practices; therefore their physiologic base and rationale should be explained. **Parents should also be taught that when their baby is well-enough to be weaned to an open crib, he**

Table 13-11	Sleep Position as a Risk Factor for SIDS: Research Basis
Supine	**Prone**
Preterm infants at 36-38 wk postconceptual age[193] • No significant difference in sleep organization based on body position • More awakenings in supine vs. prone • Standard deviations of heart rate increase during quiet sleep in supine; low and high frequency of heart rate higher in supine vs. prone in both active and quiet sleep states[194]	• Prone position reduces spontaneous arousals from sleep in term infants[256] • First quiet sleep after feedings significantly longer, fewer number of awakenings, and decrease in overall heart rate variability in prone vs. supine[193] • Above characteristics of prone sleep constitute a higher arousal threshold, thus increased vulnerability to SIDS in prone position[194] • In preterm infants at 1 month corrected age, duration of daytime nap sleep is becoming more variable, a trend of more total sleep and the percentage of active sleep during prone position[4,5]
More sleep transitions, a lower arousal threshold and higher heart rate variability while sleeping supine contributes to decrease vulnerability to SIDS[5]	• Sixty-two healthy growing LBW infants (26-37 wk gestational age; birth weight 750-1600 g). Sleeping prone—a shift of EEG activity toward slower frequency, which may be related to mechanisms associated with a decrease in behavioral arousal in prone position[445]
Full-term (10) infants in prone/supine sleep positions given 0.4 cc water infusion resulted in airway protective responses of swallowing (95%) and arousal (54%)[252] • Swallow rate rapid in supine position in response to small infusions of fluid, while respiratory rate remains largely unaffected. When supine, term infants can coordinate rapid swallowing while maintaining breathing	• A significant decrease in swallowing and breathing in active sleep in prone vs. supine position; airway protection is compromised in prone sleeping position during active sleep in healthy term infants exposed to minute pharyngeal fluid

will be physiologically and developmentally mature to tolerate supine sleep position in preparation for discharge.[300] Since the "Back to Sleep" campaign the rate of SIDS has decreased in many countries.[133] In term infants supine sleep position may delay some motor milestones by 1 month, but does not delay walking. Increased amounts of time in supervised prone play encourages earlier motor milestone attainment in supine sleepers.[116]

Head molding (i.e., bilateral flattening of the head and elongation of the face) is a significant problem in preterm infants; it results from flattening of the skull as it lies against the firm incubator mattress. To parents this head flattening is concerning, and they may find the infant less cute and desirable than a term infant with a rounded head. To prevent head molding, preterm infants are often placed on water beds, water pillows, or air or Eggcrate mattresses, with varying results.[86,89,165,276,461] Preterm infants (less than 32 weeks' gestation with birth weight less than 1500 g) who are turned every 3 hours, repositioned in one of six positions, and never placed in the same position twice in 8 hours had significantly rounder head shapes from 9 to 13 weeks of life than infants repositioned according to a standard NICU procedure.[232]

A combination of vestibular and tactile stimulation increases quieting behaviors, decreases apneic and bradycardic episodes, entrains respirations, increases visual and auditory fixation, and increases brain growth.[272,273,449] Waterbeds provide contingent stimuli, because they move in response to the infant's movement; oscillating waterbeds provide rhythmic motion. Kinesthetic stimulation is provided by rocking chairs, hammocks, baby swings, and baby carriers whose effects have not been investigated. Upright positioning in a car seat or infant seat encourages symmetry and spatial orientation. Soft rolls or foam padding maintains flexion; a rolled blanket in a horseshoe configuration around the infant's head and shoulders prevents lateral slouching.[394] Carrying quiets the infant, provides sensory communication with the caregiver, changes the infant's environment, and provides visual and auditory as well as tactile stimuli. A nasal cannula (see Chapter 23) and portable tank enable mobility for an infant receiving oxygen.

Rather than standardized protocols, tactile interventions must be individualized by assessing each infant's physiologic and behavioral responses before, during, and after touch (see Table 13-7). **While an infant is acutely ill, tactile intervention should** include (1) minimal handling, (2) containment, and (3) gentle touch (without stroking). As the infant matures and becomes physiologically stable, stroking, rocking, and holding are integrated based on the individual infant's tolerance and preferences. In healthy preterm infants a program of range-of-motion exercises with passive resistance, 5 to 10 minutes daily, 5 days a week is associated with an increase in weight gain, bone mass, and density and a decreased risk of osteopenia.[375]

Co-bedding. Co-bedding, the practice of placing medically stable twins and higher order multiples together in the same open warmer, incubator, or crib, was initiated after the observed stress response in separated siblings. Postulated advantages of co-bedding are (1) improved stability of temperature, heart rate, and respirations (i.e., fewer episodes of apnea and bradycardia, better temperature regulation), (2) enhanced physiologic status: improved rates of growth (better weight gain) and development, (3) decreased length of hospitalization and thus cost effectiveness, (4) improved parent-infant bonding and easier transition to home, and (5) improved staff-parent communication, individual care, and teaching of the family.[174,313,314]

The major reluctance to co-bed is the potential risk of increased infection rates. To date, increased infection rates in co-bedded infants have not been reported. Infection concerns are addressed by good handwashing and color coding of equipment. Other safety concerns include proper identification for medication administration and medical emergencies and maintenance of temperature stability for all co-bedded infants. Nesting and swaddling infants together and close monitoring of ambient temperature are necessary to achieve and maintain stable temperatures. Choosing medically stable infants (i.e., infants not requiring ventilator, CPAP, or oxygen hood therapy) and separating infants if one or more become unstable may prevent potential morbidity from co-bedding.[174,313,314]

The practice of co-bedding has spread based on anecdotal information, because there is limited research to support or refute its use. In a recent study of seven sets of preterm twins (less than 37 weeks' gestation), the only physiologic parameter that was changed by co-bedding was the occurrence of apnea. The decrease in apneic episodes may be caused either by a change in sleep pattern (i.e., more frequent arousal by the co-bedded twin) or a more regular breathing pattern reflective of a positive

physiologic response to skin-to-skin contact between the twins.[519] Another study found that co-bedded infants were placed in open cribs sooner (a mean of 6.44 days), had a shorter length of stay (a mean of 3.2 days), and weighed less (an average of 90 g) at discharge than controls.[303] Co-bedded multiples showed no statistically significant difference in improvement in growth, physiologic stability, or adverse events during hospitalization.[303] Clearly, the practice of co-bedding needs RCT to establish its safety and efficacy.[319]

Auditory Intervention
The NICU is a noisy environment that has no diurnal rhythm; it is as noisy at night as in the daytime* (Table 13-12). A NICU infant is exposed to an onslaught of noise 24 hours a day for days, weeks, or months. At follow-up, preterm infants exhibit a lower threshold for sound.[248] Neonatal illnesses, drug therapies, and possibly acoustic insult account for the increased risk (i.e., 10% to 12% of LBW) for sensorineural hearing loss in NICU infants (regardless of gestational age).[28,198,285,356] An increased risk of sensorineural hearing loss in VLBW infants is related to more than 90 days of oxygen therapy, a maximum Fio_2 of 0.90, minimum plasma Na less than 125 mm/L, or maximum pH above 7.60.[289] In another study, moderate to severe conductive hearing loss occurred in 42% of VLBW infants.[524]

The first goal in auditory intervention is to assess the current level of noise in the NICU† and to decrease the noise decibels wherever possible.[198,409] The noise environment of an individual infant depends on the ambient sounds in the nursery, on the type of incubator and support equipment, and on the baby's own behavior (i.e., quiet or crying). Noise measurement protocols must sample multiple noise sources and sites. Sources of noise include heating, ventilation, and air-conditioner flow units (noise levels may decrease by 2.5 to 10.5 dBA when these units are turned off).[11,439] The greatest contributor to loud noise in the NICU is talking and conversation by the staff.‡ Noise levels vary with location, time of day, and day of week within the NICU, so that various locations or various times and days should be measured.[385,440a,497]

Increased environmental noise levels are a stressor to all NICU infants—preterm as well as ill term

---

*References 120, 195, 408, 440, 439, 497.
†References 26, 198, 201, 407, 440a.
‡References 137, 198, 302, 440, 440a, 497.

Table 13-12	NOISE LEVELS IN THE NICU
LEVEL (dB)	**COMMENTS**
48-69	Humidifiers and nebulizers[367]
50-60	Normal speaking voice
50-73.5*†	Incubator (motor noise)
53	Median noise level on conventional ventilator[54]
55-88	Bradycardia alarm
58-85‡	Noise in NICU (talking, equipment alarms, telephones, radio)
59	Median noise level on high frequency oscillator[54]
65-80†	Life support equipment (ventilator, IV pumps)
66-76	Sink on/off
67	Incubator alarm
70	Background noise mean level should not exceed[26]
85	Noise level at which hearing damage is possible for adult; (?) neonatal effects
90	Peak sound intensity in NICU should not exceed[26]
90§	Adult exposure for 8 hours requires protective device and hearing conservation program
92.8†	Opening incubator porthole
84-108	Placing a plastic bottle of formula on top of the incubator
96-117†	Placing a glass bottle of formula on top of incubator
70-116†	Closing one or both cabinet doors
80-124†	Closing one or both portholes
120	Threshold for pain[201]
130-140†	Banging incubator to stimulate apneic premature infant
160-165	Recommendations for peak, single noise level not to exceed to prevent (adult) hearing loss; (?) neonatal effects

Modified from Mitchell SA: Noise pollution in the neonatal nursery, *Semin Hear* 5:17, 1984; Thomas KA: How the NICU environment sounds to a preterm infant, *Am J Matern Child Nurs* 14:249, 1989.
*Modern incubators generate <60 dBA; exceeds hourly recommendation of 50 dBA (see Table 13-13).
†Measures from inside the incubator.
‡Noise levels do not vary from morning to night.
§Occupational Safety and Health Administration (OSHA) standard. (No safety standards for neonates have been established.)

Box 13-6	EFFECTS OF LOUD NOISE*

Increase in stress behaviors
  State lability
  Arousal state
  Avoidance behaviors—more fussy, more startles, etc. (see Table 13-8)
Decrease in approach behaviors (see Table 13-8)
Cardiorespiratory changes
  Increased heart rate
  Increased respiratory rate
  Increased apnea or bradycardia
  Increased hypoxemia (decreased pulse oximeter)
  Increased peripheral and arterial vasoconstriction
    Increased systemic blood pressure
    Increased intracranial pressure
  Increased sensory neural hearing loss
  Abnormal auditory development
  Prevents habituation
Alters development of sleep-wake cycles
  Disturbs sleep; interrupts light sleep
  Increases wakefulness
Increased risk of intraventricular hemorrhage
  Increase in cerebral blood flow

*References 36, 80, 88, 98, 189, 190, 192, 198, 255, 302, 306, 372, 396, 405-407, 409, 450, 563, 564, 565.

not only to the infants but also to parents and care providers in the NICU.[440a] Three years after their NICU experience mothers recall the noise level in the NICU as a stressor.[544] NICU noise is stressful to care providers and has the potential to damage hearing, cause physiologic responses (e.g., increase blood pressure, alter immune response, increase stress hormone secretion, disturb sleep), cause fatigue, irritability, "burnout," interfere with communication with co-workers and parents, alter concentration, and increase errors.[516]

Although the AAP recommends that noise levels be below 45 dBA,[26] most NICUs' noise levels range from 38 dBA to 75 dBA,[405,407] or 57 to 90 dBA,[406] with higher noise bursts (see Table 13-12). To protect sleep, support stable vital signs, and improve speech intelligibility, recommended standards for noise criteria have been established.[101,408] **Table 13-13 presents the research basis for specific noise criteria.** Parents and care providers must be involved in planning and developing quiet hospital nurseries.[144]

Strategies to minimize external auditory stimuli include quieting alarms with suction (and remembering to reset them); not taking a shift report over, or allowing medical rounds near, the infant's incubator

infants (e.g., infants with persistent pulmonary hypertension of the newborn [PPHN] or drug withdrawal) (Box 13-6). The sudden high-pitched, shrill, dysrhythmic noise of equipment alarms alerts the care provider but it also results in infants manifesting an extreme hypersensitivity to sound (as a learned conditioned response).[248] **Noise is stressful**

Table 13-13	RATIONALE FOR SPECIFIC NOISE CRITERIA: RESEARCH BASIS[408]	
NOISE CRITERIA	**RATIONALE**	**RESEARCH**
Hourly Leq (equivalent sound level) of 50 dBA	Preserves sleep for healthy term infants most of the time.	<5% infants disturbed or awakened by 12 min. of noise at 50 dBA[171]
Hourly L₁₀ of 55 dBA (sound levels may exceed 55 dBA only 10% of the time or a total of 6 min/hr)	Preserves sleep for infants. Enables caregivers to speak at normal conversational levels and be clearly understood 12 feet away, approximately 90% of the time.	5% of infants disturbed/awakened by 55 dB; 20% infants disturbed/awakened by 60 dB[171] Term newborn wakened from light sleep by a mean sound level of 55 dB[541]
L$_{max}$ of 70 dBA (maximum decibel sound level ≤1 sec in duration—transient bursts of noise)	Minimizes rousing babies and causing startle responses.	25% infants disturbed/awakened by 65 dB; 45% infants disturbed/awakened at 70 dB; startle reflex at 70-75 dB[171] 55% infants startled 2% of time by 55 dBA; 78% infants startled 10% of time by 70 dBA; 100% startled 25% of time by 85 dBA[489] Infant wakened from a light sleep: 40% of time by 2 min at 78 dBA against a 58-dBA ambient background[358] Term infant in deep sleep wakened by 2-5 sec pure tones at 70-75 dB

(one study shows no difference in noise levels during rounds/report[440a]); having noisy equipment repaired immediately; emptying sloshing water in ventilator or nebulizer tubing; maintaining cardiac monitors in a quiet state with alarms on and purchasing quieter equipment.* Choosing heated humidifiers (48 dB) rather than nebulizers (69 dB) and keeping the containers full of water, rather than low, decreases noise from respiratory equipment.[367] Nursery design changes include smaller cubicles rather than one large room, soundproofing materials, lights for phones and alarm systems, and minimizing equipment noise. Placing a blanket on top of the incubator or using an incubator cover muffles the noise of equipment placement; gentle, considerate (to the infant) placement of equipment on or in the incubator muffles sound; and closing portholes and drawers gently decreases the structural noises of caregiving. Prohibiting placement of equipment (e.g., clipboards, stethoscopes, formula bottles) on top of the incubator prevents such noises.

No tapping (by parents or siblings) or banging (by medical, nursing, or ancillary personnel) on the incubator Plexiglas should ever be permitted. This (along with a brisk startle reflex from the infant) is an opportunity to teach about the noise levels generated by such activity. Infants should be kept in in-

cubators as long as necessary to maintain heat balance. **Older incubators do *not* protect the infant from noise—a well-managed NICU environment may be much quieter than the continuous noise of an incubator. Noise in modern incubators varies according to incubator model.**[54,440] Sound sources within an incubator include its motor, infant sounds, equipment sounds inside the incubator, equipment sounds transmitted from outside the incubator, and ambient nursing noise (e.g., personnel and phones).[440] **Modern incubator walls attenuate impulse noises from the NICU and may decrease the infant's noise exposure.**[54,137,440] Inside modern incubators, motor noise does not exceed 60 dBA,[440] but this level exceeds the more recent recommendation of 50 dBA.[101,406] However, impulse noises from the incubator (i.e., doors, latches) are louder on the inside of the incubator (see Table 13-12). Prolonged stays in an incubator not only expose the infant to repeated caregiving noises, but also mean there will be a dearth of kinesthetic stimulation (e.g., carrying, holding, rocking, swinging, and sitting upright in an infant seat) and socially relevant speech patterns. Both the internal noise generated by the incubator and how well the incubator attenuates external noise should be considered in incubator purchases.[54,101,440]

Conductive hearing loss is attributed to endotracheal intubation, poor eustachian tube function, and increased otitis media in preterm in-

*References 53, 54, 101, 408, 439, 440.

fants. Noise levels in the NICU may interfere with development of other sensory systems and influence the development of hearing and language delay.[405,407] Radios have been banned in many NICUs. If music is played, it should be on a low volume (below the dB range of normal speech), should not be rock music, and preferably should be classical (infants prefer Brahms, Bach, and Beethoven). Full-term newborns exposed to soothing music spend less time in high arousal states and had fewer behavioral state changes.[258] Full-term infants with bronchopulmonary dysplasia/chronic lung disease (BPD/CLD) and agitation were more able to calm themselves after a stressful procedure while listening to music.[83] Day-night cycles (nap time; nighttime) when auditory stimulation is decreased should be established in the NICU.[56] Institution of a quiet time or rest period through reduction of (1) noise from talking, equipment, telephones, and so on; (2) light by dimming overhead light; and (3) procedures to only emergency treatment has resulted in enhanced infant sleep (from 34% to 85%), less crying (from 14% to 2.4%) and less parental and caregiver stress.[497] On discharge NICU infants often will not sleep[560] in a quiet room. Softly playing a radio facilitates sleep, and the infant is gradually weaned from it. Signs such as "Quiet . . . baby sleeping" or "Do not disturb—I'm asleep (talk to my nurse)" ensure undisturbed sleep—provided they are heeded.

The "in-turning" premature infant (see Table 13-4) of less than 34 weeks' gestation probably receives enough auditory input from the NICU—auditory enhancement at this stage is probably overstimulation. Just as high-frequency sounds arouse, low-frequency ones, such as the heartbeat, respiratory sounds, and vacuum cleaners, quiet and facilitate sleep.[128,214,406] One study showed less behavioral response and less salivary cortisol release by infants who were presented with a heartbeat sound or white noise (both at 85 dB) during and after heelstick.[261]

Although music has been shown to sooth full-term babies, the use of music with preterm infants has not been well studied. Presentation of in utero sounds and a female voice to agitated, intubated preterm infants has resulted in improved oxygen saturation and behavioral states.[100,288] Although the use of tape recordings of music or family voices has been advocated and widely practiced, some investigators have recently recommended that such recordings not be used. Among the reasons cited against the use of recordings are that their benefits and long-term consequences have not been established, their use places a nonresponsive machine between a caring person and the preterm infant, and recordings may replace exposure of the preterm to the contingent human voice.[198,407] However, if used with preterm infants, auditory stimuli should be (1) kept at a reasonable distance from the infant's ear (never use earphones); placed inside/outside the incubator, (2) played at levels below 55 dBA, (3) played for brief periods, and (4) used if the infant is soothed and discontinued if infant becomes stressed, restless, or agitated.[198] However, because preterm infants are less able to habituate to sound than term babies, they may be unable to tolerate any added sound and may become exhausted by such stimuli.[405]

The human voice is the most preferred sound.[159,406] **The preterm in an incubator may be isolated from important exposure to his mother's voice.** The degree of attenuation of the higher frequency of mother's voice by the lower frequency of incubator noise, the incubator walls and the ambient noise of the NICU has not been measured.[440]

Teach parents the neonate's preference for high-pitched voices speaking in typical speech patterns (not baby talk). Role model and teach parents to gently talk to the infant while touching and giving care.[198,407] Teach parents to talk to their infant while presenting their faces in the infant's range of vision. Many explanations for the preference of mothers to cradle their babies on their left side have been postulated (i.e., hand dominance, importance of maternal heartbeat, left breast sensitivity, and advantage in monitoring the infant). A more recent hypothesis proposes that maternal affective signals (both auditory and visual) are given to the infant's free left ear and are processed by the more advanced right cerebral hemisphere.[479] Watch for infant tolerance and increase or decrease talk time to avoid overload. Imitate the infant's coos and babbles—this reinforces and encourages vocalizations.

For a neonate, hearing is more important than vision for attachment and bonding to the parents.[294] **Within seconds after birth, newborns are able to discriminate and prefer their mother's face—they have connected her familiar voice with her unfamiliar face.**[66] A high index of suspicion regarding hearing loss is warranted if caregivers do not observe normal responses to sound stimulation. All newborns, especially those with a history of familial hearing loss; hyperbilirubinemia (total serum bilirubin level greater than 15 mg in a preterm infant; greater than 20 mg in a term infant); congenital viral infections; defects of the ear, nose, and throat; small preterm infants (less than 1500 g); those with bacterial sepsis or meningitis; severe asphyxia at birth, prolonged (more than 10 days) mechanical ventilation, stigmata, and other syndromes; and those receiving ototoxic drugs are at increased risk of hearing loss.[30]

Because screening by these high-risk factors alone identifies only about 50% of newborns with significant hearing loss,[28,30] universal newborn hearing screening is the standard of care.[28] The first population-based study on the association between congenital hearing impairment and birth weight in the United States showed an increase in the incidence of sensorineural loss with a decrease in birth weight (i.e., infants of less than 1500 g had the highest risk and an increased risk of coexisting developmental delays), a higher rate was found in black male infants of less than 2500 g, and approximately 19% of all childhood cases of preschool congenital hearing loss were associated with low birth weight.[533] The children in this study were born between 1981 and 1990. Another study of children born between 1995 and 1997 showed no increased incidences of hearing loss resulting from low birth weight or prematurity, with a 50% incidence of high-risk infants having pathologic hearing screens.[356] This change in incidence of hearing loss may be because of different study methods, different populations, and/or the influence of quieter, more developmentally appropriate NICUs.

Visual Intervention
The NICU is lit with bright, cool-white fluorescent lights 24 hours a day. Light levels vary between and within various NICUs.[184] There is a trend toward decreasing NICU illumination: a 1990 study showed a range from 400 to 1000 lux during the day to 50 to 100 lux at night[441]; a more recent study showed 184 lux during the day and 34 lux at night.[81] However, the light levels in the LIGHT-ROP study were 399 and 447 lux, with and without goggles.[434] **The amount of light to which the preterm infant is exposed is influenced by (1) location in the NICU, (2) seasonal/climatic variations, (3) use of phototherapy, (4) opthalmoscopic exams (e.g., at birth and for ROP follow-up), and (5) infant related factors (e.g., maturity and amount of eye opening, head position, eye shielding).[158]** Ambient light levels in the NICU should be adjustable through a range of 10 to 600 lux (approximately 1 to 60 foot-candles) at every bedside.[29,101] Other light recommendations for newly built NICUs are outlined in Table 13-14.

Although decreased light levels and response to bright light have not been shown to reduce the incidence of ROP, ophthalmic sequelae of preterm birth are common (see Chapter 23 for a discussion of ROP). The three broad categories of ophthalmic sequelae are (1) decreased visual function, (2) strabismus, and (3) eye size (arrested growth) and refractive state (increased myopia).[158] In addition, there is abundant animal, child, and adult research documenting negative biochemical and physical effects (change in endocrine function, increased hypocalcemia, cell transformations, immature gonadal development, and chromosome breakage).[195] **Exposure to bright lights in the NICU is associated with (1) decreased oxygenation, (2) increased incidence of retinopathy, (3) poorer circadian rhythms, (4) altered sleep patterns, (5) skin changes (e.g., tanning, rashes), and (6) alteration of nutrients in total parenteral nutrition**

Table 13-14	LIGHT RECOMMENDATIONS IN THE NICU[29,101]
ILLUMINATION LEVEL	**PURPOSE**
High levels: 60-100 foot-candles	Evaluate and assess skin color and perfusion.
Lower levels: 10-20 foot-candles	Recommendations of Illuminating Engineering Society[295]—safe and adequate. Because of concerns over retinal/ocular damage from continuous exposure to high levels (60-100 foot-candles)
Nighttime levels: 0.5 foot-candles	Diurnal variation in light levels
Procedure light	Available at every bedside to temporarily increase lighting for infant assessment/procedure without increasing light exposure to all other babies.
Support areas	For charting, medication preparation, etc., should provide adequate and separate light to accommodate sleeping babies and working health care providers.
Daylight	One source visible from care areas for its psychologic benefit for staff and families.

(TPN) solution, formula, and breast milk.[*] Rapid increase in the intensity of ambient light causes a decrease in oxygen saturation in younger, mature preterm infants.

The first goal in visual intervention is to assess the current level of light and decrease it wherever possible. A very immature preterm infant is accustomed to the muted light of the uterus—light filtered through the abdominal and uterine walls—and has fused eyelids (if the infant is less than 26 weeks' gestation). Draping blankets on top of the incubator or using a commercial incubator cover[506] decreases the light at the infant's level but allows immediate maximal illumination when the cover is pulled back. Because infants are continuously monitored, not all infants need to be maximally illuminated at all times.[195]

Cycled light, dimming the lights in day-night cycles, is associated with positive effects (Box 13-7). The Stanford cycled light trials consisted of a comparison of the development of circadian rhythms in two groups of preterm infants: (1) a dim

---

[*]References 22, 69, 75, 110, 153, 169, 174.

Box 13-7	EFFECTS OF CYCLED LIGHT[*]

Behavior
  Decreases movement or motor activity
  Increases motor coordination
  Increases sleep time
  Decreases crying
  More eye opening
Cardiorespiratory changes
  Decreases heart rate
  Decreases respiratory rate
Feeding behavior
  Quicker progression to oral feedings
  Feeds more efficiently and in less time
  Increased weight gain
Circadian rhythm development
  Melatonin
  Temperature
  Heart rate
Decreased cortisol levels
Decreased incidence and severity of retinopathy of
  prematurity (ROP)
Decreased parental or care provider stress
Decreased infant handling and noise levels

---

[*] References 56, 180, 213, 264, 319, 343, 358, 402, 442, 475, 497, 506, 554.

---

group—incubator or crib covered with a thick blanket except during feeding or other interventions and (2) a cycled group—exposed to a regular light-dark cycle (e.g., a covered incubator/crib from 7 PM to 7 AM). At 36 weeks' postconceptual age, or 1 month and 3 months' corrected age, there was a significant maturation in circadian rhythms of both temperature and sleep, but neither was benefited by cycled light. The researchers concluded that these circadian rhythms in preterm infants develop endogenously as a factor of postconceptual age (e.g., maturation), independent of prematurity and/or environmental intervention.[364] Despite their findings, these researchers, citing sufficient data (see Box 13-7) and recommendations in the current AAP/ACOG Guidelines for Perinatal Care[29] to introduce regular day-night cycles, state that "there is no rationale for continuing a chaotic noncircadian environmental approach in the neonatal nursery for the care of the prematurely born infant."[364]

Visual attentiveness is correlated with birth weight and gestational age: the more mature the infant, the more the infant is able to fix and follow. An infant at 28 weeks' gestation fixes and follows but may become apneic as a result. Visual stimulation is very tiring and taxing (increases the heart rate) for the immature infant: those of less than 34 weeks' gestation probably receive enough stimulation from the NICU environment. When these infants reach the "coming-out stage" (see Table 13-4), they may signal their readiness for visually enhancing activities.

Infants receiving phototherapy are deprived of visual sensory stimuli because of their protective eye pads. These should be removed during care and feeding and interaction with parents and professionals. Providing interesting visual stimuli includes inanimate objects (e.g., toys, black and white faces and patterns, pictures of family members, artwork from siblings, and mobiles) and animate objects (faces of parents, siblings, and professionals) (Figure 13-7). Infants prefer the human face as a visual stimulus, especially the talking face, which stimulates both visual and auditory pathways. Parents often need to be encouraged that their faces and voices, rather than all the infant's toys, are what their infant prefers to watch and listen to.

Teach parents the abilities of the infant and appropriate methods of visual stimulation:
- Place mobiles, pictures, and faces within the visual range of the newborn—8 to 12 inches for term infants, a little closer for preterm infants.

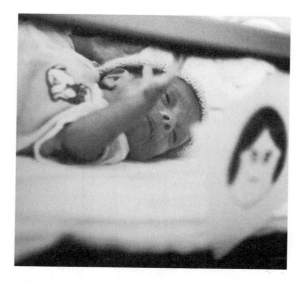

FIGURE 13-7 Premature infant fixing on a black-and-white face

- Quiet alert is the best state for visual encounters—after feedings, if awake; swaddle the infant to quiet or unwrap the infant to arouse; hold infant upright.
- Place the infant on the abdomen with objects of various sizes and shapes within visual range.
- Change toys and visual stimuli—infants become bored with the same thing.
- When the preterm infant tolerates multiple stimuli, hold him or her in *en face* position (see Chapter 29) to feed, talk to, and rock. Whether the infant is nipple or gavage fed, alternate sides so the infant sees both sides of the care provider's face (especially important if the preterm infant exhibits the common preference for right-sided head turning).
- Place the infant at varied heights (in a baby carrier, crib, swing, infant seat, on the floor) so the infant sees the world from various angles.
- Place the infant so that he or she is able to bring the hands to midline and can the see hands and fingers and eventually reach for toys.

Infants who exhibit gaze aversion should not be "pursued" by the face of the parent or professional, because this only potentiates the time "spent away" with their gaze to protect themselves from overload. Gaze aversion, flat facial affect, and absence of a smile may cast doubt on the ability of these infants to see, because there is no eye language or caregiver feedback of preference, recognition, and delight. These infants *do* see, but they fix only fleetingly. Minimizing the number of care providers is crucial for these babies so that the infant deals with as few caregiver cues, styles, and ways of being handled as possible.

Smell/Taste Intervention

The neonate's well-developed sense of smell is not stimulated in the NICU with pleasant odors. A high-risk infant is stimulated by the smell of forgotten alcohol, skin prep, or povidone-iodine (Betadine) pads inside the incubator. Because a premature infant is unable to respond by crying or moving away, **the infant responds to noxious smells by a decrease in respiratory rate, transient apnea, and/or an increase in heart rate.** Removal of noxious odors from the incubator is as critical as removal of sharp instruments after a procedure. Even the smell of NICU detergent is detected, elicits a response that differs from the response to a pleasant odor, and decreases cerebral blood flow to the right hemisphere.[47]

Enhancing the olfactory environment includes having parents hold the infant, or sit close if the infant cannot yet be held. The smell of the mother's breast milk is especially pleasant and elicits more suckling than the smell of formula.[1] Olfactory stimulation of sucking in preterm infants increases with increasing postnatal age.[1] Placing a drop of milk on the infant's lips with a cotton ball or gauze sponge helps the infant to recognize the mother's smell[534] and to associate that smell with food and feeding when the infant is able to nipple feed.

Nonnutritive suckling (during gavage and between feedings) is associated with better oxygenation; quieter, more restful behavior; increased readiness for nipple feedings; decreased tension and increased insulin and gastrin secretion that may stimulate digestion and storage of nutrients; and decreased length of hospital stay. Sucking on a pacifier satisfies the infant's sucking needs and may facilitate early learning that satiety and sucking are associated. However, nutritive and nonnutritive suckling are not alike (see Chapter 19); the fact that an infant vigorously sucks on a pacifier does not mean the infant will be able to suckle nutritively, because the expressive and swallow phases have not been present in nonnutritive suckling, and coordination of suck, swallow, and breathing[102,281]

---

*References 38, 122, 139, 166, 187, 199, 321, 335, 358, 410-412, 416, 419, 460, 521, 562.

has not been necessary. This is very confusing to most parents and many professionals.

High-risk infants often undergo prolonged periods during which an NPO[38] status has been ordered, and during these times their sensation of hunger is not relieved. Although pacifiers are soothing, these infants may learn that sucking and satiety are not related. NICU infants also undergo many aversive stimuli around and within the mouth[492] (e.g., oral intubation, oral and endotracheal tube suction, and intermittent gavage) that result in touch aversion of the mouth and a hypersensitive gag reflex. Feeding difficulties may result from the following:

- Neurologic damage (e.g., IVH).[38,40,108,109,181]
- Structural abnormalities[40,181,281,462,492] (e.g., cleft palate or submucous cleft, recessed chin).
- Prematurity: the infant is too neurologically immature and tires easily with "work" of feeding. **Neural maturation (34 to 35 weeks' gestation) is the developmental guideline for initiation of oral feedings**[38,265,287] **(see Table 13-2), although some infants are ready at an earlier age (30 to 34 weeks' gestation)* (see Table 19-4). Maturation of feeding skills occurs because of developmental changes in the CNS, coupled with experiential learning.†** However, preterm infants may exhibit periods of apnea and tachypnea with bottlefeeding, because consistent coordination of breathing with sucking and swallowing does not occur until 37 weeks' gestation[38,82] (see Table 13-2).
- Aversive feeder[40,181] (acquired or developmental sucking defect, psychologic—"hospitalitis," rumination).
- A combination of these types.‡

Preterm infants may not be at risk for chronic feeding problems if they are changed from nonoral methods (TPN and tube feeding) to oral methods by the end of the first month of life.[265] Severe behavioral eating difficulties are associated with prematurity, low birth weight, distress during feeding in the first 6 months of life, and regular or frequent vomiting.[125] Aversive feeding experiences may be the basis for early childhood eating difficulties.[125]

Because criteria for discharge include full oral feedings with adequate weight gain,[27] transition to full oral feedings is being investigated. **Longer transition time to full oral feedings is signifi-**

cantly influenced by (1) apnea, (2) birth weight/ gestational age, (3) younger age at first oral feeding, (4) BPD/CLD, (5) number of days being tube fed/receiving ventilatory therapy, and (6) desaturations of oxygen with feeding.*** Shorter transition time to complete oral feeding is associated with (1) greater weight and (2) older postconceptual age at initiation of nipple feeding.[82,287,318,421] Postconceptual age at first nippling indicates that neurodevelopmental maturation (e.g., state arousal, neuromotor skills, and respiratory control) is a factor in transition time.[108,109,287,421-424]

For infants with BPD/CLD, the more days receiving positive pressure ventilation and supplemental oxygen, the older (in PCA) the infant when he or she is first fully nipple fed.[424] For these infants transition time to full nipple feeding may be lengthened because of the increased work of breathing[2] and the precedence of breathing (at an increased rate) over feeding.[373] This study also showed an association between length of time to full enteral feeding (but not full nipple feeding) and mental (but not motor) developmental delays at 24 months.[373] Surprisingly, in this same study severe intracranial pathologic conditions such as grade 3 and 4 IVH and PVL did not influence the length of time needed to reach full enteral and full nipple feedings.[373]

The goals of intervention include (1) a safe feeding (i.e., diminished risk of aspiration); (2) a functional feeding (i.e., adequate caloric intake for optimal growth and development[282,492] **with minimal energy expenditure); and (3) a pleasant, social interactive experience for the infant and parents or caregivers. Box 13-8 outlines intervention strategies to facilitate oral feeding.**

The use of individualized developmental care may assist VLBW and preterm infants with BPD/ CLD in obtaining/maintaining an optimal condition for progression to oral feedings. **Use of skin-to-skin kangaroo care improves weight gain, supports and promotes breastfeeding, and shortens length of stay (see Box 13-3).** In one study the use of developmental care enabled VLBW preterm infants to initiate the first oral feeding and have the last gavage feeding at an earlier age than VLBW infants not receiving developmental care.[51] Another study

---

*References 38, 84, 187, 209, 283, 287, 347, 350, 351.
†References 108, 109, 281, 349, 413, 492.
‡References 38, 40, 177, 178, 181, 282.

*References 318, 373, 413, 423, 471, 476.

Box 13-8   **STRATEGIES TO FACILITATE ORAL FEEDING**

I. Minimize noxious stimuli to the mouth
  A. Suction only as needed (not routinely)
  B. Consider indwelling gastric tube rather than intermittent gavage (an infant fed every 2 hours would have gavage tube passed 12 times a day)
  C. Pass intermittent gavage tube
    1. Down mouth through hole in pacifier nipple
    2. If infant has hypersensitive gag, passing smaller tube down nose stimulates gag reflex less than passing tube down mouth
  D. Perioral and intraoral stimulation techniques[38]
    1. Are only *more aversive*, rather than therapeutic, on babies with touch aversion at mouth area
    2. When performing oral exercises, do so with care—do not stimulate aversive reflexes (e.g., gag reflex)

II. Enhance pleasant stimuli to the mouth (first experiences with suckling have lasting neurobehavioral effects[114])
  A. Have infant smell or taste breast milk[1,534]
  B. Provide nonnutritive suckling with tube feeding
  C. Facilitate hand-to-mouth behaviors
  D. Nipple with proper flow rate.[330] If flow rate too fast—increased flow, stimulates anxiety and/or gag reflex, and causes bradycardia—promotes incoordination. If flow rate is too slow—increased fatigue and frustration; inadequate consumption/growth failure.[38]
  E. Perioral and intraoral stimulation—(?) facilitates development of normal sucking behaviors
  F. Use Lact-Aid nursing supplementer (see Chapter 19)
    1. Never frustrate infant with a dry breast
    2. Positive reinforcement for infant to nurse

    3. Calorically and energy efficient method
    4. Oral therapy—teaches infant proper nutritive suckle
  G. For infants with difficulty in coordination of respiration with suck or swallow (prevents stress of apnea and hypoxia and enhances pleasure of feeding experience)[320,462] (see Chapter 19)
    1. Assess feeding pattern (e.g., continuous or intermittent suck), pulse oximeter, muscle tone, breathing pattern, heart rate
    2. Remove nipple from mouth to enable infant to breathe[470]
    3. Begin breastfeeding before bottlefeeding (see Table 19-4)
    4. Use of orthodontic nipple results in physiologic stability and more effective feeding behavior in some infants.[126]

III. Positioning—use proper position to facilitate swallow and improve suction—symmetric positioning with predominance of flexion.[181]
  A. Hold with feedings (even gavage) as much as possible
  B. Consistent caregivers[530]—parents, primary nurses, foster grandparents
  C. Swaddle
    1. Decreases startles
    2. Infant may become too warm and sleepy
  D. Facilitate swallowing
    1. Position with chin tucked
    2. If breastfeeding, turn infant's whole body toward mother so head and trunk are in alignment (infant is not trying to swallow with head turned to one side)

---

showed that preterm infants successfully completing oral feeding spent significantly more time in awake states than preterm infants who were unsuccessful in their feeding.[336]

Using developmental principles, health care providers are able to facilitate both the preterm infant and parents in effective feeding experiences. **A self-regulating preterm infant shows signs of stability during feeding: (1) smooth, regular respirations (no or minimal increase in respiratory rate/effort), (2) consistent postural control—flexed, hands near face, maintains muscle tone, calm/organized behavior, (3) maintains optimal color, (4) quiet, alert state, focuses on feeding, and (5) coordinates suck-swallow-breathe.**[287,466] Coordination of feeding is facilitated by (1) im-

posing breaks (e.g., removing the nipple from the mouth; tipping the bottle so that the nipple is empty but remains in the infant's mouth), (2) limiting bolus size (the fewer the number of sucks, the smaller the bolus size) by limiting the number of successive sucks before the infant becomes stressed, and (3) slowing the flow rate (e.g., using low-flow rate nipples[126,330] and upright positioning to decrease hydrostatic pressure and gravitational flow).[181,281,466]

Signs of stress during nipple feeding, their significance, and appropriate interventions are listed in Table 13-15. Parents must be taught how to interpret their infant's cues of stability and stress so that they can modify their behavior and learn to intervene to help their infant safely and successfully

Box 13-8	STRATEGIES TO FACILITATE ORAL FEEDING—cont'd

3. Upright position with neck, shoulders, and back supported[38]—slows gravitational flow[251] of formula from nipple (as when infant is in semireclined position); restricted milk flow (e.g., milk flows only with active sucking, not with gravity) beneficial (e.g., more efficient; more volume obtained)[281,283]
4. Cuddling, semireclined position—increases flow of formula by gravity[251]—may be too fast, regardless of nipple chosen; results in increased gags, choking, and bradycardia
5. Prone with neck extended (slightly)
    a. Keeps tongue forward and airway unobstructed
    b. Good for aversive feeder who chokes
6. Gentle, upward pressure under chin (chin support) or at base of tongue facilitates swallowing, because it mimics upward thrust of tongue with swallowing
E. Improve formation of suction
    1. Semireclining (greater than 45-degree angle) on lap of caregiver—frees both hands to work with infant on oral control
    2. Cupping both cheeks (cheek support) with fingers of free hand (i.e., hand not holding bottle) improves lip closure and suction formation[557]
    3. Gentle tugging at nipple (as if to take it out of mouth) may smooth and strengthen suck[38]
IV. Timing
    A. Do not allow infant to cry to exhaustion before feeding—infant will be too tired to eat

B. Keep external stimuli to a minimum in immature preterm infants (<34 weeks) for optimal intake and weight gain
C. If satiated, infant will not suck
    1. Feed on demand or when alert[38] (demand feeding reinforces sleep-wake cycle) and the development of self regulation.[422]
    2. If feeding on schedule, note whether infant gives cue of hunger: fussiness/crying, hand-to-mouth behaviors and/or rooting, hiccups. Infants as young as 32 to 33 weeks can provide cues so that feeding can be individualized.*
    3. If feeding on schedule, space time and see whether infant exhibits cues of hunger (as above).
    4. First, nipple what infant is able to feed; then tube feed (presence of an indwelling nasogastric tube may result in compromised respirations, oxygen desaturation, and bradycardia in the VLBW infant)[470,472]
D. Try to nipple feed for no longer than 20 to 30 minutes (infant becomes too tired and uses up energy and calories to feed instead of to grow)
E. Infants of advanced age (around 6 months) may be unable to nipple if they have never had the opportunity[40,249]; it may be more developmentally appropriate to cup or spoon-feed infant because normal infants begin cup drinking between 6-8 mo of age.[38]

*References 35, 38, 84, 187, 209, 283, 287, 347, 350.

feed.[466,517] For parents, learning to feed their infant is viewed as (1) a significant symbol of parenting, (2) an opportunity to read and react to infant cues, and (3) as a co-regulator of feeding.[517]

A feeding plan must be individualized for each infant and posted at the bedside. All care providers must adhere to the plan for consistency of stimuli and to promote infant learning.

CASE STUDY

Tommy was a 28-week preterm infant with severe RDS, prolonged ventilation, and now BPD. He is now 38 weeks' postconceptual age, receiving hood and nasal cannula oxygen, and trying to learn to nipple feed. In the morning report, the night nurse says that Tommy "has bradycardia with tube passage so that 24 hours ago he had a cardiorespiratory arrest that required resuscitation. He also has bradycardia and tachypnea with bottlefeeding."

Tommy's nurse evaluated his initial attempts to bottlefeed (after waiting for him to demand) and wrote the care plan (Box 13-9) after feeding him 45 ml in 20 minutes without tachypnea, cyanosis, or bradycardia.

Crying/Smiling Intervention
Crying is the infant's innate care-eliciting behavior—a signal that he or she needs attention. The energy expenditure of a crying infant is

Table 13-15	STRESS DURING NIPPLE FEEDING	
SIGN	**SIGNIFICANCE**	**INTERVENTION**
Color change Pallor, dusky, gray, central cyanosis—perioral/periorbital	Oxygen desaturation[181,327,417,476] a. Feeding too rapidly with brief, shallow breaths b. Low hematocrit level c. Breath-holding	Assess baseline color before feeding Periodic removal of nipple to facilitate deep-breathing Monitor changes in color during feeding Use pulse oximeter during feeding to maintain saturation $\geq$92%[225,226]
Changes in state of alertness	Quiet alert state optimal for successful feeding[287,336,465,466] a. Increased infant focus on feeding b. Increased organization of oropharyngeal muscle movements	Offer preterm opportunity to suck on pacifier before feeding—encourages awake/alert behavior[336]
	Increasing drowsiness, falls asleep: a. Respiratory fatigue resulting from rapid feeding, desaturation, increased respiratory rate, and/or work of breathing b. Fatigue resulting from behavior/energy expenditure (e.g., crying; bathing, etc.) before feeding	Pulse oximeter monitoring during feeding—give and/or adjust oxygen to maintain saturations $\geq$92% during nippling efforts Unwrap if sleepy
	Fussiness/restlessness—resulting from oxygen desaturation (e.g., hypoxia) because of the work of breathing and nippling; disorganized behavioral state	Periodic rest periods and pace energy expenditure with nipple feeding Swaddle/rock if fussy
Breathing	Increased respiratory effort resulting from work/exercise of feeding[181,327,467]	
1. Respiratory fatigue[181]: Falls asleep, ceases feeding before adequate volume obtained	Work of breathing (WOB) before feeding is increased further with effort of feeding Infants with poor endurance may be unable to feed or demonstrate poor weight gain despite acceptable intake[181]	Pulse oximeter monitoring with feeding to ensure adequate oxygenation; give oxygen prn to keep sats $\geq$92%
2. Tachypnea Respiratory rate >60/min	WOB increases with feeding; respiratory rate increases with work of feeding[181] Increased incoordination of suck-swallow-breathe with feeding; predisposes to aspiration[181] Increased risk of aspiration if gasping for breath[181]	Brief and/or frequent breaks in feeding to enable deep breaths and to reorganize breathing patterns
3. Nasal flaring	Attempts to increase oxygen intake because of hypoxia and/or increased WOB	Pulse oximeter; supply adequate oxygen Brief breaks to reorganize breathing
Nasal blanching	Distress of breathing/hypoxia Incoordination of suck-swallow-breathe with possible aspiration if flaring/blanching occur	
4. Chin tugging/head bobbing/"catch up" breathing/grunting	Attempting to increase air entry because of "air hunger"/hypoxia/WOB/decreased tidal volume Incoordination of suck-swallow-breathe; increased risk for aspiration[181]	As above

Modified from Shaker C: Nipple feeding preterm infants: an individualized, developmentally supportive approach, *Neonatal Netw* 18 :15, 1999.

Table 13-15	STRESS DURING NIPPLE FEEDING—cont'd	
SIGN	**SIGNIFICANCE**	**INTERVENTION**
5. Crowing sounds—high-pitched stridorous noise on inspiration	Incoordination of opening/closing of vocal cords that increases the risk of aspiration into the trachea[557]	As above
Swallowing 1. Drooling	Primary swallowing dysfunction predisposes to aspiration[181]; swallowing may be evaluated by videofluoroscopy[181] Loss of bolus control due to: a. Inability of tongue to collect and hold fluid that is flowing too fast b. Rapid respiratory rate, excessive WOB that shortens time for swallowing to occur, so that only part of bolus is swallowed	Give fewer sucks in a row, followed by brief break so that bolus is smaller and more able to be completely swallowed
2. Gulping	Use of prolonged sucking pattern or long sucking bursts (especially at the beginning of feeding) without deep breathing at the appropriate intervals[181] Results in oxygen desaturation, bradycardia, apnea resulting from suppression of respiration Increases incoordination of suck-swallow-breathe and stimulates pharyngeal stretch receptors, resulting in vagally stimulated apnea	Give brief breaks to assist the infant in slowing down the feeding
3. Gurgling sounds in the pharynx (breathing sounds are wet/noisy)[181]	Fluid collecting in the throat, pharynx, or supraglottal space above vocal cords Noisy respirations caused by breathing through fluid in hypopharynx because bolus is too large or too fast	Brief break from feeding to enable extra swallow/dry swallow to clear fluid from throat
4. Swallowing (several times) in succession	Deliberate swallows in succession to clear bolus (that is too large/too fast) from pharynx Breathing is delayed with successive swallowing and may result in apnea/bradycardia[329]	Break from feeding to clear throat and regain control of respiration
5. Coughing/choking/gagging/spitting up	Fluid has entered (or nearly entered) the airway[327,328] Changes in color, heart rate, respiratory rate suggest swallowing problems[181] Occurrence toward end of feeding suggests gastroesophageal reflux; frequent or intense spitting up may also indicate reflux[181]	Can usually be prevented by close attention and intervention to previous signs of feeding difficulty Breaks from feeding to clear airway, regain control of respiration and state-organization Ability to cough enables infant to clear airway Inability to cough, color change, hypotonia, bradycardia, and apnea are symptoms of airway obstruction that may require suction and CPR

Box 13-9   TOMMY'S FEEDING PLAN

1. *Sit upright.* This decreases the flow of formula from the bottle and thus decreases
    a. His gag reflex, which causes the bradycardia.
    b. His anxiety caused by a bolus of formula in his mouth.
2. *Use a blue nipple.* This is the shortest nipple and decreases stimulation of his hypersensitive gag reflex, which causes his bradycardia. (All other nipples stimulated him to gag.)
3. *Gently push up under his chin when he gets a mouthful of formula.* This pushes his tongue upward against his palate, the same way the tongue moves during swallowing. (Reader, swallow and watch your tongue motion.) He becomes frightened (i.e., eyes wide open and fearful; increased respiratory rate; arching and struggling) when he has a mouthful of formula, because he is used to only sucking on a dry pacifier and having nothing to swallow. His fear raises his heart rate, his respiratory rate, and his gag reflex, which causes bradycardia.
4. *Talk to him.* Softly and gently, tell him he can swallow and praise him when he does.
5. *Nipple.* Have him do this as much as possible (he will only get better with practice) and supplement feeding with the indwelling NG tube (no more intermittent tube passage).

---

increased by 7.5% compared with the resting state.[428] Immediate response decreases the infant's physiologic stress, increases the infant's trust in the environment, and enhances the sense of self and of control over the world. The infant's need to escalate to "out of control" crying is decreased with immediate response, so that infants are easier to soothe. Consoling the crying infant also helps the infant change states so he or she is able to attend to and interact with the environment.

Term infants vocalize, cry, and look at their caregiver more than do preterm and ill infants.[195] Although preterm infants are more irritable than full-term infants, preterm infants cry less throughout the day than do full-term infants.[239,515] **NICU infants exhibit fewer care-eliciting behaviors (some preterm infants in one study never cried, vocalized, or looked at their caregiver).**[195] Preterm infants are thus less responsive to the caregivers (both parents and professionals), who receive less positive feedback from the infant and hence are less rewarded. In one study those NICU infants who were able to cue the care provider (cry, look, vocalize) were consistently responded to 80% to 100% of the time.[195]

Intubated infants who are unable to produce an au-dible cry signal their needs by agitation, heart rate changes, and changes in oxygenation. Preterm infants (less than 32 weeks' gestation) may recover better from agitation when left alone, because active consolation is overstimulating.[192] How caregivers attempt to soothe a crying infant while giving NICU care includes no response to cries (58.1% of the time), response by talking (29.2% of the time), response by social touching (5.5% of the time), and response by talk and social touching (7.2% of the time).[195]

Parents and staff should use graduated interventions in quieting a crying infant by:

- Soothing with gentle high-pitched talking (loud enough that the infant is able to hear it above his or her crying)
- Placing the palm of the hand across the infant's chest or holding arms on chest with the palm of the care provider's hand
- Swaddling with blankets to decrease self-upsetting startles
- Picking up infant, holding (upright is the most soothing position), and rocking
- Offering a pacifier

Most stimulation in the NICU is procedural. The lack of social stimulation in the NICU not only affects the infant, but also teaches parents that their infant is too weak for, too fragile for, uninterested in, or incapable of social interaction. Again, social stimulation must be paced according to the stage of development and stability of the infant[88,134,135,290] (see Table 13-4). Enhancing the infant's social environment includes presenting the smiling, moving, talking care provider's face to the alert infant; touching and stroking; and soothing and consoling the distressed infant.

In many busy NICUs, parents and a foster grandparent program provide this sensory integrated social experience. If the infant has been transported to a referral center, parents may live some distance away and be unable to visit daily. A chronically ill 4- to 5-month-old infant who begins to recognize the foster grandmother may smile, relax, and feed better for her and is often fussier and more irritable on her day off. A foster grandparent program benefits both infants and seniors—the infant receives love and socialization, and the senior "has a reason to get up in the morning."

If at all possible, parents should be encouraged to perform the "firsts" with their infant (e.g., first nipple feeding, first bath, first time out of the incubator). Because parents are not always present, they will miss some important milestones for their infant (e.g., extubation). Many NICUs have developed baby diaries (or calendars) where the nurses, physicians, and foster grandparents write important information about the infant's day (as if the infant were the author). The text is accompanied by self-developing pictures with humorous captions (e.g., "Look at me—I've got my tube out!"). Staff are very creative in relating "what's been happening," so that the parents not only have a verbal report (that over time will be forgotten) but also a keepsake of NICU progress.

LONG-TERM CARE IN THE NICU

Because smaller, more immature preterm infants are now surviving, some infants spend months in the NICU. To facilitate the development of these chronically hospitalized infants, parents and professionals must have realistic expectations of their developmental levels. A preterm infant who reaches 40 weeks' postconceptual age is not as mature in sleep-wake cycles, attentiveness, or soothability as a 40-week term infant.[73] **In evaluating the developmental performance of a preterm infant, one must correct for the weeks of prematurity.** For example, Susie is chronologically 8 months old; she was 32 weeks' gestation at birth, so her developmental age would be calculated as follows:

8 months − 8 weeks (2 months) preterm = 6 months

Susie will be developmentally appropriate in performance if she functions at a 6-month level; developmental delay would be functioning below the 6-month level.

OUTCOME

Even though the survival rate of preterm infants, including VLBW preterm infants, has dramatically improved as a result of education of care providers, regionalization of care, and improved technology, there has not been a corresponding change in neonatal morbidity. Historically, extremely few VLBW infants and other NICU survivors have received comprehensive, long-term follow-up.[140,215] Many of these infants received no follow-up at all or were followed for only a few years.[140,215] Indeed, follow-up studies of the outcomes of NICU care vary in (1) reporting and defining handicapping conditions (e.g., serious versus minor), (2) lack of full-term infants as a control group, (3) retrospective versus prospective,

---

Box 13-10	OUTCOMES IN FOLLOW-UP STUDIES

Mortality rate increases with decreasing gestational age:
References 10, 14, 41, 96, 106, 111, 163, 188, 196, 208, 229, 246, 266, 267, 277, 279, 296, 443, 496, 535, 561.

Males have higher mortality than females:
References 106, 279, 433, 561.

Intact survival increases with increasing gestational age:
References 208, 246, 267, 277, 427, 446, 535.

Morbidity rates increase with decreasing gestational age:
References 10, 14, 75, 113, 124, 163, 185, 188, 204, 208, 246, 296, 338, 427, 433, 496, 509, 535.

Only the severest impairments can be diagnosed in the first 1-2 years of life:
References 43, 106, 152, 561.

50% of ELBW infants have morbidities serious enough to be diagnosed in the first 2 years of life:
Reference 254.

Even nonhandicapped VLBW infants have significant, multisystem, pervasive problems that may not be evident till school age:
References 43, 106, 152, 212.

Males have higher morbidity than females:
References 106, 233, 279, 433, 561.

"Normal" neonatal head sonograms are not necessarily correlated with lack of long-term morbidity (e.g., later CP; later diagnosable brain abnormalities correlated with neurodevelopmental and behavioral outcomes):
References 113, 403.

Socioeconomic status of the parents may have either a positive or a negative impact on long-term outcomes:
References 39, 43, 75, 339, 433, 559.

---

(4) impartiality (e.g., blinding) of evaluators, (5) population-based study of birth weight/gestational age morbidities, (6) definition of outcome measures, and (7) study length.[140,203,215] These study variations often make it difficult (if not impossible) to compare outcome results. **However, some outcomes appear in follow-up studies as recurring themes (Box 13-10).**

Recent national and international studies of outcomes of ELBW/VLBW infants show similar findings (Table 13-16). A recent review of the world literature on the outcomes of ELBW (less than 800 g) and gestational age (less than 26 weeks' gestation) infants reveals mortality and morbidity statistics (Table 13-17). These infants

Table 13-16	NATIONAL AND INTERNATIONAL OUTCOME STUDIES	
STUDY	**DESIGN**	**FINDINGS**
Bavarian Longitudinal Study[559]	Population: $n = 264$ (<32 weeks' ga) at 6 yr of age Strength: • Late preschool years—better identification of problems compared to infancy follow-up • Multiple centers-large geographic area • Matched (full-term) controls • Low drop-out rate	1. Preterm infants scored significantly lower on cognitive, language and prereading skills 2. Preterm infants 31 times more likely to have specific deficit in processing simultaneous information 3. Preterm infants experienced deficits in wide range of abilities 4. Preterm infants had more multiple cognitive problems, a higher incidence of serious impairment (26%), and serious deficits 10-35 times more than full-term infants 5. Preterm birth had more effect on cognitive ability than did socioeconomic status, which had an independent and additive effect to the deficits.
Epicure Study[106,561]	Population: $n = 283$ (≤25 ga) at 30 mo of age (2½ yr) Strength: • Prospective, births Mar-Dec 95 • Population based • Stratified by ga, not BW	1. Severe disability common in extreme prematurity: Overall = 49% had disability: 19%: Severe developmental delay 11%: Moderate developmental delay 10%: Severe neuromotor disability 14%: Other neuromotor disability 2%: Blind 3%: Hearing loss
National Institute of Child Health and Human Development[535]	Population: $n = 1151$ (ELBW 401-1000 g) at 18-22 mo corrected age. Strength: • Large cohort • Multicenter (12) • Prospective: 1993-1994 • 90% ELBW >600 g	1. Overall: One or more major neurodevelopmental abnormalities occurred in 49% of ELBW survivors: 25% abnormal neurologic examination result (CP 17%; seizures 5%; hydrocephalus 4%) 37% Bayley mental score <70 (more in lower BW group) 29% psychomotor development Index <70 (more in lower BW group) 9% vision impairment 11% hearing impairment 2. Abnormalities increased as BW decreased: 43% abnormal neurologic exam in 401-500 g group As ga decreased, increased risk of cognitive deficits. 3. Factors associated with neurodevelopmental morbidity: CLD/BPD; steroid use for CLD/BPD; IVH grades 3 and 4; PVL; NEC; male gender
American Psychological Association[43]	Population: $n = 118$ (24-31 ga) at 10 years of age Strength: • Matched (full-term) controls • School age follow-up	1. "Academic failure to thrive"[43] Lower scores on IQ and achievement tests: IQ <80: 18% preterm infants Lower scores on social and behavioral functioning—more behavior problems Increased need for special education services—60% compared with full-term children Increased learning disabilities: 24% preterm compared with 9% full-term Increased ADHD: 16% preterm compared with 4% controls—four to six times more ADHD in preterm infants than national estimate (e.g., 3%-5% of general population) 2. Preterm infants have apparent pervasiveness of dysfunction: ≥3 areas of dysfunction in 43% of preterm infants 3. Preterm infants without major handicaps have more subtle developmental delays (e.g., social, behavioral, cognitive) that are not detected until school age

Table 13-17	MORTALITY* AND MORBIDITY RATES FOR ELBW (>800 g) AND GESTATIONAL AGE (<26 WEEKS) INFANTS			
GESTATIONAL AGE (WK)	MORTALITY (%)*	CEREBRAL ULTRASONOGRAPHIC ABNORMALITIES (%)	BPD/CLD (%)	NEURODEVELOPMENTAL DISABILITY (%)
23	2-35	10-83	57-70	30
24	17-58	17-64	33-89	17-45
25	35-85	10-22	16-71	12-35

Modified from Hack M, Fanaroff A: Outcomes of children of low birth weight and gestational age in the 1990's, *Early Hum Dev* 53:193, 1999.
*Survival around the limits of viability (e.g., <28 weeks' gestation) may be overestimated in outcome studies because of selection bias. (Evans D, Levene M: Evidence of selection bias in preterm survival studies: a systematic review, *Arch Dis Child Fetal Neonatal Educ* 84:F79, 2001.)

are at increased risk for a multitude of physical and psychosocial emotional disabilities (Box 13-11). Appropriate follow-up care for the preterm is discussed in Chapter 32.

There is an increased incidence of failure to thrive and child abuse and neglect in preterm infants.[291] Separation of infants and parents at birth disrupts the parent-infant attachment process and increases the risk of parenting disorders (see Chapters 29 and 30). In the first year of life, preterm infants are often more "difficult" and less "easy" to care for, they are difficult to soothe, less adaptive, less able to habituate, state labile, negative in mood, and withdrawn.* **Many families (40% to 45%) of VLBW infants experience feeding difficulties in the first years of the infant's life.†** A parent who finds the preterm infant "too difficult" may become less responsive to and less involved with the infant and thus may escalate the infant's difficult behavior. Although an unsupportive environment may increase the difficult behavior, a supportive parent-infant interaction benefits the infant, who then makes developmental gains.[43,75,433,559] The impact on the family of VLBW infants is long lasting and includes financial burden, familial and social impact, personal strain, and mastery.[97,110,216,324]

The increased risk of cognitive impairment with decreasing birth weight may diminish with time and a supportive environment or may persist until school age (see Box 13-11). **Preterm infants are more likely to function below their genetic potential because of increased incidence of mental retardation, cerebral palsy, and learning disabil-**

ities (see Box 13-11). **Children who were preterm infants require more special education, repeat grades, and do less well on reading and math achievement tests than children who were born at term.** Even when NICU graduates perform well on developmental tests, they may have neurosensory difficulties (e.g., problems with visual-motor integration, spatial relationships, and speech and language development) and passive, withdrawn behavior that negatively affects school accomplishment (see Box 13-11). Although early identification of cognitive or learning difficulties enables the infant, toddler, and preschool years to be the optimal time for intervention,[508] a more recent follow-up of extensive post-NICU intervention cites negligible effects on these infants at school age.[39,337]

Just as the ability of parents to attach to and care for their infant is disrupted by illness and hospitalization (see Chapters 29 and 30), **the ability of the newborn to form a symbiotic attachment to the parents is disrupted by the NICU experience. The unattached child results when the infant internalizes the rage associated with unmet needs.**[315,488] Because of a lack of contingent, reliable, and consistent caregiving, these infants do not develop a sense of trust in parents, self, or humankind. Unmet needs may be a result of (1) lack of parental attachment and caregiving, (2) asynchrony between caregivers and the infant, so that the infant's cues are not interpreted and responded to appropriately, (3) neglect and abuse, or (4) having multiple caregivers.

The emotional disruptions of an unattached child are the same as the psychologic outcomes of a battered child[315,420,435,488]:

- The infant's ego development is derived primarily from sensations from the body surface.
- When the body suffers pain, there is a decrease in the pleasure principle as a guide to

*References 15, 43, 75, 175, 304, 317, 344, 345, 377, 494, 498, 501, 556.
†Reference 40, 109, 131, 281, 283, 348, 373, 423, 498, 556.

Box 13-11	SEQUELAE ASSOCIATED WITH PREMATURITY

Physical

1. Respiratory
(References 15, 121, 131, 160, 208, 268, 324, 373, 395, 498)
   a. Bronchopulmonary dysplasia/chronic lung disease (BPD/CLD)
   b. Reactive airway disease/asthma
   c. Complications of intubation (see Table 23-5)
   d. Complications of steroid use (see Box 23-7)
   e. Rehospitalizations—pneumonia, respiratory syncytial virus (RSV)
   f. Sudden infant death syndrome (SIDS)

2. Cardiovascular
(Reference 131)
   a. Hypertension
   b. Right ventricular hypertrophy
   c. Superior vena cava syndrome
   d. Congestive heart failure

3. Hematologic
(Reference 131)
   a. Anemia

4. Gastrointestinal
(Reference 132)
   a. Gastroesophageal reflux disease (GERD)
   b. Short gut syndrome
   c. Failure-to-thrive
      (References 112, 131, 190, 486, 556)
      (1) Organic (e.g., physiologic cause)
         • Feeding difficulties
         (References 38, 40, 108, 109, 177, 178, 348, 462, 498)

Physical—cont'd

   • Growth failure
      (References 40, 106, 121, 138, 177, 178, 235, 373, 377, 403, 498, 561)
   (2) Nonorganic (e.g., attachment problems; abuse/neglect)
      (References 38, 40, 104, 109, 160)

5. Sensorineural deficits
   a. Visual disorders (poor visual acuity; strabismus; blindness; astigmatism; myopia)
      (References 24, 48, 106, 131, 188, 207, 208, 228, 297, 403, 418, 433, 480, 535)
   b. Hearing (sensorineural and/or conductive loss)
      (References 24, 106, 131, 179, 188, 208, 480, 535, 561)

6. Developmental delay in gross/fine motor skills
   (References 14, 15, 24, 48, 51, 60, 62, 95, 106, 109, 113, 131, 152, 163, 185, 208-210, 214, 242, 275, 297, 304, 317, 322, 348, 392, 395, 414, 480, 481, 495, 535, 553, 561)
   a. Neurologic impairment (e.g., IVH; CP; seizures)
      (References 45, 451)
   b. Nursery-acquired positioning malformations
      (References 51, 127, 151, 205, 214, 374, 451)
   c. Difficulty in balance; clumsiness
      (Reference 451)

Psychosocioemotional

1. Cognitive impairment—decrease in intelligence quotient (IQ) and developmental quotient
   (References 10, 15, 24, 43, 48, 60, 152, 163, 188, 207, 208, 212, 233, 242, 250, 275, 296, 297, 304, 334, 354, 377, 389, 403, 418, 433, 447, 448, 451, 468, 480, 493, 499, 502, 535, 536, 553, 555, 559)

---

development and an increase in violent, aggressive tendencies, because the caregiver, who should comfort, is inflicting pain.

• The infant identifies with and incorporates the abusive caregiver into the infant's own ego development.
• The caregiver's control in the relationship negates the needs, feelings, and states of the infant, who also learns to discount himself or herself and inhibits self-initiated activity—is passive with learned helplessness.

Unattached and battered children exhibit poor self-esteem; difficulty or inability in developing close, intimate relationships; lack of a social conscience; and a preoccupation with or increase in violent tendencies.*

---

*Reference 35, 43, 64, 257, 304, 315, 323, 392, 420, 435, 488, 501.

NICU infants are at risk for being unattached because (1) they have multiple caregivers, (2) the parents are not always present and after a prolonged stay of the infant may be "strangers" to the infant, (3) the needs of the multiple caregivers and infant may be asynchronous (e.g., it is "care time," but the infant is asleep), (4) lifesaving care in the NICU is intrusive, noxious, and painful, and (5) these experiences give the infant a history independent of his or her parents. Rather than receiving the soothing, pleasurable nurturing of family, the NICU infant is constantly bombarded with painful touch, handling, and stimuli. From the infant's perspective, the altruistic pain of lifesaving care is indistinguishable from the pain of child abuse.[488] The infant is cognitively unable to distinguish or be taught the difference—he or she merely subjectively experiences the pain. As one mother stated, "To Joshua, cauterizing his gastrostomy site with a silver nitrate stick

---

Box 13-11   SEQUELAE ASSOCIATED WITH PREMATURITY—cont'd

Psychosocioemotional—cont'd

2. **Learning disorders**
   (References 10, 43, 76, 78, 204, 212, 242, 354, 418, 433, 448, 480, 493, 494, 498, 502, 553, 555, 559)
   a. Mathematics, reading, spelling disabilities
      (References 78, 242, 418, 448, 494, 505)
   b. Visual and/or auditory perceptual difficulties
      (References 74, 152, 197, 204, 210, 228, 275, 285, 389, 483, 495, 498, 533)
   c. Visual and/or auditory motor incoordination
      (References 74, 197, 204, 312, 483)
   d. Executive function deficits (planning; sequencing; inhibition)
      (Reference 223)
   e. Normal or delayed acquisition of speech or language
      (References 15, 76, 403, 462, 505, 560)
3. **Difficult behavioral style**
   (References 15, 38, 43, 75, 210, 304, 317, 344, 345, 377, 403, 447, 494, 495, 498, 501)
   a. Difficult to soothe
   b. Less adaptive—difficulty in habituation; state lability; dysrhythmic; attention
      (References 257, 389)
   c. Negative mood; separation anxiety
      (Reference 550)
   d. Withdrawn or highly active (ADHD)
      (References 43, 64, 306, 323, 339, 388, 550, 553)
4. **Emotional sequelae—(the "unattached child")**
   (References 315, 423, 435, 488)
   a. Feelings of powerlessness—learned helplessness
      (References 257, 339)

Psychosocioemotional—cont'd

   b. Poor ego development—low self-esteem, insecurity, oriented outside the self for cues and guidance
   c. Lack of trust in self and others
   d. Needy dependence
   e. Prone to depression; anxiety; suicide ideation
      (References 64, 323)
   f. Difficulty or inability in establishing and maintaining intimate relationships with others
   g. Increased irritability
5. **Social sequelae**
   (References 43, 257, 304, 315, 420, 435, 488)
   a. Lack of social conscience: violent or aggressive behaviors toward self and others; no guilt or remorse for behavior
      (References 35, 64, 257, 323)
   b. Difficulty or inability in developing intimate relationships with others
      (References 35, 392, 501)
6. **School difficulties/special education services**
   (References 43, 65, 124, 210, 212, 317, 334, 339, 389, 433, 446, 493, 494)
7. **Impact on family**
   (References 39, 97, 216)
   a. Financial stress
      (References 110, 324)
   b. Individual, marital, and familial stress
      (References 15, 110, 324)
   c. Mastery
      (References 97, 110, 216, 324)

---

was no different than if I'd burned him with a cigarette." To him, his mother was causing him pain.[20,136]

It is unclear whether developmental delays are caused totally by organic insults, the effect of the NICU environment on an immature CNS, or a combination of insults. Because the NICU environment does not by itself ensure optimal developmental outcome, research into the environmental characteristics of the NICU and strategies to minimize its negative effect continue.[191]

The effect on the neonate's experience of hospitalization may be ameliorated or exacerbated by such variables as maturity at birth, severity of illness, length of hospital stay, primary nursing, genetic endowment, temperament, maternal socioeconomic group, education and caregiving, and postdischarge follow-up and interventions. Because keeping parents involved is so important to outcome, parents need anticipatory guidance about

"taking their premie home." Instead of telling parents that preterm infants are "more difficult," a more positive statement, such as "Preterm infants need more help from parents in the first year of life," is warranted. Concrete techniques to soothe, feed, and interact with their infant and "rooming-in" practice help parents be more confident in caregiving. Absolving parental guilt ("What am I doing wrong?") by teaching parents that the infant has a problem helps keep parents involved with the infant. Teaching appropriate play activities assists parents in enjoying their infant while providing the infant with vital sensory and social experience for development.

Care of preterm infants began with a minimal handling policy. Research and knowledge of the unique anatomy and physiology of the neonate preceded the development of high-technology devices and high touch to manage both machines and newborns. Observation and research has documented the effect of the NICU environment on its vulnerable inhabitants. Individualized developmental interventions in the NICU and beyond have resulted in decreased developmental delay as well as medical benefits and cost savings (see Table 13-5). Because individualized developmental care improves outcomes, several recommendations have been proposed: (1) third party reimbursement may favor NICUs that are cost effective, (2) NICUs choosing not to use developmental care should have clear reasons and consider randomized trials to disprove its effectiveness, and (3) the American Academy of Pediatrics should critically evaluate developmental care and make recommendations regarding its use.[355] Positive long-term effects and benefits of individualized developmental care continue to be documented at school age.[18] Long-term complications and poor outcomes of prematurity may be prevented by use of individualized developmental care.[559]

REFERENCES

1. Abbasi S, Sivieri E, Finnegan K et al: Olfactory reinforcement of sucking in preterm infants, *Pediatr Res* 47:382a, 2000.
2. Abman S, Groothuis J: Pathophysiology and treatment of BPD, *Pediatr Clin North Am* 41:277, 1994.
3. Abrams R, Gerhardt K: The acoustic environment and physiologic responses of the fetus, *J Perinatol* 20:531, 2000.
4. Adams M, Mirmiran M, Boeddiker M et al: Effects of prone and supine position on sleep in preterm infants at one month corrected age, *Pediatr Res* 45:180A, 1999.
5. Adams M, Mirmiran M, Dubin A et al: Influence of prone-supine position on sleep and heart rate variability in preterm infants at one month corrected age, *Pediatr Res* 47:383A, 2000.
6. Adamson-Macedo E: Effects of tactile stimulation on low and VLBW infants during the first week of life, *Curr Physiol Res Rev* 4:305, 1985-1986.
7. Aebi V, Nelson J, Sidiropoulos, D et al: Outcome of 100 randomly positioned children of VLBW at two years, *Child Care Health Dev* 17:1, 1991.
8. Affonso D, Wahlberg V, Persson B: Mother's reactions to kangaroo method of prematurity care, *Neonatal Netw* 7:43, 1989.
9. Affonso D, Bosque E, Wahlberg V et al: Reconciliation and healing for mothers through skin-to-skin contact provided in American tertiary level intensive care nursery, *Neonatal Netw* 12:25, 1993.
10. Agustines LA, Lin YG, Rumney PJ et al: Outcomes of extremely low-birth-weight infants between 500 and 750 g, *Am J Obstet Gynecol* 182:1113, 2000.
11. Aitken R: Quantitative noise analysis in a modern hospital, *Arch Environ Health* 37:361, 1982.

12. Alberts J: Learning as adaptation of the infant, *Acta Paediatr Suppl* 397:77, 1994.
13. Allen MC, Capute AJ: Tone and reflex development before term, *Pediatrics* 85:393, 1990.
14. Allen MC, Donahue PK, Dusman AE et al: The limit of viability: neonatal outcome of infants born at 22-25 weeks gestation, *N Engl J Med* 329:1597, 1993.
15. Allen M, Baker S, Donohue P et al: Delayed neuromotor maturation in extremely preterm severely growth restricted infants, *Pediatr Res* 45:235A, 1999.
16. Als H: Toward a synactive theory of development: promise for assessment and support for infant individuality, *Infant Ment Health J* 3:229, 1982.
17. Als H: Infant individuality: assessing patterns of very early development. In Call JD, Galenson MD, Tyson R, eds: *Frontiers of infant psychiatry,* New York, 1983, Basic Books.
18. Als H, Gilkerson L: The role of relationship-based developmentally supportive newborn intensive care in strengthening outcome of preterm infants, *Semin Perinatol* 21:178, 1997.
19. Als H, Tronick E, Adamson L et al: The behavior of the full-term yet underweight newborn infant, *Dev Med Child Neurol* 18:590, 1976.
20. Als H, Lawhon G, Brown E et al: Toward a research instrument for the assessment of preterm infant's behavior (APIB). In Fitzgerald HE, Lester BM, Yogman MW, eds: *Theory and research in behavioral pediatrics,* vol 1, New York, 1982, Plenum Press.
21. Als H, Lawhon G, Brown E et al: Individualized behavioral and environmental care for the VLBW preterm infant at high risk for BPD: neonatal intensive care unit and developmental outcome, *Pediatrics* 78:1123, 1986.
22. Als H, Lawhon G, Brown et al: Individualized behavioral and environmental care for the VLBW preterm infant at high risk for BPD and IVH. Study II: NICU outcome. Paper presented at the annual meeting of the New England Perinatal Association, Woodstock, Vt, 1988.
23. Als H, Lawhon G, Duffy FH et al: Individualized developmental care for VLBW preterm infants, *JAMA* 272:853, 1994.
24. Ambalavanan N, Nelson KG, Alexander G et al: Prediction of neurologic morbidity in extremely low birth weight infants, *J Perinatol* 20:496, 2000.
25. Amemiya F, Vos J, Prechtl H: Effects of prone and supine position on heart rate, respiratory rate and motor activity in full-term newborn infants, *Brain Dev* 13:148, 1991.
26. American Academy of Pediatrics: Noise: a hazard for the fetus and newborn, *Pediatrics* 100:724, 1997.
27. American Academy of Pediatrics: Hospital discharge of the high-risk neonate—proposed guidelines, *Pediatrics* 102:411, 1998.

28. American Academy of Pediatrics: Task force on newborn and infant hearing: newborn and infant hearing loss: detection and intervention, *Pediatrics* 103:427, 1999.

29. American Academy of Pediatrics and American College of Obstetricians and Gynecologists: *Guidelines for perinatal care,* ed 5, Elk Grove Village, Ill, 2002.

30. American Academy of Pediatrics, Joint Committee on Infant Hearing: Position statement, *Pediatrics* 95:152, 1995.

31. American Academy of Pediatrics Task Force on Infant Position and SIDS: Positioning and sudden infant death syndrome (SIDS): update, *Pediatrics* 98:1216, 1996.

32. Anders TF, Keener M: Developmental course of nighttime sleep-wake patterns in full-term and preterm infants during the first year of life, *Sleep* 8:173, 1985.

33. Anderson G: Current knowledge about skin-to-skin (kangaroo) care for preterm infants, *J Perinatol* 11:216, 1991.

34. Anderson G: Kangaroo care of the premature infant. In Goldson E, ed: *Nurturing the premature infant: developmental interventions in the neonatal intensive care unit,* New York, 1999, Oxford University Press.

35. Anderson SW, Bechara A, Damasio H et al: Impairment of social and moral behavior related to early damage in human prefrontal cortex, *Nature Neurosci* 2:1032, 1999.

36. Anderssen S, Nicoliasen R, Gabrielsen G: Autonomic response to auditory stimulation, *Acta Paediatr* 82:913, 1993.

37. Appleton S: "Handle with care": an investigation of the handling received by preterm infants in intensive care, *J Neonatal Nurs* 31:23, 1997.

38. Arvedson J: Dysphagia in pediatric patients with neurologic damage, *Semin Neurol* 16:371, 1996.

39. Avon Premature Infant Project: Randomized trial of parental support for families with very preterm children, *Arch Dis Child Fetal Neonatal Educ* 79:F4, 1998.

40. Babbitt RL, Hoch TA, Coe DA et al: Behavioral assessment and treatment of pediatric feeding disorders, *J Dev Behav Pediatr* 15:278, 1994.

41. Bahado-Singh RO, Dashe J, Deren O, et al: Prenatal prediction of neonatal outcome in the extremely low-birth-weight infant, *Am J Obstet Gynecol* 178:462, 1998.

42. Bakeman R, Brown J: Analyzing behavioral sequences: Differences between preterm and full-term infant-mother dyads during the first months of life. In Sawin D, Hawkins R, Walker L et al, eds: *Exceptional infant,* vol 4, *Psychosocial risks in infant-environment transactions,* New York, 1980, Brunner-Mazel.

43. Barlow J, Lewandowski L: Ten-year longitudinal study of preterm infants: outcome and predictors. Paper presented at the American Psychological Association, Washington, DC, August 8, 2000.

44. Barnard KE, Bee HL: The impact of temporally patterned stimulation on the development of preterm infants, *Child Dev* 54:1156, 1983.

45. Barnes P: Neuroimaging and the timing of fetal and neonatal brain injury, *J Perinatol* 21:44, 2001.

46. Barr R: Reflections on measuring pain in infants: dissociation in responsive systems and "honest signaling," *Arch Dis Child Fetal Neonatal Educ* 79: F152, 1998.

47. Bartocci M, Serra G, Papiendieck G et al: Cerebral cortex response in newborn infants after exposure to the smell of a detergent used in NICU: a near infrared spectroscopy study, *Pediatr Res* 47:388A, 2000.

48. Bass W, Jones M, White L: Ultrasonographic differential diagnosis and neurodevelopmental outcome of cerebral white matter lesions in premature infants, *J Perinatol* 19:330, 1999.

49. Bauer K, Uhrig C, Sperling P et al: Body temperature and oxygen consumption during skin-to-skin (kangaroo care) in stable preterm infants weighing less than 1500 grams, *J Pediatr* 130:240, 1997.

50. Becker PT, Grunwald PC, Moorman J et al: Effects of developmental care on behavioral organization of very-low-birth-weight infants, *Nurs Res* 42:214, 1993.

51. Becker PT, Grunwald PC, Moorman J et al: Outcomes of developmentally supportive nursing care for very low birth weight infants, *Nurs Res* 40:150, 1991.

52. Bell SM, Ainsworth MD: Infant crying and maternal responsiveness, *Child Dev* 43:1171, 1972.

53. Berens R, Weigle C: Noise measurements during high-frequency oscillatory and conventional mechanical ventilation, *Chest* 108:1026, 1995.

54. Berens R, Weigle C: Noise analysis of three newborn infant isolettes, *J Perinatol* 17:351, 1997.

55. Blackburn S: The use of orally directed behaviors by VLBW infants, *Neonatal Netw* 12:61, 1993.

56. Blackburn S, Patteson D: Effects of cycled light on activity state and cardiorespiratory function in preterm infants, *J Perinat Neonatal Nurs* 4:47, 1991.

57. Blanchard Y, Pedneault M, Doray B: Effects of tactile stimulation on physical growth and hypoxemia in preterm infants, *Phys Occup Ther Pediatr* 11:37, 1991.

58. Blaymore-Bier JA, Ferguson AE, Morales Y et al: Comparison of skin-to-skin contact with standard contact in low-birth-weight infants who are breastfed, *Arch Pediatr Adolesc Med* 150:1265, 1996.

59. Bolton D, Herman S: Ventilation and sleep state in the newborn, *J Physiol* 64:429, 1974.

60. Bonnett A, Pimm J, Bauer C: Bayley behavior rating scale at 18 mo in a population of VLBW infants, *Pediatric Res* 45:238A, 1999.

61. Boone O et al: Sound levels in incubators: a laboratory and clinical evaluation. The physical and developmental environment of the high risk infant (abstract), Orlando, Fla, 1995, University of Southern Florida College of Medicine.

62. Bos AF, van Loon AJ, Hadders-Algra M et al: Spontaneous motility in preterm, small-for-gestational age infants. II. Qualitative aspects, *Early Human Dev* 50:131, 1997.

63. Bosque E, Brady J, Affonso D et al: Physiologic measures of kangaroo vs. incubator care in a tertiary-level nursery, *J Obstet Gynecol Neonatal Nurs* 24:219, 1995.

64. Botting N, Powls A, Cooke R: Attention deficit hyperactivity disorders and other psychiatric outcomes in VLBW children at 12 years, *J Child Psychol Psychiatry* 38:931, 1997.

65. Botting N, Powls A, Cooke R et al: Cognitive and developmental outcome of VLBW children in early adolescence, *Dev Med Child Neurol* 40:652, 1998.

66. Bower TGR: *The rational infant: learning in infancy,* New York, 1989, WH Freeman.

67. Bowlby J: *Attachment,* New York, 1973, Basic Books.

68. Bowlby J: *Separation,* New York, 1973, Basic Books.

69. Bowlby J: *Loss,* New York, 1980, Basic Books.

70. Bozynski ME, Naglie RA, Nicks JJ et al: Lateral positioning of the stable very-low-birth-weight infant: effect on transcutaneous oxygen and carbon dioxide, *Am J Dis Child* 142:200, 1988.

71. Brackbill Y, Douthitt T, West H: Neonatal posture: psychophysiological effects, *Neuropadiatrie* 4:145, 1973.

72. Bradley RM, Mistretta CM: Fetal sensory receptors, *Physiol Rev* 3:353, 1975.

73. Brazelton TB: *Neonatal behavioral assessment scale,* ed 2, Philadelphia, 1984, Spastics International Medical Publishers/JB Lippincott.

74. Breton S, Humphries T, Schmidt M et al: Neonatal brain lesions and associated subtle deficits in 4 year old children who were ELBW, *Pediatr Res* 45:238A, 1999.

75. Briet J, Van Wassenaer A, Dekker F et al: Risk factors of behavior problems at two years of age in children born <30 weeks' gestational age, *Pediatr Res* 45:238A, 1999.

76. Briscoe J, Gathercole S, Marlow N: Short-term memory and language outcomes after extreme prematurity at birth, *J Speech Lang Hear Res* 41:654, 1998.

77. Brown LD, Heermann JA: The effect of developmental care on preterm infant outcome, *Appl Nurs Res* 10:190, 1997.

78. Brown S, Kilbride H, Turnbull W et al: Health status and educational outcome at 14-15 years of age for infants <801 grams BW, *Pediatr Res* 45:239A, 1999.

79. Browne J: Considerations for touch and massage in the NICU, *Neonatal Netw* 19:61, 2000.

80. Buehler DM, Als H, Duffy FH et al: Effectiveness of individualized developmental care for low-risk preterm infants: behavioral and electrophysiologic evidence, *Pediatrics* 96:923, 1995.

81. Bullough J, Rea M: Lighting for NICUs: some critical information for design, *Lighting Res Technol* 28:189, 1996.

82. Bulock F, Woolridge M, Baum J: Development of coordination of sucking, swallowing, and breathing: ultrasound study of term and preterm infants, *Dev Med Child Neurol* 32:669, 1990.

83. Burke M, Walsh J, Oehler J, Gingras J: Music therapy following suctioning, *Neonatal Netw* 14:41, 1995.

84. Cagan J: Feeding-readiness behavior in preterm infants, *Neonatal Netw* 14:82, 1995.

85. Campos R: Soothing pain-elicited distress in infants with swaddling and pacifiers, *Child Dev* 60:781, 1989.

86. Cartlidge P, Rutter N: Reduction of head flattening in preterm infants, *Arch Dis Child* 63(7 Spec No):755, 1988.

87. Casaer P, O'Brien M, Prechtl H: Postural behavior in human newborns, *Agressologie* 14B:49, 1973.

88. Catlett AT, Holditch-Davis D: Environmental stimuli of the acutely-ill premature infant: physiologic effects and nursing implications, *Neonatal Netw* 8:19, 1990.

89. Chan J, Kelley M, Khan J: The effects of a pressure relief mattress on postnatal head molding in VLBW infants, *J Neonatal Nurs* 12:19, 1993.

90. Charpak N, Ruiz J, Figueroa Z et al: Kangaroo mother care (KMC): a method of protecting high-risk premature infants, *Pediatr Res* 45:240A, 1999.

91. Christensson K: Fathers can effectively achieve heat conservation in healthy newborn infants, *Acta Paediatr* 85:1354, 1996.

92. Christensson K, Bhat GJ, Amadi BC et al: Randomised study of skin-to-skin versus incubator care for rewarming low risk hypothermic neonates, *Lancet* 352:1115, 1998.

93. Christensson K, Cabrera T, Christensson E et al: Separation distress call in the human neonate in the absence of maternal body contact, *Acta Paediatr* 84:468, 1995.

94. Christensson K, Siles C, Moreno L et al: Temperature, metabolic adaptation and crying in healthy full-term newborns cared for skin-to-skin or in a cot, *Acta Paediatr* 81:488, 1992.

95. Clark R: High-frequency ventilation, *J Pediatr* 124:661, 1994.

96. Clark R, Whitfield J, Thomas P et al: Factors associated with survival in infants +500 gms, *Pediatr Res* 47:392A, 2000.

97. Cole FS: Extremely preterm birth: defining the limits of hope, *N Engl J Med* 343:429, 2000.

98. Cole JG: Infant stimulation reexamined: an environmental- and behavioral-based approach, *Neonatal Netw* 3:24, 1985.

99. Cole JG, Begish-Duddy A, Judas ML et al: Changing the NICU environment: the Boston City Hospital model, *Neonatal Netw* 9:15, 1990.

100. Collins SK, Kuch K: Music therapy in the NICU, *Neonatal Netw* 9:23, 1991.

101. Committee to Establish Recommended Standards for Newborn ICU Design: Recommended standards for newborn ICU design, *J Perinatol* 19(part 2):2, 1999.

102. Conway A: Instruments in neonatal research: measuring preterm infant feeding ability. Part I: bottle feeding, *Neonatal Netw* 13:71, 1994.

103. Coons S, Guilleminault C: Development of consolidated sleep and wakeful periods in relation to the day/night cycle in infancy, *Dev Med Child Neurol* 26:169, 1984.

104. Cooper R, Aslin R: Preference for infant-directed speech in the first month after birth, *Child Dev* 61:1584, 1990.

105. Corff KE, Seideman R, Venkataraman PS et al: Facilitated tucking: a nonpharmacologic comfort measure for pain in preterm neonates, *J Obstet Gynecol Neonatal Nurs* 24:143, 1995.

106. Costeloe K, Hennessey E, Gibson AT et al: The EPICure study: outcomes to discharge from hospital for infants born at the threshold of viability, *Pediatrics* 106:659, 2000.

107. Costello A, Chapman J: Mother's perceptions of the care-by-parent program prior to hospital discharge of their preterm infants, *Neonatal Netw* 17:37, 1998.

108. Craig C, Lee D: Neonatal control of nutritive sucking pressure: evidence for an intrinsic T-guide, *Exp Brain Res* 124:371, 1999.

109. Craig C, Grealy M, Lee D: Detecting motor abnormalities in preterm infants, *Exp Brain Res* 131:359, 2000.

110. Cronin C: Impact of VLBW infants on the family is long-lasting, *Arch Pediatr Adolesc Med* 149:151, 1995.

111. Dachesky J, Rogido M, Chow L et al: Is neonatal resuscitation effective for infants born at 23-27 weeks of gestation? *Pediatr Res* 47:394A, 2000.

112. Daily DK, Kilbride HW, Wheeler R et al: Growth patterns of infants weighing less than 801 grams at birth to 3 years of age, *J Perinatol* 14:454, 1994.

113. Dammann O, Leviton A: Brain damage in preterm newborns: might enhancement of developmentally regulated endogenous protection open a door for prevention? *Pediatrics* 104:541, 1999.

114. Danford DA, Miske S, Headley J et al: Effects of routine care procedures on transcutaneous oxygen in neonates: a quantitative approach, *Arch Dis Child* 58:20, 1983.

115. Dangeman BC et al: The variability of Pao$_2$ in newborn infants in response to routine care, *Pediatr Res* 10:149, 1976.

116. Davis B, Moon R, Sachs H: Effects of sleep position on infant motor development, *Pediatrics* 102: 1135, 1998.

117. DeCasper AJ, Fifer WP: Of human bonding: newborns prefer their mother's voices, *Science* 208: 1175, 1980.

118. DeCasper AJ, Spence MJ: Prenatal maternal speech influences newborn's perception of speech sounds, *Infant Behav Dev* 9:133, 1986.

119. DeLeeuw R, Colin E, Dunnebier E et al: Physiological effects of kangaroo care in very small preterm infants, *Biol Neonate* 59:149, 1991.

120. DePaul D, Chambers S: Environmental noise in the NICU: implications for nursing practice, *J Perinat Neonatal Nurs* 8:71, 1995.

121. deRegnier R, Roberts D, Ramsey D et al: Association between the severity of chronic lung disease and first-year outcomes of very low birth weight infants, *J Perinatol* 17:375, 1997.

122. DiPietro J, Cusson R, Caughy M et al: Behavioral and physiologic effects of nonnutritive sucking during gavage feeding in preterm infants, *Pediatr Res* 36:207, 1994.

123. Dobbing J, Sands J: Quantitative growth and development of the human brain, *Arch Dis Child* 48:757, 1973.

124. Donlevy S, Lee E, Wells N, Wheeler T: Are perinatal factors predictive of optimal school age outcome in the ELBW infant? *Pediatr Res* 48:213A, 1998.

125. Douglas J, Byron M: Interview data on severe behavioral eating difficulties in young children, *Arch Dis Child* 75:304, 1996.

126. Dowling D: Physiological responses of preterm infants to breastfeeding and bottlefeeding with the orthodontic nipple, *Nurs Res* 48:78, 1999.

127. Downs JA, Edwards AD, McCormick DC et al: Effect of intervention on development of hip posture in very preterm babies, *Arch Dis Child* 66:797, 1991.

128. Dreyfus-Brisac C: Organization of sleep in preterms: implications for caretaking. In Lewis M, Rosenblum LA, eds: *The effect of the infant on its caregiver,* New York, 1974, John Wiley & Sons.

129. Dreyfus-Brisac C: Ontogenesis of brain bioelectric activity and sleep organization in neonates and infants. In Faulkner F, Tanner JM, eds: *Human growth,* vol 3, New York, 1979, Plenum Publishing.

130. Duffy F, Als H, McAnulty G: Behavioral and electrophysiological evidence for gestational age effects in healthy preterm and full-term infants studied two weeks after expected due date, *Child Dev* 61:1271, 1990.

131. Dusick A: Medical outcomes in preterm infants, *Semin Perinatol* 21:164, 1997.

132. Duxbury ML, Henly SJ, Broz LJ et al: Caregiver disruptions and sleep of high-risk infants, *Heart Lung* 13:141, 1984.

133. Dwyer T, Ponsonby A: Sudden infant death syndrome: after the "back to sleep" campaign, *Br Med J* 313:180, 1996.

134. Eckerman C, Oehler J, Hannan T et al: The development prior to term age of very prematurely born newborns' responsiveness in En Face exchanges, *Inf Behav Dev* 18:283, 1995.

135. Eckerman C, Oehler J, Medvin M et al: Premature newborns as social partners before term age, *Inf Behav Dev* 17:55, 1994.

136. Eickner S: Personal communication, 1987.

137. Elander G, Hehlstrom G: Reduction of noise levels in intensive care units for infants: evaluation of an intervention program, *Heart Lung* 24:376, 1995.

138. Embleton N, Pang N, Cooke R: Postnatal nutrition and growth retardation: an inevitable consequence of current recommendations in preterm infants? *Pediatrics* 107:270, 2001.

139. Engebretson J, Wardell D: Development of a pacifier for LBW infants' nonnutritive sucking, *J Obstet Gynecol Neonatal Nurs* 26:660, 1997.

140. Escobar G, Littenberg B, Petitti D: Outcome among surviving very low birth weight infants: a meta-analysis, *Arch Dis Child* 66:204, 1991.

141. Evans J: Incidence of hypothermia associated with caregiving in premature infants, *Neonatal Netw* 10:17, 1991.

142. Evans J: Reducing the hypoxemia, bradycardia and apnea associated with suctioning in LBW infants, *J Perinatol* 7:137, 1992.

143. Evans J: Comparison of two NICU patterns of caregiving over 24 hours for preterm infants, *Neonatal Netw* 13:87, 1994.

144. Evans J, Philbin M: Facility and operations planning for quiet hospital nurseries, *J Perinatol* 20:105, 2000.

145. Evans J, McCartney E, Roth-Sautler C: Desaturation and/or bradycardic events following caregiving in the NICU, *Neonatal Intens Care* 4:20, 2000.

146. Evans J, Roth-Sautter C, McCartney E et al: Preterm infant "apneic/ bradycardic" events following clustered caregiving in the NICU. Proceedings of the Sigma Theta Tau 9th International Nursing Research Congress, 66A, 1997, Vancouver, BC.

147. Evans J, Vogelpohl D, Bourguignon C et al: Pain behaviors in LBW infants accompanying some "nonpainful" caregiving procedures, *Neonatal Netw* 16:33, 1997.

148. Eyler FD, Courtway-Meyers C, Edens MJ et al: Effects of developmental intervention on heart rate and transcutaneous oxygen levels in LBW infants, *Neonatal Netw* 8:17, 1989.

149. Fajardo B, Browning M, Fisher D et al: Emergence of state regulation in VLBW premature infants, *Inf Behav Dev* 13:287, 1990.

150. Fantz RL, Fagan JF, Miranda SB: Early visual selectivity as a function of pattern variables, previous exposure, age from birth and conception and expected cognitive deficit. In Cohen L, Salaptic P, eds: *Infant perception,* vol 1, New York, 1975, Academic Press.

151. Fay MJ: The positive effects of positioning, *Neonatal Netw* 6:23, 1988.

152. Fazzi E, Orcesi S, Telesca C et al: Neurodevelopmental outcome in very low birth weight infants at 24 months and 5 to 7 years of age: changing diagnosis, *Pediatr Neurol* 17:240, 1997.

153. Fearon I, Kisileusky B, Hains S et al: Swaddling after heel lance: age-specific effects on behavioral recovery in preterm infants, *J Dev Behav Pediatr* 18:222, 1997.

154. Field T: Infant massage therapy. In Goldson E, ed: *Nurturing the premature infant,* New York, 1999, Oxford University Press.

155. Field T, Scafidi F, Schanberg S: Massage of preterm newborns to improve growth and development, *Pediatr Nurs* 13:385, 1987.

156. Field TM: Interaction patterns of preterm and term infants. In Field TM, ed: *Infants born at risk,* New York, 1979, Spectrum Books.

157. Field TM, Schanberg SM, Scafidi F et al: Tactile/kinesthetic stimulation effects on preterm neonates, *Pediatrics* 77:654, 1986.

158. Fielder A, Moseley M: Environmental light and the preterm infant, *Semin Perinatol* 24:291, 2000.

159. Fifer W, Moon C: The role of mother's voice in the organization of brain function in the newborn, *Acta Paediatr Suppl* 397:86, 1994.

160. Fitzgerald DA, Mesiano G, Brousseau L et al: Pulmonary outcome in extremely low birth weight infants, *Pediatrics* 105:1209, 2000.

161. Fleisher BE, VandenBerg K, Constantinou J et al: Individualized developmental care for very-low-birth-weight premature infants, *Clin Pediatr* 34:523, 1995.

162. Fohe K, Kropf S, Avenardius S: Skin-to-skin contact improves gas exchange in premature infants, *J Perinatol* 20:311, 2000.

163. Forfar O, Hime R, McPhail F et al: Low birth-weight: a 10-year outcome study of the continuum of reproductive casualty, *Dev Med Child Neurol* 36:1037, 1994.

164. Foster R: Shedding light on the biological clock, *Neuron* 20:829, 1998.

165. Fowler K, Kum-Nji P, Wells P et al: Waterbeds may be useful in preventing scaphocephaly in preterm VLBW neonates, *J Perinatol* 17:397, 1997.

166. Franck L, Lawhon G: Environmental and behavioral strategies to prevent and manage neonatal pain, *Semin Perinatol* 22:434, 1998.

167. Franck L, Quinn D, Zahr L: Effect of less frequent bathing of preterm infants on skin flora and pathogen colonization, *J Obstet Gynecol Neonatal Nurs* 29:584, 2000.

168. Franco P, Pardou A, Hassid S et al: Auditory arousal thresholds are higher when infants sleep in the prone position, *J Pediatr* 132:240, 1998.

169. Freedman DG: Ethnic differences in babies, *Hum Nature* 2:36, 1979.

170. Fukuda K, Ishihara K: Development of human sleep and wakefulness rhythm during the first six months of life: discontinuous changes at the 7th and 12th week after birth, *Biol Rhythm Res* 28:94, 1997.

171. Gadeke R, Doring B, Keller F et al: Noise levels in a children's hospital and wake-up thresholds in infants, *Acta Paediatr Scand* 58:164, 1969.

172. Gale G, Vandenberg K: Kangaroo care, *Neonatal Netw* 17:69, 1998.

173. Gale G, Franck L, Lund C: Skin-to-skin (kangaroo) holding of the intubated premature infant, *Neonatal Netw* 12:49, 1993.

174. Gannon J: So happy together—co-bedding multiples boosts growth and development, enhances bonding, *Neonatal Netw* 18:39, 1998.

175. Garcia-Coll C: Behavioral responsivity in preterm infants, *Clin Perinatol* 17:113, 1990.

176. Gardner LI: Deprivation dwarfism, *Sci Am* 227:76, 1982.

177. Gardner S, Hagedorn M: Physiologic sequalae of prematurity: the nurse practitioner's role. Part V. Feeding difficulties and growth failure (pathophysiology, cause and data collection), *J Pediatr Health Care* 5:122, 1991.

178. Gardner S, Hagedorn M: Physiologic sequalae of prematurity: the nurse practitioner's role. Part VI. Feeding difficulties and growth failure (prevention, intervention, parent teaching, and complications), *J Pediatr Health Care* 5:306, 1991.

179. Gerhardt K, Abrams R: Fetal exposures to sound and vibroacoustic stimulation, *J Perinatol* 20:S21, 2001.

180. Glass P, Avery GB, Subramanian KM et al: Effect of bright light in the hospital nursery on the incidence of ROP, *N Engl J Med* 313:401, 1985.

181. Glass R, Wolf L: A global perspective on feeding assessment in the NICU, *Am J Occup Ther* 48:514, 1994.

182. Goltzbach S, Edgar D, Ariagno R: Biological rhythmicity in preterm infants prior to discharge from neonatal intensive care, *Pediatrics* 95:231, 1995.

183. Glotzbach S, Sollars P, Pagano M: Development of the human retinohypothalamic tract, *Soc Neurosci* 18:857, 1992.

184. Glotzbach SF, Rowlett EA, Edgar DM et al: Light variability in the modern neonatal nursery: chronobiologic issues, *Med Hypotheses* 41:217, 1993.

185. Goepfert AR, Goldenberg RL, Hauth JC et al: Obstetrical determinants of neonatal neurological morbidity in < or = 1000-gram infants, *Am J Perinatol* 16:33, 1999.

186. Goldberg S, DeVitto B: Parenting children born preterm. In Bornstein M, ed: *Handbook of parenting,* vol 1: children and parenting, Mahway, NJ, 1995, Lawrence Erlbaum.

187. Goldson E: Non-nutritive sucking in the sick infant, *J Perinatol* 7:30, 1987.

188. Goldson E: The micropremie: infants with birth weight less than 800 g, *Infants Young Child* 8:1, 1996.

189. Goldson E: The environment of the neonatal intensive care visit. In Goldson E, ed: *Nurturing the premature infant,* New York, 1999, Oxford University Press.

190. Gorski PA: Premature infant behavioral and physiological responses to caregiving interventions in the intensive care nursery. In Call JD, Galenson E, Tyson RL, eds: *Frontiers in infant psychiatry,* New York, 1983, Basic Books.

191. Gorski PA: Developmental intervention during neonatal hospitalization—critiquing the state of the science, *Pediatr Clin North Am* 38:1469, 1991.

192. Gorski PA, Davison MF, Brazelton TB: Stages of behavioral organization in the high risk neonate: theoretical and clinical considerations, *Semin Perinatol* 3:61, 1979.

193. Goto K, Mirmiran M, Adams M et al: More awakenings and heart rate variability during supine sleep in preterm infants, *Pediatrics* 103:603, 1999.

194. Goto K, Mirmiran M, Adams M et al: Effects of prone and supine sleeping position on heart rate variability in preterm infants, *Pediatric Res* 45:199A, 1999.

195. Gottfried AW, Gaiter JL: *Infant stress under intensive care: environmental neonatology,* Baltimore, 1985, University Park Press.

196. Gould JE, Benitz WE, Liu H: Mortality and time to death in very low birth weight infants: California, 1987 and 1993, *Pediatrics* 105:628, 2000.

197. Goyen T, Lui K, Woods R: Visual-motor, visual-perceptual and fine motor outcomes in VLBW children at 5 years, *Dev Med Child Neurol* 40:76, 1998.

198. Graven S: Sound and the developing infant in the NICU: conclusions and recommendations for care, *J Perinatol* 20:S88, 2000.

199. Gray K, Dostal S, Ternullo-Retta C et al: Developmentally supportive care in a neonnatal intensive care unit: a research utilization project, *Neonatal Netw* 17:33, 1998.

200. Gray L: Properties of sound, *J Perinatol* 20:56, 2000.

201. Gray L, Philbin M: Measuring sound in hospital nurseries, *J Perinatol* 19:5100, 2000.

202. Gretebeck R, Shaffer D, Bishop-Kurylo D: Clinical pathways for family-oriented developmental care in intensive care nursery, *J Perinat Neonatal Nurs* 12:70, 1998.

203. Gross S, Slagle T, D'Eugenio D et al: Impact of a matched term control group on interpretation of developmental performance in preterm infants, *Pediatrics* 90:681, 1992.

204. Grunau R, Whitfield M, McConnell D et al: Prediction of written output ability in ELBW (<800 g) children from age 4-8½ years, Poster Session III, Pediatric Academic Societies' Annual Meeting, May 1999, San Francisco, Calif.

205. Grunwald P, Becker P: Developmental enhancement: implementing a program for the NICU, *Neonatal Netw* 9:29, 1991.

206. Gunderson LP, Kenner C: Neonatal stress: physiologic adaptation and nursing implications, *Neonatal Netw* 6:37, 1987.

207. Gupta U, Urrutia J, Adams C et al: Long-term outcome in ELBW infants (<1000 grams), *Pediatr Res* 45:245A, 1999.

208. Hack M, Fanaroff A: Outcomes of children of extremely low birthweight and gestational age in the 1990's, *Early Human Dev* 53:193, 1999.

209. Hack M, Estabrook M, Robertson S: Development of the sucking rhythm in preterm infants, *Early Human Dev* 11:133, 1985.

210. Hack M, Taylor HG, Klein N et al: School-age outcomes in children with birth weights <750 g, *N Engl J Med* 331:753, 1994.

211. Hall J: Development of the ear and hearing, *J Perinatol* 20:512, 2000.

212. Halsey C, Collin M, Anderson C: Extremely LBW children and their peers, *Arch Pediatr Adolesc Med* 150:790, 1996.

213. Hao H, Rivkees S: The biological clock of very premature primate infants is responsive to light, *Proc Natl Acad Sci U S A* 96:2426, 1999.

214. Harris MB et al: Joint range of motion development in premature infants, *Pediatr Phys Ther* 2:185, 1990.

215. Harrison H: The principles for family-centered neonatal care, *Pediatrics* 92:643, 1993.

216. Harrison H: Making lemonade: a parent's view of the "quality of life" studies, *J Clin Ethics*. In press.

217. Harrison L: Research utilization: handling preterm infants in the NICU, *Neonatal Netw* 16:65, 1997.

218. Harrison L, Woods S: Early parental touch and preterm infants, *J Obstet Gynecol Neonatal Nurs* 20:299, 1991.

219. Harrison L, Leeper J, Yoon M: Effects of early parent touch on preterm infants' arterial oxygen saturation and heart rate levels, *J Adv Nurs* 15:877, 1990.

220. Harrison L, Leeper J, Yoon M: Preterm infants' physiologic responses to early parent touch, *West J Nurs Res* 13:698, 1991.

221. Harrison L, Olivet L, Cunningham K et al: Effects of gentle human touch on preterm infants: results of a pilot study, *Infant Behav* Special ICIS Issue 15:12, 1992.

222. Harrison L, Olivet L, Cunningham K et al: Effects of gentle human touch on preterm infants: pilot study results, *Neonatal Netw* 15:35, 1996.

223. Harvey J, O'Callaghan M, Mohay H: Executive function of children with ELBW: a case control study, *Dev Med Child Neurol* 41:292, 1999.

224. Hashimoto T, Hirua K, Endo S: Postural effects on behavioral states of newborn infants: a sleep polygraphic study, *Brain Dev* 5:286, 1983.

225. Hay W: Physiology of oxygenation and its relation to pulse oximetry in neonates, *J Perinatol* 7:309, 1987.

226. Hay W: The uses, benefits and limitations of pulse oximetry in neonatal medicine: consensus on key issues, *J Perinatol* 7:347, 1987.

227. Hays JA: Tac-Tic therapy: a non-pharmacological stroking intervention for premature infants, *Complement Ther Nurs Midwif* 4:25, 1998.

228. Hebbandi S: Ocular sequelae in extremely premature infants at 5 years of age, *J Paediatr Child Health* 33:339, 1997.

229. Hein H, Lofgren M: The changing pattern of neonatal mortality in a regionalized system of perinatal care: a current update, *Pediatrics* 104:1064, 1999.

230. Hein H, Pettit S: Back to sleep: good advice for parents but not for hospitals? *Pediatrics* 107:537, 2001.

231. Heller S, Constantinou JC, VandenBerg K et al: Sedation administered to very low birth weight premature infants, *J Perinatol* 17:107, 1997.

232. Hemingway M, Oliver S: Preterm infant positioning, *Neonatal Intens Care* 13:18, 2000.

233. Hindmarsh G, O'Callaghan M, Mohay H et al: Gender differences in cognitive abilities at 2 years in ELBW infants, *Early Hum Dev* 60:115, 2000.

234. Hirata T, Bosque E: When they grow up: the growth of ELBW (< or = 1000 gm) infants at adolescence, *J Pediatr* 132:1033, 1998.

235. Hofer M: Early relationships as regulators of infant physiology and behavior, *Act Paediatr Suppl* 387:9, 1994.

236. Holditch-Davis D: The development of sleeping and waking states in high-risk preterm infants, *Infant Behav Dev* 13:513, 1990.

237. Holditch-Davis D, Edwards L: Modeling development of sleep-wake behaviors, II, results of two cohorts of preterms, *Physiol Behav* 63:319, 1998.

238. Holditch-Davis D, Miles M: Mothers' stories about their experiences in the NICU, *Neonatal Netw* 19:13, 2000.

239. Holditch-Davis D, Thoman E: Behavioral states of premature infants: implications for neural and behavioral development, *Dev Psychobiol* 20:25, 1987.

240. Holditch-Davis D, Barham LN, O'Hale A et al: Effect of standard rest periods on convalescent preterm infants, *J Obstet Gynecol Neonatal Nurs* 24:424, 1995.

241. Holditch-Davis D, Torres C, O'Hale A et al: Standardized rest periods affect the incidence of apnea and rate of weight gain in convalescent preterm infants, *Neonatal Netw* 15:87, 1996.

242. Holsti L, Grunau R, Whitfield M: Developmental coordination disorder in ELBW children (<800 grams) at 8-9 years, Poster session III, Pediatric Academic Societies' Annual Meeting, May 1999, San Francisco, Calif.

243. Horne R, Sly D, Cranage S et al: Effects of prematurity on arousal from sleep in the newborn infant, *Pediatr Res* 47:468, 2000.

244. Horton J, Walderstrom U, Bowman E: Touch of LBW babies in NICU: observations over a 24 hour period, *J Neonatal Nurs* 4:24, 1998.

245. Hughes D, Murphy JF, Dyas J et al: I. Blood spot glucocorticoid concentrations in ill preterm infants, *Arch Dis Child* 62:1014, 1987.

246. Hussain N, Galal M, Ehrenkranz RA et al: Predischarge outcomes of 22-27 weeks gestational age infants born at tertiary care centers in Connecticut: implications for perinatal management, *Conn Med* 62:131, 1998.

247. Hutchinson A, Ross K, Russell G: Effect of posture on ventilation and lung mechanisms in preterm and light-for-date infants, *Pediatrics* 64:429, 1979.

248. Hyde BB, McCown DE: Classical conditioning in neonatal intensive care nurseries, *Pediatr Nurs* 12:11, 1986.

249. Illingworth R, Lister M: The critical or sensitive period with special reference to certain feeding problems in infants and children, *J Pediatr* 65:839, 1964.

250. Inder T, Huppi P, Warfield S et al: Periventricular white matter injury in the premature infant is associated with a reduction in cerebral cortical gray matter volume at term, Poster Session, Pediatric Academic Societies' Annual Meeting, May 1999, San Francisco, Calif.

251. Jain L, Sivieri E, Abbasi S et al: Energetics and mechanics of nutritive sucking in the preterm and term neonate, *J Pediatr* 111:894, 1987.

252. Jeffrey H, Megevand A, Page M: Why the prone position is a risk factor for sudden infant death syndrome, *Pediatrics* 104:263, 1999.

253. Jemerin J, Boyce W: Psychobiological difference in childhood stress responses. II, Cardiovascular markers of vulnerability, *J Dev Behav Pediatr* 11:140, 1990.

254. Jobe A: Overview for prevention of IVH: why are <1 kg infants normal? Paper presented at the Ross Special Conference: Hot Topics in Neonatology, Washington, DC, December 5, 2000.

255. Jurkovicova J, Aghova L: Evaluation of the effects of noise exposure on various body function in LBW newborns, *Acta Nerv Super* 31:228, 1989.

256. Kahn A, Grosswasser J, Sottiaux M et al: Prone or supine body position and sleep characteristics in infants, *Pediatrics* 91:1112, 1993.

257. Kamaya V, Moddemann D, Casiro O: Emotional and behavioral adjustment of "normal" VLBW children compared to controls at 7 years of age, *Pediatr Res* 39:269A, 1996.

258. Kaminski J, Hall W: The effect of soothing music on neonatal behavioral states in the hospital newborn nursery, *Neonatal Netw* 15:45, 1996.

259. Karl D: The interactive newborn bath: using infant behavior to connect parents and newborns, *MCN Am J Matern Child Nurs* 24:280, 1999.

260. Kattwinkel J, Nearman HS, Fanaroff AA et al: Apnea of prematurity. Comparative therapeutic effects of cutaneous stimulation and nasal continuous positive airway pressure, *J Pediatr* 86:588, 1975.

261. Kawakami K, Takai-Kawakani K, Kurihara H et al: The effect of sounds on newborn infants under stress, *Infant Behav Dev* 19:375, 1996.

262. Keene D, Wimmer J, Mathew O: Does supine positioning increase apnea, bradycardia and desaturation in preterm infants? *J Perinatol* 1:17, 2000.

263. Kemp J, Thach B: Sudden death in infants sleeping on polystyrene filled cushions, *N Engl J Med* 324:1858, 1991.

264. Kennaway D, Stamp G, Gable F: Development of melatonin production in infants and the impact of prematurity, *J Clin Endocrinol Metab* 75:367, 1992.

265. Kennedy C, Lipsitt L: Temporal characteristics of non-oral feedings and chronic feeding problems in premature infants, *J Perinat Neonat Nurs* 7:77, 1993.

266. Kilbride H, Daily D: Survival and subsequent outcome to 5 years of age for infants with birth weights (<801 grams) born from 1983-1989, *J Perinatol* 18:102, 1998.

267. Kilpatrick SJ, Schlueter MA, Piecuch R et al: Outcome of infants born at 24-26 weeks' gestation. I. Survival and cost, *Obstet Gynecol* 90:803, 1997.

268. Kitchen W, Campbell M, Charlton C et al: Eight year outcome in infants with BW 500-999 grams: continuing regional study of 1979-1980 births, *J Pediatr* 118:761, 1991.

269. Kleberg A, Westrup B, Stjernqvist K: Developmental outcome, child behavior and mother-child interaction at 3 years of age following NIDCAP intervention, *Early Hum Dev* 60:123, 2000.

270. Klinnert M, Bingham R: The organizing effects of early relationships, *Psychiatry* 57:1, 1994.

271. Korones S: Disturbances and infant's rest. In Moore T, ed: *Iatrogenic problems in neonatal intensive care. Report of the 69th Ross Conference on Pediatric Research,* Columbus, Ohio, 1976, Ross Laboratories.

272. Korner AF: The effect of the infants state, level of arousal, sex and ontogenetic stage on the caregiver. In Lewis M, Rosenblum LA, eds: *The effect of the infant on its caregiver,* New York, 1974, John Wiley & Sons.

273. Korner AF: The use of waterbeds in the care of preterm infants, *J Pediatr* 6:142, 1986.

274. Korner AF: Infant stimulation: issues of theory and research, *Clin Perinatol* 17:173, 1990.

275. Krageloh-Mann I, Toft P, Lunding J et al: Brain lesions in preterms: origin, consequences and compensation, *Acta Paediatr* 88:897, 1999.

276. Kramer L, Peirpoint M: Rocking waterbeds and auditory stimuli to enhance growth of preterm infants, *J Pediatrics* 88:297, 1976.

277. Kramer WB, Saade GR, Goodrum L et al: Neonatal outcome after active perinatal management of the very premature infant between 23 and 27 weeks' gestation, *J Perinatol* 17:439, 1997.

278. Kuhn CM, Schanberg SM, Field T et al: Tactile kinesthetic stimulation effects on sympathetic and adrenocorticol function in preterm infants, *J Pediatr* 199:434, 1991.

279. LaPine T, Felix S, Tarczy-Harnoch P et al: Outcome trends of infants weighing <800 grams at birth, *Pediatr Res* 45:247A, 1999.

280. Langor V: Minimal handling protocol for the intensive care nursery, *Neonatal Netw* 9:23, 1990.

281. Lau C, Hurst N: Oral feeding in infants, *Curr Prob Pediatrics* 29:105, 1999.

282. Lau C, Schanler R: Oral motor function in the neonate, *Clin Perinatol* 23:161, 1996.

283. Lau C, Sheena H, Shulman R et al: Oral feeding in low birth weight infants, *J Pediatr* 130:561, 1997.

284. Lawson B, Anday E, Guillet R: Brain oxidative phosphorylation following alteration in head position in preterm and term infants, *Pediatr Res* 22:302, 1987.

285. Lefebure F, Glorieux J, St. Laurent-Gagnon T: Neonatal survival and disability rate at age 18 months of infants born between 23 and 28 weeks of gestation, *Am J Ob Gyn* 174:833, 1996.

286. Leitch D: Mother-infant interaction: achieving synchrony, *Nurs Res* 48:55, 1999.

287. Lemons P: From gavage to oral feedings: just a matter of time, *Neonatal Netw* 20:7, 2001.

288. Leonard J: Music therapy: fertile ground for application of research in practice, *Neonatal Netw* 12:47, 1993.

289. Leslie GI, Kalaw MB, Bowen JR et al: Risk factors for sensorineural hearing loss in extremely premature infants, *J Pediatr Child Health* 31:312, 1995.

290. Lester BM, Tronick EZ: Guidelines for stimulation with preterm infants, *Pediatr Clin North Am* 17:31, 1990.

291. Leventhal JM, Garber RB, Brady CA et al: Identification during the postpartum period of infants who are at high risk of child maltreatment, *J Pediatr* 114:481, 1989.

292. Lewis M, Michalson L: The socialization of emotional pathology, *Infant Ment Health J* 3:125, 1984.

293. Liaw J: Tactile stimulation and preterm infants, *J Perinat Neonatal Nurs* 14:84, 2000.

294. Lickliter R: Atypical perinatal sensory stimulation and early perceptual development: insights from developmental psychobiology, *J Perinatol* 20:545, 2000.

295. *Lighting for health care facilities,* RP29, New York, 1995, Illuminating Engineering Society of North America.

296. Ling E, Battin M, Whitfield M: Has the 18 month outcome for extremely low gestational age infants of 23-25 weeks gestation improved? *Pediatr Res* 41:271A, 1997.

297. Lipper EG, Ross GS, Auld PA et al: Survival and outcome of infants weighing less than 800 grams at birth, *Am J Obstet Gynecol* 163:146, 1990.

298. Litovsky R: Stimulus differentiation by preterm infants can guide caregivers, *Prenat Perinatal Psychol J* 5:41, 1990.

299. Liu D, Diorio J, Tannenbaum B et al: Maternal care, hippocampal glucocorticoid receptors and hypothalamic-pituitary-adrenal responses to stress, *Science* 277:1659, 1997.

300. Lockridge T, Taquino L, Knight A: Back to sleep: is there room in that crib for both AAP recommendations and developmentally supportive care? *Neonatal Netw* 18:29, 1999.

301. Long J, Philip A, Lucey J: Excessive handling as a cause of hypoxemia, *Pediatrics* 65:203, 1980.

302. Long JG, Lucey JF, Philip AG et al: Noise and hypoxemia in the intensive care nursery, *Pediatrics* 65:143, 1981.

303. Longobucco D, Bernstein B, Rossi D: To co-bed or not to co-bed? A comparative study of co-bedded vs. individually bedded multiple birth infants in the NICU, *Pediatr Res* 47:413A, 2000.

304. Losse A, Henderson SE, Elliman D et al: Clumsiness in children—do they grow out of it? A 10-year follow-up study, *Dev Med Child Neurol* 33:55, 1991.

305. Lotas M, Walden M: Individualized developmental care for VLBW infant: a critical review, *J Obstet Gynecol Neonatal Nurs* 25:681, 1996.

306. Lou H: Etiology and pathogenesis of Attention-Deficit Hyperactivity Disorder (ADHD): significance of prematurity and perinatal hypoxic-haemodynamic encephalopathy, *Acta Paediatr* 85:1266, 1996.

307. Ludington-Hoe S: Energy conservation during skin-to-skin contact between premature infants and their mothers, *Heart Lung* 19:445, 1990.

308. Ludington-Hoe S, Swinth J: Developmental aspects of kangaroo care, *J Obstet Gynecol Neonatal Nurs* 25:691, 1996.

309. Ludington-Hoe S, Ferreira C, Goldstein M: Kangaroo care with a ventilated preterm infant, *Acta Paediatrica* 87:711, 1998.

310. Ludington-Hoe S, Hadeed A, Anderson G: Physiologic responses to skin-to-skin contact in hospitalized premature infants, *J Perinatol* 11:19, 1991.

311. Ludington-Hoe SM, Thompson C, Swinth J et al: Kangaroo care: research results and practice implications and guidelines, *Neonatal Netw* 13:19, 1994.

312. Luoma L, Herrgard E, Martikainen A: Neuropsychological analysis of the visuomotor problems in children born preterm at <32 weeks of gestation: a 5 year prospective follow-up, *Dev Med Child Neurol* 40:21, 1998.

313. Lutes KA, VandenBerg MA: Developmental care: bedding twins/multiples together, *Neonatal Netw* 15:61, 1996.

314. Lutz L, Altimier L: Co-bedding twins and higher-order multiples, *Central Lines* 16:10, 2000.

315. Magid K, McKelvey CA: *High risk: children without a conscience,* New York, 1989, Bantam Books.

316. Maichuk G, Zahorodny W, Marshall R: Use of positioning to reduce the severity of neonatal narcotic withdrawal syndrome, *J Perinatol* 19:510, 1999.

317. Majnemer A, Riley P, Shevell M et al: Severe bronchopulmonary dysplasia increases risk for later neurological and motor sequelae in preterm survivors, *Dev Med Child Neurol* 42:53, 2000.

318. Mandich M, Ritchie S, Mullet M: Transition times to oral feeding in premature infants with and without apnea, *J Obstet Gynecol Neonatal Nurs* 25:771, 1996.

319. Mann NP, Haddow R, Stokes L et al: Effect of night and day on preterm infants in a newborn nursery: randomized trial, *Br Med J* 292:1265, 1986.

320. Mantangos S, Moustogiannis A, Vagenakis A: Diurnal-variation of plasma-cortisol levels in infancy, *J Pediatr Endocr Metab* 11:549, 1998.

321. Marchini G, Lagercrantz H, Feuerberg Y et al: The effect of non-nutritive sucking on plasma insulin, gastrin and somatostatin levels in infants, *Acta Paediatr Scand* 76:753, 1987.

322. Marlow N, Roberts B, Cooke R: Motor skills in ELBW children at the age of 6 years, *Arch Dis Child* 64:839, 1989.

323. Marlow N, Botting N, Powls A et al: Psychiatric outcomes in adolescent VLBW children. Paper presented at thePediatric Academic Societies Annual Meeting, May 1997, Washington, DC.

324. Maroney D: Realities of a premature infant's first year: helping parents cope, *J Perinatol* 15:418, 1995.

325. Martin RJ, Herrell N, Rubin D et al: Effect of supine and prone positions on arterial oxygen tension in the preterm infant, *Pediatrics* 63:528, 1979.

326. Martin R, DiFiore JM, Korenke CB et al: Vulnerability of respiratory control in healthy preterm infants placed supine, *J Pediatr* 127:609, 1995.

327. Mathew O: Respiratory control during nipple feeding in preterm infants, *Pediatr Pulmonol* 5:220, 1988.

328. Mathew O: Breathing patterns of preterm infants during bottle feeding: role of milk flow, *J Pediatr* 119:960, 1991.

329. Mathew O, Bhatia J: Sucking and breathing patterns during breast- and bottle-feeding in term newborns, *Am J Dis Child* 143:588, 1989.

330. Mathew O, Belan M, Thoppil C: Sucking patterns of neonates during bottle feeding: comparison of different nipple units, *Am J Perinatol* 9:265, 1992.

331. Masterson J, Zucker C, Schulze K et al: Prone and supine positioning effects on energy expenditure and behavior of low birth weight neonates, *Pediatrics* 80:689, 1987.

332. Mattia F, deRegnier R: Chronic physiologic instability is associated with neurodevelopmental morbidity at one and two years in extremely premature infants, *Pediatrics* 102:e35, 1998.

333. Mayes L: A developmental perspective on the regulation of arousal states, *Semin Perinatol* 24:267, 2000.

334. Mazurier E, Lefebure F, Tessier R: Educational achievement and intelligence at 16-21 years of ex-prematures born at <1000 gm, *Pediatr Res* 45:250A, 1999.

335. McCain G: Promotion of preterm infant nipple feeding with nonnutritive sucking, *J Pediatr Nurs* 10:3, 1995.

336. McCain G: Behavioral state activity during nipple feeding for preterm infants, *Neonatal Netw* 16:43, 1997.

337. McCarton CM, Brookes-Gunn J, Wallace IF et al: Results at age 8 years of early intervention for LBW premature infants, *JAMA* 277:126, 1997.

338. McCormick M: Conceptualizing child health status: observations from studies of very premature infants, *Perspect Biol Med* 42:372, 1999.

339. McCormick M, Workman-Daniels K, Brooks-Gunn J: The behavioral and emotional well-being of school-age children with different birth weights, *Pediatrics* 97:18, 1996.

340. McGehee L, Eckerman C: The preterm infant as a social partner: responsive but unreadable, *Infant Behav Dev* 6:461, 1983.

341. McGrath J, Conliffe-Torres S: Integrating family-centered developmental assessment and intervention into routine care in the NICU, *Nurs Clin North Am* 31:367, 1996.

342. McGraw K, Hoffmann R, Harker C et al: The development of circadian rhythms in a human infant, *Sleep* 22:303, 1999.

343. McMillen I, Kok J, Adamson T et al: Development of circadian sleep-wake rhythms in preterm and full-term infants, *Pediatr Res* 29:381, 1991.

344. Medoff-Cooper B, Schraeder BD: Developmental trends and behavioral styles in VLBW infants, *Nurs Res* 31:68, 1982.

345. Medoff-Cooper B: Temperament in VLBW infants, *Nurs Res* 35:139, 1986.

346. Medoff-Cooper B: The effects of handling on preterm infants with BPD, *Image* 20:132, 1988.

347. Medoff-Cooper B: Changes in nutritive sucking patterns with increasing gestational age, *Nurs Res* 40:245, 1991.

348. Medoff-Cooper B, Gennaro S: The correlation of sucking behaviors and Bayley Scales of Infant Development at six months of age in VLBW infants, *Nurs Res* 45:291, 1996.

349. Medoff-Cooper B, Ray W: Neonatal sucking behaviors, *Image* 27:195, 1995.

350. Medoff-Cooper B, Verklan T, Carlson S: The development of sucking patterns and physiologic correlates in VLBW infants, *Nurs Res* 42:100, 1993.

351. Meier P: Bottle- and breast-feeding: effects on transcutaneous oxygen and temperature in preterm infants, *Nurs Res* 37:36, 1988.

352. Mellien A: Incubators vs. mother's arms: body temperature conservation in VLBW premature infants, *J Obstet Gynecol Neonatal Nurs* 30:157, 2001.

353. Meltzoff AN, Moore MK: Imitation of facial and manual gestures by human neonates, *Science* 198(4312):74, 1977.

354. Ment LR, Vohr B, Allan W et al: The etiology and outcome of cerebral ventriculomegaly at term in very low birth weight preterm infants, *Pediatrics* 104:243, 1999.

355. Merenstein G: Individualized developmental care: an emerging new standard for neonatal intensive care units? *JAMA* 272:890, 1994.

356. Meyer C, Witte J, Hildmann A et al: Neonatal screening for hearing disorders in infants at risk: incidence, risk factors and follow-up, *Pediatrics* 104:900, 1999.

357. Michelson K, Sirvio P, Wasz-Hockert O: Pain cry in full-term asphyxiated newborn infant correlated with late finding, *Acta Paediatr Scand* 66:611, 1977.

358. Miller C, Byrne J: Psychophysiologic and behavioral response to auditory stimuli in the newborn, *Infant Behav Dev* 6:369, 1983.

359. Miller C, White R, Whitman T et al: The effects of cycled and noncycled lighting on growth and development in preterm infants, *Infant Behav Dev* 18:87, 1995.

360. Miller D, Holditch-Davis D: Interactions of parents and nurses with high-risk preterm infants, *Res Nurs Health* 15:187, 1992.

361. Miller H, Anderson G: Nonnutritive sucking: effects on crying and heart rate in intubated infants requiring assisted mechanical ventilation, *Nurs Res* 42:305, 1993.

362. Miranda SB, Fantz RL: Visual abilities and pattern preference of preterm infants and full-term neonates, *J Exp Child Psychiatry* 10:189, 1970.

363. Mirmiran M: The function of fetal/neonatal rapid eye movement sleep, *Behav Brain Res* 69:13, 1995.

364. Mirmiran M, Ariagno R: Influence of light in the NICU on the development of circadian rhythms in preterm infants, *Semin Perinatol* 24:247, 2000.

365. Mirmiran M, Kok J: Circadian rhythms in early human development, *Early Hum Dev* 26:121, 1991.

366. Mirmiran M, Kok JH, de Kleine MJ et al: Circadian rhythms in preterm infants: a preliminary study, *Early Hum Dev* 23:139, 1990.

367. Mishoe S, Brooks C, Dennison F et al: Octave waveband analysis to determine sound frequencies and intensities produced by nebulizers and humidifiers used with hoods, *Respir Care* 40:1120, 1995.

368. Modrein-McCarthy M: The physiological and behavioral effects of a gentle human touch nursing intervention on preterm infants. Doctoral dissertation, Knoxville, 1993, Dissertation Abstracts Int, AAC9319218, University of Tennessee,

369. Montagu A: Prenatal influences, Springfield, Ill, 1962, Charles C Thomas.

370. Montagu A: *Touching,* New York, 1971, Harper & Row.

371. Moon C, Fifer W: Evidence of transnatal auditory learning, *J Perinatol* 20:S37, 2000.

372. Morris B, Philbin M, Bose C: Physiological effects of sound on the newborn, *J Perinatol* 20:555, 2000.

373. Morris BH, Miller-Loncar CL, Landry SH et al: Feeding, medical factors and developmental outcome in premature infants, *Clin Pediatr* 38:451, 1999.

374. Mouradian L, Als H: The influence of neonatal intensive care unit caregiving practices on motor functioning of preterm infants, *Am J Occup Ther* 48:527, 1994.

375. Moyer-Mileur L, Leutkemeier M, Boomer L et al: Effect of physical activity on bone mineralization in premature infants, *J Pediatr* 127:620, 1995.

376. Munson K, Bare D, Hoath S et al: A survey of skin care practices for premature low birth weight infants, *Neonatal Netw* 18:25, 1999.

377. Nadeau L, Tessier R, Boivin M: New model to explain behavior problems of extremely preterm VLBW children at school age, *Pediatr Res* 45:251A, 1999.

378. National Association of Neonatal Nurses: Draft position statement: co-bedding of twins and higher order multiples, *Central Lines* 17:7, 2001.

379. National Association of Neonatal Nurses Practice Committee: *Infant & family centered developmental care guidelines,* Petaluma, Calif, 1995, The Association.
380. Neu M: Parents perceptions of skin-to-skin care with their preterm infant requiring assisted ventilation, *J Obstet Gynecol Neonatal Nurs* 28:157, 1999.
381. Neu M, Browne J: Infant physiologic and behavioral organization during swaddled vs. unswaddled weighing, *J Perinatol* 17:193, 1997.
382. Neu M, Browne J, Vojir C: The impact of two transfer techniques used during skin-to-skin care on the physiologic and behavioral responses of preterm infants, *Nurs Res* 49:215, 2000.
383. Norris S, Campbell LA, Brenkert S: Nursing procedures and alterations in transcutaneous oxygen tension in premature infants, *Nurs Res* 31:330, 1982.
384. Northern J, Downs MA: *Hearing in children,* ed 4, Baltimore, 1991, Williams & Wilkins.
385. Nzama N, Nolte A, Dorfling C: Noise in a neonatal unit: guidelines for the reduction and prevention of noise, *Curationis* 18:16, 1995.
386. Oehler J: Examining the issue of tactile stimulation of preterm infants, *Neonatal Netw* 4:24, 1985.
387. Oehler J, Eckerman C, Wilson W: Social stimulation and the regulation of premature infants' state prior to term age, *Infant Behav Dev* 11:333, 1988.
388. Olsen P, Paakko E, Vainionpaa L et al: Magnetic resonance imaging of periventricular leukomalacia and its clinical correlation in children, *Ann Neurol* 41:754, 1997.
389. Olsen P, Vainionpaa L, Paakko E et al: Psychological findings in preterm children related to neurologic status and MRI, *Pediatrics* 102:329, 1998.
390. Orenstein SR, Whitington PF: Positioning for prevention of gastroesophageal reflux, *J Pediatr* 103:534, 1983.
391. Ottenbacher KJ, Muller L, Brandt D et al: The effectiveness of tactile stimulation as a form of early intervention: a qualitative evaluation, *J Dev Behav Pediatr* 8:68, 1987.
392. Palta M, Sadek-Badawi M, Evans M et al: Functional assessment of a multicenter very-low-birth-weight cohort at age 5 years. Newborn Lung Project, *Arch Pediatr Adolesc Med* 154:23, 2000.
393. Parmalee AH: Sleep states in premature infants, *Dev Med Child Neurol* 9:70, 1967.
394. Pelletier-Sehnar J, Palmeri A: High-risk infants. In Clark-Pratt PN, Allen AS, eds: *Occupational therapy for children,* ed 2, St Louis, 1989, Mosby.
395. Pena I, Dehmer E, deLemos R: The neurodevelopmental outcome of the ELBW infant remains precarious in the 1990's, *Pediatr Res* 39:275A, 1996.
396. Perlman J, Volpe J: Episodes of apnea and bradycardia in the preterm newborn: impact on cerebral circulation, *Pediatrics* 76:333, 1985.
397. Peters K: Does routine nursing care complicate the physiologic status of the premature neonate with RDS? *J Perinat Neonatal Nurs* 6:67, 1992.
398. Peters K: Dinosaurs in the bath, *Neonatal Netw* 15:71, 1996.
399. Peters K: Selected physiologic and behavioral responses of the critically ill premature neonate to a routine nursing intervention, *Neonatal Netw* 15:74, 1996.
400. Peters K: Bathing premature infants: physiological and behavioral consequences, *Am J Crit Care* 7:90, 1998.
401. Peters K: Neonatal stress reactivity and cortisol, *J Perinat Neonatal Nurs* 11:45, 1998.
402. Peters K: Infant handling in the NICU: does developmental care make a difference? An evaluative review of the literature, *J Perinat Neonatal Nurs* 13:83, 1999.
403. Peterson B, Vohr B, Staib LH et al: Regional brain volume abnormalities and long-term cognitive outcome in preterm infants, *JAMA* 248:1939, 2000.
404. Petryshew P, Stevens B, Hawkins J et al: Comparing nursing costs for preterm infants receiving conventional vs. developmental care, *Nurs Econ* 15:138, 1997.
405. Philbin M: The influence of auditory experience on the behavior of preterm newborns, *J Perinatol* 20:577, 2000.
406. Philbin M, Klaas P: Hearing and behavioral responses to sound in full-term newborns, *J Perinatol* 20:568, 2000.
407. Philbin M, Lickliter R, Graven S: Sensory experience and the developing organism: a history of ideas and view to the future, *J Perinatol* 20:2, 2000.
408. Philbin M, Robertson A, Hall J: Recommended permissible noise criteria for occupied, newly constructed or renovated hospital nurseries, *J Perinatol* 19:559, 1999.
409. Philbin M, Taber C, Hayman L: Preliminary report: changes in vital signs of term newborns during MRI, *Am J Neuroradiol* 17:1033, 1996.
410. Pickler R, Frankel H: The effect of non-nutritive sucking on preterm infant's behavioral organization and feeding performance, *Neonatal Netw* 14:83, 1995.
411. Pickler R, Frankel H, Walsh K et al: Effects of non-nutritive sucking on behavioral organization and feeding performance in preterm infants, *Nurs Res* 45:132, 1996.
412. Pickler R, Higgins K, Crummette B: The effect of nonnutritive stress in preterm infants, *J Obstet Gynecol Neonatal Nurs* 22:230, 1993.
413. Pickler R, Mauck A, Geldmaker B: Bottle-feeding histories of preterm infants, *J Obstet Gynecol Neonatal Nurs* 26:414, 1997.

414. Piechuch R, Leonard C, Schlueter M et al: Neurodevelopmental outcome of premature infants inborn at 24, 25 and 26 weeks gestation, *Pediatr Res* 39:275A, 1996.

415. Pinella T, Birch L: Help me make it through the night: behavioral entrainment of breast-fed infants' sleep patterns, *Pediatrics* 91:436, 1993.

416. Pinelli J, Symington A: How rewarding can a pacifier be? A systematic review of nonnutritive sucking in preterm infants, *Neonatal Netw* 19:41, 2000.

417. Poets C, Langner M, Bohnhorst B: Effects of bottle feeding and two different methods of gavage feeding on oxygenation and breathing patterns in preterm infants, *Acta Paediatrica* 86:419, 1997.

418. Powls A, Botting N, Cooke RW et al: Visual impairment in very low birthweight children, *Arch Dis Child* 76:F82, 1997.

419. Premji S, Paes B: Gastrointestinal function and growth in premature infants: is non-nutritive sucking vital? *J Perinatol* 1:46, 2000.

420. Prescott J: Body pleasure and the origins of violence, *Futurist* 2:64, 1975.

421. Pridham K, Brown R, Sondel S et al: Transition time to full nipple feeding for premature infants with a history of lung disease, *J Obstet Gynecol Neonatal Nurs* 27:533, 1998.

422. Pridham K, Kosorok MR, Greer F et al: The effects of prescribed versus ad libitum feedings and formula caloric density on premature infants dietary intake and weight gain, *Nurs Res* 48:86, 1999.

423. Pridham KF, Martin R, Sondel S et al: Parental issues in feeding young children with bronchopulmonary dysplasia, *J Pediatr* 4:177, 1989.

424. Pridham K, Sondel S, Chang A, et al: Nipple feeding for preterm infants with BPD, *J Obstet Gynecol Neonatal Nurs* 22:147, 1993.

425. Provence S, Lipton RC: *Infants in institutions,* New York, 1962, International Universities Press.

426. Quillen S: Infant and mother sleep patterns during 4th postpartum week, *Issues Compr Pediatr Nurs* 20:115, 1997.

427. Ramin S, Gilstrap L: Other factors/conditions associated with cerebral palsy, *Semin Perinatol* 24:196, 2000.

428. Rao M, Blass E, Brignol M et al: Effects of crying on energy metabolism in human neonates, *Pediatr Res* 33:309A, 1993.

429. Rauh VA, Nurcombe B, Achenbach T et al: The Mother-Infant Transaction Program. The content and implications of an intervention for the mothers of low-birthweight infants, *Pediatr Clin North Am* 17:31, 1990.

430. Renaud M et al: Neonatal outcomes in a modified NICU environment, *Neonatal Netw* 15:6, 1996.

431. Reppert S, Weaver D, Rivkees S: Maternal communication of circadian phase to the developing mammal, *Psychoneuroendocrinology* 13:63, 1988.

432. Resnick MB, Armstrong S, Carter RL et al: Developmental intervention program for high-risk premature infants: effects on development and parent-infant interactions, *J Dev Behav Pediatr* 9:73, 1988.

433. Resnick MB, Gomatam SV, Carter RL et al: Educational disabilities of neonatal intensive care graduates, *Pediatrics* 102:308, 1998.

434. Reynolds JD, Hardy RJ, Kennedy KA et al, for the Light Reduction in ROP (LIGHT-ROP) Cooperative Group: Lack of efficacy of light reduction in preventing ROP, *N Engl J Med* 338:1572, 1998.

435. Rice R: Infant stress and the relationship to violent behavior, *Neonatal Netw* 5:39, 1985.

436. Rivkees S, Hao H: Developing circadian rhythmicity, *Semin Perinatol* 24:232, 2000.

437. Rivkees S, Hofman P, Fortman J: Newborn primate infants are entrained by low intensity lighting, *Proc Natl Acad Sci U S A* 94:292, 1997.

438. Roberts KL, Paynter C, McEwan B: A comparison of kangaroo mother care and conventional cuddling care, *Neonatal Netw* 19:31, 2000.

439. Robertson A, Cooper-Peel C, Vos P: Contribution of heating, ventilation and conversation to the ambient sound in a neonatal intensive care unit, *J Perinatol* 19:362, 1999.

440. Robertson A, Cooper-Peel C, Vos P: Sound transmission into incubators in the NICU, *J Perinatol* 19:494, 1999.

440a. Robertson A, Kohn J, Vos P et al: Establishing a noise measurement protocol for NICU, *J Perinatol* 18:126, 1998.

441. Robinson J, Moseley M, Fielder A: Illuminence of neonatal units, *Arch Dis Child* 65:679, 1990.

442. Robinson J, Moseley MJ, Thompson JR et al: Eyelid opening in preterm neonates, *Arch Dis Child* 64:943, 1989.

443. Rosen T, Misra S: Morbidity and mortality in the extremely premature infant, *Pediatr Res* 47:429A, 2000.

444. Sadeh A: Sleep and melatonin in infants: a preliminary study, *Sleep* 20:185, 1997.

445. Sahni R, Lando T, Ohira-Kist K et al: Effects of sleeping position on electrocortical activity during quiet and active sleep in LBW infants, *Pediatr Res* 47:430A, 2000.

446. Saigal S, Hoult LA, Streiner DL et al: School difficulties at adolescence in a regional cohort of children who were extremely low birth weight, *Pediatrics* 105:325, 2000.

447. Saigal S, Rosenbaum P, Stoskopf B et al: Comprehensive assessment of the health status of VLBW children at 8 years of age: comparison with a reference group, *J Pediatr* 125:411, 1994.

448. Saigal S, Szatmari P, Rosenbaum P et al: Cognitive abilities and school performance of extremely low birth weight children and matched term control children at age 8 years: a regional study, *J Pediatr* 118:751, 1991.

449. Sammon M, Darnell R: Entrainment of respiration to rocking in premature infants: coherence analysis, *Appl Physiol* 77:1548, 1994.

450. Sampers J: The effect of noise on the behavior of preterm infants in a neonatal intensive care unit. The physical and developmental environment of the high-risk infant (abstract), Orlando, Fla, 1995, University of South Florida College of Medicine.

451. Samsom J, deGroot L: The influence of postural control on motility and hand function in a group of high risk preterm infants at 1 year of age, *Early Hum Dev* 60:101, 2000.

452. Sarnat HB: Olfactory reflexes in newborn infants, *J Pediatr* 92:624, 1978.

453. Saunders RB, Friedman CB, Stramoski PR: Feeding preterm infants: schedule or demand? *J Obstet Gynecol Neonatal Nurs* 20:212, 1991.

454. Scafidi F, Field T: Massage therapy improves behavior in neonates born to HIV positive mothers, *J Ped Psychol* 21:889, 1996.

455. Scafidi F, Field T, Schanberg S: Factors that predict which preterm infants benefit more from massage therapy, *J Dev Behav Pediatr* 14:176, 1993.

456. Scafidi FA, Field T, Schanberg S: Effects of tactile/kinesthetic stimulation on the clinical course and sleep-wake behavior of preterm neonates, *Infant Behav Dev* 9:91, 1986.

457. Scafidi F, Field T, Schanberg S et al: Massage stimulates growth in preterm infants: a replication, *Infant Behav Dev* 13:167, 1990.

458. Schanberg S, Field T: Maternal deprivation and supplemental stimulation. In Field T, McCabe P, Schneiderman N, eds: *Stress and coping across development,* Hillsdale, NJ, 1988, Lawrence Erlbaum.

459. Schwartz R: Effect of position on oxygenation, heart rate, and behavioral state in the transitional newborn infant, *Neonatal Netw* 12:73, 1993.

460. Schwartz R, Moddy L, Yarandi H et al: A meta-analysis of critical outcome variables in non-nutritive sucking in preterm infants, *Nurs Res* 36: 292 1987.

461. Schwirian P, Easley T, Cuellar L: Use of water pillows in reducing head shape distortion in preterm infants, *Res Nurs Health* 9:203, 1986.

462. Selley W, Ellis R, Flack F et al: Coordination of sucking, swallowing and breathing in the newborn: its relationship to infant feeding and normal development, *Br J Disord Comm* 25:311, 1990.

463. Serenius F, Lindberg T, Stuge E et al: Early kangaroo care in sick very preterm infants, *Pediatr Res* 45:244A, 1999.

464. Seron-Ferre M, Duscay C, Valensula G: Circadian rhythms during pregnancy, *Endocr Rev* 14:594, 1993.

465. Shaker C: Nipple feeding premature infants: a different perspective, *Neonatal Netw* 8:9, 1990

466. Shaker C: Nipple feeding preterm infants: an individualized, developmentally supportive approach, *Neonatal Netw* 18:15, 1999.

467. Shananhan T, Czeisler C: Physiological effects of light on the human circadian pacemaker, *Semin Perinatol* 24:299, 2000.

468. Sharp M, French N, Hagan R: Survival and outcome at very short gestation (22-25 w) in Western Australia, *Pediatr Res* 45:255A, 1999.

469. Sheagren TG, Mangurten HH, Brea F et al: Rumination: a new complication of neonatal intensive care, *Pediatrics* 66:551, 1980.

470. Shiao S-Y: Comparison of continuous vs. intermittent sucking in VLBW infants, *J Obstet Gynecol Neonatal Nurs* 26:313, 1997.

471. Shiao S, Brooker J, DiFiore T: Desaturation events during oral feedings with and without a nasogastric tube in VLBW infants, *Heart Lung* 25:236, 1996.

472. Shiao S-Y, Youngblut J, Anderson G et al: Nasogastric tube placement: effects on breathing and sucking in VLBW infants, *Nurs Res* 44:82, 1995.

473. Shimada M, Segawa M, Higurashi M et al: Development of the sleep and wakefulness rhythm in preterm infants discharged from a neonatal care unit, *Pediatr Res* 33:159, 1993.

474. Shimada M, Takahashi K, Segawa M et al: Emerging and entraining patterns of the sleep-wake rhythm in preterm and term infants, *Brain Dev* 21:468, 1999.

475. Shiroiwa Y, Kamiya Y, Uchibori S et al: Activity, cardiac and respiratory responses of blindfold preterm infants in a neonatal intensive care unit, *Early Hum Dev* 14:259, 1986.

476. Shivpuri C, Martin R, Carlo W et al: Decreased ventilation in preterm infants during oral feeding, *J Pediatr* 103:285, 1983.

477. Short MA, Brooks-Brunn JA, Reeves DS et al: The effects of swaddling versus standard positioning on neuromuscular development in very low birth weight infants, *Neonatal Netw* 15:25, 1996.

478. Siegfried E, Shah P: Skin care practices in the neonatal nursery: a clinical survey, *J Perinatol* 19: 31, 1999.

479. Sieratzki J, Woll B: Why do mothers cradle babies on their left? *Lancet* 347:1746, 1996.

480. Simon N: Long-term neurodevelopmental outcome of asphyxiated newborns, *Clin Perinatol* 26:767, 1999.

481. Simons C, Mandich M, Ritchie S et al: Assessment of motor development in VLBW infants, *J Perinatol* 3:172, 2000.

482. Skadberg B, Markestad T: Behavior and physiologic responses during prone and supine sleep in early infancy, *Arch Dis Child* 76:320, 1997.

483. Skranes JS, Vik T, Nilsen G et al: Cerebral magnetic resonance imaging and mental and motor function of VLBW children at six years of age, *Neuropediatrics* 28:149, 1997.

484. Solkoff N et al: Effects of handling on the subsequent development of premature infants, *Dev Psychol* 1:461, 1969.

485. Solkoff N, Matuszak D: Tactile stimulation and behavioral development among low birth weight infants, *Child Psychiatry Hum Dev* 6:33, 1975.

486. Spitz R: Hospitalism, *Psychoanal Study Child* 1:53, 1945.

487. St. James-Roberts I, Conroy S, Hurry J: Links between infant crying and sleep-waking at six weeks of age, *Early Hum Dev* 48:143, 1997.

488. Steele BF: The effect of abuse and neglect on psychological development. In Call JD, Galenson E, Tyson RL, eds: *Frontiers of infant psychiatry,* New York, 1983, Basic Books.

489. Steinschneider A, Lipton E, Richmond J: Auditory sensitivity in the infant: effect of intensity on cardiac and motor responsivity, *Child Dev* 37:233, 1966.

490. Stevens B, Johnston C, Franck L et al: The efficacy of developmentally sensitive interventions and sucrose for relieving procedural pain in VLBW infants, *Nurs Res* 48:35, 1999.

491. Stevens B, Petryshen P, Hawkins J et al: Developmental vs. conventional care: a comparison of clinical outcomes for very low birth weight infants, *Can J Nurs Res* 28:97, 1996.

492. Stevenson R, Allaire J: The development of normal feeding and swallowing, *Pediatr Clin North Am* 38:1439, 1991.

493. Stewart A, Kirkbride V: Very preterm infants at fourteen years: relationship with neonatal ultrasound brain scans and neurodevelopmental status at one year, *Acta Paediatr Suppl* 416:44, 1996.

494. Stewart AL, Rifkin L, Amess PL et al: Brain structure and neurocognitive and behavioral function in adolescents who were born very preterm, *Lancet* 353:1653, 1999.

495. Stjernquist K, Svenningsen N: Extremely LBW infants less than 901 gm: development and behavior after four years of life, *Acta Paediatr* 84:500, 1995.

496. Stoll B, Bauer C, Bobashev G et al: Infants at the limit of viability: 401-700 grams at birth, *Pediatr Res* 45:255A, 1999.

497. Strauth C, Brandt S, Edwards-Beckett J: Implementation of a quiet hour: effect on noise levels and infant sleep states, *Neonatal Netw* 12:31, 1993.

498. Suave R, Robertson C, Etches P et al: Before viability: a geographically based outcome study of infants weighing 500 grams or less at birth, *Pediatrics* 101:438, 1998.

499. Sumida Y, Fujimura M: Brain white matter area quantified by MRI correlates with IQ of school children born <1000 gm: Poster Session III, Pediatric Academic Societies' Annual Meeting, May 1999, San Francisco, Calif.

500. Swaab D: Development of the human hypothalamus, *Neurochem Res* 20:509, 1995.

501. Sykes DH, Hoy EA, Bill JM et al: Behavioural adjustment in school of very low birth weight children, *J Child Psychol Psychiatry* 38:315, 1997.

502. Synnes AR, Ling EW, Whitfield F et al: Perinatal outcomes of a large cohort of extremely low gestational age infants (twenty-three to twenty-eight completed weeks of gestation), *Pediatrics* 125:952, 1994.

503. Tappin DM, Ford RP, Nelson KP et al: Breathing, sleep state and rectal temperature oscillations, *Arch Dis Child* 74:427, 1996.

504. Taquino L, Blackburn S: The effects of containment during suction and heelstick on physiological and behavioral responses of preterm infants, *Neonatal Netw* 13:55, 1994.

505. Taylor H, Hack M: Achievement in children with birth weights <750 gms with normal cognitive abilities: evidence for specific learning disabilities, *J Pediatr Psychol* 20:703, 1995.

506. Tenreiro S, Dowse HB, D'Souza S et al: The development of ultradian and circadian rhythms in premature babies maintained in constant conditions, *Early Hum Dev* 27:33, 1991.

507. Tessier R, Cristo M, Velez S et al: Kangaroo mother care and the bonding hypothesis, *Pediatrics* 102:390, 1998.

508. The Infant Health and Development Program: Enhancing the outcome of low birth weight premature infants: a multisite randomized trial, *JAMA* 263:3035, 1990.

509. The Victorian Infant Collaborative Study Group: Outcome at 2 years of children 23-27 weeks' gestation born in Victoria in 1991-92, *J Pediatr Child Health* 33:161, 1997.

510. Thoden C, Koivisto M: Acoustic analysis of the normal pain cry. In Murry M, Murry J, eds: *Infant communication: crying and early speech,* Houston, 1980, College Hill Press.

511. Thoman E: The breathing bear and the remarkable premature infant. In Goldson E, ed: *Nurturing the premature infant,* New York, 1999, Oxford University Press.

512. Thoman EB, Ingersol EW, Acebo C: Premature infants seek rhythmic stimulation and the experience facilitates neurobehavioral development, *Dev Behav Pediatr* 12:11, 1991.

513. Thomas K: Biorhythms in infants and role of the care environment, *J Perinat Neonatal Nurs* 9:61, 1995.

514. Thomas K: Differential effects of breast-and-formula feeding on preterm infants' sleep-wake patterns, *J Obstet Gynecol Neonatal Nurs* 29:145, 2000.

515. Thomas K, Burr R: Preterm infant thermal care: differing thermal environments produced by art vs. skin servo-control incubators, *J Perinatol* 19:264, 1999.

516. Thomas K, Martin P: NICU sound environment and the potential problems for caregivers, *J Perinatol* 20:594, 2000.

517. Thoyre S: Mothers' ideas about their role in feeding their high-risk infants, *J Obstet Gynecol Neonatal Nurs* 29:613, 2000.

518. Torres C, Holditch-Davis D, O'Hale A et al: Effect of standard rest periods on apnea and weight gain in preterm infants, *Neonatal Netw* 16:35, 1997.

519. Touch S, Epstein M, Pohl C et al: Impact on sleep patterns of co-bedding multiple gestation infants, *Pediatr Res* 47:436A, 2000.

520. Treas L: Incubator covers: health or hazard? *Neonatal Netw* 12:50, 1993.

521. Treolar D: The effect of non-nutritive sucking on oxygenation in healthy, crying, full-term infants, *Appl Nurs Res* 2:52, 1994.

522. Tribotti S: Effects of gentle touch on the premature infant. In Gonzenhauser N, ed: *Advances in touch: new implications in human development,* Skillman, NJ, 1990, Johnson & Johnson.

523. Tronick EZ, Scanlon KB, Scanlon JW: Protective apathy: a hypothesis about the behavioral organization and its relation to clinical and physiologic status of the preterm infant during the newborn period, *Clin Perinatol* 17:125, 1990.

524. Tudehope D, Smyth V, Scott J et al: Audiological evaluation of VLBW infants, *J Pediatr Child Health* 28:172, 1992.

525. Updike C, Schmidt RE, Macke C et al: Positional support for premature infants, *Am J Occup Ther* 40(10):712, 1986.

526. Uvnas-Moberg K, Widstrom A, Marchine G et al: Release of GI hormone in mothers and infants by sensory stimulation, *Acta Paediatr Scand* 76:851, 1987.

527. Valesco-Whetsell M, Evans J, Wang M: Do postsuctioning transcutaneous Po2 values change when a neonate's movements are restrained? *J Perinatol* 12:333, 1992.

528. Vandenberg KA: Revising the traditional model: an individualized approach to developmental interventions, *Neonatal Netw* 3:32, 1985.

529. Vandenberg K: Nippling management of the sick neonate in the NICU: the disorganized feeder, *Neonatal Netw* 9:9, 1990.

530. Vandenberg K: Developmental care: is it working? *Neonatal Netw* 15:67, 1996.

531. Vandenberg K: What to tell parents about the developmental needs of their baby at discharge, *Neonatal Netw* 18:57, 1999.

532. Vandenberg KA: Basic principles of developmental caregiving, *Neonatal Netw* 16:69, 1997.

533. VanNaarden K, Decoufle P: Relative and attributable risks for moderate to profound bilateral sensorineural hearing impairment associated with lower birth weight in children 3-10 years old, *Pediatrics* 104:905, 1999.

534. Varendi H, Porter R, Winberg J: Does the newborn baby find the nipple by smell? *Lancet* 344:989, 1994.

535. Vohr BR, Wright LL, Dusick MM et al: Neurodevelopmental and functional outcomes of Child Health and Human Development Neonatal Research Network, 1993-1994, *Pediatrics* 105:1216, 2000.

536. Volpe J: Cognitive deficits in premature infants, *N Engl J Med* 325:277, 1991.

537. Volpe J: Brain injury in the premature infant from pathogenesis to prevention, *Brain Dev* 19:519, 1997.

538. Volpe J: Neurologic outcome of prematurity, *Arch Neurol* 55:297, 1998.

539. Wagaman MJ, Shutack JG, Moomjian AS et al: Improved oxygenation and lung compliance with prone positioning of neonates, *J Pediatr* 94:787, 1979.

540. Watt JE, Strongman KT: The organization and stability of sleep states in full-term, preterm and SGA infants: a comparative study, *Dev Psychobiol* 18:151, 1985.

541. Wedenberg E: Auditory tests on new-born infants, *Acta Otolaryngol* 46:446, 1956.

542. Weiss S: Psychophysiologic and behavioral effects of tactile stimulation on infants with congenital heart disease, *Res Nurs* 15:93, 1992.

543. Weiss S: Predictors of neurobehavioral response during tactile stimulation of infants with congenital heart disease, *Infant Behav Dev* 16:261, 1993.

544. Wereszczak J, Miles M, Holditch-Davis D: Maternal recall of the NICU, *Neonatal Netw* 16:33, 1997.

545. Werner L, Marean G: *Human auditory development,* Boulder, 1996, Westview Press.

546. Werner N, Conway A: Caregiver contacts experienced by premature infants in the neonatal intensive care unit, *Matern Child Nurs* 19:21, 1990.

547. Westrup B, Kleberg A, Wallin L et al: Evaluation of the Newborn Individualized Developmental Care and Assessment Program (NIDCAP) in a Swedish setting, *Prenat Neonatal Med* 2:366, 1997.

548. Westrup B, Kleberg A, von Eichwald W et al: A randomized, controlled trial to evaluate the effects of the Newborn Individualized Developmental Care and Assessment Program in a Swedish setting, *Pediatrics* 105:66, 2000.

549. Wheeden A, Scafidi FA, Field T et al: Massage effects on cocaine-exposed preterm neonates, *J Dev Behav Pediatr* 14:318, 1993.

550. Whitaker AH, Van Rossem R, Feldman JF et al: Psychiatric outcomes in low-birth-weight children at age 6 years: relation to neonatal cranial ultrasound abnormalities, *Arch Gen Psychiatry* 54:847, 1997.

551. Whitelaw A, Heisterkamp G, Sleath K et al: Skin-to-skin contact for very low birth weight infants and their mothers, *Arch Dis Child* 63:1377, 1988.

552. White-Traut RC, Nelson MN, Silvestri JM et al: Responses of preterm infants to unimodal and multimodal sensory intervention, *Pediatr Nurs* 23:169, 1997.

553. Whitfield M, Grunau R, Holsti L: Extremely premature (<800 gm) school children: multiple areas of hidden disability, *Arch Dis Child* 77:F85, 1997.

554. Whitman T, O'Callaghan M, Maxwell S: The effects of cycled vs. noncycled lighting on growth and development in preterm infants, *Infant Behav Dev* 18:87, 1995.

555. Whyte HE, Fitzhardinge PM, Shennan AT et al: Extreme immaturity: outcome of 568 pregnancies of 23-25 weeks gestation, *Obstet Gynecol* 82:1, 1993.

556. Wingert WA, Teberg A, Bergman R et al: PNPs in follow-up care of high risk infants, *Am J Nurs* 80:1485, 1980.

557. Wolf L, Glass R: *Feeding and swallowing disorders in infancy: assessment and management,* Tucson, 1992, Therapy Skill Builders.

558. Wolff P: The natural history of crying and other vocalizations in early infancy. In Foss B, ed: *Determinants of infant behavior,* ed 4, London, 1969, Metheum.

559. Wolke D, Meyer R: Cognitive status, language attainment and prereading skills of 6 year old very preterm children and their peers: the Bavarian Longitudinal Study, *Dev Med Child Neurol* 41:94, 1999.

560. Wolke D, Meyer R, Ohrt B et al: The incidence of sleeping problems in preterm and full-term infants discharged from neonatal special care units: an epidemiological longitudinal study, *J Child Psychol Psychiatry Allied Discip* 36:203, 1995.

561. Wood N, Marlow N, Costeloe K: Neurologic and developmental disability after extremely preterm birth, *N Engl J Med* 343:378, 2000.

562. Woodson R, Drinkwin J, Hamilton C et al: Effects of non-nutritive sucking on state and activity: term-preterm comparisons, *Infant Behav Dev* 8:435, 1985.

563. Zahr L, Traversay J: Premature infant responses to noise reduction by earmuffs: effects on behavioral and physiologic measures, *J Perinatol* 15:448, 1995.

564. Zahr L, Balian S: Responses of premature infants to routine nursing interventions and noise in the NICU, *Nurs Res* 44:179, 1995.

565. Zaramella P, Freato F, Salvadori S et al: Brain auditory activation measured by near-infrared spectroscopy (Nirs) in neonates, *Pediatr Res* 47:442A, 2000.

RESOURCES FOR PARENTS

Dorner A: Prematurely yours (video), Boston, 1983, Polymorph Films.

Dorner A: To have and not to hold: helping parents cope (video), Boston, 1983, Polymorph Films.

Flushman B et al: *My special start: a guide for parents in the neonatal intensive care unit,* Palo Alto, Calif, VORT.

Healy T: *Guiding your child through preterm development,* Alexandria, Va, 1988, Parent Care.

Hussey B: *Understanding my signals,* Palo Alto, Calif, 1988, VORT.

Institute for Family-Centered Care: Newborn intensive care: changing practice, changing attitudes (video), Bethesda, Md, 1996, The Institute.

Ludington-Hoe S, Golant S: *Kangaroo care: the best you can do to help your preterm infant,* New York, 1993, Bantam Books.

Rosenberg S: Kangaroo care: a parent's touch (video), Chicago, 1996, Prentice Women's Hospital.

PART III

METABOLIC AND NUTRITIONAL CARE OF THE NEONATE

14 | Fluid and Electrolyte Management

David D. Berry, Eugene W. Adcock III, Alisa Starbuck

Although advances in the management of specific neonatal disorders have contributed to a remarkable decline in morbidity and mortality in newborns, fluid and electrolyte therapy, thermal regulation, and maintenance of oxygenation remain the central features of modern, supportive neonatal intensive care. Thus it is assumed that all infants requiring tertiary care (and most infants requiring so-called intermediate, level II, or secondary care) will initially receive parenteral fluid and electrolytes. Much useful information has accumulated about full-term infants, but some crucial information is still missing, especially about VLBW infants. For example, it is now clear that the restrictive fluid policies of the 1950s (which were aimed at reducing the observed postnatal diuresis) were misguided efforts that eventuated in hyperosmolality, hyperbilirubinemia, and hypoglycemia. On the other hand, the degree to which initial fluid, electrolyte, and glucose administration should be "liberalized" remains unsettled,[1,5,6] largely because of suggestions that in VLBW infants patent ductus arteriosus, necrotizing enterocolitis, bronchopulmonary dysplasia (BPD), intraventricular hemorrhage (IVH), and hyperglycemia are associated with larger volumes of fluid, electrolyte, and glucose administration.[3] At best, approximations for therapy are necessary in many clinical situations.

This chapter is based on implementing these fundamental principles: (1) rapidly assessing the infant's initial condition, (2) developing a short-term, time-oriented, management plan, (3) initiating therapy, and (4) monitoring the infant and modifying the plan based on clinical and biochemical data.

PHYSIOLOGY

Neonates show dramatic physiologic differences when compared on a per-kilogram basis with older children and adults: (1) their basic metabolic rate is at least double, (2) their water requirements are four to five times greater, and (3) their sodium excretion is only 10% of that in older children and adults. The subdivisions of total body mass (TBM) are illustrated in Figure 14-1. TBW as a percentage of TBM demonstrates a curvilinear decline with increasing age (Figure 14-2). Intracellular fluid (ICF) and extracellular fluid (ECF) as percentages of TBM change in opposite directions as gestation advances.

These physiologic and body composition phenomena result in a narrow margin of safety in calculating fluids and electrolytes for small infants, especially those weighing less than 1250 g. Caregivers should independently calculate all requirements and compare calculations with each other. **IV fluid should be administered by a special infusion pump that can regulate fluid at a precision of 0.1 ml or greater. Intake should be measured hourly and output measured as soon as it occurs. The balance of intake and output should be assessed at least every 8 to 12 hours using a standard form (Figure 14-3).** Once clinical signs of fluid overload or deficit occur, it may be extremely difficult to regain balance. Fluid balance should be viewed prospectively. A similar procedure should be a part of every initial care plan.

The effect of gestational age on body composition is striking (Figure 14-4). Because gestational age is an important determinant of the percentage and distribution of TBW, accurate assessment is important. Changes in distribution and percent of body water may also depend on intrauterine growth, maternal fluid balance, postnatal age, diet, daily water intake, and changing metabolism. Furthermore, it now seems clear that at least part of the initial (first 1 to 3 days) weight loss of both healthy term (up to 5% to 10% of TBM) and preterm (up to 10% to

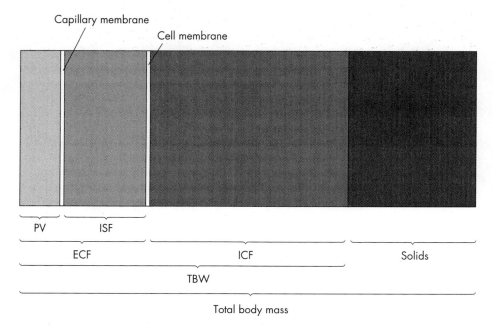

FIGURE 14-1   Major subdivisions of total body mass. *ECF,* Extracellular fluid; *ICF,* intracellular fluid; *ISF,* interstitial fluid; *PV,* plasma volume; *TBW,* total body water. (From Winters RW, ed: *The body fluids in pediatrics,* Boston, 1973, Little, Brown.)

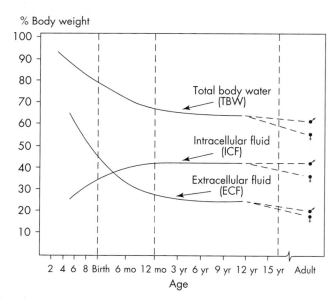

FIGURE 14-2   Effects on age of TBW, ICF, and ECF. Note curvilinear changes that are maximal during perinatal period. (From Winters RW, ed: *The body fluids in pediatrics,* Boston, 1973, Little, Brown.)

Output

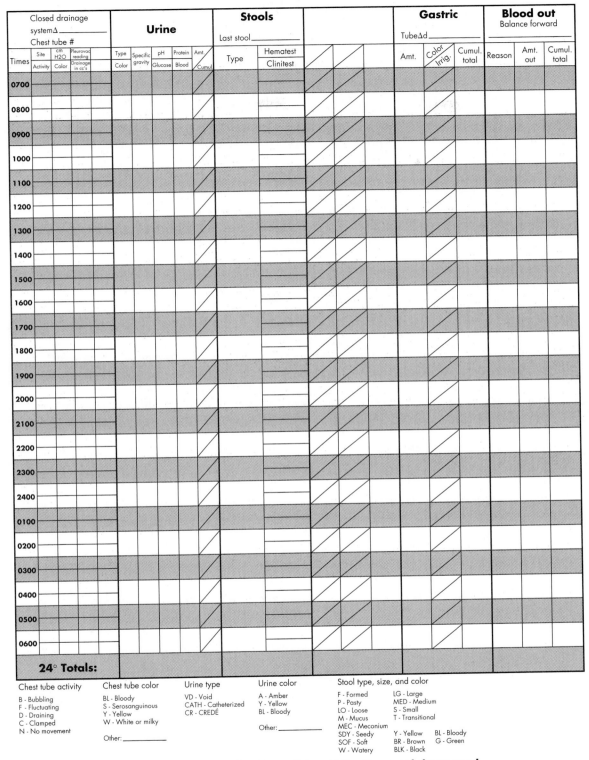

FIGURE 14-3   Model intake and output sheet. (Courtesy Brenner Children's Hospital, Winston-Salem, North Carolina.)

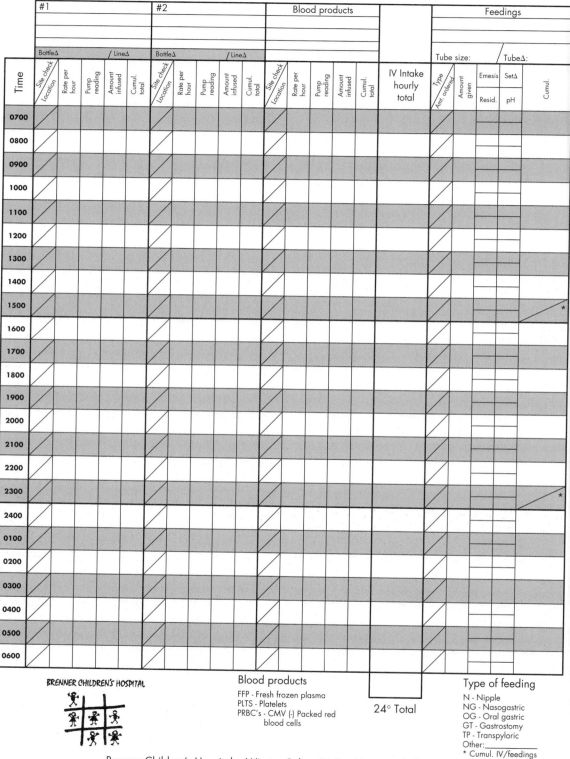

FIGURE 14-3, cont'd Model intake and output sheet. (Courtesy Brenner Children's Hospital, Winston-Salem, North Carolina.)

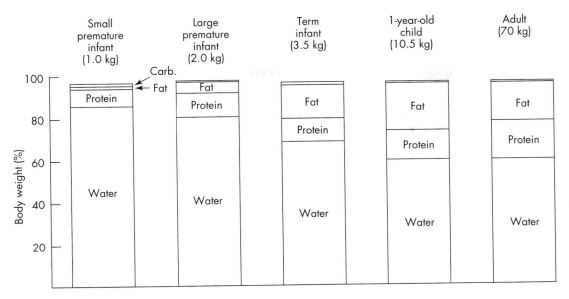

FIGURE 14-4   Effects of gestational age on body composition compared with older children and adults. (From Heird WC, Driscoll JM Jr, Schullinger JN et al: Intravenous alimentation in pediatric patients, *J Pediatr* 80:351, 1972.)

15% of TBM) infants should be considered a normal physiologic loss of fluid from the interstitial fluid (ISF), rather than a pathophysiologic catabolism of body tissues.[2]

Reviewing the maternal history and the intrapartum course may be helpful in calculating the infant's fluid and electrolyte requirements. For example, if the mother received large amounts of electrolyte-free fluids in the intrapartum period, the neonate may be hyponatremic and have expanded extracellular (ECF) at birth. Because SGA infants have reduced amounts of fat, body water (as a percentage of TBM) increases. Conversely, LGA infants have a smaller percentage of TBW because of an increased amount of body fat.

Sodium is the major cation in ECF (both ISF and plasma) and is easily measured. Potassium, the major cation in ICF, cannot be measured readily, because ICF is not clinically accessible. Because 90% of the total body potassium is intracellular, when plasma potassium is low, it is assumed that the total body potassium is invariably low. Electrolyte composition of ISF and plasma is similar, but strikingly different from ICF (Figure 14-5).

Osmotic force or pressure is a phenomenon that is a colligative property of any solution. Osmotic phe-

Table 14-1	EXAMPLES OF OSMOTIC FORCE		
	MM	N	MOSM
NaCl	1	2	2
Glucose	1	1	1
CaCl₂	1	3	3

nomena depend on the number (N) of particles (regardless of size or charge) in a solution and are measured in milliosmoles, according to the equation:

$$mOsm = (mM) \times (N)$$

Table 14-1 shows three examples. **Unfortunately, two physical chemistry terms are used interchangeably in clinical medicine: (1) osmolality (milliosmole per kilogram of water) and (2) osmolarity (milliosmole per liter of solution).** In most laboratories, osmotic forces are determined by the technique of freezing point depression, so osmolality is the correct term (normally 280 to 300 mOsm/kg water). The difference in terms is usually unimportant, because the total solid content per liter of plasma is small.

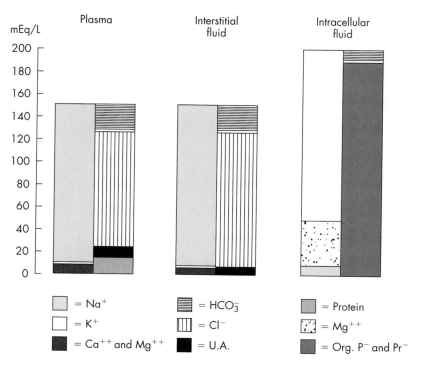

FIGURE 14-5 "Gamblegram" of plasma ISF and ICF. (From Winters RW, ed: *The body fluids in pediatrics,* Boston, 1973, Little, Brown.)

Osmotic forces can be satisfactorily estimated (Figure 14-6)[12] in many clinical settings by the following formula:

$$2(Na^+) + \frac{BUN\ (mg/dl) \times 10}{28} \times \frac{Glucose\ (mg/dl) \times 10}{180}$$

The molecular weights of two nitrogen atoms and glucose are 28 and 180, respectively; BUN is blood urea nitrogen.

Osmotic forces are responsible for apparently low plasma electrolyte concentrations in some common clinical settings. In hyperglycemia, the plasma sodium concentrate reported by the laboratory is usually low, but the total effective osmolality may be normal, as seen in this example:

Glucose = 720 mg/dl
(Na^+) = 120 mEq/L
mOsm/L = 280
$\frac{720 \times 10}{180} + 120 \times 2 = 280$

Although hyperlipidemia is less frequent, an analogous situation exists (Figure 14-7). Low laboratory values for plasma sodium occur because the increase in plasma solids (lipids) causes a lower plasma water content and hence a lower sodium concentration per liter of whole plasma. In this case the plasma water sodium concentration may be normal.

Osmotic forces largely determine shifts in the internal redistribution of water in hydration disturbances. Four pure disturbances of hydration exist: (1) too much electrolyte, (2) too little electrolyte, (3) too much water, and (4) too little water. Combinations of these disturbances may also occur.

Neonatal renal "immaturity" influences fluid and electrolyte needs. Various renal functions do not develop at the same rate. The glomerular filtration rate (GFR) is low at birth and, despite the initial gestational age, characteristically rises rapidly during the first 6 weeks of life. A VLBW infant in satisfactory condition at 6 weeks may have an adequate GFR. These observations correlate with the infant's obtaining a full complement of nephrons (about 34 weeks' gestation) and the continued increase in glomerular surface area (beyond 40 weeks' gestation).[5,6]

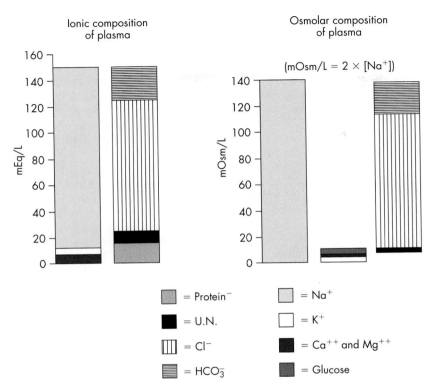

FIGURE 14-6 Ionic and osmolar composition of plasma. (From Winters RW, ed: *The body fluids in pediatrics,* Boston, 1973, Little, Brown.)

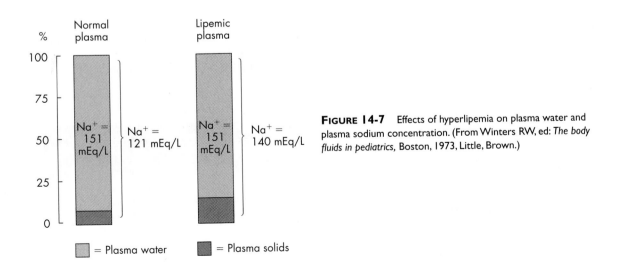

FIGURE 14-7 Effects of hyperlipemia on plasma water and plasma sodium concentration. (From Winters RW, ed: *The body fluids in pediatrics,* Boston, 1973, Little, Brown.)

Urinary sodium excretion increases slowly during the first 2 years of life. Urine sodium losses are influenced by sodium intake and gestational age. Urine sodium may rise when moderately increased amounts of sodium are given to more mature infants. VLBW infants, however, tend to lose urine sodium, which may be greater per kilogram than that of term infants, when receiving the normal (1 to 4 mEq/kg) sodium intake.

The capacity to dilute and concentrate urine appears limited but can be influenced by gestational age and nutrient intake. The immature concentrating ability (maximum of approximately 600 mOsm/L; Figure 14-8) coupled with the inability to excrete rapidly either an acute water or sodium load results in a narrow margin of safety in prescribing fluid and electrolytes, especially in the VLBW infant.[1,2,5,6]

Urea is usually the major component of urine osmolality (and hence specific gravity), whereas electrolytes quantitatively contribute less. When total parenteral nutrition is being provided, urine specific gravity may rise because of the low renal threshold for glucose and amino acids. When specific gravity rises, therefore, the cause must be ascertained before altering the fluid infusion rate. A diagnostic test (Multistix 10-SC or Chemstrip) can screen for glucose and protein but misses amino acids, which must be detected by amino acid chromatography when necessary.

Neonatal urinary acidification is limited, and the bicarbonate threshold is reduced. Both physiologic and pathophysiologic factors can contribute to an alkaline urine. For example, VLBW infants have a limited capacity for hydrogen ion excretion, whereas other infants may have acute illnesses such as bicarbonate-losing tubular necrosis or urinary tract infection.

The roles of hormones, such as antidiuretic hormone, aldosterone, atrial natriuretic factor, and parathormone, in regulating neonatal fluid and electrolyte balance are not well defined. Hormonal influences can be primary, such as in the syndrome of inappropriate secretion of antidiuretic hormone and in some cases of hypocalcemia. Secondary hormonal influences can be caused by certain drugs, such as spironolactones, which are aldosterone antagonists.

Insensible water loss (IWL) occurs by both pulmonary and cutaneous routes and is influenced by the factors listed in Table 14-2. Because clinical states and environmental factors influence water needs, there is normally a wide range (30 to 60 ml/kg/24 hr) of IWL in healthy term infants. Factors that decrease IWL may do so by as much as one third in VLBW infants and should be given consideration in each patient (Table 14-2). When operative concomitantly, several of these factors can increase IWL by as much as 300%, such as when phototherapy is used and a VLBW infant is under a radiant warmer.[5,6] This can be avoided, however, by using a bili-blanket on an infant in a double-walled isolette. For every 1° C rise in body temperature, metabolism and fluid needs increase approximately 10% (the

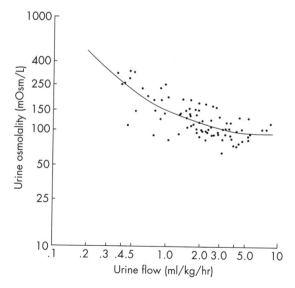

FIGURE 14-8 Normal urine flow rates. (From Jones MD, Gresham EL, Battaglia FC: Urinary flow rate and urea excretion rates in newborn infants, *Biol Neonate* 21:322, 1972.)

Table 14-2	FACTORS THAT INFLUENCE INSENSIBLE WATER LOSS (IWL)	
DECREASE IWL	**INCREASE IWL**	
Heat shield or double-walled incubators	Inversely related to gestational age and weight	
Plastic blankets	Respiratory distress	
Clothes	Ambient temperature above thermoneutral	
High relative humidity (ambient ventilator gas)	Fever	
	Radiant warmer	
	Phototherapy	
	Activity	

"Q-10 effect"). These expected increases must be recognized in calculating fluid requirements.

ETIOLOGY

The causes of common electrolyte problems and common clinical syndromes are discussed in the section on treatment.

PREVENTION

Prevention of fluid and electrolyte imbalance in neonates begins with knowing how to calculate fluid and electrolyte requirements properly. The estimated metabolic rate forms the reference base for all calculations. The metabolic rate (and hence oxygen consumption) normally increases steadily over the first weeks of life, so increases in water and probably electrolyte needs should be anticipated.

If the caloric requirement is approximately 100 cal/kg/day, the physiologic basis of metabolic rate may be used in calculating needs; however, most institutions use the 100 ml/kg basis, which will be modified by factors that influence IWL and be adjusted depending on body weight, clinical composition, and urine volume and composition (Figure 14-9 and Table 14-3).

Preterm infants usually have slightly lower metabolic rates per kilogram than term infants do. SGA infants may have higher metabolic rates than those of preterm infants of similar weight; this is thought to be related to their relatively large brain/body mass ratio. Both SGA and preterm infants, especially VLBW infants, are expected to require more frequent modification of requirements.

Preterm infants, however, often are subject to other problems that may make this physiologic fact less crucial in calculating needs. SGA infants may require more water per kilogram than either preterm or term, normally grown infants. Input should be recorded every hour, and output should be recorded as it occurs. VLBW infants require frequent monitoring of fluid balance, so if output is unusually large, intake must be adjusted immediately. If fluid intake decreases, critically ill infants may not tolerate "catching up." Continuous monitoring is necessary to ensure that fluid is infusing in appropriate amounts. Infusion pumps that accurately register 1 ml/hr or less must be used.

Requirements for fluid and electrolytes can be divided into maintenance and deficit needs. Maintenance needs keep the baby in a zero balance state and can be subdivided into (1) normal loss, which consists of water and electrolyte loss through sweat, stool, urine, and insensible (lung and skin) routes and (2) abnormal or ongoing losses, such as diarrhea, ostomy, or chest tube drainage.

All diapers should be preweighed on a gram scale and marked with dry weight. After each stool or void the diaper is reweighed; the difference equals the amount of loss. For example, if the dry weight is 20.7 g and the wet weight is 26.4 g, the difference is 5.7 g, or 5.7 ml of stool or urine. All losses should be calculated to the nearest milliliter.

The term *deficit needs* refers to previously incurred losses. These should be extremely rare in the newborn but are common in older neonates with disorders that have an insidious or delayed onset, such as renal tubular dysfunction or nonvirilizing congenital adrenal hyperplasia.

Deficits are best estimated by body weight comparisons. A weight loss greater than 10% to 15% in 1 week should be considered excessive. VLBW infants

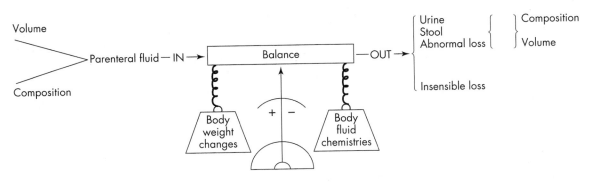

FIGURE 14-9 Basic scheme for monitoring and modifying therapy.

Table 14-3	GUIDELINES FOR FLUID (ML/KG/DAY) AND SOLUTE PROVISION BY PATIENT WEIGHT AND DAYS OF AGE				
WEIGHT (G)	RANGES OF WATER LOSS		DAY 1*	DAY 2-3*	DAY 4-7*
<1250	IWL†	40-170			
	Urine	50-100			
	Stool	5-10			
	TOTAL	95-280	120	140	150-175
1250-1750	IWL†	20-50			
	Urine	50-100			
	Stool	5-10			
	TOTAL	75-160	90	110	130-140
>1750	IWL†	15-40			
	Urine	50-100			
	Stool	5-10			
	TOTAL	70-150	80	90	100-200

Increment for phototherapy: 20-30 ml/kg/day
Increment for radiant warmer: 20-30 ml/kg/day
Maintenance solutes: Glucose: 7-12 g/kg (4-8 g/kg in VLBW infants)
Na: 1-4 mEq/kg (2-8 mEq/kg in VLBW infants)
K: 1-4 mEq/kg
Cl: 1-4 mEq/kg
Ca: 1 mEq/kg

*Adjustment based on a urine flow rate of 2 to 5 ml/kg/hr with a specific gravity of 1.002 to 1.010 and stable weight.
†May be reduced by 30% if the infant is on a ventilator.
IWL, Insensible water loss; *VLBW*, very-low-birth-weight.

are particularly difficult to maintain within 10% to 15% of birth weight during the first week of life.

The initial choice of parenteral solutions depends on the weight and postnatal age of the infant (see Table 14-3). Another important consideration is whether the infant is in an incubator or under a radiant warmer without a plastic blanket or heat shield. IWL of 170 ml/kg/day has been demonstrated in VLBW infants under radiant warmers.[5] **Maintenance of water needs in larger infants on the first day of life can usually be met by a 10% glucose solution infused at 80 ml/kg/day. The infusion rate should be increased gradually to 100 to 120 ml/kg/day using principles of monitoring discussed later.**

All sick infants require IV access for fluid administration[11] **The IV equipment should include (1) a needle or catheter, (2) connecting tubing, and (3) an infusion pump.**

Electrolytes such as sodium and potassium are usually omitted the first day and then added as chloride salts in amounts of 1 to 4 mEq/kg. Mildly acidotic and VLBW infants may be given their sodium requirements as sodium bicarbon-ate or acetate. Hypocalcemia also may be a frequent finding in tertiary care patients.

Potassium should never be added to IV fluid until urine flow and renal function have been assessed. The maintenance requirement for calcium is 0.5 to 1 mEq (100 to 200 mg)/kg given as calcium gluconate. This maintenance is most important in VLBW infants and those who are severely ill.

Factors that influence IWL must be identified early and maintenance needs adjusted appropriately to prevent problems with water and electrolyte balance. Management of VLBW infants presents special, complex problems, and further research is needed. We have observed the following:

- **Water requirements should start at 110 to 120 ml/kg at birth and often need to be increased by 20 to 40 ml/kg/day over days 2 to 4 of life, at which time they plateau at 150 to 175 ml/kg/day.**
- **Sodium requirements (including medications) are 2 to 3 mEq/kg/day after 24 hours of age and may reach a maximum of 7 mEq/ kg/day on days 5 and 6.**

- **Cumulative weight loss plateaus at 11% to 13% of birth weight (95% confidence limits) by day 3.**
- Maintaining normal serum glucose concentrations (less than 150 mg/dl) in VLBW infants requires relatively less glucose (4 to 8 g/kg/day) than in term infants. As anticipated, infants weighing 900 g or less are the most difficult to manage without causing either excessive weight loss or hypernatremia.

VLBW infants, especially infants kept under radiant warmers, may have greatly increased IWL. Hence their fluid requirements may be 175 to 200 ml/kg/day. By the end of the first week of life, as the epithelium becomes more cornified, the requirements decrease toward 120 to 150 ml/kg/day.

Neonates requiring administration of maintenance fluids when significant oral caloric intake is low (less than 50 kcal/kg/day) for more than 3 to 5 days should be given parenteral nutritional support with increased glucose, amino acids, lipids, vitamins, and micronutrients (see Chapter 17).

DATA COLLECTION

All parenteral therapy should be based on the following principles: (1) assessing the patient, including maintenance needs, factors that modify IWL, and specific medical or surgical disorders, (2) calculating short-term (12 to 24 hours) fluid and electrolyte needs, (3) initiating therapy at the proper site and rate, and (4) monitoring and modifying therapeutic measures based on clinical and biochemical data.

History

A history of factors that influence IWL (see Table 14-2) includes gestational age, birth weight, and postnatal age.

Signs and Symptoms

Weight, urine output, and serum sodium concentration are the best overall clinical guides to assessing the adequacy of therapy. Weight is the most sensitive index of IWL and must be accurately determined at least every 24 hours. Accurate daily weights in VLBW infants require special nursing efforts and often the use of electronic bed scales.

Urine output should be 2 to 5 ml/kg/hr with a specific gravity of 1.002 to 1.010 (60 to 300 mOsm) (Figure 14-10 [note the nonlinear relationship as specific gravity exceeds 1.010]; see also Figure 14-8).

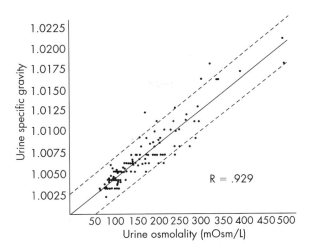

FIGURE 14-10 Urine specific gravity compared with osmolality. Solid line represents mean; broken line represents 95% confidence limits. (From Jones MD, Gresham EL, Battaglia FC: Urinary flow rate and urea excretion rates in newborn infants, *Biol Neonate* 21:322, 1972.)

Blood pressure and peripheral perfusion may reflect changes in vascular volume and cardiac output. Normal capillary refill occurs within 3 seconds, but hypothermia may falsely delay capillary refill.

Loss of skin turgor is a late and variable sign and is usually not helpful in assessing therapy, but vital signs (heart and respiratory rate and skin and core temperature) provide helpful clues about metabolic rate and stress. Drainage from ostomy sites, chest tubes, and nasogastric or other tubes must be quantitated accurately. These types of drainage represent abnormal or ongoing maintenance requirements that must be added to the calculation of normal maintenance needs (abnormal + normal = total maintenance).

Laboratory Data

Tests for concentrations of electrolytes (Na^+, K^+, Cl^-, Ca^{++}), red blood cells (hematocrit), glucose, BUN or creatinine, and acid-base status should be performed serially. Occasionally serum osmolality and protein concentrations are helpful in assessing the neonate's condition.

Urine specific gravity and volume must be measured as soon as voiding occurs. Urine osmolality and electrolyte concentration help clarify fluid and electrolyte balance when glucose, protein, or unusual solutes appear in the urine.

The water content of urine evaporates rapidly under a radiant warmer. Glucosuria and proteinuria (greater than 2+) cause modest elevations in specific gravity, whereas radiographic dyes excreted in the urine cause extreme increases in the specific gravity. All urine should be screened with a diagnostic test (Multistix or Chemstrip).

All drainage must be collected and measured, so that the concentration of solutes can be determined. Collections every 4 to 6 hours are preferable to a single "spot" collection, which is commonly misleading. Occasionally, determining trace elements, hematocrit, and protein content of urine or drainage can be crucial to management.

TREATMENT

Techniques of IV Therapy

Peripheral veins are the most easily accessible and have the least adverse effects for parenteral therapy. Scalp vein infusion sets are most commonly used in the foot, hand, or scalp veins. However, the advent of extremely small catheter and introducer sets (Quick-Cath, Angiocath, and others) has permitted prolonged (5 to 7 days) use of a single peripheral infusion site.

Often, a rubber band is the most effective tourniquet for the extremity of a small infant. The area of skin should be cleaned with an antiseptic, and efforts should be made to avoid shaving the head, because parents often find this upsetting. Before puncturing the skin, have the "setup" (as described previously) and the appropriate fluid ready.

It is important to recognize the high potential of infiltration and skin sloughs with peripheral IVs. The risk is greatest in the foot, less with the hand, and the least on the scalp. Calcium-containing solutions present an added risk. Although the needle or catheter must be taped in place, the tape must not prevent adequate visualization. **At least every hour the fluid administered should be recorded, and the site should be observed for any sign of infiltration.** The arm or leg can be positioned on a padded tongue blade (armboard or footboard) to prevent catheter displacement. A "flap" of tape can be made at the end of the board, which can be pinned or tied to the bed for further immobilization. Padded sandbags can be used to hold an infant's head or extremity still for a period of time but must be removed regularly to allow some movement. The need for immobilization is less with catheters than with scalp vein sets. However, the board may need to be removed after several hours for additional assurance of no infiltration, as well as mobilization of the limb.

Deep and central veins can be approached by two techniques. Percutaneous insertion using Silastic catheters can be accomplished readily only after much experience. Saphenous, antecubital, axillary, basilic, cephalic, or external jugular vein insertion while advancing the catheter to a deep vein is a relatively simple technique (long lines), and even subclavian cannulation of VLBW infants can be accomplished with appropriate training and experience.[4] The risk of infection and thrombosis is probably no greater than with peripheral infusion, but the consequences may be much more serious (see Chapter 17).

The second technique, venesection or cutdown, can also be performed readily with appropriate training. Catheterization for total parenteral nutrition, however, requires special consideration (see Chapter 17). The catheter is advantageous because patient mobility is greater, but the risks of infection and thrombosis may be greater than those with percutaneous techniques.

Umbilical vessel catheterization should be limited to several days' duration until a central catheter can be placed (see Chapter 7).

Common Problems

In NICUs virtually all patients initially receive IV fluid therapy, so conventional rules of pediatric fluid therapy, which estimate losses and project deficit replacement, are not completely satisfactory. Weight, urine output and concentration, and the concentration of various solutes in serum and other body fluids are usually known. The correct diagnosis usually rests on clinical and laboratory measurements (not estimates), which are supported by the clinical setting. A pure disorder of hydration is rarely encountered, but mixed disorders or syndromes usually are.

For example, one can compute the amount of sodium required to correct a deficit by the following formula:

Sodium required =
(Sodium desired − Sodium observed) × ECF

This calculation considers that the sodium will be given as a "dry salt." The total amount and the rate given is a matter of clinical judgment. In practice, the care giver usually begins sodium deficit therapy, measures serum sodium, and modifies the IV solution. The cause of the deficit must be identified while these conditions are being corrected, or it is likely to recur.

Common Electrolyte Disorders

Hypocalcemia (Infants With Less Than 7 mg/dl Serum Calcium)

Clinical findings may correlate poorly with biochemical data (total or ionized calcium). Jitteriness and twitching are nonspecific, and serum calcium (and probably glucose) should be measured. Hypocalcemia is strongly associated with infants of diabetic mothers, asphyxia, and prematurity (especially VLBW infants). "Early" hypocalcemia (occurring in the first 72 hours) can be prevented by the inclusion of 18 mg/kg of elemental calcium as 200 mg/kg of calcium gluconate in maintenance IV solution (1 mEq = 2 ml of 10% calcium gluconate).

Bolus infusion (also associated with dysrhythmias) and slow infusion for 2 to 3 minutes are not as successful as more gradual attempts to correct hypocalcemia. Either repeated (every 6 hours), slow infusion or continuous infusion is best. Additional elemental calcium should be given intravenously at 18 to 75 mg/kg for 4 to 6 hours if seizures or biochemical abnormality persists. "Late" hypocalcemia (occurring at more than 7 days of age) usually has a specific cause, such as high phosphate intake, malabsorption and postdiarrhea state, hypomagnesemia, hypoparathyroidism, or rickets and should be evaluated in detail.

Care should be taken in administering the IV calcium: (1) the infant should be placed on a cardiac monitor to detect bradycardia, (2) calcium administration should be discontinued immediately if bradycardia occurs, and (3) the peripheral IV site should be checked for patency before and during administration because of the potential for sloughing, calcification, and necrosis caused by infiltrated calcium.

Hypernatremia (Infants With More Than 150 mEq/L Serum Sodium)

Clinical signs of hypernatremia are rare, except for late-occurring seizures. The most common causes of hypernatremia are (1) dehydration (usually caused by too little "free water" administration), (2) injudicious use of sodium-containing solution (sodium bicarbonate bolus infusion and sodium-containing medications can be overlooked), and (3) congenital reduction in antidiuretic hormone. Both nephrogenic and central diabetes insipidus are uncommon. Cerebral palsy and intracranial bleeding correlate strongly with hypernatremia. Management is directed toward the causes, and serum sodium should be reduced slowly to prevent seizures.

Hyponatremia (Infants With Less Than 130 mEq/L Serum Sodium)

Hyponatremia is usually asymptomatic because of chronic rather than acute development of imbalance, but a late clinical sign is seizures. The most common causes include (1) overhydration as a result of maternal or neonatal administration of electrolyte-free solutions, (2) renal loss of sodium (common in VLBW infants) in any neonate receiving diuretic therapy, and (3) the syndrome of inappropriate antidiuretic hormone secretion (SIADH) that is suspected clinically when decreased serum sodium and increased urine specific gravity occur. This syndrome is associated with CNS and lung pathologic conditions. Criteria include (1) low serum sodium, (2) continued urine sodium loss, (3) urine osmolality greater than plasma, and (4) normal adrenal and renal function. Management is by water restriction until diuresis follows and is directed toward the etiology.

Hyperkalemia (Infants With More Than 7 mEq/L Serum Potassium)

Causes of hyperkalemia include (1) acidosis with or without tissue destruction, (2) renal failure (water overload may limit management), and (3) adrenal insufficiency (relatively uncommon). Table 14-4 outlines clinical signs and ECG changes. Management is directed toward the causes and nonspecific treatment, depending on the severity of the hyperkalemia:

- Stop all potassium administration.
- Infuse 100 to 200 mg of calcium gluconate to lower the cell membrane threshold (this is transient but may be lifesaving).
- Infuse sodium bicarbonate, 1 to 2 mEq/kg, which is another transient therapy aimed at enhancing intracellular sodium and hydrogen exchange for potassium.
- Administer 1 g/kg cation exchange resin (sodium polystyrene-sulfonate [Kayexalate]) as an oral or rectal solution. Little experience has

Table 14-4	HYPERKALEMIA (INFANTS WITH >7 mEq/L SERUM POTASSIUM)
CLINICAL SIGNS	**ELECTROCARDIOGRAPHIC CHANGES**
Muscular weakness	Short QT interval
Cardiac dysrhythmias	Widening QRS
Ileus	Sine wave QRS/T

been reported in neonates, and technical problems of retention can be substantial.

- Perform peritoneal dialysis, but frequently sodium bicarbonate must be added to dialysate to prevent acidosis.

Hypokalemia (Infants With Less Than 3.5 mEq/L Serum Potassium)

Clinical signs of hypokalemia are related to muscular weakness and cardiac dysrhythmias. Ileus may occur also. Electrocardiographic changes include a decreased T wave and ST depression. The most common causes of hypokalemia are (1) increased gastrointestinal losses from an ostomy and a nasogastric tube and (2) renal losses common in diuretic therapy.

About 90% of total potassium is intracellular. Management is directed toward the causes: (1) low serum potassium always implies significant intracellular depletion, (2) intracellular potassium can be low with normal serum potassium, and (3) **IV solutions should usually not exceed 40 mEq/L potassium.**

Common Clinical Syndromes

Acute renal failure is most often caused by (1) extrinsic factors such as asphyxia, shock, and heart failure; (2) intrinsic factors, such as congenital or acquired lesions; and (3) obstructive uropathy, including urethral or extragenitourinary mass. Oliguria or anuria usually occurs initially. Electrolyte-free glucose infusion should be limited to IWL and urine output. Elevations of BUN often do not occur, because protein intake is commonly low. Recovery is usually associated with natriuresis and osmotic diuresis. This may develop rapidly, and sodium loss as high as 20 mEq/kg/day may occur. Body weight and fluid losses must be carefully and frequently measured, at least every 12 hours. Nonrenal losses, such as gastrointestinal drainage, must also be measured. Ideally, balance treatment is directed toward no weight gain or a weight loss of 1%/day until recovery is nearly complete. Any weight gain demands careful reevaluation of the fluid plan.

Asphyxia is frequently associated with the following:

- Hypotension
- Renal failure (tubular necrosis is suggested by proteinuria and hematuria)
- Respiratory failure (ventilators reduce IWL from lungs)
- Myocardial ischemia (echocardiography can often assess ventricular function)

- SIADH early or late in the clinical course
- Cerebral edema (usually after 24 hours)

An asphyxiated neonate should be managed by prospectively reducing the initial fluid estimates by 30% to 60%. IWL and urine output may be the best initial plan, although volume expansion to treat hypotension may be a greater priority.

Major Surgery

Surgical trauma is superimposed on the normal metabolic responses of the neonate and determined by both gestational and postnatal age. In healthy term infants, negative balance of water, electrolytes, nitrogen, and calories with associated weight loss occurs during the first 3 to 5 days, with transition to positive balance and weight gain by 7 to 10 days. Similar transition times for preterm infants vary enormously. Deficits may exist as a result of delayed diagnosis, with external loss or internal loss. "Third space" (especially peritoneal) loss is a notorious source of deficit underestimation.

The exactness of the metabolic response to surgery is not resolved and varies widely among individual patients, even with similar lesions. Perhaps too many uncontrollable variables exist to define a normal postoperative physiologic response of neonates, especially those weighing less than 2 kg. Negative nitrogen balance always occurs postoperatively but is considerably less than in adults. The control of this tendency to minimize nitrogen loss is unknown. Thermal regulation is almost never controlled as well in an operating room as in an intensive care unit, but transport incubators, warmed operating rooms, radiant warmers, and prewarmed solutions should be used in an attempt to achieve thermoneutrality. Intraoperative fluid balance is rarely precise despite the best efforts. Blood loss on sponges, drapes, and other objects should be measured, but IWL from open body cavities is difficult to estimate.

The principles of postoperative management are (1) serial monitoring of clinical and chemical variables, and meticulously and frequently (every 4 to 6 hours) watching fluid balance, including drainage; (2) providing 30 to 40 kcal/kg as glucose and planning a zero balance of water and electrolytes for 1 to 3 days; and (3) using total parenteral nutrition if significant enteral feedings (less than 50 kcal/kg) cannot be achieved by 3 to 5 days. Gastrointestinal motility returns rapidly in term infants as compared with adults. Almost all VLBW infants require total parenteral nutrition after surgery.

Water intoxication (hypotonicity) is common in neonates because of small volumes of urine and relatively high volumes per kilogram of infusates. A high index of suspicion and meticulous attention to the details of IV therapy prevent hypotonicity. Increased antidiuretic hormone secretion commonly occurs and may progress to a syndrome of inappropriate antidiuretic hormone. Water intoxication may be hard to distinguish from hypotonic dehydration. Water restriction and continued sodium administration should be instituted only after the diagnosis is established. Fresh frozen plasma (10 to 20 ml/kg) given with a diuretic (1 to 2 mg/kg furosemide [Lasix]) may be used to make the diagnosis, because a good diuresis suggests dehydration or decreased plasma volume.

COMPLICATIONS

Increased fluid administration ($>$180 ml/kg) has been associated with (1) BPD, (2) necrotizing enterocolitis, and (3) patent ductus arteriosus (PDA). Reduced fluid administration (to prevent increased fluid administration) has been associated with (1) hypertonicity; (2) CNS damage, including bleeding and cerebral palsy; and (3) renal failure and tubular damage.

PARENT TEACHING

The need for and presence of an IV line in a newborn may be frightening for the parents. Clear, physiologically sound explanations of the need for fluid and electrolyte support for their sick neonate help to allay their fears. Scalp vein IVs are particularly of concern (1) if the hair must be shaved and (2) because a common fantasy is that the needle is in the infant's brain. Explain to parents that scalp vein IVs are in the large veins of the head and not the brain, and that an IV in the head stays in longer, thus decreasing the need for multiple vein puncture and allows the infant mobility of all four extremities. In answer to the question, "Does it hurt?" a truthful answer is "Yes, when it is put in, but not after it is in the vein."

Infiltrates at peripheral IV sites should be addressed prospectively with parents. Erythema and edema are expected. Sloughing of the skin is not infrequent in VLBW infants and is more common on the feet and hands than on the scalp. If extravasation occurs, the infusion should be stopped and any residual fluid in the IV tubing or cannula and local subcutaneous blebs should be aspirated.[8] Injection of the affected area with hyaluronidase is indicated if the infiltrate contained hyperalimentation fluid. The affected extremity should then be elevated to limit swelling.[10]

Including parents in the care of their sick neonate requires an explanation about the importance of measuring intake and output. Inadvertent disposal of diapers and giving fluids that are not recorded are prevented by emphasizing the importance of saving them for the infant's nurse. "A little spitting up" after feeding may seem insignificant if parents are not instructed in the importance of telling the nurse and saving it for inspection or testing.

REFERENCES

1. Aiken CG, Sherwood, Kenney IJ et al: Mineral balance studies in sick preterm intravenously fed infants during the first week after birth: a guide to fluid therapy, *Acta Pediatr Scand Suppl* 355:1, 1989.
2. Bauer K, Bovermann G, Roithmaier A et al: Body composition, nutrition, and fluid balance during the first two weeks of life in preterm neonates weighing less than 1500 grams, *J Pediatr* 118:615, 1991.
3. Bell EF, Warburton D, Stonestreet BS et al: Effect of fluid administration on the development of symptomatic patent ductus arteriosus and congestive heart failure in premature infants, *N Engl J Med* 302:598, 1980.
4. Chathas MK, Paton JB, Fisher DE et al: Percutaneous central venous catheterization, *Am J Dis Child* 144: 1246, 1990.
5. Costarino AT Jr, Gruskay JA, Corcoran L et al: Sodium restriction versus daily maintenance replacement in very low birth weight premature neonates: a randomized, blind, therapeutic trial, *J Pediatr* 120: 99, 1992.
6. El-Dahr SS, Chevalier RL: Special needs of the newborn infant in fluid therapy, *Pediatr Clin North Am* 37:323, 1990.
7. Heird WC, Driscoll JM Jr, Schullinger JN et al: Intravenous alimentation in pediatric patients, *J Pediatr* 80:351, 1972.
8. Jameson J, O'Donnell J: Guidelines for extravasation of intravenous drugs, *Infusion* 7:157, 1983
9. Jones MD, Gresham EL, Battaglia FC: Urinary flow rate and urea excretion rates in newborn infants, *Biol Neonate* 21:322, 1972.
10. MacCara ME: Extravasation: a hazard of intravenous therapy, *Drug Intell Clin Pharm* 17: 714, 1983.
11. Wilson D: Neonatal IVs: practical tips, *Neonatal Netw* 2:49, 1992.
12. Winters RW: *The body fluids in pediatrics,* Boston, 1973, Little, Brown.

15 | Glucose Homeostasis

Jane E. McGowan, Mary I. Enzman Hagedorn, William W. Hay, Jr.

During intrauterine life the fetus depends on the constant transfer of glucose across the placenta to meet its glucose requirements. After birth neonates must maintain their own glucose homeostasis by producing and regulating their own glucose supply. This requires activation of a number of metabolic processes, including gluconeogenesis (synthesis of glucose from endogenous substrates) and glycogenolysis (release of glucose via breakdown of glycogen stores), as well as intact regulatory mechanisms and an adequate supply of metabolic substrates.

PHYSIOLOGY

Throughout gestation maternal glucose provides the principal source of energy for the fetus via facilitated diffusion across the placenta. Fetal glucose concentration varies directly with maternal concentration and is usually approximately 70% of the maternal value. Changes in maternal metabolism, including increased caloric intake and decreased sensitivity of the maternal tissues to insulin, provide the additional substrate necessary to meet fetal energy demands. During maternal normoglycemia the fetus produces little, if any, glucose, although the enzymes for gluconeogenesis are present by the third month of gestation.[43] If fetal energy demands cannot be met, however, as is the case in maternal starvation with resultant maternal hypoglycemia, the fetus is capable of adapting both by using alternate substrates, such as ketone bodies, and by "turning on" its endogenous glucose production.[42] There is additional evidence that even in the basal state the fetus relies on fuels other than glucose to meet some of its energy demands. These include lactate and amino acids.

Fetal glycogen synthesis begins as early as the ninth week of gestation. Most fetal glycogen is synthesized from glucose, directly or through a three-carbon intermediate, such as lactate. The major sites of glycogen deposition are liver, lung, heart, and skeletal muscle. Rates of hepatic glycogen deposition vary with different species, depending on the length of gestation; in the human, with a relatively long gestation, hepatic glycogen increases slowly throughout the first two trimesters of pregnancy, with a more rapid rate of deposition during the third trimester.[48] By 40 weeks' gestation, hepatic glycogen stores are two to three times adult levels. Skeletal muscle glycogen content also increases during the third trimester to as much as five times adult levels. By contrast, lung and cardiac muscle glycogen stores decrease as the fetus approaches term, although these stores are still of physiologic significance. Survival after asphyxia, for example, has been shown to be directly related to cardiac glycogen content. The decrease in lung glycogen, which begins at 34 to 36 weeks' gestation, may be related to ongoing developmental processes that require utilization of stored energy (e.g., synthesis of surfactant).

Several factors can affect rates of glycogen accumulation. Decreased availability of substrate, as in maternal malnutrition, placental insufficiency, or multiple gestations, has been associated with a decreased rate of glycogen synthesis. Acute intrauterine hypoxia does not appear to produce a measurable change in glycogen content, but chronic hypoxia, as is seen in maternal preeclampsia, does result in lower tissue glycogen content as compared with normoxic fetuses.

In addition to glycogen, the human fetus also stores energy as fat in adipose tissue. Most triglyceride synthesis occurs during the third trimester. By 40 weeks' gestation the human fetus has a fat content of about 16%, making it the fattest of all terrestrial newborn mammals. The human placenta transports some free fatty acids, although the amount transported has not been well quantified. Preliminary studies suggest that the maternal fatty acids transported to the fetus are not sufficient to account for the amount of adipose tissue present; therefore the fetus must also synthesize triglycerides directly from glucose. Again, conditions in which fetal glucose supply is reduced will result in less adipose tissue accumulation.

Insulin, considered a major stimulus for fetal growth, is present in the fetal pancreas by 8 to 10 weeks' gestation. Pancreatic insulin content increases in late gestation, exceeding adult levels by the time the infant reaches term.[33] However, the fetal pancreas seems to be less sensitive than the adult pancreas to the insulin secretion–stimulating effects of increased glucose concentration. Nevertheless, insulin secretion is augmented by higher glucose concentrations; increased concentrations of amino acids add to this effect, although this may only be true for pharmacologic, not physiologic, concentrations of amino acids. The elevated insulin concentration increases both fetal glucose utilization and glucose oxidation rates without increasing total fetal oxygen consumption.[16,28] This implies that other substrates (e.g., amino acids) become available for nonoxidative metabolism, which may promote tissue accretion and growth. Animal studies have demonstrated increased rates of protein synthesis and glucose uptake with increased insulin concentration and, conversely, decreased cell numbers and DNA content with insulin deficiency, supporting insulin's role as a growth-promoting factor. The fetuses of diabetic mothers who have very unstable plasma glucose concentrations during late gestation have an increased islet cell response to hyperglycemia compared with controls, releasing more insulin than normal fetuses at any given blood glucose concentration.[33] The higher insulin levels in turn lead to increased growth consisting primarily of adipose tissue, producing the macrosomia typically seen in infants of diabetic mothers (IDMs).

The related pancreatic hormone glucagon, which, like insulin, does not cross the placenta, has been detected as early as 15 weeks' gestation. The role of glucagon in regulating fetal glucose metabolism remains unclear. The concentration of glucagon in fetal blood is relatively low, even though pancreatic content is higher than in the adult. The high insulin-to-glucagon ratio in the fetus may be important in preferentially maintaining glycogen synthesis and suppressing gluconeogenesis, because glucagon is a potent inducer of gluconeogenic enzymes.[43]

At birth an infant is removed abruptly from its glucose supply, and blood glucose concentration falls. Several hormonal and metabolic changes occur at birth that facilitate the adaptation necessary to maintain glucose homeostasis. Catecholamine levels increase markedly at birth, possibly as a response to the decrease in environmental temperature as well as to the loss of the placenta, which in utero may remove as much as 50% of circulating fetal epinephrine.[53] Glucagon concentrations also increase, reversing the relatively low fetal glucagon/insulin ratio.[50] The elevated glucagon and norepinephrine levels activate hepatic glycogen phosphorylase, which induces glycogenolysis. Simultaneously the falling glucose concentration and the perinatal surge in fetal cortisol secretion stimulate hepatic glucose-6-phosphatase activity. Together these changes lead to an increase in hepatic glucose release.[12] Increased catecholamines also stimulate lipolysis, releasing fatty acids that can be metabolized to provide precursors for gluconeogenesis as well as providing energy in the form of adenosine triphosphate (ATP) and cofactors such as nicotineamide adenine dinucleotide phosphate (NADPH) that enhance the activity of gluconeogenic enzymes. Reversal of the insulin/glucagon ratio induces synthesis of phosphoenolpyruvate carboxykinase (PEPCK), which is considered the rate-limiting enzyme in hepatic gluconeogenesis. The concentrations of PEPCK and other gluconeogenic enzymes continue to increase with postnatal age during the first 2 weeks of life, regardless of gestational age. These changes act in concert to provide glucose to replace the supply previously received via the placenta.

Studies in normal infants using several different methods have determined that the steady state glucose production/utilization rate in a term neonate is 4 to 6 mg/min/kg[15]—approximately twice the weight-specific rate measured in adults. As in the fetus, it appears that approximately half of this glucose is oxidized to CO_2 during normal metabolic processes, whereas the remainder is used in nonoxidative pathways, such as glycogen and fat synthesis.

Maintenance of glucose homeostasis depends on the balance between hepatic glucose output and peripheral glucose utilization. Hepatic glucose output is a function of rates of glycogenolysis and gluconeogenesis, which are regulated by the factors discussed above. Peripheral glucose utilization varies with the metabolic demands placed on the neonate. This utilization may increase during hypoxia resulting from the inherent inefficiency of anaerobic glycolysis; hyperinsulinemia, which increases glucose uptake by insulin-sensitive tissues; respiratory distress from increased muscle activity; and cold stress, leading to increased sympathetic nervous system activity with release of norepinephrine and epinephrine and increased thyroid hormone secretion. If rates of glycogenolysis and gluconeogenesis do not match the rate of glucose utilization because of failure of the hormonal control mechanisms or variability of substrate supply, disturbances of glucose homeostasis occur. These disturbances are recognized clinically by the presence of hypoglycemia or hyperglycemia.

DEFINITIONS

Hypoglycemia

The absolute blood glucose concentration that corresponds to hypoglycemia in a neonate remains difficult to establish. Published definitions of hypoglycemia range from a blood glucose concentration of less than 20 mg/dl in preterm infants and less than 30 mg/dl in term infants to a plasma level of less than 45 mg/dl; some sources have even suggested raising the lower limit of normal to 60 mg/dl. A number of current references use 40 to 45 mg/dl as the lower limit of "normal" plasma glucose values in the first 72 hours of life.[28,51]

These latter values are derived from data on plasma glucose values measured in large populations of infants; thus they represent a statistical definition of hypoglycemia—that is, a glucose concentration more than two standard deviations below the mean for the population.[29] For example, Srinivasan et al[51] found that 95% of normal term infants had a blood glucose value of greater than 30 mg/dl in the first 24 hours of life and greater than 45 mg/dl after 24 hours (Figure 15-1). However, it is important to recognize that such data depend not only on the physiology of the infant's adaptation to postnatal life, but also on the character of the patient population (e.g., maternal nutrition status, percent of high-risk infants) as well as the standard feeding practices in place at the time the data were collected. Thus older studies generally concluded that normal blood glucose levels were lower than the levels that are found in more recent studies, reflecting the now-discarded practice of delaying feedings in healthy infants for periods of 6 to 12 hours. The higher "normal" values in more recent studies do not mean that neonatal physiology has changed, but rather reflect better management of high-risk pregnancies, early identification and management of at-risk neonates, implementation of early feeding protocols, and other changes in perinatal

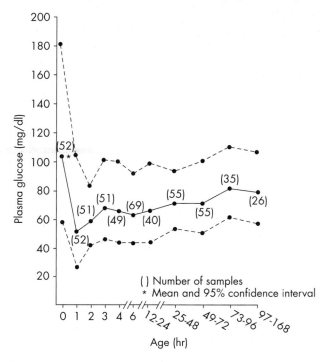

FIGURE 15-1   Plasma glucose concentrations during the first week of life in healthy appropriate-for-gestational age (AGA) term infants. (From Srinvasan G et al: *J Pediatr* 109:114, 1986.)

care. Using these definitions of hypoglycemia, the overall incidence has been estimated at 1.3 to 4.4/1000 live births. Differences in incidence figures probably reflect the fact that that some studies reported only symptomatic infants, whereas others evaluated data from screening measurements on all infants, thus including those with asymptomatic hypoglycemia. In preterm infants the incidence of hypoglycemia is increased; estimates range from 1.5% to 5.5% (Figure 15-2). The incidence of hypoglycemia in term infants with intrauterine growth retardation may be as high as 25%, with an even higher rate seen in preterm small-for-gestational-age (SGA) infants.[39]

Hypoglycemia may also be defined clinically as the glucose concentration in a neonate that is associated with symptoms that resolve when glucose is administered. However, this value is difficult to determine, because the symptoms of hypoglycemia are nonspecific and may not be noticed initially. From a physiologic point of view, an infant may be said to be hypoglycemic when glucose supply is inadequate to meet demand. Unfortunately, there is no currently available method to establish this value in a given infant. However, consideration of the physiologic basis for hypoglycemia suggests that infants with increased demand or limited capability to alter glucose delivery (which is a function of both blood supply and glucose concentration) are at increased risk for impaired organ function at low blood glucose levels.

Based on recent studies, it is clear that **the overall metabolic and physiologic status of the infant must be considered when determining acceptable blood glucose concentrations.** Some infants may undergo metabolic derangements at glucose concentrations above the "hypoglycemic" threshold, whereas others may be able to tolerate lower levels of blood glucose without developing metabolic stress. An infant with polycythemia, for example, may have a normal blood glucose concentration but decreased cerebral delivery of glucose because of reduced plasma flow. By contrast, breastfed infants may do well with "hypoglycemic" blood glucose values as a result of an increased rate of ketone body production. Preterm infants have a lower capacity for generating alternate brain energy substrates such as ketones, increasing the vulnerability of such infants to cerebral energy deficits when glucose concentrations in plasma are decreased. Further, measurements of cord blood glucose concentrations in normal human fetuses show that from midgestation through late gestation, fetal glucose concentration is above 50 mg/dl and may be as high as 70-90 mg/dl.[42] Such data indicate that the normal fetal brain develops in the presence of glucose concentrations that are significantly higher than the lower limit of normal, as defined statistically from postnatal data, raising the concern that even prolonged or repeated episodes of "low-normal" glucose concentrations could lead to altered function in the immature brain. In support of this concern is the data from Lucas et al[40] showing an association between decreased neurodevelopmental scores (mental and motor) at 18 months of age and exposure to multiple episodes of hypoglycemia (less than 2.6 mM [less than 47 mg/dl]) in preterm infants over several weeks of life. However, these abnormalities did not persist into school age, and other studies have failed to detect long-term effects of asymptomatic hypoglycemia in term or preterm infants (see below).

In summary, the definition of the blood glucose concentration at which intervention is indicated must be tailored to the clinical situation and the particular characteristics of a given infant. Kalhan and Peter-Wohl[31] recently suggested that further investigation

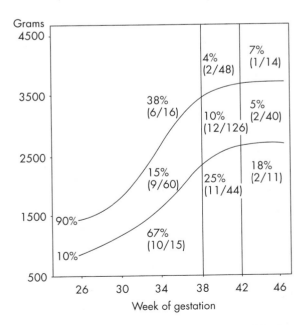

FIGURE 15-2 Incidence of neonatal hypoglycemia (blood glucose less than 30 mg/dl) by birth weight and gestational age. (From Lubchenco LO, Bard H: Incidence of hypoglycemia in newborn infants classified by birth weight and gestational age, *Pediatrics* 47:831, 1971.)

and treatment should be instituted in the symptomatic infant at blood glucose concentrations of less than 45 mg/dl, whereas asymptomatic term infants with known risk factors should be treated if their blood glucose level is less than 36 mg/dl. Several authors suggest that these thresholds for intervention should be higher in preterm infants and lower in breast-fed full-term infants.[7,26] However, it is important to recognize that at present there have been no systematic studies to demonstrate the risks or benefits of using a specific blood glucose concentration as a threshold for intervention in neonatal hypoglycemia.

Hyperglycemia

Hyperglycemia in newborns is usually defined, based on population data, as a blood glucose concentration of greater than 125 mg/dl in a term infant or greater than 150 mg/dl in a preterm infant. Incidence is difficult to determine; estimates range from 5.5% of all infants receiving IV infusions of 10% $D_{10}W$ to as high as 40% in infants weighing less than 1000 g.

ETIOLOGY

Hypoglycemia

The causes of hypoglycemia can be divided into several broad categories based on the mechanisms producing the hypoglycemia. These include inadequate substrate supply, abnormal endocrine regulation of glucose metabolism, and increased rate of glucose utilization. There are also a number of etiologies whose mechanisms are not well defined.

Inadequate Substrate Supply

If substrate availability is inadequate, hepatic glucose output will not meet metabolic demands. Most often this is due to subnormal fat and glycogen stores, which therefore do not provide enough energy to maintain glucose homeostasis until gluconeogenesis reaches adequate levels. Because most hepatic glycogen is accumulated during the third trimester, infants born prematurely will have diminished glycogen stores. An infant with IUGR secondary to placental insufficiency is also at risk for decreased glycogen accumulation, presumably because of diminished transfer of precursors across the placenta. The limited supply is then used for oxidative metabolism and tissue growth, rather than fat or glycogen accretion. Postnatally, catecholamine- and glucagon-stimulated lipolysis and glycogenolysis rapidly deplete the already less than adequate supplies at a time when gluconeogenesis is still im-

paired because of low levels of PEPCK and other gluconeogenic enzymes, and hypoglycemia results. These infants may be asymptomatic with the initial episode of hypoglycemia, but they can become symptomatic if the hypoglycemia persists.

Although inadequate stores of glycogen and lipid have been cited as the major etiologic factor in hypoglycemia in premature and SGA infants, a number of other factors may also play a role. A preterm infant with RDS, for example, has increased metabolic demands because of the increased work of breathing. Infants with IUGR and hypoglycemia have been shown to have an increased rate of glucose disappearance when receiving an IV glucose infusion, as well as reduced fat mobilization in response to hypoglycemia, when compared with normoglycemic SGA newborns. Because of the increased brain weight/liver weight ratio in an infant with asymmetric growth restriction, cerebral glucose requirements are high relative to the liver's capacity to respond, even if glycogen stores are normal for size[34] (Figure 15-3). Inappropriately elevated insulin/glucose ratios also have been observed in some SGA infants. These findings suggest that other disturbances in glucose metabolism in addition to lower-than-normal energy stores may be present in some growth-restricted infants.[32]

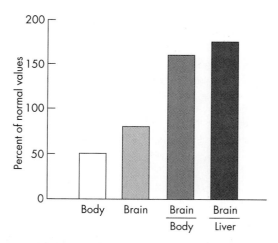

FIGURE 15-3   Differences in organ/body weight ratios in small-for-gestational-age (SGA) infant compared with appropriate-for-gestational-age (AGA) counterpart. (From Lafeber HN, Jones CT, Rolph TP: Some of the consequences on intrauterine growth retardation. In Visser HKA, ed: *Nutrition and metabolism of the fetus and infant,* Boston, 1979, Martinus Nijhoff Publishers.)

A much rarer but related problem occurs in several types of glycogen storage disease. In these inherited disorders hypoglycemia result not from inadequate glycogen stores, but rather from the inability to utilize stored glycogen as a result of one of several enzyme deficiencies. Several other inborn errors of metabolism, including proprionic and methylmalonic acidemia and glutaric aciduria, may present with hypoglycemia in the first week of life.[44]

Abnormalities of Endocrine Regulation

Hyperinsulinemia is the most common endocrinologic disturbance resulting in neonatal hypoglycemia and may be the most common cause of the infrequent cases of persistent hypoglycemia in infants. Excessive insulin secretion in the newborn increases glucose utilization by stimulating cellular glucose uptake in insulin-dependent tissues. At the same time, the high circulating insulin concentration promotes continued glycogen synthesis and inhibits both glycogenolysis and gluconeogenesis, impairing the infant's glucogenic response to the increased glucose demand and decreasing plasma glucose concentration.

The most common clinical situation in which hyperinsulinemia occurs is in an IDM. In utero, the fetus becomes hyperglycemic because of increased transfer of glucose across the placenta during episodes of maternal hyperglycemia. The fetal pancreatic beta cells are stimulated by the elevated fetal glucose concentration to produce increased quantities of insulin. As mentioned, the islet cells seem to become abnormally sensitive to increases in glucose concentration after repeated hyperglycemic stimuli as well as time-averaged hyperglycemia. Before delivery the increase in cellular glucose uptake in response to the increased insulin secretion is matched by the increased availability of glucose from the mother. After delivery, however, the source of glucose is abruptly removed while the hyperinsulinemia persists, producing hypoglycemia. The decrease in glucose concentration postpartum is a result of insulin-stimulated peripheral glucose uptake as well as inhibition of gluconeogenesis and glycogenolysis by the high insulin concentrations. Although some studies have reported other abnormalities in glucose metabolism in IDMs, Cowett et al[9] found no difference in glucose kinetics in IDMs versus controls. This may reflect the fact that maternal diabetic control was well maintained during pregnancy in the group studied, although a large review of pregnancies in diabetic mothers found no association between the incidence of neonatal hypoglycemia and the number of episodes of maternal hyperglycemia (a reflection of the degree of control) late in pregnancy.[27] Recent studies have found that the incidence of neonatal hypoglycemia in IDMs correlates better with intrapartum, rather than antepartum, maternal glucose concentrations.[10] The incidence of hypoglycemia in IDMs ranges from 15% to 75%; these infants are usually asymptomatic. A number of other neonatal complications are associated with maternal diabetes, including polycythemia, which may add to disturbances of glucose homeostasis, hypocalcemia, dystocia secondary to macrosomia, and congenital anomalies. Infants of mothers with severe diabetic vasculopathy, in contrast to most IDMs, may have IUGR caused in part by decreased placental blood flow, with hypoglycemia resulting from inadequate glycogen and fat stores rather than hyperinsulinemia.

As with IDMs, infants with Beckwith-Weidemann syndrome are also macrosomic and hyperinsulinemic; in addition, they have other associated anomalies, including macroglossia, which may cause airway obstruction, and omphalocele. Asymptomatic hypoglycemia may occur in 30% to 50% of infants with Beckwith-Weidemann syndrome and usually resolves in the first 3 days of life. However, up to 5% of affected infants may have persistent, frequently symptomatic hypoglycemia.[13] Although the specific mechanisms responsible for the syndrome and the associated hyperinsulinemia are not known, infants with Beckwith-Weidemann syndrome have been found to have mutations in the same region of the short arm of chromosome 11 where mutations associated with other hyperinsulinemic syndromes have been identified (see below).

Other causes of islet cell hyperplasia and resultant hyperinsulinemia include severe erythroblastosis fetalis,[2] possibly resulting from inactivation of insulin by glutathione released from hemolyzed red blood cells; exchange transfusion,[46] in which insulin release is stimulated by the high dextrose content of commonly used blood preservative agents; and in utero exposure to drugs such as beta-agonist tocolytics.[45] In utero exposure to valproate and postnatal exposure to indomethacin may also result in hypoglycemia, but the mechanisms responsible are not known.

Idiopathic hyperinsulinemia (i.e., increased, persistent insulin secretion without a known predisposing factor) may occur as a result of altered regulation of insulin secretion in pancreatic beta cells.[24] Mutations in several regions on the short arm of chromosome 11 have been found in approximately 50% of infants with hyperinsulinemic hypoglycemia

(HIHG); these mutations are most often inherited in an autosomal recessive pattern. Further, mutations in genes coding for glucokinase and glutamate dehydrogenase, two enzymes that regulate cellular metabolism and production of ATP, have also been associated with HIHG, usually expressed in an autosomal dominant pattern. The pancreatic abnormalities observed may be diffuse or focal, depending on the mutation present. Although the overall incidence of HIHG is low (approximately 1 in 50,000 births), the incidence of the inherited forms may be as high as 1 in 2500 infants in certain genetically homogeneous populations. Depending on the degree of hyperinsulinemia in utero, these infants, like others described earlier, may be macrosomic at birth. Most often, infants with HIHG present with severe, recurrent hypoglycemia within the first few days of life.

In addition to hyperinsulinemia, global endocrine disturbances can also result in hypoglycemia. These disturbances include a range of abnormalities of the hypothalamic-pituitary axis, the most severe being panhypopituitarism. Such infants frequently have growth hormone deficiency and hypothyroidism in addition to severe hypoglycemia. If pituitary dysfunction has resulted from a structural CNS lesion, other neurologic problems, including abnormal muscle tone and neonatal seizures, may be present. Adrenal failure and hypoglycemia can occur as a result of adrenal hemorrhage, often in association with neonatal sepsis. Isolated endocrine defects, including primary hypothyroidism and cortisol deficiency, may also be associated with hypoglycemia.

Increased Glucose Utilization

Some term infants may have normal energy stores at birth and intact regulating mechanisms but may be stressed by one of several conditions so that the available supplies do not meet the neonate's energy requirements. An asphyxiated newborn is one common example. After asphyxia and subsequent tissue ischemia, the neonate relies largely on anaerobic metabolism for energy production. Because this process is relatively inefficient, more glucose is metabolized to produce the amount of energy required than would be used under aerobic conditions. As a result, glucose produced by lipolysis and glycogenolysis is rapidly consumed. Hypoxic-ischemic damage to the liver may further impair synthesis of gluconeogenic enzymes and thus delay the normal postnatal onset of gluconeogenesis. Elevated insulin levels may also be present, providing an additional cause for the hypoglycemia.[11] Other conditions in neonates that lead

to a shift from aerobic to anaerobic metabolism, thus predisposing the infant to hypoglycemia, include hypotension, severe lung disease with hypoxemia and hypoventilation, and septic shock.

Hypothermia may result in hypoglycemia through rapid depletion of brown fat stores for nonshivering thermogenesis and secondary breakdown and exhaustion of glycogen stores. Hypothermia is most often seen in infants born at home, but milder degrees may occur in the delivery room. Hypoglycemia also has been observed in some infants with sepsis. A study done in several such infants found that they had an increased rate of glucose disappearance in response to an IV glucose infusion, suggesting an increased rate of glucose utilization.[35] Stimulation of glucose utilization may be a result of circulating endotoxins, which increase the rate of glycolysis. In addition, increased catecholamine levels in response to the stress of acute infection may play a role.

Hyperglycemia

Most often a neonate with hyperglycemia is an LBW infant (less than 32 weeks' gestation and less than 1200 g birth weight) who cannot tolerate an IV glucose infusion at the usual rate of 4 to 8 mg/kg/min (i.e., $D_{10}W$ at 60 to 100 ml/kg/day). This relative glucose intolerance is probably caused by general immaturity of the usual regulatory mechanisms, including decreased insulin release in response to glucose.[19] Some investigators have also reported that unlike fetuses and adults, most preterm and some term infants fail to suppress endogenous glucose production despite the administration of an adequate exogenous supply (e.g., IV infusion)[8]; however, other investigators did not measure any glucose production in premature infants receiving IV glucose at a rate of more than 2 mg/kg/min.[56] Hyperglycemia may also be iatrogenic in an ELBW infant (less than 750 g) who requires excess water to replace fluid lost through insensible water losses, and who receives excess glucose along with the infused water because it is necessary to provide an isotonic IV solution. The risk of developing hyperglycemia is significantly increased with decreasing birth weight, as well as with an increasing rate of glucose infusion, even within the accepted range of glucose infusion rates. Delay in initiating enteral feedings may be an additional risk factor. The incidence of hyperglycemia is higher in LBW infants receiving all of their nutrition parenterally than in those who receive at least a part of their nutrition enterally. The rate at which the glucose concentration is increased in IV solutions, including hyperalimentation, may also play a role. The presence of RDS, which requires mechanical ventilation, is associated with an increased risk of developing hyperglycemia. This may be because of increased circulating catecholamines, leading to increased lipolysis and glycogenolysis.

Although SGA infants are more commonly hypoglycemic, a few cases of what has been called *transient diabetes mellitus* have been reported, primarily in growth-restricted infants. In these cases hyperglycemia is thought to be a result of partial insulin insensitivity, but increased levels of catecholamines and other stress-related hormones may play an important role. Recent studies have identified mutations in chromosome 6 in some infants with neonatal diabetes.[49] However, in transient diabetes mellitus, unlike true diabetes mellitus, ketosis does not develop. Most cases self-resolve or respond to decreasing the glucose administration rate; occasionally insulin therapy may be required, but this should be reserved for infants with severe hyperglycemia (blood glucose concentration greater than 300 mg/dl, despite decreasing IV glucose infusion rate) that is persistent and associated with clinically significant hyperosmolality and glucosuria.

There are several other etiologic factors that must be considered in infants with hyperglycemia. Increased blood glucose concentrations have been reported in association with gram-negative sepsis.[30] Intravenous lipid infusions may also produce hyperglycemia if given rapidly at rates of more than 0.25 g/kg/hr; however, this exceeds the rate at which lipids are usually given.[54] Methylxanthines are frequently used to treat apnea in preterm infants and may be a cause of hyperglycemia. This problem has been well documented after theophylline overdose but may also occur with appropriate dosing. One study, for example, found that blood glucose concentrations in infants with therapeutic theophylline levels were higher than in untreated control subjects, with glucose concentrations in the hyperglycemic range in two treated infants.[52] Neonates undergoing surgical procedures also are at increased risk for hyperglycemia, probably because of a combination of the large quantities of glucose-containing fluids and blood products that may be administered during the procedure and the effects of stress-related hormones.

PREVENTION

Recognition of those infants at risk for disturbances in glucose homeostasis is the most important step in preventing both hypoglycemia and hyperglycemia. In infants with conditions predisposing to hypoglycemia, such as SGA infants or IDMs, early feeding and hourly monitoring of blood glucose concentrations until the infant is stable may prevent a decrease in blood glucose concentration or at least reduce the severity of the hypoglycemia. Maintenance of a neutral thermal environment is especially critical to minimize energy expenditure in those infants at risk for hypoglycemia. Other conditions associated with hypoglycemia, such as asphyxia and hypothermia, may be avoided through appropriate obstetric and neonatal intervention.

Hyperglycemia occurs most often in preterm infants receiving IV glucose. In a VLBW infant, hyperglycemia may be avoided by starting IV glucose infusions at rates of 2 to 3 mg/kg/min and checking blood glucose concentrations frequently (as often as every 3 to 4 hours) while the infant continues to receive IV glucose. However, hyperglycemia may be unavoidable in a very immature infant.

DATA COLLECTION

History

The history of any neonate must include a detailed prenatal and family history. Important maternal risk factors are listed in Box 15-1. Other important data include a history of family members with hypoglycemia or metabolic disease and previous unexplained stillbirths.

The most important information to be obtained from the infant's history is gestational age, Apgar scores, and details of events in the delivery room, especially any findings that would suggest the presence of significant perinatal asphyxia. An infant with a history of any of the conditions listed in Table 15-1 or Box 15-2 should be considered at high risk for developing a problem with glucose homeostasis.

Box 15-1	MATERNAL RISK FACTORS FOR NEONATAL HYPOGLYCEMIA

Presence of diabetes or abnormal result to glucose tolerance test
Pregnancy-induced or essential hypertension
Previous macrosomic infants
Substance abuse
Treatment with beta-agonist tocolytics
Antepartum administration of IV glucose

Table 15-1	NEONATAL HYPOGLYCEMIA: ETIOLOGIES AND TIME COURSE	
MECHANISM	**CLINICAL SETTING**	**EXPECTED DURATION**
Decreased substrate availability	Intrauterine growth restriction	Transient
	Prematurity	Transient
	Glycogen storage disease	Prolonged
	Inborn errors (e.g., fructose intolerance)	Prolonged
Endocrine disturbances		
Hyperinsulinemia	Infant of diabetic mother	Transient
	Beckwith-Wiedemann syndrome	Prolonged
	Erythroblastosis fetalis	Transient
	Exchange transfusion	Transient
	Islet cell dysplasias	Prolonged
	Maternal beta-agonist tocolytics	Transient
	Improperly placed umbilical artery catheter	Transient
Other endocrine disorders	Hypopituitarism	Prolonged
	Hypothyroidism	Prolonged
	Adrenal insufficiency	Prolonged
Increased utilization	Perinatal asphyxia	Transient
	Hypothermia	Transient
Miscellaneous/multiple mechanisms	Sepsis	Transient
	Congenital heart disease	Transient
	CNS abnormalities	Prolonged

Box 15-2	ETIOLOGIC FACTORS IN NEONATAL HYPERGLYCEMIA

Iatrogenic (e.g., during IV glucose infusion)
Decreased insulin sensitivity (e.g., VLBW infant or transient diabetes mellitus)
Sepsis
Methylxanthine side effect

Physical Examination

Careful measurement of birth weight and head circumference in combination with accurate gestational age assessment will establish whether the infant is preterm, LBW, SGA, or LGA and thus at increased risk for hypoglycemia. IDMs frequently have small heads relative to their general macrosomia and have been described as having "tomato facies" because of plethora and increased buccal fat. The physical findings associated with Beckwith-Wiedemann syndrome have already been described. The presence of midline facial defects, such as cleft lip or hypertelorism, suggests the presence of a CNS malformation with associated pituitary dysfunction.

Signs and Symptoms

Signs of neonatal hypoglycemia are nonspecific and extremely variable. They include general findings, such as abnormal cry, poor feeding, hypothermia,

and diaphoresis; neurologic signs, including tremors and jitteriness, hypotonia, irritability, lethargy, and seizures; and cardiorespiratory disturbances, including cyanosis, pallor, tachypnea, periodic breathing, apnea, and cardiac arrest. These findings may also be seen in premature infants and in neonates with sepsis, intraventricular hemorrhage, asphyxia, hypocalcemia, congenital heart disease, and structural CNS lesions, among other causes. In the presence of any of the above signs, however, hypoglycemia should always be considered, because the diagnosis can be made relatively easily and prompt treatment is essential.

Hyperglycemia is usually asymptomatic and is most often diagnosed on routine screening of the infant at risk.

Laboratory Data

When hypoglycemia is suspected, the plasma or blood glucose concentration must be determined immediately. **Ideally this determination should be made with one of the laboratory enzymatic methods, such as the glucose oxidase or hexokinase method, but even bedside reagent test strip glucose analyzers (i.e., glucometers) can be used if the test is performed carefully with awareness of the more limited accuracy of these devices.** In the clinical setting early and rapid determination of glucose concentrations in the high risk or sympto-

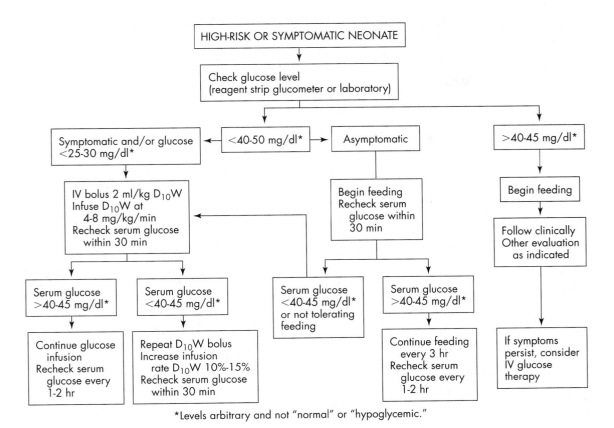

FIGURE 15-4   Decision tree for management of neonate with hypoglycemia

matic neonate is essential.[21] Prompt detection of hypoglycemia permits early treatment and potentially helps to avoid long-term neurologic sequelae.[6] Although laboratory measurements of glucose concentrations are the most effective methods for detecting hypoglycemia, results may not be available for up to 1 hour, far longer than appropriate for diagnosing hypoglycemia (Figure 15-4), thereby delaying the initiation of treatment. Rapid measurement methods available to the clinician at the bedside include several different systems using a handheld reflectance colorimeter, electrochemical detector, or ion-selective electrode methods (e.g., Glucometer, I-STAT). The sample of blood can be obtained from a warmed heelstick or venipuncture specimen.

These methods can be useful in screening infants in whom abnormal glucose concentrations are suspected if the user is aware of their limitations. The accuracy of test strip results depends in part on the technique used. An adequate sample must be placed on the test strip pad, and the timing of reading the

result is critical. Recently developed devices automatically read the result at the appropriate time, reducing one source of error. Hospital personnel should be trained and certified in the use of test strip methods and the bedside instruments used to quantify glucose concentration. **With proper technique, test strip results demonstrate a reasonable correlation with actual blood glucose concentrations, but the variation from the actual blood glucose value may be as much as 10 to 20 mg/dl.** A number of studies have compared the results obtained with specific commercial products to results obtained with laboratory methods.[1,23,41] Regardless of the test strip or instrument used, correlations with actual blood glucose concentrations are lowest at the lower glucose concentrations at which neonatal hypoglycemia must be accurately determined. **Several studies have shown that use of test strips alone may fail to detect as much as 11% to 67% of infants with statistically defined hypoglycemia.**[22,23,36] **There is also a significant incidence of false-positive results.**

Because of the limitations of these methods, whenever a diagnosis of hypoglycemia is indicated by test strip or glucometer results, the blood glucose concentration should be confirmed by a specimen sent to the chemistry laboratory for prompt (STAT) determination and reporting. Although laboratory results are more accurate and reliable than screening methods, a long delay in processing the specimen can result in a falsely low level as the erythrocytes in the sample metabolize the glucose in the plasma. This problem can be avoided by transporting blood in a tube containing a glycolytic inhibitor. Treatment of suspected hypoglycemia should not be postponed until confirmation is obtained from the laboratory, because this could mean a delay of 1 to 2 hours or more. Conversely, if hypoglycemia is suspected on the basis of clinical symptoms, initial treatment should be instituted even if the test strip result is "normal." If the actual value is abnormal, a delay in therapy could be harmful; if the actual value is within the normal range, therapy can be stopped without serious side effects.

Most cases of neonatal hypoglycemia have an identifiable cause (such as in an IDM or an SGA infant). In a term infant with no known risk factors for hypoglycemia, sepsis must be considered as the most likely cause of hypoglycemia, and an appropriate evaluation should be performed. Of those infants without an identifiable cause, most will have idiopathic hypoglycemia, which will resolve spontaneously within 2 to 5 days, and no further evaluation is needed. However, in rare cases hypoglycemia will persist beyond the first week of life with no obvious cause detected. The diagnostic evaluation of these infants should include simultaneous determination of glucose and insulin concentrations as well as alternate substrates, such as ketones and free fatty acids; evaluation of pituitary function, including measurement of TSH, thyroxine (T_4), adrenocorticotropic hormone (ACTH), cortisol, and growth hormone levels; and appropriate studies to diagnose inborn errors of metabolism, such as lactate and pyruvate concentrations. Ideally these studies should be obtained during an episode of hypoglycemia.

TREATMENT

Hypoglycemia

Anticipation and prevention are the key elements of intervention and management. Early identification of an infant at risk for developing hypoglycemia and institution of prophylactic measures to prevent its occurrence constitute the best treatment for this disorder. In infants in whom hypoglycemia does occur, the treatment goals are twofold: to return the glucose concentration to normal levels and, once normalized, to maintain levels within the normal range.

A decision tree suggesting guidelines for management of infants with hypoglycemia is shown in Figure 15-4. Although some asymptomatic infants can be managed with frequent formula feedings, most asymptomatic and all symptomatic neonates will require therapy with an IV dextrose infusion to provide glucose at an initial rate of 4 to 6 mg/kg/min. In some circumstances it may be useful to use a "minibolus" of 200 mg/kg dextrose (2 ml/kg of $D_{10}W$) plus the dextrose infusion regimen originally described by Lilien et al.[37] Advantages of the minibolus regimen include the following: (1) there is a lower incidence of hyperglycemia immediately after the bolus than occurred with use of boluses using solutions with higher dextrose concentrations, (2) the slower rate of administration decreases the insulin response to glucose infusion, thus lowering the risk of rebound hypoglycemia after the bolus, and (3) glucose concentration reaches the normal range more quickly than if continuous infusion is started without a preceding bolus (Figure 15-5). The rapid normalization

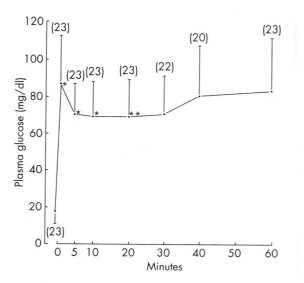

FIGURE 15-5 Plasma glucose response to glucose "minibolus" followed by continuous glucose infusion (8 mg/min/kg) as therapy for neonatal hypoglycemia. (From Lilien LD, Pildes RS, Srinivasan G et al: Treatment of neonatal hypoglycemia with minibolus and intravenous glucose infusion, *J Pediatr* 97:295, 1980.)

of blood glucose is particularly beneficial in symptomatic infants. The suggested infusion rates cover the range of hepatic glucose production in normal term newborns. In IDMs the initial minibolus and the infusion rate should be kept at the minimum necessary to produce and maintain normal blood glucose concentrations to prevent an excessive insulin response. When glucose infusion rates are being calculated, it is important to remember that commercially prepared glucose solutions actually contain glucose in its hydrated form (MW 198 versus MW 180 for anhydrous glucose), which lowers the actual glucose content of the solution by approximately 8%. Thus $D_{10}W$ contains approximately 9.2 g of glucose per deciliter.

Once the infant's glucose requirement has been determined, the glucose infusion should be maintained at that level until blood glucose concentrations are stable. The target blood glucose concentration during IV therapy should be well above the "hypoglycemic threshold" defined for that particular infant; for example, if hypoglycemia is defined as 40 mg/dl, glucose concentrations should be maintained in the 50 to 70 mg/dl range or even higher in a significantly preterm infant. If the infant was being fed before IV therapy was instituted, feedings may be continued. However, the calculated minimum glucose requirement should be provided by the IV infusion alone rather than by the combination of glucose infusion and feedings. In infants who were not previously fed, feedings can be instituted when clinically indicated. There are several advantages to feeding a hypoglycemic infant during treatment with IV glucose. In the hyperinsulinemic infant, galactose (one of the components of lactose) stimulates less insulin release than glucose and therefore helps stabilize blood glucose concentrations. Continuation of oral feedings also aids in the process of weaning off IV glucose. When feedings are well tolerated, the IV infusion generally can be slowly tapered if the glucose concentration and clinical status remain stable. However, enteral feeding also has the theoretic risk of augmenting insulin secretion and subsequent hypoglycemia as a result of the food-stimulated release of gut peptides that may potentiate insulin release from the pancreas. Thus in a few infants, typically those with hyperinsulinemic hypoglycemia, feedings may need to be stopped until glucose concentrations have been stabilized.

Adjunctive Therapy
Glucagon. Glucagon, 30 µg/kg IV or IM, will release glycogen from hepatic stores when insulin concentrations are normal. However, IDMs and other infants with hyperinsulinemia may require much larger doses, up to 300 µg/kg, to produce a response. Administration of glucagon may be useful diagnostically, because failure to respond to glycogen administration with an increase in serum glucose concentration suggests depletion of hepatic glycogen stores. Glucose infusion should be maintained after glucagon is administered, because there is a risk of increased insulin secretion in response to the glucagon-produced surge in glucose production. In addition, the rapid but transient increase in glucose concentration immediately after glucagon injection may produce a false sense that the hypoglycemia has resolved, even though the underlying cause still exists. Continuous infusions of glucagon have been used to treat refractory hypoglycemia[5]; however, this mode of administration has been associated with adverse side effects, including hyponatremia and thrombocytopenia.[3]

Other Agents. Steroids, somatostatin, and diazoxide have been used to treat hypoglycemia in refractory cases. Use of steroids to reduce peripheral glucose utilization and increase gluconeogenesis should be limited to those infants requiring more than 15 to 18 mg/kg/hr glucose infusion to maintain normal glucose concentrations. Somatostatin and diazoxide, which suppress insulin release, are most often used in infants with islet cell dysplasias who have persistent hypoglycemia after a partial pancreatectomy.

Miscellaneous. In infants with hypoglycemia caused by a specific medical problem, therapy should be directed toward alleviating the underlying illness. This includes administration of antibiotics to treat sepsis, partial exchange transfusion to relieve hyperviscosity, hormone replacement in cases of hypopituitarism, and dietary intervention for metabolic disorders. However, medical therapy alone fails to control hypoglycemia in 40% to 90% of infants with severe, persistent HIHG; partial or subtotal pancreatectomy is usually performed in these infants to decrease insulin secretion.[14]

Hyperglycemia
Glucose
Most cases of hyperglycemia can be treated by reducing the neonate's intravenous glucose infusion rate. Many LBW infants will tolerate glucose infusions at rates of up to 4 mg/kg/min, although Zarif et al[55] reported that more than 40% of infants weighing less than 1000 g had a blood glucose concentration

higher than 125 mg/dl while receiving glucose at an average rate of 4.4 mg/kg/min. In addition, a VLBW infant, with high fluid requirements resulting from large insensible water losses through the skin, may require a combination of water and glucose intake that could only be administered by using a hypotonic solution such as $D_{2.5}W$. The use of a low glucose concentration necessitates the addition of sodium (e.g., $D_{2.5}W$ has approximately 130 mOsm/L, requiring the addition of sodium chloride to produce an isotonic solution with 280 mOsm/L), which may further complicate management of fluids and electrolytes. A VLBW infant needs adequate caloric intake (50 to 60 kcal/kg/day) to avoid a negative nitrogen balance and tissue catabolism. These needs often cannot be met without resultant hyperglycemia. If the glucose is only mildly elevated (e.g., concentrations of 150 to 250 mg/dl) and the infant has no evidence of adverse effects such as osmotic diuresis, there may be no need to reduce the rate of IV glucose administration.

Insulin Infusion

Because of the above considerations, some authors[4,17] have suggested the use of a continuous insulin infusion in the infant who cannot tolerate infusion of glucose solutions with concentrations greater than 5 g/dl (i.e., D_5W). Infusion of insulin at rates of 0.2 to 0.8 mU/kg/min (0.01 to 0.05 U/kg/hr) for 12 to 24 hours may result in improved glucose tolerance. Hypoglycemia can be avoided by starting with a low infusion rate and increasing the rate by 10% to 20% every 60 to 90 minutes until the glucose concentration is less than 150 mg/dl. Blood glucose concentrations should be monitored every 15 to 20 minutes during initiation of the insulin infusion, and an IV glucose infusion should be maintained to avoid any abrupt changes in blood glucose.

Use of insulin infusion has been reported to improve tolerance to glucose infusion, resulting in increased carbohydrate intake and weight gain. However, this therapy has not been evaluated in a randomized prospective study and must be used cautiously given the role of insulin as a potent fetal and neonatal growth hormone. Further, episodes of hypoglycemia may occur even with careful monitoring during the insulin infusion.

Miscellaneous

In addition to specific measures to lower the blood glucose concentration, close attention must be paid to fluid balance in the hyperglycemic infant, because hyperglycemia can induce an osmotic diuresis. However, this is rarely seen at blood glucose concentrations less than 400 mg/dl. Finally, as in hypoglycemia, efforts should be made to treat any underlying etiology, such as sepsis.

COMPLICATION

Hypoglycemia

The outcome for infants with neonatal hypoglycemia appears to be related to the duration and severity of the hypoglycemia, as well as the underlying etiology. Those with asymptomatic hypoglycemia usually have a normal neurodevelopmental outcome, although minor abnormalities such as learning disabilities and abnormal electroencephalograms (EEGs) without seizure disorder occasionally have been reported.[25] Symptomatic infants, typically those with a plasma glucose concentration of less than 25 mg/dl for several hours or more, have a poorer prognosis, with abnormalities ranging from learning disabilities to cerebral palsy and seizure disorders, as well as mental retardation of varying degrees.[20] Prompt initiation of treatment is thought to be associated with a more positive outcome, although this has not been well documented.

In preterm infants recent data[18,40] suggest that hypoglycemia may adversely affect long-term outcome. A follow-up study of more than 600 former preterm infants found significantly lower mental and motor indices in those infants with five or more documented episodes of moderate hypoglycemia (defined as a blood glucose concentration of less than 45 mg/dl) during the neonatal period. This difference remained significant even when confounding factors such as IVH, need for ventilator support, and asphyxia were taken into consideration. However, differences in cognitive function were less apparent at school-age follow-up in the same cohort of patients. Preterm infants who were also small for gestational age were found to have lower scores on psychometric tests at both 3 years and 5 years of age, with a greater effect seen in those infants with recurrent hypoglycemia. These results suggest that further long-term studies in preterm infants are needed.

The incidence of neurodevelopmental abnormalities in IDMs ranges from 0% to 35%; the lower figures are from more recent studies and may represent improvement in obstetric and neonatal care. None of the long-term follow-up studies has shown an association between the presence of neonatal hypoglycemia and later neurodevelopmental impairment.[27,47] Instead, outcome has been related to such factors as prematurity, presence of congenital anomalies, congenital iron deficiency, and degree of control of maternal disease.

Adverse neurologic outcomes have been reported in as many as 40% to 50% of infants with HIHG, possibly because these infants cannot effectively generate ketone bodies, which could serve as an alternative source of energy for cerebral metabolism during periods of hypoglycemia. In addition, infants with HIHG who require a greater than 95% pancreatectomy often develop glucose intolerance or even frank diabetes mellitus later in life.[38] Hypoglycemia secondary to hypopituitarism is also associated with a poor outcome; often this is due to other CNS or endocrine dysfunction rather than the hypoglycemia itself.

Hyperglycemia

Although there is little direct evidence, it has been postulated that hyperglycemia in the preterm infant may increase the risk of IVH by causing rapid changes in osmolarity with resultant rapid fluid shifts within the brain and germinal matrix. One study did report an increased mortality in hyperglycemic premature infants as compared with their normoglycemic counterparts, although hyperglycemia may have been a marker for those infants with more severe illness rather than a direct cause of the increased mortality. Increased morbidity may be seen in the form of greater difficulty with fluid and electrolyte management, as well as problems establishing adequate nutrition.

Infants with transient diabetes mellitus usually recover spontaneously within the first week; persistent insulin resistance is extremely rare. However, those infants with chromosomal mutations have an increased incidence of adult-onset diabetes later in life.[49] No neurologic sequelae have been directly attributed to the presence of transient hyperglycemia in these neonates.

PARENT TEACHING

Parent teaching should begin before delivery, with emphasis placed on good nutrition and early and regular prenatal care. Teaching also should include information about those conditions that increase the risk of hypoglycemia (e.g., IUGR associated with maternal cigarette smoking and poor maternal nutrition). Regular prenatal care assures the early detection of potentially serious problems, including preeclampsia, gestational diabetes, and abnormal fetal growth.

Prenatal teaching is especially important in the woman with known diabetes mellitus, because overall outcome (although not necessarily the incidence of hypoglycemia) is directly related to the degree of control before and during pregnancy. In addition, the possibility of neonatal hypoglycemia and requirement for IV therapy can be discussed with the parents before delivery so that they will be aware that the infant may require a longer hospital stay even if delivered at term.

If IV therapy is selected to treat neonatal hypoglycemia, regardless of cause, a thorough explanation of the treatment plan must be given to the parents at the time therapy is instituted. Frequent progress reports should be provided to resolve unanswered (and often unasked) questions and relieve parental anxiety. Parents of children with islet cell dysplasias need to be aware of the symptoms of hypoglycemia and emergency treatment measures that can be instituted, because recurrent hypoglycemia may occur in these cases. Parents of infants with inborn errors of metabolism also need counseling with regard to prognosis, as well as genetic counseling about risks of recurrence in future pregnancies.

ACKNOWLEDGMENT

Supported by NIH grants HD 20337, HD20761, DK52138, and RR00069.

REFERENCES

1. Altimier L, Roberts W: One Touch II hospital system for neonates: correlation with serum glucose values, *Neonatal Netw* 15:15, 1996.
2. Barrett CT, Oliver TK: Hypoglycemia and hyperinsulinism in infants with erythroblastosis fetalis, *N Engl J Med* 278:1260, 1968.
3. Belik J, Musey J, Trussell RA: Continuous infusion of glucagon induces severe hyponatremia and thrombocytopenia in a premature neonate, *Pediatrics* 107: 595, 2001.
4. Binder N, Raschko PK, Benda GI et al: Insulin infusion with parenteral nutrition in extremely low birth weight infants with hyperglycemia, *J Pediatr* 114: 273, 1989.
5. Carter P, Lloyd D, Duffy P: Glucagon for hypoglycaemia in infants small for gestational age, *Arch Dis Child* 63:1264, 1988.
6. Cornblath M, Schwartz R: Hypoglycemia in the neonate, *J Pediatr Endocrinol* 6:113 , 1993.

7. Cornblath M, Hawdon JM, Williams A et al: Controversies regarding definition of neonatal hypoglycemia: suggested operational thresholds, *Pediatrics* 105:1141, 2000.

8. Cowett RM, Oh W, Schwartz R: Persistent glucose production during glucose infusion in the neonate, *J Clin Invest* 71:467, 1983.

9. Cowett RM, Susa JB, Gill DL et al: Glucose kinetics in infants of diabetic mothers, *Am J Obstet Gynecol* 146:781, 1983.

10. Curet LB, Izquierdo LA, Gilson GJ et al: Relative effects of antepartum and intrapartum maternal blood glucose levels on incidence of neonatal hypoglycemia, *J Perinatol* 17:113, 1997.

11. Davis DJ, Creery WD, Radziuk J: Inappropriately high plasma insulin levels in suspected perinatal asphyxia, *Acta Paediatr Scand* 88:76, 2000.

12. Dawkins MJ: Biochemical aspects of developing function in newborn mammalian liver, *Br Med Bull* 22:27, 1966.

13. DeBaun MR, King AA, White N: Hypoglycemia in Beckwith-Weidemann syndrome, *Semin Perinatol* 24:164, 2000.

14. DeLonlay-Debeney P, Poggi-Travert F, Fournet J et al: Clinical features of 52 neonates with hyperinsulinism, *N Engl J Med* 340:1169, 1999.

15. Denne SC, Kalhan SC: Glucose carbon recycling and oxidation in human newborns, *Am J Physiol* 251: E71, 1986.

16. DiGiacomo JE, Hay WW Jr.: Effect of hypoinsulinemia and hyperglycemia on fetal glucose utilization, *Am J Physiol* 259:E506, 1990.

17. Ditzenberger GR, Collins SD, Binder N: Continuous insulin intravenous infusion therapy for VLBW infants, *J Perinatal Neonatal Nurs* 13:70, 1999.

18. Duvanel CB, Fawer CL, Cotting J et al: Long-term effects of neonatal hypoglycemia on brain growth and psychomotor development in small-for-gestational age infants, *J Pediatr* 134:492, 1999.

19. Farrag HM, Cowett RM: Glucose homeostasis in the micropremie, *Clin Perinatol* 27:1, 2000.

20. Fluge G: Neurological findings at follow-up in neonatal hypoglycaemia, *Acta Paediatr Scand* 64: 629, 1975.

21. Gardner S, Hagedorn M: High risk neonatal care: level III nursery. In Gardner S, Hagedorn M, eds: *Legal aspects of maternal-child nursing practice*, Menlo Park, 1997, Addison-Wesley.

22. Garland J, Alex C, Gleisberg D et al: Clinical utility of a glucose reflectance meter for screening neonates for hypoglycemia, *J Perinatol* 16:250, 1996.

23. Giep TN, Hall RT, Harris K et al: Evaluation of neonatal whole blood versus plasma glucose concentration by ion-selective electrode technology and comparison with two whole blood chromogen test strip methods, *J Perinatol* 16:244, 1996.

24. Glaser B: Hyperinsulinism of the newborn, *Semin Perinatol* 24:150, 2000.

25. Griffiths AD, Bryant GM: Assessment of effects of neonatal hypoglycaemia, *Arch Dis Child* 46:819, 1971.

26. Hawdon JM: Hypoglycaemia and the neonatal brain, *Eur J Pediatr* 158 (Suppl 1):9, 1999.

27. Haworth JC, McRae KN, Dilling LA: Prognosis of infants of diabetic mothers in relation to neonatal hypoglycaemia, *Dev Med Child Neurol* 18:471, 1976.

28. Hay WW Jr., Meznarich HK, DiGiacomo JE et al: Effects of insulin and glucose concentrations on glucose utilization in fetal sheep, *Pediatr Res* 23:381, 1988.

29. Heck LF, Erenberg A: Serum glucose levels during the first 48 hours of life in the healthy full-term neonate, *Pediatr Res* 17:317A, 1983.

30. James T III, Blessa M, Boggs TR Jr: Recurrent hyperglycemia associated with sepsis in a neonate, *Am J Dis Child* 133:645, 1979.

31. Kalhan S, Peter-Wohl S: Hypoglycemia: what is it for the neonate? *Am J Perinatol* 17:11, 2000.

32. Kinnala A, Manner T, Nuutila P et al: Differences in respiratory metabolism during treatment of hypoglycemia in infants of diabetic mothers and small-for-gestational-age infants, *Am J Perinatol* 15:363, 1998.

33. Ktorza A, Bihoreau M, Nurjhan N et al: Insulin and glucagon during the perinatal period: Secretion and metabolic effects on the liver. *Biol Neonate* 48:204, 1985.

34. Lafeber HN, Jones CT, Rolph TP: Some of the consequences of intrauterine growth retardation. In Visser KHA, ed: *Nutrition and metabolism of the fetus and infant,* Boston, 1979, Marinus Nijhoff Publishers.

35. Leake RD, Fiser RH, Oh W: Rapid glucose disappearance in infants with infection, *Clin Pediatr* 20:397, 1981.

36. Leonard M, Chessall M, Manning D: The use of a Hemocue blood glucose analyser in a neonatal unit, *Ann Clin Biochem* 34:287, 1997.

37. Lilien LD, Pildes RS, Srinivasan G et al: Treatment of neonatal hypoglycemia with minibolus and intravenous glucose infusion. *J Pediatr* 97:295, 1980.

38. Lovvorn HN III, Nance ML, Ferry RJ Jr et al: Congenital hyperinsulinism and the surgeon: lessons learned over 35 years, *J Pediatr* 34:786, 1999.

39. Lubchenco LO, Bard H: Incidence of hypoglycemia in newborn infants classified by birth weight and gestational age, *Pediatrics* 47:831, 1971.

40. Lucas A, Morley R, Cole TJ: Adverse neurodevelopmental outcome of moderate neonatal hypoglycaemia, *Br Med J* 297:1304, 1988.

41. Maisels MJ, Lee C: Chemstrip glucose test strips: correlation with true glucose values less than 80 mg/dl, *Crit Care Med* 71:457, 1983.

42. Marconi AM, Daviani E, Baggiani AM et al: An evaluation of fetal glucogenesis in intrauterine growth-retarded pregnancies, *Metabolism* 42:860, 1993.

43. Neonatal hypoglycemia and the development of gluconeogenetic enzymes, *Nutr Rev* 35:54, 1977.

44. Ozand PT: Hypoglycemia in association with various organic and amino acid disorders, *Semin Perinatol* 24:172, 2000.

45. Procianoy RS, Pinheiro CEA: Neonatal hyperinsulinism after short-term maternal beta sympathomimetic therapy, *J Pediatr* 101:612, 1982.

46. Schiff D, Aranda JV, Colle E et al: Metabolic effects of exchange transfusion. II. Delayed hypoglycemia following exchange transfusion with citrated blood, *J Pediatr* 79:589, 1971.

47. Sells CJ, Robinson NM, Brown Z et al: Long-term developmental follow-up of infants of diabetic mothers, *J Pediatr* 125:S9, 1994.

48. Shelley HJ: Glycogen reserves and their changes at birth and in anoxia, *Br Med Bull* 17:137, 1961.

49. Shield JP: Neonatal diabetes: new insights into aetiology and implications, *Horm Res* 53(Suppl)1:7, 2000.

50. Sperling MA, Ganguli S, Leslie N et al: Fetal-perinatal catecholamine secretion: role in perinatal glucose homeostasis, *Am J Physiol* 247:E69, 1984.

51. Srinivasan G, Pildes RS, Caughy M et al: Plasma glucose values in normal neonates: a new look, *J Pediatr* 109:114, 1986.

52. Srinivasan G, Singh J, Cattamanchi G et al: Plasma glucose changes in preterm infants during oral theophylline therapy, *J Pediatr* 103:473, 1983.

53. Tenenbaum D, Cowett RM: Mechanisms of beta sympathomimetic action on neonatal glucose homeostasis in the lamb, *J Pediatr* 107:588, 1985.

54. Vileisis RA, Cowett RM, Oh W: Glycemic response to lipid infusion in the premature neonate, *J Pediatr* 100:108, 1982.

55. Zarif MA, Pildes RS, Vidyasagar D: Insulin and growth-hormone responses in neonatal hyperglycemia, *Diabetes* 25:428, 1976.

56. Zarlengo KM, Battaglia FC, Fennessey PV et al: Relationship between glucose utilization rate and glucose concentration in preterm infants, *Biol Neonate* 49:181, 1986.

SELECTED READINGS

Aynsley-Green A: Glucose: a fuel for thought, *J Paediatr Child Health* 27:21, 1991.

Cornblath M, Schwartz R, eds: *Semin Perinatol* 24(2), 2000 (entire issue is devoted to topics pertaining to glucose homeostasis in the newborn and infant).

Cowett RM: Neonatal glucose metabolism. In Cowett RM, ed: *Principles of perinatal-neonatal metabolism,* New York, 1991, Springer Verlag.

DiGiacomo JE, Hay WW Jr: Disorders of metabolic adaptation: abnormal glucose homeostasis. In Sinclair JC, Bracken MB, eds: *Effective care of the newborn infant,* Oxford, 1992, Oxford University Press.

Hay WW Jr: Reliability of blood glucose analysis. In Schwartz R, Cornblath M, eds: *Hypoglycemia in infancy: the need for a rational definition,* 1990, Ciba Symposium Report.

Kalhan S, Saker F: Metabolic and endocrine disorders. Part I: Disorders of carbohydrate metabolism. In Fanaroff AA, Martin RJ, eds: *Neonatal-perinatal medicine: diseases of the fetus and newborn,* ed 6, St Louis, 1997, Mosby.

McGowan JE: Neonatal hypoglycemia, *Neo Rev* 1:e6-e15, 1999. Ogata ES: Carbohydrate metabolism in the fetus and neonate and altered glucoregulation, *Pediatr Clin North Am* 33:25, 1986.

Stokowski L: Metabolic disorders (glucose homeostasis). In Deacon J, O'Neil P, eds: *Core curriculum for neonatal intensive care nursing,* ed 2, Philadelphia, 1999, WB Saunders.

Williams AF: Hypoglycaemia in the newborn: a review, WHO Publications #5778, 1997.

16 Enteral Nutrition

Marianne S. Anderson, Cynthia B. Johnson, Susan F. Townsend, William W. Hay Jr.

Providing adequate nutritional support to sick newborns in the intensive care unit is an important challenge: maturational, functional, and physical disturbances to the normal postnatal transition and ultimately to future health and development may result if this challenge is not met. Optimal nutrition after birth enhances future neurodevelopmental outcome in preterm infants.[46,47] Good nutrition improves surgical outcome, decreases morbidity, and shortens hospital stays. Thus it is critical to adapt feeding practices and the composition of feedings to achieve optimal nutrition in hospitalized neonates. Special attention must be given to the unique needs of individual patients, such as ELBW infants and patients with congenital heart disease, short bowel syndrome, or chronic lung disease. To meet the requirements for metabolic homeostasis, growth, and development, a combination of parenteral and enteral nutritional support is often provided. A goal of any nutritional support strategy must also be parental involvement, both to facilitate and encourage eventual breastfeeding, as well as to initiate educational interventions promoting healthy long-term nutrition practices. We view nutritional support of the newborn in the hospital as part of a continuum of care from birth through the first months at home after discharge, where ongoing attention to optimal nutrition may further enhance long-term outcome.

In this chapter we provide an overview of the physiology of nutrition and growth, with a brief discussion of gastrointestinal maturation and function. We elaborate fundamentals of neonatal nutritional requirements and monitoring and discuss techniques and strategies for enteral nutrition in hospitalized term and preterm infants, with emphasis on those infants requiring unique or special attention. Finally, we detail elements of enteral nutrition after hospital discharge in recovering infants.

PHYSIOLOGY

Growth

Fetal growth is regulated by complex genetic, nutritional, hormonal, and physical factors. Maternal nutritional factors exert some influence: weight gain during pregnancy is well correlated with fetal growth rate,[38,75] and the quality of the maternal diet (protein, energy, vitamins, and minerals) directly affects fetal growth.[38,64] However, a large maternal reserve of nutrients is available to the fetus in most circumstances, and in general, maternal diet is not the rate-limiting factor in fetal growth. Many aspects of placental function are important determinants of fetal growth. For example, there are strong correlations among placental size, uteroplacental blood flow, and fetal size. Provision of oxygen and essential nutrients by the placenta is largely responsible for determining the rate of tissue accretion and composition in the fetus over the course of gestation.[79]

In addition to maternal nutritional factors and placental function, certain hormones and growth factors play increasingly recognized roles in regulating intrauterine growth. Insulin is one of the most influential growth-promoting hormones in the fetus.[31] Apancreatic infants, who have no circulating insulin, are among the most severely growth restricted of all newborns (Figure 16-1), whereas infants of diabetic mothers (IDM) who respond to increased maternal-fetal glucose delivery with increased insulin secretion are among the fattest (Figure 16-2). Other peptide growth factors have been implicated in fetal growth and maturation, including the insulin-like growth factors, epidermal growth factor, transforming growth factors, and fibroblast growth factors.[79] Some of these factors may in turn be nutritionally regulated. Infants with other endocrine disturbances, such as those resulting from anencephaly, panhypopituitarism, or hypothyroidism, are near normal in age-specific size at birth. Thus there is a complex interplay between provision

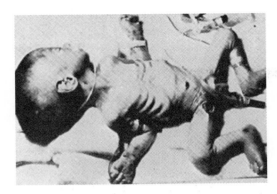

FIGURE 16-1 Term newborn (birth weight 1280 g) with pancreatic agenesis confirmed at autopsy. Plasma insulin was absent. Note marked deficiency of adipose tissue and muscle development. (From Hill D: Effect of insulin on fetal growth, *Semin Perinatol* 2:319, 1978.)

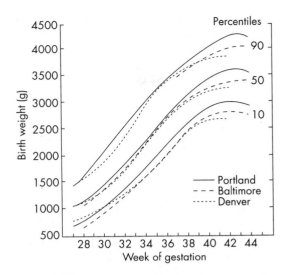

FIGURE 16-3 Comparisons of fetal weight curves for different populations in the United States. These growth curves suggest that maternal socioeconomic status and race may influence fetal growth rate as much as altitude. (From Babson SG, Behrman RE, Lessel R: Fetal growth: liveborn birth weights for gestational age of white middle class infants, *Pediatrics* 45:937, 1970.)

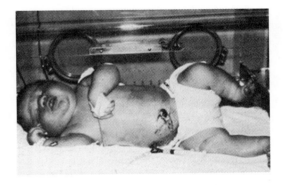

FIGURE 16-2 Characteristic large-for-gestational-age (LGA) infant of diabetic mother. (Courtesy Newborn Service, University of Health Sciences Center, Denver, 1981.)

of nutrients across the placenta to the fetus and the fetal endocrine milieu that influences intrauterine growth.

Understanding intrauterine growth is important for developing a standard by which to judge postnatal growth in preterm infants.[78] In the absence of other standards, **it is generally accepted as a nutritional goal to seek a postnatal growth rate approximating normal intrauterine growth (Figure 16-3). For the average growing preterm infant, this translates into an expected weight gain of approximately 15 to 20 g/kg/day.** It is often difficult to achieve normal rates of intrauterine growth during early extrauterine life, however, because most infants develop changes

in metabolic state and are exposed to quite different environmental influences on energy utilization and metabolic rate than occur in utero. Important environmental factors influencing infant energy expenditure include exposure to varying temperature and humidity and radiant and convective heat losses. In addition, the transition from the continuous delivery of elemental nutrients by the placenta to the intermittent provision of complex nutrient mixtures to the gut requires maturation and adaptation of GI function. Infants facing the increased energy-consuming demands of temperature maintenance, breathing, resistance to gravity, and so on might not be expected to grow well initially. Also, because of the excretion of excess extracellular salt and water after birth, resulting in significant shifts in body water content, infants born at all gestational ages often lose fluid weight initially. **Term infants may lose as much as 5% of birth weight by the third day of life, and ELBW infants (less than 1000 g) may lose 6% to 8% of birth weight.** These many postnatal factors usually preclude feeding infants sufficiently to produce normal in utero growth rates. Meeting this challenge is one of the most important aspects of future neonatal nutritional and medical practice.

Box 16-1 GROWTH MONITORING

I. Weight

Weight is subject to large variations based on fluctuations in fluid balance (e.g., presence or absence of edema, congestive heart failure, renal failure) and attached equipment (e.g., IV lines and boards, endotracheal tubes). Infant weight should be measured daily as follows:

A. Use the same scale and weigh infant with minimal or no clothing. Remove "attached" equipment if possible, or weigh similar items separately and subtract from total weight. In-bed scales are useful for the ELBW infant or infants who become unstable with handling. An electronic scale that averages several measurements reduces movement artifact and may be useful for active infants.

B. Reference standards for the weights of nursery equipment (such as diapers, IV boards, tubing, endotracheal tubes) should be available for nursery use.

C. Weigh the infant at the same time daily, preferably before a feeding.

D. Record the infant's weight, the time of weight measurement, and the scale used on the chart. Energy (calories) and fluid intake should be recorded on the same chart. This information combined with biochemical parameters (such as serum electrolytes, hemoglobin, and albumin) and the physical examination provides the best overview of the infant's nutritional status. Daily weight should be plotted on the appropriate preterm or term growth chart. Weekly review of the infant's weight change provides useful information on trends in overall growth or weight loss that may be overlooked in the daily charting.

II. Crown-heel length and head circumference

These are measured and recorded on admission and at least weekly thereafter. Accurate length measurements are difficult to obtain without special equipment such as a stadiometer, but accuracy can be improved by repeat measurements and use of the tonic-neck reflex to straighten the hip and knee.[56] Increase in head circumference is used as an indicator of brain growth.

A. To measure the crown-heel length, place the infant supine on a firm surface with the knees extended and the ankles flexed 90 degrees. Measure the length from the top of the head (crown) to the bottom of the heel.

B. Head circumference is obtained using a paper or soft tape measure. Record the largest measurement obtained with the tape placed over the frontal, parietal, and occipital prominences.

III. Ponderal index

The ponderal index (or weight-length index; see Figure 16-4) is used to assess "quality" of growth. The index is calculated as the weight in grams times 100, divided by the cube of the length in centimeters. True organ growth and tissue accretion is accompanied by increases in both weight and length and can partly be evaluated using the ponderal index.

IV. Biochemical monitoring

Monitoring of the growing infant may include periodic measurement of serum electrolytes, calcium, phosphorus, alkaline phosphatase, total protein, albumin, and hemoglobin. These data can be used to help prevent specific deficiencies in the diet, such as hyponatremia in preterm infants with excessive renal solute losses or hypophosphatemia with increased alkaline phosphatase as seen in rickets and osteopenia.

Monitoring Growth

The normal intrauterine growth rate of 15 to 20 g/kg/day usually is not seen in the first 1 to 2 weeks of life in sick preterm infants in the intensive care nursery. Most of the weight change seen in ELBW infants during this period probably represents fluid management strategies to replace insensible losses and limit fluid overload to prevent development of a patent ductus arteriosus. Stressed and sick term infants will not gain weight at a rate comparable to their healthy peers. In both cases, the most important reason for this early postnatal growth delay is inadequate nutrition, particularly protein. Nonetheless, increase in body length can usually be documented in the early newborn period without increase in weight, demonstrating new tissue accrual and the need for adequate provision of nutrients.[9] Early provision of both adequate calories and protein to sustain optimal nutrition is difficult without the addition of some parenteral nutrition for extremely preterm, LBW immature infants, and sick infants of all gestational ages (see Chapter 17).

Assessing Growth and Nutritional Status

We lack good methods for assessing nutritional adequacy in very small infants. Rates of change in anthropometric measurements provide some retrospective information, but they do not tell us what an infant needs at any one time (Box 16-1 and Figure 16-4). All too often they simply document failure to provide adequate nutrition during the previous days to weeks. Indirect calorimetry offers some advantage, but instruments that are physically practical and sufficiently accurate to quantify nutrient metabolism in

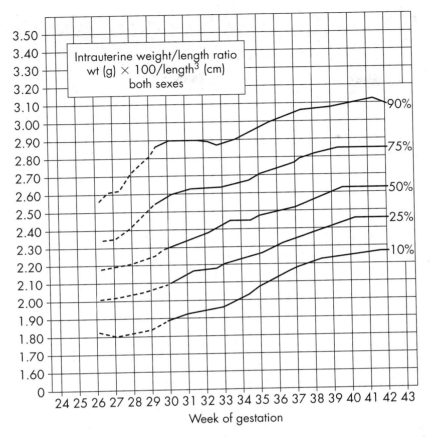

FIGURE 16-4   Ponderal index. (From Lubchenco L, Hansman C, Boyd E: Intrauterine growth in length and head circumference as estimated from live births at gestational ages from 26 to 42 weeks, *Pediatrics* 37:403, 1996.)

tiny infants are not yet available. This is particularly true for infants who are on ventilatory therapy and receiving high mixtures of oxygen. Similarly, application of stable isotope methodology to measure utilization and oxidation rates of individual nutrients remains confined to large medical centers with expensive and sophisticated mass spectrometry facilities. Evaluation of an individual infant's immediate nutrient requirements and responses to the administration of different mixtures and amounts of nutrients remains an elusive but essential goal.

Gastrointestinal Development and Function

The GI tract must adapt in the immediate postnatal period to meet the nutritional and metabolic needs of extrauterine life. In utero, the gut has been somewhat prepared for this role through the passage of large volumes of amniotic fluid (up to 300 ml/day

at term) that contains enzymes, immunoglobulins, growth factors, and hormones.[89] The human GI tract is fully developed anatomically by 20 weeks' gestation, but many functional abilities develop later (Table 16-1). Thus infants delivered prematurely will have some limitations in GI function. After birth at term, GI function also continues to develop; for example, full pancreatic function is limited until late infancy. Some GI functions may be "switched on" at birth (such as decrease in intestinal permeability, increase in mucosal lactase activity) regardless of gestation. However, others seem to be intrinsically "programmed" to occur at a certain postconceptional age (such as the onset of peristalsis at 28 to 30 weeks and the coordination of suck and swallow at 33 to 36 weeks).[89] Environmental influences, including colonization of the gut by bacteria and introduction of nutrients into the gut also affect postnatal GI development.[4] Initiation of

Table 16-1	DEVELOPMENT OF THE GASTROINTESTINAL TRACT IN THE HUMAN FETUS: FIRST APPEARANCE OF DEVELOPMENTAL MARKERS	
	DEVELOPMENTAL MARKER	WEEKS OF GESTATION
Anatomic Part		
Esophagus	Superficial glands	20
	Squamous cells	28
Stomach	Gastric glands	14
	Pylorus and fundus	14
Pancreas	Differentiation of endocrine and exocrine tissue	14
Liver	Lobules	11
Small intestine	Crypt and villi	14
	Lymph nodes	14
Colon	Increased diameter	20
	Villi	20
Functional Ability		
Sucking and swallowing	Mouthing only	28
	Immature suck-swallow	33-36
Stomach	Gastric motility and secretion	20
Pancreas	Zymogen granules	20
Liver	Bile metabolism	11
	Bile secretion	22
Small intestine	Active transport of amino acids	14
	Glucose transport	18
	Fatty acid absorption	24
Enzymes	Alpha-glucosidases	10
	Dipeptidases	10
	Lactase	10
	Enterokinase	26

From Lebenthal E: The impact of development of the gut on infant nutrition, *Pediatr Ann* 16:211, 1987.

enteral feedings in the hospitalized infant must take all these diverse factors into account.

The GI tract of a preterm newborn handles multiple nutrients in a variety of ways. Protein digestion and absorption are remarkably efficient in preterm infants despite the fact that enterokinase, the rate-limiting enzyme in the activation of pancreatic proteases, has only 10% of the adult activity. Carbohydrate absorption is limited by a relative deficiency of lactase, which splits lactose into glucose and galactose. Lactase in the infant of less than 34 weeks' gestation is present at only about 30% of the activity found in a normal term infant, although lactose intolerance is not common in these infants, particularly when they are fed human milk.[50] Preterm infants may malabsorb 10% to 30% of dietary fat because of a small bile acid pool size and relative lack of pancreatic lipase. Nonetheless, despite relative deficiencies in many enzymes important in nutrient processing, a preterm infant is usually able to digest and absorb complex nutrient mixtures, such as human milk, quite effectively.

In addition to growth of the intestine and maturation of intestinal absorption, motile function of the gut changes during gestation and after birth. Coordination of suck and swallow patterns is absent before about 34 weeks' gestation, gastroesophageal sphincter pressure increases from 28 weeks' gestation through the first week of life, and peristalsis of the small intestine improves during the third trimester of gestation. The rate of gastric emptying is slowed in preterm infants.[55] **A measure of GI motility is provided by the passage of stool within 24 hours of birth in more than 95% of full-term infants. However, the more premature the infant, the greater the delay in passing the first stool. Enteral feeding promotes gastric emptying and the release of hormones that may improve peristalsis in both the term and preterm infant.**

Table 16-2	ESTIMATED DAILY ENERGY REQUIREMENT (KCAL/KG) FOR PREMATURE INFANTS		
FACTOR	AMERICAN ACADEMY OF PEDIATRICS	EUROPEAN SOCIETY OF GASTROENTEROLOGY AND NUTRITION	
		AVERAGE	RANGE
Energy expenditure			
Resting metabolic rate	50	52.5	45-60
Activity	15	7.5	5-10
Cold stress	10	7.5	5-10
Energy cost of digestion	8	17.5	10-25
Energy stored	25	25	20-30
Energy excreted	12	20	10-30
TOTAL REQUIREMENTS	120	130	95-165

Modified from American Academy of Pediatrics, Committee on Nutrition: *Pediatrics* 112:622, 1988; Committee on Nutrition of the Preterm Infant, European Society of Pediatric Gastroenterology and Nutrition: *Nutrition and feeding of the preterm infant*, Oxford, UK, 1987, Blackwell Scientific Publications.

Nutritional Requirements

Nutritional requirements may be considered in three general categories: energy (or calories), minerals and solutes, and vitamins. Water requirements also must be considered when designing nutrition support strategies. The source, complexity, and constituents of these nutrients are important, as well as the route of administration. Enteral nutritional requirements are discussed here. (See Chapter 17 for parenteral nutrition and Chapter 19 for breastfeeding.)

Energy

Energy requirements are determined by an infant's total energy expenditure, energy excretion, and energy stored in new tissue as growth. Total energy expenditure can be subdivided into contributions of basal metabolic rate, activity, requirements for thermoregulation, and the energy costs of digestion and metabolism. Energy excretion is composed of fecal and urinary losses as well as heat lost by radiation and evaporation. Estimates of energy requirements for growing preterm infants are shown in Table 16-2.[3,14] The large variability of these estimates reflects largely the variability of infant activity and environmental conditions. Therefore it is important to adjust nutrient delivery to individual requirements. For example, if an infant is particularly active and is showing poor growth, nutrient delivery should be adjusted upward accordingly. **Caloric requirements for the healthy term infant average 110 kcal/kg/day, much lower than the energy requirements of preterm infants.**[67] **Increased en-**

Box 16-2	CALCULATING DAILY CALORIC INTAKE (KCAL/KG/DAY)

Conversion Factors

20 kcal/oz = 0.67 kcal/ml
24 kcal/oz = 0.80 kcal/ml
1 kcal = 1 Calorie
1 oz = 30 ml

Calculation

1. Add total daily feeding intake (in ml)
2. Divide total intake (ml) by the infant's weight (kg)
   This equals enteral intake: ml/kg/day
3. Multiply ml/kg/day intake by kcals per ounce of feeding
4. Multiply by 1 oz/30 ml
   This equals enteral intake as kcal/kg/day

ergy requirements can be anticipated during recovery from surgery, sepsis, and respiratory distress. Daily caloric intake should be calculated for each infant growing or recovering from illness in the nursery. Useful approaches for calculating caloric intake are shown in Box 16-2. Major components of energy (calorie) delivery are derived from protein, carbohydrate, and fat.

Protein. Protein accretion is critical for normal growth. The amount and type of protein necessary for optimal growth in preterm infants have been difficult to establish. Metabolic balance studies support a need for higher protein intakes in the growing preterm infant than in the term infant. Human milk provides adequate protein to meet the recommended

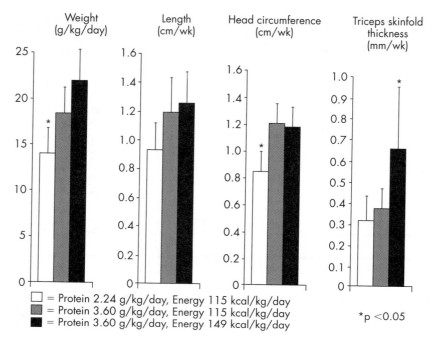

Weight (g/kg/day) | Length (cm/wk) | Head circumference (cm/wk) | Triceps skinfold thickness (mm/wk)

□ = Protein 2.24 g/kg/day, Energy 115 kcal/kg/day
▨ = Protein 3.60 g/kg/day, Energy 115 kcal/kg/day
■ = Protein 3.60 g/kg/day, Energy 149 kcal/kg/day

*p <0.05

FIGURE 16-5 Growth rates with varying protein and energy intakes. (From Kashyap S, Schulze KF, Forsyth M, et al: Growth nutrient retention and metabolic response in low birth weight infants fed varying intakes of protein and energy, *J Pediatr* 113:713, 1988; and Kennaugh JM, Hay WW Jr: Nutrition of the fetus and newborn, *Western J Med* 147:435, 1987.)

Table 16-3	NUTRIENT COMPOSITION OF HUMAN MILK FORTIFIERS	
	ENFAMIL HUMAN MILK FORTIFIER* (AMOUNT PER FOUR PACKETS)	**SIMILAC HUMAN MILK FORTIFIER† (AMOUNT PER FOUR PACKETS)**
Calories (kcal)	14	14
Protein (g)	1.1	1
Fat (g)	0.65	0.36
Linoleic acid	90	0
Linolenic acid	11	0
Carbohydrate (g)	1.1	1.8
Calcium (mg)	90	117
Phosphorus (mg)	45	67
Sodium (mg)	11	15
Chloride (mg)	9	38
Vitamin A (IU)	950	620
Vitamin D (IU)	150	120
Vitamin E (IU)	4.6	30
Vitamin K (μg)	4.4	8.3
Vitamin C (IU)	12	3.2
Iron (mg)	1.44	0.35

This table lists the major constituents; refer to product inserts for a complete listing of vitamins, minerals, and trace elements.
*Mead Johnson Nutritionals, Evansville, Indiana.
†Ross Products Division, Abbott, Columbus, Ohio.

goals of 2.0 to 2.5 g/kg/day for term infants, but it is inadequate to meet the goals of 3.5 to 4.0 g/kg/day for preterm infants.[45] Preterm infants receiving both protein and energy supplementation during enteral feedings (to as much as 3.6 g/kg/day protein and 149 kcal/kg/day) had increased gains in weight, length, head circumference, and triceps skinfold thickness compared with infants receiving 2.24 g/kg/day protein and 115 kcal/kg/day energy (Figure 16-5).[34] **Studies of preterm infants maintained on diets fortified in protein and energy have shown improved neurodevelopmental outcome at 9 months of corrected age.**[1] **Neurodevelopmental outcome appears to be even better when human milk is supplemented with protein and energy.**[2,47,48] Because of this and the other benefits of human milk feeding in preterm infants, including provision of antimicrobial factors and improved feeding tolerance, protein and energy supplementation of human milk (e.g., with Human Milk Fortifier, by Mead Johnson Nutritionals, or Natural Care, by Ross Products Division) at reasonable milk volumes is recommended (Table 16-3).

The type of protein in the newborn diet is as important as the amount provided. Conditionally, or developmentally, essential amino acids may be particularly important to the infant, especially a preterm infant. Normal growth, energy metabolism, and immune function are dependent on appropriate availability of these amino acids. In a rapidly growing infant requirements may not be met by intake of essential amino acids and biosynthesis of conditionally essential amino acids. Studies are ongoing to determine nutritional needs and benefit or risk of supplementation of such amino acids, including glutamine, taurine, cysteine, and tyrosine.[27,57,58,85]

Human milk from an infant's own mother is the preferred source of protein for the newborn. Human milk is a whey-predominant food (whey/casein ratio of 80:20), whereas cow's milk has a whey/casein ratio of 18:82. Whey protein is particularly rich in essential and conditionally essential amino acids. **Milk expressed from mothers of preterm infants is somewhat higher in protein than milk from mothers of term infants. Nonetheless, supplementation of preterm maternal milk with protein (as well as calcium, phosphorus, sodium, potassium, and lipid) is usually necessary to promote growth rates approximating that of normal-gestation human fetuses, particularly in VLBW preterm infants. An intake of 3.0 to 3.5 g/kg/day is recommended in preterm infants. Protein requirements may be higher (4.0 g/kg/day) in ELBW infants (i.e., less than 1000 g).** Growth should be monitored and supplementation provided expectantly. Term infants in general will not require protein or energy supplementation unless their dietary fluid is restricted because of illness (e.g., congestive heart failure).

Fat. Human neonates are unique among animals in having a relatively high white fat content of 16% to 18% of body weight at term.[79] Brown fat, which is necessary for thermogenesis, is also present at term. Fat deposition occurs predominantly during the last 12 to 14 weeks of gestation. Thus infants born prematurely will be significantly deficient in fat stores, both for use as energy and for thermogenesis. In addition, deposition of specific lipids is deficient in VLBW infants. An example is docosahexaenoic acid, or DHA, a long-chain polyunsaturated fatty acid (22 carbons with 6 double bonds) necessary for normal brain and retinal development.[12]

Newborn infants absorb fat less efficiently than older children. Preterm infants demonstrate even greater deficiencies in fat digestion and metabolism. Pancreatic lipase and bile acids are less available for fat digestion and absorption. Lingual and gastric lipases, present in newborn secretions, compensate for deficient pancreatic lipase, as does mammary gland lipase, if the infant is receiving breast milk.[30,49] **Current recommendations for dietary fat consist of provision of 30% to 54% of total calories (3.3 to 6.0 g/100 kcal), with at least 3% of total calories as linoleic acid.** Human milk contains considerable quantities of linolenic acid, the precursor to DHA and other long-chain fatty acids that are important for normal brain development and nerve function. Preterm infants can synthesize DHA from its precursor, linolenic acid, but whether the amount synthesized is sufficient remains uncertain. Small amounts of DHA are present in human milk and in at least one commercially available formula (Enfamil LIPIL).

Medium-chain triglycerides (MCTs) do not require bile salts for absorption and can be directly absorbed into the portal venous circulation. This offers theoretical advantages for preterm infants, although there is little evidence that inclusion of MCTs improves growth of healthy preterm infants.[59] The routine use of MCTs is therefore not recommended, although they can improve fat absorption and energy intake in infants with hepatic dysfunction or short bowel syndromes.

Although there is concern that overfeeding of infants may lead to adult obesity and therefore fat intake should be restricted, it is important to remember that fats are essential for normal infant growth. Fats provide a concentrated source of energy and are also important components of cell membranes, particularly significant for the developing nervous system. **Therefore there is no place for "fat restriction" in the nutritional support of preterm or term infants within the guidelines given above.** Areas of ongoing research include the supplementation of formulas for preterm infants with fish oil emulsions to provide n3 and n6 long-chain polyunsaturated fats, which are necessary for optimal brain and retinal development in animals, and the relationship of neonatal fat composition to the development of atherosclerosis in later life.

Carbohydrate. Carbohydrate reserves begin to accumulate as glycogen in the developing fetus as early as the start of the second trimester. This glycogen serves local organ needs, and hepatic glycogen is used by other glucose-dependent tissues, primarily the brain. Immediately after birth, with cessation of glucose supply from the placenta, the neonate must use this stored glycogen for energy. **The newborn can exhaust this supply of stored glucose from the liver within 12 hours of birth if food or**

IV glucose is not provided. The normal glucose utilization rate in a term newborn is 4.0 to 6.0 mg/kg/min. The brain accounts for most of the glucose use, especially in preterm and asymmetrically growth-restricted infants who have a larger than normal brain/body weight ratio.

The predominant carbohydrate in human milk is lactose, a disaccharide composed of glucose and galactose. Glucose has a central role in energy metabolism. Galactose provides 50% of the calories derived from lactose; its major metabolic role is in energy storage, because the newborn liver readily incorporates galactose from the portal circulation into hepatic glycogen.[35]

Provision of 40% to 60% of total caloric intake as carbohydrate (12 to 14 g/kg/day) will pre-

Table 16-4 FORMULA COMPARISON PER DECILITER

| | MATURE HUMAN MILK | COW'S MILK | | | |
		SIMILAC 20	ENFAMIL 20	LACTO FREE 20	NEOCARE 22
Protein Source					
Whey/casein	80:20	18:82	60:40	—	60:40
Amount (g)	1	1.45	1.5	1.5	1.5
Calories (%)	6	9	9	9	9
Fat Source					
Medium-chain triglycerides (%)	—	—	8.1	—	—
Polyunsaturated (linoleate [olive]) (%)	16	37	29	—	—
Saturated (coconut) (%)	38	45	47.3	—	—
Monounsaturated (oleate [safflower]) (%)	42	18	15.5	—	—
Amount (g)	4.5	3.6	3.8	3.7	4.1
Calories (%)	55	48	50	49	49
Cholesterol (mg)	14.5	1.1	1.1	—	—
Vitamin E/PUFA (mg/g)	0.4	1.1	1.9	—	—
Carbohydrate Source					
Lactose (%)	100	100	100	—	Lactose
Glucose polymers (%)	—	—	—	100	Corn syrup
Amount (g)	7.1	7.2	6.9	7	7.7
Calories (%)	39	43	41	42	41
Calories	73	68	68	68	74
Minerals					
Calcium (mg)	33	49	53	55	78
Phosphorus (mg)	15	38	36	37	46
Ca/P ratio	2.2:1	1.3:1	1.5:1	1.5:1	1.7:1
Sodium, mg (mEq)	16 (0.7)	18 (0.8)	18.1 (0.8)	20 (0.9)	25 (1.1)
Potassium, mg (mEq)	51 (1.3)	71 (1.8)	72 (1.84)	74 (1.9)	105 (2.7)
Chloride, mg (mEq)	39 (1.1)	43 (1.2)	42 (1.19)	43 (1.3)	56 (1.6)
Magnesium (mg)	4	4.1	5.4	5.4	6.7
Zinc (mg)	0.16	0.5	0.7	0.7	0.9
Iron (mg)	0.021	1.2	1.2	1.2	1.3
Iodine (μg)	30	6.1	6.8	10.1	11.2
Copper (μg)	25-40	61	51	50.7	89.3
Manganese (μg)	7-15	3.4	10.5	10.1	7.4
Osmolality (mOsm/kg)	300	300	300	200	290
Estimated renal solute load (mOsm/L)	71	96.3	95.5	100	130.8

*24 kcal/oz preterm formulas.

vent accumulation of ketone bodies and other adverse metabolic effects (e.g., hypoglycemia) in the newborn. This amount of carbohydrate is generally supplied as lactose in human milk or commercial formulas. If there are signs of lactose intolerance, such as frequent loose stools, abdominal distention or apparent cramping, or positive stool-reducing substances (as indicated by Clinitest), a portion of the carbohydrate may be given as sucrose or as glucose polymers. Glucose polymers have the added advantage of keeping formula osmolality low. Lactose-free infant formulas are commercially available (e.g., Lacto Free, by Bristol-Myers Squibb; Table 16-4). Use of such nonlactose products should be reserved for those rare infants with clinically proven lactose intolerance.

Table 16-4   FORMULA COMPARISON PER DECILITER—cont'd

| COW'S MILK* PRETERM | | | CASEIN HYDROLYSATE | SOY | |
Similac Special Care 24	Enfamil Premature 24	Premie SMA 24	Pregestimil 20	Prosobee 20	Isomil 20
60:40	60:40	60:40	1.9	2	1.7
2.4	2.4	2	11	12	10
11	12	10			
50	40	11	3	—	—
21	23	15.4	36.2	29.1	37
66	25.7	48	9.1	47.3	46
13	11.7	35	17.1	15.5	17
4.4	4.1	4.4	3.8	3.6	3.6
47	44	48	48	48	49
2.5	—	2-4	—	0	0
2.5	3.9	1.6	1.6	0.5	1.1
50	40	50	—	Sucrose	Sucrose
50	60	50	100	Corn syrup	Corn syrup
8.6	8.9	9.0	6.9	6.8	6.96
42	44	42	41	40	41
81	81	81	68	68	68
146	134	75	63	71	71
73	68	40	42	56	51
2.0:1	2.0:1	1.9:1	1.5:1	1.3:1	1.4:1
35 (1.5)	32 (1.4)	32 (1.4)	32 (1.4)	24 (1.0)	30 (1.3)
105 (2.7)	90 (2.3)	75 (1.9)	74 (1.9)	82 (2.1)	73 (1.9)
66 (1.9)	69 (1.9)	53 (1.5)	58 (1.6)	54 (1.5)	42 (1.2)
10	6.1	7	7.4	7.4	5.1
1.2	1.27	0.8	0.6	0.8	0.5
1.5	1.52	0.3	1.3	1.2	1.2
5	6.4	8.3	4.8	10	10
203	130	70	63	51	51
10	10.6	20	21	16.9	20
280	300	280	320	200	230
149	230	128	125	127	110

Table 16-5	RECOMMENDED DAILY VITAMIN INTAKE FOR INFANTS			
	ENTERAL		PARENTERAL	
VITAMIN	FDA MINIMUM (UNITS/100 KCAL)	RDA: 0-6 MO (UNITS/DAY)	PRETERM (UNITS/KG/DAY)	TERM (UNITS/DAY)
C (mg)	8	30	25	80
Thiamine (μg)	40	300	350	1200
Riboflavin (μg)	60	400	150	1400
B_6 (μg)	35	300	180	1000
Niacin (mg)	0.25	5	6.8	17
Biotin (μg)	1.5	10*	6	20
Panthothenic acid (mg)	0.3	2	2	5
B_{12} (μg)	0.15	0.3	0.3	1
Folate (μg)	4	25	56	140
A (IU)	250	1250	1665	2330
D (IU)	40	300	400†	400
E (mg)	0.5	3	2.8	7
K (μg)	4	5	80	200

Modified from Lucas A, Hudson G: Preterm milk as a source of protein for low birth weight infants, *Arch Dis Child* 59:831, 1984.
*Estimated safe and adequate intake.
†Units/day.

Table 16-6	VITAMIN CONTENT OF HUMAN MILK AND COMMERCIAL INFANT FORMULAS		
VITAMIN	HUMAN MILK* (UNITS/100 KCAL)	STANDARD MILK-BASED FORMULAS† (UNITS/100 KCAL)	PRETERM FORMULAS‡ (UNITS/100 KCAL)
C (mg)	6-7.8	8.1-9	10.5-37
Thiamine (μg)	13.4-31	78-100	120-250
Riboflavin (μg)	40.1-60	150-156	190-620
B_6 (μg)	9.3-30	60-63	75-250
Niacin (mg)	0.22-0.31	0.75-1.25	0.93-5
Biotin (μg)	0.6-1.0	2.2-4.4	2-37
Pantothenic acid (mg)	265-340	315-470	530-1900
B_{12} (μg)	0.03-0.15	0.2-0.25	0.3-0.55
Folate (μg)	4-7.4	7.5-15.6	15-37
A (IU)	73-323	300-310	475-1200
D (IU)	3-12	60-63	75-270
E (IU)	0.2-0.6	1.4-3.1	2.2-4.6
K (μg)	0.3-3	8-8.6	10.5-13

Modified from Reidel BD, Greene HL: Vitamins. In Hay WW Jr, ed: *Neonatal nutrition and metabolism*, St Louis, 1991, Mosby.
*Human milk composition varies greatly (with gestation, stage of lactation, individually, etc.).
†20 kcal/oz, Enfamil (Mead Johnson), Similac (Ross Laboratories).
‡20 kcal/oz, Enfamil Premature, Similac Special Care.

Vitamins

Vitamins are organic substances, present in trace amounts in natural food sources, that are essential to normal metabolism. Lack of vitamins in the diet produces well-recognized deficiency states in adults. The biologic roles of many vitamins are incompletely understood, and recognition of clinical deficiency states in infants is often difficult. Certain vitamins have received close attention in neonatology,[68,83] in particular vitamin C for its role in enhancing iron absorption from the GI tract, vitamin K for prevention of hemorrhagic disease of the newborn, and vitamins A and E as antioxidants. Vitamin A supplementation may have a role in decreasing chronic lung disease in ELBW infants.[84] Because vitamins have a central role in many metabolic

Table 16-7	MINERALS AND TRACE ELEMENTS IN NEONATAL NUTRITION		
MINERAL OR ELEMENT	BIOLOGIC ROLE	DEFICIENCY STATE	RECOMMENDED INTAKE FOR GROWING PRETERM INFANTS
Sodium	Growth and tissue accretion, body fluid equilibrium, cellular energy, electrical charge balance	Poor growth, fluid imbalance, neurologic dysfunction, lethargy, seizures	3-5 mEq/kg/day
Potassium	Growth and tissue accretion, acid-base balance, cellular energy, electrical charge balance	Myocardial damage, dysrhythmia, hypotonia, muscle weakness	2-3 mEq/kg/day
Chloride	Growth and tissue accretion, cellular energy, electrical charge balance	Failure to thrive, muscle weakness, vomiting	3-5 mEq/kg/day
Calcium	Bone and tooth formation, fat absorption, nerve conduction, muscle contraction	Bone demineralization, tetany, dysrhythmias, seizures	200 mg/kg/day
Phosphorus	Bone and tooth formation, energy transfer compounds	Bone demineralization, weakness	100-140 mg/kg/day
Magnesium	Metalloenzymes, cellular electrical charge balance	Neurologic dysfunction, anorexia, diarrhea, renal disease	5-10 mg/kg/day
Iron	Hemoglobin formation, metalloenzymes	Anemia, apathy	2 mg/kg/day after 1 month of age
Zinc	Metalloenzymes, DNA-RNA synthesis, wound healing, host defenses	Growth restriction, dermatitis, alopecia, diarrhea, delayed wound healing	1.2-1.5 mg/kg/day
Copper	Metalloenzymes, protein metabolism	Neurologic dysfunction, anemia, neutropenia, bone demineralization	100-200 µg/kg/day
Manganese	Metalloenzymes, carbohydrate metabolism, antioxidants, hemostasis	Neurologic dysfunction, defects in lipid metabolism, reduced coagulants, growth restriction in animals	10-20 µg/kg/day
Chromium	Carbohydrate metabolism, component of nucleic acids	Impaired glucose tolerance, impaired growth	2-4 µg/kg/day
Selenium	Metalloenzymes, antioxidants	Cardiomyopathy	1.5-3 µg/kg/day
Iodine	Thyroid hormone synthesis	Hypothyroidism	1 µg/kg/day
Molybdenum	Metalloenzymes	Neurologic and visual dysfunction, growth restriction in animals	2-3 µg/kg/day

Modified from Forbes SB: *Pediatric nutrition handbook,* Elk Grove Village, Ill, 1985, American Academy of Pediatrics; and Tsang R, ed: *Vitamin and mineral requirements of preterm infants,* New York, 1985, Marcel Dekker.

processes, signs of vitamin deficiency can be nonspecific, such as lethargy, irritability, and poor growth. **Table 16-5 summarizes the recommended daily vitamin intake for enterally and parenterally fed infants. For comparison, the average vitamin content of human milk and commercial infant formulas is given in Table 16-6.**[68] Routine supplementation of vitamins above recommended levels cannot be advised at present because of possible toxicity and lack of clearly demonstrated benefits. Supplementing vitamin D above the recommended dose of 400 IU/day does not prevent osteopenia in preterm infants.[22]

Minerals and Trace Elements
Mineral requirements for preterm infants have been largely estimated from in utero accretion rates. **Published recommendations for daily intakes in healthy, enterally fed preterm infants are shown in Table 16-7. Supplementation with calcium and phosphorus to achieve the recommended intakes (with a Ca/P ratio of 2:1) has been shown to decrease the incidence of metabolic bone disease in preterm infants. Mineral supplementation of human milk or use of an enriched preterm formula is usually necessary to achieve the intakes recommended in Table 16-7.**

FEEDING TECHNIQUES AND STRATEGIES

Composition of Human Milk and Commercial Formula

Human Milk

The ideal enteral diet for almost all (Box 16-3) term newborn infants is human milk, providing sufficient energy, protein, fat, carbohydrate, micronutrients, and water for normal growth. In addition, human milk, unlike formulas, provides a variety of antimicrobial factors that may protect against infection, such as secretory immunoglobulins (IgA), leukocytes, complement, lactoferrin, and lysozyme.[33] Human milk also contains hormones and growth factors such as epidermal and nerve growth factors, insulin-like growth factor I, erythropoietin, prolactin, calcitonin, steroids, thyrotropin-releasing hormone (TRH), and thyroxine.[79] The role of these milk hormones and trophic factors has not clearly been established, but they may play a role in organ maturation and growth. Several essential and conditionally essential amino acids are present in high concentra-

tions in human milk. The protein and fat components of human milk are readily digestible, and human milk contains large numbers of enzymes that may aid in nutrient digestion and processing (e.g., lipase). The risk of developing later food allergies are reduced in infants receiving human milk in infancy.[25] Finally, there are obvious psychological benefits to a mother who provides her own milk for her sick infant (see Chapter 19).

Human milk is the recommended basis of nutrition for preterm infants.[17] A preterm infant may not grow appropriately on human milk alone because of the special nutritional requirements addressed previously.[44] Recommended daily requirements for energy, protein, calcium, sodium, phosphorus, magnesium, iron, zinc, and several vitamins necessary to meet the normal rate of in utero growth usually will not be achieved in a growing "healthy" preterm infant who is fed with unsupplemented human milk. A preterm infant with respiratory distress, infection, excessive heat losses, or increased activity will have even greater nutritional needs. Nonetheless, milk from mothers of preterm infants has more protein and sodium than milk obtained at term, and occasionally will provide for adequate growth in larger and healthier preterm infants.[80] **The nutrient content of term (mature) human milk is compared with standard and preterm formulas in Table 16-4. The nutritional composition of preterm human milk is compared with term human milk in Table 16-8. Use of commercially available supplements to human milk that provide additional energy, protein, vitamins, and minerals is rec-**

Box 16-3	CONTRAINDICATIONS TO THE USE OF HUMAN MILK

Maternal miliary tuberculosis
Galactosemia
Maternal drug abuse
Some maternal medications (see Chapter 19)
Maternal HIV infection

Table 16-8	NUTRITIONAL COMPOSITION OF PRETERM AND TERM BREAST MILK							
	7 DAYS		**14 DAYS**		**28 DAYS**		**>56 DAYS**	
NUTRIENT	**PRETERM**	**TERM**	**PRETERM**	**TERM**	**PRETERM**	**TERM**	**PRETERM**	**TERM**
Calories	73.86	73.62	74.59	71.81	73.33	72.71	70.10	76.33
(kcal/dl)	±1.81	±3.32	±1.96	±3.57	±2.14	±1.88	±1.424	±2.34
Protein	2.76	2.55	2.39	1.97	1.90	1.76	1.99	1.96
nitrogen (g/L)	±0.18	±0.18	±0.16	±0.14	±0.09	±0.08	±0.10	±0.10
Sodium	17.23	9.54	12.36	9.37	9.56	7.04	8.85	7.14
(mEq/L)	±1.88	±1.30	±1.42	±1.95	±0.70	±0.96	±0.80	±0.51
Calcium (mg/L)	293	293	266	274	282	267	310	314
	±16	±8	±15	±13	±12	±13	±16	±12
Fat (g/dl)	3.1	2.98	3.42	3	3.24	3.07	3.43	3.46
	±0.71	±0.28	±0.18	±0.26	±0.16	±0.21	±0.16	±0.32
Lactose (g/dl)	6.38	6.43	6.86	6.63	6.79	6.92	7.21	6.68
	±0.22	±0.13	±0.16	±0.23	±0.17	±0.36	±0.11	±0.22

Modified from Lemons JA, Moye L, Hall D: Difference in the composition of preterm and term human milk during early lactation, *Pediatr Res* 16:113, 1982.

ommended.[69] **Nutrient composition of these fortifiers is shown in Table 16-3.**

Formula

Cow's milk–derived formulas have been designed to mimic human milk to provide biologically available protein mixtures with appropriate protein/energy ratios for normal growth. In general, formulas designed for term infants contain 20 kcal/oz and are adequate to meet the needs of term and larger preterm infants (greater than 1800 g) with an intact GI tract and "normal" fluid requirements. A whey and casein mixture approximating that of human milk is usually preferred. All preterm formulas contain whey/casein ratios of 60:40 and have higher protein contents than term formulas. Preterm formulas also contain less lactose as a carbohydrate source and substitute glucose polymers to provide approximately 50% of the calories derived from carbohydrate. Most preterm formulas provide some of the fat in the form of medium-chain triglycerides because of the ease with which they are absorbed. Calcium and phosphorus content is increased, with a Ca/P ratio of 2:1, which provides for improved bone mineralization. Other minerals and vitamins are also present in higher concentrations in preterm formulas to reflect the special nutritional needs of the VLBW infant. Preterm formulas are available in 20-, 22-, and 24-kcal/oz preparations, with similar osmolalities and renal solute loads.

Soy protein formulas should be reserved for infants with a strong family history of allergy who are not being fed human milk. Soy-derived formulas should not be used for long periods in VLBW infants because of the poorer quality of protein and lower calcium and zinc accretion rates seen with these formulas. Formulas derived from protein hydrolysates should be reserved for infants who are clearly allergic to cow's milk proteins and are not breast-fed or do not tolerate soy-derived formulas. In general, families with a strong history of cow's milk protein allergy should be strongly encouraged to breast-feed. For infants requiring soy or protein hydrolysate formulas, careful attention should be paid to monitoring long-term growth, and amino acid, vitamin, and trace mineral balance.

Elemental formulas are used in infants with malabsorption, abnormal GI tracts, or severe protein allergy. The protein source in these formulas is derived from casein hydrolysates, and the fat is largely from MCT oil. The composition of Pregestimil (Mead Johnson) is shown as an example of an elemental formula in Table 16-4. Use of elemental formulas is generally indicated in the infant with severe liver disease and fat malabsorption, with short bowel syndrome (such as after necrotizing enterocolitis with surgical resection), or with dysmotility syndromes (such as in gastroschisis). Occasionally formulas derived from protein hydrolysates are useful after a severe episode of infectious gastroenteritis with mucosal injury and resulting protein or lactose intolerance. A lactose-free formula may also be used in this setting. It is not necessary to use an elemental formula in the routine care of VLBW infants. A variety of other modified formulas are available for infants with special needs (e.g., lactose-free and protein-free formulas).

In some circumstances infants require fluid restriction (e.g., because of pulmonary edema, congestive heart failure, or renal failure) while receiving full enteral feedings. Caloric delivery and nutritional support can be maintained by increasing the caloric density of feedings when feeding volumes cannot be tolerated or fluid intake must be limited. This can be done by adding powdered formula, milk fortifiers, glucose polymers, corn oil, microlipids (e.g., a lipid emulsion), or MCT oil to the formula or milk as desired to achieve acceptable concentrations and intakes of these nutrients. Caloric densities of 27 to 30 kcal/oz can be achieved in this way, although infants tolerate these supplements in a highly individual fashion and should be monitored for signs of feeding intolerance (e.g., abdominal distention, increased stooling, and the presence of fat or sugar in the stool). Increasing caloric density of feedings necessitates less water delivery to the infant and generally leads to an increase in formula osmolality as well. Careful monitoring of feeding tolerance and fluid balance (renal function) is therefore necessary on a high caloric density feeding regimen.

In the future, human milk fortifiers and formulas engineered for preterm infants are likely to include a more complex mixture of fatty acids, including long-chain polyunsaturated fatty acids important for brain and retinal development. Immunoglobulins, such as IgA, may be added to decrease the incidence of necrotizing enterocolitis (NEC), and trophic factors, such as epidermal growth factor (EGF) or other hormones, may be added after their role in human milk has been established. Specific amino acids, carnitine, nucleotides, and other complex organic compounds may be supplemented or provided at unique rates as our understanding of GI maturation and optimal

Box 16-4	SPECIAL NUTRITIONAL CONDITIONS IN ELBW INFANTS

1. Minimal energy reserves (both carbohydrate and fat)
2. Intrinsically higher metabolic rate (greater relative mass of more metabolically active organs: brain, heart, liver)
3. Higher protein turnover rate (especially when growing)
4. Higher glucose needs for energy and brain metabolism
5. Higher lipid needs to match the in utero rate of fat deposition
6. Excessive evaporative rates (immature skin)
7. Occasionally very high urinary water and solute losses (depending on intake and renal maturation)
8. Low rates of gastrointestinal peristalsis
9. Limited production of gut digestive enzymes and growth factors
10. Higher incidence of stressful events (hypoxemia, respiratory distress, sepsis)
11. Metabolic effects of medications used frequently (steroids, antibiotics, sedatives, catecholamines)
12. Abnormal neurologic outcome if not fed adequately

Modified from Thureen P, Hay WW Jr: Conditions requiring special nutritional management. In Tsang RC et al, eds: *Nutritional needs of the preterm infant*, Baltimore, 1993, Williams & Wilkins.

growth-promoting substrates for the developing preterm infant evolves.

Preterm Infants

There is an urgent need to address the nutrition of ELBW (less than 1000 g) and VLBW (less than 1500 g) preterm infants. The nutritional requirements of these very small infants are marked, unique, poorly understood, and inadequately provided for, including both the quality and the quantity of nutrients in currently used IV and enteral nutrient regimens (Box 16-4). Also, many of these infants are growth restricted at birth. Thus their nutritional needs for "catch-up" growth and for normal rates of metabolism and growth are very likely to differ from those of normally grown infants. Furthermore, in spite of increasingly aggressive in-hospital nutritional management, the majority of these infants remain growth restricted and are small for postconceptual age at the time of discharge.[21,40] In fact, the fraction of these infants who are small for gestational age at discharge is several fold greater than at birth. **There is increasingly strong evidence that inadequate nutrition of preterm and growth-restricted in-**

fants can have lasting consequences resulting in neurologic and developmental impairment.[40] Many previous studies in humans and animals have documented that prolonged postnatal undernutrition and malnutrition add far greater insult than does prenatal undernutrition alone. Such observations have important implications. First, we cannot now think of "early" nutrition of these small infants simply in terms of providing immediate nutrient needs just for metabolic maintenance (such as glucose to prevent hypoglycemia); we also must consider that early nutrition has biologic effects that have lasting or lifelong significance. Second, we can no longer regard nutritional practices in preterm infants as simply a matter of personal choice.

The major impact of sufficient early nutritional support on long-term outcome should be a stimulus to new research that defines consistent approaches to the nutrition of preterm infants to optimize their future health and development. **Although concerns about the safety of enteral feeding of preterm infants have frequently delayed the initiation of feedings, evidence is accumulating to suggest that early initiation of low-volume enteral feedings ("minimal enteral nutrition"), especially with human milk, may improve GI development and function in preterm infants**[7,19] **and protect against NEC and systemic infection.*** Enteral feedings are associated with surges in gut hormone production that may mediate trophic effects on GI growth and mucosal maturation.[89] Absorption of nutrients may be improved with increased amount and length of villous absorptive surface.[13] **Providing only small quantities of milk into the neonatal GI tract promotes the production of locally acting gut hormones, such as gastrin, enteroglucagon, and motilin, that are thought to be very important for normal intestinal maturation.**[6,41,42,53] **Feeding tolerance is improved and full enteral feedings are achieved earlier in these infants.**[6,19,51,53,77] **Minimal enteral feedings also have been shown to improve nutritional outcome (weight gain and bone mineralization) in preterm infants.**[19,51] **The potential advantages of minimal enteral feeding are listed in Box 16-5.** Failure to provide any enteral nutrition for prolonged periods of time to the newborn infant should be avoided, unless there is a specific contraindication for feeding.

---

*References 7, 36, 43, 51, 61, 72, 86.

Box 16-5	ADVANTAGES OF MINIMAL ENTERAL NUTRITION

No increase in incidence of NEC[36,40,61]
Decreased sepsis[51]
Decreased permeability of mucosa to foreign antigens[72]
Increased intestinal peptides and hormones[6,43,53]
Increased mucosal thickness and villi[13]
Maturation of intestinal motor activity[6,7]
Improved feeding tolerance[6,51,53,77]
Improved bone mineralization[19]
Earlier achievement of full enteral feedings[6,20,51]
Improved weight gain[51]
Shorter hospital stay[6,7,51]
Reduced requirement for supplemental oxygen[51]

During the acute phase of a preterm infant's illness, aggressive nutrition should be provided by the parenteral route (see Chapter 17), but recent studies have shown that minimal enteral feedings can safely be started by day of life 2 or 3, even in very small or ill infants. **Feedings from 6 to 20 ml/kg/day divided into every 2 to 3 hour slow (over 30 to 60 minutes) bolus feeds are given without advancement for several days.** The transition to nutritive enteral feedings can then proceed slowly (as discussed next), with continuous assessment of feeding tolerance to avoid complications such as NEC. **Human milk is the preferred initial feeding choice, but full-strength term formula may be used as an alternative for minimal enteral feeding.** Although most infants will benefit from early enteral feeding, those who are asphyxiated, hypotensive, severely hypoxemic, or symptomatic with patent ductus arteriosus (PDA), and those with evidence of NEC should not be fed enterally. These infants should be managed with aggressive parenteral nutrition.

Few controlled trials have been conducted that support a specific feeding strategy, although rapid advances to large feeding volumes are poorly tolerated by preterm infants. There is some evidence of calorie loss from expressed human milk and increased bacterial contamination during continuous gavage feeding.[11,18] **Benefits of continuous feedings may include decreased energy expenditure and improved growth in the premature infant.**[28,82] **Similar growth has usually been achieved whether infants are fed intermittently or continuously.**[2,71,74] **Recent studies indicate that an intermittent "slow" infusion (e.g., 3 hours of volume given over 1 hour out of 3) improves gastric emptying and duodenal motility.**[5,16]

The following guidelines reflect just one approach to enteral feedings; caution and flexibility must be used in following any feeding schedule. In general, the smaller the infant, the greater the attention that must be paid to feeding tolerance, although larger infants can certainly develop serious feeding intolerance and NEC.

Following a period of gut priming with minimal enteral feedings, advancement to full nutritive enteral feedings for a less than 2000 g infant should proceed in increments not greater than 15 to 20 ml/kg/day. Full feedings of human milk or formula (approximately 150 ml/kg/day) are achieved over 7 to 10 days. In most cases breast milk should be fed to the infant in the order in which it is collected, with the colostrum given first. An alternative for infants who cannot tolerate large volumes of feedings is hindmilk, which has increased fat content and may be given preferentially to increase energy delivery while adequate protein is provided by IV protein infusion.[1] **Once the infant is tolerating 100 ml/kg/day of enteral nutrition, breast milk can be fortified by the gradual addition of liquid or powdered human milk fortifiers (see Table 16-3). Thus progression to full enteral feedings of fortified human milk or 24 kcal/oz of preterm infant formula occurs over a minimum of 2 weeks.** During this time parenteral nutritional support is tapered to maintain from birth 3.5 g/kg/day or more of protein, 30% to 54% of total calories from fat, and 40% to 60% of total calories from carbohydrate. In general, infants weighing 1000 to 1500 g are fed every 2 hours and those weighing more are fed every 3 hours, if bolus feedings are tolerated without emesis or residuals.

A suggested enteral feeding strategy is presented in Table 16-9. It is important to appreciate that firm experimental support for any feeding guidelines for preterm infants is sorely lacking. The suggested approach is both arbitrary and conservative. Individualization of feeding strategy will be necessary for either more sick and physiologically unstable infants or more well and stable infants.

Changes in Nutritional Requirements With Illness

Studies in adult patients have shown dramatic changes in nutritional requirements depending on type of illness, degree of illness, surgery, and premorbid nutritional status. Although these changes

Table 16-9	SUGGESTED GUIDELINES FOR FEEDING PRETERM INFANTS*			
DAY OF LIFE	TYPE OF FOOD	VOLUME	FREQUENCY	INCREASES
BW <1000 g				
3 to 9	Human milk or term formula	0.5-1.5 ml/kg	2 hours	None
10 to 16	Human milk or term formula	1 ml/kg	2 hours	15 ml/kg/day
17 to 19	Fortified human milk or preterm formula	8 to 9 ml/kg	2 hours	20 ml/kg/day
20 to 21	Fortified human milk or preterm formula (22 kcal/oz)	12 to 13 ml/kg	2 hours	For increasing weight
22 to 23	Fortified human milk or preterm formula (24 kcal/oz)	12 to 13 ml/kg	2 hours	For increasing weight
BW 1001-1500 g				
2 to 6	Human milk or term formula	1 ml/kg	2 hours	None
7 to 11	Human milk or term formula	2 ml/kg	2 hours	20 ml/kg/day
12 to 14	Fortified human milk or preterm formula	8 to 9 ml/kg	2 hours	20 ml/kg/day
15	Fortified human milk or preterm formula (22 kcal/oz)	12 to 13 ml/kg	2 hours	For increasing weight
17	Fortified human milk or preterm formula (24 kcal/oz)	12 to 13 ml/kg	2 hours	For increasing weight
BW 1501-2000 g				
1 to 3	Human milk or term formula	2 ml/kg	3 hours	None
4 to 5	Human milk or term formula	3 ml/kg	3 hours	None
6 to 9	Human milk or term formula	3 ml/kg	3 hours	20 ml/kg/day
10 to 12	Fortified human milk or preterm formula	12 to 14 ml/kg	3 hours	20 ml/kg/day
13	Fortified human milk or preterm formula (22 kcal/oz)	18 to 20 ml/kg	3 hours	For increasing weight

Infants must be supported with parenteral nutrition during enteral feeding advances.
*Should be individualized for more unstable or well infants.

are not well studied in neonates, preliminary data and clinical experience indicate similar changes may be expected in ill infants.[66,81,88] In fact, these patients may have even greater nutritional needs because of their requirements for growth and development. **The overriding observation from all studies, however, is that ELBW and VLBW preterm infants are underfed during the early postnatal period and that this undernutrition, combined with additional stresses from various diseases, increases the risk of long-term adverse neurologic sequelae.** The value of achieving a specific body composition and growth rate is less certain. There remains a critical need for determining the right quality as well as quantity of nutrients for these infants. **The effects of common disease states on the nutrient requirements in preterm and term infants are shown in Figure 16-6.**

Acute and chronic respiratory diseases are the most common illnesses in neonates. **Acute respiratory problems, such as respiratory distress syndrome, pneumonia, and aspiration all increase the infant's metabolic needs for energy and protein. Energy requirements are met by increasing carbohydrate and fat delivery.** However, the metabolism of excessive carbohydrate feeding (greater than 12.5 mg/kg/min) may be detrimental to pulmonary status by increasing oxygen consumption and carbon dioxide production, increasing respiratory work and adding to respiratory failure. Lipid is a good alternative source of concentrated energy, because its metabolism has a lower respiratory quotient and produces less carbon dioxide. Lipids provide dense calories for volume and prevent essential fatty acid deficiency. **Protein wasting and catabolism with illness increases the infant's requirement for exogenous support.** Adequate provision of amino acids, especially branch chain amino acids, prevents catabolism of body protein stores, including respiratory and diaphragmatic muscle protein, and may improve minute ventilation by decreasing carbon dioxide production.

Infants with chronic lung disease and bronchopulmonary dysplasia present difficult nutritional problems. Poor nutrition is associated with abnormal lung development, increased toxic effects of oxygen, decreased surfactant production, and increased risk of infection. Although energy

	Normal Requirements		Likely Changes in Requirements With Illness						
	Well Term	Well Preterm	RDS	CLD	CHD Cyanotic	CHF	Sepsis	NEC/SBS	IUGR
Free water (ml/kg)	100 to 120	120 to 140	↓	↓	∅	↓	↑	↑	↑
Energy (kcal/kg)	100	120	↑	↑↑	↑	↑↑	↑↑	↑↑	↑
Carbohydrate (g/kg)	10	12 to 14	↑	↓	↑	↑	↑	↑	↑
Protein (g/kg)	1.5 to 2.2	3.0 to 4.0	∅	↑	↑	↑	↑↑	↑	↑
Fat (g/kg)	3.3 to 6	4 to 7	∅	↑	↑	↑	∅	↑↑*	↑
Calcium (mg/kg)	45 to 60	120 to 230	∅	↑↑•♦	↑◊	↑•◊	∅	↑*	↑
Iron (mg/kg)	1	2 to 4	∅	↑♦	↑	∅	∅	↑	↑
Vitamin A (IU/kg)	333	700 to 1500	↑◊	↑◊	∅	∅	∅	∅	∅

∅ No change.
* Particularly with loss of the terminal ileum.
• Particularly with calciuric diuretics, such as furosemide.
◊ Particularly if postoperative.
♦ In <1500-g preterm infants.

RDS, Respiratory distress syndrome; CLD, chronic lung disease; CHD, congenital heart disease; CHF, congestive heart failure; NEC, necrotizing enterocolitis; IUGR, intrauterine growth restriction; SBS, short bowel syndrome.

FIGURE 16-6 Daily nutritional requirements and changes with illness. (From Premmer DM, Georgieff MK: Nutrition for ill neonates, *Neo Reviews*, September, e56, 1999; Thureen P, Hay WW Jr: Conditions requiring special nutritional management. In Tsang RC et al, eds: *Nutritional needs of the preterm infant*, Baltimore, 1993, Williams & Wilkins.)

and metabolic demands are increased in these patients, many routine management strategies may make the disease process worse. Excessive fluid volumes may increase pulmonary edema and contribute to lung injury. Increased work of breathing may limit intake. Steroid therapy and chronic disease have negative effects on protein balance. Diuretic use can waste calcium and potassium. Decreasing the proportion of energy provided by carbohydrates may decrease lipogenesis and therefore carbon dioxide production. Vitamin supplementation should be provided as needed to maintain normal serum levels.

Congenital heart disease, especially when accompanied by cyanosis or congestive heart failure, significantly impairs nutritional status and growth. **These infants have increased metabolic needs and may experience the catabolic stress of early palliative surgery.** Nutritional management is additionally complicated by underlying cyanosis, diuretic therapy, respiratory distress, malabsorption, and delicate fluid balance. Mineral derangement is common postoperatively, with diuretic therapy, and with suboptimal intake. Iron supplementation is

necessary to provide for increased erythropoesis with chronic cyanosis.

Good nutritional status can decrease the risk of infection and sepsis as well as improve recovery in neonates. Normal immune response depends on adequate protein energy, micronutrients, and trace elements. Although not well studied in this population, it appears that the metabolic requirements of septic infants, especially for energy and amino acids, are much greater than otherwise similar, but not infected, infants.

An infant with NEC or short bowel syndrome is at additional risk for malnutrition resulting from malabsorption and increased nutrient losses. During the acute illness, such an infant must receive adequate parenteral nutrition. Recovery needs to be supported by gradual increases in enteral nutrition and slowly decreasing parenteral supplementation. Of particular concern are excessive water losses, with electrolyte imbalance and malabsorption of fats and fat-soluble vitamins.

Any infant recovering from asphyxia or shock should probably not receive enteral feedings for 24 to 72 hours to allow recovery of the bowel

from the ischemic injury and decrease the risk for NEC.

Neonates who have undergone surgery are at increased risk for nutritional deficiencies as a result of the stresses of illness and surgery and possible abnormal nutrient and water losses. In these infants enteral feedings are preferred, because they are safe, more economical, preserve the integrity of the intestinal mucosa, and promote continued development of the GI tract.[20,63] **After an operative procedure, the infant is often NPO for 3 to 14 days until the return of intestinal motility and function (e.g., stooling, lack of abdominal distention, decreased gastric aspirates, and absence of bilious aspirates).**[63] The method of feeding chosen, rapidity of feeding advancement, formula composition, and type of feeding depend on the infant's general medical condition, GI function, and the type of surgery. The choice of formula for a neonate following surgery depends on bowel integrity. An infant recovering from mild NEC may be started on human milk or regular formula. With serious or surgically treated NEC, human milk is preferred but a dilute formula, or in the most severe cases an elemental formula, may be used.[63]

Nipple feedings should be started postoperatively in a term infant if the infant is awake, hungry, and able to suck, swallow, and gag and has normal intestinal motility and no respiratory distress. Preterm infants may need gavage feeding. Daily and weekly growth should be monitored and assessed relative to caloric intake. Inadequate growth may be treated with increased volumes, increased caloric density, or a less stressful method of feeding (e.g., a combination of nipple and gavage feedings).

IUGR Infants

Nutritional support for SGA infants requires separate consideration, because decreased size for dates may result from various pathologic conditions or no pathology at all. The physical finding of small size at birth may be caused by any number of diseases or abnormalities, both intrinsic and extrinsic to the fetus and newborn. **Early events in gestation may manifest in the infant as symmetric growth restriction. These infants may have limited growth potential as a result of chromosomal and genetic abnormalities or early infection. Asymmetrically growth restricted infants, by contrast, may show growth abnormality that results from late pla-**cental insufficiency or other insults more amenable to recovery in the postnatal period.

Completely healthy and normal infants may present with constitutionally small size. Complicating these issues is the fact that infants with growth restriction of any cause may be born preterm and require still more individualized management. Also, the influence of abnormal intrauterine growth and postnatal nutritional management on adult diseases, such as obesity, insulin resistance, diabetes, and cardiovascular disease, is currently the subject of much debate and study.

In general, growth-restricted infants are likely to have increased energy needs and low stores of energy, nutrients, and minerals.[15,60,65] Hypoglycemia,[32] hyperglycemia, increased need for heat production,[76] and increased risk of GI ischemia are more likely in the early postnatal period in these infants than in their normally grown peers. These problems require anticipatory nutritional monitoring and management. Early parenteral glucose, protein, and energy supplementation may be necessary while cautious enteral feedings are started.

Gavage Feeding

Gavage feedings (Box 16-6) provide a method of feeding an infant who is too immature to allow for safe nipple feeding or who is too sick to take adequate nourishment. Gavage feedings are indicated in infants requiring endotracheal intubation or those with an immature, weak, or absent suck, swallow, or gag reflex. Most infants tolerate intermittent bolus feedings delivered slowly. Continuous feedings may be initiated in infants recovering from NEC, with short bowel syndrome, with congenital heart disease, or with intolerance of bolus feedings. There is some evidence that infants fed continuously may have better absorption of nutrients and therefore improved growth.[62] Caregivers should monitor the number and consistency of stools or stoma output. Stools should be tested (e.g., Clinitest) for blood or reducing substances (to detect undigested or partially digested carbohydrate) when feeding intolerance or malabsorption is suspected. If short bowel syndrome is present, transition from continuous to bolus feedings should proceed slowly and cautiously. This may be accomplished by infusing feedings over gradually shorter periods of time, with increasing intervals between feedings until bolus feedings every 3 to 4 hours are tolerated. **Prolonged**

Box 16-6 **GAVAGE FEEDING GUIDELINES**

Equipment

1. Breast milk/formula in syringe (4-hour amount, or unit protocol, maximum)
2. Tape, optional transparent dressing
3. Lubricant—optional
4. Stethoscope
5. For intermittent feeding: infant feeding set with syringe, medicine cup, 8 Fr gavage tube
6. For indwelling feeding tubes: infant <1 kg, 4 Fr tube; >1 kg, 5/6 Fr tube; >2.5/3 kg, 8 Fr tube (tube size may also depend on placement, oral or nasal, amount of feeding, and rate of delivery of feeding)
   Short-term feeding tube (generally made of polyvinyl-chloride [PVC]) should be changed every 24-72 hr
   Long-term feeding tube (made of polyurethane) should be changed every 4 wk
   NOTE: always follow manufacturers' recommendations
7. Syringe pump and extention tubing as needed

Feeding Tube Insertion

1. Wash hands and assemble equipment in a clean area.
2. Measure for tube placement by placing tip of feeding tube at the tip of nose, draw to base of ear, then to halfway between the xiphoid process and the umbilicus.
3. Mark tube with indelible ink pen to indicate the distance from the tip of the tube to the corner of the mouth or edge of the nares.
4. Insert tube (swaddling the infant may help with tolerance of this procedure).
   NEVER FORCE THE TUBE.
   Oral placement (usually for infants <1 kg, those on nasal continuous positive airway pressure (NCPAP) or ventilator, high oxygen need, or with excoriated nares): insert tip into the oropharynx, gently pushing tube in a downward arc into the esophagus until reaching the premeasured mark.
   Nasal placement (generally preferred for infants >1 kg with mature or strong gag reflex and infants who are breastfeeding or nippling): moisten tip with water or lubricant. Insert tip gently into one nostril and advance slowly as above.
5. Gastric tube tip placement is verified by injecting 1-2 ml of air while auscultating with a stethoscope over the abdomen for the sound (swoosh) of air entry. Then gently aspirate air and stomach contents. If no air or stomach contents are aspirated, advance tube 1 cm and repeat placement verification procedure. The tube landmark should be checked with every caregiving to determine that it is still visible and at the correct location.
6. Soft Silastic tubes are generally used for transpyloric feedings and require the use of a stylet for insertion. The tube must be inspected visually and by flushing with water prior to insertion to ensure that it has not been perforated by the stylet. The stylet is removed after insertion and is stored in package by the bedside. Tip placement is usually verified by radiographic imaging.

Securing Feeding Tube

1. Intermittent feeding tubes can be taped to the cheek
2. Indwelling tubes must be taped securely to the face, leaving the landmark visible. For tubes placed nasally, a narrow piece of tape may be placed along the tubing on the upper lip, with a transparent dressing applied over tube on the cheek.

Feeding

1. Aspirate entire stomach contents to assess quantity as well as color and appearance.
2. To prevent loss of electrolytes, slowly return aspirate to the stomach. Exceptions to this include aspirates that are bloody or "coffee ground," green or bright yellow, fecal appearing, or contain large amounts of mucus. Do not refeed, and discuss feeding plan with physician/practitioner. Also report aspirates of undigested formula if amount is more than half of the feeding, occurs more than once, or if there is a change in abdominal assessment. Reducing the feeding by the amount of the refed aspirate is recommended for 1 or 2 feedings.
3. Instilling breast milk/formula with intermittent gavage feeding:
   Detach syringe from feeding tube and remove plunger; reattach syringe to feeding tube. Pour the predetermined amount of milk into the syringe. Flow may begin spontaneously or require a gentle nudge from the plunger. Allow feeding to run in slowly by gravity. *Never push a feeding.* The higher the syringe is held, the faster the feeding will flow (about 8 inches is ideal). Gavage sets may be rinsed carefully and used for up to 24 hr unless labeled "single-use only" or manufacturer's directions indicate otherwise.
4. Intermittent gavage feeding with an indwelling feeding tube:
   Check aspirate and feed as above. If feeding is to be given over a period of time (e.g., 30-60 min), use appropriate-sized syringe and pump. When feeding is complete, cap tube or close off by attaching syringe with plunger.
5. Continuous drip feedings with an indwelling feeding tube:
   Check feeding tube placement and feeding residuals every 2-4 hr using stopcock which is placed between the feeding tube and the extension tubing. Check ink landmark on feeding tube hourly to assure proper placement of the tube.
   Prepare up to 4 hours of breast milk or formula (or amount according to institutional studies of bacterial growth). Fill syringe with predetermined feeding amount plus enough to prime the extension tubing. Place syringe into syringe pump and program to deliver feeding at desired rate. To help prevent loss of milkfat by settling, place syringe in an upward vertical position and use mini-bore tubing.

Continued

Box 16-6 GAVAGE FEEDING GUIDELINES—cont'd

Care, Assessment, and Documentation

1. Assess infant's tolerance of feeding tube placement. If gagging occurs, attempt to insert tube down one side of the oropharynx rather than down the middle. If the infant becomes apneic, bradycardic, or cyanotic during feeding tube placement, pause to allow recovery or remove the tube and allow infant to rest before trying again. If these symptoms occur during the feeding, stop the feeding by lowering the syringe or stopping the pump. If recovery occurs quickly, resume feeding slowly and observe. If distress continues or recurs, stop feeding and inform the physician/practitioner.

Care, Assessment, and Documentation—cont'd

2. Use new short-term PVC feeding tube every 24-72 hr (or follow manufacturers' recommendations).
3. Change long-term polyurethane nasal feeding tube to opposite nostril weekly. Discard and replace tube after 4 wk (or follow manufacturers' recommendations).
4. Document all details of the feeding and the infant's tolerance, proper placement of the indwelling feeding tube, and when feeding tube and/or equipment is to be changed.

---

oral or nasogastric tube feedings may cause adverse oral stimulation and promote gastroesophageal reflux.[63] After certain surgical procedures, some term neonates will require gastrostomy tube placement (see Chapter 28).

It remains controversial whether intragastric or transpyloric feedings are more successful. **In general, intragastric feedings are preferred to the transpyloric feedings because the transpyloric route may have increased mortality without proven benefits. Intestinal perforations and other complications have been reported with transpyloric feeding tubes, so their use might be restricted to infants who cannot tolerate gastric feedings because of excessive regurgitation or other feeding intolerance.**

Precautions

Feeding intolerance may be the first symptom of illness (e.g., hypoxia, dyspnea, congestive heart failure, sepsis, and NEC). At first symptoms may be subtle, so the caregiver should be constantly aware of any change in the infant's overall condition and feeding tolerance.

Aspiration is of major concern in any infant of gestational age who does not have a neurologically mature swallow, gag, or cough reflex (less than 34 to 36 weeks). Any tachypneic infant with labored respirations or with an endotracheal tube is also at increased risk for aspiration. Gavage tube position must be carefully checked, feedings should run in slowly, and these infants should not be overfed. Gavage feedings should never be pushed.

Nipple Feeding

Development of appropriate neuromuscular coordination is necessary to successfully initiate nipple feedings. Criteria for initiating nipple feeding must be individualized. Coordination of suck, swallow, and breathing emerges at about 34 weeks' gestation, regardless of postnatal age.[89] Respiratory illness leads to energy depletion. Nipple feeding is not usually possible unless respiratory rate is less than 60 breaths/min, and the oxygen required is less than 40%. Neonates with craniofacial malformation (e.g., cleft lip or palate, choanal stenosis or atresia, and mandibular hypoplasia) are at increased risk for aspiration. Use of different nipple shapes and sizes and sitting the infant in the upright position facilitates safe oral feeding. Gastrostomy tube placement may be necessary if oral feedings are not adequately established (see Chapter 28).

The ability to suck on a pacifier, fingers, or a gavage tube does not ensure the infant's ability to perform nutritive sucking. A preterm infant without a gag reflex is at risk for aspiration with nipple feedings. An infant who is successful at nipple feeding should exhibit an active suck, coordinated swallow, minimal fluid loss around the nipple, and completion of feeding within 15 to 30 minutes.[73] A preterm infant in the NICU has usually been exposed to many unpleasant oral sensations, such as endotracheal tubes, suction catheters, gavage tubes, and facial tape. These infants often become "disorganized feeders."[87]

When nipple feedings are initiated in a recovering ill preterm infant, they may last only minutes. Coordination of sucking with breathing is the first lesson for the premature infant. Stress behaviors (e.g., increase or decrease in respiratory or heart rate, decreased oxygen saturation, color change, gagging, choking, emesis, fatigue, irritability, or a "panicked look") should cue the caregiver to pause for a rest period or end the feeding.

An infant receiving supplemental oxygen should be monitored by pulse oximetry to determine oxygen requirement during nipple feedings. Different types of nipples may be used for different infants. Strategies to facilitate oral feedings include a relaxed caregiver, a quiet environment with subdued light, and a snugly wrapped infant (see Chapter 13).

Nipple feedings should begin slowly at one feeding per day, then increase as tolerated to once every 8 hours, then once every third feeding, then every other feeding, and finally to full nipple feedings. Scheduling nipple feedings for parent visits enables them to actively participate in their infant's care. A too rapid change to nipple feeding results in weight loss; the infant tires with feedings and is unable to take in caloric requirements or needs gavage supplementation after nippling to meet caloric needs (with inherent danger of vomiting the nippled feeding and aspiration—when intermittent tube placement and gavage are used). Diligent attention is warranted, and a decrease in nipple feedings may be necessary to prevent dehydration, malnutrition, and a worsening of the infant's condition.

Feeding a Former Preterm Infant After Hospital Discharge

Many premature infants are still preterm when they are discharged, and most are small for their corrected gestational age despite aggressive in-hospital nutritional therapy. Continued attention to increased nutrient requirements in these infants after hospital discharge seems appropriate as a continuum of support. **Therefore efforts to wean infants to 20 kcal/oz formula before discharge may be counterproductive. In fact, providing premature infants with a formula containing a higher energy and protein content after discharge until a corrected age of 9 months has resulted in improved growth.**[46-48]

The ideal composition of feedings in "recovering" premature infants has yet to be determined; however, efforts to continue feeding with a 22- or 24-kcal/oz infant formula with a higher protein and mineral content for several months after hospital discharge are supported by studies, even for premature infants who do not have significant chronic illness. **Infants with significant chronic lung disease who will be receiving home oxygen therapy are particularly likely to need 24 kcal/oz formula after discharge to maintain adequate growth at home. Oxygen supplementation itself also improves growth in these infants when normal oxygen saturation is maintained.**[29] Infants who are discharged on breast feedings can be supplemented with a 24-kcal/oz formula or fortification of mother's milk if growth is suboptimal. Demand feeding should be initiated before discharge to document adequate growth on the chosen feeding regimen.

FEEDING INTOLERANCE AND COMPLICATIONS

Assessment for signs of feeding intolerance is imperative, because although some feeding complications can be mild and respond to nursing interventions, others are more serious and require medical intervention.[10]

Residuals
The feeding tube is aspirated every 2 to 4 hours, before a feeding, to determine whether gastric emptying is adequate. Incompletely digested aspirates of 2 to 4 ml/kg or a 1-hour volume if the infant is on continuous feedings are considered normal, and these residuals should generally be returned to the infant (Figure 16-7). Increasing residuals is a sign of feeding intolerance and may necessitate decreasing feeding volumes, slowing the rate of instillation, or slowing the rate of feeding advance. Occasionally, medications such as metoclopramide or cisapride have been used to accelerate bowel motility and improve feeding tolerance,[52] but data from other good clinical trials do not confirm this outcome. Cisipride has been removed from use by the FDA because of its side effect of prolonged cardiac arrhythmias; metoclopramide has limited, if any, evidence of efficacy. **The presence of bile or blood in the gastric aspirate warrants further investigation and consideration of NEC.**

Emesis
Emesis may be caused by an overdistended stomach, gastroesophageal reflux, a poorly positioned feeding tube, gastric irritation from enterally administered medications, infection,

Assessment of Gastric Residuals

>50% of amount of feeding given in 3 hr or >2-4 ml/kg

Evaluate Infant
Activity
Abdominal examination and girth measurement
Increased apnea or bradycardia
Increased oxygen requirement

Normal or No Change
Check feeding tube position
Position infant right side down
Check stooling pattern
Consider glycerine suppository
↓
Refeed residual
↓
Continue feedings

Abnormal or Second Residual in 24 hr
Evaluate with abdominal radiograph
Consider infection screen
Discard residual
Hold feedings
Reevaluate frequently
↓
Normal findings
↓
Restart feedings after 24 hr
Consider reducing feeding volumes by 20%

FIGURE 16-7   Gastric residuals.

obstruction, metabolic disorders, increased intracranial pressure, drug withdrawal, or overstimulation in a very small infant. Interventions include allowing the feeding to flow more slowly by use of a smaller gavage tube, instilling the feeding over a longer period of time, decreasing feeding volumes, prone positioning, giving medications at the end of the feeding, or modifying a stressful environment (see Chapter 13). Abdominal radiography to assess feeding tube position may be warranted.

Gastroesophageal reflux may be suspected in an infant with irritability, emesis, apnea and bradycardia, respiratory deterioration, refusal to eat, or otherwise unexplained blood in the stools. Postoperative emesis and abdominal distention may indicate a stricture, partial obstruction, or inflammatory abscess (see Chapter 28).

Abdominal Distention

Abdominal distention with or without palpable or visible loops of bowel may be a sign of poor gastric motility, ileus, constipation, or "gas." Variations in abdominal circumference of up to 1.5 cm may occur and without other clinical signs of illness may be normal.[8] If the abdomen remains soft and nontender, prone positioning and gentle rectal stimulation with a glycerin sliver may be helpful to relieve gas and enable stooling. Persistent abdominal distention can be a sign of a pathologic condition (e.g., anatomic obstruction or infection), and requires investigation. An abdominal x-ray examination is indicated in these patients. Abdominal girth is measured every 4 to 8 hours to document increased distention. Paper or cloth tape is placed around the abdomen at a consistent point marked on the abdomen.

Diarrhea

Diarrhea, or frequent water-loss stools, may signify transient lactase deficiency or another pathologic state. Stool culture for bacterial or viral pathogens and a stool Clinitest may be obtained. In lactose malabsorption, short-term use of a non–lactose-containing formula should result in return to normal stools.

Apnea and/or Bradycardia

Apnea and/or bradycardia frequently occurs during or after feeding. These symptoms may be vagally mediated by the passage of a feeding tube, gastric distention, or gastroesophageal reflux or may occur with abdominal distention and compromise of lung volumes or airway obstruction. Interventions to decrease vagal stimulation include changing to an indwelling gavage tube, decreasing feeding volume, and feeding more slowly.

Poor Growth

The first response to poor growth may be to increase feeding volume and calories. Factors that increase caloric expenditure (e.g., thermal instability or overstimulation) should also be considered. As feeding volumes are slowly advanced, feeding tolerance must be closely assessed. Use of a heat shield, plastic wrap, hat or other clothing, supportive positioning, and grouping of care to conserve energy may result in better growth. Although these interventions intuitively make sense, convincing data supporting success for these maneuvers are hard to find.

Danger Signs

Bile in the gastric aspirate is generally a sign of significant ileus or obstruction. The presence of blood in the stools or gastric aspirate, a tense or tender abdomen, and abdominal wall erythema are more ominous signs of feeding intolerance and may indicate frank NEC. The presence of these signs and symptoms warrants a careful physical examination and usually further investigation including x-ray examinations. Feedings should be postponed while these signs and symptoms are being investigated. Other useful studies include a complete blood cell count with differential to evaluate the extent of blood loss, presence of thrombocytopenia (a marker of necrotic bowel), and change in white blood cell count as evidence of infection. Although feeding human milk may help protect against developing NEC, and 5% to 10% of cases of NEC occur in infants who have never been fed enterally, necrotizing enterocolitis can occur in any infant. **Abnormal abdominal distention or bilious or bloody gastric aspirates should be investigated carefully regardless of feeding status.**

PARENT TEACHING

Parents of a sick NICU patient may feel overwhelmed by the infant's illness, appearance, and uncertain future. Loss of control of the infant's care and unclear parental roles may make bonding difficult and add to feelings of helplessness, frustra-

tion, and isolation. **It is imperative that the health care team and especially the bedside nurse be supportive of the parents as caregivers. This support can begin with education about early feeding practices in the nursery and anticipated infant growth and development. Feeding is an excellent way to involve parents in their infant's care.** Parents should be involved in discussions of feeding practices and formula choices. During gavage feedings parents should be encouraged to hold their infant and support the pacifier to encourage nonnutritive sucking.[23,90] Frequent communication about the ups and downs of feeding the sick newborn as well as weekly progress updates on growth charts is helpful.

A mother's ability to provide breast milk remains something she alone can do for her infant. Prematurity and prolonged illness, as well as the inability to breastfeed the infant directly, are major barriers to breastfeeding. Lactation support in the NICU has been shown to increase mothers' success at maintaining lactation through discharge from the NICU.[54,70] Guidelines for expression and collection of human breast milk, gavage feeding of human milk, and identification of oral feeding readiness are all important elements of lactation support (see Chapter 19).

REFERENCES

1. Adamkin DH: Nutrition in very very low birthweight infants, *Clin Perinatol* 13:419, 1986.
2. Akintorin SM, Kamat M, Piledes RS et al: A prospective randomized trial of feeding methods in very low birth weight infants, *Pediatrics* 100:e4, 1997.
3. American Academy of Pediatrics, Committee on Nutrition: Nutrition needs of low-birthweight infants, *Pediatrics* 112:622, 1988.
4. Aynsley-Green A: Hormones and postnatal adaptation to enteral nutrition, *J Pediatr Gastroenterol Nutr* 2:418, 1983.
5. Baker JH, Berseth CL: Duodenal motor responses in preterm infants fed formula with varying concentrations and rates of infusion, *Pediatr Res* 42:618, 1997.
6. Berseth CL: Effect of early feeding on maturation of the preterm infant's small intestine, *J Pediatr* 120:947, 1992.
7. Berseth CL, Nordyke C: Enteral nutrients promote postnatal maturation of intestinal motor activity in preterm infants, *Am J Physiol* 264:G1046, 1993.
8. Bhatia P, Johnson KJ, Bell EF: Variability of abdominal circumference of premature infants, *J Pediatr Surg* 25:543, 1990.
9. Bishop JH, King FJ, Lucas A: Linear growth in the early neonatal period, *Arch Dis Child* 65:707, 1990.

10. Bragdon DB: A basis for the nursing management of feeding the premature infant, *J Obstet Gynecol Neonatal Nurs* 12(Suppl 3):51, 1983.

11. Brennan-Behan M, Carlson G, Meier P et al: Calorie loss from expressed mother's milk during continuous gavage infusion, *Neonatal Netw* 13:27, 1994.

12. Carlson SE: Very long chain fatty acids in the developing retina and brain. In Polin RA, Fox WW, eds: *Fetal and neonatal physiology,* Philadelphia, 1992, WB Saunders.

13. Castillo RO, Pittler A, Costa F: Intestinal maturation in the rat: the role of enteral nutrients, *J Parenter Enteral Nutr* 12:490, 1988.

14. Committee on Nutrition of the Preterm Infant, European Society of Paediatric Gastroenterology and Nutrition: *Nutrition and feeding of preterm infants,* Oxford, 1987, Blackwell Scientific Publications.

15. Davies PSW, Clough H, Bishop NJ et al: Total energy expenditure in small for gestational age infants, *Arch Dis Child Fetal Neonatal Educ* 74:F208, 1996.

16. De Ville K, Knapp E, Al-Tawil Y et al: Slow infusion feedings enhance duodenal motor responses and gastric emptying in pretern infants, *Am J Clin Nutr* 68:103, 1998.

17. Dewey KG, Heinig J, Nommsen-Rivers LA: Differences in morbidity between breast-fed and formula-fed infants, *J Pediatr* 126:696, 1995.

18. Dodd V, Freman R: A field study of bacterial growth in continuous feedings in a NICU, *Neonatal Netw* 9:17, 1991.

19. Duffy B, Pencharz P: The effect of feeding route (I.V. or oral) on the protein metabolism of the neonate, *Am J Clin Nutr* 43:108, 1986.

20. Dunn L, Hulman S, Weiner J et al: Beneficial effects of early hypocaloric enteral feeding on neonatal gastrointestinal function: preliminary report of a randomized trial, *J Pediatr* 112:622, 1988.

21. Embleton NE, Pang N, Cooke RJ: Postnatal malnutrition and growth retardation: an inevitable consequence of current recommendations in preterm infants? *Pediatrics* 107:270, 2001.

22. Evans JR, Allen AC, Stinson DA et al: Effect of high-dose vitamin D supplementation on radiographically detectable bone disease of very low birth weight infants, *J Pediatr* 115:779, 1989.

23. Field T, Ignatoff E, Stringer S et al: Nonnutritive sucking during tube feedings: effects on preterm neonates in an intensive care unit, *Pediatrics* 70:381, 1982.

24. Forbes GB: *Pediatric nutrition handbook,* Elk Grove Village, Ill, 1985, American Academy of Pediatrics.

25. Foucard T: Development of food allergies with special reference to cow's milk allergy, *Pediatrics* 75:177, 1985.

26. Frank AL, Taber LH, Glezen WP et al: Breast-feeding and respiratory virus infection, *Pediatrics* 70:239, 1982.

27. Gaull GE: Taurine in milk: growth modulator or conditionally essential amino acid? *J Pediatr Gastroenterol Nutr* 2(suppl 1):266, 1983.

28. Grant J, Denne SC: Effect of intermittent versus continuous enteral feeding on energy expenditure in premature infants, *J Pediatr* 118:928, 1991.

29. Groothuis J, Rosenberg A: Home oxygen promotes weight gain in infants with bronchopulmonary dysplasia, *Am J Dis Child* 141:992, 1987.

30. Hamosh M: Lipid metabolism. In Hay WW Jr, ed: *Neonatal nutrition and metabolism,* St Louis, 1991, Mosby.

31. Hill D: Effect of insulin on fetal growth, *Semin Perinatol* 2:319, 1978.

32. Holtrop PC: The frequency of hypoglycemia in full-term large and small for gestational age newborns, *Am J Perinatol* 10:150, 1993.

33. Howie PW, Forsyth JS, Ogston SA et al: Protective effect of breast feeding against infection, *Br Med J* 300:11, 1990.

34. Kashyap S, Schulze KF, Forsyth M et al: Growth, nutrient retention, and metabolic response in low birth weight infants fed varying intakes of protein and energy, *J Pediatr* 113:713, 1988.

35. Kliegman RM, Morton S: Sequential intrahepatic metabolic effects of enteric galactose alimentation in newborn rats, *Pediatr Res* 24:302, 1988.

36. LaGamma EF, Ostertag SG, Birenbaum H: Failure of delayed oral feedings to prevent necrotizing enterocolitis, *Am J Dis Child* 139:385, 1985.

37. Lemons PM, Miller K, Eitzen H et al: Bacteria in human milk during continuous feedings, *Am J Perinatol* 1:76, 1983.

38. Lin CC, Evans MI: *Intrauterine growth retardation: pathophysiology and clinical management,* New York, 1984, McGraw Book Co.

39. Lubchenco LO, Hansman C, Boyd E: Intrauterine growth in length and head circumference as estimated from live births at gestational ages from 26 to 42 weeks, *Pediatrics* 37:403, 1966.

40. Lucas A, Cole TJ: Breast milk and neonatal necrotizing enterocolitis, *Lancet* 336:1519, 1990.

41. Lucas A, Hudson G: Preterm milk as a source of protein for low birth weight infants, *Arch Dis Child* 59:831, 1984.

42. Lucas A, Bishop NJ, Cole TJ: Randomised trial of nutrition for preterm infants after discharge, *Arch Dis Child* 67:324, 1992.

43. Lucas A, Bloom SR, Aynsley-Green A: Postnatal surges in plasma gut hormones in term and preterm infants, *Biol Neonate* 41:63, 1982.

44. Lucas A, Bloom SR, Aynsley-Green A: Gut hormones and "minimal enteral feeding," *Acta Paediatr Scand* 75:719, 1986.

45. Lucas A, Gore SM, Cole TJ et al: A multicenter trial on feeding low birthweight infants: effects of diet on early growth, *Arch Dis Child* 59:722, 1984.

46. Lucas A, Morley R, Cole TJ et al: Early diet in preterm babies and developmental status in infancy, *Arch Dis Child* 64:1590, 1989.

47. Lucas A, Morley R, Cole TJ et al: Early diet in preterm babies and developmental status at 18 months, *Lancet* 335:1477, 1990.

48. Lucas A, Morley R, Cole TJ et al: Breast milk and subsequent intelligence quotient in children born preterm, *Lancet* 339:261, 1992.

49. MacLean WC, Fink BB: Lactose malabsorption by premature infants: magnitude and clinical significance, *J Pediatr* 97:383, 1980.

50. Manson WG, Weaver LT: Fat digestion in the neonate, *Arch Dis Child Fetal Neonatal Ed* 76:F206, 1997.

51. McClure RJ, Newell SJ: Randomised controlled study of clinical outcome following trophic feeding, *Arch Dis Child Fetal Neonatal Educ* 82:F29, 2000.

52. Meadow WL, Bui KC, Strates E et al: Metoclopramide promotes enteral feeding in preterm infants with feeding intolerance, *Dev Pharmacol Ther* 13:38, 1989.

53. Meetze WH, Valentine C, McGuigan JE et al: Gastrointestinal priming prior to full enteral nutrition in very low birth weight infants, *J Pediatr Gastroenterol Nutr* 15:163, 1992.

54. Meier PP, Engstrom JL, Mangurten HH et al: Breastfeeding support services in the neonatal intensivecare unit, *J Obstet Gynecol Neonatal Nurs* 22:338, 1993.

55. Milla PJ, ed: *Disorders of gastrointestinal motility in childhood,* New York, 1988, John Wiley & Sons.

56. Miller HC, Hassanein K: Diagnosis of impaired fetal growth in newborn infants, *Pediatrics* 48:511, 1971.

57. Neu J: Glutamine: role in the fetus and low-birthweight infant, *Neo Reviews,* 1:e215, 2000.

58. Neu J, Roij JC, Meetze WH et al: Enteral glutamine supplementation for very low birth weight infants decreases morbidity, *J Pediatr* 131:691, 1997.

59. Okamoto E, Muttart CR, Zucker CL et al: Use of medium-chain triglycerides in feeding the low-birthweight infant, *Am J Dis Child* 136:428, 1982.

60. Olivares M, Llaguno S, Marin V et al: Iron status in low-birth-weight infants, small and appropriate for gestational age. A follow up study, *Acta Paediatr* 81:824, 1992.

61. Ostertag SG, LaGamma EF, Reisen CE et al: Early enteral feeding does not affect the incidence of necrotizing enterocolitis, *Pediatrics* 77:275, 1986.

62. Parker P, Stroop S, Greene H: A controlled comparison of continuous versus intermittent feeding in the treatment of infants with intestinal disease, *J Pediatr* 99:360, 1981.

63. Periera GR, Ziegler E: Nutritional care of the surgical neonate, *Clin Perinatol* 16:233, 1989.

64. Phillips C, Johnson NE: The impact of quality of diet and other factors on birth weight of infants, *Am J Clin Nutr* 30:215, 1977.

65. Pohlandt F, Mathers N: Bone mineral content of appropriate and light for gestational age preterm and term infants, *Acta Paediatr Scand* 78:835, 1989.

66. Premmer DM, Georgieff MK: Nutrition for ill neonates, *Neo Reviews,* September, e56, 1999.

67. Prentice AM, Lucas A, Vasquez-Valasquez L et al: Are current dietary guidelines for young children a prescription for overfeeding? *Lancet* 2:1066, 1988.

68. Reidel BD, Greene HL: Vitamins. In Hay WW Jr, ed: *Neonatal nutrition and metabolism,* St Louis, 1991, Mosby.

69. Reis BB, Hall RT, Schanler RJ et al: Enhanced growth of preterm infants fed a new powdered human milk fortifier: a randomized, controlled trial, *Pediatrics* 106:581, 2000.

70. Schanler RJ: Use of human milk and breastfeeding in premature infants, *Clin Perinatol* 26:379, 1999.

71. Schanler RJ, Schulman RJ, Lau C, Smith EO, Heitkemper MM: Feeding strategies for premature infants: randomized trial of gastrointestinal priming and tube-feeding, *Pediatrics* 103:434, 1999.

72. Shulman RJ, Schanler RJ, Lau C et al: Early feeding, antenatal glucocorticoids, and human milk decrease intestinal permeability in preterm infants, *Pediatr Res* 44:519, 1998.

73. Shaker CS: Nipple feeding premature infants: a different perspective, *Neonatal Netw* 8:9, 1990.

74. Silvestre MA, Morbach CA, Brans YW et al: A prospective randomized trial comparing continuous versus intermittent feeding methods in very low birth weight neonates, *J Pediatr* 128:748, 1996.

75. Simpson JW, Lawless RW, Mitchell AC: Responsibility of the obstetrician to the fetus. II. Influence of pre-pregnancy weight gain on birth weight, *Obstet Gynecol* 45:481, 1975.

76. Sinclair JC: Heat production and thermoregulation in the small-for-date infant, *Pediatr Clin North Am* 17:147, 1970.

77. Slagle TA, Gross SJ: Effect of early low-volume enteral substrate on subsequent feeding tolerance in very low birth weight infants, *J Pediatr* 113:526, 1988.

78. Sparks JW, Cetin I: Intrauterine growth. In Hay WW Jr, ed: *Neonatal nutrition and metabolism,* St Louis, 1991, Mosby.

79. Sparks JW, Girard J, Battaglia FC: An estimate of the caloric requirements of the human fetus, *Biol Neonate* 38:113, 1980.

80. Steichen JJ, Krug-Wispe SK, Tsang RC: Breastfeeding the low birth weight preterm infant, *Clin Perinatol* 14:131, 1987.

81. Thureen P, Hay WW Jr: Conditions requiring special nutritional management. In Tsang RC, Lucas A, Uauy R et al, eds: *Nutritional needs of the preterm infant,* Baltimore, 1993, Williams & Wilkins.

82. Toce SS, Keenan WJ, Homan SM: Enteral feeding in very-low-birth-weight infants, *Am J Dis Child* 141:439, 1987.

83. Tsang RC, ed: *Vitamin and mineral requirements of preterm infants,* New York, 1985, Marcel Dekker.

84. Tyson JE, Wright LL, Oh W et al: Vitamin A supplementation for extremely-low-birth-weight infants, *N Engl J Med* 340:1962,1999.

85. Uauy R, Greene HL, Heird WC: Conditionally essential nutrients: cysteine, taurine, tyrosine, arginine, glutamine, choline, inositol, and nucleotides. In Tsang RC, Lucas A, Uauy R et al, eds: *Nutritional needs of the preterm infant,* Baltimore, 1993, Williams & Wilkins.

86. Unger A, Goetzman BW, Chan C et al: Nutritional practices and outcome of extremely premature infants, *Am J Dis Child* 140:1027, 1986.

87. VandenBerg KA: Nippling management of the sick neonate in the NICU: the disorganized feeder, *Neonatal Netw* 9:9, 1990.

88. Wahlig TM, Georgieff MK: The effect of illness on neonatal metabolism and nutritional management, *Clin Perinatol* 22:77, 1995.

89. Weaver LT, Lucas A: Development of gastrointestinal structure and function. In Hay WW Jr, ed: *Neonatal nutrition and metabolism,* St Louis, 1991, Mosby.

90. Widstrom AM, Marchini G, Matthiesen AS et al: Nonnutritive sucking in tube-fed preterm infants: effects on gastric motility and gastric contents of somatostatin, *J Pediatr Gastroenterol Nutr* 7:517, 1988.

17 | Total Parenteral Nutrition

Howard W. Kilbride, Mary Kay Leick-Rude, Nancy H. Allen

Total parenteral nutrition (TPN) support for critically ill newborns was first reported three decades ago.[18] Currently, LBW infants comprise the largest group of pediatric patients receiving TPN. For preterm infants, duration of TPN therapy is inversely related to birth weight, with those weighing less than 1500 g receiving, on average, about 3 weeks of TPN.[21]

In this chapter we will discuss the nutritional needs of the newborn, specific indications for TPN, and guidelines for formulation and administration of IV nutritional solutions. We also provide an overview of mechanical, infectious, and metabolic complications, with emphasis on prevention and early identification.

PHYSIOLOGY

Fuel Stores

During periods of fasting, tissue stores of energy provide the major source of fuel for the body. Carbohydrate is stored in the liver and muscle as glycogen. Stable blood sugar levels are maintained by hormonal regulation of glycogen production (glycogenesis) and break down to glucose (glycogenolysis). Newborns, particularly those who are growth retarded or preterm, have low glycogen stores and often have insufficient regulatory mechanisms.[67]

The body's greatest energy stores are in the form of fat, which provides a calorie yield of 9 kcal/g when metabolized. In addition to normal deposits of adipose tissue, newborns (and hibernating adult animals) have unique stores called *brown fat*. These stores, which are anatomically located between the scapulae, in the axillae and mediastinum, and around the adrenal glands, protect the body from hypothermia through nonshivering thermogenesis[50] (see Chapter 6).

Protein makes up lean body mass. Although protein is not used as an energy store, it may be oxidized for this purpose during periods of starvation. Extended periods of protein catabolism may lead to body dysfunction, as noted later.

The Effects of Insufficient Nutrition

The last trimester of gestation is a time of rapid fetal growth, with active transplacental transport of most nutritional substrates. Preterm delivery interrupts the nutritional supply, and abruptly results in a catabolic state, which, if prolonged, may alter growth potential. It is unclear whether it is possible or desirable to achieve in utero growth rates for the postnatal preterm infant, but reestablishment of an anabolic state and maintenance of micronutrient sufficiency are necessary.[80] During this period of neonatal life, the rapidly growing brain is responsible for much of the nutritional requirements. Slow fetal or postnatal head growth may be indicative of poor nutrition, which will have implications for long-term neurodevelopmental outcome.[26]

Additionally, postnatal malnutrition may cause immediate clinical problems. These include muscle wasting, hypotonia, loss of ventilatory drive, apnea, and difficulty weaning from the ventilator. Immune responses may be depressed with increased susceptibility to infection[78] (see Chapter 22).

Nutritional Requirements of the Neonate

Caloric

Caloric requirements for term or near-term infants are 105 to 120 kcal/kg/day. These estimates are based on enteral intake (see Chapter 16). Parenteral requirements are about 20% less, or approximately 85 to 100 kcal/kg/day. Requirements are greater for VLBW infants, whether extremely preterm or SGA, but optimal intakes have not yet been determined.[40]

Other factors affecting caloric requirements include the infant's activity level, body temperature, and degree of stress. Physical activity, which is usually infrequent in preterm infants, contributes less than 10% to the energy needs.[40] However, in pathologic states, such as with repetitive seizures or neonatal abstinence syndrome, increased activity may result in additional caloric needs. An elevation of body temperature increases caloric expenditure by approximately 12% for each degree centigrade above 37.8° C (100.2° F). Metabolic demands of surgery or severe cardiac or pulmonary distress may increase caloric requirements by 30% and chronic failure to thrive by 50% to 100%. In addition, postnatal dexamethasone therapy may slow weight and linear growth rates[10] and potentially affect brain growth.[59]

Water

Water requirements vary with gestational and postnatal age (postconceptual age) and environmental conditions (e.g., care in an incubator versus radiant heat warmer, use of phototherapy) (see Chapter 14).

Mineral

Sodium requirements are minimal for the first days of life. After 1 week, the average requirement is 3 to 4 mEq/kg/day. Large renal losses (more than 5 mEq/kg/day) may occur in very immature infants (less than 28 weeks' gestation) in the first weeks of life.

Potassium and chloride requirements are approximately 2 mEq/kg/day and 3 to 4 mEq/kg/day, respectively. Glucosuria with resulting osmotic diuresis may increase sodium and potassium urinary losses.

Calcium is an important cofactor in hemostasis, enzyme function, and cell membrane stability. In the newborn, 98% of calcium is stored in the bone. The initial calcium requirement is 1 mEq/kg/day to maintain calcium homeostasis and to avoid irritability and tetany associated with low serum ionized calcium levels. In utero, the accretion rate is 4 to 5 mEq/kg/day, which the growing preterm infant should receive in addition to adequate phosphorus and vitamin D to avoid osteopenia, rickets, and bone fractures.[30] Excess calcium intake may cause CNS depression or signs of renal toxicity.

The phosphorus requirement for the growing preterm infant is 40 to 60 mg/kg/day (31 mg = 1 mmol). Bone contains 80% of the body's phosphorus. Low phosphorus intake will cause increased renal calcium excretion and a depletion of bone calcium phosphate. Low phosphorus intake or chronic furosemide diuretic therapy may also lead to hypercalciuria and nephrolithiasis.[15] Because phosphorus is a major constituent of cellular energy function (adenosine triphosphate, 2,3-disphosphoglycerate, creatinine phosphate), severe depletion may result in muscle paralysis, respiratory failure, and interruption of important cellular functions, such as the hemoglobin-oxygen dissociation curve and leukocyte activity.

Magnesium is essential for intracellular enzyme systems. The requirement is 0.25 to 0.5 mEq/kg/day.[36] Magnesium deficiency states mimic hypocalcemia, manifesting as irritability, tremulousness, tetany, and cardiac dysrhythmias. Magnesium excess may present as lethargy, hypotonia, and delayed stooling.

Carbohydrate

During fetal life, glucose is the primary source of energy.[71] At birth the preterm infant has only a small supply of glycogen, the storage form of glucose (equivalent to about 200 kcal of energy). Glucose is particularly important for the CNS, because other substrates are not available. Initially a glucose infusion rate (GIR) of 6 mg/kg/min is sufficient to meet metabolic needs of the newborn infant. Requirements are greater for infants who are stressed (e.g., from sepsis or hypothermia) or hyperinsulinemic (e.g., IDMs or infants with Beckwith-Wiedemann syndrome). **With long-term parenteral nutrition, at least 50% of caloric requirement should be provided as carbohydrate (GIR 8 to 10 mg/kg/min), generally as dextrose (calculated as 3.4 kcal/kg of hydrated carbohydrate). To avoid metabolic consequences of excessive glucose loads, one should avoid a GIR of more than 12 mg/kg/min (18 g/kg/day of glucose).**

Protein

The quantity of daily nitrogen required by a term newborn infant, based on estimates from breast milk intake, is approximately 325 mg/kg/day (approximately 2 g/kg/day of protein).[21] Requirements for preterm infants are much higher, as indicated by in utero accretion rates during the latter half of pregnancy. At 28 weeks' gestation the fetus requires 350 mg/kg/day of nitrogen. This figure declines to 150 mg/kg/day by term gestation. **When the estimated accretion rate is added to the obligatory postnatal nitrogen excretion, the requirement for a 28-week gestation preterm may be calculated to be approximately 495 mg/kg/day (3.1 g/kg/day of protein). If one assumes parenterally administered amino acids are converted to body proteins at 75% efficiency, the estimated parenteral amino acid requirement would be as high as 3.7 g/kg/day.[31]**

In fetal life protein is actively transported from mother's circulation across the placenta in quantities greater than needed for accretion, with the excess being oxidized for energy.[70] Clinicians have found that increasing protein intake postnatally at all energy intake levels above 40 kcal/kg/day results in increased protein accretion. Further investigations are needed to determine appropriate markers of protein toxicity and safe upper limits for maximum protein administration. **In the absence of more data, clinicians are concerned about providing protein intake in excess of 4 g/kg/day because of risk of toxicity including azotemia, acidosis, and hyperaminoacidemia.**[3]

Recent studies have shown that administration of amino acids shortly after birth will decrease protein catabolism, which may be extremely important for VLBW infants.[57,71,75,76] Balance studies indicate that a minimum of 1 to 1.5 g/kg/day of protein is needed to achieve protein synthesis. Investigations have suggested that this level or higher levels (up to 3 g/kg/day) may be given even to ill preterm infants in the first 3 days of life without apparent negative metabolic side effects.[71,75] Further studies are needed to determine whether early protein supplementation will have an impact on long-term growth and development.

The quality of the amino acid mixture infused is important for efficacy and safety.[1] **Although there is no formulation specifically for preterm infants, pediatric solutions provide greater quantities of essential amino acids and result in plasma amino acid levels similar to that of postprandial breast-fed infants.**[32] An essential amino acid is one that cannot be synthesized in adequate quantity to meet the requirements for normal growth and development. The differentiation between essential and nonessential amino acids is not clear in newborn infants, because the ability to synthesize some amino acids may vary with clinical situation or stage of maturity. Lysine and threonine are essential in their entirety. The requirement for other amino acids may be met by providing ketoanalogues, which may accept a nitrogen group during transamination. There is a high requirement for branched amino acids (leucine, isoleucine, and valine) in the growing newborn. These are primarily metabolized in skeletal muscle.

Methionine is an essential sulfur-containing amino acid that is metabolized to cysteine and taurine. **For preterm infants of less than 32 weeks' gestation, cystathionase activity is insufficient for cysteine synthesis.**[77] **Some investigators have found cysteine supplementation results in greater nitrogen retention.**[57] **For now, at least high-risk infants should receive cysteine-supplemented parenteral amino acid infusions.** Taurine is a nonprotein amino sulfonic acid that is converted from cysteine by cysteine sulfonic acid decarboxylase. Taurine concentrations are low in infants who have received nonsupplemented TPN infusions. Taurine deficiency may have a detrimental effect on the developing nervous system. One study suggests taurine may prevent cholestasis in newborns by more effectively conjugating bile salts and creating soluble end-products.[33] Tyrosine is another amino acid which appears to be essential in the newborn period. It is present in small amounts in most amino acid solutions, although one manufacturer uses a soluble form, N-acetyl-L-tyrosine, which infants slowly metabolize to tyrosine.[32] Tyrosine is a byproduct of phenylalanine metabolism, so supplementation will have an effect on the phenylalanine requirement. Histidine is considered to be an essential amino acid for newborns, with the lowest levels evident in preterm infants. Arginine may be essential only for the newborn with reduced arginine synthetase activity. This amino acid is thought to facilitate clearance of nitrogenous waste products by "priming the urea cycle." Use of amino acid infusates with deficient arginine has been associated with hyperammonemia.[28] Glutamine has also been considered a conditionally essential amino acid. It is not currently available in any amino acid solution. Glutamine serves as a fuel for intestinal epithelial cells and lymphocytes. Preliminary evidence suggests supplementation may decrease morbidity in VLBW infants, and a large controlled study is underway.[51]

Nonessential amino acids make up the largest percentage of the amino acid pool in the fetal body. The desired quantities of these amino acids for parenteral solution are not known. It is thought they should be provided in a balanced formulation. Pediatric solutions differ from adult solutions by providing glutamic acid and aspartic acid with lower glycine concentrations.

Fat

Long-chain fatty acids are essential in the newborn for brain development and appear to be important for gene expression and other molecular mechanisms.[74] Essential fatty acids (EFA) include linoleic and linolenic, and in the newborn, arachidonic acid.[3] Biochemical evidence of EFA deficiency may be seen in less than a week in VLBW infants receiving a deficient diet, and the administration of parenteral glucose and amino acids may accelerate these abnormalities.[20] EFA deficiency results in an imbalance in fatty acid production with an overproduction of nonessential fatty acids. **Clinical manifestations appearing at variable times after biochemical** changes of EFA deficiency include scaly dermatitis, poor hair growth, thrombocytopenia, failure to thrive, poor wound healing, and increased susceptibility to bacterial infection. Clinical manifestations of EFA deficiency can be avoided if 3% to 4% of caloric intake is supplied as linoleic acid (approximately 0.5 g/kg/day of intravenous lipid).[20]

In addition to preventing EFA deficiency, lipid emulsion is a concentrated source of nonprotein calories, which promotes nitrogen retention. Preterm infants appear to have limited capability to oxidize fatty acids. This limitation may be related to deficiency of carnitine, which, in the form of acylcarnitine, promotes transfer of fatty acids into mitochondria, where oxidative metabolism occurs.[11] Some authors recommend carnitine supplementation of 8 to 10 mg/kg/day for preterm infants receiving long-term TPN, although there is no documentation of physiologic benefit.[55]

Vitamins

The biologic role of vitamins, signs and symptoms of deficiency states, and recommended oral requirements are available in Chapter 16. The American Society for Clinical Nutrition (ASCN) has suggested that preterm infants receive 40% to 65% of the daily recommended vitamin doses for term infants and children.[24] These guidelines may result in excessive intakes of some water-soluble vitamins, particularly pyridoxine and riboflavin. Although preterm infants have limited stores of lipid-soluble vitamins because of low body fat, potential toxicity from excess administration is a concern. Vitamin A is a lipid-soluble vitamin important for tissue growth, protein synthesis, and epithelial differentiation. Vitamin A may be more effectively administered in lipid emulsion rather than dextrose amino acid solutions.[3,13] Additional supplementation will result in increased serum retinol levels and has been associated with a decreased incidence of BPD in some studies.[64] However, vitamin A supplementation has only been proven to be effective in lowering chronic lung disease rates when given by intramuscular injections three times per week.[73]

Vitamin E is a lipid-soluble, biologic antioxidant that is deficient in preterm infants. However, daily parenteral intake of 2 to 3 mg/kg has been associated with serum levels generally in the recommended range of 1 to 2 mg/dl. Pharmacologic doses have been tried unsuccessfully for prevention of BPD and ROP. Recent experience suggests that vitamin E sup-

plementation to achieve serum levels as high as 4 to 5 mg/dl may be used in combination with cryotherapy to decrease the sequelae of ROP.[34] Vitamin K production by intestinal flora is impaired by insufficient enteral feedings and use of broad-spectrum antibiotics in infants on long-term TPN. Vitamin K is provided at the recommended dosage through parenteral pediatric multivitamin solutions.[25]

Trace Minerals

Although trace minerals are relatively scarce (less than 0.01% of the weight of the human body by definition), they play an important role in normal growth and development. Deficiencies of both zinc and copper have been identified in infants on long-term TPN not supplemented with trace minerals. Manifestations of deficiency and recommendations for intake are provided in Chapter 16. Parenteral recommendations are lower than oral based on physiologic requirements. For infants not receiving frequent blood transfusions, iron therapy may be necessary by 2 months of age. Infants receiving erythropoietin therapy need additional iron supplementation, given either enterally or parenterally.[47]

INDICATIONS

Clinical indications for parenteral nutrition include any situation in which there will be a delay in establishing adequate enteral nutrition. For extremely low birth weight (ELBW) infants, use of modified parenteral nutrition even in the first days of life may be considered to prevent catabolism.[71] **When parenteral nutrition is administered through a peripheral vein, caloric intake is limited by the concentration of carbohydrate (usually less than 12.5% dextrose) and amino acids (less than or equal to 2%) or required fluid volume. Using lipid emulsions, a caloric intake of 70 to 80 kcal/kg/day and a protein intake of 2.5 g/kg/day may be realized.** This intake will prevent catabolism and, in some cases, result in moderate growth. Peripheral parenteral nutrition (PPN) is usually adequate for term newborns with transient bowel disease (such as may be seen after the repair of a small omphalocele) or for preterm infants whose enteral feedings are delayed for 1 week. PPN is also commonly used to supplement nutrition in newborns who are receiving partial enteral feedings. When caloric needs can be met by PPN, this route is preferred to the central route, because the catheter insertion risks are avoided and generally the risk of infection is less. If parenteral nutritional duration is greater than 1 week, administration of TPN through a central line is recommended. The placement of a central line for parenteral nutrition allows a higher carbohydrate load to be used, giving more calories with less fluid. In preterm infants at risk for a patent ductus arteriosus and pulmonary edema, diminishing fluid intake and improving nutritional status may be important aspects of management. **Specific indications for TPN by a central catheter include the following:**

- **ELBW infants (less than 1000 g BW) and others who do not tolerate oral feedings after a week of age or who cannot receive adequate caloric intake by PPN**
- **Infants who have had gastrointestinal surgery and will have a significant delay in enteral nutrition, such as an infant with a gastroschisis, bowel resection after NEC, or meconium peritonitis**
- **Infants with chronic gastrointestinal dysfunction, such as intractable diarrhea**

DATA COLLECTION

Monitoring Growth

Weight loss or insufficient weight gain is the initial effect of inadequate caloric intake. Linear growth, although less affected, will be diminished after long periods of poor nutrition. Because of "brain-sparing," head circumference growth is the least affected.

Fetal weight gain in utero at each week of gestation is currently used as the standard to assess adequacy of postnatal growth. In the midtrimester (24 to 27 weeks' gestation) expected weight gain is 1.5% of body weight.[71] Growth curves are available to allow comparison of postnatal weight gain with expected weight acquisition.[79]

Adequacy of nutrition may be better assessed by evidence of fat and muscle acquisition in the neonate. Triceps skinfold thickness may be used to estimate fat accretion, and the midarm circumference measurement to approximate muscle acquisition.[22] The need for these measurements should be weighed against the importance of protecting the fragile skin of the preterm infant.

Minimum monitoring of growth should consist of the following:

- **Weight measured daily, or more frequently in ELBW infants with rapidly changing extracellular fluid states. Maintenance of a warm environment with minimal handling**

of ELBW infants can be achieved through the use of in-bed scales. Strict attention to consistency of technique during the weighing process is essential to obtain accurate, reliable measurements.[72]
- **Length measured weekly.**
- **Head circumference measured weekly.**

Measurements should be obtained in a standardized fashion and recorded weekly, using the same equipment each time and the appropriate growth curve for premature infants.

Biochemical Monitoring

In addition to anthropometric measurements, biochemical parameters may be monitored to assess nutritional adequacy. Periodic assessment of calcium, phosphorus, and alkaline phosphatase levels is important to detect metabolic disturbances associated with osteopenia.[36] Tests for protein malnutrition include serum total protein, albumin, transferrin, retinol-binding protein, and transthyretin (prealbumin), the latter two suggested primarily for preterm infants.[21] Routine clinical use of these measurements awaits greater definition of normal variation and independent effects of systemic illness and medications.

Biochemical monitoring of the infant's physiologic status is necessary to avoid complications of TPN. Usefulness of the laboratory data should be balanced with the economic costs and risks from iatrogenic blood losses for the infant (Table 17-1).

Table 17-1	METABOLIC MONITORING FOR INFANTS RECEIVING PARENTERAL NUTRITION	
	FREQUENCY	
VARIABLE	**ACUTE PHASE**	**STABLE**
Electrolytes (Na$^+$, K$^+$, Cl, CO$_2$), BUN	Daily	2 ×/wk
Calcium, phosphorus	Weekly	Biweekly
Alkaline phosphatase	—	Biweekly
Serum glucose screen	q 8 hr	Daily
Urine glucose	q 8 hr	Daily
Hemoglobin/hematocrit	Daily	Weekly
Liver function		
Bilirubin	2 ×/wk	prn
Transaminases	Weekly	Biweekly
Triglyceride*	—	Weekly

*When on lipid emulsion.

TREATMENT

Vascular Access
UACs and UVCs

Umbilical artery catheters (UAC) and umbilical vein catheters (UVC) are commonly placed in sick newborns to provide vascular access for intravenous fluids, blood samplings, and blood pressure monitoring. Because of the risks of thromboembolic and infection complications, these lines are generally removed by one week of age.[23]

Peripheral and Midline Catheters

If continued venous access is required after this time, a peripheral, midline, or peripherally inserted central catheter (PICC) can be placed. The type of line used is determined by the anticipated length of time needed and the osmolarity of the substances to be infused. Peripheral IVs are indicated for short-term IV access. A midline catheter, which is threaded to the proximal portion of an extremity or neck, can provide longer intravenous access than a peripheral IV when prolonged peripheral strength TPN is indicated.[41,69] Midline catheters appear to be associated with lower rates of phlebitis than short peripheral catheters and lower rates of infection and cost than central lines.[41,46,69] Midline catheters can only be used to administer fluids appropriate for peripheral infusion therapy.

PICCs

Percutaneous placement of a 20- to 24-gauge (1.9 to 2.6 Fr) Silastic (silicone) or polyurethane catheter can be routinely performed in even the smallest of neonatal patients by trained nurses and physicians.[39,60] The catheter is usually placed in the antecubital or axillary veins in the arms; however, leg, scalp, or external jugular veins may be used to achieve central access. Veins that may be needed for percutaneous central line placement should not be sites for routine venipuncture (see Chapter 7).

Percutaneous line placement involves stabilization of the vein, maximal barrier precautions (sterile gloves, gown, large drape, masks) and antiseptic preparation of the skin with 2% chlorhexidine or povidone-iodine and alcohol product.[43,60] Fully equipped prepackaged kits are available for this procedure from a number of manufacturers. Most kits include an 18- or 19-gauge insertion needle. Use this needle to puncture and tunnel through the subcutaneous tissue

before entering the vein. Once the needle is within the vein, pass the catheter, which has been flushed with heparinized saline solution, through the needle into the vein and advance it a premeasured distance to the approximate location of the superior vena cava. (If the basilic vein is used, turn the infant's head to face the insertion site to minimize the risk of the catheter entering neck vessels.) The catheter tip position should be documented radiographically. Remove the needle carefully from the skin and discard it. A Steri-strip should be placed over the catheter insertion site to maintain its position before the dressing is completed. Heparinized flush solution should be periodically instilled to maintain patency.

The length of tubing outside the infant's body should be measured and recorded. Excess may be carefully curled at the site of insertion and covered with a sterile, transparent dressing. If an arm board was used for stabilization, it may be removed. Arm restraints should not be necessary.

Broviac Catheter

Large-bore Silastic catheters (Broviac) are placed surgically in infants in whom the percutaneous method is not technically possible and long-term access is anticipated. Generally the catheters are placed in the internal or external jugular veins or common facial vein by cutdown and threaded to a central venous site. The distal end is tunneled subcutaneously and exited through the anterior chest wall. The catheter must be secured and dressed sterilely.[66]

Other Vascular Access Options

Other sites that may be used for TPN infusion on a short-term basis, include subclavian, jugular, or femoral veins. Some centers use a UVC for short-term parenteral nutrition when another site is not feasible.

Composition of Infusate
Carbohydrate

The prime source of calories for the neonate is usually dextrose. Peripherally, 10% to 12% solution is used. When central access is obtained, a 15% to 30% dextrose concentration may be used. The glucose load will be increased if either the infusion rate or glucose concentration of the infusate is increased. Too rapid an increase in glucose load may exceed an infant's carbohydrate tolerance and result in hyperglycemia. A rapid decrease in the infusion rate or the glucose concentration of the infusate may result in hypoglycemia.

When calculating caloric intake, use the following:

$$1 \text{ g dextrose} = 3.4 \text{ kcal}$$

or

$$100 \text{ ml/kg of } D_{10}W = 34 \text{ kcal/kg}$$

or

$$100 \text{ ml/kg of } D_{30}W = 102 \text{ kcal/kg}$$

The glucose infusion rate (GIR) can be calculated:

$$\text{GIR (mg/kg/min)} = \frac{\text{g glucose/day} \times 1000}{1440 \text{ (min/day)}} \times \text{weight (kg)}$$

Generally, a newborn of 28 weeks' gestation or more (more than 1000 g BW) will initially tolerate a GIR of about 6 mg/kg/min. Daily increases in dextrose concentration or fluid volume to increase carbohydrate administration by 1.5 to 2.0 mg/kg/min usually are tolerated. ELBW infants may be carbohydrate intolerant, and initial GIR should be lower (4 or 5 mg/kg/min) for these infants.

Blood sugar determinations and screening for glucosuria should be performed several times each day when glucose delivery is initiated or altered.

Lipids

Lipid emulsion at a rate of 0.5 to 1 g/day/100 kcal is sufficient to prevent EFA deficiency; however, additional lipids may be provided to supplement nonprotein caloric intake and support growth. Lipids should never make up more than 50% of total caloric intake. Fat emulsions should be given cautiously, beginning with 0.5 g/kg/day and advanced 0.5 g/kg every 1 to 2 days as tolerated to 3 g/kg/day maximum.[56] Lipids should be infused over a 24-hour period, because this usually results in a well-tolerated infusion rate.[54] There appears to be no advantage to a rest period to allow for lipid clearance.[3] Fat emulsions are available as either 10% or 20% concentrations. The 20% concentration is beneficial for VLBW infants, because its lower phospholipid concentration results in lower plasma levels of triglyceride and cholesterol[29] (Table 17-2).

Emulsified fat particles are similar in size and metabolic rate to naturally occurring chylomicrons. Most are cleared through passage in the adipose and

Table 17-2	COMPOSITION OF FAT EMULSIONS	
COMPOSITION	INTRALIPID (CLINITEC) 20%	LIPOSYN II (ABBOTT) 20%
Fatty Acid Distribution (%)		
Linoleic acid	50	65.8
Oleic acid	26	17.7
Palmitic acid	10	8.8
Linolenic acid	9	4.2
Stearic acid	3.5	3.4
Components (%)		
Soybean oil	20	10
Safflower oil	—	10
Egg phospholipid	1.2	1.2
Glycerin	2.25	2.5
Caloric contents (kcal/dl)	200	200
Osmolarity (mOsm/L)	268	258

muscle tissue. The capillary endothelial lipoprotein lipase hydrolyzes triglycerides and phospholipids, generating free fatty acids (FFAs), glycerol, and other glycerides. Most of the FFAs diffuse into the adipose tissue for reesterification and storage. A small portion circulates to be used by other tissues for fuel or for conversion by the liver into very low-density lipoprotein. **Extremely immature and SGA infants with decreased adipose tissue have delayed clearance of fat emulsion. Rates of administration should be slowest in these infants.** The rate-limiting step for lipid clearance is the metabolism by lipoprotein lipase. The use of heparin stimulates the release of this enzyme and may enhance clearance of IV lipids. The use of 0.5 to 1.0 U of heparin per milliliter of TPN is common in many nurseries to increase duration of catheter patency.[2,66] Carbohydrate must also be administered with fat to provide the necessary substrates for fatty acid oxidation and to promote FFA clearance.[12]

Amino Acid Solution

The compositions of two crystalline amino acid solutions available for neonatal parenteral use are presented in Table 17-3. The maximum concentration of the amino acid solution is generally 2% for peripheral use and 3% for central use. Each solution supplies an excess of nonessential amino acids, although more recently available solutions have sought to balance the nonessential amino acid profile.

Table 17-3	**CONCENTRATIONS (MG/DL) OF AMINO ACIDS ADJUSTED TO 3% SOLUTION**	
	SOLUTIONS	
AMINO ACID	**AMINOSYN-PF (ABBOTT)**	**TROPHAMINE (KENDALL MCGAW)**
Essential		
L-Leucine	356	420
L-Phenylalanine	129	144
L-Methionine	54	102
L-Lysine	204	246
L-Isoleucine	228	246
L-Valine	194	234
L-Histidine	94	144
L-Threonine	154	126
L-Tryptophan	54	60
Nonessential		
L-Alanine	210	162
L-Arginine	369	360
L-Proline	244	204
L-Tyrosine	19	69
L-Cysteine	*	<10*
L-Serine	149	114
L-Glycine	116	108
L-Glutamine	—	—
L-Taurine	21	7.5

*Cysteine hydrochloride supplement may be added.

Cysteine, which is an essential amino acid in preterm infants, is not stable for long periods in solution. This amino acid is commercially available to be added immediately before the solution is administered. Trophamine and Aminosyn-PF include taurine, which is not available in other solutions.

A minimum quantity of energy substrates must be provided for effective utilization of parenteral protein. For ELBW infants, approximately 40 kcal/kg/day of carbohydrates or fat and 1 g protein/kg/day are required for resting metabolic needs to prevent catabolism (breakdown of endogenous substrates). For each gram of protein above the basal amount used for growth, approximately 10 kcal of energy is needed.[71] Thus a minimum of 50 kcal/kg of energy is needed for an infant receiving 2 g/kg/day of protein.

Electrolytes

Sodium is given in an estimated maintenance quantity (3 to 4 mEq/kg/day) as long as the serum sodium is 135 to 140 mEq/L and there are no excessive losses. Potassium is given in main- tenance amounts (2 to 3 mEq/kg/day) unless there are excessive losses or renal dysfunction. Potassium needs may increase with anabolism. Sodium and potassium requirements may be further evaluated by monitoring urinary electrolyte levels (i.e., if body sodium is depleted, low urine concentration would be expected).

Sodium and potassium may be supplied with chloride, acetate, or phosphate anions. The daily chloride requirement is approximately 3 mEq/ kg/day and should be balanced with acetate to avoid alkalosis or acidosis (acetate is converted to bicarbonate). Amino acid preparations also supply anions that must be recognized to calculate a balanced anion solution. For example, Trophamine supplies 1 mEq of acetate per gram of protein. On the other hand, cysteine addition to the TPN solution will reduce the pH, necessitating additional acetate supplementation.[38]

Minerals

Phosphorus may be provided as sodium or potassium phosphate. Calcium may be provided as 10% calcium gluconate (9.7 mg of elemental calcium/100 mg of salt). When one is preparing a solution with both calcium and phosphate, care must be taken to avoid calcium phosphate precipitation. Magnesium is supplied as magnesium sulfate.

When one is using a potassium phosphate solution at pH 7.4, 4.4 mEq of potassium supplies 93 mg of elemental phosphorus. When a solution of sodium phosphate is used at pH 7.4, 4.0 mEq of sodium is given with each 93 mg of elemental phosphorus.

Calcium

- **Because of increased risk of precipitation, calcium chloride should not be used.**
- **An elevation in ambient temperature, increased storage time, rise in pH, and decrease in protein or glucose concentration may increase the likelihood of precipitation. The addition of cysteine, which lowers solution pH, may enhance calcium and phosphate solubility.[2]**
- When one is preparing the solution, calcium and phosphate salts should be added separately, but not in sequence, during the last stages of solution mixing. The solubility of the added calcium should be calculated from the volume at the time the calcium is added, not the final volume.[49]
- The use of a physiologic ratio of calcium to phosphorus (1.8:1) in the TPN solution allows for increased concentration of these minerals.[53]

Vitamins

A preparation approximating the AMA's recommended formulation of IV vitamins is available (MVI-Peds). The daily recommended dose is 1 vial for infants greater than 3 kg, 65% vial for infants 1 to 3 kg, and 30% vial for infants less than 1 kg.[3]

Trace Elements

Commercially available amino acid solutions contain trace elements as contaminants, but variability even within the same brand means they cannot be relied on to meet trace element requirements.

Generally, zinc is supplied as zinc sulfate. Serum zinc levels usually approximate the maternal levels at birth and decline over the first week of life. By the second week of life, neonates not receiving dietary zinc should have supplementation. It may be necessary to initiate zinc intake earlier in neonates with intestinal loss, such as after gastrointestinal surgery.

Copper is supplied as cupric sulfate. Approximately two thirds of stored copper is accumulated during the last trimester. Therefore a preterm infant may need early supplementation but a term infant will have adequate hepatic stores for at least several weeks. Because copper is excreted through the biliary system, this mineral should be removed from parenteral fluids for infants with cholestasis.[81]

Manganese, chromium, and selenium salts should be provided for long-term parenteral nutrition. Manganese supplementation should not be provided to infants with cholestasis. The chromium dose may be reduced or discontinued in an infant with impaired renal function.

Small traces of aluminum are incorporated into parenteral solutions during processing with no known physiologic role.[35] Aluminum toxicity has been associated with bone disease, encephalopathy, anemia, and hepatic cholestasis. Renal elimination of aluminum is incomplete in newborn infants. Levels should be monitored in infants receiving long-term TPN, especially those with renal failure.

Table 17-4 outlines a suggested composition for a TPN solution (guideline only).

CASE STUDY

The following case example illustrates the preceding points regarding writing orders for TPN.

Table 17-4 SUGGESTED COMPOSITION FOR INTRAVENOUS NUTRITION REGIMEN

COMPONENT	DAILY AMOUNT
Calories	
Dextrose 3.4 kcal/g	10-15 g/kg
Lipids 2.0 kcal/ml (20%) solution	1-3 g/kg
Nitrogen	0.48-0.64 g
Protein (6.25 g protein = 1 g N$_2$)	3-4 g/kg
Electrolytes	
Sodium	3 mEq/kg
Potassium	2-3 mEq/kg
Chloride	3-4 mEq/kg
Acetate	3 mEq/kg
Phosphate	2 mM/kg
Calcium	3 mEq/kg
Magnesium	0.3 mEq (20 mg)/kg
Vitamins	
MVI = Ped	1 vial*
Vitamin A	700 µg
Thiamine (B$_1$)	1.2 mg
Riboflavin (B$_2$)	1.4 mg
Niacin	17 mg
Pyridoxine (B$_6$)	1 mg
Ascorbic acid (C)	80 mg
Ergocalciferol (D)	400 IU
Vitamin E	7 IU
Pantothenic acid	5 mg
Cyanocobalamin	1 µg
Folate	140 µg
Vitamin K	200 µg
Trace Elements	
Zinc (zinc sulfate)†	400 µg/kg
Copper (cupric sulfate)†	20 µg/kg
Manganese sulfate†	1 µg/kg
Chromium chloride†	0.2 µg/kg
Selenium	2 µg/kg
Molybdenum	0.25 µg/kg
Iodide	1 µg/kg

*MVI Pediatric (Astra Pharmaceuticals), reduced amount provided for VLBW infants (see text).
†As Multitrace-4 Neonatal (American Regent Laboratories, Inc.).

History

A male infant born at 29 weeks' gestation at 1300 g is now 14 days old and unable to be fed because he has undergone bowel resection after NEC. Because there will be a prolonged delay in enteral alimentation, a central vein catheter is placed for TPN. He is currently receiving $D_{10}W$ at 120 ml/kg with maintenance electrolytes. His current weight is 1100 g. Serum electrolytes and blood glucose are normal. The approach to calculating TPN requirements is as follows:

Caloric Requirement

Because the patient has already had a significant postpartum period without adequate nutrition, achieving caloric intake necessary for growth is a very important part of his care. The infant will probably require 100 kcal/kg or more for tissue repair and growth. We will begin with 60 kcal/kg (the birth weight is used until weight gain established) and advance the intake daily to reach this level.

Carbohydrate

Initially a dextrose load just above what has been previously tolerated should be used. Thus the patient should receive $D_{12.5}W$ at perhaps 130 ml/kg/day, depending on the infant's fluid requirements. Overhydration, with risks of cardiovascular and pulmonary complications, should be avoided.

This represents

12.5 g glucose/dl $\times$ 130 ml/kg =
$$16.2 \text{ g glucose/kg}$$
16.2 g glucose/kg $\times$ 3.4 kcal/g glucose =
$$55.1 \text{ kcal/kg}$$

Fat

Lipid emulsion should be added to increase the caloric intake, starting with 0.5 g/kg/day.

2.5 ml/kg 20% lipid emulsion (0.5 g) $\times$
$$2 \text{ kcal/ml} = 5 \text{ kcal/kg/day}$$

Thus the total nonnitrogen calories on the first day of TPN will be 60 (55 + 5).

Protein

Calculate the quantity of protein by using the ratio 150 kcal/1 g nitrogen; 0.4 g of nitrogen/kg may be given with 60 calories: (60/150 $\times$ 1 g). This quantity of nitrogen represents 2.5 g protein/kg (0.4 g/nitrogen $\times$ 6.25 g protein/g nitrogen).

Electrolytes

The patient should receive maintenance sodium ion (2 to 3 mEq/kg) and potassium ion (2 to

3 mEq/kg) unless there are excessive renal or gastrointestinal losses.

Anions

Balancing anions is the next consideration. The 2.5 g/kg of amino acids, if given as Trophamine, will add approximately 2.5 mEq/kg of acetate to the solution (1 mEq acetate/1 g amino acids). If 2.5 mEq/kg of sodium is provided as sodium chloride, the solution will have balanced anions. Giving 2.5 mEq/kg of potassium as potassium phosphate will provide approximately 53 mg/kg of elemental phosphorus:

$$(2.5 \text{ mEq K}^+/\text{kg}) \times \frac{93 \text{ mg (P)}}{4.4 \text{ mEq K}^+}$$

Minerals, Vitamins, and Trace Elements

Calcium, magnesium, vitamins, and trace elements should be ordered at this point. Calcium initially should be started at 2 to 3 mEq/kg/day, but may be increased as tolerated with growth to 4 to 5 mEq/kg/day.

TPN Orders

Thus the TPN orders would be written for this patient as follows:

$D_{12.5}W$ With the Following per Liter to Run 7 ml/hr (130 ml/kg/day)	Quantity per Kilogram
1.9 g % amino acids	2.5 g AA
19.2 mEq sodium as sodium chloride	2.5 mEq Na$^+$
19.2 mEq potassium as potassium phosphate	2.5 mEq K$^+$
13.2 mM phosphate as potassium phosphate	1.7 mM Phos
23.1 mEq calcium	3 mEq Ca$^+$
2.3 mEq magnesium	0.3 mEq
19.2 ml MVI-Ped	3.25 ml/day
2.3 mg Zinc*	0.3 mg Zn
150 μg copper*	20 μg Cu
38 μg manganese*	5 μg Mn
1.3 μg chromium*	0.17 μg Cr
15 μg selenium	2 μg Se

*Commercially available in trace element solution (Multitrace −4 Neonatal, 0.2 ml/kg/day).

Progression

On subsequent days the dextrose concentration and lipids would be advanced slowly to increase the caloric intake to requirement as tolerated. The quantity of protein would also be increased to about 3.5 g/kg/day.

Preparing the Solution

Solutions should be prepared in the hospital pharmacy under a laminar flow hood in a work area isolated from traffic and contaminated supplies. There should be quality control checks to monitor for sterility breaks in equipment, personnel, environment, and solutions.

Because many additives potentially can be insoluble in combination, a mixing sequence should be established that separates the most incompatible ingredients. Storage increases the risk of microbial contamination; therefore, TPN solutions should be prepared on the day they are needed.[45]

Administering the TPN Solution

Proper administration of the TPN solution is as important as its preparation in preventing complications. The label on the solution should always be checked for correct patient identification and current formulation order.

Standardized procedures must be established to avoid infectious complications from solution contamination. Solutions on the nursing units may be returned to the pharmacy for additives before hanging, but no additives should be placed in the solution once it is hanging. The bag or bottle of TPN solution should be changed every 24 hours, and the tubing administration sets should be changed at least every 72 hours. Lipid emulsions and tubing should be changed every 24 hours.[44,52]

Changes in TPN infusion rates result in changes in glucose delivery to the newborn and may lead to hypoglycemia or hyperglycemia if the glucose homeostatic mechanisms do not adjust fast enough. Reactive hypoglycemia may occur if the glucose load is abruptly discontinued.[7] Parenteral nutrition solutions must infuse at a constant rate via an infusion pump. Attempts to rush or slow down solutions should not occur. If the parenteral nutrition infusion is suddenly discontinued because of a clotted catheter or accidental removal, an appropriate solution with dextrose should be infused via a peripheral vein, and blood glucose should be monitored.

Use of parenteral nutrition may increase an infant's risk of hyperglycemia during surgery. Because rapid fluid infusions may be necessary during operative procedures, the TPN solution should be discontinued and replaced with a physiologic infusate during the perioperative period. After surgery TPN should be resumed when the patient is euglycemic.

Tapering of the TPN solution occurs as the infant begins to tolerate enteral feedings. When the patient is taking approximately two thirds of the required calories enterally, the central line may be removed. The length of the indwelling portion of the percutaneous catheter should be measured and compared with that stated in the original procedure note, and the appearance of the tip should be observed. Careful attention to this detail will alert the clinician to the unlikely occurrence of catheter fragmentation, in which a portion is left in the tissue or vessel.

Administering Fat Solution

Rapid infusion of the fat emulsion may exceed its clearance rate from the body and accentuate complications; therefore, fat emulsions should not be infused faster than 0.15 g/kg/hr.[3,56] Lipids generally are given through a Y-site connection to bypass the filter in the TPN line. However, some hospitals use a combined dextrose, amino acid, and lipid solution known as "three-in-one" or total nutrient admixture (TNA).[16,58] A 1.2-micron filter is used with this solution to remove certain drug precipitates (Ca/PO_4), air, and *Candida,* but it is not effective in removing bacteria. The decision to use TNA should be approached with caution in infants. Lipid emulsions increase the pH of the TPN solution, limiting the amount of calcium and phosphorus that can be delivered because of the risk of precipitation. Precipitates are particularly difficult to detect in TNA, which is a milky solution. High concentrates of calcium and low pH of the solution can also disrupt TNA, causing it to "crack," leading to separation of oil from the rest of the solution.

COMPLICATIONS

Mechanical Complications

Pneumothorax, hemothorax, hydrothorax, air embolism, thromboembolism, catheter misplacement, and cardiac perforation are recognized complications of Broviac, subclavian, and/or jugular catheter insertions. Potential mechanical complications of percutaneous central lines include catheter occlusion, accidental dislodgment, erythematous tracking, phlebitis, superior vena cava syndrome, catheter migration, and catheter entrapment or breakage. Chest x-ray examination to document correct catheter placement is necessary before a hypertonic solution is instilled.

The preceding complications may occur at any time as long as the catheter is present. Documentation of catheter position should be repeated if there is any history of pulling or tension on the catheter or any apparent change in its external position.

If the line is malfunctioning, it must be properly checked to avoid the possibility of complications from release of a clot into the bloodstream. If a clotted line is suspected, the line may be aspirated using strict sterile technique. If good blood return occurs or a clot is aspirated and removed, the catheter may be irrigated with sterile, dilute heparin solution.

Some clinicians will flush a partially occluded line with a thrombolytic agent, such as recombinant tissue plasminogen activator (rt-PA).[6,27] The risk of this practice must be weighed against the benefits of maintaining the central line. In most cases, if the catheter is a temporary line, it may be better to remove it and place a new line in another site.

A pleural effusion may be blood or chyle or may signal that the catheter has eroded into the pleural space. The effusion may be the infusate.

Infectious Complications

Infections associated with the central line may occur from contamination of the solution, tubing connections, or hubs. Although organisms may contaminate the solution during preparation, usually colonization occurs with entry into the line or bag. Intermittent administration of medications, removal of blood samples through the line, or multiple tubing changes provide opportunity for organisms to contaminate the solution.

Rigid criteria for sterile preparation of the solutions are mandatory (see previous section on solution preparation).

An in-line 0.22-μm membrane filter, which is incorporated into the IV tubing, is capable of trapping bacteria and fungi (although not endotoxin) and should be helpful in minimizing the risk of septicemia from a contaminated IV bag. Additionally, filters lessen the risk of an air embolism. An in-line filter setup is available that decreases the number of connections.

Nothing should be added to the TPN after it leaves the pharmacy.

Avoiding Line Colonization

- **Blood should not be drawn or given through smaller than 24-gauge (1.9 Fr) catheters because it increases formation of a fibrin sleeve and clots.**
- **When changing IV fluids, one should take care to avoid bleed-back into the catheter.**
- **Generally, medications should not be given into injection ports in the IV tubing, but**

should rather be given into a dedicated heparin-locked Y-site entry port. Stopcocks are not recommended.

- **The source of an infection is usually contamination with an organism that has colonized the hub or surrounding skin.[48] Scrupulous attention to hand hygiene and disinfection of catheter tubing, hubs, ports, and connections by vigorous rubbing with 70% alcohol before tubing changes or entry are critical infection prevention strategies.[42,61,65]**

Dressings are not routinely changed on PICC lines. If the dressing becomes nonocclusive or moistened, the site should be cleaned according to hospital protocol and redressed with a sterile transparent dressing. This should be performed using sterile gloves. The exposed catheter should be remeasured to ensure that it was not inadvertently moved during this process. Dressings are changed routinely on Broviac, subclavian, jugular, and femoral catheters. Dressing changes are recommended at least weekly or more frequently if drainage is noted or the dressing is no longer occlusive.

Evaluating Infants for Infectious Disease Complication

Central line–associated bacteremia represents an important source of nosocomial infections in the intensive care nursery. The prevalence of this complication varies by unit, based on patient demographics, including birth weight, gestational age, diagnoses (proportion of surgery and medicine), and care practices.

Bacteremia must be considered in a newborn with a central line in place who presents with signs of sepsis (temperature instability, lethargy, poor skin perfusion, increased cardiopulmonary distress, or apnea). Some infants may be treated successfully with the line in place. However, if the infant remains systemically ill, even if the blood culture result is negative, the central line should be removed.

Guidelines for management of an infant with a central line in place with suspected sepsis are as follows:

- **The infant should be evaluated for potential sources of infection, including a general physical examination looking for non–TPN-related sources and inspection of peripheral and central venous sites for erythema.**
- **Laboratory assessment should include (1) complete blood cell count with platelet count, (2) aerobic blood cultures, and (3) se-**

rial C-reactive protein levels.[8] Other cultures, including urine, tracheal aspirate, and cerebrospinal fluid, may be indicated, based on clinical findings. A blood fungal culture should be obtained if the infant has had preceding antibiotic treatment or signs of fungal infection.[9]

- A chest x-ray evaluation should be performed if the infant demonstrates signs of respiratory distress or there is a need to reassess catheter position.
- Consider discontinuing lipid infusion until the infection has been treated for 24 to 48 hours.[4]
- If the infant is critically ill, the central line should be removed immediately. If the infant is stable, treatment may be considered through the line.
- A positive blood culture is generally considered to indicate bacteremia or sepsis in a newborn with a central line in place. However, coagulase-negative staphylococcus, an opportunistic organism that is a common cause of catheter-related sepsis, also is normal skin flora and frequently contaminates blood cultures. Use of ancillary diagnostic tools, such as the CRP and CBC, are helpful to distinguish false-positive results from true infections. Some clinicians also recommend obtaining two cultures (two peripheral, or one peripheral and one from the line) before starting antibiotics. If both yield positive results, catheter-related sepsis is confirmed.
- If bacteremia is documented but the infant's signs are improved, the catheter may continue in place while being used for antibiotic treatment. One should be sure that the antibiotics that are used are compatible with the TPN (to avoid stopping the TPN during the antibiotic infusion). A follow-up blood culture and close clinical monitoring are necessary to document that the infection has been adequately treated.

If a central line is pulled because of sepsis, a new central line should not be placed for 48 to 72 hours.

Metabolic Complications

Glucose Metabolism

Hyperglycemia may occur with increased carbohydrate load, especially in ELBW infants who may have inadequate endogenous insulin production or

decreased sensitivity to insulin. Elevated blood sugar may lead to hyperosmolality and osmotic diuresis, resulting in hyperosmolar dehydration. Manifestations include polyuria, glucosuria, and dry, hot, flushed skin. Serum sodium is not a reliable measure of serum osmolality if there is hyperglycemia. Direct measurement or estimate by use of the following formula is necessary:

$$\text{Serum osmolality} = (1.86)\,Na^+ + BUN/2.8 + Glucose/18$$

Transient glucose intolerance may be seen with stress. If hyperglycemia occurs without apparent change in glucose infusion, the possibility of sepsis, pain, hypoxemia, intraventricular hemorrhage (especially if the infant is of less than 34 weeks' gestation), or inadvertent increase in carbohydrate administration (mistake in preparation or rate of infusion) should be considered. Glucose intolerance may also be accentuated during infusions of lipid emulsion, especially in an ELBW infant. Discontinuation of the lipid infusion without alteration of the carbohydrate load will often eliminate hyperglycemia in this situation. Some ELBW infants remain hyperglycemic even on reduced carbohydrate intakes. These infants may benefit from a continuous insulin infusion to attain adequate caloric intake. Treatment varies but the usual infant dose is 1.0 mU/kg/min.[19] Routine use of insulin to promote growth in the preterm infant is not advised because of side effects.[55]

Hypoglycemia may result from an abrupt interruption of glucose infusion or excessive exogenous insulin administration. Manifestations of hypoglycemia include tachycardia or apnea, lethargy, jitteriness, and seizures. If these occur immediately after an interruption of the TPN infusion, an IV glucose infusion must be initiated at once, followed by close monitoring of the blood glucose to allow appropriate glucose administration. The glucose concentration of the infusate may usually be safely decreased by 5 g/dl every 12 hours. Blood glucose values should be monitored hourly until stable after each change.

Amino Acid Metabolism

Hyperammonemia may be seen in preterm infants given excessive protein loads. Hyperammonemia will also occur in an infant with a congenital metabolic disturbance, such as a urea cycle defect, when challenged with an amino acid load. Hyperammonemia may be manifested as somnolence, lethargy, seizures, and coma. Biochemical screening is necessary to identify this complication before there are symptoms.

Azotemia may occur before hyperammonemia, depending on the hepatic ability to convert ammonia to urea. Azotemia may also be a sign of dehydration.

Initially the BUN should be monitored daily. When there are no further changes in amino acid administration and the BUN is stable, monitoring two times per week is adequate.

Cholestasis

Infants receiving TPN for more than 2 weeks will frequently develop cholestatic jaundice (direct bilirubin greater than 2 mg/dl).[17] **The risk appears greatest for the least mature infants and those receiving the longest period of TPN without enteral feeding.**[68] The cause appears to be multifactorial, including lack of bile flow stimulation, malnutrition, and amino acid toxicity or deficiency. Fat emulsions have been associated with cholestasis, but objective evidence of an etiologic role has not been provided. An increase in serum bile acid concentration usually precedes elevated conjugated bilirubin levels. Serum amino transferases are often normal early in the clinical course. Serum albumin and prealbumin levels usually remain normal. An abnormality in hepatic synthetic function or early rise in isoenzyme levels should lead the clinician to investigate other forms of liver disease. The differential of cholestatic jaundice includes the following:

- Bacterial sepsis
- Congenital viral infection
- Postpartum acquisition of cytomegalovirus
- Neonatal hepatitis
- Bile duct obstruction, such as biliary atresia or choledochal cyst
- Galactosemia
- Cystic fibrosis
- Alpha-1-antitrypsin deficiency

Management of cholestatic jaundice should include (when possible) the following:

- **Increase enteral feedings as tolerated and decrease proportionately the parenteral nutrition**
- **Reduction of parenteral protein to 1 to 2 g/kg/day**
- **Reduction of dextrose concentration to 10%**
- **Eliminate copper and manganese from trace minerals in TPN**
- **Protect solutions from light by covering the bag and IV tubing to reduce levels of light-induced toxic peroxides**[37]

Lipid Metabolism

Infants with decreased adipose tissue may demonstrate intolerance to fat emulsion infusions. Lipids may be poorly tolerated by SGA infants and extremely preterm infants in the first week of life. Parenteral fats should be used cautiously in these infants. Hyperlipidemia may result, causing elevation of triglyceride, FFA, and lipoprotein levels. To monitor for hyperlipidemia, serum may be checked for evidence of visible lactescence (increased plasma turbidity). A triglyceride level should be checked after initiation of therapy and then periodically as indicated. Steroid therapy may elevate the triglyceride level.[63] Triglyceride and fatty acid levels should be obtained at least weekly, and doses should be adjusted accordingly. Transient hyperglycemia may result from lipid infusion. This complication is usually dose-related and rarely requires treatment.[12]

Hyperlipidemia is responsible for the known and theoretical complications of fat emulsion infusions. Competitive displacement of bilirubin by FFA may theoretically increase the risk of kernicterus in preterm infants with hyperbilirubinemia. Therefore, hyperbilirubinemia requiring therapy is a relative contraindication to lipid infusion. Based on the AAP recommendation for preterm infants with hyperbilirubinemia, intravenous lipids infusion should be reduced to the lowest dose to avoid EFA deficiency.[3]

Altered immune function by lipid deposition in macrophages and the reticuloendothelial system must be considered in infants with sepsis. *Malassezia furfur* is a lipophilic fungus that has been reported as an opportunistic organism in infants receiving long-term lipid infusions.[14] Discontinuation of the central line and lipid infusion eliminates the infection. Coagulase-negative staphylococcal bacteremia has also been reported in association with lipid infusions, but the relationship remains controversial.[4]

PARENT TEACHING

In-Hospital TPN

Clinicians caring for an ill newborn must be attentive to the involvement and emotional state of the parents. There is a higher incidence of child abuse, foster placement, and relinquishment among infants who have been cared for in the NICU compared with healthy, full-term newborns.

Clinical conditions or policies that promote separation of parents from their infant will increase the risk of bonding problems. When a newborn infant cannot be fed orally, an important, normal part of the infant's care is no longer available for the parents. The placement of a central line may be frightening to parents and result in less handling and caregiving. **Infants requiring continuous care including TPN should have primary nursing (one regular nurse) and one physician who communicates regularly with the parents. Care providers should attempt to keep the parents involved in other parts of the infant's care, because the parents are unable to feed the infant. Parents should be fully informed regarding the purpose and appropriate care of the infant's central line so they will feel comfortable handling their infant with the line in place.**

A neonatal service that uses TPN has the best results if there is an experienced "nutrition team," including pediatrician, surgeon, nutrition support nurse, pharmacist, dietitian, and social worker, with each member playing a vital role to make TPN a safe and effective therapy.

Home TPN

Home parenteral nutrition has been used in infants with congenital intestinal anomalies or after massive bowel resection for NEC.

TPN is initiated in the hospital. If growing and otherwise well, the infant may be a candidate for TPN at home. Issues to be addressed include ability and willingness of parents to care for the infant at home, available financial support, adequate home setting, and additional skilled nursing care needed at home. The infant should have a more permanent central line placed as early in the discharge process as possible. Parent teaching should begin early, including verbal and written instruction and hands-on demonstrations.

Administration of TPN at home is different from hospital administration of TPN. Infants often go home on cyclic TPN (12 hr/day). An ambulatory pump improves the mobility and flexibility of the parent and infant and allows for a more normal life.

Compliance with home TPN is greatly increased when the parents understand TPN, the need for it, and the need for strict adherence to sterile technique.

REFERENCES

1. Adamkin DD, Radmacher P, Rosen P: Comparison of a neonatal versus general-purpose amino acid formulation in preterm neonates, *J Perinatol* 15:108, 1995.
2. Alpan G, Eyal F, Springer C et al: Heparinization of alimentation solutions administered through peripheral veins in premature infants, a controlled study, *Pediatrics* 74:375, 1984.
3. American Academy of Pediatrics Committee on Nutrition: Parenteral nutrition. In Kleinman RE, ed. *Pediatric Nutrition Handbook,* ed 4, Elk Grove Village, Ill. 1998, The Academy.
4. Avila-Figueroa C, Goldmann DA, Richardson DC et al: Intravenous lipid emulsion are the major determinant of coagulase-negative staphylococcal bacteremia in very low birth weight newborns, *Pediatr Infect Dis J* 17:10, 1998.
5. Baeckert PA, Greene HL, Fritz et al: Vitamin concentrations in very low birth weight infants given vitamins intravenously in a lipid emulsion: measurement of vitamins A, D, and E and riboflavin, *J Pediatr* 113:1057, 1988.
6. Bell SG: Recombinant tissue plasminogen activator. *Neonatal Netw* 15:13, 1996.
7. Bendorf K, Friesen CA, Roberts CC: Glucose response to discontinuation of parenteral nutrition in patients less than 3 years of age, *J Parenter Enteral Nutr* 20:120, 1996.
8. Benitz WE, Han MY, Madan A et al: Serial serum C-reactive protein levels in the diagnosis of neonatal infection, *Pediatrics* 102:E41, 1998.
9. Benjamin DK, Ross K, McKinney RE et al: When to suspect fungal infection in neonates: a clinical comparison of *Candida albicans* and *Candida parapsilosis fungemia* with coagulase-negative staphylococcal bacteremia, *Pediatrics* 106:712, 2000.
10. Bloomfield FH, Knight DB, Harding JE: Side effects of 2 different dexamethasone courses for preterm infants at risk of chronic lung disease: a randomized trial, *J Pediatr* 133:395, 1998.
11. Bonner CM, DeBrie KL, Hug G et al: Effects of parenteral L-carnitine supplementation on fat metabolism and nutrition in premature neonates, *J Pediatr* 126:287, 1995.
12. Cooke RJ, Yeh YY, Gibson D et al: Soybean oil emulsion administration during parenteral nutrition in the preterm infant: effect of essential fatty acid, lipid, and glucose metabolism, *J Pediatr* 111:767, 1987.
13. Dahl GB, Svensson L, Kinnander NJ et al: Stability of vitamins in soybean oil fat emulsion under conditions simulating intravenous feeding of neonates and children, *J Parenter Enteral Nutr* 18:234, 1994.
14. Dankner WM, Spector SA, Fierer J et al: Malassezia fungemia in neonates and adults: complications of hyperalimination, *Rev Infect Dis* 9:743, 1987.
15. Downing GJ, Egelhoff JC, Daily DK et al: Kidney function in very low birth weight infants with furosemide-related renal calcifications at ages 1 to 2 years, *J Pediatr* 120:599, 1992.
16. Driscoll DF: Total nutrient admixtures: theory and practice, *Nutr Clin Pract* 10:114, 1995.
17. Drongowski RA, Coran AG: An analysis of factors contributing to the development of total parenteral nutrition-induced cholestasis, *J Parenter Enteral Nutr* 13:586, 1989.

18. Dudrick SJ, Wilmore DW, Vars HM et al: Long term total parenteral nutrition with growth, development, and positive nitrogen balance, *Surgery* 64:134, 1968.

19. Farrag HM, Cowett RM: Glucose homeostasis in the micropremie, *Clin Perinatol* 27:1, 2000.

20. Farrell PM, Gutcher GR, Palta M et al: Essential fatty acid deficiency in premature infants, *Am J Clin Nutr* 48:220, 1988.

21. Fomon SJ: Requirements and recommended dietary intake of protein during infancy, *Pediatr Res* 30:391, 1991.

22. Georgieff MK, Amarnath UM, Mill MM: Determinants of arm muscle and fat accretion during the first postnatal month in preterm newborn infants, *J Pediatr Gastroenerol Nutr* 9:219, 1989.

23. Green C, Yohannan MD: Umbilical arterial and venous catheters: placement, use, and complications, *Neonatal Netw* 17:23, 1998.

24. Greene HL, Hambidge KM, Schanler R et al: Guidelines for use of vitamins, trace elements, calcium, magnesium, and phosphorus in infants and children receiving total parenteral nutrition, *Am J Clin Nutr* 48:1324, 1988.

25. Greene HL, Moore ME, Phillips B et al: Evaluation of a pediatric multiple vitamin preparation for total parenteral nutrition. II. Blood levels of vitamins A, D, and E, *Pediatrics* 77:539, 1986.

26. Hack M, Breslau N, Weissman B et al: Effect of very low birth weight and subnormal head size on cognitive abilities at school age, *N Engl J Med* 325:231, 1991.

27. Haire WD, Atkinson JB, Stephens LC et al: Urokinase versus recombinant tissue plasminogen activator in thrombosed central venous catheters: a double-blinded, randomized trial, *Thromb Haemost* 72:543, 1994.

28. Hanning RM, Zlotkin SH: Amino acid and protein needs of the neonate: effects of excess and deficiency, *Semin Perinatol* 13:131, 1989.

29. Haumont D, Deckelbaum RJ, Richelle M et al: Plasma lipid and plasma lipoprotein concentrations in very low birth weight infants given parenteral nutrition with twenty or ten percent lipid emulsion, *J Pediatr* 115:787, 1989.

30. Hay WW: Nutritional needs of the extremely low-birth-weight infant, *Semin Perinatol* 15:482-492, 1991.

31. Heird WC: Amino acid and energy needs of pediatric patients receiving parenteral nutrition, *Pediatr Clin North Am* 42:765, 1995.

32. Heird WC, Hay W, Helms RA et al: Pediatric parenteral amino acid mixture in low birth weight infants, *Pediatrics* 81:41, 1988.

33. Howard D, Thompson DF: Taurine: an essential amino acid to prevent cholestasis in neonates? *Ann Pharmacother* 26:1390, 1992.

34. Johnson L, Quinn GE, Abbasi S et al: Severe retinopathy of prematurity in infants with birth weights less than 1250 grams: incidence and outcome of treatment with pharmacologic serum levels of vitamin E in addition to cryotherapy from 1985 to 1991, *J Pediatr* 127:632, 1995.

35. Klein GL: Aluminum in parenteral solutions revisited—again, *Am J Clin Nutr* 61:449, 1995.

36. Koo WWK, Tsang RC: Mineral requirements of low-birth-weight infants, *J Am Coll Nutr* 10:474, 1991.

37. Laborie S, Lavoie JC, Pineault M et al: Protecting solutions of parenteral nutrition from perioxidation, *J Parenter Enteral Nutr* 23:104, 1999.

38. Laine L, Shulman RJ, Pitre D et al: Cysteine usage increases the need for acetate in neonates who receive total parenteral nutrition, *Am J Clin Nutr* 54:565, 1991.

39. Leick-Rude MK: Use of percutaneous silastic intravascular catheters in high-risk neonates, *Neonatal Netw* 9:17, 1990.

40. Leitch CA, Denne SC: Energy expenditure in the extremely low-birth-weight infant, *Clin Perinatol* 27:181, 2000.

41. Lesser E, Chhabra R, Brion LP et al: Use of midline catheters in low birth weight infants, *J Perinatol* 16:205, 1996.

42. Maas A, Flament P, Pardou A et al: Central venous catheter-related bacteraemia in critically ill neonates: risk factors and impact of a prevention programme, *J Hosp Infect* 40:211, 1998.

43. Maki DG, Ringer M, Alvarado CJ: Prospective, randomised trial of povidone-iodine, alcohol and chlorhexidine for prevention of infection with central venous and arterial catheters, *Lancet* 338:339, 1991.

44. Matlow AG, Kitai I, Kirpalani H et al: A randomized trial of 72- versus 24-hour intravenous tubing set changes in newborns receiving lipid therapy, *Infect Control Hosp Epidemiol* 20:487, 1999.

45. McKinnon BT: FDA safety alert: hazards of precipitation associated with parenteral nutrition, *Nutr Clin Pract* 11:59, 1996.

46. Mermel LA, Parenteau S, Tow SM: The risk of midline catheterization in hospitalized patients. A prospective study, *Ann Intern Med* 123:841, 1995.

47. Meyer MP, Haworth C, Meyer JH et al: A comparison of oral and intravenous iron supplementation in preterm infants receiving recombinant erythropoietin, *J Pediatr* 129:258, 1996.

48. Mueller-Premru M, Gubina M, Kaufmann ME et al: Use of semi-quantitative and quantitative culture methods and types for studying the epidemiology of central venous catheter-related infections in neonates on parenteral nutrition, *J Med Microbiol* 48:451, 1999.

49. National Advisory Group on Standards and Practice Guidelines for Parenteral Nutrition: Safe practices for parenteral nutrition formulations, *J Parenter Enteral Nutr* 22:49, 1998.

50. Nedergaard J, Cannon B: Brown adipose tissue: development and function. In Polin RA, Fox WW, eds: *Fetal and neonatal physiology,* Philadelphia, 1998, WB Saunders.

51. Neu J, Roig JC, Meetze WH et al: Enteral glutamine supplemental for very low birth weight infants decreases morbidity, *J Pediatr* 131:691, 1997.

52. Pearson ML: Guideline for prevention of intravascular device-related infections. Part II. Recommendations for the prevention of nosocomial intravascular device-related infections. The Hospital Infection Control Practices Advisory Committee, *Am J Infect Control* 24:277, 1996.

53. Pelegano JF, Rowe JC, Carey DE et al: Simultaneous infusion of calcium and phosphorus in parenteral nutrition for premature infants: use of physiologic calcium/phosphorus ratio, *J Pediatr* 114:115, 1989.

54. Phelps SJ, Cochran EB: Effect of the continuous administration of fat emulsion on the infiltration of intravenous lines in infants receiving peripheral parenteral nutrition solutions, *J Parenter Enteral Nutr* 13:628, 1989.

55. Poindexter BB, Karr CA, Denne SC: Exogenous insulin reduces proteolysis and protein synthesis in extremely low birth weight infants, *J Pediatr* 132:948, 1998.

56. Putet G: Lipid metabolism of the micropremie, *Clin Perinatol* 27:57, 2000.

57. Rivera A, Bell EF, Bier DM: Effect of intravenous amino acids on protein metabolism of preterm infants during the first three days of life, *Pediatr Res* 33:106, 1993.

58. Rollins CJ: Total nutrient admixtures: stability issues and their impact on nursing practice, *J Intraven Nurs* 20:299, 1997.

59. Romagnoli C, Zecca E, Vento G et al: Effect on growth of two different dexamethasone courses for preterm infants at risk of chronic lung disease: a randomized trial, *Pharmacology* 59:266, 1999.

60. Ryder MA: Peripherally inserted central venous catheters, *Nurs Clin North Am* 28:937, 1993.

61. Salzman MB, Rubin LG: Relevance of the catheter hub as a portal for microorganisms causing catheter-related bloodstream infections, *Nutrition* 13(suppl): 15, 1997.

62. Sentipal-Walerius J, Dollberg S, Mimouni F et al: Effect of pulsed dexamethasone therapy on tolerance of intravenously administered lipids in extremely low birth weight infants, *J Pediatr* 134:229, 1999.

63. Shenai JP, Kennedy KA, Chytil F et al: Clinical trial of vitamin A supplementation in infants susceptible to bronchopulmonary dysplasia, *J Pediatr* 111:269, 1987.

64. Sitges-Serra A, Hernandez R, Maestro S et al: Prevention of catheter sepsis: the hub, *Nutrition* 13(4 suppl):30S, 1997.

65. Stovroff M, Teague WG: Intravenous access in infants and children, *Pediatr Clin North Am* 45:1373, 1998.

66. Sunehag A, Gustafsson J, Ewald U: Very immature infants (≤30 wk) respond to glucose infusion with incomplete suppression of glucose production, *Pediatr Res* 550, 1994.

67. Teitelbaum DH: Parenteral nutrition-associated cholestasis, *Curr Opin Pediatr* 9:270, 1997.

68. Thiagarajan RR, Bratton SL, Gettmann T et al: Efficacy of peripherally inserted central venous catheters placed in noncentral veins, *Arch Pediatr Adolesc Med* 152:436, 1998.

69. Thureen PJ, Hay WW: Intravenous nutrition and postnatal growth of the micropremie, *Clin Perinat* 27:197, 2000.

70. Thureen PJ, Anderson AH, Baron KA et al: Protein balance in the first week of life in ventilated neonates receiving parenteral nutrition, *Am J Clin Nutr* 68:1128, 1998.

71. Torrence CR, Horns KM, East C: Accuracy and precision of neonatal electronic incubator scales, *Neonatal Netw* 14:35, 1995.

72. Tyson JE, Wright LL, Oh W et al: Vitamin A supplementation for extremely-low-birth-weight infants, *N Engl J Med* 340:1962, 1999.

73. Uauy R, Hoffman DR: Essential fat requirements of preterm infants, *Am J Clin Nutr* 71(Suppl):245, 2000.

74. Van Goudoever JB, Colen T, Wattimena JL et al: Immediate commencement of amino acid supplementation in preterm infants: effect on serum amino acid concentrations and protein kinetics on the first day of life, *J Pediatr* 127:458, 1995.

75. Van Lingen RA, Van Goudoever JB, Luijendijk IH et al: Effect of early amino acid administration during total parenteral nutrition on protein metabolism in pre-term infants, *Clin Sci* 82:199, 1992.

77. Viña J, Vento M, Garcia-Sala F et al: L-cysteine and glutathione metabolism are impaired in premature infants due to cystathionase deficiency, *Am J Clin Nutr* 61:1067, 1995.

78. Wilmore DW: Catabolic illness. Strategies for enhancing recovery, *N Engl J Med* 325:695, 1991.

79. Wright K, Dawson JP, Fallis D et al: New postnatal growth grids for very low birth weight infants, *Pediatrics* 91:922, 1993.

80. Ziegler EE, O'Donnell AM, Nelson SE et al: Body composition of the reference fetus, *Growth* 40:329, 1976.

81. Zlotkin SH, Atkinson S, Lockitch G: Trace elements in nutrition for premature infants, *Clin Perinatol* 22:223, 1995.

18 | Skin and Skin Care

Carolyn Houska-Lund, David J. Durand

The skin is a large organ in premature and term infants, comprising at least 13% of body weight in contrast to 3% of the body weight in adults.[58] Skin functions include thermoregulation; barrier against toxins and infections, water and electrolyte excretion, fat storage and insulation, and tactile sensation.

Like many other organs, the skin of a premature infant is immature. The combination of immaturity with the need for intensive care monitoring and procedures places premature infants at risk for skin trauma and loss of skin integrity. Skin trauma and skin immaturity have serious consequences for infants in the NICU, including problems in thermoregulation, fluid and electrolyte balance, diversion of calories for tissue repair, discomfort, potential toxicity from absorbed substances, and increased risk for infection.

In this chapter we will review the physiology of term and premature infants' skin, the differences in structure and function related to skin immaturity, and prevention and treatment strategies to promote optimal skin integrity for infants in the NICU.

PHYSIOLOGY

There are three layers to the skin: the epidermis, the dermis, and the subcutaneous layer (Figure 18-1). The epidermis is comprised of the stratum corneum, a nonliving layer, and the basal layer. The stratum corneum is formed of lipids and protein in "brick and mortar" configuration. The basal layer of the epidermis replaces the stratum corneum with cells called keratinocytes. Approximately every 26 days, keratinocytes migrate from the basal layer to the exfoliated layers of the stratum corneum. In addition to keratinocytes, melanocytes are also found in the basal layer.

The dermis, a woven layer of collagen and elastin fibers, is 2 to 4 mm thick at birth. It contains nerves, blood vessels, and hair follicles. Sensations of heat, touch, pressure, and pain originate in the dermal layer. Sebaceous glands and sweat glands are located in the dermis, as well as in the subcutaneous layer of the skin. Sweat glands become mature in term infants during the first week of life, whereas maturation in premature infants occurs between 21 and 33 days and perhaps even longer in extremely premature infants. Full adult sweat gland function does not occur until the child is 2 to 3 years of age.[28]

The subcutaneous layer is composed of fatty connective tissue, with fat deposition occurring primarily during the last trimester of pregnancy. This layer provides heat insulation and functions as a calorie reservoir.

The skin of a normal term infant is covered with vernix caseosa, a cheesy substance composed of sebum from sebaceous glands, broken off lanugo, and desquamated cells from the amnion. The vernix accumulates during the last month of pregnancy and protects the fetus against maceration from the amniotic fluid and chafing caused by crowding in utero.[84] After delivery excessive vernix is either worn off or removed, and a desquamation process begins that results in visible peeling over the first week of life. Vernix may contribute to the development of epidermal barrier function and may help to regulate surface adhesion properties, heat flux, and surface electrical activities.[48]

The skin of premature infants is thinner than that of term infants and may appear transparent or even gelatinous in extremely immature infants. There is usually a ruddy, red appearance caused by the underdeveloped stratum corneum, making skin color a poor tool for assessing the oxygenation status of very immature infants. There are fewer wrinkles on skin surfaces than in term infants, and the skin is covered by lanugo to varying degrees, depending on maturity; these fine hairs cover the upper back, arms, and forehead. The subcutaneous layer in premature infants is often edematous because of an excess of cutaneous water and sodium[103] (Figure 18-2) (see Chapter 14).

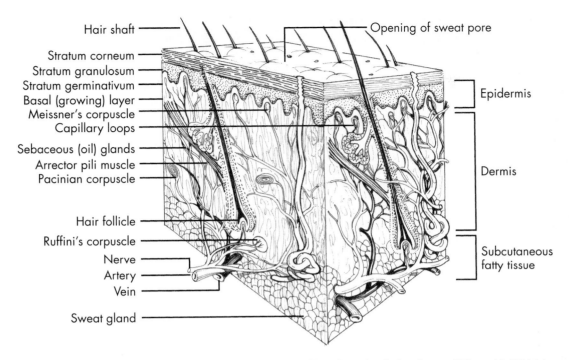

Hair shaft

Stratum corneum
Stratum granulosum
Stratum germinativum
Basal (growing) layer
Meissner's corpuscle
Capillary loops

Sebaceous (oil) glands
Arrector pili muscle
Pacinian corpuscle

Hair follicle

Ruffini's corpuscle
Nerve
Artery
Vein

Sweat gland

Opening of sweat pore

Epidermis

Dermis

Subcutaneous
fatty tissue

FIGURE 18-1   Cross section of skin layers and anatomic structures. (From *Principles of infant skin care*, Skillman, NJ, 1994, Johnson & Johnson.)

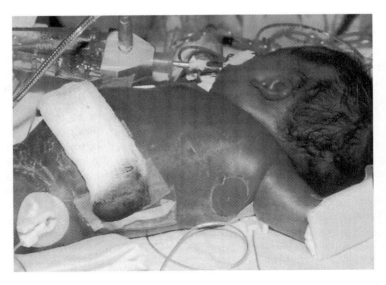

FIGURE 18-2   Edema in a premature infant caused by excess cutaneous water and sodium.

Table 18-1	NORMAL VARIATIONS OF TERM NEWBORN SKIN
Linea nigra	Line of increased pigmentation from umbilicus to genitalia
Mongolian spots	Irregular, blue-gray, bruiselike spots
	Usually seen over sacrum and buttocks, may extend over back and shoulders
	Caused by pigmented cells in dermis
	Most common in infants with darker pigmentation
Lanugo	Fine, downy hair over back, shoulders, and face
	Shed at 32 to 36 weeks' gestation
Milia	White, pinhead-sized bumps over chin, cheeks, nose, and forehead
	Tiny, epidermal cysts
	If on palate, called Epstein's pearls
Miliaria	Caused by retention of sweat from edema in stratum corneum that blocks sweat glands
	Most common is rubra (prickly pear), but there are clear versions as well
Harlequin sign	Color of half of body turns deep red while the other half is pale
	Caused by immature autoregulation of blood flow
Vernix caseosa	Gray-white, cheesey substance that protects fetal skin in utero
	Gradually diminishes near term
Cutis marmorata	Mottling caused by vasomotor immaturity
Erythema toxicum	Small, firm white or yellow pustules with erythematous margin
neonatorum	Most often seen on trunk, arms, and perineal area
	Benign condition seen in 30% to 70% of newborns
Acne neonatorum	Acne-like rash seen in newborns at several weeks of age
	Caused by stimulation of sebaceous glands by maternal hormones
	More common in males
	Instruct caregivers not to use creams, lotion, or ointments since they can worsen the rash
Transient neonatal	Resembles miliaria but present at birth
pustular melanosis	Most frequently found on face, palms of hands, soles of feet
	Not infectious or contagious
Cafe au lait spots	Irregularly shaped oval lesions
	If large size (>4 × 6 cm), or if greater than 6 in number, associated with neurofibromatosis

ETIOLOGY

Term Newborn Skin Variations

Although the basic skin structures are the same in all term newborns without dermatologic disease, there may be cutaneous variations seen on physical examination. These variations (Table 18-1) are not considered pathologic, but it is useful for clinicians to know them, because many parents will ask the significance of physical variations as they examine their newborn.

Physiologic and Anatomic Differences in Premature Skin

There are, however, developmental differences in skin physiology and anatomy in premature infants. In this section we discuss these differences and identify the implications for care.

Underdevelopment of the Stratum Corneum

The stratum corneum, the nonliving layer of the epidermis that is responsible for controlling evaporative heat loss and transepidermal water loss (TEWL), contains 10 to 20 layers in adults and term infants. **Premature infants have fewer layers of stratum corneum depending on their gestational age; at less than 30 weeks' gestation, it may contain only two or three layers (Figure 18-3), and extremely premature infants of less than 24 weeks' gestation may have virtually no stratum corneum.**[47,87] Another function of the stratum corneum—protection against toxins and infectious agents such as bacteria and viruses—is minimal in premature infants, leaving them vulnerable to transcutaneously transmitted infections and toxicity from topically applied substances.

The transition from the aquatic, intrauterine environment to the atmospheric, external environment has been thought to result in accelerated maturation of the stratum corneum and more mature function after the first 10 to 14 days of life.[34,45] **However, other authors cite a slower process in premature infants less than 27 weeks' ges-**

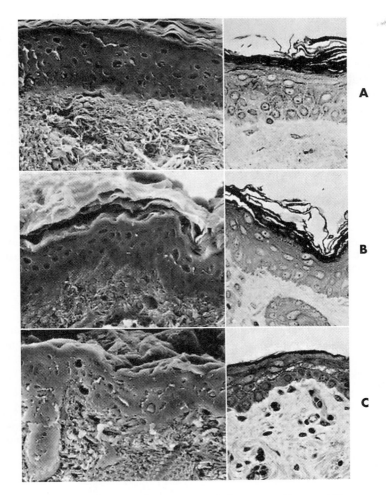

FIGURE 18-3   Photomicrograph of the stratum corneum in **A,** an adult, **B,** a term newborn, and **C,** a premature infant of 28 weeks' gestation. Note fewer layers of stratum corneum in the premature infant. (From Holbrook KA: A histological comparison of infant and adult skin. In Maibach HI, Boisits EK, eds: *Neonatal skin: structure and function,* New York, 1982, Marcel Dekker.)

tation, with rates of TEWL nearly double adult levels even at 28 days of life.[100] Premature infants of 23 to 25 weeks' gestation have losses 10 times higher than term infants initially, and they continue to have elevated heat and water loss resulting from immature barrier function for a longer period.[1] The maturation process can take as long as 8 weeks in an infant of 23 weeks' gestation.[56]

Dermal Instability

Collagen deposition in the dermis increases with advancing gestational age, preventing fluid from accumulating in this layer. Premature infants have a tendency to become edematous, because they have less collagen and fewer elastin fibers in the dermis.[28] They may be prone to necrotic injury, because edema in the dermis reduces blood flow to the epidermis. In addition, they may need protection from pressure and ischemic injury, including injuries caused by routine turning; the use of water beds and gelled mattresses or pads to minimize pressure points is helpful.

Diminished Cohesion Between Epidermis and Dermis

Numerous fibrils connect the epidermis to the dermis at the dermo-epidermal junction. These fibrils are more widely spaced and fewer in number in the premature infant[47] (Figure 18-4) but become stronger with advancing gestational and postnatal age. Genetically abnormal fibrils at this junction result in the dermatologic disorder epidermolysis bullosa, a blistering skin condition that occurs with even minimal trauma. **Premature infants are also prone to blistering from injury, although this decreases as they mature. This diminished cohesion places premature infants at risk for injury from adhesive removal as well. Particularly if extremely aggressive adhesives are used, there may be a stronger bond of the adhesive to the epidermis than of the epidermis to the dermis, and epidermal stripping may result during adhesive removal.**

Skin pH

The ability of the skin surface to form and maintain an acid surface is a function of various chemical and biologic processes. Acid skin surfaces with a pH less than 5 have been documented extensively in adults and children.[10] This *acid mantle* has protective qualities against some pathogens and other microorganisms. Because microbial colonization begins with delivery, the acid skin surface helps to keep a state of equilibrium; if the pH shifts from acidic to neutral, there may be an increase in total numbers of bacteria and a shift in species.[101] There may also be an increase in TEWL when skin pH rises.[109]

Term newborns are born with a relatively alkaline skin surface, measuring a mean pH of 6.34. Within 4 days the pH declines to a mean of 4.95.[10] Skin pH measurements have been reported in premature infants of varying gestational ages, and the pH was above 6.0 on the first day, decreasing to 5.5 during the first week, and gradually declining to 5.0 during the first month.[36] Bathing and other skin care practices alter skin pH; it may take an hour or longer to regenerate the acid mantle after bathing with an alkaline soap.[90]

Nutritional Deficiencies

Fat and zinc accumulate in the fetus during the last trimester of pregnancy. Because these nutritional components are necessary for maintaining an intact,

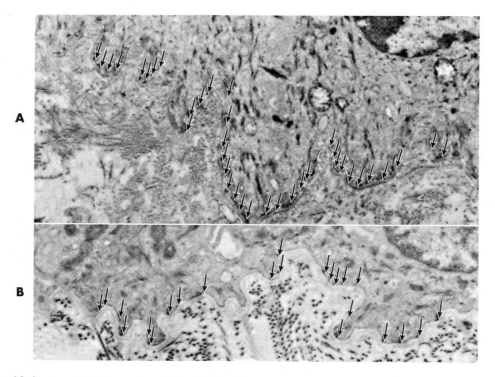

FIGURE 18-4 **A** and **B,** Arrows indicate fibrils called hemidesmosomes, which anchor the epidermis to the dermis. They are fewer in number and more widely spaced in the premature infant **(B).** (From Holbrook KA: A histological comparison of infant and adult skin. In Maibach HI, Boisits EK, eds: *Neonatal skin: structure and function,* New York, 1982, Marcel Dekker.)

healthy skin surface, premature infants born before the last trimester may develop skin problems caused by deficiencies in either of these nutrients. Problems may also be seen in infants who are unable to receive adequate enteral nutrition unless appropriate parenteral supplements are employed.

EFA deficiency can be seen in premature and postmature infants because of decreased fat stores (see Chapter 16). In this condition there is a superficial scaling and occasionally desquamation and irritation in the neck, groin, or perianal areas. There may be decreased serum levels of EFAs, thrombocytopenia, and impaired platelet aggregation, because EFAs are needed to promote platelet function.[38]

Providing adequate EFA prevents skin manifestations of EFA deficiency. In infants who are receiving small amounts of enteral nutrients or none at all, administration of IV lipid solutions at a total dose of 0.5 g/kg/day can prevent EFA deficiency (see Chapter 17). Once EFA deficiency occurs, IV lipids can reverse the process in 1 to 2 weeks. Dietary replacement takes longer and is effective only if gastrointestinal function is good. Topical therapy with sunflower seed oil, which is rich in linoleic acid, promotes transdermal absorption of EFA and raises serum levels but is variable in the rate of absorption. In a study of topical application, researchers found that safflower oil failed to yield improvements in patients with EFA deficiency.[50]

Zinc, an essential trace mineral, is a cofactor in many areas of metabolism, including lymphocyte transformation and metabolism of protein, nucleic acids, and mucopolysaccharides of skin and subcutaneous tissues and is required for normal wound healing.[29] Two thirds of the transfer of zinc from mother to fetus occurs in the last 10 weeks of pregnancy.

Zinc deficiency occurs when there are abnormal losses of zinc in stool or urine; when there are low or absent stores, as in premature birth; or during increased demands, such as during rapid growth, stress, or tissue healing. Thus premature infants and infants with pathologic conditions of the intestine (including chronic diarrhea, short bowel syndrome, intestinal diversions such as ileostomy, or intestinal resection) are at increased risk for zinc deficiency. In addition, any infant receiving total parenteral nutrition should receive trace minerals to prevent zinc deficiency (see Chapter 17).

Symptoms of zinc deficiency include erythematous, scaly skin and excoriations of the groin and perianal areas, neck folds, circumoral area, and at sites of trauma, such as areas of adhesive removal.[33]

Other clinical features include lethargy, poor growth, alopecia, and diarrhea. Serum zinc levels of less than 68 μg/ml accompanied by a low alkaline phosphatase and clinical symptoms are diagnostic of zinc deficiency. Prevention of zinc deficiency for term infants receiving total parenteral nutrition includes zinc supplementation with 100 to 200 μg/kg/day; premature infants require higher levels of supplementation, 400 μg/kg/day.[113] Premature infants have also been reported to develop zinc deficiency while fed breast milk; they may require an oral zinc sulfate supplement.[112]

PREVENTION

During daily skin care practices such as bathing, lubrication, antimicrobial skin disinfection, and adhesive removal, the skin of newborns is at risk for trauma or disruption of normal barrier function. This is particularly true of newborns in the NICU, who may have been born prematurely or may be critically ill or require surgery.

In this section we review basic skin care practices in terms of impact on skin integrity, preventing potential toxicity, and reducing exposure to potentially sensitizing chemical. We present recommendations for preventing trauma, protecting immature barrier function, and promoting skin integrity supported by scientific evidence. These recommendations are also integrated into an evidence-based skin care guideline for health professionals.[7]

Bathing

Among the purposes of bathing the newborn are overall hygiene, aesthetics, and protection of health care workers by removing blood and body fluids. Bathing, however, is not an innocuous procedure. During the immediate postbirth period bathing can result in hypothermia, increased oxygen consumption, and respiratory distress. The first bath should be delayed until the infant's temperature has been stabilized in the normal range for 2 to 4 hours,[91] or at 1 hour if radiant heat is provided during the bath.[107] Bathing has also been shown to destabilize vital signs and temperature in premature infants.[92]

Bathing with antiseptic soaps and cleansers is still practiced in some nurseries. Studies have shown that although hexachlorophene reduced the number of *Staphylococcus aureus* strains present on the skin, toxicity was reported, especially in premature infants, associated with absorption through the skin; it should not be used.[3,60,98] Both povidone-iodine and chlorhexidine are sometimes used for the initial bath in newborn nurseries, although the effect on bacterial colonization is transient.[26] Chlorhexidine has proved effective in reducing colonization for up to 4 hours[26] but can also be absorbed.[25] Although toxicity from chlorhexidine has not been identified, many nurseries do not use chlorhexidine for routine bathing because of the potential risk. There are no guidelines from the Centers for Disease Control and Prevention or the AAP recommending that antimicrobial cleansers be used for the newborn's first or subsequent baths.[3,20]

Soaps made with lye and animal fats are alkaline, with a pH above 7.0. Cleansing bars and liquids made with synthetic detergents are formulated to a more neutral pH of 5.5 to 7.0. All soaps and cleansers are at least mildly irritating and drying to skin surfaces[37,101,105,106] and disrupt the skin surface pH.[43] In addition, the degree to which the skin is irritated also depends on the length of contact and the frequency of bathing.

The wisest method is to select cleansers that have a neutral pH and minimal dyes and perfumes to reduce risk of future sensitization to these products and to bathe the infant only two or three times per week. Even reducing the frequency of bathing to every 4 days does not increase colonization with pathogens or result in infections, even in healthy premature infants.[37] For premature infants of less than 32 weeks' gestation, skin surfaces can be cleaned with warm water for the first week, using soft materials such as cotton balls or cloth. A rinsing technique should be used during cleansing, because rubbing is irritating to immature skin and potentially uncomfortable. If areas of skin breakdown are evident, warm sterile water is used.

When clinically feasible, immersion bathing may be beneficial from a developmental perspective.[2,4] Immersion bathing places the infant's entire body, except the head and neck, into warm water (38° C [100.4° F]), deep enough to cover the shoulders. Stable premature infants, after umbilical catheters are removed, and term infants with umbilical clamp in place can safely be bathed in this way.[7] Bathing is also an excellent time to educate parents about how to physically care for their baby and may also integrate information about their baby's neurobehavioral status and social characteristics.[57]

Emollients

The skin surface of term newborns is drier than that of adults but becomes gradually better hydrated as the eccrine sweat glands mature during the first year of life.[84,97] Maintaining the hydration of the stratum corneum is necessary for an intact skin surface and normal barrier function. Skin that is dry, scaly, or cracking is not only uncomfortable but can also be a portal of entry for microorganisms. Products used to counteract dryness are called *moisturizers, emollients,* or *lubricants.* Common emollients include mineral oils, petrolatum, and lanolin and its derivatives. Emollients are sometimes divided into oil-in-water or water-in-oil emulsions.

Emollient use to prevent dermatitis and improve skin integrity in premature infants has been studied extensively. In one report[62] premature infants of 29 to 36 weeks' gestation were treated with Eucerin cream daily and had less dermatitis as measured by a visual grading scale but no differences in direct measurements of TEWL with an evaporimeter. In a later study premature infants of both younger gestation and postnatal age were treated with Aquaphor ointment, a water-miscible oil-in-water preparation that contains neither dyes nor perfumes. In this study there was improvement in both TEWL and visual scale dermatitis. No increases in skin surface temperatures or thermal burns were seen, even when the emollient was applied to infants under radiant heaters or phototherapy lights. In addition, cutaneous cultures revealed no increase in bacterial or fungal colonization on skin treated with emollients. A statistically significant smaller number of treated infants had positive blood or cerebrospinal fluid culture results compared with control subjects.[88]

A large, randomized controlled trial of 1191 infants with birthweights of 501 to 1000 g was conducted to determine whether twice-daily application of Aquaphor ointment would reduce combined outcome measures of mortality and sepsis. **Although skin integrity appeared improved with routine emollient use, there was no effect seen in the outcomes of sepsis plus mortality. Of note, an increase in coagulase-negative *Staphylococcus epidermidis* bloodstream infections was seen in infants with birthweights below 750 g, although the mechanism and relationship to emollient use are not clearly understood.[32] Although a small case-control study had previously associated petrolatum-based emollients with a higher incidence of fungal infections,[18] this was not seen in the larger trial.[32] The effects of emollients on TEWL or fluid balance were not studied in this trial.**

The benefits of emollient use must be carefully weighed against the risk of infection. In general, emollients can be safely used to treat skin with excessive drying, skin cracking, and fissures. They may also be beneficial in reducing TEWL and evaporative heat loss, although other methods, such as using a high-humidity environment or transparent adhesive dressings, are also available for this purpose. Avoiding products with perfumes or dyes is prudent, because these can be absorbed and are potential contact irritants.[21] Small tubes or jars for single patient use are recommended to prevent contamination with microorganisms.

Skin Disinfectants

Decontamination of skin before invasive procedures such as venipuncture and placement of umbilical catheters and chest tubes is common practice in neonatal intensive care nurseries. However, there are anecdotal reports of skin injury, including blistering, burns, and sloughing from both isopropyl alcohol and povidone-iodine use in premature infants.[46,99] There have also been case reports of high iodine levels, iodine goiter, and hypothyroidism associated with povidone-iodine use in premature infants.[22,54,93] Several prospective studies of routine povidone-iodine use in intensive care nurseries[67,89,102] and one study of presurgical skin preparation of infants under 3 months of age[82] found alterations in iodine levels and potential thyroid effects from povidone-iodine exposure as a result of absorption through the skin. Although one study did not find thyroid effects from iodine absorption in neonates,[42] the study period (10 days) may be too short a period of time to see the effect.

Another important aspect of skin disinfection is the efficacy of the solutions used. During skin preparation before blood culture sampling in children and adults, lower rates of microbial colonization were seen with povidone-iodine compared with isopropyl alcohol.[24] A larger study of blood culture sampling in adults found fewer contaminated cultures when chlorhexidine had been used compared with cultures from povidone-iodine–cleansed subjects.[83]

Two studies in premature infants compared skin and peripheral intravenous catheter colonization with bacteria after skin preparation with either chlorhexidine or povidone-iodine. Malathi et al[76] found the rate of colonization was no different between disinfectants, but the technique of application was important: the authors recommended longer periods of cleansing (more than 30 seconds) or two consecutive cleansings for maximum reduction of colonization. Garland, Buck, and Maloney[40] reported that

chlorhexidine reduced catheter colonization: 4.3% with chlorhexine compared with 9.3% with povidone-iodine. A comparison of isopropyl alcohol, povidone-iodine, and 2% chlorhexidine aqueous solution for disinfection of 668 central venous catheters in adults during insertion and routine dressing changes showed chlorhexidine to be significantly more effective in reducing catheter-related infections.[75]

Recommended skin disinfectants for newborns include both chlorhexidine or povidone-iodine solutions. Chlorhexidine is available as a tincture (0.5% in isopropyl alcohol) or as a surgical scrub (2% or 4% in an aqueous solution). A single-use applicator of 2% chlorhexidine in isopropyl alcohol has recently been approved for preoperative skin preparation in adults. Other chlorhexidine products must be poured from bottles or packages onto sterile gauze for application. Chlorhexidine should not be used as a preoperative skin disinfection agent on the face or head, because misuse has been reported to result in injury if it remains in contact with either the eye or ear during surgical procedures. However, careful use before scalp intravenous or central line insertion is acceptable, if splashing or using excessive amounts of chlorhexidine is avoided. **Chlorhexidine is applied in two consecutive wipings, or for a 30-second scrubbing period, then is removed with sterile water or saline solution when the procedure is completed.**

Povidone-iodine is available in a 10% aqueous solution in a variety of single-use applications. It is also applied in two consecutive wipings, or for a 30-second scrubbing period, and then is allowed to dry for at least 30 seconds before the procedure. Any solution should be completely removed after the procedure using sterile water or saline solution to prevent any further absorption. Disinfection with isopropyl alcohol is questionable in the NICU, because it is less effective than either povidone-iodine or chlorhexidine and can be irritating and drying to skin surfaces.

Use of disinfectants for umbilical cord care is debatable. The use of antibiotic ointments and antiseptics can prolong the time to cord separation, and it seems to have no beneficial effect on the frequency of infection.[5,55,114] A study of 1811 newborns randomized to receive either routine isopropyl alcohol with each diaper change or natural drying found no umbilical infections in either group, and time to cord separation was reduced from 9.8 days in the alcohol-treated group to 8.16 days in the natural-drying group.[31] Therefore routine use of

alcohol for cord care is not helpful in facilitating cord separation or reducing risk of infection.

Adhesive Application and Removal

One of the most common practices in the NICU is the application and removal of adhesives that secure endotracheal tubes, IV devices, and monitoring probes and electrodes. **A research utilization project involving 2820 premature and term newborns found that adhesives were the primary cause of skin breakdown among NICU patients.**[74] Changes in TEWL and skin barrier function are seen in adults after 10 consecutive removals of adhesive tape[68] and after one removal of adhesive tape in premature infants.[45] Types of damage from adhesive removal include epidermal stripping, tearing, maceration, tension blisters, chemical irritation, sensitization, and folliculitis.[49]

Solvents are sometimes used to prevent discomfort and skin disruption from adhesive removal. They contain hydrocarbon derivatives or petroleum distillates that have potential or proven toxicities. Toxicity is a major concern, especially in premature infants with their underdeveloped stratum corneum, increased skin permeability, larger surface area/body weight ratio, and immature hepatic and renal function. A case report of toxic epidermal necrosis in a premature infant resulted from the use of a solvent.[53] **Mineral oil or petrolatum products may be helpful in removing adhesives but cannot be used if the site must be used again for reapplication of adhesives, such as with the retaping of an endotracheal tube.**

Skin bonding agents promote adherence. Unfortunately, they may create a stronger bond between adhesive and epidermis than the fragile cohesion of the epidermis to the dermis; when the adhesive is removed, epidermal stripping may result. Plastic polymers have been studied and are reported to reduce skin trauma.[35] An alcohol-free skin protectant is available that is less irritating to skin surfaces in adults than comparable products containing alcohol.[44] This product has been approved for infants over 30 days of age to treat mild diaper dermatitis and to prevent skin injury from adhesive removal.[104] Although a single study from England reports positive effects when using this skin protectant to tape intravenous lines in newborns,[52] it has not yet been approved for use in premature infants or term newborns in the United States.

Skin barriers such as karaya rings and pectin products have been used to protect the peristomal skin in adult ostomy patients. A comparison of regular adhesive electrodes and karaya electrodes found less skin disruption, as measured by TEWL, from the karaya electrodes in premature infants.[19] However, some premature infants developed skin irritation from the karaya electrodes, and they are no longer available. **Pectin barriers (Hollihesive, Duoderm, Comfeel) have been used beneath adhesives in premature infants and are reported to leave less visible skin trauma when removed.**[30,72,81] **However, a controlled trial of pectin barrier (Hollihesive), plastic tape (Transpore), and hydrophilic gelled adhesive found that significant skin disruption, as measured by TEWL and visual inspection, occurred after removal of both the pectin barrier and plastic tape.**[73] Because the adhesives were left in place 24 hours before removal in this study, there may be a time effect of peak adhesive aggressiveness that was reached. It is interesting to note that significant changes were identified after a single adhesive removal in all three weight groups studied (less than 1000 g, 1001 to 1500 g, and greater than 1501 g), indicating that even larger premature infants are at risk for skin injury from tape removal.

Prevention of skin trauma from adhesive removal includes minimizing tape use when possible by using smaller pieces, backing the adhesive with cotton, and delaying tape removal until adherence is reduced. Pectin barriers and hydrocolloid adhesives may prove helpful, because they mold and adhere well to body contours and often attach better in moist conditions. As with tape, removal of pectin barriers and hydrocolloid should be delayed, if possible, until the adherence lessens. The use of soft gauze wraps to secure probes and hydrogel ECG electrodes and hydrogel tapes are helpful. Adhesives should be removed slowly and carefully with warm water and cotton balls. Mineral oil or an emollient may facilitate adhesive removal if reapplication of adhesives at the site of removal is not necessary.

DATA COLLECTION

History

The gestational age and postnatal age of neonates in the NICU are both important considerations for determining appropriate skin care practices. Premature infants of lower gestational ages have underdeveloped skin layers and function. With advancing postnatal age and maturation, skin integrity and skin barrier function results.

Reviewing the maternal history for any dermatologic diseases is also important. Many of the most severe skin diseases, such as forms of congenital ichthyosis or epidermolysis bullosa, are inherited disorders. A positive family history will alert the clinician to the potential for developing these rare disorders.[6,51,64,66]

Signs and Symptoms

A thorough daily examination of all skin surfaces will reveal the state of skin integrity for neonates in the NICU. Early signs such as skin abrasions or small excoriations may call for either diagnostic or treatment procedures. A scoring tool, such as the Neonatal Skin Condition Score (NSCS) (Box 18-1), used in the AWHONN/NANN research-based practice project, may be beneficial when assessing skin condition.[70,74] **Identifying risk factors for skin injury for individual patients may include a gestational age of less than 32 weeks, edema, use of paralytic agents and vasopressors, multiple tubes and lines, numerous monitors, surgical wounds, ostomies, and technologies that limit patient movement such as high-frequency ventilation and extracorporeal membrane oxygenation (ECMO).** In the first week of life in ELBW infants (less than 30 weeks, under 1000 g), there may be problems with thermoregulation (see Chapter 6) and dehydration (see Chapter 14) because of the large evaporative heat losses and transepidermal water losses through the immature stratum corneum

Laboratory Data

With the many skin excoriations in both small and large neonates that result from traumatic events such as adhesive removal or pressure necrosis, there is the potential for infection through this portal of entry in the skin. In VLBW infants it may be useful to obtain a skin culture, Gram stain, or potassium hydroxide (KOH) preparation[8,9] for early detection of microorganisms that can lead to systemic illness in these immunocompromised patients. A skin surface culture is helpful if the skin breakdown cannot be traced to a traumatic injury, because the origin of the breakdown is often linked to infection, especially with fungal infections[96] or staphylococcal scalded skin syndrome. A more comprehensive workup for infection may be indicated if there is evidence of clinical deterioration in infants with extensive skin breakdown (see Chapter 22).

TREATMENT

Skin Excoriations

Skin excoriations are cleansed with warmed sterile water or half-normal saline solution; a 20- or 30-ml syringe with a Teflon IV catheter attached can be used to gently debride the excoriation. This technique is effective in flushing out debris and dead tissue from an infected or "dirty" wound, allowing a better surface for healing. Moistening the tissue every 4 to 6 hours aids the healing process, because drying of tissue actually impedes the migration of cells. Once the wound surface is clear, other dressings or ointments can be used.

Ointments are sometimes used because of their antibacterial or antifungal properties and also because covering the wound with a semiocclusive layer promotes healing by facilitating the migration of epithelial cells across the surface. Only if extensive bacterial colonization is suspected, Polysporin, Bacitracin, or Bactroban ointment is used sparingly every 8 to 12 hours. Many dermatologists do not recommend the use of Neosporin because of the potential for developing later sensitization to this ointment, although sensitization to Bacitracin is being reported with increasing frequency.[80] Overuse of antimicrobial ointments can be a problem in promoting more resistant strains of

Box 18-1	THE NEONATAL SKIN CONDITION SCORE (NCSC)

Dryness

1 = Normal, no sign of dry skin
2 = Dry skin, visible scaling
3 = Very dry skin, cracking/fissures

Erythema

1 = No evidence erythema
2 = Visible erythema <50% body surface
3 = Visible erythema >50% body surface

Breakdown

1 = None evident
2 = Small localized areas
3 = Extensive

NOTE: Perfect score = 3; worst score = 9.

From Lund CH, Osborne JW, Kuller J et al: *Neonatal skin care: clinical outcomes for the AWHONN/NANN evidence based clinical practice,* Washington DC, 2001, Association of Women's Health, Obstetric, and Neonatal Nurses.

bacteria. If fungal infection is suspected, Nystatin ointment is used, and it can also be applied to surrounding intact skin to prevent extension of the infection. In general, ointments are preferable to creams in this application because of better adherence and healing properties.

Transparent adhesive dressings are made from a polyurethane film backed with adhesive that is impermeable to water and bacteria but allows air flow. There must be a rim of intact skin around the wound to attach the dressing. Uses include wound care, dressings for IV devices including central venous lines and percutaneous silicone catheters, and prevention of friction injuries to areas such as the knees or sacrum.

When used for wound care, transparent adhesive dressing promotes "moist healing" that allows the rapid migration of epithelial cells across the site. These dressings should only be used on "clean" (uninfected) wounds since bacteria and fungus can proliferate under the dressing. When placed over a clean wound, there is often a serous or milky exudate that forms that is composed of leukocytes that actually aid in the prevention of infection. The dressings can be left in place for days at a time or until they become loose. Removing and reattaching the dressings on a daily basis is not recommended since the adhesive can injure the intact skin around the wound and further impede healing.

Another use of transparent adhesive dressings in the NICU is the prevention of excessive TEWL in premature infants.[16,59,78,108] **TEWL, as measured by an evaporimeter, can be reduced by as much as 50% by the creation of this "second skin."** In one study[78] a nonadherent transparent dressing (not commercially available) was used, and the skin under the dressing not only had a lower TEWL while covered but actually had lower TEWL when removed, suggesting that perhaps a faster maturation of the skin barrier function had occurred. Cultures were obtained both on covered and uncovered skin and showed no increase in either bacterial or fungal colonization under the dressings. Unfortunately, nonadherent dressings are not commercially available, and transparent adhesive dressings can cause a significant amount of skin trauma when removed. Alternative ways to reduce TEWL in VLBW infants can be used, including double-walled incubators, heated humidity (see Chapter 6), and emollients such as Aquaphor ointment.

Other types of dressings used in wound management include hydrogel dressings (Vigilon) and hy-drocolloid, pectin dressings (Duoderm), both of which promote moist healing.[61,69] Hydrogel dressings can be used after irrigation of the wound and in conjunction with either antibacterial or antifungal ointment if the wound is infected. These dressings must be changed every 8 to 12 hours, because they can dry out. There is no adhesive that attaches these dressings. It is best to avoid placing hydrogel dressings on intact skin surfaces, because they can macerate the skin and actually reduce barrier function. Hydrocolloid dressings are used over uninfected wounds and can be left in place for 5 to 7 days while healing takes place.

Surgical wounds that open or dehisce are infrequent but require expert wound management. Nutrition is often a part of the process in getting these wounds to heal, as is the prevention of infection.[41] Often the surgeon or an enterostomal therapist will design the appropriate wound management program for these situations.

Intravenous Extravasations

Prevention of tissue injury from IV extravasations includes taping IV devices with transparent dressings or plastic tape so that the insertions site is clearly visible (Figure 18-5) and observing the site with appropriate documentation every hour. If the IV device is placed in a limb, the tape that secures it to the rigid board should be placed loosely over a bony prominence, such as the elbow or knee, and not on skin in close proximity to the insertion site. This allows extravasated fluid and medications to expand over a larger surface and not remain in a small, constricted area, which can result in greater tissue injury. It may be wise to avoid poorly perfused extremities in favor of scalp veins, except the forehead. Using central venous lines such as percutaneous catheters to infuse highly irritating solutions and medications is also recommended. Many nurseries limit the glucose concentrations in peripheral lines to 12.5% and the amino acid concentrations to 2%; calcium and potassium concentrations are also more dilute than those used in central lines.

If IV fluid has extravasated into surrounding tissue, the IV device should be removed and the extremity elevated. Use of moisture, heat, or cold is not recommended, because the tissue is vulnerable at this point to further injury.[13] Hyaluronidase (Wydase) can be extremely helpful if administered within an hour of extravasation (see Chapter 9). This medication is an enzyme that

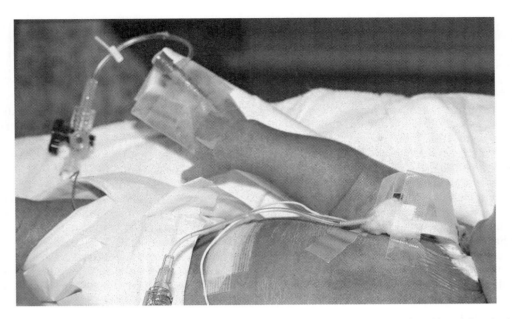

FIGURE 18-5   An appropriately taped peripheral intravenous catheter with the insertion site clearly visible and the infant's arm anchored at the joint to prevent obstruction of venous return.

causes a breakdown of interstitial barrier and allows the diffusion of the extravasated fluid over a larger area to prevent tissue necrosis.[63,95,110] The dose of hyaluronidase is 15 U diluted to 1 ml, although in one study using an animal model, 150 U was used without harmful effects.[63] It is administered in five injections, inserted subcutaneously around the periphery of the extravasation site (Figure 18-6), and should be administered within 1 to 2 hours of the extravasation. **Extravasations that may benefit from administration of hyaluronidase include any with evidence of blanching, discoloration, or blistering, or extravasations involving hypertonic or calcium-containing solutions, even if the site appears relatively undisturbed.** Calcium-containing solutions may cause deep tissue injury even when epidermal tissues are not involved. If hyaluronidase is not available, multiple puncture holes over the area of swelling and gently squeezing or letting the extravasated fluid leak out can facilitate the removal of the infiltrate and prevent skin sloughs.[23]

Hyaluronidase is not recommended in the extravasation of vasoconstrictive medications such as dopamine, because the vasoconstriction could extend with its use. Phentolamine (Regitine) is used in this case, because it directly counteracts the action

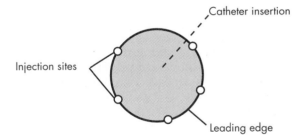

FIGURE 18-6   Technique for administration of both hyaluronidase (Wydase) and phentolamine (Regitine). A total volume of 1 ml is administered at five sites subcutaneously (0.2 ml each) around the periphery of the intravenous extravasation.

of dopamine. The method of delivery is the same as for hyalurondiase, with the total dose (0.5 mg) diluted to 1 ml, injected in five sites subcutaneously around the periphery of the extravasation.[111]

When tissue injury occurs after extravasation, covering the wound with ointment and petrolatum gauze will facilitate healing. For deeper wounds, irrigation in conjunction with either ointments or dressings may be used. In the most severe cases, surgical or plastic surgical consultation is necessary, and skin grafts may be required. In all cases of tissue injury, open wounds should be considered a portal of entry for infection, and topical or systemic treatment should be considered.

Diaper Dermatitis

Diaper dermatitis, which has a multitude of causes in infants, affects the perineum, groin, thighs, buttocks, and anal regions. The underlying skin condition of the infant contributes to the degree of diaper dermatitis that occurs.

Another factor that influences the development of diaper dermatitis is the degree of wetness of the skin, because skin that is moist and macerated becomes more permeable and susceptible to injury.[11,12] In addition, skin that is moisture laden becomes more heavily colonized with microorganisms. Skin pH also has an effect; when the skin is exposed to urine, the pH can rise from acid to alkaline ranges and tissues become more vulnerable to injury and penetration by microorganisms.[12,65] The alkaline pH can also activate enzymes found in stool, protease, and lipase, which break down protein and fat, the building blocks of the stratum corneum.[15] This is the primary mechanism for direct contact dermatitis from exposure to stool, the most common form of diaper dermatitis.

Strategies for preventing diaper dermatitis include maintaining a skin surface that is dry and has a normal (acidic) skin pH. Superabsorbent gelled diapers have been introduced that keep skin surfaces dry by "wicking" the moisture away from the skin.[18,27] Use of powders is discouraged because of the risk of inhalation of particles into the respiratory tract.

After skin injury from diaper dermatitis has occurred, protecting injured skin to prevent reinjury is the primary goal of treatment. Generous application of protective skin barriers that contain zinc oxide can prevent further injury while allowing skin to heal. Once skin excoriations occur, keeping skin open to air may not be effective, because the already impaired tissue may be reinjured with fecal contact, and dryness is counterproductive to healing. It is not necessary or desirable to completely remove skin barrier products with diaper changes, because this may disrupt healing tissue. Instead, remove as much waste material as possible and reapply the barrier generously to the affected areas with each diaper change.

If _Candida albicans_ is involved in the diaper dermatitis, it is necessary to use an antifungal ointment or cream. Antifungal preparations include Mycostatin, miconazole, chlortrimazole, and ketoconozale in ointment, cream, or powder forms. If the dermatitis is both fungal and a contact irritant dermatitis, it may be necessary to layer the ointment with the antifungal preparation.

Occasionally infants may experience extremely severe diaper dermatitis from intestinal malabsorption syndromes or if there is constant dribbling of stool, as in the case of infants with spina bifida. In the case of malabsorption, the stool may have a pH that is higher than normal because of rapid transit through the small intestine, and there may be significant amounts of undigested carbohydrates and stool enzymes, as well as increased stool frequency. Severe diaper dermatitis in this case can be a symptom of a more severe nutritional deficiency, or even dehydration, and needs thorough medical evaluation. Stools in these infants should be regularly tested for pH, carbohydrates, and occult blood, in addition to measuring their number and total volume.

While optimal nutritional therapy is being addressed with special diets or parenteral nutrition, skin protection from injury should be initiated. Products such as pectin-based powders or pectin paste without alcohol (such as Ilex, a nonalcohol pectin paste) are often better barriers for these infants than zinc oxide preparations are. The skin should be thoroughly cleansed before a very thick application of the pectin paste. It is then necessary to apply a greasy ointment over this, because the pectin-based paste may adhere to the diaper. When the infant has a stool, it is not necessary to completely remove the barrier paste; the stool can be wiped away as much as possible before reapplying the thick paste barrier. The skin will heal under this protective covering as long as it is protected from reinjury.[69] If fungal infection is a component of the dermatitis, antifungal therapy must be instituted in addition to the protective barriers. In this case, Mycostatin powder attached with alcohol-free skin protectant is the first layer, then the barrier cream is applied.

COMPLICATIONS

Improper handling of newborn skin (and injudicious use of products) can cause damage, prevent healing, and interfere with normal maturation processes. Compromised skin integrity can lead to infection, pain and discomfort, and diversion of calories for tissue repair. Other dangers include toxicity from topically applied substances that are readily ab-

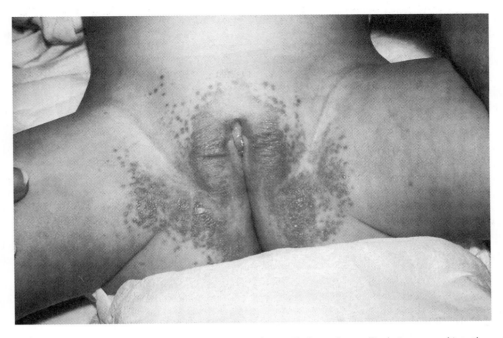

FIGURE 18-7   Diaper dermatitis caused by a *Candida albicans* infection. Red pustular satellite lesions extend into the periphery.

sorbed by small infants with a large surface area/ body weight ratio as well as immature renal and hepatic function that cannot detoxify chemicals readily.

Injury from infiltrated IV solutions can cause skin injury and occasionally deep tissue necrosis with both muscle and nerve damage. Factors that increase the risk of injury from IV extravasations include length of time between extravasation and treatment; hypertonic solutions, such as those with high calcium, potassium, amino acid, or glucose solutions; medications such as nafcillin that are irritating to veins; and the use of mechanical pumps for infusions. There may be an added risk for injury in patients with poor perfusion to extremities and in limbs that have been secured with restricting adhesives that obstruct venous return.

If the epidermis has been injured, it can easily become a portal of entry for infection. Thus a contact irritant diaper dermatitis can progress to a fungal or staphylococcal infection. *Staphylococcus aureus* can cause pustule formation at hair follicles and is a rare complication of diaper dermatitis. The mechanism for fungal diaper dermatitis is still debated. Some researchers believe that *Candida albicans* is a secondary invasion to skin that has been previously injured, whereas others see this organism as a primary cause of skin disruption.[94]

Candida albicans diaper dermatitis causes an intense inflammation that is bright red and sharply demarginated in the inguinal folds, buttocks, thighs, abdomen, and genitalia, often with satellite lesions that extend the rash over the trunk (Figure 18-7). *Candida albicans* can be harbored in the gastrointestinal tract, necessitating oral therapy if lesions are found in the mouth.

PARENT TEACHING

It is the responsibility of professionals to teach parents informally during caregiving procedures such as bathing, cord care, and diaper changes and to prepare written materials regarding appropriate skin care practices for their infant after discharge from the NICU. Parents will need education about the normal mechanisms of cord healing, including the range of appearance in umbilical cords, because some cords can appear very moist and soggy. The cord can be cleansed with water if it becomes soiled with urine or stool.[7] Inform parents that minimal use of skin care products is optimal, and may reduce the incidence of contact sensitization to chemicals.[14,21,79] It is also extremely useful to educate parents about the mechanisms that are involved in diaper dermatitis so that prevention is stressed and appropriate interventions are selected depending on the underlying cause.

Developmental differences in the anatomy and physiology of neonatal skin affect skin integrity for term and premature infants in the NICU. Prevention is the primary focus of care, and decisions about the best way to provide basic skin care and hygiene based on current research are essential for care providers, both professionals and parents.

REFERENCES

1. Agren J, Sjors G, Sedin G: Transepidermal water loss in infants born at 24 and 25 weeks of gestation, *Acta Paediatr* 87:1185, 1998.
2. Als H, Lawhon G, Brown E et al: Individualized behavioral and environmental care for the very low birth weight preterm infant at high risk for bronchopulmonary dysplasia: neonatal intensive care unit and developmental outcome, *Pediatrics* 78:1123, 1986.
3. American Academy of Pediatrics: *Red book: report of the committee on infectious diseases,* ed 24, Elk Grove Village, Ill, 1997, The Academy.
4. Anderson GM, Lane A, Chang H: Axillary temperature in transitional newborn infants before and after tub bath, *Appl Nurs Res* 8:123, 1995.
5. Arad I, Eyal F, Fainmesser P: Umbilical cord care: a study of bacitracin ointment vs. triple dye, *Arch Dis Child* 56:887-888, 1981.
6. Artnak K, Moore L, Clements C: Epidermolysis bullosa: an inherited skin disorder, *Am J Nurs* 81:1837, 1981.
7. Association of Women's Health, Obstetric and Neonatal Nurses: *Evidence-based clinical practice guideline: neonatal skin care,* Washington, DC, 2001, AWHONN.
8. Baley J, Silverman R: Systemic candidiasis: cutaneous manifestations in low birth weight infants, *Pediatrics* 82:211, 1988.
9. Baley J, Kliegman RM, Boxerbaum B et al: Fungal colonization in the very low birth weight infant, *Pediatrics* 78:225, 1986.
10. Behrendt H, Green M: *Patterns of skin pH from birth through adolescence,* Springfield, Ill, 1971, Charles C Thomas.
11. Berg R: Etiologic factors in diaper dermatitis: a model for development of improved diapers, *Pediatrician* 14:27, 1987.
12. Berg R, Buckingham K, Stewart R: Etiologic factors in diaper dermatitis: the role of urine, *Pediatr Dermatol* 3:102, 1986.
13. Brown A, Hoelzer D, Piercy S: Skin necrosis from extravasation of intravenous fluids in children, *Plast Reconstr Surg* 64:145, 1979.
14. Bruckner A, Weston W, Morelli J: Does sensitization to contact allergens begin in infancy? *Pediatrics* 105:E3, 2000.
15. Buckingham K, Berg R: Etiologic factors in diaper dermatitis: the role of feces, *Pediatr Dermatol* 3:107, 1986.
16. Bustamante S, Steslow J: Use of a transparent adhesive dressing in very low birth weight infants, *J Perinatol* 9:165, 1989.
17. Campbell J, Zaccaria E, Baker C: Systemic candidiasis in extremely low birth weight infants receiving topical petrolatum ointment for care: a case control study, *Pediatrics* 105:1041, 2000.
18. Campbell R, Seymour JL, Stone LC et al: Clinical studies with disposable diapers containing absorbent gelling materials: evaluation on infant skin condition, *J Am Acad Dermatol* 17:978, 1987.
19. Cartlidge P, Rutter N: Karaya gum electrocardiographic electrodes for preterm infants, *Arch Dis Child* 62:1281, 1987.
20. Centers for Disease Control: Leads from the MMWR. Update: universal precautions for prevention of transmission of human immunodeficiency virus, hepatitis B virus, and other bloodborne pathogens in health care settings, *JAMA* 260:462, 1988.
21. Cetta F, Lambert G, Ros S: Newborn chemical exposure from over-the-counter skin care products, *Clin Pediatr* 30:286, 1991.
22. Chabrolle J, Rossier A: Goiter and hypothyroidism in the newborn after cutaneous absorption of iodine, *Arch Dis Child* 53:495, 1978.
23. Chandavasu O, Garrow E, Valsa V et al: A new method for the prevention of skin sloughs and necrosis secondary to intravenous infiltration, *Am J Perinatol* 3:4, 1986.
24. Choudhuri J, McQueen R, Inoue S et al: Efficacy of skin sterilization for a venipuncture with the use of commercially available alcohol or iodine pads, *Am J Infect Control* 18:82, 1990.
25. Cowen J, Ellis S, McAinsh J: Absorption of chlorhexidine from the intact skin of newborn infants, *Arch Dis Child* 54:379, 1979.
26. Davies J, Babb J, Ayliffe A: The effect on the skin flora of bathing with antiseptic solutions, *J Antimicrob Chemother* 3:473, 1977.
27. Davis J, Leyden J, Grove G et al: Comparison of disposable diapers with fluff absorbent and fluff plus absorbent polymers: effects on skin hydration, skin pH, and diaper dermatitis, *Pediatr Dermatol* 6:102, 1989.
28. Dietel K: Morphological and functional development of the skin. In Stave U, ed: *Perinatal physiology,* New York, 1978, Plenum Press.
29. Dixon A: Think zinc, *Neonatal Netw* 5:29, 1987.

30. Dollison E, Beckstrand J: Adhesive tape vs. pectin-based barrier use in preterm infants, *Neonatal Netw* 14:35, 1995.

31. Dore S, Buchan D, Coulas S et al: Alcohol versus natural drying for newborn cord care, *J Obstet Gyencol Neonatal Nurs* 27:621-627, 1998.

32. Edwards W, Conner J, Gerdes J, Hoath S et al: The effect of Aquaphor emollient ointment on nosocomial sepsis rates and skin integrity in infants of birthweights 501-1000 grams. Paper presented at the Hot Topics Neonatology Conference, Washington, DC, December 2000.

33. Esterly N, Spraker M: Neonatal skin problems. In Moschella S, Hurley H, eds: *Dermatology,* vol 2, ed 2, Philadelphia, 1985, WB Saunders.

34. Evans N, Rutter N: Development of the epidermis in the newborn, *Biol Neonate* 49:74, 1986.

35. Evans N, Rutter N: Reduction of skin damage from transcutaneous oxygen electrodes using a spray on dressing, *Arch Dis Child* 61:881, 1986.

36. Fox C, Nelson D, Wareham J: The timing of skin acidification in very low birth weight infants, *J Perinatol* 18:272-275, 1998.

37. Franck L, Quinn D, Zahr L: Effect of less frequent bathing of preterm infants on skin flora and pathogen colonization, *J Obstet Gyencol Neonatal Nurs* 29:584, 2000.

38. Friedman Z: Essential fatty acids revisited, *Am J Dis Child* 134:397, 1980.

39. Frosch PJ, Kligman AM: The soap chamber test, *J Am Acad Dermatol* 1:35, 1979.

40. Garland J, Buck R, Maloney P: Comparison of 10% povidone-iodine and 0.5% chlorhexidine gluconate for the prevention of peripheral intravenous catheter colonization in neonates: a prospective trial, *Pediatr Infect Dis J* 14:510-516, 1995.

41. Garvin G: Wound healing in pediatrics, *Nurs Clin North Am* 25:181, 1990.

42. Gordon C, Rowitch D, Mitchell M et al: Topical iodine and neonatal hypothyroidism, *Arch Pediatr Adolesc Med* 149:1336, 1995.

43. Gfatter R, Hackl P, Braun F: Effects of soap and detergents on skin surface pH, stratum corneum hydration and fat content in infants, *Dermatology* 195:258, 1997.

44. Grove G, Leydon J: Comparison of the skin protectant properties of various film-forming products, Broomall, Pa, 1993, Sin Study Center, KLG, Inc.

45. Harpin V, Rutter N: Barrier properties of the newborn infant's skin, *J Pediatr* 102:419, 1983.

46. Harpin V, Rutter N: Percutaneous alcohol absorption and skin necrosis in a preterm infant, *Arch Dis Child* 57:825, 1982.

47. Holbrook KA: A histological comparison of infant and adult skin. In Maibach HI, Boisits EK, eds: *Neonatal skin: structure and function,* New York, 1982, Marcel Dekker.

48. Hoath S, Narendran V, Visscher M: The biology and role of vernix, *Newborn Infant Nurs Rev* 1:53, 2001.

49. Hoath S, Narendran V: Adhesives and emollients in the preterm infant, *Semin Neonatol* 5:112, 2000.

50. Hunt C, Engel RR, Modler S et al: Essential fatty acid deficiency in neonates: inability to reverse deficiency by topical applications of EFA-rich oil, *J Pediatr* 92:603, 1978.

51. Hymes D: Epidermolysis bullosa in the neonate, *Neonatal Netw* 1:36, 1983.

52. Irving V: Reducing the risk of epidermal stripping in the neonatal population: an evaluation of an alcohol free barrier film, *J Neonatal Nurs* 7:5, 2001.

53. Ittman P, Bozynski ME: Toxic epidermal necrolysis in a newborn infant after exposure to adhesive remover, *J Perinatol* 13:476, 1993.

54. Jackson H, Sutherland R: Effect of povidine-iodine on neonatal thyroid function, *Lancet* 2:992, 1981.

55. Johnson J, Malachowshi N, Vosti K et al: A sequential study of various modes of skin and umbilical care and the incidence of staphylcoccal colonization and infection in the neonate, *Pediatrics* 58:354, 1976.

56. Kalia Y, Nonato L, Lund C et al: Development of the skin barrier function in premature infants, *J Invest Dermatol* 111:320, 1998.

57. Karl D: The interactive newborn bath: using infant behavior to connect parents and newborns, *Am J Matern Child Nurs* 24:280-286, 1999.

58. Klaus MH, Fanaroff AA: *Yearbook of perinatal/ neonatal medicine,* Chicago, 1987, Year Book.

59. Knauth A, Gordin M, McNelis W et al: Semipermeable polyurethane membrane as an artificial skin for the premature neonate, *Pediatrics* 83:945, 1989.

60. Kopelman AE: Cutaneous absorption of hexachlorophene in low-birth-weight infants, *J Pediatr* 82:972, 1973.

61. Krasner D, Kennedy K, Rolstad B: The ABCs of wound care dressings, *Ostomy Wound Manage* 39:68, 1993.

62. Lane A, Drost S: Effects of repeated application of emollient cream to premature neonates' skin, *Pediatrics* 92:415, 1993.

63. Laurie S, Wilson K, Kernahan D et al: Intravenous extravasation injuries: the effectiveness of hyaluronidase in their treatment, *Ann Plast Surg* 13:191, 1984.

64. Lawlor F: Progress of a Harlequin fetus to nonbullous ichthyosiform erythroderma, *Pediatrics* 82:870, 1988.

65. Leydon J: Urinary ammonia and ammonia-producing micro-organisms in infants with and without diaper dermatitis, *Arch Dermatol* 113:1678, 1977.

66. Lin A, Carter DM: Epidermolysis bullosa: when the skin falls apart, *J Pediatr* 114:349, 1989.

67. Linder N, Davidovich N, Reichman B et al: Topical iodine-containing antiseptics and subclinical hypothyroidism in preterm infants, *J Pediatr* 131:434, 1997.

68. Lo J, Oriba H, Maibach H et al: Transepidermal potassium, ion, and water flux across delipidized and cellophane tape-stripped skin, *Dermatologica* 180:66, 1990.

69. Lund C: Prevention and management of infant skin breakdown, *Nurs Clin North Am* 34:907, 1999.

70. Lund C, Kuller J, Lane A et al: Neonatal skin care: evaluation of the AWHONN/NANN research-based practice project on knowledge and skin care practices, *J Obstet Gyencol Neonatal Nurs* 30:30, 2001.

71. Lund C, Kuller J, Lane A et al: Neonatal skin care: the scientific basis for practice, *J Obstet Gyencol Neonatal Nurs* 28:241, 1999.

72. Lund C, Kuller JM, Tobin C et al: Evaluation of a pectin-based barrier under tape to protect neonatal skin, *J Obstet Gynecol Neonat Nurs* 15:39, 1986.

73. Lund C, Nonato L, Kuller J et al: Disruption of barrier function in neonatal skin associated with adhesive removal, *J Pediatr* 131:367, 1997.

74. Lund C, Osborne J, Kuller J et al: Neonatal skin care: clinical outcomes of the AWHONN/NANN evidence-based clinical practice guideline, *J Obstet Gyencol Neonatal Nurs* 30:41, 2001.

75. Maki D, Ringer M, Alvarado C: Prospective randomized trial povidone-iodine, alcohol, and chlorhexidine for prevention of infection associated with central venous and arterial catheters, *Lancet* 338: 339, 1991.

76. Malathi I, Millar M, Leeming et al: Skin disinfection in preterm infants, *Arch Dis Child* 69:312, 1993.

77. Malloy-McDonald M: Skin care for high-risk neonates, *J Wound Ostomy Continence Nurs* 22: 177, 1995.

78. Mancini A, Sookdeo-Drost S, Madison K et al: Semipermeable dressings improve epidermal barrier function in premature infants, *Pediatr Res* 36:306, 1994.

79. Manzini B, Ferdani G, Simonetti V et al: Contact sensitization in children, *Pediatr Dermatol* 15:12, 1998.

80. Marks J, Belsito D, DeLeo V, Fowler J et al: North American Contact Dermatitis Group: standard tray patch test results, *Am J Contact Derm* 6:160, 1995.

81. McLean S, Kirchoff KT, Kriynovich K et al: Three methods of securing endotracheal tubes in neonates: a comparison, *Neonatal Netw* 11:17, 1992.

82. Mitchell I, Pollock JC, Jamieson MP et al: Transcutaneous iodine absorption in infants undergoing cardiac operation, *Ann Thorac Surg* 52:1138, 1991.

83. Mimoz O, Karim A, Mercat A et al: Chlorhexidine compared with povidone-iodine as skin preparation before blood culture, *Ann Intern Med* 131:834, 1999.

84. Mize M, Vila-Coro A, Prager T: The relationship between postnatal skin maturation and electrical skin impedance, *Arch Dermatol* 125:647, 1989.

85. Moore K: *The developing human,* ed 4, Philadelphia, 1988, WB Saunders.

86. Morelli J, Weston W: Soaps and shampoos in pediatric practice, *Pediatrics* 80:634, 1987.

87. Nonato L: Evolution of skin barrier function in neonates. Unpublished doctoral dissertation, 1998, University of California: Berkeley, Calif, UMI Publication Number AAT9827176.

88. Nopper A, Horii K, Sookdeo-Drost S et al: Topical ointment therapy benefits premature infants, *J Pediatr* 128:660, 1996.

89. Parravicini E, Fontana C, Paterlini G et al: Iodine, thyroid function, and very low birth weight infants, *Pediatrics* 98:730, 1996.

90. Peck S, Botwinick J: The buffering capacity of infants' skin against an alkaline soap and neutral detergent, *J Mt Sinai Hosp* 31:134, 1964.

91. Penny-MacGillivray T: A newborn's first bath: when? *J Obstet Gyencol Neonatal Nurs* 25:481, 1996.

92. Peters K: Bathing premature infants: physiological and behavioral consequences, *Am J Crit Care* 7:90, 1998.

93. Pyati SP, Ramamurthy RS, Krauss MT et al: Absorption of iodine in the neonate following topical use of povidone-iodine, *J Pediatr* 91:825, 1977.

94. Rasmussen J: Classification of diaper dermatitis: an overview, *Pediatrician* 14:6, 1987.

95. Raszka W, Kueser T, Smith F et al: The use of hyaluronidase in the treatment of intravenous extravasation injuries, *J Perinatol* 10:146-149, 1990.

96. Rowen JL, Atkins JT, Levy ML et al: Invasive fungal dermatitis in the < or = 1000-gram neonate, *Pediatrics* 95:682, 1995.

97. Saijo S, Tagami H: Dry skin of newborn infants: functional analysis of the stratum corneum, *Pediatr Dermatol* 8:155, 1991.

98. Sarkany I, Arnold L: The effect of single and repeated applications of hexachlorophene on the bacterial flora of the skin of the newborn, *Br J Dermatol* 82:261, 1970.

99. Schick JB, Milstein JM: Burn hazard of isopropyl alcohol in the neonate, *Pediatrics* 68:587, 1981.

100. Sedin G et al: Measurements of transepidermal water loss in newborn infants, *Clin Perinatol* 12:79, 1985.

101. Shalita A: *Principles of infant skin care,* Skillman, NJ, 1981, Johnson & Johnson.

102. Smerdely P et al: Topical iodine-containing antiseptics and neonatal hypothyroidism in very-low-birth weight infants, *Lancet* 16:661, 1989.

103. Solomon L, Esterly N: Neonatal dermatology. In Schaffer A, ed: *Major problems in clinical pediatrics,* vol 9, Philadelphia, 1973, WB Saunders.

104. 3M Health Care: *3M Cavilon No Sting Barrier Film* (brochure), St Paul, Minn, 2001, 3M.
105. Tupker RA, Pinnagoda J, Nater JP: The transient and cumulative effect of sodium lauryl sulphate on the epidermal barrier assessed by transepidermal water loss: inter-individual variation, *Acta Derm Venererol* 70:1, 1990.
106. Tupker RA, Pinnagoda J, Coenraads PJ et al: Evaluation of detergent-induced irritant skin reactions by visual scoring and transepidermal water loss measurement, *Dermatol Clin* 8:33, 1990.
107. Varda K, Behnke R: The effect of timing of initial bath on newborn's temperature, *J Obstet Gyencol Neonatal Nurs* 29:27, 2000.
108. Vernon H, Lane AT, Wischerath LJ et al: Semipermeable dressing and transepidermal water loss in premature infants, *Pediatrics* 86:357, 1990.
109. Wilhelm K, Maibach H: Factors predisposing to cutaneous irritation, *Dermatol Clin* 8:17, 1990.
110. Zenk K: Management of intravenous extravasations, *Infusion* 5:77, 1981.
111. Zenk K, Sills J: Management of dopamine-induced perivascular blanching and extravasation in LBW infants, *J Perinatol* 6:82, 1986.
112. Zimmerman A: Acrodermatitis in breast-fed premature infants: evidence for a defect in mammary gland zinc secretion, *Pediatrics* 69:176, 1982.
113. Zlotkin S, Buchanan B: Meeting zinc and copper intake requirements in the parenterally fed preterm and full-term infant, *J Pediatr* 103:441, 1983.
114. Zupan J, Garner P: Topical umbilical cord care at birth, *Cochrane Database Syst Rev* 2:CD001057, 2000.

Human milk has been recognized as the gold standard for human infants for centuries. Published studies from 1918 on have confirmed that problems develop when human milk is replaced with artificial formulas made from the milk of other species. Milk of other species that is fed to human infants has been known to contribute to increased infant mortality. Over the years increasing research has confirmed the presence of the antiinfective properties of human milk, which provide protection against infections of the gastrointestinal tract, the upper and lower respiratory tracts, and the urinary tract, as well as against, otitis media, bacteremia, bacterial meningitis, botulism, and necrotizing enterocolitis (NEC).* In numerous studies human milk has also been shown to have a protective effect against sudden infant death syndrome (SIDS), insulin-dependent diabetes, Crohn's disease, ulcerative colitis, lymphoma, allergic diseases, and chronic digestive disorders.† In preterm infants, human milk provides both short- and long-term advantages (Table 19-1).

Because of a lack of experience and knowledge about breastfeeding, a new mother who is discharged early (24 to 48 hours) (see Chapter 5) from the hospital may find it challenging to initiate breastfeeding for her healthy newborn infant. The mother of a newborn with special needs, such as a preterm infant, a sick term newborn, or an infant with a congenital anomaly, may have even more difficulty in establishing breastfeeding because of the stress of separation and concerns about the infant's well-being. The tremendous benefits of providing human milk for all infants, but especially the premature, outweigh any apparent difficulties.

Healthy People 2010,[244] the health policy statement for the United States, states the following goal regarding breastfeeding: 75% of women breastfeeding in the early postpartum period, at least 50% still breastfeeding their infant at 6 months, and 25% breastfeeding at 1 year of age. In addition, a report published by the Institute of Medicine from the Subcommittee on Nutrition during Lactation,[104] the AAP Work Group on Breastfeeding,[5] and the U.S. Surgeon General's *Blueprint for Action on Breastfeeding*,[243] respectively, state: (1) that all infants in the United States should be breastfed, (2) that "human milk is uniquely superior for infant feeding," and (3) that "breastfeeding is the ideal method of feeding and nurturing infants."

The goal of this chapter is to give the health care provider the skill and knowledge to support the breastfeeding dyad, especially when it involves the neonate with special needs.

PHYSIOLOGY

Nutritional Value of Breast Milk

The components of breast milk vary with the (1) stage of lactation, (2) time of day, (3) sampling time during a feeding, and (4) maternal nutrition. In addition, there is variation among individuals.*

Colostrum is produced immediately at delivery and over 5 to 7 days, gradually changing to transitional and finally mature milk. It contains a higher ash content, including higher concentrations of sodium, potassium, chloride, protein, fat-soluble vitamins, and minerals than mature milk does. Colostrum has a lower fat content, especially of lauric and myristic acids, than mature milk does. This milk is

---

*References 5, 9, 11, 24, 47, 53, 57, 60, 129, 134, 190, 197, 249, 256.
†References 69, 75, 117, 137, 176, 204, 214, 225, 254.

*References 120, 127, 129, 183, 184, 208.

Table 19-1	ADVANTAGES OF BREASTFEEDING AND HUMAN MILK INTAKE FOR PRETERM INFANTS
BENEFIT	**COMMENT**
Protection from necrotizing enterocolitis (NEC)	Formula-fed infants developed NEC 6-10 times more often than infants receiving only human milk. Infants ≥30 weeks' gestation: incidence of NEC 20 times more in formula-fed than human milk–fed infants.[134,219] Lower incidence of intestinal perforations and less severity of NEC with human milk intake before NEC.[48a]
Protection from infection or sepsis	Lowered incidence and severity of infections in hospitalized LBW infants fed human milk.* Decreased protection if formula feeding added to human milk feedings.[244] Increased rehospitalizations: 7 for formula-fed compared with 0-1 for infants who are breastfed (both partially and completely).[84]
Increased feeding tolerance	Whey protein in human milk is more easily digested, which results in more rapid gastric emptying and less gastric residual.[30,73,238] Fat globule that provides optimal absorption.[10,219] It is possible to achieve complete enteral feedings by 6 weeks of age in VLBW infants fed own mother's milk (compared with VLBW infants fed donor milk or formula-fed).[135] Formula-fed infants: increased vomiting, gastric residuals, and longer time to achieve complete enteral feedings.[135]
Decreased risk of later allergy	Lower incidence of allergic symptoms (especially eczema) at 18 mo in human milk–fed preterm infants.[137]
Improved retinal function	Better retinal function, depending on omega-3 fatty acid concentration (found in human milk, but not previously in formula) in enteral feedings.[42,43,240] Less retinopathy of prematurity (ROP) and less severe ROP in human milk–fed compared with formula-fed infants.[101]
Improved neurocognitive development	Long-term advantages: higher intelligence quotients (IQ) at 7-8 yr of age[8,97,140] and better developmental outcomes at 18 mo of age.[136,141] Faster brainstem maturation—resulting in better control of breathing.[6]

Modified from Meier P, Brown L: Breastfeeding for mothers and low birth weight infants, *Nurs Clin North Am* 31:351, 1996.
*References 63, 101, 103, 216, 219, 221.

yellowish, thick, and rich in antibodies, has a specific gravity between 1.040 and 1.060, and contains 67 kcal/dl. Multiparas and women who have previously breastfed have more colostrum during the first few days than women who have not.

Transitional milk is produced between 7 and 10 days postpartum, remains high in protein and lower in fat, and has a dramatic increase in water content compared with colostrum. Among mothers, the high variability of transitional milk accounts for 67 to 75 kcal/dl.

Mature milk is produced after 10 days postpartum and contains 75 kcal/dl. By the second week of life, maternal milk production averages about 30 ml/hr (e.g., 750 to 800 ml/day).[183] During a feeding the relative content of protein and the absolute content of fat increase. Morning feedings have a higher fat content than afternoon and evening feedings. Foremilk is lower in fat than hindmilk. Severely malnourished mothers have been shown to produce less milk, and water-soluble vitamins may be affected by deficient diets, as may occur in strict vegetarians.

Human Milk Versus Cow's Milk

Cow's milk has significant differences from human milk. Cow's milk has 18 parts whey to 82 parts casein, whereas human milk has 60 parts whey to 40 parts casein. Casein is composed of proteins with ester-bound phosphate, high proline content, and low solubility at a pH of 4 to 5. Casein forms curd by combining with calcium caseinate and calcium phosphate. The cysteine and taurine content is low in cow's milk but high in human milk, whereas the methionine content is high in cow's milk and low in human milk (the human infant lacks the enzyme to digest methionine). Human milk also has lower aromatic amino acids, phenylalanine, and tyrosine. Human milk contains 6.8 g/dl of lactose, and cow's milk contains 4.9 g/dl of lactose. Sodium, phosphorus, calcium, magnesium, citrate, and total ash content are higher in cow's milk, but potassium and the calcium/phosphorus ratio are higher in human milk. Formula attempts to mimic human milk but still lacks cholesterol, omega-3 fatty acids, enzymes, antibodies, lactoferrin, and other protective antiinfective properties.

Human milk contains more iron than unsupplemented cow's milk but less iron than supplemented cow's milk. Only 10% of iron is absorbed from formula, whereas about 80% is absorbed from human milk. Iron in formula encourages the growth of *Escherichia coli* and inactivates lactoferrin. Cow's milk has a mean pH of 6.8, osmolality of 350 mOsm, and 221 mOsm renal osmolar load. Human milk has a mean pH of 7.1, osmolality of 286 mOsm, and 79 mOsm renal osmolar load.

Cow's milk forms curd much more easily and thus delays gastric emptying. The newborn cannot handle certain proteins well because of lack of specific enzymes required for metabolism. However, 95% of human milk protein is nutritionally available to term infants, whereas the gastrointestinal immaturity of the preterm infant enables four to six times higher daily losses of human milk protein.[120] Iron is more bioavailable in human milk, and iron absorption from human milk is more efficient, but cow's milk has a higher concentration of zinc and contains more fluorine than human milk. Human milk, however, contains a ligand specific to zinc absorption and has been used as a therapy for zinc deficiency (see Chapter 16 for other human milk components).

Preterm Versus Term Breast Milk

Significant evidence exists that there are many differences in the breast milk that a mother produces when she has a preterm infant compared with breast milk produced for a term infant: (1) there is increased protein content in preterm breast milk[13,14]; (2) the types of protein, predominantly whey, have a more physiologic balance of amino acids and contain many antiinfective properties; (3) the lipid content in preterm breast milk is more specific for the preterm neonate (i.e., an increased supply of medium- to intermediate-chain[74] fatty acids); and (4) lactose, the major carbohydrate in breast milk, has increased absorption in preterm infants (see Chapter 16 for a comparison of preterm and term breast milk).

The Immunologic Value of Breast Milk

Because human milk protects neonates through its many antiinfective properties, breastfed infants have decreased morbidity compared with bottlefed infants.* The main defense factors in human milk

---

*References 57, 72, 78, 89, 120, 182, 208.

are (1) antimicrobial agents, (2) antiinflammatory factors, and (3) immunomodulators and leukocytes.[72,208] In addition to providing protective agents, the components in human milk also modulate the development of the newborn's own immune functions.[89] Bioactive factors in human milk and their functions are listed in Table 19-2. Because the highest concentration of some of these factors is found in colostrum,[89,153,216] this early milk should be pumped, preserved, and fed to a neonate with special needs. Reduction of antiinfective activity occurs with the addition of formula but not breast milk fortifier to the diet.[128,138,189,221] Yet in one study, when infection and NEC were combined, preterm infants fed fortified breast milk had more infectious events than did a partial-supplement group.[138,217,221] Continued surveillance in the use of fortifiers is recommended.[217,221]

Normal Lactation

Breast development during pregnancy is stimulated by luteal and placental hormones, lactogen, prolactin, and chorionic gonadotropin.[182] Estrogen stimulates growth of the milk collection (ductal) system, whereas progesterone stimulates growth of the milk production system. There is great variation in breast growth during pregnancy, and it is unclear how much breast tissue is necessary to support full lactation. Many factors other than breast size affect milk production, such as stress and fatigue, both of which are increased when a preterm infant is born.

If a woman aborts as early as 16 weeks, her breasts will secrete colostrum. Therefore mothers are capable of breastfeeding any viable infant.

Estrogen and progesterone function as inhibitors to actual milk production. Therefore stimulation of the breast before delivery will not create milk. Once the infant and placenta are delivered, stimulation of the nipple becomes effective in producing milk.

Stimulating the nipple by the infant's sucking action causes an increase in the prolactin released in the bloodstream and induces the synthesis and release of oxytocin (Figure 19-1).[107,157] The amount of prolactin is directly related to the quantity and quality of nipple stimulation; because prolactin stimulates the synthesis and secretion of milk, the surges in prolactin levels are related to the quantity of milk. A decrease in the quality of stimulation causes a decrease in prolactin surges and thus a decrease in milk production.[184]

Adequate prolactin secretion controls the maintenance of milk supply. The sooner the infant nurses, the sooner the milk comes in and becomes established. Initially production of milk is on a more consistent basis, because the basal level of prolactin is very high immediately after birth. Maintenance of milk depends on adequate stimulation of the breast and removal of milk on a regular and frequent basis.[191] Initially a newborn needs to nurse for a longer time to stimulate milk production and letdown. As the infant grows, sucking becomes more efficient, with the infant stimulating sequential letdowns early in the nursing period, thereby shortening the length of nursing. Establishing a generous milk supply is critical in long-term maintenance. Research has demonstrated that for mothers who are separated from their infants, pumping both breasts simultaneously stimulates a higher prolactin surge with increased milk supply than single breast pumping.[1,93,179,259]

Table 19-2	BIOACTIVE FACTORS IN HUMAN MILK
COMPONENT	**FUNCTION**
Antibodies	
Secretory IgA (sIgA)	Attaches to mucosal epithelium of digestive tract, thus preventing attachment of pathogens[120,208]; sIgA against enteric, respiratory, and viral pathogens, as well as specific pathogens to which the mother has been exposed; highest concentration in colostrum, peaks during first 3-4 days postpartum, present in mature milk through first year of life[126,153,216]; antiallergic properties: inhibits absorption of macromolecular antigens from neonatal small intestine.
Major Nutrients	
Protein	
sIgA;IgM;IgG	Immune protection
Lactoferrin	Binds iron, thwarts growth of pathogens (e.g., bactericidal, antiviral), modulates cytokine function and is antiinflammatory; highest levels in colostrum; present in mature milk through first year of life.[72,120,208]
Lysozyme	Destroys pathogens (e.g., gram-positive and few gram-negative bacteria) by cell wall lysis; human milk contains 300 times the concentration in cow's milk; concentration increases with prolonged lactation.[208]
Casein	Inhibits microbial adhesion to mucous membranes of respiratory and gastrointestinal tracts. Promotes growth of *Lactobacillus bifidus,* the normal intestinal flora for breastfed infants, and inhibits pathogens; by one month of age, bifidobacterium level in infants fed human milk is 10 times that of formula-fed infants.
Fibronectin	Enhances antimicrobial activity of macrophages[72,208]; assists in repair of intestinal tissue damage by immune reactions.
Carbohydrate	
Oligosaccharides	Binds to microorganisms (microbial ligands), thus preventing pathogens from attaching to respiratory mucosal surfaces.[120,219]
Glycoconjugates Mucin; lactadherin	Microbial and viral ligands.[88,120,193]
Fat	
Free fatty acids (FFA)	Disrupt and destroy lipid-enveloped virus, bacteria, and protozoa.[88]
Minor Nutrients	
Nucleotides	Enhance T-cell maturation, antibody response to vaccines, intestinal maturation, repair after diarrhea and natural killer cell activity; promote growth of *Lactobicillus bifidus.*
Vitamins	
A, C, E	Antiinflammatory: scavenges oxygen radicals.

Modified from Hamosh B: Bioactive factors in human milk, *Pediatr Clin North Am* 48:69, 2001

Continued

Table 19-2	BIOACTIVE FACTORS IN HUMAN MILK—cont'd
COMPONENT	**FUNCTION**

Minor Nutrients—cont'd

Enzymes

Component	Function
Bile salt–dependent lipase	Production of FFA with antibacterial/protozoan activity.
Catalase	Antiinflammatory: degrades H_2O_2.
Glutathione peroxidase	Antiinflammatory: prevents lipid peroxidation.
Platelet-activating factor (PAF) acetylhydrolase	Degrades PAF, a potent cause of ulceration; protects against NEC.

Growth Factors

Component	Function
Epithelial growth factors	Enhances maturation of gut epithelial barrier, limiting penetration by foreign antigens, thus decreasing immune stimulation.[208]
Transforming growth factors	Alpha: promotes epithelial cell growth Beta: suppresses lymphocyte function: antiinflammatory.

Hormones

Component	Function
Prolactin	Enhances B- and T-lymphocyte development; affects differentiation of intestinal lymphoid tissue.
Cortisol, thyroxine, insulin	Promotes maturation of neonatal intestine and development of intestinal host-defense mechanisms.[120]

Cells

Component	Function
Blymphocytes	Synthesize IgA and other antibodies targeted against specific pathogens.
Macrophages	90% of cells in breast milk; phagocytize microorganisms and kill bacteria in neonatal intestine; produce lysozyme, lactoferrin, and complement.
Neutrophils	Phagocytize bacteria in neonatal gastrointestinal tract.
T-lymphocytes	Phagocytosis against organisms in GI tract; mobilizes other host defenses; antigens introduced into maternal respiratory and/or gastrointestinal systems stimulate development of antibodies in breast milk; incorporation into neonatal tissue bestows short-term adoptive immunity.[72,78,129]
Cytokines	Modulate functions and maturation of immune system.[41,72]
Proinflammatory: Interleukin 1b, 6, 8, 12; interferon-gamma; tumor necrosis factor-alpha	Enhances inflammation.
Antiinflammatory: Interleukin 10; tumor growth factor-beta	Suppresses function of macrophages, natural killer and T-cells.

Modified from Hamosh B: Bioactive factors in human milk, *Pediatr Clin North Am* 48:69, 2001

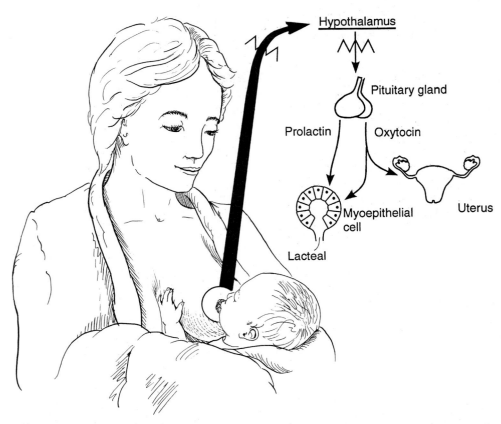

FIGURE 19-1   Ejection reflex arc, or letdown reflex. Infant suckling stimulates mechanoreceptors in the mother's nipple and areola that send the stimuli along the nerve pathways to the hypothalamus. Stimulation of the posterior pituitary releases oxytocin that (a) stimulates myoepithelial cells of the breast to contract and eject milk and (b) stimulates the uterus to contract. Stimulation of the anterior pituitary releases prolactin, which is responsible for milk production in mammary alveoli. (Modified from Lawrence R: *Breastfeeding, a guide for the medical profession,* ed 5, St Louis, 1999, Mosby.)

PSYCHOLOGIC VALUES OF BREASTFEEDING

The short-term advantage of breastfeeding is early mother and infant contact.[219] The *en face* position of breastfeeding enhances this contact. During the first 1 to 2 hours after birth, the infant's suckling and touching of the mother's areola increases maternal attentiveness to the baby's needs for at least the first week of life.[251] Because several studies show that maternal analgesia alters the infant's initial breastfeeding behavior,[185,186] the mother's behavior may also be altered. In a sick neonate early contact, whether by breastfeeding or another physical means, sometimes must be delayed or modified.

The long-term psychologic effect for the mother of unrestricted nursing appears to be a more even mood cycle as a result of elevated prolactin and endorphin levels,[219] which enhance coping mechanisms associated with caring for a new family member. Providing her own milk, including pumping and gavaging breast milk and eventual feeding at the breast, enhances maternal attachment and maternal behaviors* and enables the mother to contribute to her infant's care (see Chapter 29).[165,219,250] Proximity of mother and infant, as well as the infant's initial

---

*References 80, 109, 167, 210, 219, 236.

experience at the breast, contribute to maternal and infant regulation and the establishment of innate behaviors and emotional and social ties between mother and infant.* A recent study described rewards to the mother from breastfeeding: (1) knowing that she is providing the healthiest nutrition, (2) enhancing closeness between mother and the preterm infant, (3) perceiving her preterm infant's contentment and tranquility during breastfeeding, (4) convenience for the mother, and (5) giving the mother a tangible claim to the preterm infant.[109]

All referring physicians and nursing personnel who admit infants to the NICU should support and assist mothers who wish to breastfeed their infants. Use of kangaroo care (see Chapter 13) in the NICU facilitates early initiation of breastfeeding, increases maternal confidence, competence, and breastfeeding duration.[25,92,95,114] If the infant is able to take oral nourishment, he or she can be breastfed at 1000 to 1200 g and about 32 weeks' gestational age.† (See Chapter 13, Strategies to Facilitate Oral Feeding.)

FACILITATING SUCCESSFUL BREASTFEEDING

Although breastfeeding is a normal, natural function, it is not a reflex, but rather a highly complex interaction and interdependence between mother and infant. To be successful, the breastfeeding dyad must synchronize their behavior and physiology and receive support from their environment. Delayed breastfeeding may be as successful as immediate feeding when (1) problems are prevented, (2) the mother receives support and encouragement in maintaining her milk supply, and (3) everyone is patient and knowledgeable about teaching the infant to suckle. Initiating breastfeeding as early as possible is important to prevent problems. Thorough evaluation of the effectiveness of the nursing couple is important in achieving adequate nutrition and breastfeeding success. Knowledgeable health care providers and licensed, certified lactation consultants, where available, can perform these evaluations.

Sucking

Sucking is a primitive reflex appearing as early as 15 to 16 weeks' gestation. Although isolated components of feeding behaviors (e.g., root, suck, swallow, gag) are all present early in gestation, they are not effectively coordinated for bottlefeedings before 32 to 34 weeks' gestational age (see Table 13-2).[79] The infant can coordinate suck and swallow while breastfeeding as early as 28 weeks' gestation. Two distinct types of sucking, nonnutritive and nutritive, develop in the human infant.

Nonnutritive Sucking
Nonnutritive sucking is sucking activity in which no fluid or nutrition is delivered to the infant. Characterized by short bursts of rapid motion, pauses, and few swallows, nonnutritive sucking has a stabilizing effect on physiologic responses (e.g., better oxygenation; quieter, more restful behavior; decreased tension; increased insulin and gastrin secretion that may stimulate digestion and storage of nutrients; and improved readiness for oral feedings; see Chapter 13). Because there is no bolus of fluid to swallow, nonnutritive sucking results in an alternation of inspiration/expiration without the regular apneic periods of nutritive sucking.[222]

Nutritive Sucking
Nutritive sucking, used by an infant when fluid or nutrition is available, is characterized by an organized, rhythmic pattern that is about half the rate of nonnutritive sucking (i.e., 1 per second). During nutritive sucking, each milk expression is followed by a reflexive swallow and an occasional brief pause. In a term neonate, rates of sucking range from 40 to 100/min.[188] Nutritive sucking provides the neonate with positive reinforcement, which encourages a steady level of behavior.[160] A variety of factors affect nutritive sucking including (1) maternal anesthesia and/or analgesia, (2) length of labor, (3) type of delivery, (4) gestational age, (5) birth weight, (6) age (in hours), (7) infant state, (8) type of fluid, (9) disorders of the CNS, and (10) individual variations.* Although nutritive sucking is associated with faster heart rate (when bottlefeeding),[51] little information is available describing energy requirements of nutritive sucking. The findings of one study suggest that during bottlefeeding, preterm infants expend significantly less energy to suck the same volume than do full-term infants.[105] Bottlefeeding requires more energy than breastfeeding in all infants.[105]

*References 32, 95, 127, 210, 229, 236, 251.
†References 29, 79, 129, 161, 162, 164, 168, 177, 230.

*References 12, 51, 52, 59, 76, 77, 123, 142, 150, 158, 185, 186, 222.

Two patterns of nutritive sucking have been identified: continuous sucking and intermittent sucking.[152,224] Continuous sucking occurs at the beginning of bottlefeeding, when the suck is strong and continuous for at least 30 seconds.[149,152,224] Intermittent sucking, an alteration of sucking bursts with periods of pause/no sucking,[149,152,224] occurs first during breastfeeding, followed by continuous sucking (with breast milk letdown).[150,164] Breathing is affected more during continuous than during intermittent sucking, even in full term infants who can exhibit apnea and bradycardia with feeding.[148]

An increasing level of organization of nutritive sucking occurs with increasing gestational age, maturity, and experience.* Preterm sucking patterns exhibit more sucking to breathing ratio (2:1 to 4:1) than well-coordinated sucking breathing ratios (e.g., 1:1) of full-term newborns.[39,116] By 32 to 34 weeks' postconceptual age, there is a change in sucking bursts (i.e., increase in number of sucks, number of suck bursts and pressure, decrease in time between sucking bursts). This developmental maturation enables nutritive sucking to take less time and is less tiring.

Nutritive sucking requires coordination between suck, swallow, and breathing. During coordinated sucking bursts, suck/swallow/breathing occur in a 1:1:1 sequential pattern.[39,222] The lack of a sucking, swallowing, and breathing ratio of 1:1:1 contributes to a preterm infant's apnea with feeding, a reflexive protection of the airway.[150,222] Although suck/swallow is achieved by 32 weeks' gestation,[79,83,159] respiration may still not be well coordinated so that the preterm infant may develop apneic episodes, with bottlefeeding.[39] With increasing postconceptual age and neuromuscular maturity *consistent* coordination of suck/swallow/breathing (with bottlefeeding) occurs by 37 weeks' postconceptual age.[39]

Human nutritive suckling is composed of five separate yet interrelated processes: (1) rooting, (2) orienting, (3) suction, (4) expression, and (5) swallowing[35] (Figure 19-2). Rooting, the tactile stimulating of the infant's face and lips, elicits the head to turn toward the stimulus. Stimulation of the center of the lower lip enables the infant to root by coming forward and latching on, rather than turning the head to one side.[127] Orienting, or latching on, occurs when the tongue draws the nipple and areola into an elongated teat and compresses it against the hard palate.[91,228] The lactiferous sinuses,

located behind the nipple and areola, must be stimulated by the infant's mouth for milk to be extracted (Figure 19-3).

Suction, the application of negative pressure in the infant's mouth, holds the nipple and areola in place.[61,91,228] At the beginning of breastfeeding, a strong suction stretches and shapes the nipple, but only moderate suction is required to maintain adequate grasp of the nipple. During the feeding, occasional bursts of suckling enable milk to be expressed. Expression of milk occurs when the peristaltic motion of the tongue[91] stimulates the myoepithelial cells surrounding the milk ducts (see Figure 19-3) to contract, and milk is ejected from the ducts. As peristaltic motion of the tongue stimulates milk ejection, the lips should be flanged out to create a seal. After maximal compression of the nipple[228] with peristaltic motion, milk is expressed from the lactiferous sinuses.

Swallowing milk occurs as the peristaltic motion of the tongue triggers peristaltic motion of the posterior pharynx (reflexive swallowing)[91,187,188] and propulsion down the esophagus (which also shows peristalsis). These peristaltic motions coordinate suck and swallow so breastfeeding infants do not choke, unless letdown reflex is excessive. Swallowing milk also reflexively initiates the expression cycle of jaw and tongue movements. Therefore nutritive suckling is primarily expression and swallowing of milk. During nursing, just enough suction to keep the nipple in proper position is used, even during the expressive phase of suckling. Breastfeeding is an infant-regulated system; milk flow depends on the active suckling by the infant. When an infant pauses to regain physiologic stability, the flow of milk from the breast ceases.

Ultrasonographic studies of full-term infants breastfeeding note (1) an elongation to twice the resting size of the maternal nipple, (2) formation of a passive seal by the neonate's oral cavity, and (3) milk ejection coinciding with the downstroke of the tongue and jaw, creating negative pressure by oral cavity enlargement.[228] Ultrasonographic studies of full-term infants bottlefeeding note (1) less elasticity and less elongation of artificial nipples (compared with human nipple), (2) similar mechanisms used to suckle artificial nipples as used to breastfeed, and (3) milk expression dependent on a vacuum phenomenon by oral cavity enlargement rather than by nipple compression.[39,61,91,187,188] Artificial nipples have also been shown to vary in their rate of milk flow.[61,145,147,149] Nipple hole size, rather than the type of nipple,[145,151] has been found to be the major determinant in the

---

*References: 39, 49, 50, 76, 143, 159, 202.

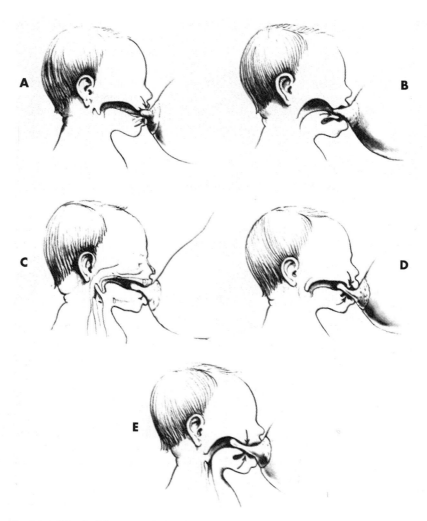

FIGURE 19-2 Normal suckling. **A,** Infant grasps breast (note arrows showing jaw action). **B,** Tongue moves forward to draw nipple in. **C,** Nipple and areola move toward palate as glottis still permits breathing. **D,** Tongue moves along nipple, pressing it against hard palate, creating pressure. **E,** Ductules under areola are milked, and flow begins because of peristaltic movement of tongue. Glottis closes and swallow follows. (From Lawrence RA: *Breastfeeding, a guide for the medical profession,* ed 5, St Louis, 1999, Mosby.)

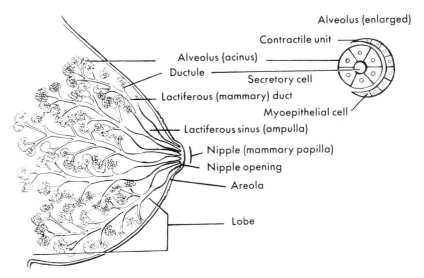

FIGURE 19-3 Structure of human breast during lactation. (From Riordan J: *A practical guide to breastfeeding*, St Louis, 1983, Mosby.)

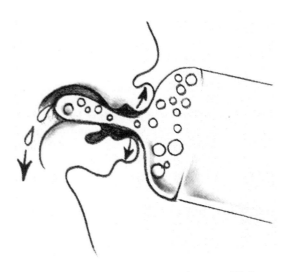

FIGURE 19-4 Artificial nipple. (From Lawrence RA: *Breastfeeding, a guide for the medical profession*, ed 5, St Louis, 1999, Mosby.)

variability in milk flow.[147] With an artificial nipple, fluid flows into the posterior oropharynx by gravity (Figure 19-4). Artificial nipples and bottles are gravity-regulated systems requiring the infant to actively inhibit milk flow to permit swallowing and breathing. In an attempt to regulate milk flow and prevent choking or gagging, infants may clench their jaws or obstruct the nipples' holes with their tongues in a thrusting motion.[39] Orthodontic nipples result in physiologic stability and more effective feeding behavior in some infants.[58]

PREVENTION

Problems with breastfeeding may be with the mother, the neonate, or arise from a combination of problems in the dyad. Lack of information regarding common problems in the early weeks of breastfeeding is a common reason for breastfeeding failure.[33,178,203,215] In descriptive studies addressing breastfeeding problems, mothers have frequently identified concerns related to sore nipples, breast discomfort, and inadequate milk supply.[22,30,122,178,199] Breastfeeding problems should be prevented. To solve a breastfeeding problem, the mother must be observed feeding the infant.

Maternal Problems

Inadequate Milk Supply

Inadequate milk supply, a major problem for both mother and infant, is the most commonly cited reason for discontinuation of breastfeeding in the NICU and after discharge.* Initially some neonates with special needs are unable to breastfeed.

---

*References 92, 108, 163, 166, 167, 170, 177, 178, 199.

In this common situation, the most compelling breastfeeding issue is establishing an adequate milk supply without the neonate's assistance[219] (Table 19-3). Developing a very early program of education and support for the mother will help her to establish an early milk supply and prevent low milk volume.

Initiating, establishing, and maintaining a milk supply must be accomplished mechanically when the infant is unable to breastfeed. Because milk production depends on adequate and frequent expression,[178,191] maternal education is the key to establishing an adequate supply[219] (see Table 19-3). The mother who wants to breastfeed should be instructed about initiating and maintaining a milk supply until the infant can breastfeed. In general, instruction includes information about pumping, which is individualized to the mother's situation. Milk production through pumping should be encouraged early and regularly to (1) collect colostrum, rich in antiinfective properties, (2) ease initial engorgement associated with lack of regular stimulation, (3) provide quality nutrition for the neonate, and (4) alleviate concerns about available volume once the infant begins breastfeeding. The early postpartal period in the hospital is the optimal time to teach pumping methods, while support and encouragement are readily available.

Breast Discomfort

Maternal problems include engorgement, painful nipples, and cracked nipples.[178,199,206] A primipara is at high risk for developing engorgement. Frequent emptying of the breast is the best prevention.

Engorgement occurring in the early postpartum period is characterized by general discomfort, usually in both breasts in a well, afebrile woman. Areolar engorgement blocks the nipple and makes grasping the areola difficult for the infant. Gentle breast massage and manual expression of a small amount of milk softens the areola so the infant is able to "latch on." When the body of the breasts and the areola are affected, the goal of management is to make the mother comfortable so that nursing may continue. Supporting the breasts is crucial, and the mother should wear a well-fitting but adjustable brassiere 24 hours a day.[128] Applying cold packs between nursing decreases pain and swelling. Pain relievers may also be prescribed. Applying heat (packs or a warm shower) and expressing some milk prior to feeding helps initiate milk flow. A nursing infant, manual expression, or an effective pump helps initiate and maintain milk flow.[178,191,199] Breast massage before and during breast pumping/feeding also facilitates milk flow.

Prenatal stimulation of the nipple by pulling or rolling (to toughen it for breastfeeding) is not recommended because of the possibility of initiating uterine contractions and premature labor.[128,173]

Sore nipples are another major discomfort and concern for the new mother. The initial grasp of the nipple by the infant or with pumping can be painful. Poor positioning of the infant

Table 19-3	FACTORS THAT INFLUENCE THE MOTHER'S MILK SUPPLY AND SUCCESSFUL BREASTFEEDING OF THE PRETERM INFANT	
ENHANCES	**REDUCES**	**COMMENTS**
Early initiation of pumping, preferably with a double-pumping setup	Immediate separation at birth,[126] delayed initiation of pumping or feeding at the breast	Initiate within 2-3 hr of birth, if possible; pumping both breasts simultaneously is associated with higher prolactin levels, milk yield, fat concentration, and maternal preference.[15,93,259]
Frequent milk expression with complete breast emptying at each session[54,96,178,191,199]	Failure to express frequently and/or incomplete emptying of the breasts	5-8 expressions/day (every 3-4 hr): duration of pumping >100 min/day (about 15-20 min with double-pump setup); longest nonpumping interval ≤6 hr.[19,96,218,219,232]
Rest, relaxation, and stress management[66,219] (see Chapters 29 and 30)	Fatigue, anxiety, stress (i.e., maternal illness; return to work; more commitments in and outside the home)	Inverse relationship between maternal anxiety scores and milk volume for mothers of preterm infants; uninterrupted sleep of at least 6 hr.[38,129,241]

Modified from Schanler R, Hurst N: Human milk for the hospitalized preterm infant, *Semin Perinatol* 18:476, 1994.

Table 19-3	FACTORS THAT INFLUENCE THE MOTHER'S MILK SUPPLY AND SUCCESSFUL BREASTFEEDING OF THE PRETERM INFANT— cont'd	
ENHANCES	**REDUCES**	**COMMENTS**
Adequate nutrition	Inadequate nutrition	At least 60% of recommended daily allowances produces milk of adequate quantity and quality to promote infant growth.[198]
Medications: Metoclopramide, oxytocin, reserpines, phenothiazines	Bromocriptine, antihistamine, oral contraceptives (especially estrogen and progesterone combination)	Knowledge of maternal medication use enables effective counseling.
Herb Fenugreek		2-3 capsules 2-3×/day: maternal diarrhea, lowers blood glucose, may increase asthma symptoms; maple syrup smell to sweat, urine, milk.[85]
Positive feedback to mother regarding infant growth; infant's condition improving	Worsening infant's condition	Mothers report feeling rewarded by infant's growth while receiving expressed mother's milk by gavage.[163]
Skin-to-skin contact (kangaroo care)[100] (see Chapter 13)	Parental separation	Maternal reinforcement of lactation, maternal behaviors, confidence, and attachment; ensures maternal exposure to pathogens in NICU so that her immune system is stimulated to produce environmentally specific antibodies that will be passed in maternal milk and protect the preterm.[218]
Educational information (e.g., video brochure) readily available	No verbal or written information for parents	Decision about type of pump, frequency; written instructions on collection and storage per NICU protocol; information about maternal rest, fluid intake, and nutrition
Knowledgeable professional care providers (e.g., nurses, lactation specialists, physicians) who educate, support, and assist through consistent, practical advice	Nonsupportive care providers and/or inconsistent advice and information	Prevention of maternal problems (e.g., inadequate supply, sore nipples, engorgement) through self-education and professional interaction and education enhances success and prevents discontinuation of breastfeeding.
Initiation of breastfeeding *before* bottlefeeding	Initiation of bottlefeeding before breastfeeding	Early breastfeeding is less stressful than early bottlefeeding* because of differences in the patterns of sucking and breathing; during bottlefeedings, preterm infants alternate short bursts of sucking with breathing and do not breathe within sucking bursts; during breastfeeding, breathing is integrated within sucking bursts.[162]
		Test weighing (i.e., weighing before and after breastfeeding, with differences in weight representing milk intake [1 g = 1 ml]) using electronic scales is a reliable method of documenting milk intake in preterm infants.[165,166]
		For specific problems, maximizing milk intake may be assisted by lactational support devices and/or breast pump stimulation of the opposite breast during infant feeding.[129,163,219]

*References 29, 161-164, 166, 173, 230, 237, 252.

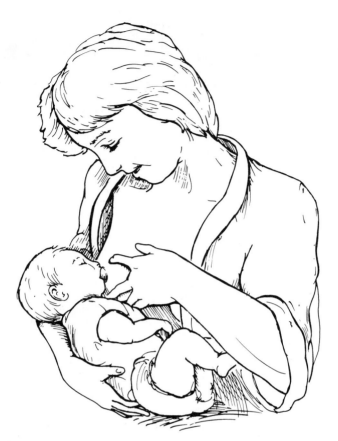

FIGURE 19-5   Proper positioning for breastfeeding infant tummy-to-tummy facing the mother.

causes painful and eventually cracked nipples. Prevention and treatment involve educating the mother about careful positioning of the infant facing the mother, looking directly at the breast, and tummy-to-tummy with her (Figure 19-5). Compression of the areola behind the nipple extracts milk from the sinuses[206] (see Figure 19-3). Changing the infant's position on the nipple at different feedings is helpful.

Positioning the infant correctly at the breast will assist in the prevention of sore nipples. There are three positions that can be used with breastfeeding: the cradle hold, the football hold, and lying down (Figures 19-5 to 19-7). Initially the cradle and/or football hold will allow the most control for the mother and infant to learn breastfeeding. Breastfeeding in the lying down position becomes easier once latch-on techniques are developed.

Nipple care involves keeping nipples clean and dry. Clear water (no soap or alcohol) is all that is necessary to keep the nipples clean. Drying nipples well, not using plastic nursing pads, and exposing nipples to air and dry heat (sunlight, light bulb sauna, or a low setting on a hair dryer) is comforting. Using ointments may be helpful, especially in dry climates. If used, a small amount (i.e., one drop) should be gently massaged into the nipple. Purified lanolin (if there is no allergy to wool), A and D ointment, or vitamin E may be used to treat but will not prevent sore nipples. A recent randomized clinical trial (RCT) found that use of breast shells (Figure 19-8) and lanolin cream to treat sore nipples promoted healing and prevented infections.[36] Severe and/or persistent nipple pain may be caused by bacterial or yeast infection, which should be promptly treated.[178]

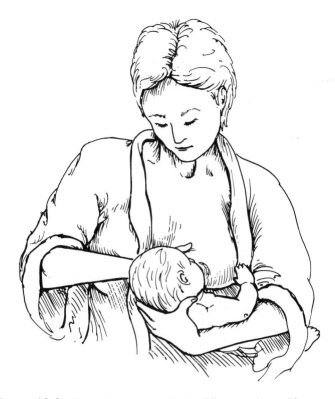

FIGURE 19-6   Football hold in breastfeeding. Pillows may be used for support.

In the past nipple shields were not recommended because they are awkward for the mother, confusing for the infant, and decrease milk production by 50%. More recently, supervised temporary use of silicone nipple shields has been found to be a useful tool in treatment of sore nipples, latch on problems and as a bridging technique to direct breastfeeding.[178,192,199,253] A recent study showed that for preterm infants, use of a nipple shield increased breast milk intake, and promoted longer duration of breastfeeding.[172] Breast pumping after use of nipple shields is necessary to express residual milk, maintain adequate milk supply, and obtain milk for supplemental feeding.[178,199]

Flat or inverted nipples may be difficult for the infant to grasp and result in maternal engorgement, decreased milk supply, and infant frustration (Figure 19-9). Inverted nipples may be treated by wearing plastic breast cups or shells, which apply pressure to the areola, averting the nipple (see Figure 19-8). In one study prenatal use of breast shells was not associated with improved likelihood of breastfeeding at 6 weeks postpartum.[142a] Drawing the nipple out with a pump just before latch-on also works well.

Neonatal Problems

Ideally no term or preterm infant who will be breastfed should ever be fed with an artificial nipple, but this is not always possible, especially for a sick premature infant who requires prolonged hospitalization. However, teaching a premature infant to suck often starts long before nutrition is obtained from a nipple. When a premature infant is gavage fed, giving a pacifier teaches the infant to equate satiety with sucking. Using a pacifier provides nonnutritive sucking that calms and soothes the preterm infant, as well as providing the opportunity to develop sucking skill. When the mother is present for gavage feeding, the infant can be given the breast instead of an artificial nipple. If it is necessary to avoid swallowing any fluid, the breast can be

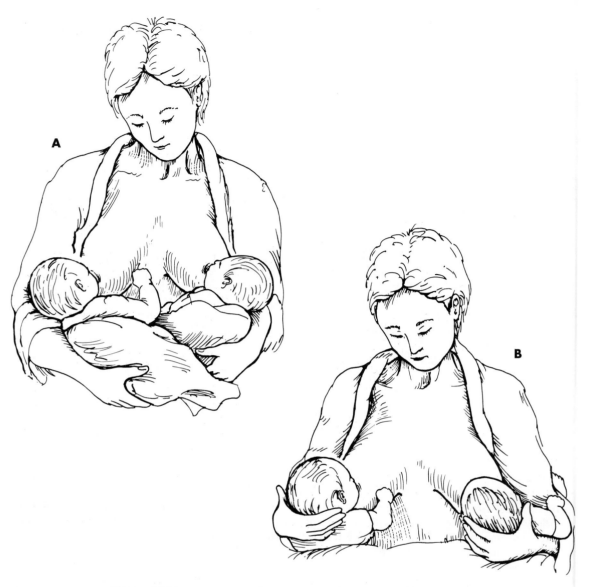

FIGURE 19-7 Breastfeeding twins. **A,** Cradle position. **B,** Football hold position.

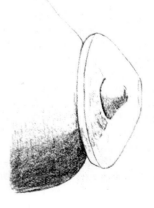

FIGURE 19-8 Breast shell. Special breast shells may be worn under the bra during the last 3 to 4 months of pregnancy. Gentle pressure at the edge of the areola gradually forces the nipple through the center opening of the shell to help increase nipple protractility. It may be used after childbirth if needed. NOTE: Milk can leak from the breasts into the shells. Because maternal body warmth can foster rapid bacterial contamination, such milk should be discarded. (Courtesy Jimmy Lynne Scholl Avery.)

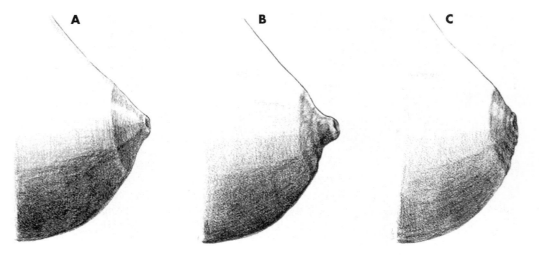

FIGURE 19-9   Inverted nipples. **A,** Normal and inverted nipples may look similar when nipple is not stimulated. **B,** Normal nipple protrudes when stimulated. **C,** Inverted nipple retracts when stimulated. (Courtesy Jimmy Lynne Scholl Avery.)

prepumped. Placing the infant in direct skin-to-skin contact with the mother's breast enables nuzzling and licking behaviors and teaches that relief from hunger and the breastfeeding position are associated. Because increased stimulation creates an increased milk supply, it is possible to breastfeed multiple infants.[199,239] In the early weeks it will be difficult and time consuming, but eventually it can become faster and more convenient than bottlefeeding. Two infants can be fed at the same time, in the cradle position or in the football hold position (see Figure 19-7). The infants should change breasts with each feeding, because one may have a stronger suck than the other and each breast should receive an equal amount of stimulation.

Understanding the mechanisms of suckling is essential to preventing, assessing, and intervening in neonatal suckling problems. *Nipple confusion* describes the difficulty of infants who have been fed with artificial nipples before learning to breastfeed. The infant who has learned to feed from a bottle nipple often sucks incorrectly at the breast, preventing milk flow. The infant's confusion creates frustration and crying, which may inhibit milk letdown. The best means for preventing nipple confusion is to enable the infant to learn breastfeeding *before* bottlefeeding is established[180] (see Table 19-3).

Assessment of the problem includes evalua-

tion of the method of feeding and possibly using alternative nutritional methods (gavage feedings) until the cause is determined. If the infant is bottlefed, choking may be a result of a soft nipple, a fast flow that the infant cannot control, or a nipple that is too long for the infant's (particularly the preterm infant's) mouth. If the mother is breastfeeding and the ejection is strong, the first rush of milk could cause choking, which may be prevented by manual expression of a small amount (several spurts) of milk before offering the nipple to the infant.

Some suckling problems result from the sequelae of perinatal events, such as low Apgar score, preterm low birth weight, SGA, LGA, IDM, and multiple births,* or of physical disorders, such as hyperbilirubinemia, hypoglycemia, cardiorespiratory conditions, sepsis, neuromotor/developmental problems, and structural abnormalities of the oral cavity,* and represent developmental delays. These suckling difficulties require diagnostic evaluation of the underlying cause and appropriate intervention.*

Some mothers may not establish or may have difficulty maintaining an adequate milk supply, yet infants with problems require an easily obtainable milk supply. The Lact-Aid Nursing Trainer system

---

*References 12, 23, 77, 129, 179, 180, 199.

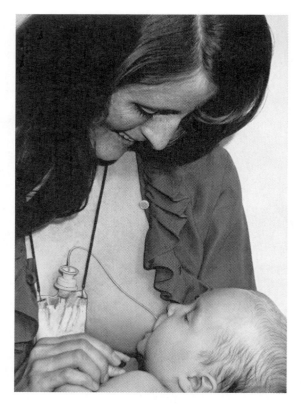

FIGURE 19-10 Lact-Aid Nursing Trainer. (Courtesy Lact-Aid International, Inc.)

(Figure 19-10) addresses a variety of breastfeeding problems, including suckling defects.[17-19] Expressed breast milk or formula is contained in a presterilized, disposable bag suspended between the mother's breasts by a cord, and the liquid is delivered by a thin, flexible tube attached to the bag. The end of the tube is placed against the mother's nipple to enable the infant to suckle the tube and nipple at the same time. This device provides the correct rate of flow and volume of liquid that elicits the reflexes of swallowing and expression. The Lact-Aid trainer provides oral therapy and nutritional supplementation for the infant and the mammary stimulus necessary to enhance the mother's lactation.[22,129] It is effective in managing low milk production in the mother that has resulted from separation, delayed breastfeeding, poor technique, or other correctable problems, and the device gives nutritional and oral therapy to an infant who is slow in gaining weight or has a suckling dysfunction.

CAUTION: To prevent the spread of serious infections, the Lact-Aid trainer should never be borrowed, rented, or loaned from another mother.

The Lact-Aid STARTrainer Nursing System introduced in 1997 (Figure 19-11) is a low-cost starter breastfeeding supplementer. It was developed especially for use when an infant needs assistance latching on to the breast, when supplementing is needed for a brief period, a trial period is desired, or a semidisposable unit is needed. The Lact-Aid trainer converts any standard infant feeding bottle, including Volufeed, Accufeed, and similar feeders, to create a breastfeeding supplementer system that is equivalent in function, safety, and effectiveness to the original Lact-Aid Nursing Trainer System. If a mother needs to switch to the original model for longer-term use, she will be able to use most of the STARTrainer components with it.

Problems with the letdown reflex may originate with the mother, the neonate, or both. The mother's emotional state may interfere with letdown: a tense mother will not have a letdown reflex.[66,219,241] Often, especially in breastfeeding a premature infant, this is because of fear of failure or a lack of privacy. Knowledge of the mechanisms of lactation can help the mother avoid a fear of failing. It is important to give the mother as much privacy and the least stressful environment possible when she is pumping her breasts and breastfeeding. If a mother experiences a weak or delayed letdown, she should massage the colostrum or milk down to the nipple before putting the infant to the breast. Infants with a poor suck, such as preterm infants or infants with Down syndrome or a neurologic deficit, understimulate the breast and do not trigger the letdown reflex. Use of the Lact-Aid trainer provides oral therapy, improves these infants' suckling ability, and facilitates a successful nursing relationship. The breast can also be stimulated with a good pump between feedings to increase the milk supply.

DATA COLLECTION AND INTERVENTION

Establishment of Breastfeeding

Available Feeding and Suckling Neonate
Infants who have been admitted to a NICU often present a dilemma to care providers as to the most favorable time to begin putting the infant to the breast.[124] The infant's current physical status, plus considerations of nutrition and energy

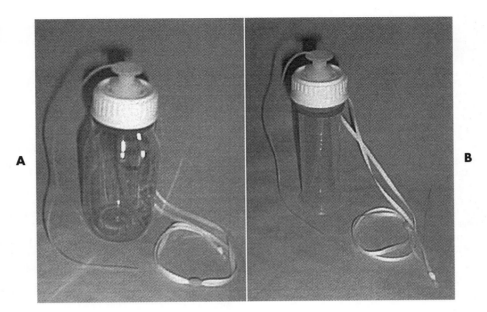

FIGURE 19-11   Lact-Aid STARTrainer Nursing System. **A,** With a standard infant feeding bottle. **B,** With a metered feeding bottle. A Lact-Aid STARTrainer Unit replaces the nipple of the infant bottle cap to make an infant feeding bottle a Lact-Aid breastfeeding supplementer and suckling aid for short-term use or whenever a semidisposable unit is desired. The adjustable neck strap raises or lowers the unit to adjust flow rate. The tip of the nursing tube fits notch of bottle holder to stop flow when not in use. The Lact-Aid STARTrainer Nursing System includes a STARTrainer Unit (Body/Nursing Tube, STARTrainer Ring, Extension Tube), STARTrainer Adjustable Neck Strap and Notched Bottle Holder, and STARTrainer Instructions. (Courtesy Lact-Aid International.)

expenditure, help determine such decisions. In a national survey criteria used to determine readiness for oral feedings included the following: (1) 75% used gestational age (e.g., 34 weeks by 60%) or weight (e.g., 1500 g by 50%) and (2) infant behavioral cues (e.g., sucking behaviors) (Table 19-4).[226] There are few empirical data to support the contention that either weight or gestational age affects the ability of a preterm infant to coordinate suck and swallow at the breast. In the same survey a majority (85% to 93%) responded that bottlefeeding is started first, before breastfeeding.[226] Professional caregivers believe and teach parents that breastfeeding is too stressful and requires more energy and exertion than bottlefeeding.[252] Contrary to physiologic evidence, progression of nutritional support for the preterm has proceeded from IV fluids → total parenteral nutrition → gavage (continuous → intermittent) → bottlefeeding (at 1500 to 1800 g or 34 to 35 weeks' postconceptual age) → breastfeeding (after bottlefeeding without distress). Problems arising from this approach include (1)

delay in initial oral feedings, (2) establishment of a sucking method that may not easily transfer to breastfeeding, and (3) initiation of breastfeeding when discharge is imminent so that the mother receives little, if any, breastfeeding assistance and support.[94,163,165,169,252]

Use of a breastfeeding protocol[232] without use of bottlefeeding (either before breastfeeding or to supplement breastfeeding) is associated with the longest duration of breastfeeding. A recent RCT of this protocol in which nasogastric (NG) supplementation was compared with bottlefeeding for a transition to feeding at the breast found that NG supplementation was associated with feeding from the breast at discharge, 3 days, 3 months, and 6 months compared with preterm infants supplemented with bottlefeeding.[115] In this same study earlier age at initiation of breastfeeding was also associated with successful and longer duration of breastfeeding.[115] After discharge from the NICU, mothers wean their preterm infants from the breast because of (1) infant resistance to latching on, (2) weak suck, (3)

Table 19-4	READINESS FOR INITIATION OF ORAL FEEDINGS: RESEARCH BASIS	
BREASTFEEDING	**CRITERIA**	**BOTTLEFEEDING**
Preterm	Gestational/post-←conceptual→ Age (PCA) ←Weight→	**Preterm**
28-36 wk: Better able to coordinate suck, swallow, and breathing.[161,162,164,168,230]		34-35 wk: PCA is a developmental guideline—based on belief that sucking pattern is similar to that of full-terms[12,110,111,125]; infants may be ready at an earlier age (i.e., 28-34 wk).[12,79,159]
		Coordination of respirations with sucking and swallowing is consistently achieved by infants >37 wk PCA.[12,39]
<1500 g: Better able to coordinate sucking, swallowing, and breathing.*		1500-1800 g: Traditional criteria without research basis.
Full-Term	Mechanics of ←Sucking→	**Full-Term**
Ultrasound study shows human nipple elongates to twice its resting length; neonatal cheeks act as a passive seal for the oral cavity.[228]		Higher maximum pressure and number of sucks or bursts; greater suck widths[160] and greater intake/suck.
		Able to alter sucking to accommodate nutrient composition, nipple, and hole size to minimize energy expenditure[61,151] and autoregulate milk flow by controlling pressure generated during sucking.[151]
		Regulates sucking pressure by coordination of various oral motor structures so that intraoral pressure is controlled to enable milk to flow in a manageable fashion.[49,61,222]
		Preterm
		Burst width (interburst and intersuck width) similar to that of full-term infant.[105,160]
		At the beginning of a feeding, preterms generate weaker sucking pressure within the oral cavity that changes over time to pressures and duration in the same range as term infants, because of neural maturation and sucking experience.[49,50]
Full-Term	←Energy→ Expenditure	**Full-Term**
50% of feeding obtained in first 2 min; 80%-90% by 4 min; last 5 min minimal obtained from each breast.[135]		86% of feeding obtained in first 4 min of sucking.[135] Generate larger negative pressure with sucks with higher energy expenditure.[105]
		Able to alter sucking to accommodate nutrient composition, nipple and hole size to minimize energy expenditure[61,151] and autoregulate milk flow by controlling pressure generated during sucking.[151]
Premature		**Preterm**
After 34 wk: 70%-80% of feeding ingested in first 6 min, then intake sluggish, rest periods increase; and sucking and nourishment decrease.[143]		40% of total volume ingested in first min,[143] less energy to suck same volume as full-term infant.[105]
At 36-37 wk: Sucking standards are similar to mature neonate.[143]		Infants born 26-29 wk GA benefit from restricted milk flow (i.e., milk is only obtained with active sucking; no milk flows to infant by gravity or high-low nipples during rest periods).[12,124,125] At initiation of oral feeding (with restricted milk flow), an intake of 1.5 ml/min and a proficiency of 30% (e.g., intake of 9 ml in first 5 min; intake of 30 ml in 20 min) is indicative of earlier attainment of full oral feeding.[124,125]
The younger the gestational age the higher the variability.[143]		
Longer duration of breast than bottlefeeding.[161,164,168]		
No difference in duration of breast vs bottlefeeding.[29]		

*References 29, 33, 114, 161-164, 168, 230, 237.

Table 19-4	READINESS FOR INITIATION OF ORAL FEEDINGS: RESEARCH BASIS—cont'd	
BREASTFEEDING	**CRITERIA**	**BOTTLEFEEDING**
Preterm Skin temperature higher (than when bottlefeeding) because of bodily contact with mother.[161,164,166,168,230] No temperature change before (ac) or after feeding (pc).[29]	←Temperature→	
Preterm Less weight gain after breastfeeding compared with bottlefeeding.[29]	←Weight Gain→	
	←Heart Rate→	**Preterm** Bradycardia occurred with bottlefeeding but not breastfeeding; bradycardia possibly related to faster milk flow and interference with breathing[161,164,166,168,230]; apnea and bradycardia with bottle feeding in otherwise healthy preterms.[82]
	←Coordination→ of Suck, Swallow, and Breathing	**Full-Term** Suck, swallow, breathe in 1:1:1 pattern.[39,222] Alteration of breathing pattern—prolongation of expiration and shortening of inspiration.[152,224] No difference in sucking frequency/pressure when bottlefeeding expressed milk or formula. Differences in sucking/breathing patterns attributed to nutrient delivery rather than nutrient composition.[150]
Preterm Different patterns of sucking bursts and better coordination, breathing is integrated within sucking bursts.[162]	←Coordination→ of Suck, Swallow, and Breathing	**Preterm** Effective coordination by 32-34 wk.[79,83] High-flow nipples result in apnea or bradycardia.[145-147,149,151,224] Do not breathe within sucking bursts but in alternate short bursts of sucking with breathing.[77,164] Consistently achieved by infants 37 wk PCA.[39] Use of orthodontic nipple results in physiologic stability and effective feeding behavior in some preterms.[58] At 34 wk PCA, sucking pattern primarily expression component; with maturation, experience, endurance/strength there is a shift to more frequent use of term sucking pattern.[125] Not necessary to wait for full-term sucking pattern for successful oral feeding to begin.[123,125]
Full-Term No desaturation with feeding.[87,224] 18% pc saturations <90%.	←Oxygen→ Saturation	**Full-Term** No desaturation with feeding.[87,224] 29% of pc saturations <90%. More oxygen desaturations (<90%) than breastfeeding.[150]
Preterm No difference in oxygenation with breast vs. bottlefeeding[161,164,166,168,230]; no pc decline of oxygenation; oxygenation more stable than with bottlefeeding—fewer desaturations.[58]		**Preterm** Decreased oxygenation during initial sustained sucking but oxygenation increased as sucking pattern modulated.[166,224] 32-36 wk: range of 94%-97% with feeding[168]; with sucking decreased saturation from 2.5%-16% (range 80%-100%).[159] Fluctuations and sharper decrease in saturation with bottlefeedings vs. breastfeeding[161,164,168,230]; 10 min pc saturation 50% below baseline.[161,164]

Continued

Table 19-4	**READINESS FOR INITIATION OF ORAL FEEDINGS: RESEARCH BASIS—cont'd**	
BREASTFEEDING	**CRITERIA**	**BOTTLEFEEDING**

BREASTFEEDING	CRITERIA	BOTTLEFEEDING
Preterm—cont'd		**Preterm—cont'd**
Desaturation (<90%) in 21% of breastfeedings.[29,33] With BPD, saturations higher than with bottlefeeding.[29,33]		Desaturation (<90%) in 38% of bottlefeedings.[29,33]
	←Hypercapnea→ ($\uparrow$Pco$_2$)	**Preterm** 34-35 wk: $\uparrow$Pco$_2$ depresses sucking and swallowing so that respirations may supercede feeding in preterms with increased respiratory drive[237] (i.e., BPD).
Preterm 32 wk: Increased feeding in active/alert and quiet/alert.[7]	←Behavioral→ Cues ←Quiet, alert→ state before and during feedings associated with more successful feeding behaviors.[155] Offer pacifier for nonnutritive suck (NNS) ac to promote awake behavior at beginning of feeding.[154] ←NNS pattern of→ sucking develops before nutritive pattern; mature NNS pattern not reliable cue for readiness to orally feed.[123] ←Cues include†:→ Oral behaviors— sucking on pacifier, fingers, feeding tube. Rooting reflex, hand-to-mouth behaviors, mouthing movements. ←Behavioral state→ changes—arousal from sleep, quiet alert state ac. ←Crying→ fussing and demanding to feed—a late sign.	**Full-Term and Preterm** Motor behavior: Change in arm posture (i.e., flexion) with feeding.[55]

†References 5, 40, 132, 154, 155, 219, 226.

refusing the breast, and (4) difficulty with latch-on.[94] If the sucking pattern learned with bottle-feeding impedes breastfeeding, health care providers should promote early, exclusive breast-feeding to prolong the duration of preterm breastfeeding after discharge.[115]

Maturation of feeding skills depends on developmental changes in the infant's central nervous system coupled with experiential learning.[132,196,231] Studies show that preterm infants are able to breastfeed far earlier (less than 1500 g or 28 to 36 weeks' gestation) than they can bottlefeed.* A comparison of studies of breastfeeding and bottlefeeding shows (1) less oxygen desaturation, (2) warmer skin temperature, (3) no bradycardia, and (4) better coordination of sucking and breathing with breastfeeding when compared with bottlefeeding (see Table 19-4). According to these research data, the ability of the preterm infant to breastfeed without alterations in homeostasis occurs *before* the ability to safely bottlefeed. Oxygenation is more stable with breastfeeding,[161] because the type of sucking pattern (e.g., intermittent) and the flow of milk at the beginning of breastfeeding may be easier for the VLBW infant to control and regulate.[146,223] In VLBW infants breathing is compromised (e.g., desaturations, increase in heart and respiratory rates) more during continuous sucking than intermittent sucking.[223] When an NG tube is in place, a VLBW infant has even poorer oxygenation, shallower breathing, and inability to increase tidal volume.[223] The postfeeding period enables recovery of oxygen saturation and end-tidal CO_2 to the prefeeding levels.[223]

Health care providers and parents should closely observe VLBW infants during the continuous sucking period (e.g., the first minute of bottlefeeding; with letdown during breastfeeding) for apnea, oxygen desaturation, and heart rate changes. Recommendations for continuous sucking periods include (1) not allowing breathing pauses of more than 10 seconds, (2) monitoring oxygen saturation and heart rate for continuous sucking of more than 30 seconds, and (3) interrupting sucking by withdrawing the nipple for breathing pauses and desaturations.[223]

Skin-to-skin (kangaroo) care provides a safe, effective alternative method of caring for pre-mature infants.[114] During skin-to-skin contact the infant may initiate nonnutritive suckling at the breast. Nonnutritive time at the breast is used to accustom both mother and baby to each other and the pleasant sensory stimuli at the breast. As the preterm matures, nonnutritive suckling is replaced by hunger cues, latching on, and effective nutritive suckling. Both AGA and SGA infants (700 to 2450 g) experience benefits from early (sometimes starting at birth) and sustained breastfeeding: (1) more mothers breastfeed and are more confident, (2) more frequent feedings are given, (3) more milk is produced, (4) infants breastfeed longer (e.g., at 1 month after discharge, breastfeeding rates increased from 11% to 50%),[34] (5) there is less bradycardia than with gavage or bottlefeeding, and (6) there is better weight gain and earlier discharge[114] (see Chapter 13).

Both maternal and neonatal responses to breastfeeding should be monitored. Adequate milk volume is available when the milk ejection (letdown) reflex occurs. Breast massage may assist in bringing down the milk, thus making it easier for the infant to obtain. Letdown may be felt by the mother and/or observed as a change in the rhythm of infant sucking and audible swallowing. After letdown is established, the infant expends little energy in sucking. He or she only needs to coordinate swallowing and breathing with an occasional burst of sucking. The nurse should be available during the initial breastfeeding to provide support to the mother, to ensure that the infant exhibits no signs of distress (e.g., color changes, bradycardia, oxygen desaturation, and drop in temperature), and to provide guidance for the mother if the infant chokes with letdown. The nurse also needs to reinforce to the mother that the infant's sucking pattern will be a pattern of bursts and pauses. The pauses are present in all infants and provide rest periods for the infant.

The infant's respiratory status should be reviewed. Infants requiring supplemental oxygen can breastfeed. If the infant requires 35% oxygen or less, oxygen may be delivered through a nasal cannula to ensure adequate, consistent oxygenation. This will eliminate another source of concern for the mother: having to worry about juggling the blow-by oxygen line. If the infant has not previously been placed on a nasal cannula, the nurse should initiate the cannula and then

---

*References 29, 161-164, 166, 168, 230.

assess oxygenation using a pulse oximeter before the feeding begins. The infant's temperature status requires review. Attention should be directed toward preventing hypothermia with infants who require significant thermal support. The infant should be swaddled, and a hat should be placed on the infant's head to prevent heat loss.

Duration of breastfeeding should be based on cues of satiety, such as sucking cessation or falling asleep or cues of physiologic instability and/or fatigue.[166] Frequency of breastfeeding can be progressed, as can frequency of bottlefeeding: from one breastfeeding per day to one per shift to every other breastfeeding. If the mother is available with this progression, bottlefeeding may be deferred until breastfeeding is well established, or bottlefeeding may be avoided altogether. When the infant is taking all nutrition orally, the mother can be encouraged to breastfeed as often as possible and to institute an ad lib schedule.[166] If the mother is available, the infant should breastfeed as often as is necessary and supplementation should not be provided. However, if the breast milk supply is insufficient, using a Lact-Aid Nursing Trainer provides nutritional supplementation and mammary stimulation to increase maternal milk supply. Total intake will need to be estimated to ensure adequate calories. If the infant weighs less than 1500 g, it may be necessary to augment calories, protein, and calcium with human milk fortifiers (see Chapter 16).

Families and staff often fear that the infant will not get enough during a breastfeeding. This concern is especially predominant when infants have been hospitalized for prematurity and fluids and calories have been scrutinized closely. Health professionals need to be sensitive to such concerns and refrain from employing methods such as weighing infants before and after feedings or using gavage tubes to attempt to determine the exact amount of breast milk ingested during the feeding. With today's electronic NICU scales, however, test weighing (before and after feeding; see Table 19-3) is accurate, if really necessary. However, health professionals need to focus on cues that can be used during and after hospitalization by both caregivers and the family. These cues include the infant's satisfaction after the feeding (asleep or fussy), the frequency of feedings, voiding pattern (minimum of six to eight wet diapers per day, weighing diapers and checking specific gravity) and palpation of the mother's breasts before and after feeding. Trends in weight gain can also demonstrate the success of the mother-infant dyad in breastfeeding.

A small infant may have difficulty taking a large nipple into the mouth. The mother should shape her nipple by compressing behind the areola to allow more of the nipple to be placed in the infant's mouth. The thumb and index finger or the first two fingers should be parallel to the infant's nose and chin. The breast must be soft enough to be compressed in this manner. It is important that the mother hold the infant close for the comfort of both, with the infant's entire body, not just the head, turned toward the mother's body (see Figure 19-5).

A nipple shield allows the infant to get a nipple in the mouth but increases the amount of sucking required to obtain milk and decreases the amount of stimulation received at the nipple. Supervised temporary use of silicone nipple shields has been found to be a successful bridging technique for the infant to transfer to direct breastfeeding (after only a few sessions of shield use).[178,192,199,253] Use of a nipple shield should be followed by breast pumping to express residual milk, maintain adequate milk supply, and obtain milk to freeze for supplemental feeding.[178,199]

Because nonnutritive suckling does not stimulate prolactin secretion and milk production, infants should not be placed on an empty breast to feed. Without positive reinforcement (i.e., milk) for their efforts, infants soon learn that the breast does not give milk, become frustrated, and refuse to feed. The Lact-Aid trainer may be used to initiate proper suckle and supplement intake in a small premature infant who is able to nurse (see Prevention).

Supplementing breastfeedings with bottlefed formula is inefficient in terms of energy and calories, because the infant expends energy, and thus calories, to feed twice. More energy-efficient and calorically efficient methods of initiating breastfeeding include offering smaller, more frequent feedings, supplementing by gavage feeding, or use of a lactation supplementing device. Breast milk fortifiers (see Chapter 16) should be used when the mother is unavailable for feedings when they are needed.

Nonavailability of a Feeding or Suckling Neonate

If premature birth or neonatal or maternal illness delays the onset of breastfeeding, the mother experiences a decrease in her milk production. Depending on how long breastfeeding has been delayed, mammary involution and the return of menstrual hormonal cycles may inhibit breastfeeding. A preterm infant or one who is ill may be weak and tire easily, so that adequate lactation is not established.

If a neonate is unable to feed at the breast, breast milk must be produced through artificial stimulation of the breast. The mother should establish a regular routine of breast massage[219] and pumping soon after the infant's birth. A comfortable chair with armrests or a pillow often helps, and the mother should be assured of privacy during breastfeeding and breast pumping. It is often necessary for the care provider to help the mother start and encourage her routine. Each breast should be pumped every 2 to 4 hours, preferably with a double pumping system in order to enhance milk supply.[93,96] Mothers should increase pumping time up to 15 to 20 minutes as her milk comes in, with the suction pressure increased as the mother tolerates. Early in pumping the mother should awaken to pump at night to establish a good milk supply. Sleep and rest are necessary for good milk supply; however, the mother should not sleep when breasts are engorged because this will decrease the supply. Mothers need to be advised that if their infant were with them, they would be feeding every 2 to 4 hours around the clock and therefore should develop that pattern to establish an adequate supply.

CAUTION: Mothers should be counseled regarding the potential risks of using breast shells or breast pump kits that have been used by other women. Breast shells, breast pump kits, and lactation aids are intimate-care items and are meant for use with one mother and one baby.

Induction Aids. Various induction aids using tactile and mechanical principles are available to assist the mother in lactating and relactating. Knowledge of the different systems and their advantages and disadvantages enables the health care provider to help the mother choose the most helpful aid.

Breast massage (gentle, tactile stimulus usually in a circular motion using increasing pressure) before breastfeeding or pumping may help unplug breast ducts and enable milk to flow more easily. Breast massage during pumping provides the important tactile stimulation that is missing without the infant's nursing and facilitates prolactin release and milk yield.[20,129,219]

Hand Expression. Once the breast milk supply has been established, hand expression (Figure 19-12) is the simplest and most cost-effective way to collect milk; however, prolactin secretion and milk yields are less than with a pulsative breast pump.[259] Some mothers find hand expression aesthetically unsatisfactory, and they should use other methods.

Mechanical Devices. Breast pumps work by application of negative pressure (e.g., -50 to -155 mm Hg) and compression in a suck-release pattern (e.g., rate of 40 to 50 suck/release cycles/min) by fitting the nipple cup (or flange) over the maternal nipple and areola.[1,28] Nonautomated pumps are regulated by the number of times the mother manually exerts and releases pressure. Three types of nonautomated pumps are available: (1) bicycle horn pumps, (2) cylinder pumps, and (3) trigger or handle pumps.[28] Nonautomated pumps are best for occasional use. Automated pumps (either fully or partially) exert more negative pressure, the greatest number of cycles per minute and are the pumps of choice for establishing and maintaining lactation for a preterm or sick infant.[28,219] A recent randomized trial comparing a novel manual breast pump (with compressive action on the areola) to a standard electric pump, used by mothers of preterm infants,

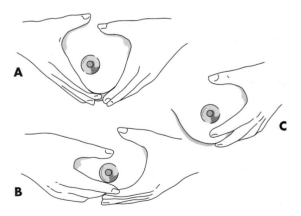

FIGURE 19-12 Breast massage. **A,** Place hands with palms toward chest at breast. Encircle breast with fingers and thumbs. **B** and **C,** Applying pressure, move hands forward, overlapping as they near nipple. Stop posterior to areola. Continue for 1 to 2 minutes or until milk is on nipple. Repeat on opposite breast. (From Bowman J, Hill R: *Pediatrics* 35:815, 1965; *Breastfeeding,* Evanston, Ill, 1981, American Academy of Pediatrics.)

found that the manual pump produced greater milk flow, resulted in greater total milk volume, was preferred by most mothers, and was more cost effective.[67] Automated pumps are available in the NICU and for home rental use. Health insurance (both public and private) may reimburse for pump rental. Innovative programs assist those unable to afford home rental.[194]

Serum prolactin levels and increased milk yield more closely approximate those of natural infant suckling when an intermittent, pulsative pump is used.[259] Just as nursing twins simultaneously results in a greater prolactin response, pumping both breasts simultaneously is more convenient[81] and provides higher prolactin release (and higher milk yield).[1,93,259]

To increase milk supply when the infant is not nursing, the pump should be used frequently (see Table 19-3). Because the breast pump is not as efficient as the suckling infant,[27] before initiating pumping the mother may find that tactile stimulation and breast massage helps to increase the milk supply. Looking at the infant's picture or listening to a tape recording of the infant's cry stimulates her milk production with a pump.

Beginning on the low or normal pump setting and carefully breaking the suction at the breast with a finger helps to prevent sore nipples. Painful engorgement is relieved by pumping each breast just enough to obtain relief. Nipple or areolar engorgement must be relieved so that the infant is able to grasp and suckle the nipple.

Lactoengineering. To increase caloric density of expressed breast milk to improve growth/weight gain in VLBW infants, the pumping process can be altered to increase lipid content. Because the lipid content of hindmilk (e.g., milk expressed after letdown or later in the pumping session) is two to three times higher than the lipid content of foremilk and hindmilk, feeding hindmilk to VLBW infants has been shown to increase growth and weight gain.[199,219,245] For VLBW infants with a consistent weight gain of less than 15 g/kg/day, hindmilk feedings may be initiated until a consistent weight gain of more than 30 g/kg/day is achieved.[245]

To express hindmilk, breast pumping is interrupted an average of 2 to 5 minutes after milk ejection has begun. This milk is collected and labeled "foremilk." Pumping is resumed until about 2 minutes after milk flow has ceased. This milk is placed in a separate container labeled "hindmilk." Another method of lactoengineering is to individualize the milk fractionation procedure by use of a creamatocrit that accurately estimates lipid and caloric content of expressed breast milk.* A small sample (less than 1.0 ml) of pumped breast milk is aliquoted into two capillary tubes that are sealed and centrifuged for 5 minutes. The lipid/cream layer rises to the top of the tubes, can be quantitated as a percentage of breast milk volume using a hematocrit reader and converted to estimates of lipid concentration and caloric density using published regression equations.[113,131,139,171] A recent study showed that mothers are able to cost-effectively and accurately perform creamatocrit assays; the mothers enjoyed the responsibility and increased involvement in their infant's care.[80] Interestingly, low-income mothers with fewer years of formal education and skilled rather than professional occupations were the most accurate in their performance of creamatocrits.

COMPLICATIONS

There are many complications other than prematurity that may pose difficulties with breastfeeding. Information on perinatal complications and breastfeeding is shown in Table 19-5.[5,128,129] Because of the significant benefits of breast milk, infants with special needs should be encouraged and mothers assisted in breastfeeding. Many principles used with the preterm and other variations of feeding styles and techniques may be helpful in facilitating these infants and their mothers in enjoying a successful breastfeeding experience. Consultation with and/or referral to a lactation consultant or specialist may also be helpful.

Drugs in Breast Milk

Table 19-6 provides information about specific drugs excreted in breast milk.[3,98,129] Protein binding, degree of ionization, molecular weight, and solubility of drugs influence the passage of drugs into milk.[98] Protein-bound drugs and drugs of large molecular weight (above 200) are less likely to pass into milk. Conversely, lipid-soluble drugs pass more easily into the milk. Because breast milk is slightly acidic when compared with plasma, weakly alkaline compounds are equal or

---

*References 80, 131, 139, 169, 171, 247, 248.

Text continued on p. 408

Table 19-5	PERINATAL COMPLICATIONS AND BREASTFEEDING		
	BREASTFEED		
COMPLICATIONS	**YES**	**NO**	**COMMENTS**
Maternal Complications			
Cesarean section	X		Regional anesthesia enables contact and feeding in recovery room. Pain medication is best given after feeding so levels peak before next feeding.
Pregnancy-induced hypertension	X		Preterm or SGA infants may be delivered, making delayed breastfeeding and pumping necessary. Maternal drugs may affect infant (see Table 19-6).
Venous thrombosis and pulmonary embolism	X		Depending on mother's ability; radioactive materials may be used for diagnosis, and anticoagulants may be used for therapy (see Table 19-6).
Bacterial Infections			
Urinary tract	X		Choice of antibiotics is important (see Table 19-6).
Mastitis	X		Continued emptying of breast (i.e., nursing baby or breast pump), bed rest, antibiotic therapy that is safe for infant, application of heat and cold, and use of analgesics are therapeutic.
Sexually transmitted diseases	X		No contraindication once mother is treated appropriately.
Tuberculosis	X	X	Culture-positive mothers must be separated from their infants regardless of mode of feeding; may pump and provide breast milk because tubercle bacillus is not passed through milk but through respiratory contact.[129]
	X		After therapy, when it is safe for mother to contact infant, then it is safe to breastfeed directly.
Diarrhea	X		Proper hand washing should be done and breastfeeding continued.
Viral Infections			
Cytomegalovirus	X		Both virus and protective antibodies occur in breast milk. For preterm infants with lower concentration of transplacental antibodies: freeze milk (which kills virus) for 7 days before feeding (for the first few weeks) until antibodies received via milk increase.[129]
Rubella	X		Isolate infected infant from other infants and susceptible personnel. Mother is not contagious postpartum and need not be isolated from infant. Rooming-in may be considered.
Rubella immunization	X		There is no known adverse effect on infant.
Herpes simplex (HSV)	X	X	May breastfeed if there is no active lesion on breast. Strict hand washing, as well as covering of genital lesions, is necessary. Rooming-in supports breastfeeding while isolating infant from others in nursery.
Varicella (chickenpox)	X	X	If mother has chickenpox within 6 days of delivery, isolate mother and do not allow her to breastfeed until she is no longer contagious. Infant should be separated regardless of mode of feeding.
Measles (rubeola)	X	X	If infant has measles, may isolate mother and infant together and allow breastfeeding. Mothers with measles postpartum have breastfed, and neonates have acquired mild disease. Secretory antibodies are probably present in milk in 45 hr. Mother exposed before delivery without active disease should be isolated from infant, because 50% of infants contract disease.
Hepatitis	X		Hepatitis A: may breastfeed as soon as mother receives gamma globulin.
	X		Hepatitis B antigen has been found in breast milk, but transmission by this route is not well documented. Both infants of chronic HBsAg carriers and those with acute hepatitis should receive high titer hepatitis B immunoglobulin and hepatitis vaccine, and breastfeeding is permitted.
	X		Hepatitis C infection rate is 4% in both breast/bottlefed infants; breastfeeding permitted: HCV-positive women do not increase the infection risk to their infants.

Modified from American Academy of Pediatrics: *Report of the committee on infectious disease,* ed 25, Evanston, III, 2000, American Academy of Pediatrics; and Lawrence RA: *Breastfeeding: a guide for the medical profession,* ed 5, St Louis, 1999, Mosby.

Continued

Table 19-5	PERINATAL COMPLICATIONS AND BREASTFEEDING—cont'd		

| | BREASTFEED | | |
COMPLICATIONS	YES	NO	COMMENTS
Viral Infections—cont'd			
HIV, AIDS		X	Breastfeeding is absolutely contraindicated in mothers who are HIV positive and living in developed countries where *safe* alternatives are available.[4,65,128,129]
Human T-cell leukemia virus type I (HTLV-I)		X	Infected lymphocytes found in breastmilk, unknown if able to cause disease. Current U.S. position: breastfeeding contraindicated.[129]
Parasitic Infections			
Toxoplasmosis	X		No transmission of toxoplasmosis has been demonstrated in humans. Antibodies are present in breast milk.
Other Infections			
Trichomoniasis		X	Metronidazole is contraindicated for infant; milk may be pumped and discarded until therapy is completed. Mother's dose can be modified so she can pump and discard milk for 24-48 hr.
Other Maternal Complications			
Diabetes	X		Lactation is antidiabetogenic. Lactosuria must be differentiated from glycosuria.
Thyroid disease	X	X	Radioisotopes and thiouracil are found in breast milk and may adversely affect infant. Mother who is taking propylthiouracil can breastfeed. Neither hypothyroidism nor hyperthyroidism is contraindication alone.
Cystic fibrosis	X	X	May cause nutritional drain on mother. Milk composition is normal. The Cystic Fibrosis Association has guidelines for lactation.
Smoking	X	X	Nicotine interferes with letdown and is excreted in milk. Of mothers who smoke, breastfed infants are healthier than bottlefed infants.
Neonatal Complications			
Medical			
Diarrhea	X	X	Maintain breastfeeding in infectious diarrhea unless milk is source of infection. Congenital lactase deficiency is rare but requires lactose-free formula.
Respiratory disease	X	X	Breast milk by gavage may be used if infant's condition permits.
Galactosemia		X	Galactose (lactose)-free diet is required.

Modified from American Academy of Pediatrics: *Report of the committee on infectious disease,* ed 25, Evanston, Ill, 2000, American Academy of Pediatrics; and Lawrence RA: *Breastfeeding: a guide for the medical profession,* ed 5, St Louis, 1999, Mosby.

Table 19-5	PERINATAL COMPLICATIONS AND BREASTFEEDING—cont'd		
	BREASTFEED		
COMPLICATIONS	**YES**	**NO**	**COMMENTS**
Neonatal Complications—cont'd			
Medical—cont'd			
Inborn errors of metabolism (such as PKU)	X	X	Combination of breast milk and special formula may sometimes be used. Careful monitoring of blood and urine levels of the amino acid is required.
Acrodermatitis enteropathica	X		Low plasma zinc levels are corrected by human milk and zinc sulfate supplementation.
Down syndrome	X		Hypotonia and poor suck reflex contribute to poor letdown and inadequate supply. Proper positioning, manual expression to begin feeding, and supporting the breast so infant does not lose nipple are helpful. Support from another mother with a Down syndrome infant is helpful.
Hypothyroidism	X		Enough T_3 may be ingested to avoid serious symptoms.
Hyperbilirubinemia	X		May have slightly higher bilirubin than bottlefed infant. There is no evidence that supplements are beneficial (see Chapter 21).
Breast milk jaundice	X	X	Uncommon occurrence; diagnosis of exclusion; if all other causes are excluded, a temporary cessation of breast milk may be indicated (see Chapter 21).
Cystic fibrosis	X		Increased losses of and lower electrolyte content of breast milk may cause electrolyte imbalance, which is less likely than with formulas.
Surgical			
Cleft lip and/or palate	X		Associated lesions, size, and position of defect influence successful feeding. Positioning and stabilizing breast in infant's mouth may help seal defect. Consult plastic surgeon.
Gastrostomy	X		If gastrostomy feedings are used, expressed breast milk is appropriate.
Partial obstruction (meconium plug, ileus, Hirschsprung's disease)	X		If oral feedings are indicated, breast milk is feeding of choice because of digestibility and mild cathartic effect.
Necrotizing enterocolitis	X		Breastfeeding may be partially protective and may be used when feeding resumes.
Gastrointestinal bleeding	X		Most common cause is maternal bleeding from nipple. Perform Apt test to differentiate fetal from adult hemoglobin.
CNS malformations	X		Weak suck and uncoordinated suck and swallow may be problems; however, may breastfeed more effectively than bottlefeed.

Table 19-6	DRUGS EXCRETED IN BREAST MILK	
DRUGS	**BREAST MILK**	**INFANT**
Analgesics		
Heroin,* codeine, meperidine, fentanyl, morphine, pentazocine, dextropropoxyphene	Appears in variable amounts.	Symptoms of depression and floppiness have been associated with these drugs.
Aspirin	Safe on a single-dose schedule, although it passes into milk in low concentration.	In a deliberate overdose, metabolic acidosis resulted from an accumulation in the infant; use cautiously because of the risk of Reye's syndrome.
Acetaminophen	Appears in small amounts.	Well tolerated.
Ibuprofen	Appears in small amounts.	Well tolerated.
Sumatripan succinate	Appears in small amounts.	Well tolerated.
Antibiotics and Sulfa Drugs		
Sulfa drugs	Appear in breast milk and may interfere with bilirubin binding in neonate; infants with G6PD deficiency may develop hemolysis.	Should not be used for breastfeeding mother in the first month if infant is jaundiced or if infant has G6PD deficiency.
Chloramphenicol	Appears in breast milk.	Contraindicated in nursing mother because infant may accumulate drug and develop "gray baby syndrome."
Penicillins (ampicillin, amoxicillin, etc.)	Small amounts in breast milk.	Disruption of GI flora, allergic sensitization/reactions. Observe for thrush, diarrhea, rash. Breast milk assists recolonization of normal gut flora.
Tetracycline	Appears in breast milk at 50% of serum level.	Infants may develop stained and mottled teeth when therapy exceeds 10 days; should only be given for life-threatening maternal infections. Discontinue breastfeeding during treatment.
Antifungals		
Metronidazole/Tinidazole	Appears in breast milk in levels equal to serum levels.	Side effects include decreased appetite, vomiting, blood dyscrasia, and animal evidence of tumorigenicity. Mother's dose can be modified (i.e., 2 g single-dose therapy) so she can pump and discard milk for 24 hr.
Antimalarial (chloroquine)	Very small amounts appear in breast milk.	Observe for GI symptoms—vomiting; diarrhea; hypotension.
Cephalosporins (cephalexin, cephalothin)	Very small amounts appear in breast milk.	Rash and sensitization are possible. May also affect bacterial flora—diarrhea, thrush.
Fluoroquinolones (levofloxacin, norfloxacine, ofloxacin, ciprofloxacin)	Varying levels in breast milk—use with caution.	Pseudomembranous colitis—observe for GI symptoms—vomiting, diarrhea. Tooth discoloration; phototoxicity. Arthropathy in animals.
Anticholinergics		
Atropine, scopolamine, synthetic quaternary ammonium derivatives	Atropine appears, but quaternary ammonium derivatives do not appear in breast milk.	The neonate of a nursing mother receiving atropine should be observed for tachycardia, constipation, and urinary retention.

Modified from Lawrence RA: *Breastfeeding: a guide for the medical profession,* ed 5, St Louis, 1999, Mosby; American Academy of Pediatrics, Committee on Drugs: *Pediatrics* 93:137, 1994; Howard C, Lawrence R: *Clin Perinatol* 26:447, 1999; Hale T: *Medications and mother's milk,* ed 9, Amarillo, TX, 2000, Pharmasoft.

*Drug of abuse; contraindicated during breastfeeding—hazardous to both mother and infant.

Table 19-6	DRUGS EXCRETED IN BREAST MILK—cont'd	
DRUGS	**BREAST MILK**	**INFANT**
Anticholinergics—cont'd		
Cimetidine	Appears in higher concentration than in serum.	No reported effects, although may suppress gastric activity, inhibit drug metabolism, and produce CNS stimulation. Use with caution until more information about antiandrogenic effects.
Anticoagulants		
Heparin and warfarin (Coumadin)	Do not appear in breast milk.	
Antithyroidal Agents		
Iodide	Passes into milk.	May affect thyroid activity and cause goiters. Not contraindicated during breastfeeding.
Thiouracil	Higher concentration in maternal milk than in blood.	Neonatal problems include suppression of thyroid activity and agranulocytosis. If breastfed, infant should be given thyroid supplement and thyroid function should be followed.
Propylthiouracil	Appears in small amounts (<0.3% of maternal dose).[37]	No reported effects on infant. Follow with T_3, T_4, and TSH.
Anticonvulsants		
Phenobarbital, phenytoin, carbamazepine (Tegretol), and valproic acid (Depakene)	All appear in small amounts.	Sedation is possible, but rarely are clinical symptoms significant enough to cause adverse effects. Due to long half-life of valproic acid, accumulation may occur.
Cardiovascular Drugs		
Digoxin	Appears only in small amounts.	Appears to be safe.
Reserpine	Appears in breast milk.	Symptoms include diarrhea, lethargy, nasal stuffiness, bradycardia, and respiratory difficulties; contraindicated in breastfeeding.
Propranolol, metaprolol, labetalol	Appear in breast milk in varying degrees. Safest beta blockers with breastfeeding.	Observe for beta blockade—respiratory depression, bradycardia, or hypoglycemia.
Nifedipine, verapamil, diltiazem	Appear in varying amounts in breast milk.	Appear to be safe.
Cathartics		
Aloin, cascara sagrada, and anthraquine preparations	Appear in breast milk.	Colic and diarrhea are possible side effects.
Contraceptives		
Birth control pills (combined; progestin only; minipill)	Appear in breast milk with peak levels 2 hr after intake.	Combined: may alter the quality and quantity of milk—suppress lactation, shorter breastfeeding, and slower weight gain. Progestin only or minipill—no alteration of milk volume or infant weight gain. Unknown long-term risk of cancer—no evidence in last 30 years.[128]
Medroxyprogesterone (Depo-Provera)	Increased prolactin levels before/after sucking.	No adverse effects—3-mo injection (increased protein and quantity of milk); 6-mo injection (increased quantity but decrease in protein, fat, calcium).[128]

Continued

Table 19-6	DRUGS EXCRETED IN BREAST MILK—cont'd	
DRUGS	**BREAST MILK**	**INFANT**
Contraceptives—cont'd		
Norplant	Steroid appears in small amount in breast milk.	No effect on milk production or infant growth and development.
Intrauterine devices	No chemicals to be excreted into breast milk.	No effects on infant.
Barrier methods (diaphragm, condoms, foams, cervical cap)	No chemicals to be excreted into breast milk.	No effects on infant.
Diagnostic Radioactive Compounds		
^{67}Ga, ^{125}I, ^{131}I, and ^{64}Cu	Appear for 24-48 hr.	Check half-life of specific compound. Pump and discard, then resume breastfeeding.
Diuretics		
Hydrochlorothiazide	May suppress lactation.	Inadequate milk; no significant risks are present—compatible with breastfeeding.
Psychotherapeutic Agents		
Lithium	Appears in breast milk; infant serum level is 10%-50% of mother.	Contraindicated in pregnancy; controversial during lactation. Cyanosis, hypotonia, ECG changes. Evaluate Lithium levels. Inhibits cyclic 3'-5' AMP, a substance significant to brain growth.
Phenothiazines	Appear in small amounts.	Evaluate each drug separately; observe for sedation.
Diazepam (Valium)	Appears in breast milk and may accumulate in infant because it is detoxified in liver.	Poor feeding, weight loss, hypoventilation, and drowsiness may be seen. Low incidence of toxicity and adverse events.[31]
Tricyclic antidepressants (amitriptyline, nortriptyline, desipramine)	Appear in minimal amounts (<1%).	Careful considerations to select the safest for the infant.
Selective serotonin reuptake inhibitors (SSRI) (fluoxetine, sertraline, paroxetine)[156]	Appear in varying amounts. Fluoxetine—high levels, highly lipid bound.	Sertraline is the drug of choice after birth because plasma levels are low (<2 ng/ml).[21,64,118,233] May alter short/long-term central nervous system development and function. Slower growth curve/weight gain with fluoxetine.[44]
Stimulants		
Caffeine	Appears in small amounts (<1%) but may accumulate in infant.	Symptoms include jitteriness, wakefulness, and irritability. May alter iron concentration in milk and iron deficiency anemia at 1 month of age.

Modified from Lawrence RA: *Breastfeeding: a guide for the medical profession,* ed 5, St Louis, 1999, Mosby; American Academy of Pediatrics, Committee on Drugs: *Pediatrics* 93:137, 1994; Howard C, Lawrence R: *Clin Perinatol* 26:447, 1999; Hale T: *Medications and mother's milk,* ed 9, Amarillo, TX, 2000, Pharmasoft.

Table 19-6	DRUGS EXCRETED IN BREAST MILK—cont'd	
DRUGS	**BREAST MILK**	**INFANT**
Stimulants—cont'd		
Theophylline	Appears in moderate amounts.	Irritability, jitteriness, and wakefulness may be seen in infant.
Cocaine*	Appears in breast milk.	Cocaine intoxication: neurotoxicity (e.g., irritability, hyperactive reflexes, tremulousness, and mood lability) and seizures have been reported[45,46] (see Chapter 4).
Other Substances		
Methadone	Appears in breast milk.	Management depends on maternal dosage—under 20 mg/24 hr probably safe. Observe for sedation, withdrawal.
Ethanol (alcohol)	Quick equilibration between serum and breast milk levels.	Large quantities associated with lethargy, drowsiness, and affected motor development.[133] May inhibit milk letdown reflex and suppress lactation.[48] Avoid nursing within 2-3 hr of alcohol intake.
Marijuana*	May reach high concentrations.	May decrease prolactin levels, milk supply, and motor development. Exposure to secondary smoke. Avoid breastfeeding for several hours after use.[126]
Nicotine	Appears in breast milk in proportion to number of cigarettes smoked/time from last cigarette.[144,174]	Irritability; failure-to-thrive may result because of suppression of lactation. Effects of secondary smoke: increased incidence of upper respiratory infections, otitis media, bronchitis, pneumonia and SIDS. Avoid smoking in the same room with the infant.
Herbal tea mixtures (containing anise, fennel, licorice, galega) used to stimulate lactation (i.e., mother's milk tea).	Essential oils found in anise and fennel appear in breast milk.	Difficulty feeding; growth failure; hypotonia; lethargy; vomiting; weak cry; poor suck; decreased reaction to painful stimuli.[211]
Fenugreek	Appears in breast milk; milk has a maple syrup smell.	Urine may have maple syrup smell.
Ginseng	No data on amount in breast milk.	May cause neonatal androgen effect and hirsutism.
Comfrey	No data on amount in breast milk. Caution use in any form.	Associated with venoocclusive disease, hepatotoxicity, and is carcinogenic. Contraindicated in breastfeeding.
Silicone breast implants	Intact implants—not necessary to check milk for silicone. Leaking of ruptured implants—amount in breast milk unknown without silicone testing of milk and urine.	No absolute contraindication to breastfeeding by women with silicone implants.[26]

greater in breast milk than in plasma. Weakly acidic compounds have a higher concentration in plasma than in breast milk.

Several factors influence the drug effect on the infant.[98] Most drugs appear in milk, but drug levels usually do not exceed 1% to 2% of the ingested dose and do not depend on the milk volume.[129] Drug transfers through breast milk may be minimized by ingestion of oral medications after nursing/feeding the infant before taking the drug.[16] Many variables, such as gastric emptying, pH, and effects of intestinal enzymes, affect absorption. Finally, the chronologic and gestational ages of the infant affect the maturity of the systems involved in excretion and detoxification (see Chapter 9).

PARENT TEACHING

Parent teaching has been discussed throughout this chapter because it is so essential to a successful breastfeeding experience for both mother and infant.

Before a premature or sick infant is actually nursed at the breast, the colostrum and breast milk are pumped and fed to the infant. If the mother's production is adequate, no supplementation is necessary. Before collecting the mother's milk, perform the following:

- Screen the mother (by history) for disease.
- Screen the mother (by history) for drugs that she has taken.
- Instruct the mother in sterile technique.

Proper collection and storage must be discussed with each family so that stored milk does not cause infections. A written handout of pumping, storing, and thawing practices is helpful. Often the mother pumps and collects the milk, and the father transports it to the NICU (see Chapter 29). Methods of treatment and storage are listed in Box 19-1. Rewarming techniques include placing frozen milk in (1) a room-temperature water bath, (2) a hot-water bath, (3) a microwave oven, or (4) under cold running water and then tepid water. Slow room-temperature rewarming is a concern because of bacterial overgrowth, especially if thawing is prolonged. Most nurseries use room-temperature water bath rewarming to avoid exposure to the high temperatures of the hot-water bath and the microwave. Microwaving is contraindicated because of the destruction of antiinfective properties (e.g., lysozyme and se-

---

Box 19-1 TREATMENT AND STORAGE OF BREAST MILK

Treatment

1. Heat: Significant loss of lysozyme, lactoferrin, immunoglobulins, lactoperoxidase, lymphocyte function, complement, phagocytosis, and macromolecules may occur. Fat content altered (~13%) by milk sterilization.[68] Pasteurization does not alter fat content or fatty acid composition, but fat absorption by small preterm infants may be reduced from inactivation of bile salt lipase.[120]
2. Lyophilization: Effects are similar to those of heat treatment.
3. Freezing: Limited information; cells are not viable, but there is no effect on IgA content. Fat content is altered by freezing and thawing.[248]

Storage

1. Use sterile glass or polypropylene containers (amount for one feeding/bag); polyethylene bags change immunologic properties of breast milk and are more difficult for mothers to handle.
2. Label with name, date, and time of collection.
3. Store in refrigerator for 24 hours (at 0° to 4° C [32° to 39.2° F]) or (−18° C [0° F]) for longer periods.

---

cretory IgA), resulting in an overgrowth of bacteria.[106,201,227] Fresh breast milk is preferable for feedings because of its immunologic properties. If the mother visits the infant at feeding time, she may pump her breasts and the breast milk immediately fed to the infant.

Human milk banks that collect, store, and distribute milk to infants other than those of the donating mother exist around the world. This support is not available to some NICUs; others intentionally choose not to store donor milk. The reservations about storing donor milk generally involve questions concerning adequate nutrition and immunologic benefit versus harm to a high-risk infant. Adequate screening of human milk donors (for cytomegalovirus [CMV], human immunodeficiency virus [HIV], and other viruses) is essential, as is informed consent. Because of the possibility of milk-borne pathogens (e.g., HIV, hepatitis C), all donor milk must be pasteurized.[129] Many nurseries do not give human milk other than the mother's. Milk banks ship human milk when necessary. For milk bank locations, contact the Human Milk Banking Association of North America, Inc. (HMBANA), c/o

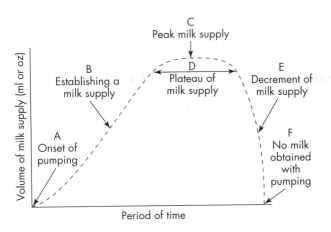

FIGURE 19-13 Establishing and maintaining milk supply by pumping. **A,** Pumping begins. **B,** Milk supply is established and increases. **C,** Peak or maximum volume of milk is established and plateaus. **D,** Gradually, supply begins to dwindle and may totally cease, **E** and **F,** The volume of milk and time period for decline in supply to begin and end in no milk production is an individual process. Some women begin and end cycle in days or weeks; others are able to pump for months. Even if the supply dwindles to no milk, nutritive suckling of the infant with a Lact-Aid Nursing Trainer in place (see Figure 19-10) will reestablish the supply.

Mother's Milk Bank, WakeMed, 3000 New Bern Avenue, Raleigh, NC 27610; phone (919) 350-8599; email mtully@wakemed.org.

A mother may be so concerned about the welfare of her infant that she spends most of her time at the hospital and receives inadequate rest, which is a common cause of milk production problems. The care plan includes encouraging, educating, and giving a mother permission to go home and rest, which may require someone to assist with the care of the newborn's siblings. The stress of having a sick infant and the time spent at the hospital may mean that the mother does not receive adequate nutrition.

It is necessary to add about 600 kcal to the non-pregnant diet and to replace elements, such as calcium, minerals, and fat-soluble vitamins, used in producing milk. The recommended dietary increases are similar to those during pregnancy. Adequate fluid intake, 6 to 8 glasses of water, skim milk, or other noncaffeine liquids, should be consumed every day. Certain components of breast milk, such as quantity, as well as protein and calcium content, do not vary with the mother's diet, whereas others (e.g., fatty and amino acids, lysine, methionine, and water-soluble vitamins) vary with maternal intake.

A mother's diet does not have much effect on the quality of the breast milk[199] (unless malnutrition intervenes) but affects the mother's overall health. She should be reminded to eat a balanced diet. Vegetarian diets should be supplemented with about 4 mg of cyanocobalamin per day.

Anticipatory guidance is essential for mothers who are breastfeeding preterm infants. Mothers must be informed in the beginning that their milk supply may dwindle, even though they closely adhere to the pumping schedule. This is normal, because no pump stimulates the breast as efficiently and physiologically as the suckling infant. When the pumping regimen begins, explaining and drawing the mother a picture (Figure 19-13) of what is commonly experienced helps alleviate guilt caused by a dwindling milk supply. A rather sparse supply of milk does not mean she cannot nurse the infant, because the milk supply will build in response to the infant's nutritive suckle. The parent should be taught that there is no correlation between the amount of breast milk expressed and the amount of milk a mother actually lets down when the infant is at the breast.

Breastfeeding problems may be particularly detrimental to the mother's perception of breastfeeding success. Disappointment with the breastfeeding experience may result from unrealistic expectations regarding breastfeeding the preterm infant. Establishing realistic parental expectations for the first time the infant breastfeeds decreases disappointment from unattainable goals. Breastfeeding, like parenting, is not instinctual but is a learned behavior for both the mother and the infant. No one, including the health care provider, should expect immediate latch-on and vigorous sucking. The first several attempts at breastfeeding may consist only of direct skin contact, nuzzling, and licking behaviors by the infant, and cuddling and positioning by the mother. Any actual sucking is an "extra" reward but should not be anticipated.

Emotional support during breastfeeding of a normal or sick infant facilitates a successful experience for both the mother and the infant.[166,178,255] In one NICU without formalized support, only 10% of mothers were still breastfeeding 2 weeks after discharge. After a breastfeeding support group was instituted, 80% of mothers continued breastfeeding 2 weeks after discharge.[255] In another NICU a breastfeeding support program resulted in breastfeeding rates of 71% at discharge.[170] Support groups with mothers who have had similar experiences are helpful in supplementing support obtained from significant others and professionals.[166,178]

The incidence and duration of breastfeeding preterm or sick newborns vary among NICUs and among countries. In the United States in 1995 only 32% to 38% of mothers of LBW infants initiated breastfeeding compared with 62% of all mothers.[212] During the same period 75% of mothers of hospitalized newborns in Switzerland succeeded in breastfeeding their infants: 50% exclusively and 25% partially breastfed.[99] There is an inverse relationship between gestational age and duration of breastfeeding, with most mothers (more than 50%) abandoning breastfeeding before their infants are discharged from the hospital.* In a recent German cohort study, the average duration of breast milk feedings in VLBW infants was one third that of a matched group of term infants.[111] Early cessation of breast milk feeding (e.g., during initial hospitalization) in VLBW infants was associated with the mother's smoking and low parental education. In the same study prolonged breast milk feeding was associated with (1) multiple pregnancy, (2) infants of less than 29 weeks' gestation, (3) maternal age greater than 35 years, and (4) spontaneous pregnancy.[111]

In a study reported by Bell, Geyer, and Jones,[25] at discharge from the NICU 40% of sick or preterm infants were receiving breast milk, but only 3% were actually feeding at the breast. Hill, Ledbetter, and Kavanaugh,[94] reported that 54% of preterm infants were receiving breast milk or breastfeeding at discharge and only 51% at 4 weeks after discharge. The most common reason cited by mothers for discontinuation of breastfeeding (both in the hospital and after discharge) is inadequate milk supply (or "not getting enough").* Early initiation and establishment of adequate feeding at the breast before discharge encourages both mothers and professionals that exclusive breastfeeding is successful. However, the early postdischarge period may be significantly stressful for mothers, because the breastfeeding pattern of a preterm infant may predispose to underconsumption (i.e., inability to compensate for inadequate intake in one feeding by increasing the number or intake of subsequent feedings), result in behaviors indicative of inadequate intake, and require nutritional supplementation.†

Education and training regarding the many facets of breastfeeding are essential for medical and nursing staff.‡ Staff attitudes and behaviors are important to breastfeeding families and affect the breastfeeding experience.§ A multidimensional approach to such education includes providing the staff with manuals, guides, and other educational materials as well as scheduling routine classes, in-service training, and workshops. Moreover, professionals with clinical expertise should be identified[258]; these resource personnel can increase the staff's competency in counseling and assisting breastfeeding families.

Protocols addressing breastfeeding can outline a consistent approach for staff, as well as provide resource material that addresses successful strategies for handling common problems. Protocols can also reduce the amount of incorrect information that is disseminated.[200,213,258]

Breast milk is the best milk, especially for a sick or premature infant. By understanding normal lactation, the health care provider can sup-

*References 92, 111, 163, 165, 166.

*References 92, 108, 163, 165, 166, 167, 178, 199.
†References 62, 86, 108, 165, 166, 178, 235.
‡References 5, 56, 70, 119, 130, 175, 195, 200, 207, 213, 220, 255, 258.
§References 56, 117, 119, 195, 207, 220, 257.

port the breastfeeding dyad when breastfeeding is delayed or disrupted.

REFERENCES

1. Alekseev N, Ilyin VI, Yaroslovski VK et al: Compression stimuli increase the efficacy of breast pump function, *Eur J Obstet Gynecol Reprod Biol* 77:131, 1998.
2. American Academy of Pediatrics: *Report of the Committee on Infectious Disease,* ed 25, Evanston, Ill, 2000, The Academy.
3. American Academy of Pediatrics, Committee on Drugs: The transfer of drugs and other chemicals into human breastmilk, *Pediatrics* 93:137, 1994.
4. American Academy of Pediatrics, Committee on Pediatric AIDS: Human milk, breastfeeding, and transmission of human immunodeficiency virus in the United States, *Pediatrics* 96:977, 1995.
5. American Academy of Pediatrics, Work Group on Breastfeeding: Breastfeeding and the use of human milk, *Pediatrics* 100:1035, 1997.
6. Amin S, Merle KS, Orlando MS et al: Brainstem maturation in premature infants as a function of enteral feeding type, *Pediatrics* 106:318, 2000.
7. Anderson G, Behnke M, Gill N et al: Self-regulatory gavage-to-bottle feeding for preterm infants: effects on behavioral state, energy expenditure, and weight gain. In Funk S, Tornquist E, Champagne M et al, eds: *Key aspects to recovery,* New York, 1990, Sprigle Publishing.
8. Anderson J, Johnstone B, Remley D: Breastfeeding and cognitive development: a meta-analysis, *Am J Clin Nutr* 70:525, 1999.
9. Aniansson G, Alm B, Andersson B et al: A prospective cohort study on breast-feeding and otitis media in Swedish infants, *Pediatr Infect Dis J* 13:183, 1994.
10. Armand M, Hamosh M, Mehta NR et al: Effect of human milk or formula on gastric function and fat digestion in the premature infant, *Pediatr Res* 40:429, 1996.
11. Arnon S: Breastfeeding and toxigenic intestinal infections: missing links in crib death? *Rev Infect Dis* 6:5193, 1984.
12. Arvedson J: Dysphagia in pediatric patients with neurologic damage, *Semin Neurol* 16:371, 1996.
13. Atkinson S, Kaufman K: Lactational performance and milk composition in relation to duration of pregnancy and lactation. In Hamosh M, Goldman A, eds: *Human lactation 2: maternal and environmental factors,* New York, 1986, Plenum Press.
14. Atkinson S, Anderson GH, Bryan MH et al: Human milk: comparison of the nitrogen component in milk from mothers of premature and full-term infants, *Am J Clin Nutr* 33:811, 1980.
15. Auerbach K: Sequential and simultaneous breast pumping: a comparison, *Int J Nurs Study* 27:257, 1993.
16. Auerbach K: Breastfeeding and maternal medication use, *J Obstet Gynecol Neonatal Nurs* 28:554, 1999.
17. Auerbach K, Avery JL: Relactation after an untimely weaning: report from a survey, *Res Hum Nurtur* (monograph 2), 1979.
18. Auerbach K, Avery JL: Relactation and the premature infant: report from a survey, *Res Hum Nurtur* (monograph 3), 1979.
19. Auerbach K, Avery JL: Relactation after a hospital-induced separation: report from a survey, *Res Hum Nurtur* (monograph 4), 1979.
20. Auerbach K, Walker M: When the mother of a premature infant uses a breast pump: what every NICU nurse needs to know, *Neonatal Netw* 13:23, 1994.
21. Austin M, Mitchell P: Use of psychotropic medications in breastfeeding women: acute and prophylactic treatment, *Aust N Z J Psychiatry* 32:778, 1998.
22. Avery JL: Relactation and induced lactation. In Riordan J, ed: *A practical guide to breastfeeding,* St Louis, 1983, Mosby.
23. Babbitt RL, Hoch TA, Coe DA et al: Behavioral assessment and treatment of pediatric feeding disorders, *Dev Behav Pediatr* 15:278, 1994.
24. Beaudry M, Dufour R, Marcoux S: Relations between infant feeding and infections during the first six months of life, *J Pediatr* 126:191, 1995.
25. Bell E, Geyer J, Jones L: A structured intervention improves breastfeeding success for ill or preterm infants, *MCN Am J Matern Child Nurs* 20:309, 1995.
26. Berlin C: Silicone breast implants and breast feeding, *Pediatrics* 94:547, 1994.
27. Biancuzzo M: *Breastfeeding the newborn: clinical strategies for nurses,* St Louis, 1999, Mosby.
28. Biancuzzo M: Selecting pumps for breast feeding mothers, *J Obstet Gynecol Neonatal Nurs* 28:417, 1999.
29. Bier JB, Ferguson A, Anderson L et al: Breast-feeding of very low birth weight infants, *J Pediatr* 123:773, 1993.
30. Billeaud C, Guillet J, Sandler B: Gastric emptying in infants with or without gastro-esophageal reflux according to the type of milk, *Eur J Clin Nutr* 44: 577, 1990.
31. Birnbaum CS, Cohen LS, Bailey JW et al: Serum concentrations of antidepressants and benzodiazepines in nursing infants: a case series, *Pediatrics* 104:e11, 1999.
32. Blass E: Behavioral and physiological consequences of suckling in rat and human newborns, *Acta Paediatr Suppl* 397:71, 1994.
33. Blaymore Bier JA, Ferguson AE Morales Y et al: Breastfed infants who were ELBW, *Pediatrics* 100(6):e3, 1997.

34. Blaymore-Bier J, Ferguson A, Morales Y et al: Comparison of skin-to-skin contact with standard contact in LBW infants who are breastfed, *Arch Pediatr Adolesc Med* 150:1265, 1996.

35. Bosma JF, ed: Oral sensation and perception, Department of Health, Education and Welfare Pub No (NIH) 73-546, Bethesda, Md, 1973, Department of Health, Education and Welfare.

36. Brent N, Rudy SJ, Redd B et al: Sore nipples in breast-feeding women: a clinical trial of wound dressings vs. conventional care, *Arch Pediatr Adolesc Med* 152:1077, 1998.

37. Briggs G, Freeman R, Yaffe S, eds: *Drugs in pregnancy and lactation,* ed 5, Baltimore, 1998, Williams & Wilkins.

38. Brown L, Hollingsworth A, Armstrong C: Factors affecting milk volume in mothers of VLBW infants. In Programs and Abstracts of the 1991 Scientific Sessions of the 31st Biennial Convention, 1991.

39. Bulock F, Woolridge M, Baum J: Development of coordination of sucking, swallowing, and breathing: ultrasound study of term and preterm infants, *Dev Med Child Neurol* 32:669, 1990.

40. Cagan J: Feeding readiness behavior in preterm infants, *Neonatal Netw* 14:82, 1995.

41. Calhoun D, Lunoe M, Du Y et al: Human milk as an enteral source of granulocyte colony-stimulating factor, *Pediatr Res* 45:187A, 1999.

42. Carlson S, Werkman S: A randomized trial of visual attention of preterm infants fed docosahexaenoic acid until two months, *Lipids* 31:85, 1996.

43. Carlson S, Werkman S, Rhodes P et al: Visual-acuity development in healthy preterm infants: effect of marine-oil supplementation, *Am J Clin Nutr* 58:35, 1993.

44. Chambers CD, Anderson PO, Thomas RG et al: Weight gain in infants breastfed by mothers who take fluoxetine, *Pediatrics* 104:1120, 1999.

45. Chaney NE, Franke J, Wadlington WB: Cocaine convulsions in a breastfeeding baby, *J Pediatr* 112:134, 1988.

46. Chasnoff IJ, Lewis DE, Squires L: Cocaine intoxication in a breastfeeding infant, *Pediatrics* 80:836, 1987.

47. Cochi S, Fleming DW, Hightower AW et al: Primary invasive *Haemophilus influenzae* type b disease: a population-based assessment of risk factors, *J Pediatr* 108:887, 1986.

48. Coiro V, Alboni A, Gramellini D et al: Inhibition by ethanol of the oxytocin response to breast stimulation in normal women and the role of endogenous opioids, *Acta Endocrinol* 126:213, 1992.

48a. Covert R, Barman N, Domanico R et al: Prior enteral nutrition with human milk protects against intestinal perforation in infants who develop NEC, *Pediatr Res* 37:305A, 1995.

49. Craig C, Lee D: Neonatal control of nutritive sucking pressure: evidence for an intrinsic τ-guide, *Exp Brain Res* 124:371, 1999.

50. Craig C, Grealy M, Lee D: Detecting motor abnormalities in preterm infants, *Exp Brain Res* 131:359, 2000.

51. Crook C, Lipsitt L: Neonatal nutritive sucking: effects of taste stimulation upon sucking rhythm and heart rate, *Child Dev* 47:518, 1976.

52. Crowell M, Hill P, Humenick S: Relationship between OB analgesia and time of effective breast-feeding, *J Nurse Midwifery* 39:150, 1994.

53. Cunningham A, Jelliffe D, Jelliffe E: Breastfeeding and health in the 1980s: a global epidemiologic review, *J Pediatr* 118:659, 1991.

54. Daly SE, Kent JC, Owens RA et al: Frequency and degree of milk removal and short-term control of human milk synthesis, *Exp Physiol* 81:861, 1996.

55. Daniels H, Casaer P: Development of arm posture during bottle feeding in preterm infants, *Infants Behav Dev* 8:241, 1985.

56. Dermer A: Breastfeeding: what you—and your patients—need to know, *Womens Health Prim Care* 1:599, 1998.

57. Dewey K, Heinig J, Nommsen-Rivers L: Differences in morbidity between breastfed and formula fed infants, *J Pediatr* 126:696, 1995.

58. Dowling D: Physiological responses of preterm infants to breast-feeding and bottle-feeding with the orthodontic nipple, *Nurs Res* 48:78, 1999.

59. Dubignon J, Campbell D, Curtis M et al: The relation between laboratory measures of sucking, food intake, and perinatal factors during the newborn period, *Child Dev* 40:1107, 1969.

60. Duncan B, Ey J, Holberg CJ et al: Exclusive breast-feeding for at least 4 months protects against otitis media, *Pediatrics* 91:867, 1993.

61. Eishima K: The analysis of sucking behavior in newborn infants, *Early Hum Dev* 27:163, 1991.

62. Elliott S, Reimer C: Postdischarge telephone follow-up program for breastfeeding preterm infants discharged from a special care nursery, *Neonatal Netw* 17:41, 1998.

63. El-Mohandes A, Picard M, Simmens S et al: Use of human milk in the intensive care nursery decreases the incidence of nosocomial sepsis, *J Perinatol* 17:130, 1997.

64. Epperson C, Anderson G, McDougle C: Sertraline and breastfeeding, *N Engl J Med* 336:1189, 1997.

65. European Collaborative Study: Risk factors for mother-to-child transmission of HIV-1, *Lancet* 339:1007, 1992.

66. Fehrer S, Berger L, Johnson D et al: Increasing breast milk production for premature infants with a relaxation/imagery audiotape, *Pediatrics* 83:57, 1989.

67. Fewtrell MS, Lucas P, Collier S et al: Randomized trial comparing the efficacy of a novel manual breast pump with a standard electric breast pump in mothers who delivered preterm infants, *Pediatrics* 107:1291, 2001.

68. Fidler N, Sauerwald TU, Koletzko B et al: Effects of human milk pasteurization and sterilization on available fat content and fatty acid composition, *J Pediatr Gastroenterol Nutr* 27:317, 1998.

69. Ford RP, Taylor BJ, Mitchell EA et al: Breastfeeding and the risk of sudden infant death syndrome, *Int J Epidemiol* 22:885, 1993.

70. Freed GL, Clark SJ, Sorensen J et al: National assessment of physicians' breast-feeding knowledge, attitudes, training and experience, *JAMA* 273:472, 1995.

71. Gartner L: Breastfeeding in the hospital, *Semin Perinatol* 18:475, 1994.

72. Garofalo R, Goldman A: Expression of functional immunomodulatory and anti-inflammatory factors in human milk, *Clin Perinatol* 26:361, 1999.

73. Garza C, Schanler R, Butte N et al: Special properties of human milk, *Clin Perinatol* 14:11, 1987.

74. Genzel B, Wahle J, Koletzko B: Fatty acid composition of human milk during the first month after term and preterm delivery, *Eur J Pediatr* 156:142, 1997.

75. Gerstein H: Cow's milk exposure and type I diabetes mellitus, *Diabetes Care* 17:13, 1994.

76. Gewolb I, Vice F, Schweitzer E et al: Developmental patterns of rhythmic suckle and swallow in preterm infants, *Pediatr Res* 45:199A, 1999.

77. Glass R, Wolf L: A global perspective on feeding assessment in the neonatal intensive care unit, *Am J Occup Ther* 48:514, 1994.

78. Goldman A, Chheda S, Garofalo R: Evolution of immunologic functions of the mammary gland and the postnatal development of immunity, *Pediatr Res* 43:155, 1998.

79. Goldson E: Nonnutritive sucking in the sick infant, *J Perinatol* 9:30, 1987.

80. Griffin TL, Meyer PP, Bradford LP et al: Mothers' performing creamatocrit measures in the NICU: accuracy, reactions and cost, *J Obstet Gynecol Neonatal Nurs* 29:249, 2000.

81. Groh-Wargo S, Toth A, Mahoney K et al: The utility of a bilateral breast pumping system for mothers of premature infants, *Neonatal Netw* 14:31, 1995.

82. Guilleminault C, Coons S: Apnea and bradycardia during feeding in infants weighing >2,000 grams, *J Pediatr* 104: 932, 1984.

83. Hack M, Estabrook M, Robertson S: Development of the sucking rhythm in preterm infants, *Early Hum Dev* 11:133, 1985.

84. Hagan R et al: Breastfeeding and very low birthweight (VLBW) infants, Abstract No 1284, *Neonatol Gen,* 1991.

85. Hale T: *Medications and mother's milk,* ed 9, Amarillo, 2000, Pharmasoft Publishing.

86. Hall R, Simon S, Smith M: Readmission of breast-fed infants in the first two weeks of life, *J Perinatol* 20:432, 2000.

87. Hammerman C, Kaplan M: Oxygen saturation during and after feeding in healthy term infants, *Biol Neonate* 67:94, 1995.

88. Hamosh M, Peterson JA, Henderson TR et al: Protective function of human milk: the milk fat globule, *Semin Perinatol* 23:242, 1999.

89. Hamosh M: Bioactive factors in human milk, *Pediatr Clin North Am* 48:69, 2001.

90. Hay WW Jr, Lucas A, Heird WC et al: Workshop summary: nutrition of the extremely low birth weight infant, *Pediatrics* 104:1360, 1999.

91. Hayashi Y, Haashi E, Nana T: Ultrasonographic analysis of sucking behavior of newborn infants: the driving force of sucking pressure, *Early Hum Dev* 49:33, 1997.

92. Hill P, Anderson J, Ledbetter R: Delayed initiation of breastfeeding the preterm infant, *J Perinat Neonatal Nurs* 9:10, 1995.

93. Hill P, Aldag J, Chatterton R: The effect of sequential and simultaneous breast pumping on milk volume and prolactin levels: a pilot study, *J Hum Lact* 12:193, 1996.

94. Hill P, Ledbetter R, Kavanaugh K: Breastfeeding pattern of low birth weight infants after hospital discharge, *J Obstet Gynecol Neonatal Nurs* 26:190, 1997.

95. Hofer M: Early relationships as regulators of infant physiology and behavior, *Acta Paediatr Suppl* 397: 9, 1994.

96. Hopkinson J, Schanler R, Garza C: Milk production by mothers of premature infants, *Pediatrics* 81:815, 1988.

97. Horwood L, Darlaw B, Mogridge N: Breast milk feeding and cognitive ability at 7-8 years, *Arch Dis Child Fetal Neonatal Ed* 84:F23, 2001.

98. Howard C, Lawrence R: Drugs and breastfeeding, *Clin Perinatol* 26:447, 1999.

99. Hunkeler B, Aebi C, Minder C et al: Incidence and duration of breast-feeding of ill newborns, *J Pediatr Gastroenterol Nutr* 18:37, 1994.

100. Hurst NM, Valentine CJ, Renfro L et al: Skin-to-skin holding in the neonatal intensive care unit influences maternal milk volume, *J Perinatol* 17: 213, 1997.

101. Hylander M, Strobino D, Dhanireddy R: Human milk feedings and ROP among VLBW infants, *Pediatr Res* 37:214A, 1995.

102. Hylander M, Strobino D, Dhanireddy R: Human milk feedings and infection among VLBW infants, *Pediatr Res* 39:295A, 1996.

103. Hylander MA, Strobino DM, Dhanireddy R et al: Human milk feedings and infection among VLBW infants, *Pediatrics* 102:630, 1998.

104. Institute of Medicine, Committee on Nutritional Status During Pregnancy and Lactation: *Nutrition during pregnancy and lactation: an implementation guide,* Washington, DC, 1992, National Academy Press.

105. Jain L, Sivieri E, Abbasi S et al: Energetics and mechanics of nutritive sucking in the preterm and term neonate, *J Pediatr* 111:894, 1987.

106. Jason JM, Jones BM, Haff BC: The effects of microwave on human milk immune components, *Pediatr Res* 20:390A, 1986.

107. Johnston JM, Amico JA: A prospective longitudinal study of the release of oxytocin and prolactin in response to infant suckling in long term lactation, *J Clin Endocrinol Metab* 62:653, 1986.

108. Kavanaugh K, Mead L, Meier P et al: Getting enough: mothers' concerns about breastfeeding a preterm infant after discharge, *J Obstet Gynecol Neonatal Nurs* 24:23, 1995.

109. Kavanaugh K, Meier P, Zimmerman B et al: The rewards outweigh the efforts: breastfeeding outcomes of mothers of preterm infants, *J Hum Lact* 13:15, 1997.

110. Kennedy C, Lipsitt L: Temporal characteristics of non-oral feedings and chronic feeding problems in premature infants, *J Perinat Neonatal Nurs* 7:77, 1993.

111. Killersreiter B, Grimmer I, Buhrer C et al: Early cessation of breast milk feeding in very low birthweight infants, *Early Hum Dev* 60:193, 2001.

112. Kinneer M, Beachy P: Nipple feeding premature infants in the NICU: factors and decisions, *J Obstet Gynecol Neonatal Nurs* 23:105, 1994.

113. Kirsten D, Bradford L: Hindmilk feedings, *Neonatal Netw* 18:68, 1999.

114. Kirsten G, Berman N, Hann F: Kangaroo mother care in the nursery, *Pediatr Clin North Am* 48:207, 2001.

115. Kliethermes PA, Cross ML, Lanese MG et al: Transitioning preterm infants with nasogastric tube supplementation: increased likelihood of breastfeeding, *J Obstet Gynecol Neonatal Nurs* 28:264, 1999.

116. Koenig J, Davies A, Thach B: Coordination of breathing, sucking, and swallowing during bottle feedings, *J Appl Physiol* 69:1623, 1990.

117. Kramer MS, Chalmers B, Hodnett ED et al: Promotion of Breastfeeding Intervention Trial (PROBIT): a randomized trial in the Republic of Belarus, *JAMA* 285:413, 2001.

118. Kristensen JH, Ilett KF, Dusci LJ et al: Distribution and excretion of sertraline and N-desmethylsertraline in human milk, *Br J Clin Pharmacol* 45:453, 1998.

119. Kuan LW, Britto M, Decolongon J et al: Health system factor contributing to breastfeeding success, *Pediatrics* 104:552, 1999.

120. Kunz C, Rodriquez-Palmero M, Koletzko B et al: Nutritional and biochemical properties of human milk. Part I: general aspects, proteins and carbohydrates, *Clin Perinatol* 26:307, 1999.

121. Lantig CI, Fidler V, Huisman M et al: Neurologic differences between 9 year old children fed breast milk or formula milk as babies, *Lancet* 344:1319, 1994.

122. Lau C: Effect of stress on lactation, *Pediatr Clin North Am* 48:221, 2001.

123. Lau C, Hurst N: Oral feeding in infants, *Curr Probl Pediatr* 29:105, 1999.

124. Lau C, Schanler R: Oral motor function in the neonate, *Clin Perinatol* 23:161, 1996.

125. Lau C, Sheena H, Shulman R et al: Oral feeding in low birth weight infants, *J Pediatr* 130:561, 1997.

126. Lawrence R: Breast milk: best source of nutrition for term and preterm infants, *Pediatr Clin North Am* 41:925, 1994.

127. Lawrence R: The clinician's role in teaching proper infant feeding techniques, *J Pediatr* 126:5112, 1995.

128. Lawrence R, Howard C: Given the benefits of breastfeeding, are there any contraindications? *Clin Perinatol* 26:479, 1999.

129. Lawrence RA, Lawrence RM: *Breastfeeding: a guide for the medical profession,* ed 5, St Louis, 1999, Mosby.

130. Lee A, Moretti M, Collantes A et al: Choice of breastfeeding and physicians' advice: a cohort study of women receiving propylthiouracil, *Pediatrics* 106:27, 2000.

131. Lemons J, Schreiner R, Gresham E: Simple method for determining the caloric and fat content of human milk, *Pediatrics* 66:626, 1980.

132. Lemons P: From gavage to oral feedings: just a matter of time, *Neonatal Netw* 20:7, 2001.

133. Little RE, Anderson KW, Ervin CH et al: Maternal alcohol use during breast-feeding and infant mental and motor development at one year, *N Engl J Med* 321:425, 1989.

134. Lucas A, Cole T: Breast milk and neonatal necrotizing enterocolitis, *Lancet* 336:1519, 1990.

135. Lucas A, Lucas P, Baum J: Differences in the pattern of milk intake between breast and bottlefed infants, *Early Hum Dev* 5:195, 1981.

136. Lucas A, Morley R, Cole TJ: Randomised trial of early diet in preterm babies and later intelligence quotient, *Br Med J* 317:1481, 1998.

137. Lucas A, Brooke OG, Cole TJ et al: Early diet of preterm infants and development of allergic or atopic diseases: randomized prospective study, *Br Med J* 300:837, 1990.

138. Lucas A, Fewtrell MS, Morley R et al: Randomized outcome trial of human milk fortification and developmental outcome in preterm infants, *Am J Clin Nutr* 64:142, 1996.

139. Lucas A, Gibbs J, Lyster R et al: Creamatocrit: simple clinical technique for estimating fat concentration and energy value of human milk, *Br Med J* 1:1018, 1978.

140. Lucas A, Morley R, Cole TJ et al: Breast milk and subsequent intelligence quotient in children born preterm, *Lancet* 339:261, 1992.

141. Lucas A, Morley R, Cole TJ et al: A randomised multicentre study of human milk versus formula and later development in preterm infants, *Arch Dis Child Fetal Neonatal Educ* 70:F141, 1994.

142. MacMullen N, Dulski L: Factors related to sucking ability in healthy newborns, *J Obstet Gynecol Neonatal Nurs* 29:390, 2000.

142a. The MAIN Trial Collaborative Group: Preparing for breastfeeding: treatment of inverted and non-protractile nipples in pregnancy, *Midwifery* 10:200, 1994.

143. Martell M, Martinez G, Gonzalez M et al: Suction patterns in preterm infants, *J Perinat Med* 21:363, 1993.

144. Mascola M, Van Vunakis H, Tager IB et al: Exposure of young infants to environmental tobacco smoke: breastfeeding among smoking mothers, *Am J Public Health* 88:893, 1998.

145. Mathew O: Nipple units for newborn infants: a functional comparison, *Pediatrics* 81:688, 1988.

146. Mathew O: Respiratory control during nipple feeding in preterm infants, *Pediatr Pulmonol* 5:220, 1988.

147. Mathew O: Determinants of milk flow through nipples, *Am J Dis Child* 144:222, 1990.

148. Mathew O: Breathing patterns of preterm infants during bottle feeding: role of milk flow, *J Pediatr* 199:960, 1991.

149. Mathew O: Science of bottle feeding, *J Pediatr* 119:511, 1991.

150. Mathew O, Bhatia J: Sucking and breathing patterns during breast- and bottle-feeding in term neonates, *Am J Dis Child* 143:588, 1989.

151. Mathew O, Belan M, Thoppil C: Sucking patterns of neonates during bottlefeeding: comparison of different nipple units, *Am J Perinatol* 9:265, 1992.

152. Mathew OP, Clark ML, Pronske ML et al: Breathing pattern and ventilation during oral feeding in term newborn infants, *J Pediatr* 106:810, 1985.

153. Mathur N, Dwarkadas AM, Sharma VK et al: Anti-infective factors in preterm human colostrum, *Acta Paediatr Scand* 79:1039, 1990.

154. McCain G: Promotion of preterm nipple feeding with non-nutritive sucking, *J Pediatr Nurs* 10:3, 1995.

155. McCain G: Behavioral state activity during nipple feedings for preterm infants, *Neonatal Netw* 16:43, 1997.

156. McCoy D, Holmberg S: Antidepressant medications during breastfeeding: safety and efficacy for mother and infant, *Am J Nurse Pract* 5:9, 2001.

157. McNeilly AS, Robinson IC, Houston MJ et al: Release of oxytocin and prolactin in responses to suckling, *Br Med J* 286:257, 1983.

158. Medoff-Cooper B, Ray W: Neonatal sucking behaviors, *Image J Nurs Sch* 27:195, 1995.

159. Medoff-Cooper B, Verklan T, Carlson S: The development of sucking patterns and physiologic correlates in very-low-birth-weight infants, *Nurs Res* 42:100, 1993.

160. Medoff-Cooper B, Weininger S, Zukowsky K: Neonatal sucking as a clinical assessment tool: preliminary findings, *Nurs Res* 40:245, 1991.

161. Meier P: Bottle and breastfeeding: effects on transcutaneous pressure and temperature in preterm infants, *Nurs Res* 37:36, 1988.

162. Meier P: Suck-breathe patterning during bottle and breastfeeding for preterm infants. In David T, ed: *Major controversies in infant nutrition,* London, 1996, Royal Society of Medicine Press.

163. Meier P: Breastfeeding in the special care nursery: prematures and infants with medical problems, *Pediatr Clin North Am* 48:425, 2001.

164. Meier P, Anderson GC: Responses of small preterm infants to bottle and breastfeeding, *Matern Child Nurs J* 12:97, 1987.

165. Meier P, Brown L: Breastfeeding for mothers and low birth weight infants, *Nurs Clin North Am* 31:351, 1996.

166. Meier P, Brown L: Strategies for assisting breastfeeding in preterm infants, *Rec Adv Pediatr* 15:137, 1997.

167. Meier P, Brown L: Breastfeeding a preterm infant after NICU discharge: reflections on Ryan's story, *Breastfeed Abstr* 3:4, 1998.

168. Meier P, Pugh EJ: Breastfeeding behavior of small preterm infants, *Matern Child Nurs J* 10:396, 1985.

169. Meier P, Brown L, Hurst N: Breastfeeding the preterm infant. In Riordan J, Averbach K, eds: *Breastfeeding and human lactation,* ed 2, Boston, 1998, Jones & Bartlett.

170. Meier PP, Engstrom JL, Mangurten HH et al: Breastfeeding support services in the neonatal intensive care unit, *J Obstet Gynecol Neonatal Nurs* 22:338, 1993.

171. Meier P, Murtaugh M, Vasan U et al: Modification of the lipid concentrations in own mother's milk feedings in the NICU: clinical application of the creamatocrit technique, *Pediatr Res* 45:287A, 1999.

172. Meier P, Brown L, Hurst N et al: Nipple shields for preterm infants: effect on milk intake and duration of breastfeeding, *Pediatr Res* 45:287A, 1999.

173. Melnikow J, Bedinghaus J: Management of common breastfeeding problems, *J Fam Pract* 39:56, 1994.

174. Menella J, Beauchamp G: Smoking and the flavor of breastmilk, *N Engl J Med* 339(21):1559, 1998.

175. Misra R, James DC: Breast-feeding practices among adolescent and adult mothers in the Missouri WIC population, *J Am Diet Assoc* 100:1071, 2000.

176. Mitchell EA, Taylor BJ, Ford RP et al: Four modifiable and other major risk factors for cot death: the New Zealand study, *J Pediatr Child Health* 28:53, 1992.

177. Narayanan I: Sucking on the "emptied" breast—a better method of non-nutritive sucking than use of a pacifier, *Indian Pediatr* 27:1122, 1990.

178. Neifert M: Clinical aspects of lactation: promoting breastfeeding success, *Clin Perinatol* 26:281, 1999.

179. Neifert M: Prevention of breastfeeding tragedies, *Pediatr Clin North Am* 48:273, 2001.

180. Neifert M, Lawrence R: Nipple confusion: toward a more formal definition, *J Pediatr* 126:5125, 1995.

181. Neville M: Physiology of lactation, *Clin Perinatol* 26:251, 1999.

182. Neville M: Anatomy and physiology of lactation, *Pediatr Clin North Am* 48:13, 2001.

183. Neville MC, Allen JC, Archer PC et al: Studies in human lactation: milk volume and nutrient composition during weaning and lactogenesis, *Am J Clin Nutr* 54:81, 1991.

184. Newton N: The relation of milk-ejection reflux to the ability to breastfeed, *Ann NY Acad Sci* 652:484, 1992.

185. Nissen E, Lilja G, Mathiesen AS et al: Effects of maternal pethidine on infants' developing breastfeeding behaviors, *Acta Paediatr* 84:140, 1995.

186. Nissen E, Widstrom AM, Lilja G et al: Effects of routinely given pethidine during labour on infants' developing breastfeeding behavior: effects of dose-delivery time interval and various concentrations of pethidine/norpethidine in cord plasma, *Acta Paediatr* 86:201, 1997.

187. Nowak A, Smith W, Erenberg A: Imaging evaluation of artificial nipples during bottlefeeding, *Arch Pediatr Adolesc Med* 148:40, 1994.

188. Nowak A, Smith W, Erenberg A: Imaging evaluation of breastfeeding and bottlefeeding systems, *J Pediatr* 126:5130, 1995.

189. Orlando S: The immunologic significance of breast milk, *J Obstet Gynecol Neonatal Nurs* 24:678, 1995.

190. Owen MJ, Baldwin CD, Swank PR et al: Relation of infant feeding practices, cigarette smoke exposure and group child care to the onset and duration of otitis media with effusion in the first two years of life, *J Pediatr* 123:702, 1993.

191. Peaker M, Wilde C: Feedback control of milk secretion from milk, *J Mammary Gland Biol Neoplasia* 1:307, 1996.

192. Pessl M: Are we creating our own breastfeeding mythology? *J Hum Lact* 12:271, 1996.

193. Peterson J, Patton S, Hamosh M: Glycoproteins of the human milk fat globule in protection of the breastfed infant against infection, *Biol Neonate* 143:162, 1998.

194. Philipp B, Brown E, Merewood A: Pumps for peanuts: leveling the field in the NICU, *J Perinatol* 4:249, 2000.

195. Philipp B, Merewood A, O'Brien S: Physicians and breastfeeding promotion in the US: a call for action, *Pediatrics* 107:584, 2001.

196. Pickler R, Mauck A, Geldmacker B: Bottle-feeding histories of preterm infants, *J Obstet Gynecol Neonatal Nurs* 26:414, 1997.

197. Pisacane A, Graziano L, Mazzerella G et al: Breast-feeding and urinary tract infection, *J Pediatr* 120:87, 1992.

198. Position of the American Dietetic Association: Promotion and support of breastfeeding, *J Am Diet Assoc* 93:467, 1993.

199. Powers N: Slow weight gain and low milk supply in the breastfeeding dyad, *Clin Perinatol* 26:399, 1999.

200. Powers N, Naylor A, Wester R: Hospital policies: crucial to breastfeeding success, *Semin Perinatol* 18:517, 1994.

201. Quan R, Yang C, Rubenstein S et al: Effects of microwave radiation on anti-infective factors in human milk, *Pediatrics* 89:667, 1992.

202. Qureshi M, Vice F, Taciak V et al: Rhythmic suckle patterns in term infants over the first month of life, *Pediatr Res* 45:219A, 1999.

203. Rentschler D: Correlates of successful breastfeeding, *Image J Nurs Sch* 23:151, 1991.

204. Rigas A, Rigas B, Glassman M et al: Breast-feeding and maternal smoking in the etiology of Crohn's disease and ulcerative colitis in childhood, *Ann Epidemiol* 3:387, 1993.

205. Riordan J: Social support and breast feeding, *Breastfeed Abstr* 8:13, 1989.

206. Riordan J, Auerbach K: *Breastfeeding and human lactation,* Boston, 1999, Jones & Bartlett.

207. Riordan J, Gill-Hopple K: Breastfeeding care in multicultural populations, *J Obstet Gynecol Neonatal Nurs* 30:216, 2001.

208. Rodriguez-Palmero M, Koletzko B, Kunz C et al: Nutritional and biochemical properties of human milk: II. Lipids, micronutrients and bioactive factors, *Clin Perinatol* 26:335, 1999.

209. Rogan W, Gladen B: Breast-feeding and cognitive development, *Early Hum Dev* 31:181, 1993.

210. Rosenblatt J: Psychobiology of maternal behavior: contribution to the clinical understanding of maternal behavior among humans, *Acta Paediatr Suppl* 397:3, 1994.

211. Rosti L, Nardini A, Bettinelli ME et al: Toxic effects of herbal tea mixture in two newborns, *Acta Paediatr* 83:683, 1994.

212. Ryan A: The resurgence of breastfeeding in the United States, *Pediatrics* 99:e12, 1997.

213. Saadeh R, Akre J: Ten steps to successful breast-feeding: a summary of the rationale and scientific evidence, *Birth* 23:154, 1996.

214. Saarinen U, Kajosaari M: Breastfeeding as prophylaxis against atopic disease: prospective follow-up study until 17 years old, *Lancet* 346:1065, 1995.

215. Samuels SE, Margen S, Schoen EJ: Incidence and duration of breastfeeding in a health maintenance organization population, *Am J Clin Nutr* 42:504, 1985.

216. Schanler R: Suitability of human milk for the LBW infant, *Clin Perinatol* 22:207, 1995.

217. Schanler R: Human milk fortification for premature infants, *Am J Clin Nutr* 64:249, 1996.

218. Schanler R, Hurst N: Human milk for the hospitalized preterm infant, *Semin Perinatol* 18:476, 1994.

219. Schanler R, Hurst N, Lau C: The use of human milk and breastfeeding in premature infants, *Clin Perinatol* 26:379, 1999.

220. Schanler R, O'Connor K, Lawrence R: Pediatricians' practices and attitudes regarding breastfeeding promotion, *Pediatrics* 103(3):e35, 1999.

221. Schanler R, Shulman R, Lau C: Feeding strategies for premature infants: beneficial outcomes of feeding fortified human milk versus preterm formula, *Pediatrics* 103:1150, 1999.

222. Selley W, Ellis R, Flack F, Brooks W: Coordination of sucking, swallowing and breathing in the newborn: its relationship to infant feeding and normal development, *Br J Disord Commun* 25:311, 1990.

223. Shiao, S-Y: Comparison of continuous versus intermittent sucking in VLBW infants, *J Obstet Gynecol Neonatal Nurs* 26:313, 1997.

224. Shivpuri CR, Martin RJ, Carlo WA et al: Decreased ventilation in preterm infants during oral feeding, *J Pediatr* 103:285, 1983.

225. Shu XO, Clemens J, Zheng W et al: Infant breastfeeding and the risk of childhood lymphoma and leukaemia, *Int J Epidemiol* 24:27, 1995.

226. Sidell E, Froman R: A national survey of neonatal intensive care units: criteria used to determine readiness for oral feedings, *J Obstet Gynecol Neonatal Nurs* 23:783, 1994.

227. Sigman M, Burke KI, Swarner OW et al: Effects of microwaving human milk: changes in IgA content and bacterial content, *J Am Diet Assoc* 89:690, 1989.

228. Smith WL, Erenberg A, Nowak A: Imaging evaluation of the human nipple during breastfeeding, *Am J Dis Child* 142:76, 1988.

229. Smotherman W, Robinson S: Milk as the proximal mechanism for behavioral changes in the newborn, *Acta Paediatr Suppl* 397:64, 1994.

230. Snell BJ: Physiologic response of the preterm infant during the early initiation of breastfeeding versus bottlefeeding, Doctoral dissertation, 1991, Oregon Health Sciences University.

231. Stevenson R, Allaire J: The development of normal feeding and swallowing, *Pediatr Clin North Am* 38:1439, 1991.

232. Stine M: Breastfeeding and the premature newborn: a protocol without bottles, *J Hum Lact* 6:167, 1990.

233. Stowe ZN, Owens MJ, Landry JC et al: Sertraline and desmethylsertraline in human breast milk and nursing infants, *Am J Psychiatry* 154:1255, 1997.

234. Temboury MC, Otero A, Polanco I et al: Influence of breast-feeding on the infant's intellectual development, *J Pediatr Gastroenterol Nutr* 18:32, 1994.

235. Thomas K: Differential effects of breast- and formula-feeding on preterm infants' sleep-wake patterns, *J Obstet Gynecol Neonatal Nurs* 29:145, 2000.

236. Thoyre S: Mothers' ideas about their role in feeding their high-risk infants, *J Obstet Gynecol Neonatal Nurs* 29:613, 2000.

237. Timms BJ, DiFiore JM, Martin RJ et al: Increased respiratory drive as an inhibitor of oral feeding of preterm infants, *J Pediatr* 123:127, 1993.

238. Tomomasa T, Hyman P, Itoh K: Gastroduodenal motility in neonates: response to human milk compared with cow's milk formula, *Pediatrics* 80:434, 1987.

239. Tyson JE: Nursing and prolactin secretion: principal determinants in the mediation of puerperal infertility. In Crosignani PG et al, editors: *Prolactin and human reproduction,* New York, 1977, Academic Press.

240. Uauy RD, Birch DG, Birch EE et al: Effect of dietary omega-3 fatty acids on retrieval function of very-low-birth-weight neonates, *Pediatr Res* 28:415, 1990.

241. Udea T, Yokohama Y, Irahara M et al: Influence of psychological stress on suckling-induced pulsatile oxytoxin release, *Obstet Gynecol* 8:259, 1994.

242. Urziee F, Gross S: Improved feeding tolerance and reduced incidence of sepsis of very low birth weight infants fed maternal milk, *Pediatr Res* 25:298A, 1989.

243. US Department of Health and Human Services: HHS Blueprint for action on breastfeeding, Washington, DC, 2000, US Department of Health and Human Services, Office of Women's Health.

244. US Public Health Service: *Healthy people 2010,* Washington, DC, 1999, US Department of Health and Human Services, US Government Printing Office.

245. Valentine C, Hurst N, Schanler R: Hindmilk improves weight gain in LBW infants fed human milk, *J Pediatr Gastroenterol Nutr* 18:474, 1994.

246. Van de Perre P, Simonon A, Hitimana DG et al: Infective and anti-infective properties of breastmilk from HIV-1-infected women, *Lancet* 341:914, 1993.

247. Vasan U, Meier P, Meier W, Kirsten D: Individualizing the lipid content of own mothers' milk: effect on weight gain for ELBW, *Pediatr Res* 43:270A, 1998.

248. Wang C, Chu P, Mellen B, Shenai J: Creamatocrit and the nutrient composition of human milk, *J Perinatol* 19:343, 1999.

249. Wang Y, Wu S: The effect of exclusive breastfeeding on development and incidence of infection in infants, *J Hum Lact* 12:27, 1996.

250. Wereszczak J, Miles M, Holditch-Davis D: Maternal recall of the NICU, *Neonatal Netw* 16:33, 1997.

251. Widstrom A, Wahlberg V, Werner S, Wingerg J: Short term effects of early suckling and touch of the nipple on maternal behavior, *Early Hum Dev* 21:153, 1990.

252. Wight N: Management of common breastfeeding issues, *Pediatr Clin North Am* 48:321, 2001.

253. Wilson-Clay B: Clinical use of silicone nipple shields, *J Hum Lact* 12:279, 1996.

254. Wold A, Hanson L: Defense factors in human milk, *Curr Opin Gastroenterol* 10:652, 1994.

255. Woldt EH: Breastfeeding support group in the NICU, *Neonatal Netw* 9:53, 1991.

256. Wright A, Holberg CJ, Taussig LM et al: Relationship of infant feeding to recurrent wheezing at age 6 yrs, *Arch Pediatr Adolesc Med* 149:758, 1995.

257. Wright A, Rice S, Wells, S: Changing hospital practices to increase the duration of breastfeeding, *Pediatrics* 97:669, 1996.

258. Ziemer MM, George C: Breastfeeding the LBW infant, *Neonatal Netw* 9:33, 1990.

259. Zinamen MJ, Hughes V, Queenan J et al: Acute prolactin and oxytocin responses and milk yield to infant suckling and artificial methods of expression in lactating women, *Pediatrics* 89(3):437, 1992.

RESOURCE MATERIALS FOR PARENTS

Danner S: *Nursing your premature infant, nursing the neurological impaired infant; nursing the infant with cleft lip and cleft palate,* 1994, Childbirth Graphics.

Eiger M, Olds S: *The complete book of breastfeeding,* ed 3, New York, 1999, Workman Publishing.

Harrison H: *The premature baby book,* New York, 1983, St Martin's Press.

Huggins K: *The nursing mother's companion,* ed 4, Boston, 1999, Harvard Common Press.

Lact-Aid International, PO Box 1066, Athens, TN 37303; (423) 744-9090.

LaLeche League International: *The womanly art of breastfeeding,* ed 6, Schaumburg, Ill, 1997, LaLeche League International.

Lauwers J, Woessner C: *Counseling the nursing mother,* ed 2, New York, 1990, Avery Publishing Group.

Pryor G: *Nursing mother, working mother,* Boston, 1997, Harvard Commons Press.

Renfrew M, Fischer C, Arms S: *Breastfeeding, getting breastfeeding right for you,* Berkeley, California, 2000, Celestial Arts.

Tomaselli KM: *Guide to breastfeeding,* New York, 1991, Childbirth Graphics.

Walker M, Watson J: *Breastfeeding your premature or special care baby: a practical guide for nursing the tiny baby,* ed 2, Boston, 1989, Lactation Associates.

World Health Organization: *Relactation: a review of experience and recommendations for practice,* Geneva, Switzerland, 1998, WHO.

PART IV

INFECTION AND HEMATOLOGIC
DISEASES OF THE NEONATE

20 | Newborn Hematology

Marilyn Manco-Johnson, Donna J. Rodden, Shannon Collins

RED BLOOD CELLS

Physiology

Red blood cells transport and deliver oxygen to vital organs and body tissues. Red blood corpuscles are simple cells composed of membrane encasing hemoglobin with an energy system to fuel the cells. Hemoglobin is the protein in red cells that carries oxygen, binding and releasing it based on concentration differences. Ex utero, red cells absorb oxygen by diffusion in the lungs, where the oxygen tension of the alveolar air is higher than that of the capillary blood, and release it from the systemic capillaries, where the oxygen tension is now higher than that of surrounding tissues. In utero, oxygen diffuses to the fetus from the placental venous circulation. Fetal red cells contain a unique hemoglobin (fetal hemoglobin) in which the two beta chains of adult hemoglobin (called *hemoglobin A_1*) are replaced by two gamma chains. Fetal hemoglobin (called *hemoglobin F*) has a higher affinity for oxygen than does adult hemoglobin, allowing fetal red cells to compete successfully for available oxygen. Normal fetal red cells are characterized by an increased mean corpuscular hemoglobin (MCH), mean corpuscular volume (MCV), hemoglobin, and hematocrit. After birth with the transition to air breathing and a higher blood oxygen tension, the hypoxic stimulus driving fetal red cell production in the bone marrow is removed. The plasma concentration of erythropoietin, the hormone that stimulates bone marrow production of red blood cells, falls. The number of circulating reticulocytes, which are young red blood cells in the circulation, decreases. Subsequently, the hemoglobin and hematocrit diminish until a new equilibrium is reached. Postnatal changes in red cell production include an increase in the ratio of hemoglobin A to hemoglobin F and an increase in levels of the red cell enzyme 2,3-diphosphoglycerate (2,3-DPG). 2,3-DPG promotes the release of oxygen to tissues by decreasing hemoglobin affinity to oxygen within tissues. Oxygen delivery in the neonate is a function both of the ratio of hemoglobin F to A and of the red cell concentration of 2,3-DPG.

The production of embryonic and fetal hematopoieic cells is first seen within the yolk sac in the 14-day embryo and disappears by the eleventh week of gestation.[13] Hematopoiesis in other tissues results from colonization by stem cells derived from the yolk sac.[6] By the fifth to sixth week, embryonic erythropoietic activity is present in the liver. The liver becomes the primary source of red cell production by 8 to 9 weeks.[9] Between the eighth and twelfth week the spleen and lymph nodes are involved in erythropoiesis.[11] Other tissues and organs involved in erythropoiesis include the kidney, thymus, and connective tissue. There is no evidence of erythropoietin production before the tenth week.[48] After the tenth week of gestation, erythropoietin production rises and seems to be involved in red cell production in the bone marrow during the third trimester.[12] Initially, production of erythropoietin is in the fetal liver, and by the last trimester, production is in the kidneys. The level of erythropoietin gradually rises to significant levels after the thirty-fourth week of gestation.[11] Elevated erythropoietin levels can be found when the fetus is hypoxic.[9] Erythropoiesis is found in the bone marrow at 10 to 11 weeks. This activity increases rapidly until the twenty-fourth week when bone marrow erythropoiesis replaces liver erythropoiesis. Changes in the blood count at the time of birth are shown in Table 20-1.[10,11]

Table 20-1	CHANGES IN ERYTHROPOIESIS AROUND THE TIME OF TERM BIRTH	
	IN UTERO	**POSTDELIVERY**
Oxygen saturation (%)	45*	95
Erythropoietin levels	High	Undetectable
Red cell production	Rapid	<10% (by day 7)
Reticulocyte count (%)	3-7	0-1 (by day 7)
Hemoglobin (g/dl)	16.8	18.4
Hematocrit (%)	53	58
MCV (fl)	107	98 (by day 7)
MCHC (g/dl)	31.7	33 (by day 7)

MCHC, Mean corpuscular hemoglobin concentration[4,7]; *MCV*, mean corpuscular volume.
*Mean values represented.

In more than 90% of healthy term infants the hematocrit range is 48% to 60% and the hemoglobin range is 16 to 20 g/dl.[11] Normally after a term birth, hemoglobin concentrations fall from a mean of 17 g/dl to approximately 11 g/dl by 2 to 3 months of age. This nadir in red blood cell values is called *physiologic anemia of the newborn* and is a normal process in the adaptation to extrauterine life.

Several factors need to be considered in the interpretation of hematocrit values in the newborn, including age of the infant (both in hours and days), site of blood collection, and method of analysis. Hematocrit changes significantly during the first 24 hours of life; it peaks at 2 hours of age and then progressively drops, with decreases occurring at 6 and 24 hours of age.[41] This drop is caused by transudation of fluid out of the intravascular space. The method used to determine hematocrit can significantly affect the value. Capillary hematocrit measurements are highly subject to variations in blood flow.[20,30] Prewarming the site minimizes the artifactual increase in the hematocrit. When obtaining blood counts, it is important to note that in both term and preterm infants there can be as much as a 20% difference between the hematocrit obtained from a capillary puncture (commonly termed heel stick) and the hematocrit drawn from a central vein.

Capillary, arterial, and venous blood reveal notably decreasing values in that order, thereby underscoring the importance of same-source serial measurements. Finally, it is crucial that a microcentrifuge or spun hematocrit measurement be obtained rather than a hematocrit determination in an automated blood cell counter (Coulter Counter), because the latter frequently gives falsely low hematocrit values in the newborn.[44]

Adult red cells circulate for an average of 120 days. Normal neonatal red blood cells have a circulating half-life reduction of 20% to 25% compared with the red blood cells of older children or adults. Survival of red cells of premature infants is reduced by approximately 50%.

Pathophysiology of Anemia

Anemia is a deficiency in the concentration of red cells and hemoglobin in the blood and results in tissue hypoxia and acidosis. Anemia is defined by a hemoglobin or hematocrit value that is greater than two standard deviations below the mean for postconceptual and postnatal age.

Determination of the cause of anemia is important to direct treatment. **Anemia in the newborn results from one or more of the following basic mechanisms:**

- **Blood loss (acute or chronic)**
- **Decreased red cell production**
- **Shortened red cell survival**

Blood Loss

Acute and chronic blood loss is the most common cause of anemia in the neonate. Blood loss can occur intrauterine, perinatally, or postnatally. Some form of fetomaternal hemorrhage occurs in 50% of all pregnancies.[10] Blood loss is usually insignificant; however, in 1% of pregnancies, blood loss can be greater than 40 ml.[22] The blood volume of the fetus is approximately 90 ml/kg. Large blood loss can cause profound anemia, asphyxia, and death. Anemia caused by chronic blood loss is better tolerated, because the neonate is able to compensate for the gradual loss in red cell mass. There is a large differential for blood loss in the neonate (Box 20-1).

Fetomaternal transfusion is a common cause of occult blood loss in the fetus. The Kleihauer-Betke acid elution test is the method used to confirm the presence of fetal blood cells in the maternal circulation.[47] The volume of fetal blood in the maternal circulation is estimated by counting fetal red cells on the maternal blood smear under light microscopy. Fetal cells retain red staining of hemoglobin after fixing, whereas adult cells (also called *ghost cells*) are very pale because hemoglobin has been eluted. Ten fetal cells per 30 fields viewed under high power are equal to 1 ml of fetal blood.

Box 20-1	CAUSES OF BLOOD LOSS IN THE NEONATE

I. Hemorrhage before birth
  A. Fetomaternal
    1. Traumatic amniocentesis of periumbilical blood sampling
    2. Spontaneous
    3. Chronic gastrointestinal
    4. Blunt trauma to the maternal abdomen
    5. Postexternal positioning
  B. Twin-to-twin
  C. External
    1. Abruptio placenta
    2. Placenta previa
II. Hemorrhage during birth
  A. Placental malformation
    1. Chorangioma
    2. Chorangiocarcinoma
  B. Hematoma of the cord or placenta
  C. Rupture of a normal umbilical cord
    1. Precipitous delivery
    2. Entanglement

  D. Rupture of an abnormal umbilical cord
    1. Varices
    2. Aneurysm
  E. Rupture of anomalous vessels
    1. Aberrant vessel
    2. Velamentous insertion of the cord
    3. Communicating vessels in the multilobular placenta
  F. Incision of placenta during cesarean section
III. Internal fetal or neonatal hemorrhage
  A. Intracranial
  B. Giant cephalohematoma, caput succedaneum
  C. Pulmonary
  D. Retroperitoneum
  E. Subcapsular liver or spleen
  F. Renal or adrenal
IV. External neonatal hemorrhage
  A. Delayed clamping of the umbilical cord
  B. Gastrointestinal
  C. Iatrogenic from blood sampling

*Modified from Luchtman-Jones L, Schwartz A, Wilson D: Hematologic problems in the fetus and neonate. In Fanaroff A: *Neonatal-perinatal medicine: diseases of the fetus and infant,* vol 2, St. Louis, 1997, Mosby.

Twin-to-twin transfusion is another cause of occult blood loss and is seen in 15% to 30% of all monochorionic twins with abnormalities of placental blood vessels.[42] The anemic twin is on the arterial side of the placental vascular malformation. The clinical significance of twin-to-twin transfusion depends on the duration of blood transfer. With chronic transfusion, a 20% weight discordance similar to that observed with placental insufficiency can be found.[32]

Intracranial bleeding associated with prematurity, later birth order of a multiple-gestation delivery, rapid delivery, breech delivery, and massive cephalhematoma can cause anemia. Other sites of neonatal hemorrhage include umbilical, retroperitoneal, adrenal, renal, and gastrointestinal bleeding, as well as ruptured liver or spleen.

Swallowed maternal blood may be confused with GI bleeding. The Apt test is used to distinguish swallowed maternal blood from neonatal blood and is based on alkali resistance of fetal hemoglobin.[2] A 1% solution of sodium hydroxide is added to 5 ml of diluted blood. Fetal hemoglobin will remain pink, but adult hemoglobin will become yellow.

Iatrogenic blood loss results from blood sampling with inadequate replacement. A survey performed in the intensive care nursery of the University of California at San Francisco found that an average of 38.9 ml of blood was removed for laboratory tests during the first week of life.[38] For premature infants, whose blood volume can be as little as 50 ml, anemia is commonly caused by blood draws. **The majority of red cell transfusions given in nurseries is directly related to frequent blood sampling.**[28]

Decreased Red Cell Production

Anemia caused by decreased production of red cells tends to develop slowly, allowing time for physiologic compensation. Affected infants may have few signs of anemia other than pallor. The reticulocyte count will be low and inappropriate for the degree of anemia.

Worldwide, iron deficiency is the leading cause of anemia in infancy and childhood. Iron-deficiency anemia can occur at any time when growth exceeds the ability of the stores and dietary intake to supply sufficient iron for erythropoiesis. Iron storage at birth is directly related to body weight. A term infant should have sufficient iron stores for 4 to 6 months of life.[31] Infants who are fed exclusively breast milk or iron-enriched formula and cereal are less likely to develop iron-deficiency anemia.

Premature infants have iron stores adequate for less than 3 months postnatally because of low birth weight, faster rate of growth, and iatrogenic blood losses. Iron supplementation is required early in preterm infants to prevent anemia (Table 20-2).

Iron deficiency causes a hypochromic, microcytic anemia. The peripheral smear shows small, pale red cells with a large variety of shapes and sizes resulting in an increased relative distribution of width (RDW). The platelet count is increased and may be greater than 1,000,000/μl.

Mild forms of iron deficiency may be confused with other causes of anemia, including infection and thalassemia. A therapeutic trial of iron can be used to diagnose iron deficiency. After 1 month of receiving ferrous sulfate at a rate of 6 mg/kg/day, the patient's hemoglobin should rise at least 1 g/dl, in the absence of ongoing blood loss.[22]

Anemia of prematurity is common in infants born at less than 35 weeks' gestation. This is a normocytic, normochromic anemia appearing between 2 and 6 weeks characterized by a low reticulocyte count and an inadequate response to erythropoietin.[39] If hemoglobin levels drop below 10 g/dl, the infant may display decreased activity, poor growth, tachypnea, and tachycardia. Randomized placebo-controlled studies that include supplemental iron demonstrate a reduction in the amount of blood transfused in infants treated with erythropoietin.[29]

Hypothyroidism, deficiency of transcobalamin II, and inborn errors of cobalamin utilization cause macrocytic anemia because of decreased and ineffective bone marrow production.

Constitutional pure red cell aplasia is also known as *Blackfan-Diamond anemia.*[21] This normocytic or macrocytic anemia presents at birth in 10% and by 1 month in 25% of affected infants. Signs and symptoms include pallor, anemia, and reticulocytopenia. In red cell aplasia the platelet count may be moderately elevated and the leukocyte count may be slightly decreased. Bone marrow examination is normocellular with few erythroid precursors. Thirty percent of affected infants demonstrate congenital anomalies, primarily of the head, face, eyes, and thumb. The syndrome can have autosomal dominant or recessive inheritance. As infants grow older characteristics of fetal erythropoiesis persist, including elevations in fetal hemoglobin, i antigen, and red cell adenosine deaminase (ADA), as well as fetal patterns of red cell enzymes. Seventy percent of affected infants respond to corticosteroid therapy, particularly if treatment is initiated early in infancy. Infants who do not respond to steroids require long-term red cell transfusion therapy and are at risk for subsequent iron overload. In Blackfan-Diamond anemia the erythrocyte progenitors do not respond to erythropoietin, but often respond to stem cell factor, and to a lesser degree IL-3, suggesting a mutation in one of the growth factors as a cause.

Fanconi's anemia is a congenital syndrome of progressive bone marrow failure with autosomal recessive inheritance.[1] At birth, infants may be recognized by one or more of the associated congenital defects, which include microcephaly; short stature; absent or abnormal thumb; and other cutaneous, musculoskeletal, and urogenital abnormalities. Thrombocytopenia and an elevated MCV are usually the first hematologic abnormalities, but they are seldom recognized in the neonatal period. The underlying defect in Fanconi's anemia is an inability to repair damaged DNA. Chromosomal breakage analyses and specific molecular diagnosis have been used for prenatal diagnosis. Blackfan-Diamond and Fanconi's anemias have been successfully treated with bone marrow transplantation.

B19 parvovirus exerts an inhibitory effect on bone marrow production of red cells.[46] Infection with B19 parvovirus during pregnancy can cause hydrops fetalis, a syndrome of congestive heart failure, massive skin edema, and severe anemia, especially during the first two trimesters. Early detection of parvovirus infection in pregnant women and serial examinations with ultrasonography are important to diagnose and monitor the condition. Affected fetuses have been successfully supported with intrauterine transfusions of red blood cells. Parvovirus effects on the bone marrow are insufficient to cause anemia in most infants with a normal red cell lifespan but may cause symptomatic anemia in infants with hemolytic anemia or immunodeficiency. In-

Table 20-2	RECOMMENDED IRON SUPPLEMENTATION FOR THE NEONATE	
GROUP	DOSE (MG/KG/DAY)	INITIATION, DURATION
Full term	1	4 mo to 3 yr
Preterm, low	2	2 mo to 1 yr, then
birth weight	1	1 yr to 3 yr
Very low birth	4	2 mo to 1 yr, then
weight	1	1 yr to 3 yr

fants with congenital or acquired immunodeficiency may become anemic because of an inability to clear parvovirus.

Infants with genetic hemoglobin mutations of alpha or gamma chains, resulting in production of hemoglobins with decreased oxygen affinity, will have lower hemoglobins without signs of tissue hypoxia.

Shortened Red Cell Survival

Senescent red cells are removed from the circulation by the reticuloendothelial system. Bilirubin is produced by degradation of the heme moiety of hemoglobin, and red cell iron is recycled. Many conditions accelerate removal of red cells from the circulation. *Hemolysis* is a term for red cell destruction that is premature in terms of expected lifespan of the red cells relative to postconceptual age. Hyperbilirubinemia is evident in most cases of hemolysis. Reticulocytosis is usually found. However, in the presence of chronic illness, nutritional deficiency, or congenital infection, the reticulocyte count may be lower than expected for the degree of anemia. In the most severe cases of intrauterine hemolysis the outcome is hydrops fetalis, a syndrome of severe anemia with congestive heart failure and diffuse skin edema (Box 20-2).

Isoimmune hemolytic anemia occurs when fetal cells, bearing antigens of paternal origin that the mother does not possess, enter the maternal circulation and stimulate production of IgG antibodies. The IgG antibodies are transferred across the placenta, coat fetal red cells, and mediate their removal from the circulation through the reticuloendothelial system.

The major fetal red cell antigens responsible for isoimmune hemolytic anemia include the Rh (also called D) antigen in an Rh-negative mother and the blood group A and B antigens in a group O mother. Kell, Duffy, and Kidd antigens can also cause isoimmune hemolytic anemia. Sources of maternal sensitization to fetal red cell antigens include chorionic villus sampling, amniocentesis, abortion, rupture of an ectopic pregnancy, maternal blood transfusion, and fetomaternal transfusion. Anti-Rh antibodies derived from plasma of previously sensitized donors are given to Rh-negative mothers at 28 weeks' gestation, at delivery, and at the time of any of the above mentioned events. These antibodies coat any fetal red cells present in the maternal circulation and prevent them from initiating the maternal immune response. Thus they provide a form of passive immunization. With widespread use of

---

Box 20-2	**CAUSES OF SHORTENED RED CELL SURVIVAL IN THE NEONATE**

I. Isoimmune-mediated hemolysis
  A. Rh incompatibility
  B. ABO incompatibility
  C. Minor blood cell antigen incompatibility
II. Infection
  A. Bacterial sepsis
  B. Campylobacter jejuni
  C. Clostridium welchii
  D. Rubella
  E. Cytomegalovirus
  F. Epstein-Barr virus
  G. Disseminated herpes
  H. Malaria
  I. Toxoplasmosis
  J. Syphilis
III. Microangiopathic and macroangiopathic
  A. Cavernous hemangioma (Kasabach-Merritt)
  B. Renal vein thrombosis
  C. Disseminated intravascular coagulation
  D. Severe coarctation of the aorta
  E. Renal artery stenosis

IV. Vitamin E deficiency
V. Congenital red cell membrane disorders
  A. Hereditary spherocytosis
  B. Hereditary elliptocytosis
    1. Hereditary poikilocytosis
    2. Hereditary pyropoikilocytosis
    3. Hereditary stomatocytosis
  C. Infantile pyknocytosis
VI. Congenital red cell enzyme disorders
  A. G6PD deficiency
  B. Pyruvate kinase deficiency
VII. Congenital hemoglobinopathies
  A. Alpha and fetal chain defects
    1. Alpha and gamma thalassemia
    2. Alpha and gamma structural abnormalities; unstable hemoglobin
VIII. Metabolic
  A. Galactosemia
  B. Organic aciduria; orotic aciduria
  C. Prolonged or recurrent acidosis
IX. Liver disease

G6PD, Glucose-6-phosphate-dehydrogenase.

Rh immune globulin (Ig) to Rh-negative mothers, the rate of anti-Rh Ig formation dropped from 17% to 9% to 13%.[3,45] The rate of Rh hemolytic disease in the United States is 10.6 per 10,000 live births.[8] The persistence of Rh isoimmunization may be attributed to failures in administering Rh Ig to all women at risk and incorrect dosing. Women who receive no prenatal care and women who develop silent antenatal sensitization compose two populations that are difficult to reach with prevention strategies.

ABO hemolytic anemia is more common than Rh hemolytic disease but less severe. Unlike Rh disease, hemolysis secondary to ABO incompatibility can occur during the first pregnancy because A and B antigens are ubiquitous in foods and bacteria, causing sensitization.

Most isoimmune hemolytic diseases that are not related to ABO or Rh incompatibility are caused by sensitization to minor blood group antigens Kell, Duffy, Lewis, Kidd, M, or S. Mothers should be screened at 34 weeks for antibodies to these minor blood group antigens.

Congenital bacterial and viral infections may cause hemolytic anemia and bone marrow suppression with reticulocytopenia. Microspherocytes may be very prominent.

The microangiopathies and macroangiopathies are characterized by red cell fragmentation, shortened red cell survival, and thrombocytopenia. Coagulation proteins are also consumed in cavernous hemangiomas and disseminated intravascular coagulation (DIC).

Vitamin E is a fat-soluble vitamin that functions as an antioxidant. Deficiency of vitamin E manifests with hemolytic anemia, reticulocytosis, thrombocytosis, and edema of the lower extremities.[39] Diets high in polyunsaturated fatty acids and iron increase requirements for vitamin E. With current supplementation of infant formulas and parenteral nutrition with vitamin E, prevention of vitamin E deficiency using a water-soluble form of tocopherol is not currently necessary.

Shortened red cell survival secondary to an intrinsic red cell defect is a rare but important cause of shortened red cell survival in the neonate. Affected infants usually present with anemia and hyperbilirubinemia. Splenomegaly develops later in infancy or early childhood. A preliminary diagnosis of constitutional red cell defect is made by family history and careful inspection of the peripheral smear. Abnormalities of red cell shape, including spherocytes, eliptocytes, pyknocytes, "bite cells," target cells, and other bizarre morphologic structures, are often characteristic of the specific red cell defect.

Constitutional defects in red cell membranes cause lifelong hemolytic anemia. Because even normal neonates have shortened red cell survival and hyperbilirubinemia, the presentation of these syndromes in the neonate is often more severe than in older affected family members. Hereditary spherocytosis is the most common red cell membrane defect and is usually inherited as an autosomal dominant trait.

Glucose-6-phosphate dehydrogenase (G6PD) is the first rate-limiting enzyme in the pentose phosphate pathway of red cell energy metabolism. This enzyme is important in the production of NADPH, which maintains cellular systems in a reduced state. G6PD deficiency is the most common inherited disorder of red blood cells and is transmitted as an X-linked recessive. There are many isoforms of abnormal G6PD enzymes. The Mediterranean type produces severe hemolysis, whereas the form found in African Americans is usually mild. Infants are asymptomatic until challenged with oxidant stresses from infections or drugs. Agents associated with hemolysis in G6PD deficient infants are shown in Box 20-3.

Hemoglobinopathies are inherited disorders resulting from defects in the quantity or function of the hemoglobin proteins. The clinical expression of a hemoglobinopathy is dependent on the affected globin chain, the developmental state of globin synthesis, and the amount and function of alternate hemoglobins. Beta chains of hemoglobin are not produced until 3 months of postnatal age; therefore defects of beta chains, including beta thalassemia and sickle cell anemia, do not present in the nursery. Hemoglobinopathies presenting at birth affect either the alpha or gamma chains of hemoglobin.

The thalassemias are disorders manifested by absence or decrease of specific globin proteins. Because there are four genes controlling alpha globin synthesis, clinical signs may range from asymptomatic (absence of hemoglobin production from one alpha hemoglobin gene) to incompatible with life (absence of production from all four alpha hemoglobin genes). Alpha globin is an essential component of both hemoglobin F and hemoglobin A. Compensatory hemoglobins include Bart's hemoglobin Barts in the neonatal period, which is composed of four gamma chains, and later hemoglobin H, which is composed of four beta chains. These he-

Box 20-3	SOME AGENTS REPORTED TO PRODUCE HEMOLYSIS IN PATIENTS WITH G6PD DEFICIENCY

Drugs and Chemicals Clearly Shown to Cause Clinically Significant Hemolytic Anemia in G6PD Deficiency:

Acetanilid
Methylene blue
Nalidixic acid (NegGram)
Naphthalene
Niridazole (Ambilhar)
Phenylhydrazine
Primaquine
Pamaquine
Pentaquine
Sulfanilamide
Sulfacetamide
Sulfapyridine
Sulfamethoxazole (Gantanol)
Thiazolesulfone
Toluidine blue
Trinitrotoluene (TNT)

Drugs Probably Safe in Normal Therapeutic Doses for G6PD-Deficient Individuals (Without Nonspherocytic Hemolytic Anemia):

Acetaminophen (Paracetamol, Tylenol, Tralgon, Hydroxyacetanillid)
Acetophenetidine (Phenacetin)
Acetylsalicylic acid (aspirin)
Aminopyrine (Pyramidone, Amidopyrine)
Antazoline (Antistine)
Antipyrine
Ascorbic acid (vitamin C)

Drugs Probably Safe in Normal Therapeutic Doses for G6PD-Deficient Individuals (Without Nonspherocytic Hemolytic Anemia):—cont'd

Benzhexol (Artane)
Chloramphenicol
Chlorguanidine (Proguanil, Paludrine)
Chloroquine
Colchicine
Diphenhydramine (Benadryl)
L-Dopa
Menadione sodium bisulfite (Hykinone)
Menaphtone
p-Aminobenzoic acid
Phenylbutazone
Phenytoin
Probenecid (Benemid)
Procaine amide hydrochloride (Pronestyl)
Pyrimethamine (Daraprim)
Quinidine
Quinine
Streptomycin
Sulfacytine
Sulfadiazine
Sulfaguanidine
Sulfamerazine
Sulfamethoxypyriazine (Kynex)
Sulfisoxazole (Gantrisin)
Trimethoprim
Tripelennamine (Pyribenzamine)
Vitamin K

From Beutler: *Hemolytic anemia in disorders of red cell metabolism.* Plenum Press, 1978.
G6PD, Glucose-6-phosphate dehydrogenase.

moglobins are poor carriers of oxygen.[43] Homozygous thalassemia of the gamma chain is incompatible with life. Heterozygotes may have a moderately severe microcytic hemolytic anemia at birth.[18] In Western societies there has been a dramatic decline in the incidence of new births with severe thalassemia syndromes, because the widespread use of molecular diagnostic techniques by couples at risk.

Methemoglobin contains an oxidized form of heme iron, ferric Fe^{+++}, which renders it incapable of reversible binding to oxygen. Constitutional methemoglobinemia is caused either by deficiency of the red cell enzyme methemoglobin reductase or by an M hemoglobinopathy. Infants with either of these disorders present with cyanosis of the skin and mucous membranes but are otherwise asymp-

tomatic. Normal newborn infants are susceptible to acquired methemoglobinemia from oxidative stresses because neonatal red blood cells contain lower levels of the enzyme NADH-methemoglobin reductase.

Data Collection

History

Information obtained should include maternal history of illness and dietary intake during pregnancy, delivery type, hemorrhage, transfusion or iron therapy, and any abnormal occurrences during birth. A careful family history includes specific questioning regarding anemia, iron or transfusion therapy, pallor, jaundice, splenomegaly, splenectomy, gall stones, cholecystectomy, or congenital malformations in the parents, grandparents, siblings, aunts, uncles, and cousins of the infant.

Signs and Symptoms

When performing a physical examination of a newborn with anemia, attention should be paid to the infant's cardiovascular function, general vigor, and signs of pallor, jaundice, skin lesions, hepatosplenomegaly, lymphadenopathy, and congenital malformations (Box 20-4).

Box 20-4	SIGNS AND SYMPTOMS OF ANEMIA IN THE NEONATE

I. Acute anemia (with hemorrhage anemia may not be present initially; hemodilution will develop over 3-4 hr)
  A. Hypovolemia, hypotension
  B. Hypoxemia, tachypnea
  C. Tachycardia
II. Chronic anemia (may be well compensated)
  A. Pallor, metabolic acidosis, poor growth
  B. High-output congestive heart failure
  C. Persistent or increased oxygen requirement
  D. Iron deficiency with hypochromia, microcytosis

Laboratory Data

The diagnosis of anemia is based on the hemoglobin and hematocrit in comparison with normal values established for postconceptual and postnatal age. The peripheral blood smear should be carefully examined in all cases of abnormal hemoglobin and hematocrit, and the red cell indices should be evaluated. A clinical decision tree in the evaluation of anemia is shown in Figure 20-1. The characterization of anemia is dependent on additional laboratory testing (Table 20-3).

Treatment

If acute blood loss is suspected and the infant is pale and limp at birth, blood pressure should be obtained and monitored, IV fluids started at 20 ml/kg, and oxygen administered. A catheter should be inserted into the umbilical artery to measure blood gases. Blood should be obtained for complete blood count (CBC), reticulocyte count, Coombs' test, blood type, and serum screen for blood group antibodies. Because infants less than 4 months of age rarely produce antibodies against blood group antigens, maternal serum can be used in the antibody screen.

Table 20-3	CHARACTERIZATION OF ANEMIA
CHARACTERIZATION	**TEST**
Blood loss	Kleihauer-Betke on maternal sample
	Apt test on gastric blood from infant as indicated
Bone marrow production	Reticulocyte count
	Platelet and white blood cell count
	Erythropoietin level
	T3, T4, TSH
	Bone marrow aspirate and biopsy
	Fetal hemoglobin iAg, MCV
Iron deficiency	Ferritin, iron, and iron-binding capacity
Antibody mediated	Maternal and infant blood type
	Direct and indirect Coombs' test
Hemolysis	Bilirubin
	Coagulation tests (if sepsis or liver disease is suspected)
	Osmotic fragility, specific determinations of red cell membrane proteins, enzymes, hemoglobin, and ceruloplasmin as indicated
Infection	Culture and serologies as appropriate
Microangiopathy, macroangiopathy	DIC screen
Vitamin E deficiency	Vitamin E level
Metabolic disorder	pH, Lactate, Pyruvate
	Galactosemia screen

DIC, Disseminated intravascular coagulation; *MCV,* mean corpuscular volume; *TSH,* thyroid-stimulating hormone.

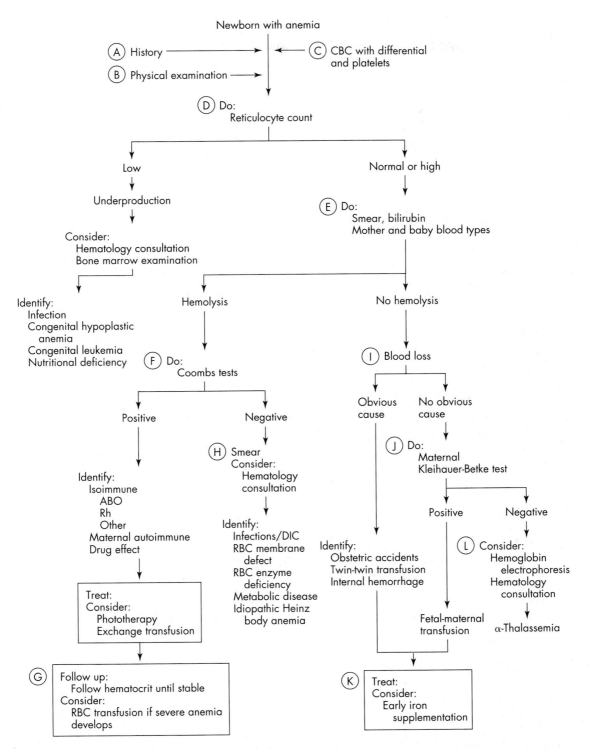

FIGURE 20-1   Clinical decision tree in evaluation of anemia. (From Lane PA, Nuss R: Anemia in the newborn. In Berman S, editor: *Pediatric decision making,* ed 3, St. Louis, 1996, Mosby.)   *Continued*

A. In the history, document any prenatal infections or drug use. Also note any history of maternal vaginal bleeding, placenta previa, abruptio placentae, or umbilical cord rupture, constriction or velamentous insertion, as well as cesarean, breech, or traumatic delivery. Obtain a family history of neonatal jaundice, anemia, splenomegaly, and unexplained gallstones.

B. In the physical examination, note tachypnea, tachycardia, peripheral vasoconstriction (acute blood loss), and hepatosplenomegaly (chronic anemia, intrauterine infection, congenital malignancy). Jaundice appearing before 24 hours of age suggests significant hemolysis.

C. A hematocrit less than 45% during the first 3 days of life is abnormal and requires explanation. The mean corpuscular volume (MCV) at birth is normally above 95. An MCV below 95 suggests α-thalassemia or chronic intrauterine blood loss (as with fetal maternal transfusion). Rarely, a low MCV may be seen with hemolytic disease caused by hereditary elliptocytosis or pyropoikilocytosis. The presence of neutropenia or thrombocytopenia suggests the possibility of infection. Except in an emergency, no anemic newborn should receive a blood transfusion before adequate diagnostic studies.

D. Normal reticulocyte values are 3% to 7% during the first day of life and 1% to 3% during the second and third days. A low reticulocyte count in the presence of significant anemia suggests bone marrow failure.

E. An indirect hyperbilirubinemia, abnormal peripheral blood smear, or ABO or Rh incompatibility between the mother and infant suggests hemolysis.

F. Perform direct and indirect Coombs tests. ABO isoimmunization is usually associated with a negative direct and a positive indirect Coombs test.

G. Infants with immune hemolysis have varying degrees of hemolysis, which may continue for 3 months. Severe, life-threatening anemia may develop in infants with Rh sensitization; such infants require close follow-up with serial hematocrit measurements until the hemolysis resolves.

H. Examine the peripheral blood smear. Spherocytes suggest ABO isoimmunization, hereditary spherocytosis, or infection (e.g., cytomegalovirus). Red cell fragmentation suggests intravascular hemolysis (infection, disseminated intravascular coagulation [DIC]). Consider infection or DIC in any ill newborn with hemolysis, particularly if thrombocytopenia is also present.

I. Review the obstetric history and examine the placenta for clues to the cause of fetal blood loss.

J. Perform a Kleihauer-Betke test to detect fetal red cells in the maternal circulation. False-negatives occur when an ABO incompatibility results in the rapid clearance of the infant's red cells from the maternal circulation.

K. Newborns with significant prenatal or perinatal blood loss are at risk for iron deficiency during the first 6 months of life.

L. Anemic infants without evidence of hemolysis or blood loss whose mothers have a negative Kleihauer test may have α-thalassemia, especially if the MCV is below 95. Ethnic groups affected most often include South and Southeast Asians, Mediterraneans, and Africans. The diagnosis of α-thalassemia may be confirmed with a hemoglobin electrophoresis that shows Bart's hemoglobin.

References

Ballin A, Brown EJ, Zipursky A: Idiopathic Heinz body hemolytic anemia in newborn infants, *Am J Pediatr Hematol Oncol* 11:3, 1989.

Blanchette VS, Zipursky A: Assessment of anemia in newborn infants, *Clin Perinatol* 11:489, 1984.

Oski FA: Anemia in the neonatal period. In Oski FA, Naiman JL, eds: *Hematologic problems in the newborn*, ed 3, Philadelphia, 1982, WB Saunders.

Oski FA: The erythrocyte and its disorders. In Nathan DG, Oski FA, eds: *Hematology of infancy and childhood*, ed 4, Philadelphia, 1993, WB Saunders.

FIGURE 20-1, cont'd Clinical decision tree in evaluation of anemia. (From Lane PA, Nuss R: Anemia in the newborn. In Berman S, editor: *Pediatric decision making*, ed 3, St. Louis, 1996, Mosby.)

Once the infant's condition stabilizes, a decision can be made regarding transfusion based on clinical status. **If the infant is anemic with signs of hypoxemia or has underlying pulmonary or cardiac disease, transfusion of 10 ml/kg of red blood cells over 2 to 3 hours may be given to increase oxygen carrying capacity.** Normally, larger quantities of blood should not be given in one transfusion. If the results of an antibody screen in the infant (or mother) are negative, major cross-matching need not be done if red cells used for transfusion are either type O or ABO, type compatible with both infant and mother, and Rh compatible.[33] **Blood used for transfusion should be less than 7 days old and negative for syphilis, hepatitis B and C, cytomegalovirus (CMV), and human immunodeficiency virus (HIV).** Irradiation of red blood cells and other blood cell products to prevent graft-versus-host disease is recommended for intrauterine transfusions or neonatal exchange transfusion and for infants with congenital or acquired immune deficiency. For infants with continuing hemorrhage requiring massive transfusion exceeding one blood volume, transfusions of fresh frozen plasma are required to replace clotting factors and prevent the consumptive coagulopathy that results from massive transfusion of stored blood. Platelet transfusions may also be needed.

An order from a physician or nurse practitioner is required for any blood transfusion. Parental consent should be obtained by the physician before transfusion. **In the neonatal intensive care nursery a policy of "double checking" blood is essential to ensure that the proper blood is being administered to the infant. Blood should be warmed and administered through a blood filter of at least 40 μm. Fresh blood can be administered through a 25-gauge needle without significant hemolysis.**

Directed donor programs are becoming more widely used in hospitals for nonemergent blood transfusions. In most cases biologic parents are able to serve as directed donors for their neonates. At this time there are no scientific data that suggest directed donor programs increase blood safety. Some immunologic incompatibilities may exist between maternal and paternal donors; therefore the following guidelines should be considered for parental donors[11]:

- Mothers should not provide blood components containing plasma. If maternal red cells are transfused, they should be washed.
- Fathers are not recommended as blood cell (red, white, or platelet) donors for their newborns unless maternal serum is shown to lack cytotoxic antibodies.
- All parental blood components should be irradiated before transfusion to the infant.

Equipment required for blood transfusion includes a filter, extension tubing, and a pump. Except in extreme emergencies, blood should be administered through a peripheral catheter rather than through a umbilical artery catheter (UAC). It is essential to confirm that the unit of blood infused matches the typed blood bank form and assigned number, patient name, and patient hospital number. The expiration date and time must be respected. IV tubing used for blood transfusion should be flushed with 0.45% normal saline solution before infusing blood products.

Blood bags should not be used for more than 4 to 6 hours after opening. Vital signs should be obtained and recorded every 15 minutes during blood transfusion. Careful observations should be made for reactions including increased temperature, diaphoresis, irregular respiration, bradycardia, restlessness, and pallor. Transfusions should be stopped promptly if any of these signs are present. All materials used for blood transfusion should be disposed of properly.

Infants who are anemic as a result of chronic blood loss or acute blood loss who do not require transfusion therapy should be treated with iron replacement 6 mg/kg/day until the blood count is normal and 2 additional months to replace stores.

Infants who are born with isoimmune hemolytic anemia are often treated with exchange transfusion. In this procedure, catheters placed in central and peripheral veins are used to remove the infant's blood in small aliquots and replace it with packed red cells usually reconstituted with fresh frozen plasma. General guidelines for aliquot volumes are as follows:

3 kg	20 ml per aliquot
2 kg	15 ml per aliquot
1 kg	5 ml per aliquot

Infants who are treated for isoimmune hemolytic anemia with intrauterine transfusions may be born with normal or near-normal hematocrit and bilirubin levels. Exchange transfusion is often used early after delivery to remove antibody and decrease postnatal hemolysis. Hyperbilirubinemia can be managed using phototherapy.

Prevention

Many forms of neonatal anemia are preventable. Improved fetal monitoring and obstetric care may prevent anemia caused by blood loss during delivery.

Administering Rh Ig to Rh-negative mothers within 72 hours of delivery of an Rh-positive infant prevents most cases of hydrops fetalis in subsequent pregnancies. For previously sensitized Rh-negative mothers carrying Rh-positive fetuses, amniocentesis performed between 20 and 22 weeks' gestation may allow for intrauterine transfusion of Rh-negative red blood cells and possible early delivery of a nonhydropic infant. For severe thalassemia syndromes and sickle cell anemia, prenatal diagnosis is possible. Intrauterine transfusions are also appropriate for infants with severe α-thalassemia. Clinical trials of prenatal and early postnatal bone marrow reconstitution with normal red cell progenitors are currently in progress.

Hemolysis may be prevented in infants with significant G6PD deficiency by avoiding administration of drugs known to present an oxidative stress to the red cells.

LBW premature infants are at high risk for late-onset anemia because of low endogenous production of erythropoietin, exacerbated by phlebotomy losses for laboratory surveillance. Inadequate nutrition and other factors may also play a significant role. Recombinant human erythropoietin (r-HuEPO) has been successfully used to decrease the severity of anemia and lessen the use of blood transfusion in small premature infants. Long-term risks are unknown at present but appear to be minimal. Benefits of therapy other than decreased exposure to blood transfusion are also unknown at present. Potential improvements in organ maturation or infant growth because of higher sustained levels of hemoglobin are speculative at present. The cost of a 6-week course of therapy with r-HuEPO is comparable in most institutions with that of conventional therapies with blood replacement.

Treatment with EPO should be considered in all infants of birth weight 800 to 1300 g. Infants with a birth weight of less than 800 g may receive so many transfusions early in their hospital course that treating with r-HuEPO may confer no substantial additional benefit. Infants with a birth weight of more than1300 g rarely require blood transfusion.

Treatment with r-HuEPO can begin when infants are stable and can tolerate iron supplementation, usually when tolerating approximately 60% of required enteral feedings. The recommended dose is 200 to 250 U/kg r-HuEPO IV or SC, three times weekly. The reticulocyte count should be monitored to document an adequate response. Oral iron supplementation should be initiated at the time of therapy, beginning with 2 mg/kg/day of elemental iron and increasing to 6 mg/kg/day as tolerated. A baseline hematocrit measurement and reticulocyte count should be obtained and followed weekly. Dosing should be adjusted to maintain a reticulocyte count above 6%. Supplemental vitamin E, 15 to 25 IU/day, and folic acid 100 μg/kg/day may be given at the start of therapy. Treatment is continued for 6 weeks or until 36 weeks' postconceptual age. Once treatment is discontinued, hematocrit levels should be monitored every other week until stable.[28,29]

The treatment of methemoglobinemia is oral methylene blue, except in the presence of G6PD deficiency in which treatment consists of ascorbic acid 200 to 500 mg/kg/day.[17,37]

POLYCYTHEMIA AND HYPERVISCOSITY

Physiology

Neonatal polycythemia is most commonly defined by a venous hematocrit greater than 65%.[14] Viscosity is related to but not identical to hematocrit. The viscosity of blood increases logarithmically in relation to the hematocrit.[23]

Although viscosity may be measured directly, hematocrit is often used as an indicator of viscosity. Blood sampling at 12 hours' postnatal age seems ideal to determine hematocrit and viscosity for diagnosis of polycythemic hyperviscosity.[45] Capillary hematocrit can be used as a screening test but should not be used alone for the diagnosis of polycythemia[20]; a venous sample should be analyzed to confirm an abnormally high capillary hematocrit.

Pathophysiology

Hyperviscosity is a syndrome of circulatory impairment resulting from increased resistance to blood flow. Complications of polycythemia and hyperviscosity include respiratory distress, congestive heart failure, hypoglycemia, hyperbilirubinemia, neurologic signs, and sequelae such as significant motor and mental retardation, cerebral infarcts, and cerebral palsy. Thromboemboli, cerebral artery thrombosis, necrotizing enterocolitis (NEC), and acute tubular necrosis are additional complications. Polycythemia can result from a large number of perinatal complications, as shown in Box 20-5.

In up to one third of monochorionic twins there is a significant transfusion of blood from one twin into the other defined as a discrepancy in the infants' blood counts of greater than 5 g of hemoglobin. Usually, the recipient twin is larger and prone to cardiorespiratory symptoms, hyperviscosity, and hyperbilirubinemia, whereas the donor twin is smaller and at risk for congestive heart failure.[42]

Blood viscosity correlates better with symptoms than does hematocrit.[34] In addition, clinical signs and symptoms may be related to an underlying condition instead of polycythemia per se. In most nurseries, because instruments to measure viscosity are not readily available, neonatal hyperviscosity is diagnosed by a combination of symptoms and an abnormally high hematocrit level.

Box 20-5	CAUSES OF NEONATAL POLYCYTHEMIA

A. Placental transfusion
   1. Delayed cord clamping (may increase the blood volume and red cell mass of the infant by as much as 55%)
   2. Twin-to-twin transfusion
B. Intrauterine hypoxia/placental vascular insufficiency
   1. Intrauterine growth restriction syndrome
   2. Maternal diabetes
   3. Maternal smoking
   4. Fetal risk factors
   5. Maternal hypertension syndromes
   6. Maternal cyanotic heart disease
C. Fetal factors
   1. Trisomy 13, 18, 21
   2. Hyperthyroidism
   3. Neonatal thyrotoxicosis
   4. Congenital adrenal hyperplasia
   5. Beckwith-Weidemann syndrome
D. High altitude
E. Idiopathic

Data Collection

History

In addition to a complete history of the pregnancy and delivery, questions should be directed to pertinent maternal medical conditions, including insulin-dependent diabetes mellitus, hypertension, and heart disease. Additional maternal risk factors include cigarette smoking and living at high altitude. Fetal risk factors include documentation of fetal growth restriction and delayed cord clamping.

Signs and Symptoms

Newborn infants with hematocrit values of greater than 65% to 70% may manifest symptoms because of increased viscosity.[45] Physical examination may be normal except for plethora and, occasionally, cyanosis. Neurologic findings may include lethargy, irritability, hypotonia, tremor, and poor suck. Tachypnea, tachycardia, and respiratory distress may be present. Poor gastrointestinal function is common with abdominal distension, decreased bowel sounds, and poor feeding.

Laboratory Data

The diagnosis of polycythemia is based on hemoglobin and hematocrit in comparison with normal values for postconceptual and postnatal age. The di-

agnosis of hyperviscosity may be based on direct viscosity measurement but usually is assigned based on polycythemia in the presence of consistent clinical signs and symptoms. Affected infants often have thrombocytopenia, hyperbilirubinemia, and hypoglycemia. Tests of thyroid and adrenal function to rule out hyperthyroidism and adrenal hyperplasia should be performed with appropriate clinical indication. Chromosome analysis should be considered for babies with dysmorphic features.

Treatment

Therapy of polycythemia is generally based on the presence of consistent signs and symptoms. Therapy, when indicated, is aimed at decreasing the hematocrit and includes removal of red cells by simple phlebotomy as well as partial exchange transfusion with replacement of removed red cell volume with volume expanders or plasma. Exchange transfusion often requires placement of a umbilical venous catheter (UVC). Risks of umbilical catheterization in polycythemic infants include portal vein thrombosis, phlebitis of the portal vein, and decreased plasma volume (if phlebotomy is used alone). In addition, infants with polycythemia and hyperviscosity are at increased risk of spontaneous large vessel thrombosis, especially renal vein thrombosis and stroke.

There is evidence that treating all infants with polycythemia may not improve outcome. In a study by Bada et al[4] symptomatic infants received partial plasma exchange transfusion, which reduced blood viscosity, improved cerebral blood flow, and ameliorated symptoms. Infants who were asymptomatic before therapy showed little or no improvement in cerebral blood flow with partial exchange transfusion.

In a randomized controlled trial, Roithmaier et al[36] showed that partial exchange transfusion using crystalloid solution (Ringer's solution) was as effective as partial exchange transfusion using a colloid (plasma) in decreasing the hematocrit of polycythemic neonates. Crystalloid solutions are preferable to colloids because they are less expensive and are infection free.

COAGULATION

Physiology

When a blood vessel is torn, blood will clot at the site of vessel injury through a series of carefully controlled enzymatic reactions. First, platelets that are small, platelike blood cells without nuclei adhere to the damaged endothelium both directly and by linkage through the von Willebrand protein to collagen, which is exposed beneath the blood vessel lining. The platelets release adenosine diphosphate (ADP) which recruits more platelets to the activation process. Activated platelets express a receptor for the blood protein fibrinogen, which binds to adjoining platelets and links them. Fibrinogen is a contractile protein that pulls platelets together, forming a tightly woven net over the vessel tear. This is known as a *platelet plug* and is responsible for the initial cessation of bleeding, especially on mucous membranes of the nose, mouth, throat, and GI and genitourinary tracts. At the same time, thromboxanes produced by the platelet prostaglandin pathway stimulate platelet aggregation, vasoconstriction, and decreased local blood flow.

Figure 20-2 shows the sequential reactions in activation of coagulation known as the "clotting cascade."[26] The coagulation proteins in the blood are inert proenzymes until they are activated. The primary activation process involves exposure of a potent membrane glycoprotein receptor for clotting activation called tissue factor. This is known as the *tissue factor pathway of coagulation activation.* Tissue factor is normally hidden in the subendothelium and becomes exposed by vascular injury or is presented on the intact surface of monocytes and endothelial cells through the inflammatory process. Activated factor VII in the plasma binds to tissue factor and forms a complex that results in the sequential activation first of factor X and then of factor II (also called prothrombin). These biochemical reactions are similar in that they take place preferentially on procoagulant phospholipid surfaces of endothelial cells and platelets at the site of injury, involve calcium-dependent binding to the surface, and can be accelerated by cofactors (factors VIII and V).

The contact activation pathway is an alternative route to factor X activation. In this pathway, factor XII is activated by contact with negatively charged subendothelial collagen or by acidosis, cold, or heat injury. Activated factor XII subsequently activates factors XI and IX. Prekallikrein and high-molecular-weight kininogen serve as cofactors of activation. Contact activation initiates clot lysis and also many inflammatory pathways, including the complement system, which is important for host defense. The tissue factor and contact pathways activate each

other and thus generally are not functioning completely independently.

Procoagulant factors II, VII, IX, and X and regulatory proteins, protein C and protein S, are biochemically related. They are all produced in the liver and require vitamin K to become functional. Vitamin K catalyzes the transfer of carboxyl groups to glutamic acid residues of vitamin K–dependent proteins; only after carboxylation can these unique proteins then bind to surfaces via calcium.

Thrombin is the terminal coagulation enzyme and functions as an important regulator of coagulation. It is a potent platelet activator. Thrombin provides positive feedback activation of factors VIII and V and initiates the regulation of factors VIIIa and Va through activation of protein C. Thrombin cleaves fibrinogen to form a sticky fibrin strand. Factor XIII is activated by thrombin and cross-links the fibrin strand, greatly increasing its strength and stability. Fibrin then contracts and forms a tight dense clot. A fibrin clot holds opposed surfaces together for about a week as thrombin and other growth factors stimulate fibroblasts to grow. Ultimately, scar tissue bridges the original injury. When a blood clot is no longer needed, it is dissolved by an enzyme system called *fibrinolysis.* The blood zymogen plasminogen is activated by tissue plasminogen activator (TPA), which is released from endothelial cells. The active enzyme plasmin cleaves the fibrin clot into fragments of various sizes, called *fibrin split products (FSPs).* Split products that contain factor XIII mediated cross-linked fibrin are called the D-*dimer fragments.* Several proteins are responsible for regulating the coagulation process and ensuring that these powerful enzymes are not activated in the systemic circulation, causing uncontrolled blood clotting. The most important of these regulatory proteins are antithrombin, protein C, and the protein C cofactor protein S. Heparin cofactor II, alpha$_2$-macroglobulin, and alpha$_1$-antitrypsin also function as coagulation regulatory proteins. Plasminogen activator inhibitor (PAI), histamine-rich glycoprotein, and fibrin binding of plasminogen regulate the activation of fibrinolysis.

Normal Values

Healthy term and preterm infants have platelet counts within the normal adult range. The coagulation system of the newborn infant is unique in that blood clotting proteins mature at different rates (Table 20-4).[16] Factors V, VIII, and fibrinogen are within the normal adult range by 20 weeks of fetal

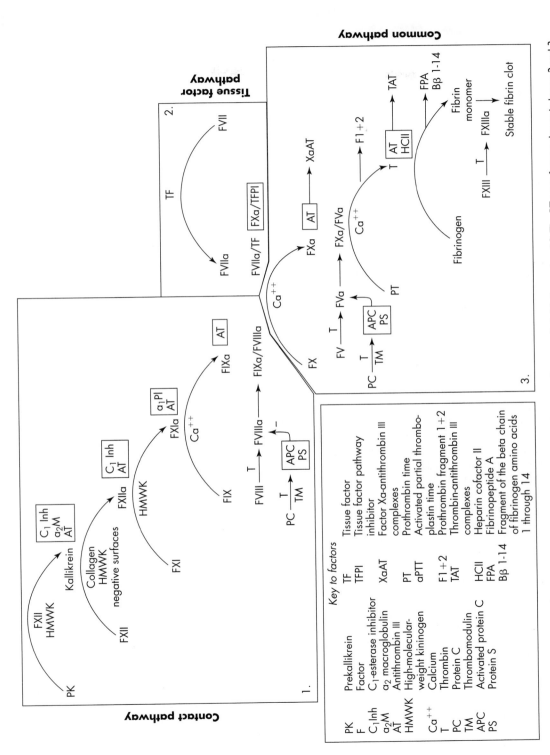

FIGURE 20-2 The clotting cascade. The aPTT screening test of coagulation tests factors included in boxes 1 and 3. The PT tests factors shown in boxes 2 and 3. Proteins encased in boxes inhibit the procoagulant reactions.

Table 20-4	COAGULATION FACTOR VALUES* FOR FETUS AND NEWBORN INFANT								
SUBJECTS	I (MG/DL)	II	V	VII	VIII:C	vWF:AG	IX	X	XI
Fetus (~20 wk)	96	0.16	0.70	0.21	0.50	0.65	0.10	0.19	—
	(40)	(0.10)	(0.40)	(0.12)	(0.23)	(0.40)	(0.05)	(0.15)	—
Preterm newborn	250	0.32	0.80	0.37	0.75	1.50	0.22	0.38	0.20
(25-32 wk)	(100)	(0.18)	(0.43)	(0.24)	(0.40)	(0.90)	(0.17)	(0.20)	(0.12)
Preterm newborn	300	0.45	0.82	0.59	0.93	1.66	0.41	0.44	—
(33-36 wk)	(120)	(0.26)	(0.48)	(0.34)	(0.54)	(1.35)	(0.20)	(0.21)	—
Term newborn	240	0.52	1.00	0.57	1.50	1.60	0.35	0.45	0.42
(37-41 wk)	(150)	(0.25)	(0.54)	(0.35)	(0.55)	(0.84)	(0.15)	(0.30)	(0.20)
Older infant (age	340	0.97	1.00	0.90	0.93	1.13	0.7	0.55	0.52
and level when	(21 days)	(45-60 days)	(1 day)	(21 days)	(1-2 days)	(1 wk)	(6 mo)	(6 wk)	(6 wk)
adult value is									
approximated)									

From Hathaway WE, Bonnar J: *Hemostatic disorders of the pregnant woman and newborn infant,* New York, 1987, Elsevier Science.
AT-III, Antithrombin III; *HMWK,* high-molecular-weight kininogen; *PK,* prekallikrein; *vWF,* von Willebrand factor.
Values (data taken from references discussed in text) are expressed in units per milliliter as compared with normal adult subject reference plasma (100% = 1 U/ml); the mean and (lower limit of range (or −2 SD) are shown.
*Clotting activity or chromogenic substrate methods (except protein C:Ag, protein S:Ag) in subjects in the first 24 hours of life.
†Cord. All other values are venous. All subjects received vitamin K at birth.

development. Low levels of these clotting proteins are never normal. The level of the von Willebrand protein is higher at birth than in an adult, and the von Willebrand protein subunits (called *multimers*) include ultralarge forms, which makes the protein more adherent to platelets and vessel walls. Fetal fibrinogen differs from the adult molecule in its content of sialic acid. This prolongs the thrombin time (TT) of the neonate. Vitamin K–dependent factors II, VII, IX, X, protein C, and protein S develop very slowly. Factor IX does not reach its full adult potential until 9 months of age; protein C may not reach adult levels until puberty. It is very difficult to determine if these proteins are genetically deficient during the neonatal period.

The clotting system is evaluated using a hemostasis screen, which includes testing for partial thromboplastin time (PTT), prothrombin time (PT), TT, fibrinogen concentration, platelet count, and a test of platelet function, such as the platelet function analyzer (PFA-100). The PTT may be within the adult range at term birth or may achieve the adult range by 2 months. The PTT of a stable preterm infant with a birth weight of less than 1000 g is often extremely prolonged, without signs of excessive bleeding. The PT is usually near normal at birth, may prolong slightly by day 3, and may

reach adult normal values by day 5. The TT is slightly prolonged because of fetal fibrinogen until 3 weeks of age. The fibrinogen and platelet concentrations are within the normal adult range at birth in stable term and preterm infants. The PFA-100 is a whole blood test that estimates platelet function. Certain tests of specific platelet activities including aggregation are somewhat decreased at birth and for the first 3 weeks of age. However, the PFA-100, which measures global platelet function, is shorter in a term neonate than in an adult, and clinically the neonate is in a hypercoagulable state.

Pathophysiology

Thrombocytopenia

Thrombocytopenia is a general term that denotes a decreased number of platelets in the infant's blood. Thrombocytopenia is the most common coagulation disorder in the neonate. It is important to determine whether the infant appears well or ill. The causes of thrombocytopenia in an otherwise well infant differ from those in an acutely ill neonate (Box 20-6).

A well-appearing infant is likely to suffer from alloimmune thrombocytopenia, in which the platelets are coated by circulating antibody and rapidly cleared from the circulation by the spleen and liver. Alloimmune thrombocytopenia develops when the mother is

Table 20-4		COAGULATION FACTOR VALUES* FOR FETUS AND NEWBORN INFANT—cont'd						
XII	PK	HMWK	XIII	PLASMINOGEN	α_2-ANTIPLASMIN	AT-III	Protein C:Ag	Protein S:Ag
—	—	—	~0.30	—	—	0.23	0.10	—
—	—	—	—	—	—	(0.12)	(0.06)	—
0.22	0.26	0.28	0.11-0.40	0.35	74	0.35	0.29	—
(0.09)	(0.14)	(0.20)		(0.20)	(~50)	(0.20)	(0.21)	—
0.25	0.33	—	—	0.38	73	0.40	0.38	—
(0.09)	(0.23)			(0.26)	(~50)	(0.25)	(0.23)	—
0.44	0.35	0.64	0.61	0.49	83	0.56	0.50†	0.24†
(0.16)	(0.16)	(0.50)	(0.36)	(0.25)	(~65)	(0.32)	(0.30)	(0.10)
1.00	0.86	0.82	1.0	1.00	1.0	0.82	0.82	—
(14 days)	(6 mo)	(6 mo)	(1 mo)	(6 mo)	(1 wk)	(3-6 mo)	(24 mo)	—

Box 20-6	CAUSE OF THROMBOCYTOPENIA IN THE NEWBORN INFANT

I. Well infant
  A. Immune
    1. Alloimmune thrombocytopenia
    2. Maternal idiopathic thrombocytopenia purpura
  B. Constitutional
    1. Thrombocytopenia absent radius
    2. Amegakaryocytic thrombocytopenia
    3. Wiskott-Aldrich syndrome
    4. Fanconi's anemia
    5. Bernard-Soulier syndrome
    6. Autosomal dominant thrombocytopenia

II. Sick Infant
  A. Respiratory distress syndrome
  B. Bacterial sepsis
  C. Viral infection
  D. Necrotizing enterocolitis
  E. Hyperviscosity
  F. Disseminated intravascular coagulation
III. May appear either well or sick
  A. Kasabach-Merritt (giant hemangioma) syndrome
  B. Trisomy 21, 18, 13
  C. Leukemia
  D. Thrombosis

negative for a platelet antigen, usually PLA-1, for which the father is positive. Fifty percent of recognized cases of alloimmune thrombocytopenia present in a mother's first infant. Subsequent infants can be more severely involved. Presentations of alloimmune thrombocytopenia range from asymptomatic infants in whom a low platelet count is detected coincidentally on a blood count to fatal cases of intracranial hemorrhage with onset in utero. Infants of mothers with idiopathic thrombocytopenic purpura (ITP) may have a low platelet count because the maternal anti-body crosses the placenta to the infant but usually does not develop life-threatening hemorrhage.

Constitutional thrombocytopenia is rare. Affected infants often manifest congenital skeletal malformations of the hands and arms. Thrombocytopenia absent radius (TAR) is a rare but well-characterized syndrome. A bone marrow examination is important to evaluate the megakaryocyte pool, which produces platelets. In Bernard-Soulier syndrome the platelet number is moderately decreased and giant platelets are seen on the peripheral smear. Infants with trisomy 21 (Down syndrome), 18, or 13 can manifest abnormal platelet counts without apparent illness. The bone marrow of infants with Down syndrome is highly reactive. Other features of trisomy 21 should be present.

Giant, cavernous hemangiomas often trap platelets in a syndrome known as Kasabach-Merritt, resulting in accelerated destruction. Clues to this syndrome include skin hemangiomas; bruits over the liver, spleen, or brain; or high-output congestive heart failure with a structurally normal heart.

Thrombocytopenia develops in most infants with respiratory distress severe enough to require mechanical ventilation. The lowest platelet counts are usually found at about day 3 of life, and normal counts recover by day 10 if the infant's course is not complicated by infection or thrombosis. Infants of less than 32 weeks' gestation with RDS and severe thrombocytopenia are at increased risk of intracranial hemorrhage.

Bacterial and viral infections must be excluded in any thrombocytopenic neonate. The infant of a mother with chorioamnionitis often demonstrates thrombocytopenia in the cord blood.

Thrombosis in a neonate often presents with an idiopathic falling platelet count. Thromboses are most commonly found at the tips of umbilical artery catheters (UACs) and UVCs and can be diagnosed with ultrasound. An infected clot should be suspected in an infant with diagnosed catheter-related thrombosis and alterations in temperature, respiratory stability, or cardiovascular stability.

Thrombocytopenia in an ill infant is often part of the larger syndrome of DIC.[26] In DIC, activation of blood-clotting proteins is initiated by tissue factor from bacterial products (endotoxin) or inflammation or through the contact system. The activation of clotting proteins leads to a hypercoagulable state and thromboses occur, especially in the small vessels of the liver, spleen, brain, lungs, kidneys, and adrenal glands. The bone marrow and liver partially compensate by releasing platelets and clotting factors into the circulation. However, the regulatory system of coagulation is immature in term and preterm neonates. The capacity to neutralize activated clotting proteins is quickly exhausted, and the resulting deficiencies of platelets and clotting factors is called *consumptive coagulopathy*. DIC predisposes a preterm infant to intracranial hemorrhage. Venous thrombosis of the germinal matrix occurs as the initial lesion, followed by postthrombotic hemorrhage. Bleeding is also seen in the skin,

around indwelling catheters, around endotracheal and chest tubes, and in the urine and stool.

Vitamin K Deficiency

The most important bleeding syndrome in the otherwise stable neonate is hemorrhagic disease of the newborn, caused by vitamin K deficiency.[19] There is a tenfold gradient in vitamin K concentration between the maternal and fetal plasma. Marginal fetal vitamin K levels are further compromised by maternal use of anticonvulsants or warfarin. Approximately 3% of cord blood samples from normal term pregnancies show biochemical evidence of noncarboxylated clotting proteins.[40] Early hemorrhagic disease of the newborn presents within the first 24 hours of life with massive cephalhematoma, GI tract bleeding, or intracranial hemorrhage. Classic hemorrhagic disease of the newborn presents between 1 and 7 days of life; late vitamin K deficiency occurs between 1 week and 2 months of life. The recommendation of the American Academy of Pediatrics is to give every neonate 1 mg of vitamin K by intramuscular injection[5]; this is adequate to prevent bleeding in most infants. Vitamin K prophylaxis can be achieved with use of an oral vitamin K preparation. However, because oral therapy requires multiple doses over the first 6 weeks of life, it is difficult to ensure compliance and protect all infants using this formulation. Vitamin K concentrations are physiologically very low in human breast milk; cow's milk contains 10 times the amount of vitamin K (1.5 and 15 mg/L, respectively). Infants fed breast milk are at increased risk of vitamin K deficiency. In addition, infants with fat malabsorption caused by cystic fibrosis, alpha$_1$-antitrypsin deficiency, or biliary atresia and infants treated with prolonged courses of antibiotics are at increased risk of vitamin K deficiency.

Hemophilia and Other Congenital Bleeding Disorders

The hemophilias are a group of lifelong bleeding disorders caused by genetic deficiencies of one or more coagulation proteins. Factor VIII deficiency causes 80% of the hemophilias, and factor IX deficiency causes most of the remainder. Both factors VIII and IX are encoded on the X chromosome; thus deficiency states are manifested in carrier mothers and affected sons. Deficiencies of other coagulation factors are inherited as autosomal traits with severe bleeding manifested with homozygous deficiency. Most infants with hemophilia appear to tolerate labor and a routine vaginal delivery with no undue problem. However, intracranial hemorrhage has been documented in approximately 1% to 4% of infants with hemophilia as a result of birth trauma.[7] Current recommendations call for vaginal delivery in the absence of complications; however, cesarean section should be elected if needed to avoid prolonged or difficult labor. Fifty percent of male infants with severe hemophilia will hemorrhage from a circumcision. The absence of procedure-related bleeding in the neonatal period does not exclude hemophilia owing to physiologically increased platelet function around birth. Prolonged bleeding from the umbilical cord stump is suggestive of factor XIII deficiency. Spontaneous intracranial hemorrhage also occurs in infants with homozygous deficiency of factors V, VII, X, XIII, or fibrinogen.

Data Collection

History

A history of maternal bleeding, medical and obstetric diagnoses, and medications should be elicited for every infant at birth. A careful family history for bleeding disorders in the parents, grandparents, siblings, aunts, uncles, and cousins of an infant should be taken as part of every admission evaluation. Specific questions must be asked about excessive bleeding with surgeries, menses, childbirth, traumas, and spontaneous bleeding events. Efforts should be made to obtain confirmatory medical records for any positive response. Procedures, including circumcision, should not be performed until the possibility of a bleeding disorder in the infant is excluded. The administration of vitamin K to the infant should be confirmed by review of the nursing notes.

Signs and Symptoms

Thrombocytopenia usually presents with small, flat hemorrhages into the skin called *petechiae* that do not blanch with pressure. Petechiae may be concentrated in skin creases of the neck and axilla and around the site of a tourniquet or may be scattered over the entire body. More severe thrombocytopenia results in large ecchymoses, which are flat bruises. Infants with severe thrombocytopenia may hemorrhage into the CNS or the gastrointestinal tract.

Bleeding with coagulation disorders causes palpable hematomas of the skin and scalp. Intracranial, retroperitoneal, intraperitoneal, gastrointestinal, and genitourinary bleeding may occur. Bleeding with surgeries or procedures may be immediate or delayed.

Laboratory Data

Any infant with bleeding signs should be evaluated with a hemostasis screen and a platelet count. The results of the hemostasis screen in the healthy infant and during many states of illness are shown in Table 20-5. The possibility of hemophilia should be excluded by specific factor assays. In addition, factors XIII, alpha$_2$-antiplasmin, and PAI-1 should be assayed in a term infant with unexplained significant hemorrhage, such as intracranial hemorrhage.

Treatment

Thrombocytopenia

Therapy for thrombocytopenia depends on the overall health and stability of the neonate. **The primary support of a thrombocytopenic infant is replacement transfusions of platelets,** which are derived from CMV-negative donors. A stable, otherwise healthy infant can tolerate a platelet count as low as 20,000/μl without undue risk of serious bleeding.

Table 20-5	COAGULATION RESULTS IN NORMAL NEONATES AND NEONATES WITH BLEEDING SYNDROMES					
DESCRIPTION	PTT	PT	TT	FIB	D-DIMER	PLT CT
Healthy term	N-↑	N-↑	↑	NL	Neg	NL
Healthy preterm	↑↑	N-↑	↑	NL	Neg	NL
Vit K deficiency	↑↑	↑↑↑	↑	NL	Neg	NL
Liver disease	↑↑	↑↑↑	↑↑-↑↑↑	↓	Pos	↓
Hemophilia	↑↑↑	N-↑	↑	NL	Neg	NL
DIC	↑↑↑	↑↑	↑↑	↓	Pos	↓↓

Fib, Fibrogen; *N*, normal; *Plt Ct*, platelet count; *PT*, prothrombin time; *PTT*, partial thromboplastin time; *TT*, thrombin time; ↑, mildly prolonged; ↑↑, moderately prolonged; ↑↑↑, severely prolonged; ↓, decreased.

However, an infant who is less than 30 weeks' gestation, mechanically ventilated, on extracorporeal membrane oxygenation (ECMO) therapy, with indwelling UACs or UVCs and chest tubes, septic or otherwise unstable, will require a platelet count of 50,000/µl to prevent or treat bleeding.

Infants with alloimmune thrombocytopenia are likely to receive incompatible platelets from a random donor. Thrombocytopenia in this disorder responds well to intravenous gamma globulin (IVIG). Platelet transfusions, when needed, should be derived from the mother, if practical, or from a type-specific donor. Infants with Kasabach-Merritt syndrome may respond to steroid therapy, antifibrinolytic agents, or interferon.

Transfusion of platelets into infants with thrombosis or DIC may aggravate the platelet consumption unless specific therapy of the underlying condition is also administered. The primary treatment of DIC is reversal of the trigger (Box 20-7). Adequate ventilation, support of circulation and perfusion, treatment of sepsis, and general supportive care usually interrupt the DIC process within 48 hours. Replacement of coagulation regulatory proteins in fresh frozen plasma or antithrombin (AT) concentrate or inhibition of coagulation activation with low dose heparin is helpful in some cases.

Bleeding Disorders

Infants with vitamin K deficiency are treated with vitamin K 1 mg by slow IV push. Fresh frozen plasma 10 to 15 ml/kg may be given to control active bleeding.

Neonates with severe liver disease can be treated for active bleeding or prepared for liver biopsy using transfusions of fresh frozen plasma and platelet concentrates. Parenteral administration of vitamin K should be confirmed; ongoing replacement may be necessary if there is fat malabsorption. A recombinant preparation of activated factor VII (VIIa, Novo-Seven, manufactured by NovoNordisk, Copenhagen, Denmark) has been used to control bleeding in the neonate with encouraging results. Concentrates of vitamin K–dependent clotting factors purified from human plasma and subjected to viral inactivation techniques are also available. Consultation with a regional hemophilia treatment center regarding use and availability of these specialized products is strongly recommended.

Treatment of congenital coagulation factor deficiencies is based on the deficient factor. Factor VIII or IX should be replaced in a bleeding neonate (or for surgery) using only recombinant proteins because they have greater viral safety than human plasma–derived proteins. Factor XIII and fibrinogen may be replaced in cryoprecipitate. The von Willebrand protein is contained both in certain viral inactivated coagulation concentrates as well as in cryoprecipitate. Replacement of other clotting proteins usually requires fresh frozen plasma. DDAVP, a synthetic vasopressin that stimulates release of endothelial stores of factor VIII and the von Willebrand protein, is generally not used in the neonate because of the possibility of seizures related to hyponatremia in this age-group. The hemophilia center should be involved in the diagnosis and management of all infants with congenital bleeding disorders.

Prevention and Parent Teaching

Mothers should be instructed during pregnancy that vitamin K deficiency is routinely prevented with an IM injection of vitamin K to the neonate. Primary care providers should be careful to document administration of vitamin K, especially for infants born at home.

Bleeding in an infant with a bleeding disorder can be minimized by exerting care to prevent undue trauma. Intramuscular injections and other invasive procedures should be avoided if at all possible. The infant should be handled in as gentle a manner as possible. Pressure for holding and placement of a tourniquet should be minimized. Extreme care should be taken with arterial puncture.

Replacement platelet or clotting factor infusions should be considered before any necessary invasive procedure. Parents should be educated about the nature of the bleeding disorder and its cause in their infant. They need to know whether this is a time-

---

Box 20-7	THERAPY OF DIC

1. Reverse the trigger; treat the underlying disorder.
2. Maintain hemostatic levels of fibrinogen (>100 mg/dl) and platelets (50,000/µl) using fresh frozen plasma and platelet concentrates (10 ml/kg).
3. If necessary, replace regulatory proteins; antithrombin concentrate (50-150 U/kg).
4. Consider low-dose heparin therapy 10 U/kg/hr if survival of infused fibrinogen and platelets is <12 hr.

DIC, Disseminated intravascular coagulation.

limited complication of the neonatal course or a long-term concern. Infants with constitutional thrombocytopenia or coagulopathy are at lifelong risk of bleeding. The risk of platelet sensitization and the consequent aim to minimize platelet exposure must be conveyed to the parents. Any other family member at risk of a genetic cause of thrombocytopenia or bleeding should be identified, screened, and counseled.

Education of families about hemophilia or constitutional thrombocytopenia begins as soon as the diagnosis is established. Nurses should instruct parents about routine infant care and recognition of possible bleeding events in coordination with the hemophilia nurse coordinator.

THROMBOSIS

Pathophysiology

Thrombosis is an uncommon problem in pediatric patients, with increased incidence noted in both the neonatal period and after puberty. Physiologic correlates of the neonate's increased predisposition to thrombosis are shown in Boxes 20-8 and 20-9.

Box 20-8	PROTHROMBOTIC CHARACTERISTICS OF NEONATAL BLOOD

Increased hematocrit values
Increased concentration and size of von Willebrand factor multimers
Low concentrations of physiologic anticoagulants, antithrombin, protein C, and protein S
Low concentration of the fibrinolytic protein plasminogen
Small caliber blood vessels

Box 20-9	PATHOLOGIC CONDITIONS PREDISPOSING TO THROMBOSIS IN THE NEONATE

Hypotension
Hyperviscosity
Severe genetic and acquired deficiencies of antithrombin, protein C, protein S, and plasminogen.[49,50]
Genetic mutations in factor V and prothrombin; hyperhomocysteinemia
Mechanical obstruction by catheters
Maternal diabetes mellitus

The most common sites of spontaneous thrombosis in the neonate are the renal veins, the central nervous system (CNS), the superior and inferior vena cava and the aorta. Catheters placed for critical care support are associated with an increased risk of thrombosis.

Purpura Fulminans

Purpura fulminans is a syndrome of skin necrosis from venous thrombosis caused by severe deficiencies of protein C or protein S.[15,24] Most cases are caused by homozygous or compound heterozygous genetic defects. Rarely, acquired deficiences from maternal lupus anticoagulants can mimic the genetic syndromes. Consumption of protein C and protein S during bacterial sepsis usually presents at a later age and is less fulminant than the genetic syndromes.

Thrombocytosis

Thrombocytosis occurs with iron-deficiency anemia. An iron-deficient neonate may have suffered from chronic blood loss in utero, either by hemorrhage into the placenta to a twin, or with GI bleeding. Neuroblastoma, a malignancy of neural crest cells, and Down syndrome may also be associated with thrombocytosis.

Data Collection

History

A history of thrombosis in the parents, grandparents, siblings, aunts, uncles, and cousins of the infant raises suspicion of genetic thrombophilia. Unfortunately, many family members affected with heterozygous deficiencies of protein C or protein S are often asymptomatic until early to mid-adult life. A history of fetal or neonatal death with thrombosis is helpful.

Signs and Symptoms

Thrombosis. Signs of decreased organ perfusion and subsequent dysfunction indicate the possibility of a thrombosis. The classic presentation of renal vein thrombosis includes hematuria, thrombocytopenia, and hypertension. Palpably enlarged kidneys may be noted on physical examination. The presence of unilateral or bilateral flank masses on the initial physical assessment indicates prenatal occurrence of renal vein thrombosis. Stroke usually presents with seizures during the first 24 hours of life. Aortic thromboses present with cool, pale extremities, decreased pulses and capillary refill, and upper extremity hypertension. Confirmation is made with ultrasound examination of the renal veins and aorta, renal scan, and computerized tomography (CT) or magnetic resonance imaging (MRI) of the brain.

Purpura Fulminans. Purpura fulminans is a dramatic syndrome that usually presents within hours of birth. Infants develop patchy areas of skin thrombosis over the trunk and buttocks, usually in dependent areas. The lesions are palpable, initially dark red, and quickly become dusky purple and then black; an eschar forms. The lesions are exquisitely painful. Most infants will manifest a white light reflex of the eyes from in utero thrombosis of the primary vitreal veins with subsequent retinal detachment, hemorrhage, and blindness. Imaging studies of the brain show evidence of CNS infarction in many infants. Renal vein thrombosis is not uncommon.

Thrombocytosis. Infants rarely manifest signs of thrombocytosis. Occasionally, platelet counts of greater than 2,000,000/μl are associated with cerebral ischemia.

Treatment

Thrombosis. The optimal therapy for neonatal thrombosis has not been determined. Two approaches include **anticoagulation with unfractionated or low molecular weight heparin to prevent propagation of the clot or fibrinolytic therapy to dissolve the clot,** as shown in Box 20-10. Fibrinolytic therapy may restore blood flow more rapidly. However, the risk of hemorrhage is greater with fibrinolytic therapy, especially CNS bleeding in an infant with brain ischemia from a previous episode of asphyxia or hypotension. Fibrinolytic therapy, if deemed acceptably safe, may be preferable for renal vein thrombosis and for life- or limb-threatening aortic thrombosis. Long-term anticoagulation with warfarin is necessary only in the small proportion of infants who have an ongoing trigger for thrombosis.

Purpura Fulminans. **The treatment of neonatal purpura fulminans is replacement of protein C or protein S.** Fresh frozen plasma should be administered while confirmatory laboratory assays are being performed, using 10 ml/kg every 8 to 12 hours. Concentrates of viral-inactivated, human plasma–

Box 20-10	**ANTITHROMBOTIC THERAPY IN THE NEONATE**

Anticoagulant Therapy

Unfractionated heparin
  50-100 U/kg bolus
  25-40 U/kg/hr maintenance; adjusted to maintain anti-Xa level of 0.3-0.7 U/ml
Low-molecular-weight heparin (Enoxiparin)
  1.7 mg/kg SC every 12 hr; adjusted to maintain anti-Xa level of 0.5-1.0 U/ml 4 hr after injection
Consider FFP 10 ml/kg or AT concentrate 50-150 U/kg q 24-48 hr to enhance heparin effect, if necessary

Fibrinolytic Therapy

Tissue plasminogen activator
  0.1-0.5 mg/kg/hr for 4-12 hr
  or 0.03 to 0.12 mg/kg/hr for 12-48 hr
Fibrinolytic therapy has been given to neonates both as higher-dose, shorter infusions and lower-dose, longer-term infusions. The higher-dose infusions may be more effective in thromboses that are acute, arterial and smaller in volume (e.g., aortic or cardiac). Lower, longer infusions may be more efficacious in larger, older, or venous thromboses (e.g., subclavian or extensive vena cava).
Tissue plasminogen activator
  0.1-0.5 mg/kg for 4-12 hr
  or 0.03-0.05 mg/kg/hr for 24-48 hr
Heparin 10 U/kg/hr (no bolus) or Enoxiparin 0.5 mg/kg q 12 h SC
Consider fresh frozen plasma 10 ml/kg q 24 h to replace plasminogen

---

Term infants show the highest dose requirements for unfractionated and low-molecular-weight heparin with increased volume of distribution and more rapid plasma elimination. Extremely preterm infants show the lowest dose requirements.

derived protein C have been developed. The hemophilia center staff members are the best resources on the availability and safety of existing replacement proteins. Children with severe genetic deficiencies of protein C or protein S require lifelong anticoagulation with warfarin sodium (Coumadin) at this time, because prophylactic replacement with the appropriate proteins is not currently available.

Infants with acquired deficiencies of protein C or protein S may respond to IVIG or steroids in addition to plasma replacement. Infants with sepsis will require fresh frozen plasma until antibiotics have successfully controlled their infection.

Prevention and Parent Teaching

Parents of infants with severe genetic deficiencies of protein C or protein S will require intensive teaching regarding administration and monitoring of warfarin, observation for early lesions of purpura fulminans, as well as care and rehabilitation of early lesions, which lead to blindness, skin necrosis, and other lesions.

REFERENCES

1. Alter BP: Fanconi's anemia: current concepts, *Am J Pediatr Hematol Oncol* 14:170, 1992.
2. Apt L, Downey WS: "Melena" neonatorum: the swallowed blood syndrome: a simple test for the differentiation of adult and fetal hemoglobin in bloody stools, *J Pediatr* 47:6, 1955.
3. Ascari WQ, Levine P, Pollack W: Incidence of maternal Rh immunization by ABO compatible and incompatible pregnancies, *Br Med J* 1:399, 1969.
4. Bada HS, Korones SB, Pourcyrous M et al: Asymptomatic syndrome of polycythemic hyperviscosity: effect of partial plasma exchange transfusion, *J Pediatr* 120:579, 1992.
5. Barness LA: *Vitamins in pediatric nutrition handbook,* Evanston, IL, 1979, American Academy of Pediatrics.
6. Boussios T, Bertles JF, Goldwasser E: Erythropoietin: receptor characteristics during the ontogeny of hamster yolk sac erythroid cells, *J Biol Chem* 148:443, 1989.
7. Bray GL, Luban NLC: Hemophilia presenting with intracranial hemorrhage, *Am J Dis Child* 141:1215, 1987.
8. Chavez GF, Mulinare J, Edmonds LD: Epidemiology of Rh hemolytic disease of the newborn in the United States, *JAMA* 265:3270, 1991.
9. Clapp DW, Shannon KM: Embryonic and fetal erythropoiesis. In Feig SA, Freedman MH, eds: *Clinical disorders and experimental models of erythropoietin failure,* Boca Raton, Fla, 1993, CRC Press.
10. Cohen A, Manno C: Anemia, Intensive care of the fetus and neonate. In Spitzer AR: *Intensive care of the fetus and neonate,* St. Louis, 1996, Mosby.
11. Dallman PR: Anemia of prematurity, *Ann Rev Med* 32:143, 1981.
12. Finne PH, Halvorsen S: Regulation of erythropoiesis in the fetus and newborn, *Arch Dis Child* 47:683, 1972.
13. Gilmore JR: Normal hematopoiesis in intra-uterine and neonatal life, *J Pathol Bacteriol* 52:25, 1941.
14. Gross GP, Hathaway WE, McGaughey HR: Hyperviscosity in the neonate, *J Pediatr* 82:1004, 1973.
15. Hartman KP, Manco-Johnson M, Rawlings J et al: Homozygous protein C deficiency: early treatment with warfarin, *Am J Pediatr Hematol Oncol* 11:395, 1989.
16. Hathaway WE, Bonnar J: *Hemostatic disorders of the pregnant woman and newborn infant,* New York, 1987, Elsevier Science.
17. Jaffe ER: The reduction of methemoglobin in erythrocytes of a patient with congenital methemoglobinemia, subjects with glucose-6-phosphate dehydrogenase deficiency, and normal individuals, *Blood* 21:561, 1963.
18. Kan YW, Forget BG, Nathan DG: Gamma-beta thalassemia: a cause of hemolytic disease of the newborn, *N Engl J Med* 286:129, 1972.
19. Lane PA, Hathaway WE: Vitamin K deficiency, *J Pediatr* 106:351, 1985.
20. Linderkamp O, Versmold HT, Strohhacker I et al: Capillary-venous hematocrit differences in newborn infants, *Eur J Pediatr* 127:9, 1977.
21. Lipton JM, Alter BP: Blackfan-Diamond anemia. In Feig SA, Freedman MH, eds: *Clinical disorders and experimental models of erythropoietic failure,* Boca Raton, FL, 1993, CRC Press.
22. Luchtman-Jones L, Schwartz A, Wilson D: Hematologic problems in the fetus and neonate. In Fanaroff A, Martin RJ, eds: *Neonatal-perinatal medicine,* ed 6, St. Louis, 1997, Mosby.
23. MackIntosh TF, Walker CHM: Blood viscosity in the newborn, *Arch Dis Child* 48:547, 1973.
24. Mahasandana C, Suvatte V, Chuansumrit A et al: Homozygous protein S deficiency in an infant with purpura fulminans, *J Pediatr* 117:750, 1990.
25. Manco-Johnson MJ: Neonatal antithrombin III deficiency, *Am J Med* 87(suppl):49, 1989.
26. Manco-Johnson MJ: Disseminated intravascular coagulation and other hypercoagulable syndromes, *Int J Pediatr Hematol Oncol* 1:1, 1994.
27. Manco-Johnson MJ, Abshire TC, Jacobson LJ et al: Severe neonatal protein C deficiency: prevalence and thrombotic risk, *J Pediatr* 119:793, 1991.
28. Mentzer WC Jr, Shannon KM, Phibbs RH: Recombinant human erythropoietin (Epoetin Alpha) in patients with the anemia of prematurity. In Ersler AJ et al, eds: *Erythropoietin, molecular cellular, and clinical biology,* Baltimore, 1991, Johns Hopkins University Press.
29. Meyer MP, Meyer JH, Commerford A et al: Recombinant human erythropoietin in the treatment of the anemia of prematurity: results on a double-blind, placebo controlled study, *Pediatrics* 93:918, 1994.
30. Oh W, Lind J: Venous and capillary hematocrit in newborn infants and placental transfusion, *Acta Paediatr* 55:38, 1966.
31. Oski FA: Iron deficiency anemia in infancy and childhood, *N Engl J Med* 329:190, 1993.
32. Paludetto R: Neonatal complications specific to twin (multiple) births (twin transfusion syndrome, intrauterine death of cotwins), *J Perinat Med* 19:246, 1964.

33. Pisciotto PT, ed: Pediatric transfusion practices. In *Blood transfusion therapy: a physician's handbook,* ed 3, Arlington, Va, 1989, American Association of Blood Banks.
34. Ramamurthy RD, Brans YW: Neonatal polycythemia. I. Criteria for diagnosis and treatment, *Pediatrics* 68:168, 1981.
35. Ramamurthy RS, Berlanga M: Postnatal alteration in hematocrit and viscosity in normal and polycythemic infants, *J Pediatr* 110:929, 1987.
36. Roithmaier A, Arlettaz R, Bauer K et al: Randomized controlled trial of Ringer solution versus serum for partial exchange transfusion in neonatal polycythemia, *Eur J Pediatr* 154:53, 1995.
37. Rosen PJ, Johnson C, McGehee WG et al: Failure of methylene blue treatment in toxic methemoglobinemia associated with glucose-6-phosphate dehydrogenase deficiency, *Ann Intern Med* 75:83, 1971.
38. Shannon KM: Anemia of prematurity: progress and prospects, *Am J Pediatr Hematol Oncol* 12:14, 1990.
39. Shannon KM, Naylor GS, Torkildson JC et al: Circulating erythroid progenitors in the anemia of prematurity, *N Engl J Med* 317:728, 1987.
40. Shapiro AD, Jacobson LJ, Armon ME et al: Vitamin K deficiency in the newborn infant: prevalence and perinatal risk factors, *J Pediatr* 109:675, 1986.
41. Shohat M, Reisner SH: Neonatal polycythemia. I. Early diagnosis and incidence relating to time of sampling, *Pediatrics* 73:7, 1984.
42. Tan KL, Tan R, Tan SH et al: The twin transfusion syndrome: clinical observation of 35 affected pairs, *Clin Pediatr* 18:111, 1979.
43. Todd D, Lai MC, Beaven GH et al: The abnormal haemoglobins in homozygous alpha-thalassemia, *Br J Haematol* 20:9, 1970.
44. Villalta IA, Pramanik AK, Diaz-Blanco J et al: Diagnostic errors in neonatal polycythemia based on method of hematocrit determination, *J Pediatr* 115:460, 1989.
45. Woodrow JC, Donohue WTA: Rh-immunization by pregnancy: results of a survey and their relevance to prophylactic therapy, *Br Med J* 4:139, 1968.
46. Yaegashi N, Shiraishi H, Takeshita T et al: Propagation of human parvovirus B19 in primary culture of erythroid lineage cells derived from fetal liver, *J Virol* 63:2422, 1989.
47. Zipursky A et al: Foetal erythrocytes in the maternal circulation, *Lancet* 1:451, 1959.
48. Zivny J, Kobilkova J, Neuwirt J et al: Regulation of erythropoiesis in fetus and mother during normal pregnancy, *Obstet Gynecol* 60:77, 1982.

SUGGESTED READINGS

Bifano EM, Ehrenkranz RA, eds: *Clinics in perinatology: perinatal hematology,* vol 22, Philadelphia, 1995, WB Saunders.
Hathaway WE, Bonnar J: *Hemostatic disorders of the pregnant woman and newborn infant,* New York, 1987, Elsevier Science.
Kulkarni R, Lusher J: Perinatal management of newborns with haemophilia, *Br J Haematol* 112:264, 2001.
Manco-Johnson MJ: Diagnosis and management of thromboses in the perinatal period, *Semin Perinatol* 14:393, 1990.
Manco-Johnson MJ: Disseminated intravascular coagulation and other hypercoagulable syndromes, *Int J Pediatr Hematol Oncol* 1:1, 1994.
Onwuzurike N, Warrier I, Lusher JM: Types of bleeding seen during the first 30 months of life in children with severe haemophilia A and B, *Haemophilia* 2:137, 1996.
Oski FA: The erythrocyte and its disorder. In Nathan DG, Oski FA, eds: *Hematology of infancy and childhood,* ed 4, Philadelphia, 1993, WB Saunders.
Polin RA, Fox WW: *Fetal and neonatal physiology,* vol 2, Philadelphia, 1992, WB Saunders.
Sutor AH, von Kries R, Cornelissen EA et al: Vitamin K deficiency bleeding (VKDB) in infancy. ISTH Pediatric/Perinatal Subcommittee. International Society on Thrombosis and Haemostasis, *Thromb Haemost* 81:456, 1999.
Zipurski A et al: Isoimmune hemolytic disease. In Nathan DG, Osk FA, eds: *Hematology of infancy and childhood,* ed 4, Philadelphia, 1992, WB Saunders.

21 | Jaundice

C. Gilbert Frank, Sharla C. Cooper, Gerald B. Merenstein

Jaundice, or hyperbilirubinemia, is an almost universal occurrence in neonates, although it is not usually of clinical significance. Past experiences have suggested the dangers of excessive levels of unconjugated bilirubin, but precise identification of what constitutes a "safe" level for an individual newborn remains elusive and is the subject of much ongoing investigation.

In this chapter we provide the reader with a basic understanding of the multiple causes and contributing factors in the development of hyperbilirubinemia; the diagnosis, clinical significance, and complications of hyperbilirubinemia; and current treatment modalities and their complications.

PHYSIOLOGY

To understand the pathophysiology and clinical significance of hyperbilirubinemia, we must review normal bilirubin metabolism in the newborn (Figure 21-1). Most of the bilirubin (75% to 85%) produced by a newborn infant comes from the breakdown of the heme portion of erythrocyte hemoglobin. The remaining 15% to 25% of bilirubin is derived from nonerythroid heme proteins found principally in the liver and heme precursors in the marrow and extramedullary hemopoietic areas that do not go on to form red blood cells (early peak or shunt bilirubin).

Bilirubin metabolism is initiated in the reticuloendothelial system, principally in the liver and spleen, as old or abnormal red blood cells are removed from the circulation. The enzymes *microsomal heme oxygenase* and *biliverdin reductase* are responsible for the production of bilirubin and carbon monoxide. This bilirubin, in its unconjugated or indirect-reacting form, is released into the plasma.

At a normal plasma pH, bilirubin is very poorly soluble and binds tightly to circulating albumin that serves as a carrier protein. Albumin contains one high-affinity site for bilirubin and one or more sites of lower affinity. Bilirubin binds to albumin in a molar ratio of between 0.5 and 1 mole of bilirubin per mole of albumin. This ratio may be somewhat lower in a sick VLBW infant. The ability of albumin to bind bilirubin is affected by a number of different factors, including plasma pH, free fatty acid levels, and certain drugs.

Bilirubin bound to albumin is carried to the liver and transported into the hepatocyte by carrier-mediated diffusion. Intracellularly, bilirubin is bound to ligandin (Y protein) and, to a lesser extent, to the Z protein. Conjugation occurs within the smooth endoplasmic reticulum of the cell. This reaction, catalyzed by the enzyme bilirubin UDP glucuronosyl transferase (UDPGT), leads to the formation of bilirubin glucuronides that are water-soluble compounds. In addition to this enzyme, conjugation requires glucuronic acid synthesized from glucose. Conjugated bilirubin is then actively secreted into bile and passes into the small intestine.

Conjugated bilirubin is not reabsorbed from the intestine, but the bowel lumen of the newborn contains the enzyme beta-glucuronidase, which can convert conjugated bilirubin back into glucuronic acid and unconjugated bilirubin, which may be absorbed. This pathway constitutes the enterohepatic circulation of bilirubin and contributes significantly to an infant's bilirubin load.[18]

The catabolism of 1 g of hemoglobin yields 35 mg of bilirubin. Because the red blood cell of a newborn has a shortened lifespan of 70 to 90 days (adult, 120 days), a significant bilirubin load is produced. The breakdown of bilirubin is the only chemical reaction in the body that results in formation of carbon monoxide (CO), a marker sometimes used in studying bilirubin production. Measurement of end-tidal CO (ETCO) could identify infants with unusually high rates of bilirubin production.[3]

Albumin binding of unconjugated bilirubin may be important in the prevention of toxicity (kernicterus). Once the high-affinity site is saturated, there is a rapid increase in potentially toxic-free (nonbound) unconjugated bilirubin. A bilirubin/albumin molar ratio of 1 corresponds to approximately 8.5 mg bilirubin/g of albumin. Kernicterus has been clinically associated with administration

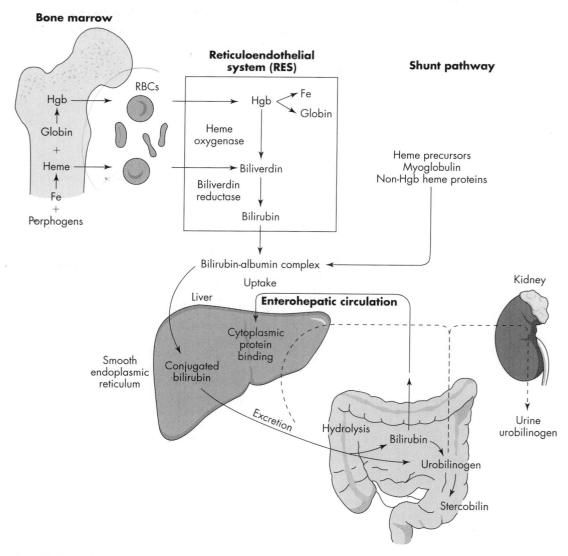

FIGURE 21-1 Pathways of bilirubin synthesis, transport, and metabolism. (From Gartner LM, Hollander M: Disorders of bilirubin metabolism. In Assali NS, ed: *Pathophysiology of gestation,* vol 3, New York, 1972, Academic Press.)

Table 21-1	FACTORS AFFECTING BILIRUBIN-ALBUMIN BINDING
FACTORS	**MECHANISM**
pH (acidosis)	Decreases binding by decreasing affinity at the binding site and increasing tissue affinity
Hematin	Competitively inhibits binding at primary site
Free fatty acid (Intralipid)	Competitively inhibits binding at primary site
Infection	Mechanism not established
Drugs such as sulfa compounds, sodium salicylate, phenylbutazone, and ceftriaxone	Primarily competitive binding; principally at secondary site; best established for sulfisoxazole
Stabilizers for albumin preparations	Competitively inhibit binding at primary site
X-ray contrast media for cholangiography	Competitively inhibit binding at primary site

of sulfisoxazole to newborns as a result of displacement of bilirubin from the primary binding site on albumin. Other drugs such as ceftriaxone also appear to displace bilirubin from this binding site (Table 21-1). The effect on bilirubin-albumin binding of some but not all drugs used in newborn medicine have been studied in vitro.[20]

In a hypoglycemic infant, glucuronide production may be limited, and thus conjugation is impaired. The presence of beta-glucuronidase in the bowel lumen during fetal life enables bilirubin to be reabsorbed and transported across the placenta for excretion by the maternal liver.

ETIOLOGY

Chemical hyperbilirubinemia occurs in virtually all newborns. The National Collaborative Perinatal Project[10] found that only about 6% of newborns weighing greater than 2500 g at birth had serum bilirubin levels greater than 12.9 mg/dl. These infants were predominantly formula fed. **With recent trends to increased breastfeeding it has been suggested that the upper limit of "physiologic" bilirubin levels may approach 17 to 18 mg/dl (95th percentile). Interpretation of bilirubin levels must also take into account the infant's age in hours.** Pathologic (non-"physiologic") hyperbilirubinemia can be the result of increased production or decreased excretion of bilirubin or occasionally a combination of these two processes (Box 21-1).

Overproduction of Bilirubin
Hemolytic Disease of the Newborn
Hemolytic disease of the newborn may occur when blood group incompatibilities such as Rh, ABO, or in rare instances minor blood groups exist between a mother and her fetus. An Rh-negative mother can become sensitized to the Rh antigen in many ways. For example, an improperly matched blood transfusion or the occurrence of fetal-maternal blood transfusion during pregnancy, delivery, abortion, or amniocentesis can cause sensitization. The presence of the Rh antigen induces maternal antibody production, and IgG crosses the placenta into the fetal circulation. There it reacts with the Rh antigen on fetal erythrocytes. These antibody-coated cells are recognized as abnormal and are destroyed by the spleen. This results in increased amounts of hemoglobin, requiring metabolic degradation as discussed previously. As the destruction of erythrocytes and production of bilirubin progress, the ability of the fetus to compensate may be surpassed.

Box 21-1	CAUSES OF HYPERBILIRUBINEMIA

Overproduction
    Hemolytic disease of the newborn
    Hereditary hemolytic anemias
        Membrane defects
        Hemoglobinopathies
        Enzyme defects
    Polycythemia
    Extravascular blood
        Swallowed
        Bruising/enclosed hemorrhage (e.g.,
            cephalohematoma)
    Increased enterohepatic circulation
Undersecretion
    Decreased hepatic uptake
        Decreased sinusoidal perfusion
        Ligandin deficiency
    Decreased conjugation
        Enzyme deficiency
        Enzyme inhibition and the Lucey-Driscoll syndrome[13]
    Inadequate transport out of hepatocyte
    Biliary obstruction
Combined
    Bacterial infection
    Congenital intrauterine infection
Breastfeeding
    Breastfeeding jaundice
    Breast milk jaundice
Miscellaneous
    Hypothyroidism
    Galactosemia
    Infant of diabetic mother
Physiologic

The wide range of clinical features is discussed elsewhere.

The classic example of hemolytic disease of the newborn has been erythroblastosis fetalis as a result of Rh incompatibility. Of the white population 15% is Rh negative. Fortunately the use of anti-D gamma globulin (RhoGAM), including antenatal administration at 26 to 28 weeks' gestation, has markedly decreased the incidence of this serious disease.

The IgG on the surface of the infant's red blood cells is the basis of a positive direct Coombs' test result. Because prior sensitization with the Rh antigen is required for antibody production, the first Rh-positive infant is usually not affected.

With the widespread use of RhoGAM, the most frequent cause of hemolytic disease of the newborn is ABO blood group incompatibility. ABO incompatibility is limited to mothers of blood group O and affects infants of blood group A or B. All group O individuals have naturally occurring anti-A and anti-B (IgG) antibodies, so previous sensitization is not necessary. Clinical disease is generally milder than that seen with Rh incompatibility.

Hereditary Hemolytic Anemias

Erythrocytes with abnormal membranes have abnormal osmotic fragility (generally increased) and an increased rate of splenic destruction. Hemoglobinopathies can be diagnosed by hemoglobin electrophoresis. Individuals with enzyme defects are unable to maintain the integrity of the red blood cells. A precipitating factor for the hemolysis is often not found in infants.

Examples of hemolytic anemias include hereditary spherocytosis and elliptocytosis. The family history may be positive in as many as 80% of cases.

G6PD deficiency is the most common enzyme defect. It is more common in certain racial and ethnic groups, including Chinese, Greeks, and blacks. Deficiency of pyruvate kinase may also occur.

Polycythemia

Polycythemia (with a central venous hematocrit value above 65) is the condition in which an increased red blood cell mass, along with the shortened lifespan of these cells found in all newborns, results in an increased bilirubin load.

Polycythemia may be idiopathic or may occur as a result of a maternal-fetal transfusion, twin-to-twin transfusion, chronic in utero hypoxia, or delayed clamping of the umbilical cord at the time of delivery.

Extravascular Blood

Red blood cells trapped in the enclosed hemorrhages are broken down as resolution occurs.

Clinically, enclosed hemorrhage includes cephalohematoma, subgaleal hemorrhage, cerebral hemorrhage, intraabdominal bleeding, or any occult bleeding. Extensive bruising is associated with higher bilirubin loads as healing occurs. Swallowed maternal blood is another source of increased bilirubin load. Supernatant fluid of stool or gastric juices can be tested by the Apt test. Fetal hemoglobin will resist denaturation by alkali.

Increased Enterohepatic Circulation

The lumen of the newborn's bowel contains the enzyme beta-glucuronidase, which can convert conjugated bilirubin back into its unconjugated (absorbable) form and glucuronic acid.

Meconium contains a substantial amount of bilirubin. It is estimated that there is about 1 mg bilirubin/g of meconium, or a total load of 100 to 200 mg. Any delay in the passage of meconium, such as can occur with Hirschsprung's disease (aganglionosis), intestinal atresia, intestinal stenosis, or the meconium plug and meconium ileus syndromes, will increase the bilirubin load that must be metabolized. Pathologic jaundice from these causes is rarely evident in the first 24 to 48 hours of life.

Undersecretion of Bilirubin

Infants with normal bilirubin production rates may be unable to remove this load for a variety of reasons.

Decreased Hepatic Uptake of Bilirubin

Diminished hepatic uptake of bilirubin may be a result of inadequate perfusion of hepatic sinusoids or deficient carrier proteins (Y and Z). Certain drugs and compounds, such as steroid hormones, free fatty acids, and chloramphenicol, may competitively bind to these proteins, creating a functional deficiency.

Inadequate perfusion of hepatic sinusoids occurs when there is a shunt through a persistent ductus venous or extrahepatic portal vein thrombosis, or with hyperviscosity and hypovolemia. This may occur in infants with severe congestive heart failure.

Although Y and Z protein are decreased in other primates, no actual deficiency has yet been demonstrated in the human newborn.

Decreased Bilirubin Conjugation

Decreased bilirubin conjugation may be a result of glucuronyl transferase deficiency, as in Crigler-Najjar syndromes I and II or Gilbert's syndrome. These disorders are caused by defects in the UDPGT1 gene complex recently identified on chromosome 2. It may also be a result of enzyme inhibition, as in the Lucey-Driscoll syndrome.[14] Serums of some women and their infants contain an increased amount of an as yet unidentified factor that inhibits hepatic conjugation. Icteric infants with pyloric stenosis appear to have inhibition of glucuronyl transferase activity and increased enterohepatic circulation.[5]

Crigler-Najjar syndrome exists in two forms with either complete or partial absence of enzymatic activity. Type I, or complete absence, is an autosomal recessive disorder. Phototherapy becomes ineffective in preventing excessive bilirubin levels and this defect can be corrected by liver transplantation. Type II, or partial enzyme deficiency, is inherited as an autosomal dominant disorder and responds to enzyme induction with phenobarbital. Gilbert's syndrome is another autosomal dominant disorder with partial enzyme activity affecting individuals out of the newborn period with mild bilirubin elevation. Infants with Lucey-Driscoll syndrome may require exchange transfusion. Bilirubin levels rapidly decrease to normal after surgery for pyloric stenosis.

Inadequate Transport Out of the Hepatocyte

Dubin-Johnson and Rotor's syndromes are genetically inherited conditions (autosomal recessive and dominant, respectively) in which individuals are able to conjugate bilirubin normally but are unable to excrete it, resulting in direct hyperbilirubinemia. Dubin-Johnson and Rotor's syndromes and generalized hepatocellular damage require specialized evaluation, including liver biopsy.

Biliary Obstruction

Biliary obstruction is often seen as a diagnostic dilemma between generalized hepatocellular damage and mechanical obstruction.

A variety of disorders can cause cellular damage, including infections such as hepatitis and metabolic disorders such as galactosemia. In the NICU the most common cause of cellular damage is the use of IV alimentation. The mechanism is not well established, but the damage takes at least 2 weeks to develop and is especially prominent in VLBW infants. Biliary atresia or, much less frequently, a choledochal cyst can cause mechanical obstruction to bile flow, resulting in a direct-reacting hyperbilirubinemia.

Combined Overproduction and Undersecretion

Bacterial infections (sepsis neonatorum) or the occurrence of intrauterine viral infections can result in increased bilirubin production and decreased hepatic clearance. Infants with NEC caused by a toxin-producing organism such as certain *Escherichia coli* may develop this form of hepatocellular damage.

Intrauterine infections, including congenital syphilis, toxoplasmosis, rubella, infection caused by CMV, herpes simplex, Coxsackie B virus, and hepatitis virus, cause clinical jaundice. Infants with these infections will often have additional clinical stigmata of their infection.

Jaundice Associated With Breastfeeding

Breastfeeding Jaundice

In general, breastfed infants have higher bilirubin levels than bottlefed infants, especially on the fifth day of life. It has been postulated that this early jaundice is related to decreased caloric and fluid intake from colostrum[7] and increased enterohepatic circulation resulting from low stool output and breast milk beta-glucuronidase.[9] In many studies there has been a relationship between the degree of hyperbilirubinemia and the amount of weight lost by the infant.

Breast Milk Jaundice

A small percentage (1% to 2%) of breastfed infants exhibit prolonged and exaggerated jaundice because of an inhibitor or inhibitory substance found in their mother's breast milk prolonging increased enterohepatic circulation.[1] The rate of recurrence in families approaches 70%.

Despite lack of supporting data that breastfed infants are underfed, it once was common practice in some institutions to supplement with glucose water or electrolyte solutions after nursing. Such supplementation should be avoided because it reduces breastfeeding frequency and maternal milk production. Supplemented infants have higher peak bilirubin levels. Optimal management of a breastfeeding mother and infant includes early and frequent nursing: eight to 12 times each day.

Clinically, infants with breast milk jaundice have an unconjugated hyperbilirubinemia (greater than 12 mg/dl) that becomes exaggerated and persistent by about the fifth day of life. Elevated bilirubin levels may persist for 4 to 14 days, followed by a very gradual decline. **For most infants it is not necessary to interrupt breastfeeding, even as the bilirubin increases to a level that may require phototherapy. Other causes of excessive jaundice must be ruled out. If it becomes necessary to temporarily interrupt breastfeeding, it is important to support the mother during this period so as not to foster feelings of guilt or inadequacy. It is strongly recommended that a trained observer evaluate all breastfed infants within 48 to 72 hours of discharge in either a home or office setting. Early discharge of breastfed infants with inadequate follow-up may result in excessive levels of bilirubin and the possibility of kernicterus.**

Physiologic or Developmental Jaundice

Physiologic or developmental jaundice is a diagnosis of exclusion. A newborn has a rate of bilirubin production of 8 to 10 mg/kg/24 hr, which is two to two and a half times the production rate in adults. Perfusion of the hepatic sinusoids may be somewhat compromised by incomplete closure of the ductus venosus or the presence of extramedullary hemopoietic tissue in the liver. Newborn monkeys have been shown to be deficient in the Y and Z proteins for the first few days of life, and this may also occur in the human newborn. Enterohepatic circulation contributes significantly to the bilirubin load.

The hormonal (estrogen) environment of the infant may inhibit liver function and bilirubin secretion. **Although a level of 12.9 may define "pathologic" jaundice in a bottlefed infant, levels of up to 17 to 18 mg/dl[4] may be physiologic in a breastfed infant (Figure 21-2).**

Physiologic jaundice is partially attributable to a relative deficiency of UDP glucuronosyltransferase activity (0.1% of adult levels at 30 weeks' gestation). Enzyme activity increases rapidly after birth independent of the infant's gestational age. A major factor in physiologic jaundice remains the increased rate of bilirubin production (Box 21-2). Certain eth-

nic groups, including Eskimo, Oriental, and American Indian, have an increased incidence and severity of physiologic jaundice for reasons that are not clearly understood.

It has been suggested that bilirubin at physiologic levels may serve as an important antioxidant and prevent oxidative membrane damage. In vitro studies have shown bilirubin to be a powerful antioxidant.

Miscellaneous Causes
Hypothyroidism
The mechanism of hyperbilirubinemia in hypothyroidism is not well understood, but in some animal studies thyroxin was needed for the hepatic clearance of bilirubin. Hypothyroid infants have unconjugated hyperbilirubinemia that may be prolonged. They may fail to show any other signs or symptoms of hypothyroidism until later in their course. There-

Box 21-2	**CRITERIA THAT RULE OUT THE DIAGNOSIS OF PHYSIOLOGIC JAUNDICE***

1. Clinical jaundice in the first 24 hours of life
2. Total serum bilirubin concentrations increasing by more than 5 mg/dl (85 μmol/L/day)
3. Total serum bilirubin concentration exceeding 12.9 mg/dl (221 μmol/L) in a full-term infant or 15 mg/dl (257 μmol/L) in a premature infant

4. Direct serum bilirubin concentration exceeding 1.5 to 2 mg/dl (26 to 34 μmol/L)
5. Clinical jaundice persisting for more than 1 week in a full-term infant or 2 weeks in a premature infant

From Maisels MJ: Neonatal jaundice. In Avery GB, ed: *Neonatology: pathophysiology and management of the newborn,* ed 2, Philadelphia, 1981, JB Lippincott.

*The absence of these criteria does not imply that the jaundice is physiologic. In the presence of any of these criteria, the jaundice must be investigated further.

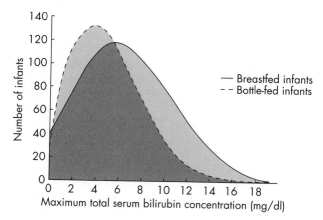

FIGURE 21-2 Distribution of maximum serum bilirubin concentration in white infants weighing more than 2500 g. Curves were computer-generated using exponential 1 knot spline regression. (From Maisels MJ, Gifford K: Normal serum bilirubin levels in the newborn and the effect of breastfeeding, *Pediatrics* 78:837, 1986.)

fore most states now require routine screening for hypothyroidism, galactosemia, and phenylketonuria.

Galactosemia

The mechanism in galactosemia may be related to a lack of substrate for glucuronidation and the accumulation of abnormal metabolic byproducts that are hepatotoxic.

Galactosemia is an autosomal recessive disorder characterized by increased jaundice in infants fed breast milk or lactose-containing formulas. The presence of non–glucose-reducing substances in the urine suggests galactosemia.

Infant of a Diabetic Mother

The cause of hyperbilirubinemia in an infant of a diabetic mother (IDM) appears to be multifactorial. In addition to prematurity and a tendency to feed poorly, an IDM may have an increased bilirubin load as a result of an expanded red blood cell mass and hypovolemia. Erythrocyte membrane composition may be altered, and macrosomic infants are often bruised during labor and delivery.

PREVENTION

Anti-D gamma globulin (RhoGAM) antibody provides passive protection, allowing destruction of fetal red blood cells and preventing maternal production of anti-Rh antibodies that might affect subsequent Rh-positive pregnancies.

Widespread use of RhoGAM has proved effective in preventing the sensitization of Rh-negative mothers after delivery or abortion of Rh-positive infants. Failures may occur if the amount of RhoGAM administered is insufficient compared with the load of fetal red blood cells received or if a significant fetal-maternal hemorrhage occurred before delivery. RhoGAM should be administered to Rh-negative women undergoing amniocentesis. Routine management of the Rh-negative mother now includes the administration of antenatal RhoGAM in the second trimester (26 to 28 weeks).

Early Feeding

The physiologic mechanism is not entirely known but may be caused by a decrease in intestinal transit time and decreased enterohepatic circulation.

When compared with infants not fed during the first 24 to 48 hours of life, infants fed earlier have lower peak bilirubin levels.

Phenobarbital

Phenobarbital acts as an inducer of microsomal enzymes, increasing the conjugation of bilirubin. It also has a direct effect to stimulate bile secretion in infants with nonobstructive cholestasis. Phenobarbital also increases the concentration of ligandin. When used in conjunction with phototherapy, it does not increase the rate of decline.

Phenobarbital is effective when given to the mother before delivery. In infants with significant hemolytic disease of the newborn, it appears to slow the rate of rise of bilirubin and decrease the incidence of exchange transfusion. It is also indicated in infants with Crigler-Najjar syndrome type II. Its use is not indicated on a routine prophylactic basis, because such use would overtreat many infants, and other effects may be detrimental.

Tin Protoporphyrin and Tin Mesoporphyrin

Clinical trials have shown that administration of tin protoporphyrin (SnPP) or tin mesoporphyrin (SnMP) to preterm infants, term and near-term infants, or infants with ABO hemolytic disease of the newborn or G6PD deficiency decreases bilirubin production. These compounds are potent competitive inhibitors of the enzyme heme oxygenase.[12,13,25] Heme is excreted directly into bile when bilirubin production is suppressed. Infants receiving a single dose of SnMP (6 µmol/kg body weight IM) have lower peak serum bilirubin levels and a decreased need for phototherapy. Side effects have been minimal and include a transient erythema in those infants requiring phototherapy after receiving SnMP. Additional studies to determine the role of these compounds in the management and prevention of neonatal jaundice are ongoing.

DATA COLLECTION

The history, physical examination, and laboratory data play an important role in the evaluation of the jaundiced newborn (Box 21-3).

History

The evaluation of a jaundiced infant begins with a good familial, perinatal, and neonatal history. The family history should include the occurrence of disorders associated with jaundice in other family members, especially siblings. The perinatal and obstetric history may provide clues or enable the

---

Box 21-3 **EVALUATION OF UNCONJUGATED HYPERBILIRUBINEMIA IN THE NEONATE**

History
    Family
    Perinatal and obstetric
    Neonatal
Physical examination
    Pallor
    Hepatosplenomegaly
    Enclosed hemorrhage
    Petechiae
    Congenital anomalies
Laboratory data
    All jaundiced infants
        Maternal and infant blood type
        Coombs' test on cord blood
        Total/direct bilirubin (serial measurements)
        Complete blood count, including hematocrit, reticulocyte and platelet counts, white blood cell differential, and peripheral smear for red blood cell morphology
        Urinalysis, test for reducing substances
    Selected cases
        Protein, total and/or albumin
        Sepsis evaluation
        IgM
        Urine cytology for cytomegalovirus
        Viral cultures
    New techniques
        Transcutaneous bilirubinometry
        Bilirubin-binding tests

---

clinician to anticipate possible hyperbilirubinemia. The infant's course since birth may be important.

Signs and Symptoms and Clinical Approach

A wide spectrum of signs and symptoms may occur in a jaundiced infant, often depending on the causes of the jaundice. In the absence of hemolysis, an infant may be asymptomatic, with dermal icterus as the only clinical sign. An infant with hemolytic disease of the newborn may show signs of jaundice and pallor in association with severe anemia and hydrops fetalis or may appear entirely normal at birth. Hepatosplenomegaly resulting from congestion and extramedullary hemopoiesis may be present. Infants affected by hemolytic disease of the newborn also have pancreatic islet cell hyperplasia and are at increased risk for hypoglycemia. Careful physical examination may reveal the presence of a cephalohematoma or other enclosed hemorrhage. The oc-

currence of petechiae or purpura raises the possibility of intrauterine infection or sepsis. Congenital anomalies should be noted.

Laboratory Data

Knowledge of the mother's and infant's blood types and Rh will establish the potential for hemolytic disease. The result of a direct Coombs' test on cord blood is positive in ABO disease. Later testing of the infant's blood in an ABO incompatibility situation may yield negative Coombs' results. In addition to hematocrit and reticulocyte determinations, a careful examination of the peripheral blood smear should be performed, looking for evidence of hemolysis such as increased numbers of nucleated red blood cells or the presence of fragmented cells, poikilocytosis, and anisocytosis.

Microspherocytosis is characteristic of ABO incompatibility and may at times be confused with hereditary spherocytosis. Knowledge of blood types and clinical course will help in differentiating these two. An abnormal white blood cell count or differential, or thrombocytopenia may suggest infection. In addition to jaundice and anemia in the first few days of life, infants with a hemolytic disease are at risk for a "late" anemia after discharge from the nursery. Obtaining fractionated (total/direct) bilirubin levels and serial levels helps to establish causes and enables the clinician to follow the rate of bilirubin rise. Protein and albumin determinations allow a gross assessment of adequacy of bilirubin binding. A great deal of clinical and laboratory research has been performed to determine the degree of and sites available for bilirubin albumin binding. This information may someday enable clinicians to assess the risk for kernicterus and perform an exchange transfusion at the appropriate time, but these determinations are not presently recommended or available for routine use.

Items of interest include possible infection during the pregnancy or the use of oxytocin induction for delivery. Also of concern is the occurrence of an asphyxial episode during labor or delivery. Premature infants have higher mean bilirubin levels and a slightly later peak. A history of asphyxia and medication should be obtained. Also of interest are the infant's feeding and stooling patterns. The time of onset or detection of jaundice may be important. Jaundice in the first 24 hours of life must always be considered abnormal.

Jaundice in a newborn can usually be detected clinically at a level of 6 to 7 mg/dl. Visible icterus

Table 21-2	MANAGEMENT OF HYPERBILIRUBINEMIA IN THE HEALTHY TERM NEWBORN*			
	TSB* LEVEL, MG/DL (µMOL/L)			
AGE (HR)	**CONSIDER PHOTOTHERAPY†**	**PHOTOTHERAPY**	**EXCHANGE TRANSFUSION IF INTENSIVE PHOTOTHERAPY FAILS‡**	**EXCHANGE TRANSFUSION AND INTENSIVE PHOTOTHERAPY**
≤24§	—	—		≥25 (430)
25-48	≥12 (170)	≥15 (260)	≥20 (340)	≥30 (510)
49-72	≥15 (260)	≥18 (310)	≥25 (430)	≥30 (510)
>72	≥17 (290)	≥20 (340)	≥25 (430)	

From American Academy of Pediatrics: Practice parameter: management of hyperbilirubinemia in the healthy term infant, *Pediatrics* 94:558, 1994.

*TSB indicates total serum bilirubin.

†Phototherapy at these TSB levels is a clinical option, meaning that the intervention is available and may be used *on the basis of individual clinical judgment.*

‡Intensive phototherapy should produce a decline of TSB of 1 to 2 mg/dl within 4 to 6 hr and the TSB level should continue to fall and remain below the threshold level for exchange transfusion. If this does not occur, it is considered a failure of phototherapy.

§Term infants who are clinically jaundiced at ≤24 hr old are not considered healthy and require further evaluation.

appears first on the head and face and progresses in a cephalocaudal manner. The extremities are the last skin surface to be affected.

Immediate exchange transfusion with type O Rh-negative red blood cells may be necessary in Rh incompatibility with a severely affected infant. Hydrops fetalis is rare in hemolytic disease as a result of ABO incompatibility.

There is an increased incidence of jaundice in trisomic syndromes. Jaundice and umbilical hernia are associated with congenital hypothyroidism.

Minimal laboratory evaluation of the jaundiced newborn should include the mother's and infant's blood types, Rh status, and Coombs' test on cord blood. A CBC to include reticulocyte and platelet counts, white blood cell count and differential, peripheral smear for red blood cell morphology, and hematocrit should be performed. Infants suspected of having bacterial sepsis should receive antibiotic treatment and a complete sepsis evaluation, including cultures of blood, urine, and cerebrospinal fluid. Bilirubin levels (total and direct) should be measured serially. Total protein and/or albumin levels may be helpful as the infant approaches exchange transfusion.

Urinalysis, including evaluation for reducing substances, may be helpful. Infants suspected of having congenital infection should have additional tests, including IgM levels. Viral cultures and urine cytology for CMV may be performed. Newborn screening should be performed for hypothyroidism, galactosemia, and PKU.

TREATMENT

Treatment is aimed at preventing the complications of kernicterus and bilirubin encephalopathy. Phototherapy and exchange transfusions are widely used; however, decisions to use these therapies are complicated by an incomplete understanding of bilirubin toxicity, especially as applied to an individual infant. **The American Academy of Pediatrics published "Practice Parameter: Management of Hyperbilirubinemia in the Healthy Term Newborn." These management guidelines are outlined in Table 21-2 and in the algorithm detailed in Figure 21-3.** Extensive review of the literature dealing with full-term infants without hemolytic disease has found little evidence of adverse effects of bilirubin on IQ, neurologic examination, or hearing.[16] Infants with hemolytic disease and premature (especially VLBW) infants should receive phototherapy and exchange transfusion at lower levels. A suggested guideline is to initiate phototherapy when the serum bilirubin is 5 mg/dl below the serum bilirubin concentration at which an exchange transfusion will be performed for that individual infant.[2] As more data become available, perhaps clearer guidelines can be established and more specific recommendations made for these infants.

Phototherapy

Phototherapy is the most commonly employed means of treatment. The indication for phototherapy is to prevent the infant from requiring an exchange

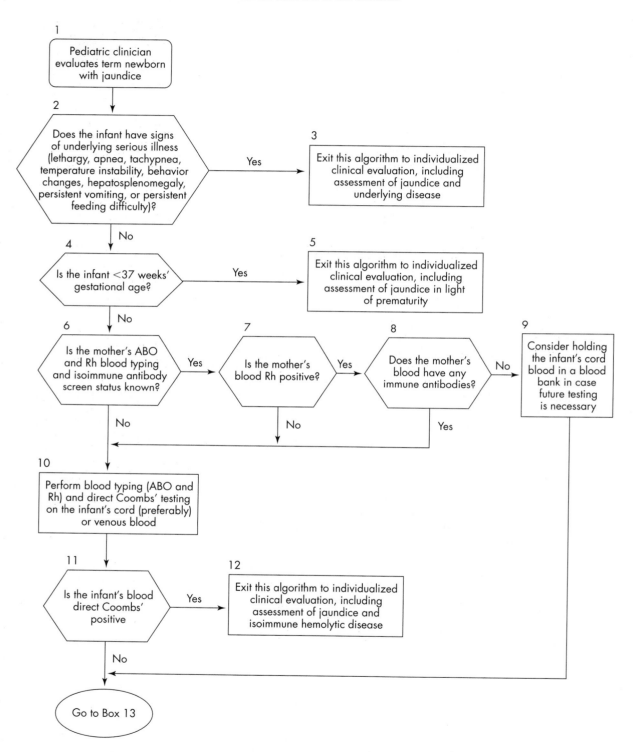

FIGURE 21-3   Algorithm for the management of hyperbilirubinemia in a healthy term infant.

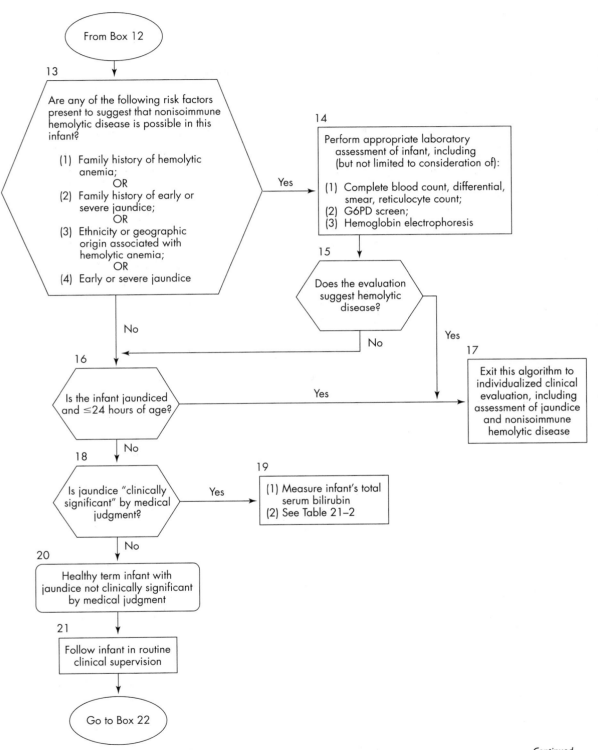

FIGURE 21-3, cont'd   Algorithm for the management of hyperbilirubinemia in a healthy term infant.

Continued

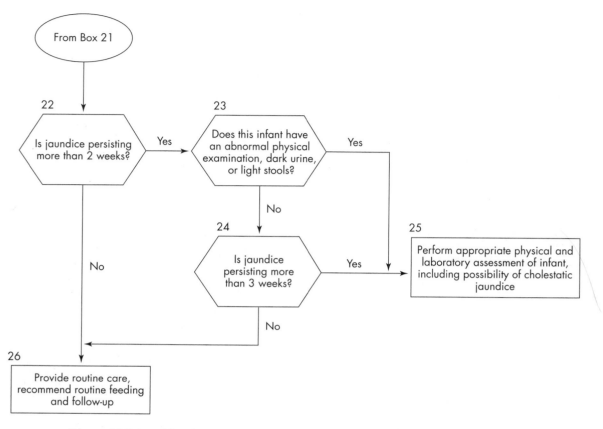

FIGURE 21-3, cont'd   Algorithm for the management of hyperbilirubinemia in a healthy term infant.

transfusion. It is estimated that 10% of newborns in the United States are treated with phototherapy.

Before the initiation of phototherapy in any infant, appropriate evaluation as to the cause of the jaundice must be performed. Indications for the initiation of phototherapy vary widely from nursery to nursery and depend on the individual infant's clinical status.

Phototherapy generally consists of a single tungsten halogen lamp or a bank of four to eight cool white, daybright, or special blue fluorescent bulbs covered by a Plexiglas shield and placed 15 to 20 cm from the patient. Manufacturers' recommendations should be followed. Fiberoptic blankets delivering phototherapy from a high-intensity light source are also available either for use by themselves or in conjunction with other sources of phototherapy. The spectrum of light at 420 to 460 nm is the most effective. The energy output (irradiance) in this spec-

trum should be checked periodically to ensure maximum efficiency.

Phototherapy by photoisomerization and photooxidation results in the formation of more polar, water-soluble bilirubin products. The most important of these reactions appears to be the formation of lumirubin,[15] a stable structural photoisomer. Lumirubin does not require conjugation and is rapidly excreted in bile and urine. The production of lumirubin is an irreversible reaction that appears to be dose related (Figure 21-4).

The efficacy of phototherapy depends on energy output (irradiance) in the blue spectrum of the lights, the distance of the light source from the infant, and the surface area of the infant exposed to those lights.

Animal studies have demonstrated a potential retinal toxicity of light. It is not established that this occurs in the human newborn, but it remains a major concern.

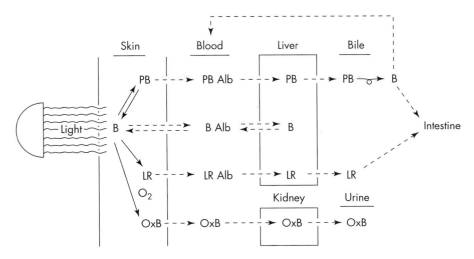

FIGURE 21-4   *General mechanisms of phototherapy for neonatal jaundice. Solid arrows represent chemical reactions; broken arrows represent transport processes. Pigments may be bound to proteins in compartments other than blood. Some excretion of photoisomers, particularly lumirubin, in urine also occurs. B, Bilirubin (Z,Z isomer); PB, photobilirubin (E,E and E,Z isomers); LR, lumirubin (E and Z isomers); OxB, bilirubin oxidation products; Alb, albumin. (From McDonagh A, Lightner D:"Like a shrivelled blood orange"—bilirubin, jaundice, and phototherapy, Pediatrics 75:443, 1985.)*

Infants exposed to phototherapy, particularly LBW infants and infants under a radiant warmer, have significant increases in their insensible water losses (IWL). These infants also have increased stool water losses and may develop temporary lactose intolerance. There are conflicting data in the literature on whether continuous or intermittent administration of phototherapy is most effective.

The concept behind phototherapy arose from the serendipitous observation that infants exposed to sunlight had less jaundice than infants positioned away from the windows. Phototherapy is not a substitute for exchange transfusion when an exchange is indicated. The decision to treat with phototherapy must be made on an individual basis.

Special blue lights are the most effective but are not widely used, because they mask the clinical signs of cyanosis and color change in the infant. Green light appears slightly less effective.[22] Many nurseries employ white fluorescent phototherapy bulbs. These are effective and permit better visual monitoring of the patient. The Plexiglas shield absorbs ultraviolet irradiation. Tungsten halogen lights are replacing fluorescent lights in many nurseries. Halogen lights cannot be as close to the infant as fluorescent tubes because of the risk of burning the infant. Fiberoptic phototherapy blankets are available. These systems (Wallaby Phototherapy System,

Fiberoptic Medical Products, Inc., Allentown, Pa.; and Biliblanket, Ohmeda, Columbia, Md.) use a high-intensity halogen light source for transmission of light by fiberoptic bundles. Irradiance and efficacy appear comparable with standard phototherapy.[21] Purported advantages of these systems are elimination of the need for eye patches, exposure of greater surface area, and provision of phototherapy outside of the nursery with less interference in mother-infant bonding. These blankets are more convenient to use when phototherapy is required in an outpatient setting. Manufacturer's recommendations should be followed when using this method of phototherapy.

A photoreaction occurs in the very outer layers (top 2 mm) of the skin, probably within superficial blood vessels or in interstitial spaces. Once phototherapy has been initiated, serum levels of bilirubin must be monitored frequently (every 4 to 12 hours), because visual assessment of icterus is no longer valid. Hematocrit must also be monitored, especially in infants with hemolytic disease.

To increase exposure, most infants are placed naked under the lights with shielding over the eyes. In a small infant, diapers may cover a significant amount of surface area, and some clinicians have found that using a tie-on surgeon's mask as a "bikini bottom" is effective in containing stool and urine.

The infant's position should be changed frequently. This permits maximum skin exposure to the lights.

Because of the potential for eye damage, the infant's eyes should be covered while phototherapy is in use. Patches should completely cover the eyes without placing excessive pressure on the eyes and be carefully positioned to avoid occluding the nares. To permit evaluation of the infant's eyes, eye patches should be removed every 4 hours. The patches should be left off during feedings and parental visits.

The infant's temperature should be monitored frequently. Infants in incubators or servocontrolled care centers may become overheated. The servocontrol probe should be shielded by an opaque covering. Infants treated in open cribs may become cold stressed. Fluid balance must be carefully monitored in an infant receiving phototherapy. Weights taken twice a day and close monitoring of intake and output such as urine volume and specific gravity may indicate a need for increased fluids, given either orally or intravenously. The presence of reducing substances in the stool can be treated with a non–lactose-containing formula. With continuous phototherapy the infant will receive 18 to 20 hours of light per day with interruptions for feeding, blood drawing, and parental visits. In some studies, intermittent schedules such as 15 minutes on and 60 minutes off appear to be as effective as continuous schedules with much less irradiation, but the occurrence of in vitro complications may be greater. After phototherapy ceases, bilirubin levels should be followed for at least 24 hours to rule out the occurrence of significant rebound. Table 21-3 outlines some of the nursing assessments and management to be performed in infants undergoing phototherapy.

Exchange Transfusion

An exchange transfusion is indicated for correction of severe anemia, removal of antibody-coated red blood cells in hemolytic disease, or removal of excessive unconjugated bilirubin regardless of its cause. Phototherapy has significantly decreased the need for exchange transfusion. Again, the indications, especially in a VLBW infant, vary from nursery to nursery.

In an infant with severe hemolytic disease, a packed red blood cell exchange transfusion using type O Rh-negative blood may save the infant's life, correct anemia and hypoxemia, and permit successful transition.

Administration of 1 g/kg of salt-poor albumin 1 hour before the exchange transfusion has been shown in some studies to increase the efficiency of exchange by about 40%.[17] Aliquot size appears to have no significant effect on the efficiency of the exchange. Smaller aliquots are less stressful to the infant.

Citrate used as part of the anticoagulant solution binds divalent ions such as calcium and magnesium.

Immediately after the exchange, the bilirubin level will be about 45% of the preexchange level. As plasma and tissue levels equilibrate, the bilirubin rises to about 60% of the preexchange level.

It must be stressed that the decision to perform an exchange transfusion must be individualized for each patient.

Central venous pressure must be carefully followed when performing an exchange transfusion with packed red blood cells. If necessary in the delivery room, a slow exchange is performed to reach a hematocrit of 45. Then the infant is transported to the NICU.

Exchange transfusion trays are commercially available and include a four-way stopcock, necessary tubing and syringes, 10% calcium gluconate, and a plastic bag for discarded blood.

Whole blood with a hematocrit of 50% to 55% is used for exchange transfusion. ABO type-specific Rh-negative blood should be used in cases with Rh incompatibility. Type O Rh-specific cells are indicated when ABO incompatibility exists. Citrate-phosphate-dextrose is the anticoagulant most widely used. Insist on fresh blood (less than 24 hours old). Albumin priming results in an expansion of plasma volume and should not be used in anemic or edematous infants.

For exchange transfusion the infant should be on a cardiac monitor and restrained in an incubator or on an infant care center with a radiant heater. Generally, 5- to 20-ml aliquots of blood are used, depending on the size and condition of the infant. The initial aliquot should be withdrawn and sent to the laboratory for bilirubin, hematocrit, calcium, and cultures. The rate of exchange is usually 2 to 4 ml/min. Blood used in the exchange should be warmed and mixed in the bag after every 50 to 100 ml. Central venous pressure measurements should be made about every 100 ml or every 50 ml in the hydropic infant.

The infant should be evaluated for hypocalcemia after each 100 ml of the exchange has been completed. Clinical signs and symptoms of hypocalcemia include irritability, tachycardia, or prolongation of the Q-oTc interval. If hypocalcemia is detected, 1 ml of a 10% calcium gluconate solution is slowly infused.

Table 21-3	NURSING MANAGEMENT OF INFANTS UNDERGOING PHOTOTHERAPY

NURSING ASSESSMENT

AREA	PARAMETER
Physical status	Intake and output
	Color
	Location of jaundice
	Skin integrity
	Stools (character, consistency)
	Vital signs
	Infant/environmental temperature
	Hydration status
	Signs of phototherapy side effects
	Eye discharge and tearing
	Position
	Activity
Neurobehavioral status	Sleep-wake states
	Sensory threshold
	Behavioral responsiveness
	Feeding behaviors
	Consoling abilities
	Stress responses
	Interactive capabilities

NURSING MANAGEMENT

NURSING DIAGNOSIS	INTERVENTION
Fluid volume deficit (actual or potential)	Monitor intake and output.
	Monitor hydration status (weight, specific gravity, urine output).
	Monitor stooling pattern, character.
	Maintain adequate fluid intake (oral or parenteral).
Alteration in nutrition	Assess feeding behavior and activity.
	Monitor fluid and caloric intake, weight, abdominal girth.
	Remove eye shields during feeding.
	Hold during oral feedings as health and thermal status permit.
	Bring to alert state before feeding.
	Feed on demand if possible.
Impaired skin integrity	Observe color, rashes, excoriation.
	Clean skin with warm water.
	Clean perineal area after stooling.
	Turn frequently (also increases skin exposure to phototherapy).
	Ensure Plexiglas shield is in place between light source and infant to reduce exposure to UV light.
Potential for injury	Observe for side effects associated with phototherapy.
	Observe for signs of sepsis.
	Provide care to minimize side effects of phototherapy.
	Shield eyes from lights with opaque patches.
	Ensure eyelids are closed when shield is applied to prevent corneal injury.
	Remove eye shield and observe eyes regularly.
	Monitor position of eye shield to prevent occlusion of nose.
	Avoid tight head band on eye shield to reduce risk of increased intracranial pressure, especially in preterm infants.
	Observe for eye discharge, tearing.
	Shield testes and possibly ovaries (data unclear about need to do this) with diaper.[23]
Alteration in thermal status	Place in warm, thermoneutral environment.
	Monitor environmental and infant temperature.
	Observe for hypothermia and hyperthermia.
	Reduce heat losses from environmental sources.
	Use servocontrol for infants in incubator or under radiant warmer.
	Shield servocontrol thermistor from direct exposure to phototherapy lights.

From Blackburn S: Hyperbilirubinemia and neonatal jaundice, *Neonatal Netw* 14:15, 1995.

The final aliquot from an exchange should be sent for CBC, fractionated bilirubin, calcium ion, electrolytes, culture, and repeat type and cross-match for potential additional exchange transfusion. In addition to the individuals performing the exchange, one person must keep an accurate record of time, volumes withdrawn and infused, vital signs, and medications administered.

COMPLICATIONS

Hyperbilirubinemia

Hyperbilirubinemia is of clinical concern because of the complication of bilirubin encephalopathy (kernicterus). Kernicterus refers to yellowish staining in nuclear centers of the CNS, particularly in the basal ganglia, cerebellum, and hippocampus.

Development of toxicity may depend on albumin-bilirubin binding, although interruption of the blood-brain barrier may also play a role. Factors that interfere with albumin-bilirubin binding appear to predispose to the development of kernicterus and have been outlined earlier in this chapter (see Table 21-1). Free unconjugated bilirubin appears to be cytotoxic for CNS cells and uncouples oxidative phosphorylation and reduces protein synthesis in vitro at the mitochondrial level. Once toxicity has occurred, it appears to be irreversible.

Phototherapy

Despite its widespread use since 1958, questions about the safety and side effects of phototherapy remain. The potential for retinal damage, increase in IWLs, loose stools, lactose intolerance, temperature elevations, or cold stress have already been discussed. Infants who have an associated cholestatic jaundice and are exposed to phototherapy may develop the *bronze baby syndrome*. This presumably is caused by retention of a bilirubin breakdown product produced by phototherapy. Increased platelet turnover and lower mean platelet counts may occur, although the mechanism is unknown. Transient skin rashes and tanning, particularly in black infants, have been reported. Tanning is a result of increased melanin production.

Cell culture studies have demonstrated DNA damage when exposed to phototherapy, especially with intermittent administration. Other potential problems include interference with biologic (circadian) rhythms and with maternal-infant bonding. Although there may be some transient, short-term growth effects, long-term growth effects and development appear unaffected by phototherapy.

Complications of phototherapy may include the following:

- Potential retinal damage if eyes are exposed
- Increased IWL
- Loose bowel movements
- Temporary lactose intolerance
- Temperature maintenance (hyperthermia or hypothermia)
- Bronze baby syndrome
- Decreased platelet count
- Transient skin rashes and tanning
- Potential cellular damage
- Potential interference with biologic rhythm
- Potential interference with maternal-infant bonding

Exchange Transfusion

Exchange transfusion is a procedure with many potential complications and carries a mortality risk of about 0.5%. Some complications are listed in Table 21-4.

Table 21-4	COMPLICATIONS OF EXCHANGE TRANSFUSION
SYSTEM	**COMPLICATIONS**
Vascular	Embolization, thrombosis, and necrotizing enterocolitis
Cardiac	Dysrhythmias, volume overload, and arrest
Electrolyte	Hypernatremia, hyperkalemia, hypocalcemia, acidosis, and alkalosis after exchange
Clotting	Thrombocytopenia, overheparinization, and bleeding
Infection	Bacteremia and bloodborne viral hepatitis
Others	Hemolysis from old donor blood or from mechanical or thermal injury, perforations of vessels and viscera, hypoglycemia from induced insulin release, and hypothermia from overexposure

Modified from Odell GB: *Neonatal hyperbilirubinemia,* New York, 1980, Grune & Stratton.

Vascular complications are related to the use of umbilical catheters (discussed in Chapter 7). NEC has been reported as a postexchange complication, probably as a result of bowel ischemia during the procedure.

Electrolyte and glucose disturbances are related to the blood preparation used during the exchange. Acid-citrate-dextrose and citrate-phosphate-dextrose blood have high levels of sodium and glucose and perhaps potassium. Initial hyperglycemia may be followed by reactive hypoglycemia as a result of an insulin response. Although acidic at the time of infusion, a postexchange alkalosis may occur as citrate is metabolized to bicarbonate in the liver.

Many of the electrolyte and acid-base disturbances may be avoided by the use of fresh, heparinized blood. Bleeding may occur in an overheparinized infant but is reversible with protamine sulfate. Thrombocytopenia may occur, especially in the infant requiring repeated exchange transfusions. Bacterial infection is rare, and routine antibiotic prophylaxis is not indicated. Most complications are avoidable if careful attention to technique is observed.

CLINICAL COMPLICATIONS

Hyperbilirubinemia

Early clinical signs of kernicterus include a poor Moro reflex with incomplete flexion of the extremities. Because of the infant's poor sucking ability, feeding may be difficult. In progressive cases the infant develops a high-pitched cry, is hypotonic, and may vomit. Opisthotonic posturing also may occur. In later life, severely affected survivors may manifest choreoathetosis, spastic cerebral palsy, mental retardation, sensory and perceptual deafness, and visual-motor incoordination. More subtle findings may occur in less severely affected infants and may not be apparent during the newborn period. There is speculation that some learning disabilities may be related to hyperbilirubinemia even at what had been previously considered "safe" levels. Unfortunately, the critical level at which bilirubin toxicity occurs in either preterm or term infants has not been established.

Phototherapy

An infant with bronze baby syndrome develops a dark gray-brown discoloration of the skin, urine, and serum. There are generally no clinical symptoms with this syndrome, but there has been at least one reported death. After phototherapy ceases, the bronzing gradu-

ally resolves. In addition to shielding the eyes, it has been recommended that the gonads be shielded.

Exchange Transfusion

The use of freshly collected blood (less than 72 hours old) will help maintain acceptable potassium levels. Infants with hemolytic disease of the newborn are already at risk for hypoglycemia because of islet cell hyperplasia. Blood glucose levels must be followed closely in the first few hours after an exchange. Heparinized blood must be used within 24 hours of preparation of the unit. In addition to other forms of viral hepatitis, CMV and HIV may be transmitted to the infant, and one must screen for these.

PARENT TEACHING

Jaundice and its treatment can be very disturbing to parents. Parents often feel guilty that perhaps something they did or failed to do resulted in their infant's jaundice. Reassurance and support are vital, especially for the nursing mother, who may question her ability to adequately nourish her infant.

Phototherapy is especially distressing and should be explained to the parents before they see the infant under the lights. Parents may tend to believe that there may be problems with the infant's eyes despite reassurances to the contrary. The lights should be turned off and eye patches removed during visits so normal parent-infant interaction can occur. Side effects of phototherapy such as loose or dark-green stools should be explained to parents.

Early discharge policies (less than 48 hours) have increased the need for outpatient evaluation and/or management of neonatal hyperbilirubinemia. Hyperbilirubinemia is the leading indication for hospital readmission in these infants.

As with many disorders in newborn infants, a little time spent in careful explanation with the parents can alleviate much fear, guilt, and occasionally anger and help to establish a normal family relationship. Causes of jaundice should be explained to the parents, emphasizing that it is usually a transient problem and one to which all infants must adapt after birth. Giving the parents a pamphlet containing information on jaundice and its therapy may help reinforce the instructive efforts.

REFERENCES

1. Alonzo EM, Whitington PF, Whitington SH et al: Enterohepatic circulation of nonconjugated bilirubin in rats fed with human milk, *J Pediatr* 118:425, 1991.

2. American Academy of Pediatrics/American College of Obstetrics and Gynecology: *Hyperbilirubinemia: guidelines for perinatal care,* ed 4, Elk Grove Village, Ill, 1997, The Academy.

3. Bartoletti AL, Stevenson DK, Ostrander CR et al: Pulmonary excretion of carbon monoxide in the human infant as an index of bilirubin production: I. Effects of gestational and postnatal age and some common neonatal abnormalities, *J Pediatr* 94:952,1979.

4. Bhutani VK, Johnson L, Sivieri EM: Predictive ability of a predischarge hour-specific serum bilirubin for subsequent significant hyperbilirubinemia in healthy term and near-term newborns, *Pediatrics* 103:6, 1999

5. Bleicher MA, Reiner MA, Rapaport SA et al: Extraordinary hyperbilirubinemia in a neonate with idiopathic hypertrophic pyloric stenosis, *J Pediatr Surg* 14:527, 1979.

6. Cole AP, Hargreaves T: Conjugation inhibitors in early neonatal hyperbilirubinemia, *Arch Dis Child* 47:415, 1972.

7. Cornwall R, Cornelius CE: Effect of fasting on bilirubin metabolism, *N Engl J Med* 283:204, 1970.

8. Gartner LM, Arias IM: Studies of prolonged neonatal jaundice in the breast-fed infant, *J Pediatr* 68:54, 1966.

9. Gourley G, Arend R: B-glucuronide and hyperbilirubinemia in breastfed and formula fed babies, *Lancet* 1:644, 1986.

10. Hardy JB, Orage JS, Jackson EC et al: *The first year of life: the collaborative perinatal project of the National Institute of Neurological and Communicative Disorders and Stroke, Baltimore,* 1979, The Johns Hopkins University Press.

11. Hargreaves T: Effect of fatty acids on bilirubin conjugation, *Arch Dis Child* 48:446, 1973.

12. Kappas A, Drummond GS, Henschke C et al: Direct comparison of Sn-mesoporphyrin, an inhibitor of bilirubin production, and phototherapy in controlling hyperbilirubinemia in term and near-term newborns, *Pediatrics* 95:468, 1995

13. Kappas A, Drummond GS, Manola T et al: Sn-protoporphyrin use in the management of hyperbilirubinemia in term newborns with direct Coombs-positive ABO incompatibility, *Pediatrics* 81:485, 1988.

14. Lucey JF, Arias I, McKay R: Transient familial hyperbilirubinemia, *Am J Dis Child* 100:787, 1960.

15. McDonagh A, Lightner D: "Like a shrivelled blood orange"—bilirubin, jaundice, and phototherapy, *Pediatrics* 75:443, 1985.

16. Newman TB, Maisels MJ: Does hyperbilirubinemia damage the brain of healthy full term infants? *Clin Perinatol* 17:331, 1990.

17. Odell GB, Cohen SN, Gordes EH: Administration of albumin in the management of hyperbilirubinemia by exchange transfusions, *Pediatrics* 30:613, 1962.

18. Poland RL, Odell GB: Physiologic jaundice: the enterohepatic circulation of bilirubin, *N Engl J Med* 284:1, 1971.

19. Poland RL, Schultz GE, Garg G: High milk lipase activity associated with breast milk jaundice, *Pediatr Res* 14:1328, 1980.

20. Robertson Odell GB, Cohen SN, Gordes EH: Administration of albumin in the management of hyperbilirubinemia by exchange transfusions, *Pediatrics* 30:613, 1962.

21. Robertson A, Karp W, Brodersen R: Bilirubin displacing effect of drugs used in neonatology. *Acta Paediatr Scand* 80:1119, 1991.

22. Rosenfeld W, Twist P, Concepcion L: A new device for phototherapy treatment of jaundiced infants, *J Perinatol* 10:243, 1990.

23. Speck W: Effect on fertilization and embryonic development, *Pediatr Res* 10:506, 1979.

24. Tan KL: Efficiency of fluorescent daylight, blue and green lamps in the management of nonhemolytic hyperbilirubinemia, *J Pediatr* 90:448, 1989.

25. Valdes T, Petmezak S, Henschke C et al: Control of jaundice in preterm newborns by an inhibitor of bilirubin production, *Pediatrics* 93:1, 1994

SELECTED READINGS

Allen FM, Diamond LK: *Erythroblastosis fetalis including exchange transfusion technique,* Boston, 1958, Little, Brown.

American Academy of Pediatrics: Practice parameter: management of hyperbilirubinemia in the healthy term infant, *Pediatrics* 94:558, 1994.

Auerbach K, Gartner L: Breastfeeding and human milk: their association with jaundice in the neonate, *Clin Perinatol* 14:89, 1987.

Blackburn S: Hyperbilirubinemia and neonatal jaundice, *Neonatal Netw* 14:15, 1995.

Broderson R: Free bilirubin in blood plasma of the newborn: effects of albumin, fatty acids, pH, displacing drugs and phototherapy. In Stern L, Oh W, Fris-Hansen B, eds: *Intensive care of the newborn,* ed 2, New York, 1978, Masson.

Brown AK, Johnson L: Loss of concern about jaundice and the reemergence of kernicterus in full-term infants in the era of managed care. In Fanaroff AA, Klaus MH, eds: *The yearbook of neonatal and perinatal medicine,* St. Louis, 1996, Mosby.

Cashore WJ, Stein L: Neonatal hyperbilirubinemia, *Pediatr Clin North Am* 29:1191, 1982.

Catz C, Hanson JW, Simpson L et al: Summary of workshop: early discharge and neonatal hyperbilirubinemia, *Pediatrics* 96:743, 1995.

Dennery PA, Seidman DS, Stevenson DK: Neonatal hyperbilirubinemia, *N Engl J Med* 344:581,2001.

Gartner LM, Herschel M: Jaundice and breastfeeding, *Pediatr Clin North Am* 48:389, 2001.

Gartner LM, Hollander M: Disorders of bilirubin metabolism. In Assali NS, ed: *Pathophysiology of gestation,* vol 3, New York, 1972, Academic Press.

Gartner LM, Lee KS: Jaundice and liver disease. In Fanaroff AA, Martin RJ, eds: *Neonatal-perinatal medicine: diseases of the fetus and infant,* ed 5, St. Louis, 1992, Mosby.

Graziani LJ, Mitchell DG, Kornhauser M et al: Neurodevelopment of preterm infants: neonatal neurosonographic and serum bilirubin studies, *Pediatrics* 89:229, 1992.

Gross SJ: Vitamin E and neonatal bilirubinemia, *Pediatrics* 64:321, 1979.

Halamek LP, Stevenson DK: Neonatal jaundice and liver disease. In Fanaroff AA, Martin RJ, eds: *Neonatal-perinatal medicine: diseases of the fetus and infant,* ed 6 St. Louis, 1998, Mosby.

Kopelman AE, Brown RS, Odell GB: The "bronze" baby syndrome: a complication of phototherapy, *J Pediatr* 8:466, 1972.

Levine R, Maisels JM, eds: *Hyperbilirubinemia in the newborn, Report of the Eighty-fifth Ross Conference on Pediatric Research,* Columbus, Ohio, 1983, Ross Laboratories.

Levine RL, Fredericks WR, Rapoport SI: Entry of bilirubin into the brain due to opening of the blood-brain barrier, *Pediatrics* 69:255, 1982.

Lucey JF: Neonatal jaundice and phototherapy, *Pediatr Clin North Am* 19:287, 1972.

Maisels MJ, ed: Neonatal jaundice, *Clin Perinatol* 17:2, 1990 (14 articles).

Maisels MJ: Phototherapy: 25 years later. In Fanaroff AA, Klaus MH, eds: *The yearbook of neonatal and perinatal medicine,* St. Louis, 1996, Mosby.

Maisels MJ: Neonatal jaundice. In Avery GB, ed: *Neonatology: pathophysiology and management of the newborn,* ed 5, Philadelphia, 1999, JB Lippincott.

Maisels MJ, Gifford K: Jaundice in full-term infants, *Am J Dis Child* 137:561, 1983.

Maisels MJ, Gifford K: Normal serum bilirubin levels in the newborn and the effect of breastfeeding, *Pediatrics* 78:837, 1986.

Odell GB: *Neonatal hyperbilirubinemia,* New York, 1980, Grune & Stratton.

Poland RL, Odell G: Physiologic jaundice: the enterohepatic circulation of bilirubin, *N Engl J Med* 284:1, 1971.

Robinson SH: The origins of bilirubin, *N Engl J Med* 279:143, 1968.

Scheidt PC, Bryla DA, Nelson KB et al: Phototherapy for neonatal hyperbilirubinemia: six-year follow-up of the National Institute of Child Health and Human Development Clinical Trial, *Pediatrics* 85:455, 1990.

Tan KL: Phototherapy for neonatal jaundice, *Clin Perinatol* 18:423, 1991.

Valaes T: Bilirubin metabolism: review and discussion of inborn errors, *Clin Perinatol* 3:177, 1976.

Volpe J: Bilirubin and brain injury. In Volpe J, ed: *Neurology of the newborn,* ed 4, Philadelphia, 2001, WB Saunders.

Yao TC, Stevenson DK: Advances in the diagnosis and treatment of neonatal hyperbilirubinemia, *Clin Perinatol* 22:741, 1995.

Young CY et al: Phenobarbitone prophylaxis for neonatal hyperbilirubinemia, *Pediatrics* 48:372, 1971.

22 | Infection in the Neonate

Gerald B. Merenstein, Karen Adams, Leonard E. Weisman

A newborn infant is uniquely susceptible to infectious diseases. In this chapter we present causes of infectious diseases with particular emphasis on prevention, history, presenting signs and symptoms, laboratory data, treatment, and parent teaching methods of prevention applicable to the care of the neonate. Abbreviations for this chapter are listed in Box 22-1.

PATHOPHYSIOLOGY AND PATHOGENESIS

An infection occurs when a susceptible host comes in contact with a potentially pathogenic organism. When the encountered organism proliferates and overcomes the host defenses, infection results. **Sources of infection in a newborn can be divided into three categories: (1) transplacental acquisition (intrauterine infection), (2) perinatal acquisition during labor and delivery (intrapartum infection), and (3) hospital acquisition in the neonatal period (postnatal infection) from the mother, hospital environment, or personnel.**

In general, most infecting organisms can, under the proper circumstances, cross the placenta or ascend from the birth canal and invade the at-risk neonate. These infections may result in abortion, stillbirth, and disease present at birth or in the neonatal period.

The main goal is to prevent infections in the fetus and newborn. Unfortunately, few proven measures exist for the prevention of transplacentally or perinatally acquired infections. These measures are important, because most nonbacterial infections (except syphilis and possibly toxoplasmosis, CMV, and herpes simplex) do not respond to current therapy.

ETIOLOGY

Thorough data collection for diagnosis of infectious diseases includes a review of the perinatal history, signs and symptoms, and laboratory data.

Intrauterine, intrapartum, or neonatal disease may be caused by a wide variety of organisms, many of which are discussed in this chapter.

SPECIFIC INFECTIOUS DISEASES

The following specific infectious diseases are divided by their source of infection.

Transplacental (Intrauterine) Acquisition

Acquired Immunodeficiency Syndrome[3,5-7,19]

Prevention. The primary risk to infants for infection with HIV, the causative agent of acquired immunodeficiency syndrome (AIDS), is intrauterine, intrapartal, and postpartal exposure to a mother with HIV infection. HIV has been isolated from blood and many body fluids. Epidemiologic evidence has implicated only blood, semen, vaginal secretions, and breast milk in transmission. In countries such as the United States, where safe alternatives exist, mothers with HIV infection should be discouraged from breastfeeding. HIV testing should be recommended and encouraged to all pregnant women.[3]

Because the medical history and examination cannot reliably identify all patients infected with HIV (or other bloodborne pathogens) and because during delivery and initial care of the infant, perinatal care providers are exposed to large amounts of maternal blood, precautions (e.g., gloves) should be consistently used for all patients when handling the placenta or infant until all maternal blood has been washed away.[3]

Data Collection

History. AIDS infection in the mother is primarily acquired sexually (from a bisexual partner, prostitution, promiscuity, and rarely, in hemophiliac partners) or by IV drug abuse. Infection may be asymptomatic. Transmission from infected mother to the fetus or infant occurs in 12.9% to 39% of births. About 30% of transmission is before birth and 70% around the time of delivery. Two thirds of

Box 22-1	ABBREVIATIONS
AIDS	Acquired immunodeficiency syndrome
CF	Complement fixation test
CIE	Counter immunoelectrophoresis
CSF	Cerebrospinal fluid
ELISA	Enzyme-linked immunosorbent assay
FA	Fluorescent antibody test
FAMA	Fluorescent antibody to membrane antigen
FTA-ABS	Fluorescent treponemal antibody absorption test
HbsAg	Hepatitis B surface antigen
HIV	Human immunodeficiency virus
IAHA	Immune adherence hemagglutination
IFA	Indirect fluorescent antibody test
IHA	Hemagglutination inhibition test
MHA-TP	Microhemagglutination test for *Treponema pallidum* infection
RPR	Rapid plasma reagin test
VDRL	Venereal Disease Research Laboratory test

infections occurring before delivery are caused by transmission within the 14 days before delivery.[3]

Signs and Symptoms.   Infants with perinatally acquired HIV infection uncommonly have symptoms in the neonatal period, but the majority of these infants will present with clinical illness by 24 months of life. These may include failure to thrive, developmental disabilities, neurologic dysfunction, hepatosplenomegaly, generalized lymphadenopathy, parotitis, persistent oral candidiasis (thrush), and chronic or recurrent diarrhea. Lymphoid interstitial pneumonia is frequently seen in these infants. HIV-infected infants commonly have osteomyelitis, septic joints, pneumonia, sepsis, meningitis, and otitis media with common organisms (e.g., *Streptococcus pneumoniae, Haemophilus influenzae* type B), and these infections are frequently recurrent.[6]

Laboratory Data.   Although hypogammaglobulinemia has been reported, hypergammaglobulinemia is usually present. **The primary serologic laboratory test for HIV antibody is the enzyme-linked immunosorbent assay (ELISA). The Western blot test is used for confirmation of positive ELISA test results.** Differentiation of the child with passively acquired antibody from the infant with active infection is critical but difficult. Acquired antibody is undetectable in 75% of infants by 12 months of age and in most infants by 15 to 18 months of age. Infants have also been described

with negative serology but active infection.[6] **Early identification is possible. HIV nucleic acid detection by PCR of DNA extracted from peripheral blood mononuclear cells is the preferred test for diagnosis of infected infants and results are available within 24 hours.** About 30% of HIV infected infants will have a positive DNA PCR from samples obtained within 48 hours of age, 93% have detectable HIV DNA by 2 weeks and almost all by 1 month. Virus isolation by culture is difficult and expensive, and both p24 antigen detection and HIV RNA PCR is specific but less sensitive.[2]

Treatment.   Zidovudine (ZDV) reduces HIV transmission from infected mothers to their newborns.[23] ZDV should be given to infants of infected women beginning at 8 to 12 hours of life and be continued for 6 weeks.[2] ZDV is administered orally at 2 mg/kg body weight/dose every 6 hours.[46] Infants who are perinatally infected with HIV are at high risk for developing *Pneumocystis carinii* pneumonia (PCP) early in the first year of life. New guidelines recommend initiating prophylaxis for the prevention of PCP for all HIV-exposed infants at 4 to 6 weeks of age, regardless of their CD4+ cell count. For children receiving ZDV, PCP prophylaxis should begin after completion of the 6-week course of ZDV. PCP prophylaxis may be provided by 5 mg of trimethoprim (TMP) and 25 mg of sulfamethoxazole (SMX)/kg body weight/day administered in two divided doses.[2] TMP + SMX prophylaxis should be continued through the first year of life or until HIV is reasonably excluded.[36]

Parent Teaching.   Care of an infant at risk for HIV requires close and long-term follow-up. Involvement of the parents is essential to this process. Education of the parents will maximize the success of such a care plan, and utilization of all available community resources should provide additional support. In addition to the rationale and importance for the medical management outlined above, the parents should be counseled concerning the need for immunizations following the American Academy of Pediatrics schedule—except the use of inactivated polio virus vaccine (IPV) is recommended instead of oral polio vaccine (OPV); rapid consultation with the child's physician if he or she is exposed to varicella (may need treatment with varicella zoster immune globulin [VZIG] within 96 hours of exposure) or measles (may need vaccination within 72 hours of exposure); or development of thrush, a diaper rash, or any other signs or symptoms of illness. Prevention of infections is important, and this requires good handwashing, regular bathing, appropriate food preparation skills (wash bottles, nipples, and pacifiers), and good skin care (changing diapers and moisturizing skin in other areas to prevent drying and cracking).[2,5]

Cytomegalovirus[12,57]

Prevention. There are no practical methods for preventing CMV. Avoiding exposure is virtually impossible because of the ubiquitous and asymptomatic nature of the infections. Avoiding unnecessary blood transfusions or using CMV serum-negative blood donors has proved to be important in minimizing the occurrence of postnatally acquired CMV, particularly in premature infants.[3]

The question frequently arises regarding assignment of staff to infants with a possible diagnosis of CMV. Staff members who may be pregnant have heightened concern regarding this issue. Staff members should be aware that many infants with CMV are often asymptomatic and therefore not identified while in the hospital. To avoid any problems, staff members should employ good handwashing technique with all infants. Wearing gloves when handling urine and other secretions is a strategy that can also be employed by staff members who are working in the NICU and are pregnant or of childbearing age. The actual risk of an infected infant's transmitting disease to a susceptible health care worker is unknown but probably small.[2]

Data Collection

History. Congenital infections are represented by a wide spectrum of disease from asymptomatic disease to profoundly symptomatic disease. Infection in the mother is usually asymptomatic.[57]

Signs and Symptoms. An infant with CMV is usually asymptomatic. Congenital manifestations include intrauterine growth restriction (IUGR), neonatal jaundice (increased direct fraction), purpura, hepatosplenomegaly, microcephaly, seizures, intracerebral calcification, chorioretinitis, and progressive sensorineural hearing loss.[12,57]

Laboratory Data. CMV may be cultured from urine, pharyngeal secretions, and peripheral leukocytes. Isolation of the virus within 2 weeks of birth

indicates transplacental acquisition. A paired sera demonstration of a fourfold titer rise or histopathologic demonstration of characteristic nuclear inclusions in certain tissues can confirm infection. Examining the urine for intranuclear inclusions is not helpful.[2]

Treatment. Currently ganciclovir, foscarnet, and cidofovir are the only licensed antiviral agents effective against CMV. These drugs are only approved for treatment of life- and sight-saving disease. A multicenter controlled study is currently under way to evaluate ganciclovir in the treatment of infants with symptomatic CMV and CNS involvement. Preliminary data suggest that treatment may significantly decrease the progression of hearing loss during the first year of life.

Parent Teaching. The need for good handwashing technique by parents and caregivers of infants with suspected CMV should be included in discharge instructions.

Rubella[2,3,21]

Prevention. Medical personnel should ensure that all mothers have a protective hemagglutination titer before conception. If the woman is susceptible, vaccinate her with rubella vaccine before conception. If a woman is found to lack immunity to rubella during pregnancy, she should receive rubella immunization in the postpartum period.[3,21]

All perinatal health care workers should have rubella titers drawn to identify immunity status, and they should be reimmunized if this is not adequate. Women of childbearing age who do not have immune titers should be encouraged to have rubella immunization.[2]

Data Collection

History. Rubella in the first 4 to 5 months of pregnancy has a high incidence of sequelae in the infant.[3] A mother with rubella may be relatively asymptomatic or mildly ill with respiratory symptoms with or without a rash.[2]

Signs and Symptoms. Congenital manifestations of rubella include IUGR, sensorineural deafness, cataracts, neonatal jaundice (increased direct fraction), purpura, hepatosplenomegaly, microcephaly, chronic encephalitis, chorioretinitis, and cardiac defects (especially PDA and pe-

ripheral pulmonic stenosis). Less frequent manifestations include bone lesions and pneumonitis.[2]

Laboratory Data. The virus may be isolated from the throat, blood, urine, and cerebrospinal fluid (CSF). A paired sera demonstration of a fourfold titer rise, such as a hemagglutination inhibition test (IHA) or a fluorescent antibody test (FA), is diagnostic.[2]

Parent Teaching. Infants with congenital rubella may secrete the virus for many years. This requires that discharge instructions include preventive strategies that need to be employed to decrease the chance of contact of susceptible pregnant women with the infant. Parents need to be informed of their responsibility to ensure that potentially seronegative women of childbearing age avoid direct contact with the infant.[2] The challenge arises to impress this on the family and at the same time avoid ostracizing the infant or negatively affecting the parent-infant attachment process. In discharge planning with these families, a collaborative approach should be employed, using community health, medical, nursing, and social work input and support.

Syphilis[2,3,41,58]

Prevention. Avoid exposing the mother to syphilis. Monitor the serum early and late in pregnancy, and treat the mother for the appropriate stage of disease. Erythromycin, previously used in penicillin-sensitive women, is not considered adequate treatment during gestation because of 30% treatment failure rates in adults and failure to establish a cure in newborns as a result of poor transplacental passage of erythromycin. Infants born to women treated with erythromycin should be considered high risk for infection and appropriately evaluated and treated.[58] If penicillin allergy is confirmed in the pregnant woman, acute desensitization is necessary.[41] Desensitization can be accomplished using increasing doses of oral penicillin over 4 to 6 hours.

Data Collection

History. A congenital infection may be manifested by a multisystem disease. A primary syphilitic chancre on the cervix or rectal mucosa in a mother may be unnoticed.[58]

Signs and Symptoms. An infant exposed to syphilis may be asymptomatic at birth or involve virtually all organ systems. Clinical findings may include hepatitis, pneumonitis, bone marrow failure, myocarditis, meningitis, nephrotic syndrome, rhinitis (snuffles), and a rash involving the palms and soles.[58]

Laboratory Data. The microscopic darkfield examination identifies spirochetes from nonoral lesions. Nonspecific, nontreponemal, reaginic tests, such as Venereal Disease Research Laboratory (VDRL) tests and rapid plasma reagin (RPR) tests, followed serially with a rise or absence of fall after birth, are diagnostic. Specific treponemal antibody serologic tests such as a fluorescent treponemal antibody absorption test (FTA-ABS) and a microhemagglutination test for *Treponema pallidum* (MHA-TP) may also be diagnostic, but an FTA-ABS IgM test is unreliable. A long-bone x-ray examination showing metaphysitis or periostitis may help in diagnosing syphilis. VDRL tests on CSF are mandatory in all infants suspected of having congenital syphilis. When the diagnosis of active congenital syphilis is equivocal, it is often best to treat and ascertain the diagnosis by serial serologic determinations.[41,58]

Treatment. Table 22-1 outlines treatment for syphilis.

Parent Teaching. Adequate follow-up of both symptomatic and asymptomatic neonates is very important. A physical evaluation should be conducted at 1, 2, 3, 6, and 12 months. Serologic testing should be performed at 3 months, and if still reactive, at 6 and 12 months. If titers fail to decline, increase, or are still present after 12 months, the infant should be reevaluated and retreated. Infants with neurosyphilis should have repeat CSF examinations every 6 months until it is normal and VDRL nonreactive. If CSF VDRL is still reactive at 6 months or CSF is abnormal at 24 months, reevaluation and retreatment is indicated.[41]

Toxoplasmosis[2]

Prevention. Women should avoid unnecessary exposure to raw meat and cat feces. Using a pair of gloves when emptying the litter box may provide protection if the pregnant woman (or a woman attempting to become pregnant) must empty the litter box.[2]

Data Collection

History. Congenital infections are represented by a wide range of disease from asymptomatic disease

Table 22-1	RECOMMENDED THERAPY FOR INDICATED CONDITIONS
CONDITION	TREATMENT*

Sepsis and/or Meningitis

Initial therapy	
Early onset	IV ampicillin and gentamicin or IV amikacin (if gentamicin-resistant organisms are present in nursery, ampicillin plus cefotaxime is a suitable alternative, particularly if meningitis is present)
Late onset	IV vancomycin plus cefotaxime or IV aminoglycoside (see early onset)
Once specific organisms are identified	
Group B streptococci	IV ampicillin and gentimicin for 10-14 days (gentamicin may be discontinued if strain is not tolerant)
Coliform species	IV ampicillin and gentimicin for 10-14 days (cefotaxime may replace gentamicin)
Listeria monocytogenes	IV ampicillin and IV gentamicin for 14-21 days
Enterococci	Same as for *Listeria monocytogenes*
Group A streptococci	IV penicillin G for 10-14 days
Group D streptococci (nonenterococcal)	Same as for group A streptococci
Staphylococcus aureus	IV nafcillin for 10-14 days, IV vancomycin for methicillin-resistant strains
Staphylococcus epidermidis	IV vancomycin for 10-14 days
Pseudomonas aeruginosa	IV mezlocillin and IV gentamicin for 10-14 days
Anaerobes	IV chloramphenicol if levels can be monitored (levels should be in 20-25 μg/ml range) or IV clindamycin

Pneumonia

Group B streptococci	Same as for sepsis (respiratory distress syndrome may mimic pneumonitis and vice versa)
Staphylococcus aureus	Same as for sepsis
Chlamydia trachomatis	PO erythromycin for 14 days
Pneumocystis carinii	PO or IV trimethoprim and sulfamethoxazole or IV pentamidine isethionate
Pertussis	PO erythromycin for 14 days (clinical course is unchanged but shedding of organism is diminished significantly)
Other organisms	Same as for sepsis

Skin and Soft-Tissue Infections

Impetigo	IV nafcillin or PO dicloxacillin for 7 days (depending on clinical severity)
Group A streptococcal infections	IV penicillin G for 7 days
Breast abscess	IV nafcillin and gentamicin for 7 days pending identification of etiologic agent (change to IV penicillin if streptococcus is etiologic) (IV ampicillin and/or gentamicin should be used for coliform species pending sensitivities); value of surgical drainage is individualized
Omphalitis and/or funisitis	IV nafcillin for 7 days (penicillin may be used if infection is caused by group A or B streptococci)

*Modified from Nelson JD: *Pocketbook of pediatric antimicrobial therapy,* ed 5, Dallas, 1983, Jodone Publishing.
See Table 22-6 for dosages.

Table 22-1	RECOMMENDED THERAPY FOR INDICATED CONDITIONS—cont'd
CONDITION	**TREATMENT***

Gastrointestinal Infections

Salmonella species	IV ampicillin for 7-10 days, IV chloramphenicol for 7-10 days, or IV gentamicin for 7-10 days depending on sensitivities (focal complications of meningitis and arthritis should be monitored closely)
Shigella species	PO trimethoprim/sulfamethoxazole or PO or IV ampicillin, depending on sensitivities
Enteropathogenic *Escherichia coli*	PO colistin, 10-15 mg/kg/day divided q 8 hr, for 5-7 days
Necrotizing enterocolitis	IV ampicillin and IV gentamicin for 2-3 weeks (if *Pseudomonas* is isolated, IV mezlocillin may be substituted for ampicillin); supportive measures (gastrointestinal suction) are appropriate

Osteomyelitis or Septic Arthritis

Group B streptococci	IV penicillin G for 21 days minimum
S. aureus	IV nafcillin for 21 days minimum
Coliform species	IV gentamicin for 21 days minimum (IV ampicillin for 21 days minimum if organism is sensitive)
Gonococcal species	IV penicillin G for 10 days
Unknown	IV nafcillin and gentamicin for 21 days minimum

Urinary Tract Infections

Suspect predisposing anatomic defect if urinary tract infection; individualize workup and follow-up

Coliform species	Gentamicin, 3 mg/kg/day divided q 8 hr for 10 days
Enterococcal species	Ampicillin, 30 mg/kg/day divided q 8 hr for 10 days

Miscellaneous Conditions

Congenital syphilis	
Without CNS involvement	IM procaine penicillin G (50,000 U/kg) daily for 10-14 days (follow-up VDRL test results should revert to negative if treatment is adequate by 1 year)
With CNS involvement	IV aqueous crystalline penicillin 100,000 to 150,000 U/kg/day divided q 8-12 hr for 10-14 days.
Toxoplasmosis	PO sulfadiazine, 100-120 mg/kg/day divided q 12 hr and PO pyrimethamine, 1 mg/kg/day divided q 12 hr (duration of treatment is debatable but should be long [i.e., months]; supplemental folic acid, 1 mg/day, should be added)
Herpes simplex infections	IV acyclovir, 30 mg/kg/day as 1-hr infusion divided q 8 hr for 10 days
Conjunctivitis	
Chlamydia species	PO erythromycin for 10 days (topical may be ineffective)
Gonococcal species	IV penicillin G for 10 days; cefoxitin for penicillin-resistant strains
Otitis media	
In otherwise normal neonate	PO amoxicillin/clavulinic acid (Augmentin), 40 mg/kg
In neonate with nosocomial infection	PO or IV ampicillin and IV gentamicin (if there is no response to treatment, consider diagnostic tympanocentesis; *S. aureus* and coliform species may be present)

to profound symptomatic disease. Mothers may have noted an influenza-like illness, posterior cervical adenitis, or chorioretinitis but usually lack accompanying signs or symptoms. A history of exposure to cat feces or ingestion of raw meat may occasionally be obtained.[2,3]

Signs and Symptoms. Manifestations in a newborn may be prematurity, IUGR, hydrocephalus, chorioretinitis, seizures, cerebral calcifications, hepatosplenomegaly, thrombocytopenia, jaundice, generalized lymphadenopathy, and a rash.[2]

Laboratory Data. Isolating *Toxoplasma gondii* from blood or body fluids is difficult and tedious. Cysts may be found in the placenta or tissues of a fetus or newborn. Most congenitally infected infants will have a Sabin-Feldman dye test titer greater than 1:1000 at birth.

Treatment. Table 22-1 outlines treatment of toxoplasmosis.

Perinatal Acquisition During Labor and Delivery

Chlamydia Trachomatis[2,3,24]

Prevention. Eye prophylaxis with erythromycin (preferred) or tetracycline ophthalmic ointment minimizes the development of conjunctivitis but has no effect on the subsequent development of pneumonitis.[2,24]

Data Collection

History. A mother with a *Chlamydia trachomatis* infection is usually asymptomatic during her pregnancy.[3,24]

Signs and Symptoms. Conjunctivitis may be manifested as congestion and edema of the conjunctiva, with minimal discharge developing 1 to 2 weeks after birth and lasting several weeks with recurrences, particularly after topical therapy. Infants with pneumonitis usually do not have a fever but have a prolonged staccato cough, tachypnea, mild hypoxemia, and eosinophilia. Otitis media and bronchiolitis may also occur.[2,24]

Laboratory Data. Definitive diagnosis is made by isolating the organism in tissue culture. Demonstrating chlamydial antigen in clinical specimens by the direct fluorescent antibody method or enzyme immunoassay is very reliable. To enhance the likelihood of obtaining an adequate sample, it is important to scrape the lower conjunctiva (for conjunctivitis) or obtain deep tracheal secretions or a nasopharyngeal aspirate (for pneumonia). Scraping conjunctival epithelial cells and demonstrating characteristic intracytoplasmic inclusion bodies by a Giemsa stain is diagnostic. Although serologic tests for conjunctivitis are unreliable, a significant titer rise in IgM specific antibody may be reliable in cases of pneumonia. Eosinophilia (greater than 300 to 400/mm^3) may be suggestive of pneumonia.[2,24]

Enterovirus (Coxsackievirus A and B, Echovirus, and Poliomyelitis)

Prevention. To prevent poliomyelitis, it is essential to maintain poliomyelitis immunity with active immunization before conception. Passive protection with pooled human serum globulin may help in selected exposures (0.2 ml/kg body weight, given IM). Routine nursery infection control procedures must be observed. **It is recommended that only IPV vaccine, not OPV vaccine, be used in the nursery.** The IPV is administered intramuscularly and contains no live virus, whereas OPV is administered orally and contains live but attenuated virus, which has been reported to cause infection in immunocompromised patients.[2]

Data Collection

History. Infection may occur year-round but is more prevalent from June to December in temperate climates. Most enterovirus infections are asymptomatic. Poliomyelitis is rare because of a high vaccine-induced immunity in most of the world.[2]

Signs and Symptoms. Mothers with enteroviral infections are usually mildly ill, with fever or diarrhea. Infants may be asymptomatic or have fever or diarrhea. Fulminating encephalomyocarditis or acute hepatic necrosis may occur within several days of birth, but their occurrence is rare.[2]

Laboratory Data. The virus may be isolated from the throat, rectum, or CSF. Isolating coxsackievirus A may require suckling mouse inoculation. Serologic screening is impractical because of the large number of serotypes.[2]

Group B Streptococcus[13,37,59]

Prevention. Intrapartum (during labor) treatment of the mother with penicillin significantly de-

creases group B *Streptococcus* (GBS) disease in the neonate and maternal postpartum endometritis.[13] Neonatal sepsis has been reported with less than 4 hours of maternal antibiotics at term and with up to 48 hours in preterm infants.[59]

Data Collection. See the section on bacterial infections and bacterial sepsis, pp. 474-481.

Treatment. See Table 22-1.

Hepatitis B*
Prevention. Prenatal screening of women for hepatitis B surface antigen (HBsAg) is indicated and is cost effective. Use of active and passive immunization in infants born of HBsAg-positive mothers is indicated (Tables 22-2 and 22-3). Use of active immunization for infants born to HBsAg-negative women is recommended.

Data Collection
History. Mothers who are HBsAg positive because of the chronic carrier state or acute disease before delivery may pass the infection to their infants at delivery.[3]

Women at high risk include women of Asian, Pacific Island, or Alaskan Eskimo descent; women born in Haiti or sub-Saharan Africa; or women with a history of liver disease, IV drug abuse, or frequent exposure to blood in a medical-dental setting.[20]

Signs and Symptoms. A neonate with hepatitis B is usually asymptomatic. Occasionally, infected infants demonstrate elevated liver enzymes or acute fulminating hepatitis.[2] Neonatal infection with subsequent chronic carriage has been implicated in the development of primary hepatocellular carcinoma later in life.

Laboratory Data. Most infants at risk of acquiring hepatitis from their mother are HBsAg negative at birth. Many untreated infants become HBsAg positive 4 to 12 weeks after birth and become lifelong asymptomatic carriers or develop hepatitis B.[2]

Herpes Simplex (Types 1 and 2)*
Prevention. The key to preventing herpes simplex is avoiding exposure. Mothers with active lesions or prodrome should have a cesarean section preferably within 4 to 6 hours of membrane rupture. Treatment with acyclovir should begin at the first sign of neonatal disease or when infants have been exposed to an active lesion.[3]

Communication is required between obstetric and neonatal staff to determine the status of a family with a history of herpes. Unnecessary restrictions should not be placed on postpartum mothers who are not actively infected.[3] Health professionals need to employ all family-centered strategies used in their institutions with these families unless these are precluded by the need for the infant's treatment.

---

*References 2-4, 8, 20, 64.

*References 3, 14, 15, 40, 51, 59a, 61.

Table 22-2	ACCEPTABLE METHODS OF PASSIVE IMMUNIZATION IN NEWBORNS			
DISEASE	**INDICATIONS FOR USE IN NEWBORNS**	**WHEN TO USE**	**PRODUCT**	**DOSE**
Hepatitis A	Active infection in mother or close family contacts	As soon as possible	HISG	0.02-0.04 ml/kg body weight given intramuscularly (IM)
Hepatitis B	Mothers with acute type B infection or mothers who are antigen positive	As soon as possible (within 12 hr)	HBIG*	0.5 ml/kg body weight given IM
Tetanus	Inadequately immunized mothers with contaminated infant (e.g., dirty cord)	As soon as possible	TIG	250 U given IM (optimal dose not established)
Varicella	Infant born to a mother who develops lesions less than 5 days before delivery or within 2 days after delivery	Within 72 hr of birth	ZIG	2 ml given IM

Modified from Remington JS, Klein JO, eds: *Infectious diseases of the fetus and newborn infant,* ed 2, Philadelphia, 1983, WB Saunders.
*Should be used in conjunction with active immunization with HBV vaccine (Table 22-3).
HBIG, Hepatitis B immune globulin; *HSIG,* human immune serum globulin; *TIG,* tetanus immuneglobulin (human); *ZIG,* zoster immune globulin.

Table 22-3	ACCEPTABLE METHODS OF ACTIVE IMMUNIZATION IN NEWBORNS			
DISEASE	INDICATIONS FOR USE IN NEWBORNS	WHEN TO USE	PRODUCT	DOSE
Hepatitis B	HBsAg-positive	3 separate doses at birth,* 1 mo, and 6 mo	Recombivax	0.5 ml IM
			Engerix-B	0.5 ml IM
	HBsAg-negative		Recombivax	0.25 ml IM
			Engerix-B	0.5 ml IM
Pertussis	To control rare outbreak in nursery	As soon as possible	Pertussis vaccine	0.25-0.5 ml administered subcutaneously
Tuberculosis	Selected infants at risk of contracting tuberculosis	As soon as possible	BCG	0.1 ml given intradermally and divided into two sites over deltoid muscle

*As soon as possible.

BCG, Calmette-Guérin bacillus; *HBsAg*, hepatitis B surface antigen.

Data Collection

History. Disease caused by type 1 herpes simplex is usually spread by the oral route, whereas disease caused by type 2 herpes simplex is usually spread by the genital route.[2]

Many mothers who transmit herpes simplex to their newborn infants are asymptomatic. The risk to the infant from recurrent lesions is minimal.[14,15]

Signs and Symptoms. Infants with herpes simplex have a spectrum of illnesses ranging from localized skin lesions to generalized infections involving the liver, lungs, and CNS. This disseminated disease has a high morbidity and mortality rate.[61]

Laboratory Data. A cytologic examination of the base of skin vesicles with a Giemsa stain (Tzanck test) may reveal characteristic but non-specific giant cells and eosinophilic intranuclear inclusions. The virus may be readily identified on a tissue culture within 24 to 48 hours from the respiratory and genital tracts, blood, urine, and CSF. Rapid viral diagnosis by fluorescent tests is widely available. Although tests of paired serology such as complement fixation test (CF), ELISA, and neutralization are available, they are of little value in an acute clinical situation.[2]

Treatment. See Table 22-1.

Parent Teaching. Families with herpes simplex require consistent and detailed teaching regarding prevention of transmission of herpes to the infant. Breastfeeding mothers can be reassured that they may continue to breastfeed as long as there are no lesions on their breasts. Emphasis should be placed on the need for breastfeeding mothers to check their breasts for lesions.[3]

Parents with active herpes simplex need to employ good handwashing technique while caring for their infants. Parents with oral herpes should avoid kissing their infants while lesions are open and draining.[3]

Listeria monocytogenes[3,26]

Prevention. Pregnant women should avoid drinking unpasteurized milk to prevent *Listeria monocytogenes* infection.[26]

Data Collection. See the section on bacterial infections and bacterial sepsis, pp. 474-481.

Treatment. See Table 22-1.

Mycobacterium tuberculosis[2,3]

Prevention. Mothers at risk for *Mycobacterium tuberculosis* infection may be identified with a tuberculin test during pregnancy. If the mother is a tuberculin converter (has had a positive skin test result within the past 2 years), a chest x-ray examination should be performed. If the mother has active tuberculosis, she should be treated with isoniazid and rifampin, with the addition of ethambutol initially until sensitivity testing is available. Pyridoxine should always be given with isoniazid during pregnancy because of the increased requirements for this vitamin in pregnant women. If the mother does not have active tuberculosis, household contacts should be screened. If the disease is identified in the mother or household contacts, the infant is at high risk for developing tuberculosis.[2]

Separate infants of mothers with active disease from the mother until the mother is not contagious (usually negative sputum). Treat high-risk infants with isoniazid (10 mg/kg/day) or a tuberculosis vaccine (Calmette-Guérin bacillus) (see Table 22-3).[2,3]

Data Collection

History. A strong history of maternal contact with tuberculosis favors the diagnosis. This is especially true in high-risk populations (Southeast Asians, American Indians, and families with a known cavitary disease). Mothers with HIV infection are at an increased risk for developing active tuberculosis.[2]

Signs and Symptoms. Mothers may be relatively asymptomatic or have signs and symptoms that are generalized (fever and weight loss) or localized to the respiratory tract.[2] A congenital infection is extremely rare.[3] Nonspecific signs and symptoms such as failure to thrive and unexplained hypothermia or hyperthermia are the most common manifestations in the neonatal period.

Laboratory Data. Acid-fast organisms found on smears of gastric aspirates, sputum, CSF, or infected tissues strongly suggest tuberculosis in the neonate. Isolating *Mycobacterium tuberculosis* by culture is diagnostic and should be aggressively sought. The tuberculin test result is usually positive (more than 10 mm induration) in active tuberculosis. However, a positive skin test result requires 3 to 12 weeks after infection to manifest itself and is usually negative in a neonate. A chest x-ray examination also usually yields a negative result in a neonate.[2]

Treatment. Because congenital tuberculosis is such a rare condition, optimal therapy has not been established. However, most recommendations suggest four-drug therapy (isoniazid, rifampin, pyrazinamide, plus either ethambutol or streptomycin).[2]

Parent Teaching. Infants who are treated with isoniazid or breastfed infants whose mothers are treated with isoniazid should receive pyridoxine supplementation.[2]

Neisseria gonorrhea

Prevention. Screening high-risk mothers before delivery may identify asymptomatic gonorrhea. Treating positive mothers before delivery or exposed infants at delivery is necessary.[2]

Administering silver nitrate, erythromycin, or tetracycline in the eyes is mandatory in all vaginal deliveries.[2]

Data Collection

History. Mothers with previous venereal disease are a high-risk group, because 80% of the infected women may be asymptomatic.

Signs and Symptoms. The predominant manifestation of gonorrhea is ophthalmia neonatorum, although a systemic bloodborne infection may rarely occur involving the joints, lungs, endocardium, and CNS. Conjunctivitis usually begins 2 to 5 days after birth. Eye prophylaxis minimizes but does not guarantee freedom from infection. Scalp abscess resulting from fetal monitoring has been reported.[2]

Laboratory Data. A gram stain of purulent eye discharge revealing gram-negative intracellular diplococci is diagnostic. Culture confirmation using fermentation or fluorescence establishes the diagnosis of gonorrhea. The organism is labile, so cultures should be taken to the laboratory and plated immediately. When gonorrhea is diagnosed, other sexually transmitted diseases may be present concomitantly (especially *Chlamydia*).[2]

Treatment. See Table 22-1.

Varicella[3]

Prevention. Table 22-2 outlines prevention of infection.

Data Collection

History. A history of varicella in the mother before conception virtually excludes the diagnosis. Varicella presents in the mother with a fever, respiratory symptoms, and characteristic vesicular rash primarily on the trunk. If this occurs within 5 days of delivery, it threatens a newborn. Preventive measures should be instituted as soon as possible.[3] Acute perinatal varicella is frequently a devastating systemic disease. Nosocomially acquired transmission of varicella is a potentially significant problem for high-risk infants: premature infants born to susceptible mothers, infants who are severely premature regardless of maternal status, and immunocompromised patients of all ages (Table 22-4).

Signs and Symptoms. Congenital varicella is rare but has followed maternal varicella in the first

Table 22-4	INFECTION CONTROL MEASURES AND ISOLATION TECHNIQUES FOR SPECIFIC DISEASES				
	RECOMMENDED PRECAUTIONS				
DISEASE/ORGANISM	HANDWASHING	PRIVATE ROOM OR COHORT	MASK	GOWN	GLOVES
AIDS/HIV	X	D	No	(X)	(X)
Adenovirus	X	X	No	(X)	No
Conjunctivitis					
Gonococcal *(Ophthalmia neonatorum)*	X	X	No	No	(X)
Chlamydia	X	No	No	No	(X)
Coxsackievirus	X	D	No	(X)	(X)
Cytomegalovirus	X	No	No	No	(X)
Diarrhea	X	D	No	(X)	(X)
Echovirus	X	D	No	(X)	(X)
Gastroenteritis	X	X	No	(X)	(X)
Hepatitis					
Type A	X	D	No	(X)	(X)
Type B	X	No	No	(X)	(X)
Herpes simplex	X	X	No	(X)	(X)
Influenza A or B	X	X	No	(X)	(X)
Meningitis					
Aseptic	X	D	No	(X)	(X)
Bacterial	X	No	No	No	No
Necrotizing enterocolitis	X	No	No	(X)	(X)
Respiratory syncytial virus	X	X	X	(X)	(X)
Rubella	X	X	X	No	No
Staphylococcal disease *(S. aureus)*	X	D	No	(X)	(X)
Streptococcal disease					
Group A	X	D	No	(X)	(X)
Group B	X	D	No	(X)	(X)
Syphilis	X	No	No	No	(X)
Toxoplasmosis	X	No	No	No	No
Varicella	X	X	X	X	X
Vancomycin-resistant organisms	X	X	No	X	X

D, Desirable but optional; X, recommended at all times; (X), recommended if soiling is likely, or if touching infective materials.

| Table 22-4 | INFECTION CONTROL MEASURES AND ISOLATION TECHNIQUES FOR SPECIFIC DISEASES—cont'd | |

INFECTIVE MATERIAL	DURATION OF ISOLATION/PRECAUTION	COMMENTS
Blood and body fluids	Duration of illness	Utmost care needed to avoid needle sticks
Respiratory secretions and feces	Duration of hospitalization	During outbreaks cohort patients suspected of having adenovirus infection
Purulent exudate	Until 24 hr after initiation of effective therapy	
Purulent exudate	Duration of illness	
Feces and respiratory secretions	7 days after onset	
Urine and respiratory secretions		Counsel pregnant personnel
Feces	Duration of illness	Identify colonized or infected infants by culture; institute cohorting
Feces and respiratory secretions	For 7 days after onset of illness	
Feces	Duration of illness	
Feces	For 7 days after onset of illness	Most contagious before symptoms
Blood and body fluids	Duration of positivity	Avoid needlesticks
Lesions, secretions, urine, and stool	Duration of illness	
Respiratory secretions	Duration of illness	Cohort patients suspected of having influenza during outbreak; staff should receive yearly influenza vaccine
Feces	Duration of illness	Cohort colonized or infected infants during a nursery outbreak
(?) Feces	Duration of illness	Cohort ill infants
Respiratory secretions	Duration of illness	Cohort suspected infants, especially premature infants, during outbreaks
Respiratory secretions	Duration of hospitalization	Infants may shed virus for as long as 2 years; seronegative women should avoid contact
Purulent exudate	Duration of illness	
Respiratory secretions	24 hr after initiation of effective therapy	
Respiratory and genital secretions		Cohort ill and colonized infants during a nursery outbreak
Lesion secretions and blood	24 hr after initiation of effective therapy	
	None	
Respiratory and lesion secretions	Until lesions are crusted	Neonates born to mothers with active chickenpox should be placed on isolation precautions at birth; persons who are not susceptible do not need to mask
Secretions	Duration of illness	

trimester of pregnancy. Congenital manifestations include limb atrophy, skin scars, and CNS and eye abnormalities.[2]

Laboratory Data. The demonstration of multinucleated giant cells containing intranuclear inclusions in skin scrapings on Giemsa stain is nonspecific but helpful. Virus can be isolated from scrapings of vesicle base during the first 3 to 4 days of the eruption. Isolating the virus from the respiratory tract is difficult. A number of serologic tests such as the fluorescent antibody to membrane antigen test (FAMA), immune adherence hemagglutination test (IAHA), ELISA, and neutralization test are available but are not helpful in the acute clinical situation. Complement fixation (CF) serologic tests are relatively insensitive.[2]

Early-Onset Bacterial Disease*
Prevention. For GBS only see p. 468.

Data Collection
History. Early-onset disease is almost always acquired perinatally and is discussed here. Late-onset disease is discussed in the section on postnatally acquired disease. **Early-onset disease presents as a fulminate multisystem illness during the first days of life. Many of these infants are premature and have a history of one or more significant obstetric complications, including premature rupture of maternal membranes, premature onset of labor, chorioamnionitis, or peripartum maternal fever, prolonged membrane rupture (18 hours or more), maternal genitourinary tract infection, fetal distress, or aspiration by the neonate.**[32] Bacteria responsible for early-onset disease are acquired from the birth canal before or during delivery and are shown in Box 22-2. Early-onset bacterial disease carries a high mortality rate.[3,53]

Signs and Symptoms. Neonatal bacterial sepsis is characterized by systemic signs of infection associated with bacteremia. Meningitis in a neonate can be a sequela of bacteremia. In addition, bloodborne bacteria may localize in other tissues, causing focal disease. Both patterns of bacterial disease, early onset and late onset, have been associated with systemic infections during the neonatal period.[2,53]

*References 3, 32, 33, 47, 54, 60.

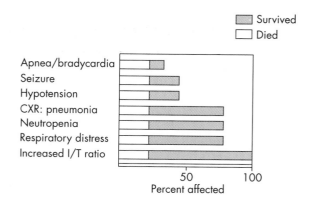

FIGURE 22-1 Clinical and laboratory findings in nine infants with signs and symptoms of early onset group B streptococcal disease. (From Nelson SN, Merenstein GB, Pierce JR: Early onset group B streptococcal disease, *J Perinatol* 6:234, 1986.)

Box 22-2	ORGANISMS CAUSING EARLY-ONSET BACTERIAL SEPSIS

Common Organisms

Group B *streptococcus*
Escherichia coli
Haemophilus influenzae (type B and nontypable)
Coagulase-negative *Staphylococcus*

Unusual Organisms

Staphylococcus aureus
Neisseria meningitidis
Streptococcus pneumoniae

Rare Organisms

Klebsiella pneumoniae
Pseudomonas aeruginosa
Enterobacter species
Serratia marcescens
Group A *Streptococcus*
Anaerobic species

In general, signs, particularly of early-onset disease, are nonspecific and nonlocalizing. Symptoms include temperature instability (hypothermia and/or hyperthermia), respiratory distress (apnea, cyanosis, and tachypnea), lethargy, feeding abnormalities (vomiting, increased residuals, and abdominal distention), jaundice (particularly increased direct fraction), seizures, or purpura (Figure 22-1).[53]

Table 22-5	NORMAL CEREBROSPINAL FLUID VALUES IN NEONATES			
	WHITE BLOOD CELLS	POLYMORPHONUCLEAR NEUTROPHILIC (LEUKOCYTES)	PROTEIN (MG/DL)	GLUCOSE (MG/DL)
Premature Infants				
Reported means	2-27		75-150	79-83
Reported ranges	0-112		31-292	64-106
Term Infants				
Reported means	3-5	2-3	47-67	51-55
Reported ranges	0-90	0-70	17-240	32-78

Modified from Remington JS, Klein JO, eds: *Infectious diseases of the fetus and newborn infant*, ed 2, Philadelphia, 1983, WB Saunders.

Laboratory Data. **Isolating bacteria from a nonpermissive site (blood, CSF, urine, closed body space) is the most valid method of establishing the diagnosis of bacterial sepsis. Surface cultures (including ear and gastric aspirates) do not establish the presence of active systemic infection but merely indicate colonization.** Bacterial antigens or endotoxins may be demonstrated in sera, CSF, urine, or body fluids by a variety of methods (counterimmunoelectrophoresis [CIE], latex agglutination [LA], and limulus lysate test). Such a demonstration is not totally definitive, nor does it allow the determination of the antibiotic sensitivity of the offending organism.[53] False-positive reactions may be caused by skin surface contamination or gastrointestinal absorption of antigen.[9] The CSF is examined in most infants suspected of sepsis, because meningitis is a frequent manifestation of sepsis in neonates, especially in symptomatic infants, and infants with GBS sepsis and with late-onset disease[53] (Table 22-5). It has been suggested that, because of the low yield and potential adverse effects from lumbar puncture, examination of CSF be deferred in asymptomatic infants being evaluated for maternal risk factors or respiratory distress.[53] **The CSF is examined in most infants suspected of sepsis, because meningitis is difficult to exclude without a lumbar puncture, and its diagnosis affects therapy and follow-up in a neonate.**[53]

Several laboratory aids are used in assessing neonatal sepsis, but it must be realized that these tests are nonspecific and occasionally may be misleading.[22] They include information obtained from the CBC (i.e., total neutrophils, immature to total neutrophil ratio, and platelet count), all of which may be associated with bacterial sepsis[24,41]

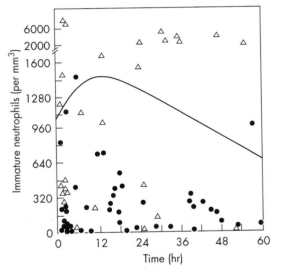

FIGURE 22-2 Total immature neutrophil counts during the first 60 hours of life in infants with sepsis (△) and those delivered of women with pregnancy-induced hypertension (•). (From Engle WD, Rosenfeld CR: Neutropenia in high risk neonates, *J Pediatr* 105:982, 1984.)

(Figures 22-2 to 22-5). The usefulness of these tests is improved if a second CBC is obtained in 12 to 24 hours.[33] Acute phase reactants, including C-reactive protein, fibrinogen, haptoglobin, and erythrocyte sedimentation rates, are occasionally useful adjunctive tests clinically, and chest x-ray examination and x-ray evaluation of specific indicated areas may also help.[53] Several other nonspecific laboratory abnormalities may accompany neonatal sepsis, including hyperglycemia, hypoglycemia, and unexplained metabolic acidosis.

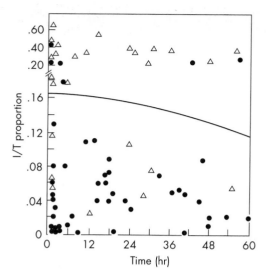

FIGURE 22-3 Immature-to-total neutrophil proportion during the first 60 hours of life in infants with sepsis (△) and those delivered of women with pregnancy-induced hypertension (•). (From Engle WD, Rosenfeld CR: Neutropenia in high risk neonates, *J Pediatr* 105:982, 1984.)

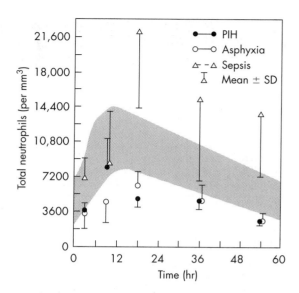

FIGURE 22-5 Distribution of absolute total neutrophil counts in first 60 hours of life in infants with sepsis (n = 13), asphyxia neonatorum (n = 12), and those delivered of women with pregnancy-induced hypertension (PIH) (n = 20). (From Engle WD, Rosenfeld CR: Neutropenia in high risk neonates, *J Pediatr* 105:982, 1984.)

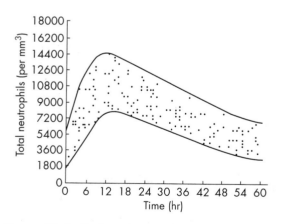

FIGURE 22-4 Total neutrophil count reference range in the first 60 hours of life. Heavy line represents envelope bounding these data. (From Manroe BL, Weinberg AG, Rosenfeld CR: The neonatal blood count in health and disease. I. Reference values for neutropenic cells, *J Pediatr* 95:89, 1979.)

Treatment. Antibiotics are the cornerstone of the treatment for presumed or confirmed infections in neonates. The indiscriminate or inappropriate use of systemic antibiotics may cause undesirable side effects, favor the emergence of resistant strains of bacteria, and alter the normal flora of the newborn. **Adequate and appropriate specimens for culture should be obtained before antibiotic therapy is initiated.**

Broad-spectrum antibiotic coverage, usually with ampicillin and an aminoglycoside for early onset sepsis, is commonly initiated pending culture and sensitivity results. Once causative organisms are identified and antibiotic sensitivities established, the most appropriate and least toxic antibiotic or antibiotic combination should be continued for an appropriate period by a suitable route. If adequate cultures are negative after a reasonable period (24 to 48 hours), antibiotic therapy may be discontinued in most situations.

It is important to realize that antibiotics are not the entire solution to treating the infected newborn. Meticulous attention to the treatment of associated conditions, such as shock, hypoxemia, thermal abnormalities, electrolyte or acid-base imbalance, adequate nutrition, anemia, drainage of pus, and removal of foreign bodies, may be as important as choosing the proper antibiotic. Further investigation is required before newer adjunctive therapies such as IV immunoglobulin and nonantibiotic therapies or preventions can be recommended.[59a] Table 22-1 provides guidelines for choosing the proper antibiotic for indicated conditions; Table 22-6 gives the

Table 22-6	ANTIBIOTIC DOSAGES FOR NEONATES		
		DAILY DOSAGE AND INTERVALS	
ANTIBIOTIC	**ROUTE**	**LESS THAN 7 DAYS OF AGE**	**MORE THAN 7 DAYS OF AGE**
Amikacin sulfate	IV, IM	15 mg/kg/day divided q 12 hr	15-20 mg/kg/day divided q 8-12 hr
Amoxicillin	PO	50 mg/kg/day divided q 12 hr	50 mg/kg/day divided q 8 hr
Amoxicillin/clavulinic acid	PO	Not recommended	40 mg/kg/day divided q 8 hr
Amphotericin B*	IV	0.1 mg/kg over 6 hr infusion initially, increase to 1 mg/kg/day in small increments	Same
Ampicillin			
Meningitis	IV	100 mg/kg/day divided q 12 hr	150-200 mg/kg/day divided q 6-8 hr
Other indications	IV, IM, PO	50 mg/kg/day divided q 12 hr	75 mg/kg/day divided q 8 hr
Carbenicillin	IV, IM	200 mg/kg/day divided q 12 hr	300-400 mg/kg/day divided q 6-8 hr
Cefazolin*	IV, IM	40 mg/kg/day divided q 12 hr	40 mg/kg/day divided q 12 hr
Cefotaxime	IV, IM	100 mg/kg/day divided q 12 hr	150 mg/kg/day divided q 8 hr
Cefoxitin	IV	15 mg/kg/day divided q 8 hr	30 mg/kg/day divided q 6 hr
Chloramphenicol succinate (not recommended unless serum concentrations are monitored)	IV, PO	25 mg/kg once daily	25-50 mg/kg/day divided q 12-24 hr
Clindamycin*	IV, PO	25 mg/kg/day divided q 8 hr	25-40 mg/kg/day divided q 6 hr
Colistin	PO	4 mg/kg divided q 6 hr	Same
Dicloxacillin*	PO	25 mg/kg twice daily	25 mg/kg divided q 8 hr
Erythromycin estolate	PO	20 mg/kg/day divided q 12 hr	20-30 mg/kg/day divided q 8-12 hr
Gentamicin	IV, IM	5 mg/kg/day divided q 12 hr	7.5 mg/kg/day divided q 8 hr
Kanamycin	IV, IM	15-20 mg/kg/day divided q 12 hr	20-30 mg/kg/day divided q 8-12 hr
Methicillin	IV, IM	50-75 mg/kg/day divided q 8-12 hr	100-150 mg/kg/day divided q 6-8 hr
Metronidazole	IV, PO	15 mg/kg loading dose; then 15 mg/kg/day divided q 12 hr	Same
Moxalactam	IV, IM	100 mg/kg/day divided q 12 hr	150 mg/kg/day divided q 8 hr
Nafcillin	IV	40 mg/kg/day divided q 12 hr	60-80 mg/kg/day divided q 6-8 hr
Neomycin	PO	25 mg/kg divided q 6 hr	Same
Nystatin	PO	400,000 units/day divided q 6 hr	Same
Mezlocillin	IV, IM	150-225 mg/kg/day divided q 8-12 hr	225-300 mg/kg/day divided q 6-8 hr
Penicillin G			
Meningitis	IV	100,000-150,000 units/kg/day divided q 8-12 hr	150,000-250,000 units/kg/day divided q 6-8 hr
Other indications	IV	50,000 units/kg/day divided q 12 hr	75,000 units/kg/day divided q 6-8 hr
Penicillin G, benzathine	IM	50,000 units/kg (1 dose only)	Same
Penicillin G, procaine	IM	50,000 units/kg/day once daily	Same
Pentamidine isethionate*	IV	4 mg/kg/day for 14 days (available from CDC, Atlanta, Ga)	Same
Ticarcillin	IV, IM	150-225 mg/kg/day divided q 8-12 hr	225-300 mg/kg/day divided q 6-8 hr
Tobramycin	IV, IM	4 mg/kg/day divided q 12 hr	6 mg/kg/day divided q 8 hr
Trimethoprim/ sulfamethoxazole (TMP/SMX)	IV, PO	10-20 mg/kg/day TMP or 50-100 kg/day SMX	Same
Vancomycin	IV	30 mg/kg/day divided q 12 hr	45 mg/kg/day divided q 8 hr

*Pharmacokinetics in newborns not well characterized. These drugs should be used with extra caution in neonates (pediatric infectious disease consultation recommended).

Table 22-7	Passage of Antibiotics Across the Placenta*	
Percentage of Antibiotic in Indicated Category		**Antibiotic**
Equal to serum concentration		Amoxicillin
		Ampicillin
		Carbenicillin
		Chloramphenicol
		Methicillin
		Nitrofurantoin
		Penicillin G
		Sulfonamides
		Tetracyclines
		Trimethoprim
50% of serum concentration		Aminoglycosides
10%-15% of serum concentration		Amikacin
		Cephalosporins
		Clindamycin
		Nafcillin
		Tobramycin
Negligible (less than 10% of serum concentration)		Dicloxacillin
		Erythromycin

*Several factors determine the degree of transfer of antibiotics across the placenta, including lipid solubility, degree of ionization, molecular weight, protein binding, placental maturation, and placental and fetal blood flow.

Table 22-8	Passage of Antibiotics into Breast Milk*	
Percentage of Antibiotic in Indicated Category		**Antibiotic**
Equal to serum concentration		Isoniazid
		Metronidazole
		Sulfonamides
		Trimethoprim
50% of serum concentration		Chloramphenicol
		Erythromycin
		Tetracyclines
Less than 25% of serum concentration		Cefazolin
		Kanamycin
		Nitrofurantoin
		Oxacillin
		Penicillin G
		Penicillin V

*Data on concentrations of antibiotics in human breast milk are sparse. Because most antibiotics are present in breast milk in microgram amounts, they are normally not ingested by the infant in therapeutic amounts.

proper dose, route, and frequency of administration of commonly used antibiotics in the newborn nursery. Table 22-7 describes the passage of antibiotics across the placenta, and Table 22-8 describes their passage into breast milk.

Parent Teaching. Transplacental infection often results in fetal abnormality and/or death. Newborns who survive may have long-term sequelae such as developmental, neurologic, motor, sensory, growth, and physical abnormalities.

Before antibiotic use, the mortality from bacterial sepsis was 95% to 100%, but antibiotics and supportive care have reduced mortality to less than 50%, but survival is highly variable and dependent upon the organism and underlying or associated conditions. Debilitated infants (preterm and sick neonates) are at greater risk and have a higher incidence of morbidity and mortality than term healthy neonates. The most common complications of bacterial sepsis are meningitis and septic shock. The outcome is influenced by early recognition and vigorous treatment with appropriate antibiotics and supportive care.

Postnatal Acquisition Late-Onset Bacterial Disease*

Prevention. The Centers for Disease Control and Prevention (CDC) defines all neonatal infections acquired intrapartum or during hospitalization as nosocomial. Infants requiring the specialized care of NICUs are highly susceptible to infections. Prematurity, stress, immature immune systems, and complicated medical and surgical problems contribute to their increased susceptibility. In addition, most infants in the NICU require a variety of invasive diagnostic, therapeutic, and monitoring procedures; many of these procedures bypass natural physical barriers that may allow colonization to occur and a nosocomial (late-onset) infection to develop.

Infection control principles and practices for the prevention of these nosocomial infections are outlined in Table 22-9.[2,3,16,30,39] Table 22-4 outlines infection control measures and isolation techniques for specific diseases.[2,18,31]

Data Collection

History. Late-onset disease may occur as early as 5 days of age but is more common after the first week of life. These infants may have a his-

*References 11, 29, 37, 43, 49, 56, 58.

Table 22-9	INFECTION CONTROL PRINCIPLES AND PRACTICES TO PREVENT NOSOCOMIAL INFECTION
PRINCIPLE	**PRACTICE**

Handwashing

Handwashing is the most important procedure for controlling infection in the NICU.

1. Before each shift, wash hands, wrists, forearms, and elbows with an antiseptic. Scrub hands with a brush or pad for 2-3 min and rinse thoroughly. Chlorhexidine, hexachlorophene, and iodophors are the preferred products.
2. Wash hands for 10-15 sec between infant contacts. Soap and water are adequate unless the infant is infected or contaminated objects have been handled.
3. Use an antiseptic for handwashing before surgical or similar invasive procedures.

Patient Placement

Overcrowding in the NICU increases risk of cross-contamination.

1. Provide 4- to 6-ft intervals between infants.

Skin and Cord Care

The skin, its secretions, and normal flora are natural defense mechanisms that protect against invading pathogens. Manipulating an infant's skin must be minimized.

No single method of cord care has been identified to prevent colonization or limit disease.

1. The American Academy of Pediatrics suggests using a dry technique:
   a. Delay initial cleansing until temperature is stable.
   b. Use sterile cotton sponges and sterile water or a mild soap to remove blood from face and head and meconium from perineal area.
   c. *Do not* touch other areas unless they are grossly soiled.
2. Local application of alcohol, triple dye, and various antimicrobial agents is currently used.

Medical Devices

Medical devices facilitate infections by the following:

1. Bypassing normal defense mechanisms, providing direct access to blood and deep tissues
2. Supporting growth of microorganisms and becoming reservoirs from which bacteria can be transmitted with the device to another patient
3. Providing a "protected site" when placed in deeper tissue, so phagocytosis or defense mechanisms cannot eradicate the organisms
4. Using sterile medical devices that are occasionally contaminated from the manufacturer or central supply

1. IV infusion devices predispose infants to phlebitis and bacteremia. Preventive measures include preparing the site with tincture of iodine (2% iodine in 70% alcohol), an iodophor, or 70% alcohol; anchoring the IV securely; performing site assessment and care every 24 hr (routine site care is not necessary with polyurethane dressings); rotating the IV site every 48-72 hr; changing the IV tubing every 24-48 hr on regular IVs; and discontinuing the IV at the first sign of complication.
2. Arterial lines predispose infants to bacteremia. Preventive measures include aseptically inserting the catheter using gloves, inspecting the site and performing site care every 24 hr, treating the catheter and stopcocks as sterile fields, and minimizing manipulation by drawing all blood specimens at the same time.
3. Intravascular pressure—monitoring systems predispose infants to septicemia. Preventive measures include replacing the flush solution every 24 hr, replacing the chamber dome, and replacing the tubing and continuous flow device (if used) at 48-hr intervals and between each patient.
4. Respiratory therapy devices increase the risk of contamination. Preventive measures include using aseptic technique during suctioning; dating opened solution for irrigation, humidification, and nebulization, and discarding after 24 hr; ensuring routine replacement and cleaning of all respiratory equipment, including Ambu bags, cascade nebulizers, endotracheal tube adaptors and tubing; and checking sputum cultures and gram stains every several days to assess the degree of colonization or infection in the intubated patient.

Continued

Table 22-9	INFECTION CONTROL PRINCIPLES AND PRACTICES TO PREVENT NOSOCOMIAL INFECTION—cont'd	
PRINCIPLE	**PRACTICE**	
Specimen Collection Improperly collected specimens cause infection at the site of collection or erroneous diagnosis, leading to the administration of the wrong antibiotic or delayed administration of the appropriate antibiotic.	1. Wash hands before collecting specimen. 2. Observe aseptic technique to reduce risk of infection and to avoid contamination of specimen. 3. Deliver specimens to the laboratory immediately. 4. *Do not use femoral sticks.*	
Nursery Attire Personal clothing and unscrubbed skin areas of personnel should not touch infants.	1. Short-sleeved scrub gowns accommodate washing to elbows. 2. Long-sleeved gowns should be worn and changed between handling of infected or potentially infected infants. 3. Sterile gowns are necessary for sterile procedures.	
Employee Health Transmission of disease among patients and employees can occur bidirectionally. Each NICU must establish reasonable guidelines for restriction of assignments based on the employee's potential to transmit disease and the potential risk of acquiring disease.	1. Conditions that commonly restrict personnel from patient care in the NICU are skin lesions and draining wounds, acute respiratory infections, fever, gastroenteritis, active herpes simplex (oral, genital, or paronychial), and herpes zoster. 2. Conditions that are transmitted from infants to personnel are a. Rubella: Obtain rubella titers from women of childbearing age; if a protective level is not present, they should be vaccinated. b. Cytomegalovirus: CMV is a potential threat to pregnant women. Adherence to good infection control practices may reduce this threat. c. Hepatitis B is usually not a major problem in the NICU, because host infants are not infectious in the early neonatal period. An effective vaccine is available and may be considered for high-risk individuals (see Tables 22-2 and 22-3). d. Use of gloves with body fluid contact will decrease the risk of transmission of HBV and HIV.	
Cohorting Cohorting is an important infection control measure used primarily during outbreaks or epidemics in the NICU. The object of cohorting is to limit the number of contacts of one infant with other infants and personnel.	1. Group together infants born within the same time frame (usually 24-48 hr) or who are colonized or infected with the same pathogen. These infants should remain together until discharged. 2. Provide nursing care by personnel who do not care for other infants. 3. After all infants in cohort are discharged, clean room before admittance of a new group of infants.	

tory of obstetric complications, but they are less common than obstetric complications in early-onset disease. Bacteria responsible for late onset sepsis and meningitis include those acquired from the maternal genital tract and organisms acquired after birth from human contact or from contaminated equipment or material[3] (Box 22-3). **Although prematurity remains the most significant factor, invasive procedures performed on a neonate, such as intubation, catheterization, and surgery, also increase the risk for bacterial infection.**

Signs and Symptoms. Similar to those of early-onset sepsis, they are nonspecific (see p. 474).

Laboratory Data. A complete set of cultures should be obtained but have similar limitations as in early-onset infection.

Treatment. Broad-spectrum antibiotic coverage, usually vancomycin and an aminoglycoside or a third-generation cephalosporin, is commonly initiated pending culture and sensitivity results

Box 22-3	ORGANISMS CAUSING LATE-ONSET SEPSIS	
Coagulase-negative *Staphylococcus*		*Malassezia furfur*
Escherichia coli		Other enteric organisms
Klebsiella species		Group B *Streptococcus*
Enterobacter species		Methicillin-resistant *Staphylococcus aureus*
Candida species		

Table 22-10	ANTIFUNGAL THERAPY	
DRUG	**DOSAGE**	**COMMENTS**
Amphotericin B	0.1 to 1 mg/kg/day IV; begin at 0.1 mg/kg and increase daily as tolerated	Nephrotoxic
5-Fluorocytosine (5-FC)	50 to 100 mg/kg/day PO q 6 hr	Hepatotoxic; bone marrow suppression

(see pp. 476-477). **However, vancomycin resistance is emerging as a potential problem in the care of sick neonates.[52] To minimize the development of these resistant organisms, the CDC has recommended prudent vancomycin use, education of medical personnel about the problem of vancomycin resistance, early detection and prompt reporting of organisms, and immediate implementation of appropriate infection control measures (see Table 22-4).**

Fungal Infection[10,11,44,49]

Fungal infections in neonates can cause significant morbidity and mortality. They are usually seen in VLBW infants, infants with congenital anomalies requiring surgery, and/or infants who require multiple or prolonged vascular catheters.

Prevention. Because these infants are often colonized at birth, strict adherence to aseptic technique when dealing with central catheters is essential. Antibiotic use should be minimized and limited to treatment of specific illnesses.

Data Collection

History. VLBW infants, infants requiring surgery, and/or infants requiring invasive procedures such as arterial or venous catheters are at increased risk for fungal infection. The use of lipids, especially excess use, may increase the risk for infection with certain organisms.[44]

Signs and Symptoms. Signs and symptoms may be nonspecific, nonlocalizing, and difficult to differentiate from infants with bacterial sepsis. Skin infections in high-risk infants can become invasive and should be closely monitored.[49]

Laboratory Data. Routine laboratory data, as may be collected based on clinical signs and symptoms, are rarely helpful in differentiating fungal from bacterial infection. A positive culture result from urine, blood, or a skin biopsy indicate systemic infection.[49] Urine and a buffy coat smear of blood from central catheters should be examined for evidence of budding yeast.[10]

Treatment.   The treatment of fungal infection will vary from infant to infant. Very few infants will respond to simple interventions such as stopping broad-spectrum antibiotics, stopping lipid infusions, or removing central catheters. Almost all will require treatment with antifungal agents such as amphotericin B and/or 5-fluorocytosine (5-FC)[49] (Table 22-10).

PARENT TEACHING

Parents who have infants with viral or bacterial infection require support and information regarding their infant's condition. Questions arise regarding treatment and prognosis, as well as possible long-range effects of the infection. Parents experience significant guilt feelings based on misperceptions regarding what role they had in causing the infection. Health care professionals need to remain sensitive to the crisis that parents are experiencing and address the issues of etiology as well as treatment and prognosis. Valid and factual data as well as information regarding complications and long-term effects should be shared with parents in a timely manner.

Controlling infection in the nursery is of prime importance but does not include excluding the parents from caring for their sick infant. Everyone must adhere to proper hand washing, gowning, and isolation techniques.[3] Educating the parents and siblings about the importance of these procedures, along with appropriate reminders, ensures cooperation. With proper precautions, there is no evidence of increased incidence of infection with parent and sibling visits.

All those entering the nursery must be screened for the presence of illness. Anyone with a fever, respiratory symptoms (cough, runny nose, sore throat), gastrointestinal symptoms (nausea, vomiting, diarrhea), or skin lesions should not come in contact with the infant. People with communicable disease (e.g., varicella) or recent exposure to a communicable disease also should not come in contact with the sick neonate.[3]

Daily cord care should be demonstrated, and a demonstration by the parents should be observed before discharging the infant. Every parent should be taught the signs and symptoms of neonatal illness, because early recognition of signs and symptoms expedites prompt treatment. Parents must be taught to take axillary temperatures and to read a thermometer. They need to be aware that both hypothermia and hyperthermia may be signs of neonatal illness.[3]

REFERENCES

1. Abzug MJ, Rotbart HA, Magliato SA et al: Evolution of the placental barrier to fetal infection by murine enterovirus, *J Infect Dis* 163:1336, 1991.
2. American Academy of Pediatrics: *Report of the committee on infectious disease,* ed 25, Elk Grove Village, Ill, 2000, The Academy.
3. American Academy of Pediatrics and American College of Obstetricians and Gynecologists: *Guidelines for perinatal care,* ed 5, Elk Grove Village, Ill, 2002, The Academy.
4. American Academy of Pediatrics Committee on Infectious Disease: Universal hepatitis B immunization, *Pediatrics* 89:795, 1992.
5. American Academy of Pediatrics Task Force on Pediatric AIDS: Perinatal HIV infection (AIDS), *Pediatics* 82:941, 1988.
6. American Academy of Pediatrics Task Force on Pediatric AIDS: Pediatric guidelines for infection control of HIV (AIDS virus) in hospitals, medical offices, schools and other settings, *Pediatrics* 82:801, 1988.
7. American Academy of Pediatrics Task Force on Pediatric AIDS: Perinatal human immunodeficiency virus (HIV) testing, *Pediatrics* 95:303, 1995.
8. Arevalo JA, Washington AE: Cost-effectiveness of prenatal screening and immunization for hepatitis B virus, *JAMA* 259:365, 1988.
9. Ascher DP, Wilson S, Mendiola J et al: Group B streptococcal latex agglutination testing in the neonate, *J Pediatr* 119:458, 1991.
10. Ascuitto RJ, Gerber MA, Cates KL et al: Buffy coat smears of blood drawn through central venous catheters as an aid to rapid diagnosis of systemic fungal infection, *J Pediatr* 106:445, 1985.
11. Bailey JE: Neonatal candidiasis: the current challenge, *Clin Perinatol* 18:303, 1991.
12. Boppanna SB, Pass RF, Britt WJ et al: Symptomatic congenital cytomegalovirus infection: neonatal morbidity and mortality, *Pediatr Infect Dis J* 11:93, 1992.
13. Boyer SM, Gotoff SP: Prevention of early onset group B streptococcal disease with selected intrapartum chemoprophylaxis, *N Engl J Med* 31:16655, 1986.
14. Brown ZA, Vontver LA, Benedetti J et al: Effects on infants of a first episode of genital herpes during pregnancy, *N Engl J Med* 317:1246, 1987.
15. Brown ZA, Benedetti J, Ashley R et al: Neonatal herpes simplex virus infection in relation to asymptomatic maternal infection at the time of labor, *N Engl J Med* 324:1247, 1991.
16. Burch SM, Chadwick JV: Use of Retroset in the delivery of intravenous medications in the neonate, *Neonatal Netw* 6:51, 1987.
17. Cairo MS: Cytokines: a new immunotherapy, *Clin Perinatol* 18:343, 1991.
18. Centers for Disease Control: *Guidelines of isolation precautions,* ed 4, Washington DC, 1983, US Government Printing Office.
19. Centers for Disease Control: Guidelines for prevention of transmission of human immunodeficiency virus and hepatitis B virus to health care and public safety workers, *MMWR Morb Mortal Wkly Rep* 38(Suppl):1, 1989.
20. Centers for Disease Control: Hepatitis B virus, a comprehensive strategy for eliminating transmission in the United States through universal childhood vaccination, *MMWR Morb Mortal Wkly Rep* 40:1, 1991.
21. Centers for Disease Control: Increase in rubella and congenital rubella syndrome—United States 1988-90, *MMWR Morb Mortal Wkly Rep* 40:93, 1991.
22. Christensen RD, Rothstein G, Hill HR et al: Fatal early onset group B streptococcal sepsis with normal leukocyte counts, *Pediatr Infect Dis J* 4:242, 1985.
23. Connor EM, Sperling RS, Gelber R et al: Reduction of maternal-infant transmission of human immunodeficiency virus type 1 with zidovudine treatment, *N Engl J Med* 331:1173, 1994.
24. Cromblehome W: Neonatal chlamydial infections, *Contemp Ob-Gyn,* p 57, 1991.

25. Engle WD, Rosenfeld CR: Neutropenia in high risk neonates, *J Pediatr* 105:982, 1984.

26. Enocksson E, Wretlind B, Sterner G et al: Listeriosis during pregnancy and in neonates, *Scand J Infect Dis* 71(Suppl):89, 1990.

27. Fakler CR, Weisman LE: Currently available non-antibiotic approaches to the prevention or adjunct therapy of neonatal bacterial infections. *Semin Pediatr Infect Dis* 10:97, 1999.

28. Fielkow S, Reuter S, Gotoff SP: Cerebrospinal fluid examination in symptom free infants with risk factors for infection, *J Pediatr* 119:971, 1991.

29. Freeman J, Platt R, Epstein MF et al: Birth weight and length of stay as determinants of nosocomial coagulase negative staphylococcal bacteremia in neonatal intensive care unit populations: potential for confounding, *Am J Epidemiol* 132:1130, 1991.

30. Fryklund B, Tullu K, Burman LG: Epidemiology of enteric bacteria in neonatal units—influence of procedures and patient variables, *J Hosp Infect* 18:15, 1991.

31. Garner JS, Simmons BP: Guidelines for isolation precautions in hospitals, *Infect Control* 4(suppl):245, 1983.

32. Gerdes JS: Clinicopathologic approach to the diagnosis of sepsis, *Clin Perinatol* 18:361, 1991.

33. Gibbs R, Duff P: Progress in pathogenesis and management of clinical intraamniotic infection, *Am J Obstet Gynecol* 164:1317, 1991.

34. Gray JG: Lues-lues: maternal and fetal considerations of syphilis, *Obstet Gynecol Surv* 50:845, 1995.

35. Greenberg DN, Yoder BA: Changes in the differential white blood count in screening for group B streptococcal sepsis, *Pediatr Infect Dis J* 9:886, 1990.

36. Grubman S, Simonds RJ: Preventing *Pneumocystis carinii* pneumonia in human immunodeficiency virus-infected children: new guidelines for prophylaxis, *Pediatr Infect Dis J* 15:165, 1996.

37. Guidelines for preventing perinatal GBS infection, *Contemp Obstet Gynecol* 84, 1996.

38. Hall SL: Coagulase-negative staphylococcal infections in neonates, *Pediatr Infect Dis J* 10:57, 1991.

39. Hargrove C: Administration of I.V. medications in the NICU: the development of a procedure, *Neonatal Netw* 6:41, 1987.

40. Hutto C et al: Intrauterine herpes simplex infections, *J Pediatr* 110:97, 1987.

41. Ikeda MK, Jensen HB: Evaluation and treatment of congenital syphilis, *J Pediatr* 117:843, 1990.

42. Kliegman RM, Clapp DW: Rational principles for immunoglobulin prophylaxis and therapy for neonatal infections, *Clin Perinatol* 18:303, 1991.

43. Landers S, Moise AA, Fraley JK et al: Factors associated with umbilical catheter-related sepsis in neonates, *Am J Dis Child* 145:675, 1991.

44. Long JG, Keyserling HL: Catheter-related infections in infants due to an unusual lipophilic yeast—*Malassezia furfur, Pediatrics* 76:8896, 1985.

45. Manroe BL, Weinberg AG, Rosenfeld CR et al: The neonatal blood count in health and disease. I. Reference values for neutropenic cells, *J Pediatr* 95:89, 1979.

46. Mofenson LM: The role of antiretroviral therapy in the management of HIV infection in women, *Clin Obstet Gynecol* 39:361, 1996.

47. Nelson SN, Merenstein GB, Pierce JR: Early onset group B streptococcal disease, *J Perinatol* 6:234, 1986.

48. Noel GJ, Kreiswirth BN, Edelson PJ et al: Multiple methicillin-resistant *Staphylococcus aureus* strains as a cause for a single outbreak of severe disease in hospitalized neonates, *Pediatr Infect Dis J* 11:184, 1992.

49. Phillips G, Golledge C: Fungal infection in neonates, *J Antimicrob Chemother* 28:159, 1991.

50. Pierce JR, Merenstein GB, Stocker JT: Immediate postpartum cultures in an intensive care nursery, *Pediatr Infect Dis J* 3:510, 1984.

51. Prober CG, Sullender WM, Yasukawa LL et al: Low risk of herpes simplex virus in neonates exposed to the virus at the time of vaginal delivery to mothers with recurrent genital herpes simplex infection, *N Engl J Med* 316:240, 1987.

52. Recommendations for preventing the spread of vancomycin disease, *MMWR Morb Mortal Weekly Rep* 44:1, 1994.

53. Remington JS, Klein JO: *Infectious diseases of the newborn infant,* ed 5, Philadelphia, Pa., 2001, WB Saunders.

54. Rusi P, Adam RO, Peterson EA et al: *Haemophilus influenzae:* an important cause of maternal and neonatal infections, *Obstet Gynecol* 77:92, 1991.

55. Schwerenski J, McIntyre L, Bauer CR: Lumbar puncture frequency and cerebrospinal fluid analysis in the neonate, *Am J Dis Child* 145:54, 1991.

56. St. Geme JW III, Harris MC: Coagulase-negative staphylococcal infection in the neonate, *Clin Perinatol* 18:281, 1991.

57. Stagno S, Pass RF, Dworsky ME et al: Congenital cytomegalovirus infection: the relative importance of primary and recurrent maternal infection, *N Engl J Med* 306:945, 1982.

58. Stoll BJ: Congenital syphilis: evaluation and management of neonates born with reactive serologic tests for syphilis, *Pediatr Infect Dis J* 13:845, 1994.

59. Weisman LE, Stoll BJ, Cruess DF et al: Early onset group B streptococcal sepsis: a current assessment, *J Pediatr* 121:428, 1992.

59a. Weisman LE, Givner L: Adjunctive therapies for the treatment or prevention of sepsis, *Semin Pediatr Infect Dis* 12, 2001.

60. Weiss MG, Ionides SP, Anderson CL: Meningitis in premature infants with respiratory distress: role of admission lumbar puncture, *J Pediatr* 119:973, 1991.

61. Whitley R, Arvin A, Prober C et al: A controlled trial comparing vidabrine with acyclovir in neonatal herpes simplex virus infection, *N Engl J Med* 324:444, 1991.

62. Whitley RJ, Cloud G, Gruber W et al: Ganciclovir treatment of symptomatic congenital cytomegalovirus infection: results of a phase II study, *J Infect Dis* 175:1080, 1997.

63. Wiswell TE, Hachey WE: Multiple site blood cultures in the evaluation for neonatal sepsis during the first week of life, *Pediatr Infect Dis J* 10:365, 1991.

64. Wittek AE, Yeager AS, Au DS et al: Asymptomatic shedding of herpes simplex virus from the cervix and lesion site during pregnancy: correlation of antepartum shedding with shedding at delivery, *Am J Dis Child* 138:439, 1984.

65. Wong VC, Ip HM, Reesink HW et al: Prevention of HBsAg carrier state in the newborn infants of mothers who are chronic carriers of HBsAg and HBeAg by administration of hepatitis-B vaccine and hepatitis-B immunoglobin, *Lancet* 1:921, 1984.

66. Yamauchi T: Nosocomial infections in the newborn, *Curr Opin Infect Dis* 4:474, 1991.

COMMON SYSTEMIC DISEASES OF THE NEONATE

23 | Respiratory Diseases

Mary I. Enzman Hagedorn, Sandra L. Gardner, Steven H. Abman

Despite the marked improvement over the past decade in the outcome of premature newborns with respiratory distress, significant mortality and high morbidity rates persist. Much of the improvement in neonatal mortality has been the result of successful treatment and management of respiratory diseases in the neonate.

In this chapter we present an overview of some of the common respiratory diseases, their treatments, and outcomes. General principles and concepts related to respiratory physiology, etiologic factors, and symptomatology are presented, followed by specific disease processes and their management.

GENERAL PHYSIOLOGY

Any discussion of general respiratory physiology must include some elements of anatomy and embryology and their significance to the clinician (Table 23-1).

Surface-active compounds such as phosphatidylcholine and phosphatidylglycerol stabilize the alveoli. Surface tension forces act on air-fluid interfaces, causing a water droplet to "bead up." The surface-active compound (e.g., soap added to a water droplet) reduces the surface tension and allows the droplet to spread out in a thin film. In the lung, surface tension forces tend to cause alveoli to collapse. A compound such as surfactant reduces surface tension and allows the alveoli to remain open.

The situation, however, is more complicated than just described. LaPlace detailed the magnitude of the pressure (P) exerted at the surface of an air-liquid interface as equaling twice the surface tension (st) divided by the radius (r) of curvature of the surface ($P = 2\ st \div r$). In the absence of surfactant, an alveolus with a small radius of curvature has a greater magnitude of pressure at its surface (tending to collapse it) than does an alveolus with a larger radius of curvature. Therefore smaller alveoli would tend to collapse and empty contained gas into larger alveoli.

Surfactant modifies surface tension by decreasing surface tension when the radius of curvature is small and increasing surface tension when the radius of curvature is greater. An alveolus with a larger radius of curvature has a greater-than-expected pressure (tending to reduce its volume), and an alveolus with a smaller radius of curvature has less-than-expected pressure. Therefore the alveoli are stabilized at a uniform radius of curvature (uniform volume).

Surfactant provides a number of useful properties in addition to reducing surface tension, which increases lung compliance, provides alveolar stability, and decreases opening pressure. It also enhances alveolar fluid clearance, decreases precapillary tone, and plays a protective role for the epithelial cell surface. Surfactant is constantly being formed, stored, secreted, and recycled. **Conditions that interfere with surfactant metabolism include acidemia, hypoxia, shock, overinflation, underinflation, pulmonary edema, mechanical ventilation, and hypercapnia. Surfactant production is delayed in infants of diabetic mothers (IDMs) of classes A, B, and C; infants with erythroblastosis fetalis; and infants who are the smaller of twins.** Surfactant production is accelerated in the following:

- IDMs of classes D, F, and R
- Infants of heroin-addicted mothers
- Premature rupture of membranes of greater than 48 hours' duration
- Infants of mothers with hypertension
- Infants subjected to maternal infection

Table 23-1	LUNG DEVELOPMENT	
STAGE AND MAJOR EVENTS	**SIGNIFICANCE**
Embryonic (Up to 5 Weeks)	
Single ventral outpocketing quickly divides into two lung buds	Airways begin to differentiate
Mesenchyme surrounds endodermal lung buds, which continue to divide and extend into the mesenchyme	
Branching of the airways begins	Branching anomalies (e.g., pulmonary agenesis and sequestered lobe) occur early in fetal life
Pulmonary arteries invade lung tissue, following the airways, and divide as the airways divide	
Pulmonary veins arise independently from the lung parenchyma and return to the left atrium, thus completing the pulmonary circuit	
Pseudoglandular (5-16 Weeks)	
Progressive airway branching begins; bronchi and terminal bronchioles form	All subdivisions that will form airways are complete by the sixteenth week
Muscle fibers, elastic tissue, and early cartilage formation can be seen along the tracheobronchial tree	
Mucous glands are found at 12 weeks and increase in number until 25-26 weeks, when cilia begin to develop	
Diaphragm develops	Herniation of the diaphragm occurs
Cannicular (13-25 Weeks)	
Airway changes from glandular to tubular and increases in length and diameter	Air conducting portion (bronchi and terminal bronchioli) continues luminal development
20 Weeks	
Fetal airways end in blind pouches lined with cuboid epithelium; a relatively large amount of interstitial mesenchyme is present; few pulmonary capillaries are present, and they are not closely associated with the respiratory epithelium	

- Infants suffering from placental insufficiency
- Infants affected by administration of corticosteroids
- Infants affected by abruptio placentae

The fetal lung is filled with a volume of liquid (20 to 30 ml/kg) equal to the functional residual capacity. This fluid is not amniotic fluid but rather a liquid that has been produced in the lung and discharged through the larynx and mouth into the amniotic fluid. Lung fluid is continuously produced at a rate of approximately 2 to 4 ml/kg/hr.

Because of the movement of lung fluid and its components (notably lecithin) into amniotic fluid, the lecithin/sphingomyelin (L/S) ratio has become a notable clinical tool. Noting a sharp increase in the L/S ratio, Gluck and Kulovich[219] found they could predict which infants were at risk for respiratory distress syndrome (RDS). In general, L/S ratios of more than 2:1 are not associated with RDS, whereas ratios of less than 2:1 are associated with it. Phosphatidylglycerol (PG), the second most common phospholipid in surfactant, appears at about 36 weeks' gestation and increases until term. The presence of PG is associated with a very low risk of RDS, whereas its absence is associated with the development of RDS. Unlike the L/S ratio, PG determination is valid in the presence of blood-contaminated amniotic fluid.

During vaginal delivery, approximately one third of the lung fluid may be removed during the thoracic "squeeze" as the infant passes through the birth canal; the remainder of the fluid is removed mainly by the pulmonary lymphatics, although pulmonary capillaries may play a role. After a cesarean section, all of the

Table 23-1	LUNG DEVELOPMENT—cont'd	
STAGE AND MAJOR EVENTS		**SIGNIFICANCE**

22-24 Weeks

Rapid proliferation of the pulmonary capillary bed, an increase of the surface area of the respiratory epithelium, and formation of alveolar ducts and sacculi occur	Development of the gas exchange portion (the respiratory bronchi and alveolar ducts) begins; pulmonary vasculature develops most rapidly
Respiratory epithelium contains cells that become differentiated into type I and type II pneumocytes	
Type I pneumocytes produce an extremely thin squamous epithelial layer that lines the alveoli and fuses to the underlying capillary endothelial cells	By the late fetal period the resulting membrane between the alveoli and capillaries allows sufficient gas exchange to support independent life
Type II pneumocytes (cuboid cells) are the site of surfactant synthesis and storage	At 22 weeks, surface-active phospholipid (lecithin) can first be detected

Terminal (24-40 Weeks)

Lung differentiation: proliferation of the pulmonary vascular bed, creation of new respiratory units (alveolar ducts and alveoli), decrease in amount of interstitial mesenchyme, and fusion of the gas exchange epithelium to the pulmonary capillary epithelium occur	Before this time the fetal lungs are incapable of supporting adequate gas exchange because of insufficient alveolar surface area and inadequate pulmonary vasculature

34-36 Weeks

Phosphatidylglycerol appears, and a dramatic increase in the principal surfactant compound phosphatidylcholine occurs	Adequate amounts of surface-active material protects against the development of respiratory distress syndrome

Alveolar (Postnatal Lung Development) (Late Fetal Life to 8-10 Years of Age)

At term the number of airways is complete; there is sufficient respiratory surface for gaseous exchange, and the pulmonary capillary bed is sufficient to carry the gases that have been exchanged	Although the infant is capable of sustaining respiratory effort and the lung is able to provide oxygenation and ventilation at birth, lung development is still incomplete
Alveoli continue to increase in number, size, and shape; they enlarge and become deeper to maximize the exposed surface area for gas exchange	Ongoing lung development implies that infants who have suffered severe lung disease at birth need not become life-long pulmonary cripples

lung fluid will be removed by the pulmonary lymphatic system and the capillaries.

The first breath of life, a response to tactile, thermal, chemical, and mechanical stimuli, initiates respiratory effort. The fluid-filled lungs, surface forces, and tissue-sensitive forces are obstacles to the first breath. At birth, gas is substituted for liquid to expand the alveoli. After the alveoli are "opened" during the first few breaths, a film of surface-active material stabilizes the alveoli.

The first breath of life requires an opening pressure of 60 to 80 cm of water to overcome the effects of the surface tension of the air-liquid interface, particularly the small airways and alveoli. Thus on each subsequent breath, less pressure is required to allow for a similar increase in air volume in the lung. The effort of breathing is lessened with subsequent breaths.

GENERAL ETIOLOGIC FACTORS

Respiratory disease may be defined as a progressive impairment of the lungs to exchange gas at the alveolar level. Although the pathologic process causing respiratory disease in the neonate may occur in any portion of the respiratory system (or in other organ systems), the final common pathway in respiratory disease is impairment of gas exchange.

Prematurity is the single most common factor in the occurrence of RDS. Its incidence is inversely proportional to gestational age and occurs most frequently in infants of less than 1200 g and 30 weeks' gestation. RDS occurs in male infants twice as frequently as in female infants (2:1).

The principal factor operating in the development of RDS in very premature infants is surfactant deficiency.

Multiple gestations increase the risk of respiratory disease related to lung maturity in the second, third, or more siblings. The second (and subsequent) infants may experience perinatal asphyxia, malpresentation, and mode of delivery (e.g., cesarean section) that contributes to respiratory disease. A recent study shows a significantly increased risk of respiratory disease associated with being the second born preterm twin, especially at 30 to 31 weeks' gestation.[240] Grand multiparity is associated with increased risk of respiratory disease, particularly when other siblings have had RDS.

Prenatal maternal complications increase the risk for respiratory disease in the infant. Maternal illnesses such as cardiorespiratory disease, hypoxia, hemorrhage, shock, hypotension, or hypertension result in decreased uterine blood flow with subsequent hypoxia or ischemia at the placental level. Severe maternal anemia causes fetal cardiac depression and respiratory depression. Maternal diabetes may result in preterm delivery because of fetal and maternal indications. There is also a greater incidence of false-positive L/S ratios in diabetic populations. There has been a propensity of IDMs to develop RDS despite documentation of L/S ratios greater than 2:1. (A combination of an L/S ratio greater than or equal to 2:1 and the presence of PG confirms fetal lung maturity.) Abnormal placental conditions (compressed umbilical cord caused by prolapse or breech delivery, placental disease such as infarcts or syphilis, or hemorrhage as a result of placenta previa or abruptio placentae) affect oxygen transfer from mother to fetus and result in an asphyxial insult to the developing fetal lung. Premature rupture of the membranes predisposes the fetus or newborn to the development of infections such as pneumonia, sepsis, or meningitis. Premature or prolonged rupture of the membranes not associated with neonatal infection accelerates fetal lung development and thereby lessens the incidence of RDS. Prenatal administration of glucocorticoids,[411] maternal toxemia, and maternal heroin addiction also hasten fetal lung maturation.

Factors affecting the fetus during the birth process may lead to respiratory distress. Depression of the respiratory center can occur as a result of maternal medications that cross the placenta. An infant delivered shortly after an analgesic or anesthetic is administered to the mother may have only minimal respiratory efforts at birth. Excessive uterine activity, usually as a result of oxytocin induction or augmentation of labor, results in decreased

uterine blood flow, late fetal heart deceleration, and respiratory depression in the infant at birth. Respiratory disease may be the result of direct trauma to the respiratory center or a cerebral hemorrhage in close proximity to it. Fetal shock caused by difficult labor or dystocia, tight nuchal cord, cerebral hemorrhage, or hemorrhage from the fetal side of the placenta results in CNS depression and hypoxia. Bleeding results in a generalized hypovolemic condition characterized by decreased oxygen-carrying capacity. Fetal or neonatal asphyxia and blood loss lead to progressive respiratory distress. Delivery by cesarean section prevents one third of the lung fluid from being expelled by the thoracic squeeze of vaginal birth. Thus after cesarean birth all lung fluid must be absorbed through circulatory and lymphatic channels; therefore a greater incidence of transient tachypnea of the newborn may occur as the increased volume of retained fluid is absorbed.

The role of cesarean section in the development of RDS is still controversial. However, the general consensus is that cesarean section delivery in the absence of fetal distress is not associated with an increased incidence of RDS. Yet a correlation appears between absence of labor and increased risk of developing RDS, but the amount of retained lung fluid may be the significant factor.

Obstruction of the airway caused by aspiration of meconium or amniotic fluid occurs either spontaneously at birth or during resuscitative efforts. Although the lungs initially fill with air, subsequent atelectasis occurs as complete airway obstruction prevents further entrance of air. Conversely, a "ball valve" effect or "air-trapping" effect may occur as air is allowed in but is unable to escape because of intermittent obstruction. The presence of amniotic debris, vernix, lanugo, and meconium in the respiratory tract increases the incidence and severity of pulmonary infection. Diaphragmatic paralysis occurs after phrenic nerve injury during birth (usually in an LGA infant) and is often associated with Erb's palsy. The paradoxic movement of the paralyzed diaphragm during inspiration and expiration results in inadequate tidal volume and impaired gaseous exchange.

Existing neonatal conditions increase the risk of respiratory disease. Congenital defects that prevent transmission of the stimulus to or from the respiratory center, prevent normal respiratory effort, reduce gas exchange surface area, or hamper the delivery of oxygen to the site of exchange will predispose the infant to respiratory embarrassment. Such defects include heart or great vessel anomalies, diaphragmatic hernia and hypoplastic lung, respiratory tract anomalies (e.g., choanal atresia or tracheoesophageal fistula), chest wall deformities, and CNS defects.

Diseases of the infant can also lead to respiratory disease. Hemolytic disease, such as ABO and Rh incompatibility, results in anemia and, if severe, in hypovolemic shock. Blood incompatibilities increase respiratory distress by decreasing the oxygen-carrying capacity of the blood. Infections stress the body's systems, increase oxygen requirements, and contribute to an impairment of surfactant production. Chronic lung disease in the form of bronchopulmonary dysplasia (BPD) occurs in 17% to 54% of VLBW infants.[383] Prolonged treatment of RDS may be necessitated by the severity of the disease but may increase the risk of developing chronic lung disease.

GENERAL PREVENTION

Antepartum

Prevention of respiratory disease begins with prevention of conditions that predispose to respiratory distress. These conditions that constitute "reproductive risks" have been identified and can be categorized as psychosocial, genetic, biophysical, or economic in nature. Once an individual is identified as being in a high-risk category, comprehensive prenatal care with immediate attention given to maternal complications that arise is crucial (see Chapters 2 and 3).

Intrapartum

Fetal well-being is assessed by using electronic monitoring of uterine activity and fetal heart rate and fetal scalp blood sampling. Electronic fetal heart rate monitoring enables instantaneous fetal heart rate tracings as opposed to the previous method of intermittent evaluation by stethoscope. Fetal heart rate monitoring allows for coincident correlation between uterine contractions and fetal response. These tools enable the practitioner to evaluate how well the fetus withstands the stresses of labor and to make decisions regarding the laboring course.

Fetal cardiac response to stress is unlike an older child's or adult's response to hypoxia, hypercapnia, and acidosis with tachycardia from sympathetic nervous system discharge. A fetus responds to these same stresses with an initial increase in heart rate.

This is quickly followed by bradycardia from parasympathetic stimulation when the hypoxia, hypercapnia, and acidosis persist (see Chapter 2).

Postpartum

After delivery an infant should be maintained in an environment that minimizes stress and thereby minimizes oxygen requirement. All infants, but particularly at-risk infants, should be maintained within the narrow parameter of physiologic homeostasis (as outlined in Part II).

GENERAL DATA COLLECTION

Because the clinical manifestations of many neonatal illnesses include respiratory symptoms (cardiac, metabolic, neurologic, and hematologic), a systematic and thorough approach to data collection is essential in evaluating an infant in respiratory distress.

History

The perinatal history (antepartum, intrapartum, and postpartum) should be reviewed for risk factors (see Chapter 2).

Signs and Symptoms

Vital signs such as temperature, pulse, respiration, and blood pressure should be evaluated. Hypothermia and hyperthermia increase oxygen requirements by altering the basal metabolic rate. Hypotension is often associated with respiratory disease.

Respiratory Examination

Respiratory effort is normally irregular in rate and depth, and is chiefly abdominal, rather than thoracic, with a rate of 30 to 60 breaths/min. Bradypnea is characterized by a rate below 30 breaths/min that is regular (as opposed to periodic or apneic) and may be caused by an insult to the respiratory center of the CNS. Tachypnea, a rate above 60 breaths/min after the first hour of life, is the earliest symptom of respiratory (and often other) diseases. As a compensatory mechanism, tachypnea attempts to maintain alveolar ventilation and gaseous exchange. As a decompensatory mechanism, tachypnea increases oxygen demand, energy output, and the "work" of breathing.

Periodic respirations are cyclic respirations of apnea (5 to 10 seconds) and ventilation (10 to 15 seconds). The average respiratory rate is 30 to 40 breaths/min. Periodic breathing is a common occurrence in small preterm infants as a result of an immature CNS. **Apnea is a nonbreathing episode lasting longer than 20 seconds and accompanied by physiologic alterations.** The syndrome of apnea is discussed later in this chapter.

Use of accessory muscles of respiration is indicative of a marked increase in the work of breathing. Retractions reflect the inward pull of the thin chest wall on inspiration. Retracting is best observed in relation to the sternum (substernal and suprasternal) and the intercostal, supracostal, and subcostal spaces. The increased negative intrathoracic pressure necessary to ventilate the stiff, noncompliant lung causes the chest wall to retract. This further compromises the lung's expansion. The degree of retraction is directly proportional to the severity of the disease.

Nasal flaring is a compensatory mechanism that attempts to take in more oxygen by increasing the size of the nares and thus decreasing the resistance (by as much as 40%) of the narrow airways. Grunting is forced expiration through a partially closed glottis. The audible grunt may be heard with or without the aid of a stethoscope. As a compensatory mechanism, grunting stabilizes the alveoli by increasing transpulmonary pressure and increases gaseous exchange by delaying expiration.[74]

Color is normally pink after the first breaths of life. Acrocyanosis, which is peripheral cyanosis of the hands and feet in the first 24 hours of life, is normal. **Pallor with poor peripheral circulation may indicate systemic hypotension. Ruddy, plethoric skin color may indicate hyperviscosity or polycythemia, or both, as causes of respiratory symptoms.** However, the lack of a deep-red coloring does not rule out polycythemia or hyperviscosity.

Cyanosis, a late and serious sign, is a blue discoloration of the skin, nail beds, and mucous membranes. Differentiation between peripheral cyanosis (of hands and feet) and central cyanosis (of mucous membranes of mouth and generalized body cyanosis) is essential. Because a large decrease in Pao_2 may be tolerated without detectable cyanosis, the lack of cyanosis does not ensure a healthy infant. When hypoxemia reaches a level that produces frank cyanosis, the insufficiency is usually in advanced stages (see Chapter 11). Therefore cyanosis or its lack is not a reliable sign in neonates.

Symmetry of the newborn chest is characterized by a relatively round or barrel shape, because the anteroposterior diameter equals the transverse diameter. With prolonged respiratory distress, there is

an increase in the anteroposterior diameter, so that the neonate becomes pigeon-chested.

Auscultation of a newborn's chest includes comparing and contrasting one side with the other and noting the quality of breath sounds and the presence or absence of rales, rhonchi, or other abnormal sounds. Because of the relatively small size of the newborn's chest, it is hyperresonant, so that breath sounds are widely transmitted. Therefore one cannot always rely on auscultation to detect pathologic conditions (e.g., pneumothorax). Percussion of the chest to determine the presence of air, fluid, or solids may not be useful in the neonate because of small chest size and hyperresonance. Palpation of the neonatal chest wall while the infant is crying may detect gross changes in sound transmission through the chest. Palpation of crepitus in the neck, around the clavicles, or on the chest wall suggests the complication of air leak.

Nonrespiratory Examination

Hypotonia is characterized by a froglike positioning and a lax, open mouth. Progressing from flexion to flaccidity indicates progression of hypoxia and exhaustion from the work of breathing. Cardiac findings such as a murmur, absence of pulses, bounding pulses, palmar or calf pulses, weight gain, hepatosplenomegaly, cyanosis, edema, bradycardia, or tachycardia indicate congestive heart failure or congenital heart defects. A scaphoid abdomen indicates a diaphragmatic hernia.

Laboratory Data

Because the clinical presentation of many respiratory and nonrespiratory diseases is the same, a chest x-ray examination may be the only way to differentiate cause and establish the proper diagnosis. X-ray evaluation helps eliminate congenital anomalies (e.g., diaphragmatic hernia with lung hypoplasia, masses, and obstruction) as the cause when acquired respiratory disease (e.g., RDS, transient tachypnea of the newborn, and pneumonia) is the cause of the distress. X-ray films confirm the presence of pneumothorax or other pulmonary air leaks.

Measurement of arterial blood gases is used to demonstrate alterations in oxygenation and acid-base balance and to differentiate between respiratory and metabolic components. Initial baseline values are followed by serial observations at least every 15 to 30 minutes after any change in therapy during the acute phase of illness. Pulse oximetry enables immediate evaluation of oxygenation status and is an adjunct to arterial blood gas sampling.[17] **A shunt study may differentiate between lung origin and cardiac origin of respiratory distress.** The symptoms of pulmonary disease (cyanosis and low PaO_2) are often alleviated with crying, increased FiO_2, and/or continuous positive airway pressure. If the same symptoms are cardiac in origin, they remain unchanged or worsen with these interventions. Administration of 100% FiO_2 for 10 minutes or longer may result in an increased PaO_2 (greater than 100 mm Hg), whereas in cardiac disease caused by right-to-left shunting there is no change in PaO_2 after 100% FiO_2 administration. CAUTION: In the presence of severe lung disease with significant right-to-left shunting, cyanosis and PaO_2 may not be changed with 100% FiO_2.

The hematocrit value is used to rule out anemia or polycythemia as the cause of the respiratory distress. In anemia, inadequate oxygen content promotes tissue hypoxia. In polycythemia, increased viscosity and sludging of blood flow adversely affect tissue oxygenation.

The white blood cell count, differential, and C-reactive protein (CRP) (see Chapter 22) aid in diagnosing sepsis as the cause of distress. A blood culture is an invaluable aid when infection is suspected and should be obtained before antibiotic therapy is initiated. Blood glucose determination to rule out hypoglycemia as a cause is particularly important in IDMs, SGA infants, LGA infants, and preterm AGA infants. An electrocardiogram (ECG), echocardiogram, and cardiac catheterization are used to rule out cardiac abnormalities.

An electroencephalogram (EEG) and ultrasonographic examination of the brain help to rule out CNS abnormalities. Serum electrolytes (calcium, sodium, and potassium) aid in eliminating metabolic aberration as the cause of the distress.

GENERAL TREATMENT STRATEGIES

Treatment of any condition should be directed at correction of its underlying cause. In meconium aspiration syndrome, if prevention of the aspiration through thorough suction is to no avail, damage to the neonatal lung results. No therapeutic measure is available at present to augment the healing process. Therapy is thus directed at preventing or alleviating the consequences of neonatal lung diseases, such as hypoxemia and acidemia, allowing healing to take place and reducing the potential for iatrogenic complications.

Respiratory support is the hallmark of treatment of neonatal respiratory disease. Respiratory support involves increasing inspired oxygen tensions and providing ventilation if required.

Supplemental Oxygen

When the neonate is unable to maintain adequate oxygenation, supplemental oxygen must be provided. Because oxygen is a drug, it must be treated as such and given only for specific indications. Biochemical criteria (PaO_2 less than 60 mm Hg) and clinical criteria such as respiratory distress, central cyanosis, apnea, asphyxia, hypotonia, and low oxygen saturation are indications to prescribe oxygen.

Regardless of the mode of delivery (hood, nasal prongs, endotracheal tube, bag, or mask), safe and effective oxygen administration follows certain principles:

- No concentration of oxygen has been proved to be "safe." A concentration (e.g., 30%, 40%, 80%, 100%) that is therapeutic for one infant may be toxic for another.
- To titrate inspired oxygen concentrations to the individual infant's need, arterial PO_2 should be measured and maintained between 60 and 80 mm Hg.
- Oxygen administration without some form of continuous monitoring of the infant's oxygenation (e.g., arterial blood gases, pulse oximetry) is dangerous and not recommended.[17]
- Delivered oxygen should be humidified (30% to 40%), because dry gases are irritating to the airways and humidity decreases insensible water losses. To prevent respiratory therapy equipment from becoming a source of infection, humidifiers and tubing should be replaced per institutional/product protocol.
- Oxygen should be warmed (31° to 34° C [88° to 94° F]) so temperature at the delivery site is the same as the incubator temperature. Oxygen delivered by endotracheal tube should be warmed to core temperature (i.e., 36.5° to 37° C [97.9° to 98.6° F]). This prevents cold stress and increased oxygen consumption from blowing cold air in the infant's face.[532]
- Oxygen concentration must be monitored by continuous or intermittent sampling (at least every hour) and recorded. Oxygen monitors and analyzers should be calibrated to room air and 100% oxygen level every 8 hours.[17]
- A stable concentration of oxygen is necessary to maintain PaO_2 within normal limits. A sudden

increase or decrease in oxygen concentration may result in a disproportionate increase or decrease in PaO_2 caused by vasodilation or vasoconstriction in response to oxygen.[532] Adjustment of supplemental oxygen (particularly lowering FiO_2) must be done slowly to avoid the *flip-flop phenomenon.* Hypoxic insult initiates pulmonary vasoconstriction, which causes hypoperfusion and increased pulmonary vascular resistance. The infant should be weaned from supplemental oxygen cautiously.[532] (Refer to Chapter 11 for a discussion of the "rule of seven," which states that the estimated percentage change in inspired oxygen is equal to the desired change in PaO_2 divided by 7.)

- Observing color, respiratory effort, activity, and circulatory response and monitoring arterial oxygen concentration aid in determining the need for oxygen therapy and for appropriate adjustments.
- Clinical observations, FiO_2 concentrations, and time of adjustments must be described, documented, and reported.
- Oxygen concentration should be returned to previous levels if clinical observations of distress and inability to tolerate decreased levels of oxygen occur.

Delivery Methods

For instructions on the bag and mask resuscitation method, see Chapter 4.

An **oxygen hood** is a clear plastic hood that fits over the infant's head to deliver a constant concentration of oxygen. If the infant has sufficient ventilation to maintain a normal arterial carbon dioxide tension, oxygenation by increased inspired oxygen tensions through an oxygen hood may be all the respiratory support that is required. This degree of support is particularly applicable in cases of mild RDS, transient tachypnea of the newborn (TTN), meconium aspiration, or neonatal pneumonia.

A **blender system** is the most reliable way to administer a fixed oxygen concentration via a hood. An appropriately sized hood should be used. If it is too large, the infant may slip out of the hood and FiO_2 may be diluted by leaks; if it is too small, pressure points may develop, especially around the neck. Another source of oxygen must be provided when the infant's head is removed from the hood because of feeding, being held, or suctioning. This secondary source may be set up from the blender source so that the infant's PaO_2 remains constant during suctioning

or feedings. The infant may need increased FiO_2 from the secondary source, and this can be easily adjusted according to assessments made with pulse oximetry; these changes should be recorded.

For both home and hospital use, **a nasal cannula is used to administer oxygen to the dependent infant who is developing social and motor skills.**[577]

- Choose the appropriately sized cannula for the infant.
- Position the cannula across the infant's upper lip. Secure it to the infant's face by first applying Stomahesive or Tegaderm (OpSite) directly to the infant's cheeks and taping the cannula to it to prevent skin irritation.

CAUTION: Neonates are obligatory nasal breathers, so that nasal obstruction (mucus or milk) will decrease the amount of oxygen actually received. Therefore nares should be suctioned as needed. **The exact concentrations of oxygen delivered by cannula cannot be measured.**[595] **Flow rates are titrated by monitoring PaO_2 and/or pulse oximetry levels and by evaluating the clinical course.** Use of nasal cannulas with oxygen rates above 0.5 L/min may result in inadvertent administration of continuous distending (positive) pressure, causing increased respiratory effort (i.e., tachypnea, retractions, exaggerated periodic breathing).[366,595] However, a newer study comparing the use of nasal cannula high flow (e.g., up to 2.5 L/min) with nasal CPAP for treatment of apnea found that the nasal cannula high flow oxygen was as effective as nasal CPAP. Preterm infants with high flow nasal cannula oxygen tolerated it well, had no drying of the nares, and no ventilation was required.[528] Oxygen tubing should be long enough to provide opportunities for social and gross motor skill development.

Continuous Distending Pressure

Application of a continuous distending pressure (CDP) to the lungs increases functional residual capacity and PaO_2. It improves oxygenation by decreasing intrapulmonary shunting and by improving the match of ventilation and perfusion. The application of CDP improves compliance of the lung and lessens the work of breathing.[229]

In RDS, where the functional residual capacity is reduced, increased respiratory oxygen tensions through an oxygen hood (Oxyhood) may not be sufficient to maintain an adequate arterial oxygen tension. More invasive techniques may be required. **CPAP or continuous negative pressure (CNP) are two methods of delivery of CDP.** If the infant

Table 23-2	CONTINUOUS POSITIVE AIRWAY PRESSURE (CPAP)	
INDICATIONS	**COMPLICATIONS**
Infant who breathes spontaneously yet has mild to moderate respiratory distress syndrome (RDS)	Respiratory difficulty secondary to narrowing of the nasal passage with prongs or trachea with the presence of an endotracheal tube
Very low birth weight (VLBW) infant with primary or secondary apnea	Pneumothorax and other air leaks
During the weaning process from ventilatory support	Nasal irritation, trauma, deformity, infection, obstruction; gastric and abdominal distention; perforation

cannot maintain a PaO_2 of 60 mm Hg in 0.6 FiO_2, a trial of CPAP through the nasal route is indicated. Initial levels of CPAP should be in the range of 4 to 5 cm of water. CPAP should be increased to 8 to 10 cm of water by 1 to 2 cm increments if required to raise the infant's PaO_2 (as measured by arterial blood gas determinations, noninvasive monitoring, or both).

Indications and complications in the use of CPAP are listed in Table 23-2. If the infant is able to maintain ventilation as indicated by normal arterial carbon dioxide tension, no further respiratory support may be required. Although early institution of nasal CPAP in the management of respiratory insufficiency may reduce the need for mechanical ventilation,[373] in one study 43% to 80% of infants with RDS eventually needed mechanical ventilation.[570]

CPAP may be delivered by face mask, nasal pharyngeal tubes, nasal prongs, or ET tube. Delivery of CPAP by nasal prongs is the most common method used. However, in much of the research literature nasal prongs are compared with nasal pharyngeal tubes for administration of CPAP. **Advantages to the use of nasal CPAP include** (1) less invasive than endotracheal tube, (2) decreases incidence, duration and complications of intubation, (3) earlier extubation, and (4) decreases the incidence and morbidity of BPD/chronic lung disease.* **Disadvantages include** (1) gaseous distention of the bowel,[290] (2) gastrointestinal perforation,[209] (3) difficulties keeping prongs in the nose, maintaining patency, and infant agitation, and (4) alteration in appearance (dilation of the nares). Placing an OG tube for decompression, PRN suctioning of the nares, comfort measures, and use of medications for sedation/pain relief may be necessary (see Chapter 12).

---

*References 27, 216, 289, 305, 373, 383, 570.

Box 23-1	CRITERIA THAT INDICATE IMPROVEMENT ON CPAP[18]

Blood Gases

- Decrease or stabilization of oxygen requirement FiO_2 $\leq$0.60 with PaO_2 >50 mm Hg or pulse oximetry >90%
- Maintenance of adequate ventilation $PaCO_2$ $\leq$50-60 mm Hg pH 7.25-7.45

Clinical

- Decreased work of breathing—decreased respiratory rate, grunting, flaring, and retracting
- Improved lung volumes and appearance on chest x-ray films
- Improved patient comfort

Criteria that indicate improvement on CPAP are listed in Box 23-1. When the infant's PaO_2 is consistently over 70 mm Hg, inspired oxygen concentration and/or CDP may be lowered. Oxygen concentration is usually lowered in 5% to 10% increments to a level of 40% to 60%. CDP is lowered in increments of 1 cm of water to a level of 2 cm of water before discontinuation. The infant may then be placed into an oxygen hood with the same FiO_2. Neonates should be closely monitored with pulse oximetry and arterial blood gases.

Pulmonary Hygiene

Pulmonary hygiene is normally maintained by ciliary activity, a covering of mucus, and narrowing and dilation of the bronchi with respiration and coughing. Anatomic and physiologic variations in the neonate alter these normal pulmonary mechanisms. The small airway of the neonate has a diameter that is four times smaller than that of the normal adult. Debris that causes only a moderate obstruction for the adult airway causes a disproportionately greater obstruction of the smaller airway of the neonate. Also, a neonate normally has an underdeveloped cough reflex. A sick neonate with insufficient respiratory effort and a weak or nonexistent cry has underventilated lungs. If a neonate who is attached to multiple life-support systems is cared for in the same position, secretions localize in the dependent pulmonary tree and predispose to hypostatic pneumonia.

Pulmonary hygiene consists of two major components: chest physiotherapy (CPT) and suctioning. The goals of pulmonary hygiene are:

- To maintain a patent airway by clearing secretions
- To promote optimal pulmonary oxygenation and ventilation
- To prevent pulmonary infection from accumulated secretions
- To facilitate removal of pulmonary debris by loosening and mobilizing secretions into the mainstem bronchi for suctioning

Pulmonary hygiene has been used as a treatment for intubated patients with conditions associated with atelectasis, increased secretions, and pulmonary debris (pneumonia, meconium aspiration, RDS, and BPD).

Chest Physiotherapy

Chest physiotherapy (CPT) consists of positioning, percussion, and vibration. Postural changes use gravity to facilitate the movement of pulmonary debris from smaller to larger bronchi. Postural changes used with pediatric and adult respiratory patients have been used for neonatal CPT. **However, most ill neonates, especially VLBW and ELBW infants, do not tolerate multiple positioning and repositioning.** Periodic (every 2 to 4 hours with care) repositioning changes the ventilation/perfusion matching in dependent lung areas and improves oxygenation.[143] Prone positioning improves lung mechanics, lung volumes, and improves oxygenation.[385,502,578]

Percussion of the chest wall creates a suction action that loosens secretions. Percussion should occur through gently tapping over the affected lung every 2 to 4 hours. **In infants with BPD, rib fractures have been documented that resulted from vigorous percussion**[168,459] **and vibrator use.**[602] Vibration of the neonate's chest may follow percussion. Even though vibration must be done on expiration to move secretions with the exhalation of air,

this is very difficult to accomplish with the neonate's rapid, shallow breathing cycle.

Any manipulation of the sick neonate has the potential for decreasing oxygenation and precipitating hypoxia.[175,368] **During CPT, bradycardia, cyanosis, hypotonia, fighting, struggling, and alterations in oxygenation are signs of stress.** Both increases[469] but more often decreases in oxygenation occur with CPT.* Pulse oximeter readings show that pulmonary hygiene lowers oxygen tension. Research into the effectiveness of CPT in preventing and treating postextubation atelectasis is also conflicting. Two recent studies and one review found that CPT is not effective in preventing and treating postextubation atelectasis.[7,63,190] Another study found that CPT does decrease postextubation atelectasis in infants with multiple intubations, PDA, and sepsis[423] and reduces the use of reintubation in the overall review of three studies.[190]

The most severe complications reportedly resulting from CPT are an increased risk of intraventricular hemorrhage (IVH) (see Chapter 26) and cerebral encephalopathy. An increased incidence of severe intraventricular/periventricular hemorrhage has been reported in preterm infants treated with early CPT.[468,470] In 1992 a previously unrecognized and distinct pattern of severe, late onset brain injury was reported in 15 neonates (24 to 32 weeks' gestational age; 600 to 1270 g birth weight). The pattern of brain injury was of extensive, dense, and cystic lesions involving the periphery of the brain bilaterally. This full-thickness cortical necrosis, called *encephaloclastic porencephaly,* resulted in 14 deaths and severe neurologic deficit in the only survivor.[121] This nursery changed their protocol to include holding the baby's head steady during CPT; no further cases of brain injury have occurred.[466]

Another study of 454 babies found 13 babies (24 to 27 weeks' gestational age; 680 to 1100 g birth weight) with lesions similar to the encephaloclastic porencephaly described above. The lesions in these infants were described as cystic with cortical and subcortical destruction, and peripheral rather than periventricular; they occurred between 2 to 3 weeks of life. These hemorrhagic infarcts are consistent with the pathologic changes in older infants from shaken-baby syndrome. The extremely immature brain of the

---

VLBW infant may be particularly vulnerable to the shaking movements of CPT.[252] Five of these infants died; seven of the eight surviving infants had handicaps (e.g., mild hemiplegia to severe spastic quadriplegia; cognitive delay) at 6 to 16 months of age. For longer than 3 years no VLBW infant in this NICU has received CPT in the first month of life; no further cases of this brain injury have occurred.[109,252]

CPT has not been studied sufficiently regarding technique, efficacy, complications, outcomes, safety, and frequency. Given the lack of data, the lack of clear evidence of benefit, and the concerns of safety for VLBW infants, recommendations include the following:

- Use CPT cautiously[190]
- Do not use CPT on VLBW infants in the first month of life[252]
- Keep the infant's head steady during CPT[466]
- CPT should only occur for definite indications when the infant is fit and able to tolerate the procedure[466]
- CPT should never be done "routinely" but on an individual basis after careful and thorough assessment[466]
- Percussion should only be used when secretions are not cleared by suction alone[466]
- Use of CPT in the delivery room lacks evidence-based research to support its use[146]
- CPT should not be included in pulmonary hygiene until research clearly substantiates its benefits[604]

Suctioning

Once secretions are loosened and mobilized, they must be removed through the nose, mouth, and/or trachea with suctioning.

Nasooropharyngeal Suctioning. When an infant has no artificial airway, suctioning the nasooropharynx serves two purposes: removing secretions and initiating a cough reflex that mobilizes secretions. With either a suction bulb or catheter, the infant is suctioned when secretions are produced. Providing an oxygen source during the procedure is necessary. Because stimulation of the nares causes reflex inspiration with possible inhalation of oropharyngeal contents, first the mouth and then the nose should be suctioned. The results should be documented.

CAUTION: Suctioning should be avoided for 30 minutes to 1 hour after feeding unless it is necessary to establish a patent airway. The catheter should be gently inserted upward and back into the nares, never forced. If the catheter is hard to pass or the nares seem blocked, this procedure should be abandoned to prevent swelling and/or trauma. **Frequent nasal suction creates trauma and edema. The catheter may initiate vasovagal stimulation with resultant bradycardia.**

Endotracheal Suctioning. An artificial airway prevents normal warming, humidifying, and cleansing of the air by the upper airway. The presence of the foreign body (the tube) also increases pulmonary secretions. **To maintain a patent airway, sterile endotracheal suction should be performed on an individual basis, never on a routine basis (e.g., on a schedule of every 2, 3, or 4 hours).** In one study suction frequency was decided based on time, patient stability, routine, desaturations, decreased air entry, and previous secretion removal. In this study there was no consensus by the nurses on even a single factor used to make this decision.[112] **Individual assessment criteria to establish that the infant "needs" suction are listed in Box 23-2.** Knowledge

---

Box 23-2 INDIVIDUAL ASSESSMENT CRITERIA FOR SUCTION

Evidence of Secretions

- Visible secretions in tube
- Audible coarse, wet, or decreased breath sounds
- Palpation of wet, coarse vibrations through chest wall

Alterations in Vital Signs

- Changes in respiratory pattern:
  Increased work of breathing (retractions, grunting, flaring)
  Tachypnea/apnea
- Change in cardiac pattern: tachycardia or bradycardia

Alteration in Neonatal State

- Increased agitation, irritability, restlessness
- Hypertonic/hypotonic
- Listless, lethargic

Alteration in Oxygenation and Ventilation

- Desaturations (<90%) or labile saturations on pulse oximeter
- Skin color changes—pale, dusky, cyanotic
- Changes in arterial blood gas values—increased PCO_2, decreased PaO_2, respiratory acidosis
- Increased PIP on mechanical ventilation and increased high-pressure alarms

PIP, Peak inspiratory pressure.

of the infant's respiratory diagnosis suggests the need and the frequency of suction. The acute phase (first 72 hours) of RDS is a restrictive disease—few secretions are produced so that minimal suctioning (every 12 to 24 hours) is required. In one study, when suction frequency was changed from every 6 to every 12 hours during the first 72 hours of RDS, there was no increase in secretions or occluded tubes.[594] Disease processes noted for secretion production (e.g., the chronic phase of RDS, BPD/CLD, meconium aspiration syndrome, or pneumonia) may require early and frequent suctioning.[604]

Endotracheal tube suctioning (ETT) is not an innocuous procedure. **ETT suction is associated with numerous physiologic alterations and complications (see Box 23-3).** Hypoxia and changes in heart rate and blood pressure alter cerebral blood flow, increase intracranial pressure, and predispose the preterm to an increased risk of IVH (see Chapter 26). Pulse oximetry is a valuable tool in assessing oxygenation status during and after suctioning. If oxygen saturation falls (below 90%) during suctioning, the infant may be hyperventilated or hyperoxygenated. Hyperventilation (e.g., increasing respiratory rate) with a bag or the manual breaths on the ventilator, after each catheter pass, minimizes hypoxia, and contributes to shortened time of stabilization and recovery.[36] Hyperoxygenation is the increase of FiO_2 above baseline concentration until recovery occurs. To avoid exposing the preterm to hyperoxic events that may predispose to retinopathy of prematurity (ROP), the FiO_2 is increased by 10% to 20% above baseline.[340,469] If baseline oxygenation is decreased or marginal, the FiO_2 should be increased to 100%.[469] More research is needed on the optimal timing of increasing the FiO_2 and the amount of oxygen to use.[36,469,473,579] Pain medication may be used to decrease the periods of hypoxia, alterations in cerebral blood flow, and increased intracranial pressure associated with the pain of suctioning (see Chapter 12).[62,69]

Most of the physiologic alterations and complications of ETT suction are the result of decreases in PEEP, lung volume, and oxygen during disconnection of the ETT from the ventilator for use of the open suction procedure. Use of closed suction systems (e.g., an adapter to suction without disconnection from the ventilator) decreases associated hypoxemia and bradycardia by enabling oxygenation and ventilation to continue during suction.* Closed suction is asso-

---

*References 114, 224, 234, 235, 300, 603.

Box 23-3   PHYSIOLOGIC ALTERATIONS AND COMPLICATIONS ASSOCIATED WITH ENDOTRACHEAL TUBE SUCTION

Hypoxia/hypoxemia—References 83, 175, 176, 318, 368, 372, 420, 448, 514
Caused by disconnection from the ventilator and oxygen as well as presence of suction catheter and application of negative pressure that partially occludes the airway; handling during the procedure.
Alterations in heart rate—References 175, 176, 300, 368
Dysrhythmias, bradycardia, asystole are precipitated by hypoxemia.
Alterations in blood pressure—References 166, 175, 368, 505, 507
Hypertension/hypotension.
Alterations in cerebral blood flow—References 50, 56, 166, 339, 372, 445, 491, 505, 507
Changes in oxygenation, heart rate, and blood pressure increase intracranial pressure.
Tissue damage—References 69, 113, 233, 336, 337, 340, 394, 409
Granuloma formation within airways; increased severity of BPD/CLD associated with colonization of lungs with gram-negative bacilli; lobar emphysema and atelectasis; bronchial stenosis.
Atelectasis—References 175, 409
Microatelectasis of lung tissue may occur during suction; positive pressure ventilation may prevent/resolve but hyperinflation (e.g., use of positive pressure greater than baseline) increases risk of pneumothorax.
Pneumothorax—Reference 80
From aggressively ventilating neonate above baseline pressures.
Infection—References 114, 534
Airway colonization with gram-positive cocci and gram-negative bacilli by 2 weeks of life despite the method of suction.
Accidental extubation.

ciated with smaller decreases in cerebral oxygenation, smaller variations in cerebral blood volume, and related hemodynamic changes particularly in ventilated preterms.[403,492] Closed suction removes secretions as effectively as open suction[601] with no increase in the rate of bacterial airway colonization (with catheter change every 24 hours), suction frequency, reintubation, duration of mechanical ventilation, length of hospitalization, incidence of nosocomial pneumonia/sepsis, severity of BPD/CLD, or mortality in 175 LBW infants.[114] Enclosure of the catheter in a clear sheath decreases the possibility of cross-contamination and environmental pollution of objects and personnel with bacterial and viral pathogens.[104] Closed suction systems are easier to use, less time consuming, better tolerated by the neonate, cost effective, and well accepted by neonatal nurses.[114,300]

The actual procedures used in closed and open suction are often not supported by research data. Table 23-3 outlines common suction techniques, research data, and recommendations to alter clinical practice.

PROCEDURE FOR CLOSED SUCTION

Equipment To Be Prepared
- Inline suction catheter (changed daily)
- Sterile normal saline (without preservative)
- Suction canister and tubing (60 to 80 mm Hg negative pressure)

Procedure
- Unlock the inline suction catheter. Press suction control valve and check suction pressure.
- Place saline solution syringe on the proximal port of the adapter to irrigate the catheter before suction, place normal saline syringe or bullet at the distal port or adapter and squeeze saline solution into the port while simultaneously applying suctioning.
- Slide the catheter through the plastic cover down the endotracheal tube to the predetermined distance.
- Apply suction while withdrawing the catheter tip to the catheter window (the plastic cover will inflate from ventilation if the catheter is pulled back too far; the catheter will completely or partially occlude the ventilatory circuit if not pulled back far enough). Only one suction attempt should be made before the infant is again ventilated. Assess tolerance of the procedure by observing pulse oximeter and infant's color, heart rate, tone, and activity. Hyperventilate the lungs with appropriate FiO_2 for 6 to 8 breaths or until adequate oxygenation has been established.
- To irrigate the catheter after suction, place a normal saline syringe at the distal port adapter and squeeze saline solution into the port while simultaneously applying suction. Remove the saline solution and close the port when the catheter has been thoroughly rinsed.
- Rotate and lock the suction control cap to discontinue suction.
- Suction the nasopharynx and oropharynx prn with a suction bulb or separate suction catheter and tubing. *Do not* disconnect the closed suction catheter from its suction line—this contaminates the setup for ETT suction.
- Check respirator settings, including alarm system in "on" position. Check tube position to be sure the tracheal tube is not strained or bent.
- Note amount and type of secretions obtained.

PROCEDURE FOR OPEN SUCTION

Equipment To Be Prepared
- Sterile suction catheter of appropriate size (discard after each suctioning)
- Sterile gloves
- Sterile normal saline solution (without preservative)
- Stethoscope
- Suction machine and tubing (60 to 80 mm Hg negative pressure)

Procedure
- The sterile catheter and glove package are opened. Sterile normal saline solution (0.25 to 0.5 ml) is drawn up in a 1-ml syringe. The resuscitation bag is connected to oxygen, and the patency is checked so that, if the neonate becomes apneic or bradycardic during the procedure, resuscitation equipment is immediately available. If the infant is on a ventilator equipped with a bag, this may be used for resuscitation if necessary.
- Disconnect and dip the suction catheter in/or wet the tip of the suction catheter with the sterile normal saline.
- Put gloves on and attach sterile catheter to suction tubing. With nondominant hand, disconnect from ventilator.
- Gently pass catheter down endotracheal tube to premeasured length.
- Occlude suction hole in catheter and withdraw. Use continuous suction so that secretions are not "released" with intermittent suction. Only one suction attempt should be made before the infant is again ventilated. Assess tolerance of procedure by observing pulse oximeter and infant's color, heart rate, tone, and activity.
- Replace on ventilator and hyperventilate with appropriate FiO_2 for six to eight breaths or until adequate oxygenation has been established. Check ventilator settings including alarm system in "on" position. Check tube position to assure that the tube is not bent or strained. Note amount and type of secretions obtained.

Table 23-3	SUCTION PROCEDURE: RESEARCH BASIS AND RECOMMENDATIONS	
COMMON TECHNIQUES	**RESEARCH DATA**	**RECOMMENDATIONS**
Instillation of 0.25-0.5 ml sterile normal saline before suction Purpose: Mobilize and thin secretions; aid catheter passage	Mucus is not miscible with saline solution so bolus saline does not thin or liquefy secretions[149]; vaporized or nebulized saline thins secretions[149] Bolus saline accumulates at the end of the ETT; <20% saline solution is retrieved with suction, remainder is absorbed by the body[251] Two studies support saline use,[49,513] whereas others cite increased hypoxia, fatigue, and infection with saline use*	Closed suction: Irrigate catheter before suction; place normal saline syringe at distal port adapter and squeeze saline solution into port while simultaneously applying suction Open suction: Dip or moisten catheter tip in sterile saline or water soluble jelly to facilitate sliding down the small diameter ETT[91]
Head turned from side to side with suction Purpose: To advance catheter down contralateral bronchus	Suction causes fluctuations in cerebral blood flow that increases ICP and the risk of IVH[445] Sharply turning the head to the side occludes the jugular vein and increases ICP, which is at its lowest when the head is in the midline or slightly elevated position[339]	Turned head position: Contraindicated secondary to data on increased ICP, jugular vein occlusion and physiologic impossibility of passing catheter into bronchi using this strategy Do not turn the infant's head during suction; keep head in midline for suction
Catheter inserted until resistance (touching the carina) is met, withdrawn slightly and suction applied	Application of both negative pressure with suction and touching the bronchial mucosa with catheter causes irritation and tissue damage†	Shallow suction does not touch the carina with the catheter tip; using the ETT markings and the length of the adapter, insert the catheter no more than 1 cm beyond the total distance[603] (e.g., if the ETT is inserted 10 cm and the length of the adapter is 1.5 cm, the suction catheter should be inserted 11.5 cm to no farther than 12.5 cm)
Catheter is inserted and removed several times	One small study (16 neonates) evaluated nurses subjective reports of amount of secretions obtained with one and two suction passes; no difference was noted[4]	Limit number of catheter passes to number needed to adequately remove secretions Do not use up and down motion while removing the catheter, since this decreases oxygenation and promotes hypoxia and tissue damage; only one suction attempt should be made before the neonate is again ventilated; every catheter passage is considered a suction event; occlude tracheal tube with catheter for no longer than 5-10 sec
No use of developmental care adjustments during the stressful procedure of suction[448]	Body containment significantly decreases the magnitude of the preterm's responses to suctioning[176,545,568]	Use the developmental care technique of containment (see Chapter 13) during suction

ETT, Endotracheal tube; *ICP*, intracranial pressure; *IVH*, intraventricular hemorrhage.
*References 5, 66, 130, 241, 526, 534, 553.
†References 69, 233, 336, 337, 340, 394, 409.

- NOTE: When two persons are available for suction one remains "sterile" and does the suctioning, while the other detaches the ETT from the ventilator and hyperventilates the infant between suctionings.

Because ETT suctioning compromises the neo- nate's physiologic homeostasis, adequate recovery time is necessary after the procedure. If CPT is used, an average of 5 minutes to a maximum of 11 minutes are required for recovery.[86] For ETT suction an average of 4.4 minutes recovery time is

Table 23-4	CHEST AUSCULTATION FOR ETT PLACEMENT
FINDING	CAUSE
No air entry bilaterally	Esophagus intubated; air leak
Air entry over left upper abdominal quadrant	Esophagus intubated; air entry heard over stomach
Diminished air entry	Endotracheal tube too high; air leak
Air entry unequal; right chest better aerated than left chest	Endotracheal tube too low; down right mainstem bronchus

necessary (6 of 25 infants in this study never returned to baseline during the observation).[420] These recovery times are also supported by other studies.[175,176,579] Use of containment, such as facilitated tucking (see Chapter 13), has been shown in 24 preterm infants to improve oxygenation after suctioning.[545,568] **These infants may need a significant rest period after suctioning before other aspects of care such as feeding are attempted.**

Endotracheal Intubation

Endotracheal intubation may be accomplished by the orotracheal route or the nasotracheal route. An endotracheal tube diameter that approximates the diameter of the infant's fifth digit generally fits snugly into the trachea. To measure for an endotracheal tube, the distance from the oral orifice to midway between the glottis and carina may be calculated by multiplying the crown-heel length by 0.2. In an emergency the distance from the lips to midway between the glottis and carina may be approximated by the 7-8-9-10 rule. The distance is 7 cm in a 1-kg infant, 8 cm in a 2-kg infant, 9 cm in a 3-kg infant, and 10 cm in a 4-kg infant.

Intubation Procedure

Endotracheal tube placement must be immediately verified by auscultation and confirmed by a chest x-ray examination. Findings on auscultation and what they suggest are listed in Table 23-4. A newly developed, disposable, end-tidal carbon dioxide (ETCO$_2$) detector (Pedi-CAP) (Figure 23-1) to immediately verify tube placement has been tested in the delivery room and NICU.[28] In the presence of exhaled CO_2 (after 6 breaths) the Pedi-CAP changes color from purple to yellow. The time required to detect proper ETT placement with the Pedi-CAP was 4 to 12 seconds versus 0 to 90 seconds by clinical evaluation. This significantly faster time enables quicker extubation and reintubation if the ETT is in the esophagus.[28]

For long-term stability, commercially available endotracheal tube anchors prevent accidental extu-

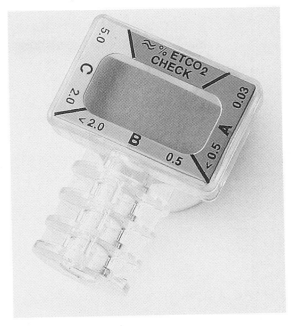

FIGURE 23-1 Pedi-CAP disposable pediatric CO_2 detector. (Courtesy Nellcor Puritan Bennett Inc., Pleasanton, Calif.)

bation. Some nurseries still prefer fixing tubes with tape or sutures.

Extubation Procedure

Assess the infant's condition by observing the heart rate, color, respiratory rate and effort, and by auscultating the chest. If the infant's condition is stable, proceed with extubation. Extubate before feeding, or empty the stomach to prevent vomiting. Because neonates are obligatory nasal breathers, the nasopharynx must also be suctioned and patent for extubation.

Hyperinflate with deep breaths with the infant's head in the midline and remove the tube on inflation[334] (to provide adequate lung expansion and prevent atelectasis), on expiration[229] (so that secretions that have accumulated around the tracheal tube are "blown away" on exhalation and tube removal), or while suctioning (to remove secretions that have accumulated around the tube). Place neonate in a warm, humidified oxygen hood at Fio_2 to keep pulse oximeter at 92% to 94%.

Reassess the infant's condition, especially for signs of increased work of breathing and distress. Document tube removal and the infant's tolerance. Check arterial blood gases 15 to 20 minutes after

extubation to assess oxygenation and ventilation status. Perform a chest x-ray examination to document atelectasis or fully expanded lungs. **Observe for complications of intubation (Table 23-5).**

Mechanical Ventilation

Mechanical ventilation is used in neonates to correct abnormalities in oxygenation ($\downarrow Pao_2$), alveolar

Table 23-5	COMPLICATIONS OF ENDOTRACHEAL INTUBATION	
COMPLICATIONS	**COMMENTS**	
Immediate		
Malposition		
Too low	Usually in right mainstem bronchus; no or diminished breath sounds in left chest or upper right lobe; asymmetrical chest movement; atelectasis (withdraw tube until breath sounds are heard bilaterally and equally)	
Too high	Inadequate ventilation bilaterally, especially at lung bases	
Esophagus	Air movement auscultated in stomach with no or inadequate breath sounds	
Obstruction		
Plug	Partial—no change or diminished breath sounds audible Complete—distant or no breath sounds audible	
Kinking of the tube		
Head position	Flexion or extension of the head results in diminished or blocked airflow	
Perforation		
Vocal cords		
Trachea		
Pharynx		
Esophagus		
Pulmonary Hemorrhage		
Infection	Colonization in the neonatal airway increases with the duration of intubation; presence of ETT >72 hr is associated with colonization; this biofilm may contribute to the chondritis that precedes subglottic stenosis[147]; MRSA tracheal infection causes subglottic stenosis[605]	
Air Leak		
Increased Intracranial Pressure		
Postextubation		
Migratory labor collapse	Prevent and treat with pulmonary hygiene	
Diffuse microatelectasis	In VLBW infants may be associated with apnea; treatable by pulmonary hygiene or nasal CPAP, or both	
Long Term		
General	Vocal cord inflammation, stenosis, and eventual dysfunction; tracheoesophageal fistula; subglottic stenosis; tracheal inflammation and stenosis; necrotizing tracheobronchitis; contributes to bronchopulmonary dysplasia	
Specific to the Type of Tube		
Orotracheal	Abnormal dentition; gingival and palatal erosion; palatal grooves	
Nasotracheal	Otitis media; erosion of alae nasae and nasal septum; nasal stenosis	

CPAP, Continuous positive airway pressure; *MRSA,* methicillin-resistant *Staphylococcus aureus.*

ventilation ($\uparrow Paco_2$), or respiratory effort (apnea, ineffectual respirations, or increased work of breathing). It may not be used to treat the primary disease, but frequently is used to support the infant until the disease is treated or resolved. **Newborns who meet the criteria listed in Box 23-4 are candidates for assisted ventilation.**

Ventilator Settings

To individualize assisted ventilation, knowledge of the ventilator capabilities is essential.

Intermittent Mandatory Ventilation. Most mechanical ventilators in common use today allow for intermittent mandatory ventilation (IMV). **IMV provides a continuous flow of gas that is available to the infant during spontaneous respirations. Periodic occlusion of the system diverts gas under pressure to the infant.** Because IMV provides for spontaneous and mechanical ventilation, only the amount of ventilatory assistance that is needed by the individual infant is provided.

Continuous Distending Pressure. **Continuous distending pressure (CDP) is expressed in centimeters of water. CDP may be given without**

Box 23-4 | CRITERIA THAT QUALIFY NEWBORNS FOR ASSISTED VENTILATION

Blood Gases

- Severe hypoxemia (Pao_2 <50-60 mm Hg with Fio_2 ≥0.60 or Pao_2 <60 mm Hg with Fio_2 >0.4 in infant <1250 g)
- Severe hypercapnia ($Paco_2$ >55-65 mm Hg with pH <7.20-7.25)

Clinical

- Apnea and bradycardia requiring resuscitation in infants with lung disease or unresponsive to CPAP, or theophylline therapy in preterm infants with normal lungs
- Inefficient respiratory effort, such as gasping respirations from asphyxia, narcosis, or primary cardiopulmonary disease
- Shock and asphyxia with hypoperfusion and hypotension
- RDS in infants weighing <1000 g, frequently making them incapable of maintaining ventilation (in these infants it has been suggested that mechanical ventilation without a trial of CPAP is appropriate)

CPAP, Continuous positive airway pressure; *RDS,* respiratory distress syndrome.

IMV (CPAP) or with it (positive end-expiratory pressure [PEEP]).

The effects of CDP include increased alveolar stability, increased functional residual capacity, decreased risk of atelectasis, increased intrathoracic pressure, and impeded passage of fluid from lung capillaries to alveolar spaces, aiding in the prevention or treatment of pulmonary edema. Effects of changes in PEEP are dependent on severity of lung disease and degree of lung inflation. High PEEP in the presence of relatively compliant lungs will cause overdistention, worsen Pao_2, and increase pulmonary vascular resistance. In addition, overdistention may increase the risk of barotrauma.[32,60,230,555] However, the use of levels of PEEP that are too low contributes to hypoxia and pulmonary hypertension because of low lung volumes. Acute lung injury is actually worsened by the failure to recruit adequate lung volume by using insufficient PEEP.

Peak Inspiratory Pressure. **Peak inspiratory pressure (PIP) is the maximum pressure measured during the delivery of gas (inspiration) during conventional mechanical ventilation.** PIP reflects the effects of the amount of gas delivered to the lungs in a given breath (tidal volume) and the underlying mechanical properties of the lungs. For example, if the same PIP is used in neonates with severe RDS (with stiff, noncompliant lungs) as in neonates ventilated for apnea with minimal lung disease, the tidal volume will be much greater in the latter group. **Recent studies suggest that overdistention of the lungs caused by excessive tidal volumes, and not pressure itself, worsens acute lung injury** (so-called volutrauma).[96,106,230] Thus adverse effects of high PIP are dependent upon the degree of lung disease.

Rate. **The rate reflects how often a volume of gas in the system is delivered to the infant. It is expressed as breaths per minute.** Too rapid a rate, especially with a poorly inflated lung, can cause lung injury caused by gas trapping ("inadvertent PEEP").

Inspiration/Expiration Ratio. **The inspiration/expiration ratio (I/E ratio) reflects the relationship between time spent in inspiration and time spent in expiration.** When the rate is 60 breaths/min and the total respiratory cycle is 1 second, an I/E ratio of 1:1 means 0.5 second is inspiration and 0.5 second is expiration. If the I/E ratio is 1:2 with a rate of 60 and the total respiratory cycle is 1 second, inspiration is 0.33 second and expiration is 0.66 second.

Prolonged inspiration may be associated with more efficient ventilation, optimal arterial oxygenation, a higher risk of air leak, and impeding of venous return. Prolonged expiration also improves oxygenation, especially in air-trapping conditions (such as rapid rate ventilation or airway disease).[64]

Mean Airway Pressure. **Mean airway pressure (MAP) is the amount of pressure transmitted to the airway throughout an entire respiratory cycle.**[64] Any change in ventilator settings affects the MAP. MAP is most affected by changes in PEEP, inspiratory time, or I/E ratio.[25] MAP is associated with optimal oxygenation ($\uparrow$Pao$_2$) and ventilation ($\downarrow$Paco$_2$) when pressures range between 6 and 14 cm of water.[64] When MAP exceeds 14 cm of water, there is a progressive deterioration of the blood gases ($\downarrow$Pao$_2$, $\uparrow$Paco$_2$).[64] The effects of any given level of MAP are dependent upon the changes in mechanical properties of the lung caused by the primary disease. For example, high MAP may be needed to improve oxygenation in severe RDS or meconium aspiration syndrome, especially in term neonates. Low MAP in this setting will cause sustained hypoxemia and atelectasis. In contrast, use of high MAP in neonates in the presence of minimal lung disease will cause overdistention and deterioration of arterial blood gas tensions. In general, the goal of increasing MAP is to improve Pao$_2$ and is usually achieved by small increases in PEEP or prolongation of inspiratory time. Repeat chest x-ray examination and continuous monitoring of blood pressure and oxygenation (by pulse oximeter) will help determine the optimal level of MAP.

Usual starting pressures for beginning ventilatory support are listed in Table 23-6.

The inspired oxygen tension is adjusted to provide an adequate arterial oxygen tension. If the infant still has difficulty maintaining an adequate carbon dioxide tension, a faster rate and/or greater inspiratory pressure would be indicated. **Table 23-7 lists the usual effects to be expected from changing specific ventilator settings.**

To evaluate the efficacy of mechanical ventilation and any adjustments made with the system, continuous monitoring with pulse oximeters (see Chapter 7) must be maintained and/or blood gases obtained. During the acute phase of illness, blood gases should be obtained 15 to 30 minutes

Table 23-6	STARTING PRESSURES FOR BEGINNING VENTILATORY SUPPORT
PARAMETER	**RANGE**
Fio$_2$	At previous level of 10% higher than previously required concentration
PEEP	4 to 6 cm water
PIP	16 to 20 cm water
Rate	40 to 60
I/E ratio	1:1 to 1:2

PEEP, Positive end-expiratory pressure; *PIP,* peak inspiratory pressure.

after beginning ventilatory support or after any change in settings, every 4 to 6 hours if no change is made in ventilator settings, and as needed based on the clinical condition of the infant.

Arterial blood gases should be maintained in the following range (see Chapter 11):

Pao$_2$	60 to 80 mm Hg
Paco$_2$	35 to 45 mm Hg
pH	7.35 to 7.45

Optimal arterial blood gas tensions are somewhat controversial. To decrease the risk of acute lung injury by minimizing lung overdistention and barotrauma, some advocate strategies that target lower Pao$_2$ and higher Paco$_2$ ("permissive hypercapnia").[204,380] The risks and benefits of such strategies depend on the specific clinical setting. If excessive ventilator settings are required to lower Paco$_2$, allowing Paco$_2$ to rise (as long as the pH is greater than 7.25) is often accepted in an attempt to avoid lung injury. Hypercapnia increases cerebral blood flow which may contribute to IVH and worsen the neonate's neurologic outcome.[204] However, hyperventilation (low Paco$_2$) decreases cerebral blood flow and oxygen delivery to the brain and may increase the risk of IVH and contribute to adverse long-term neurologic sequelae.[204] In addition, because the goal of respiratory care is to optimize oxygen delivery to tissues, the effect of a given Pao$_2$ is partly dependent on cardiac function (see Chapter 24) and hemoglobin level (see Chapter 20). Accepting lower Pao$_2$ and O$_2$ saturation may lead to worse outcomes in the setting of systemic hypotension and poor cardiac function (e.g., sepsis).

Recognizing that aggressive ventilator management (e.g., intubation, high PIP, high MAP) is associated with increased lung injury and BPD/CLD,

Table 23-7	USUAL EFFECTS OF CHANGING CONVENTIONAL MECHANICAL VENTILATOR SETTINGS				
				CAUSES	
INCREASING	**Pao$_2$**	**Paco$_2$**	**pH**	**COMPLICATIONS**	
Fio$_2$	↑	0	0	Oxygen toxicity (bronchopulmonary dysplasia, retrolental fibroplasia); absorption atelectasis; Fio$_2$ may have no effect on oxygenation in the presence of severe R → L (right to left) shunt (PPHN), congenital heart disease, or marked intrapulmonary shunting as a result of severe parenchymal lung disease	
CPAP/PEEP	↑	0/↑	0/↓	Hypoventilation with respiratory acidosis; decreased cardiac output with metabolic acidosis; air leaks	
PIP	↑	↓	↑	Barotrauma with air leaks and bronchopulmonary dysplasia; respiratory alkalosis	
Rate	↓	↓	↑	Respiratory alkalosis	
I/E ratio (1:1 to 1:2)	↑	0	0	Increased intrapleural pressure; decreased venous return	

CPAP, Continuous positive airway pressure; *PEEP,* positive end-expiratory pressure; *PIP,* peak inspiratory pressure.

gentler ventilator techniques and management have been developed and are being used.[106,367,500] Many gentler strategies incorporate relinquishment of traditional ventilator controls (from the health care provider) to patient control of ventilator parameters. Facilitated by computer-assisted technology, newer types of ventilators are being utilized.

Patient-Triggered Ventilation

Asynchrony between the infant's respiratory efforts and the ventilator causes increased barotrauma, which contributes to lung injury (e.g., BPD/CLD).[158] Altered cerebral blood flow may contribute to IVH. **Patient-ventilator synchrony occurs when patient-triggered ventilation (PTV) responds to the neonate's signal representing spontaneous respiratory effort and delivers a mechanical breath, timed to the onset of inspiration.** Patient triggered ventilation[106,158,367,500]:

- Decreases asynchrony
- Improves gaseous exchange
- Creates respiratory support that is more synergistic with the neonate's respiratory efforts
- Decreases the need for ventilatory support

Studies comparing PTV with conventional mechanical ventilation (CMV) have found no proven benefit in[46,52,106]:

- Decreasing the incidence in severity of BPD/CLD
- Mortality
- Head ultrasound abnormalities

These studies did show an increased rate of pneumothorax, worsening arterial blood gas values, desaturations, and need for increased ventilatory support.[46,52]

No studies comparing PTV to high-frequency ventilation (HFV) have been conducted.[106]

Modes of PTV include the following:
- Synchronized intermittent mandatory ventilation (SIMV)
- Assist/Control ventilation—oxygenation, volume guarantee, and minute ventilation
- Pressure support ventilation (PSV)
- Proportional assist ventilation (PAV)

Synchronized Intermittent Mandatory Ventilation.

Synchronized intermittent mandatory ventilation (SIMV), a commonly used form of patient-triggered ventilation, delivers mechanical breaths at a fixed rate.[367] **SIMV enables synchronization of ventilation breaths by sensing (through an airway or diaphragmatic sensor) the neonate's initiation of respiration, then triggering of a mechanical breath.** Synchronized ventilation prevents the generation of excessive pressure within the respiratory tract when infant exhalation coincides with mechanical ventilation. Use of SIMV is associated with a decrease in (1) oxygen need, (2) duration of ventilator therapy, (3) incidence of BPD, and (4) severity of IVH.[57,272,395,575] Use of SIMV is also associated with fewer episodes of hypoxia and better oxygenation as a result improved ventilation/perfusion and increased resting lung volume (FRC) when compared with IMV ventilation of VLBW infants.[185]

Assist/Control Ventilation

Newer neonatal ventilators are equipped with computer technology with rapid digital feedback circuits. **Computer-assisted control enables adjustments** of FiO₂, PIP to control tidal volume, and ventilatory rate to control minute ventilation.[500] Small studies have reported that computer-assisted maintenance of a target oxygen saturation is as effective as manual FiO₂ adjustments.[102,500] Larger RCTs on safety and efficacy are warranted.

In volume guarantee a preset target tidal volume is maintained by the ventilator as the pressure limit varies inversely with lung compliance and the neonate's respiratory effort. In preliminary studies VLBW infants had lower MAP on volume guarantee when compared with VLBW infants treated with SIMV.[87,266,267,362] Less ventilator support for the VLBW infant was required, because volume guarantee enables an increase in the infant's respiratory effort while guaranteeing a physiologic tidal volume (about 4 to 5 ml/kg) in contrast to SIMV, which delivers a constant PIP regardless of tidal volume delivered.[87,266] Larger RCTs are required.[266,500]

Minute ventilation (e.g., the volume of gas moving in and out of the lungs over time, expressed in milliliters per kilogram per minute) is a successful predictor of readiness to wean, extubate, and establish optimal pulmonary mechanics.[593] Mandatory minute ventilation (MMV), a new ventilator mode in the NICU, provides mechanically generated breaths only if the neonate's spontaneous breathing doesn't meet a minimum level of minute ventilation (chosen by the health care provider). If the infant's spontaneous pressure-supported breaths exceed the minimum minute ventilation, no additional breaths are delivered by the ventilator. If the infant fails to meet the specified minute ventilation, intermittent mandatory breaths are delivered at the preset tidal volume.[156] MMV enables the infant to control the rate, flow, and inspiratory time of the ventilator, which enhances synchrony and ensures a "backup" system to assume the work of breathing if the infant is unable to maintain adequate minute ventilation. MMV's role in weaning infants from mechanical ventilation and as a ventilator mode of the future awaits RCTs for safety and efficacy.[156]

Pressure Support Ventilation

Pressure support ventilation (PSV) complements the infant's respiratory effort by triggering a mechanical breath, preset to a specific pressure. PSV decreases the work of breathing created by airway resistance (e.g., narrowed diameter of neonatal ETT) and ventilator circuit resistance. PSV also decreases work of breathing by assisting the activity of the infant's respiratory muscles. PSV is used alone (if the infant has effective respiratory drive) or in conjunction with SIMV. PSV is useful in chronic and acute situations as well as weaning chronically ventilator-dependent infants.[517] In a study of 10 preterm infants with BPD/CLD who had been unable to wean before the use of PSV, all were extubated at a mean time of 7 days after PSV use.[157] In another study of 50 randomized preterm infants, those infants weaned using SIMV/PSV were extubated significantly sooner and with fewer IVH/PVL than the control group.[518] Choosing ventilator settings for the use of PSV has been characterized as "a significant amount of guesswork" and a "challenge," even by experienced clinicians.[156] More studies on the use of PSV with neonates and the potential to expedite weaning are needed.[158,500]

Proportional Assist Ventilation

In proportional assist ventilation (PAV) ventilator pressure increases in proportion to inspiratory volume (e.g., inspiratory flow varies to match the neonate's respiratory effort).[106,500] Both volume and flow proportional assist relieves the neonate of both elastic (e.g., respiratory muscles) and resistive work of breathing. During PAV, the infant's breathing completely controls all variables of the ventilator breathing pattern through exceptionally fast computer-controlled feedback circuitry.[500] In the only published trial using PAV in infants, less MAP and transpulmonary pressure were used to effectively oxygenate and ventilate infants with mild to moderate respiratory insufficiency.[501] Clinically, respiratory rates were 50 to 80/min with a fast and shallow pattern, and tidal volumes less than 5 cc/kg. Although PAV was found to be as safe and effective as CMV, it has not been evaluated as a sole ventilator modality or used in other types of cardiorespiratory conditions.[500]

High-Frequency Ventilation

Barotrauma/volutrauma is a major contributing factor to the development of chronic lung disease or death from progressive lung injury in newborns treated with conventional mechanical ventilation. The goal of high-frequency ventilation (HFV) is to reduce barotrauma by its application early in the course of RDS, or to reduce the progression of injury in infants already having advanced pulmonary interstitial emphysema, recurrent pneumothoraxes, or bronchopleural fistula. In addition to minimizing lung injury, the goal of HFV is to enhance oxygenation more effectively than conventional ventilation. For example, the use of high-frequency oscillating ventilators (HFOV) has been shown to reduce the need for ECMO in term neonates,[81] results in better survival,[581] and in combination with other therapies, especially inhaled nitric oxide (iNO), may contribute more to improved clinical outcome than either therapy used alone.[3]

HFV differs from conventional modes of ventilator support in that it uses smaller tidal volumes at supraphysiologic frequencies, allowing for generation of lower intrathoracic pressure. At high frequencies the calculated tidal volume is less than dead space. Thus the physics of gas flow and exchange are different from the traditional teaching of lung mechanics and are related to augmented diffusion. Reduction in barotrauma occurs by allowing for ventilation with a very small pressure amplitude around the mean airway pressure in the distal airway. Therefore at high frequencies (commonly 10 to 15 Hz), the peak inspiratory and expiratory pressures approach MAP (i.e., lower downstream pressures). Because of this effect, higher MAP can be used to improve oxygenation without worsening lung injury.

HFV can be achieved by jet ventilators or by oscillators. Jet ventilators deliver short bursts of high-flow gases directly into the proximal airway via a small cannula and have a passive exhalation cycle. Oscillators vibrate columns of air and have active exhalation cycles. Although clinical comparisons of these two methods are still pending, a high incidence of necrotizing tracheitis has been reported with high-frequency jet ventilation. This problem, however, appears to be related more to insufficient humidification during jet ventilation.[92] Early use of HFJV in one study decreased the incidence of BPD/CLD and neurologic injury, but may worsen neurodevelopmental outcome if not used properly.[319]

HFOV is used both as a rescue therapy when CMV is unsuccessful and electively as a primary mode of ventilation. HFOV is in widespread use with all centers (100%) in one survey using it for rescue and 40% using it electively.[67] Early elective use of HFOV (compared with CMV) has been studied and found to (1) decrease surfactant replacement requirements,[400] (2) decrease days on oxygen and ventilation,[474] (3) decrease the incidence of BPD/CLD,[96,215,286,319,474] (4) fail to decrease the incidence of BPD/CLD, (5) not increase the risk of PVL,[96,215,319,424,552] (6) have a similar incidence of air leak,[215,424,471] (7) be associated with an increased incidence of severe (grade 3 or higher) IVH,[6,269,270,400] and (8) be associated with hydrocephalus after prolonged use.[250] Discordance in study findings may be attributed to (1) maturity/immaturity of preterm infants, (2) time to initiation of HFOV, (3) use of antenatal steroids, (4) use of surfactant replacement, (5) differences in techniques used (e.g., presence/absence of lung volume recruitment strategy), (6) level of MAP, (7) duration of use, and (8) variations in CBF secondary to P_{CO_2}.[400] Some researchers recommend that CMV be the first choice in treatment of preterm infants with RDS and HFOV be reserved for rescue therapy if CMV is unsuccessful.[400] Further research is needed to clarify which ventilator should be used initially.

Inhaled Nitric Oxide

Inhaled NO (iNO) is one of the exciting new developments in the treatment of hypoxemic newborns. Based on the initial discovery that vascular endothelial cells endogenously produce a potent vasodilator substance ("endothelium-derived relaxing factor"),[182,326,476] which was later identified as nitric oxide,[284] clinical research into the use of iNO in neonates, infants, children, and adults began. Because NO could be delivered as a gas, its potential role for clinical treatment of pulmonary hypertension and hypoxemia was quickly recognized and tested in adults with primary pulmonary hypertension.[442] **Experimental animal studies demonstrated that low doses of iNO caused potent, selective, and sustained pulmonary vasodilation in the perinatal pulmonary circulation.**[327] The vasodilator response occurs as a result of iNO stimulation of soluble guanylate cyclase activity, increasing cyclic guanosine monophosphate (GMP) in vascular smooth muscle and causing vasorelaxation. Selectivity of iNO for the pulmonary circulation is based on direct delivery of NO into the lung; because NO is avidly bound by hemoglobin in red blood cells and inactivated after metabolism to nitrite and nitrate, there are no direct effects on systemic arterial pressure.[476]

Inhaled NO has been approved by the FDA for treatment for near-term (more than 34 weeks' gestational age) and term neonates with PPHN (see PPHN section). A randomized control trial of iNO in preterm infants found (1) improved oxygenation, (2) decreased need for mechanical ventilation, (3) improved survival without increase in IVH, and (4) a trend toward a decrease in BPD/CLD.[96,332] In a metaanalysis of iNO use in preterm infants, no RCT has been able to demonstrate a benefit in mortality or incidence of BPD/CLD.[181,276] **Potential toxicities and research outcomes in use of iNO are listed in Table 23-8.** Use of iNO in preterm infants remains experimental.[15,181,326] Variations in use of iNO include (1) dosing, (2) duration, (3) early versus later use, (4) best candidates, and (5) outcomes.[93,181] **Recommendations for use of iNO are listed in the PPHN section (see Table 23-22).**

Extracorporeal Membrane Oxygenation/Extracorporeal Life Support

Extracorporeal membrane oxygenation/extracorporeal life support (ECMO/ECLS) is a modification of cardiopulmonary bypass that allows for more prolonged therapy than is traditionally performed in the operating room for cardiac surgery. ECMO/ECLS establishes a pulmonary bypass circuit, allowing gas exchange to occur outside of the lung by perfusion of blood through a membrane oxygenator. Blood is drawn from a catheter in the right internal jugular vein or right atrium, oxygenated as it crosses the membrane, and then returned to the patient via the right common carotid artery (venoarterial ECMO/ECLS) or the femoral vein (venovenous ECMO/ECLS). The pump produces a continuous, nonpulsatile flow through the membrane oxygenator as the patient is kept heparinized and continues to be ventilated at low pressures, rates, and oxygen tensions. The goal of this therapy is to "buy time" for the severely injured lung to heal while attenuating ongoing lung injury by decreasing exposure to hyperoxia and barotrauma. Therapy can be continued for several days, until lung recovery appears sufficient to maintain adequate gas tension without ECMO/ECLS.

A multicenter randomized trial of ECMO/ECLS therapy in the United Kingdom has demonstrated improved survival in term neonates with severe hypoxemic respiratory failure and PPHN.[561] ECMO/ECLS is used as a treatment of last option[581] when

Table 23-8	POTENTIAL TOXICITIES AND OUTCOMES OF INHALED NITRIC OXIDE (iNO)	
TYPE	**RESEARCH DATA**
Decrease platelet aggregation[210,213]	30-min exposure to 40 ppm of iNO does not inhibit ADP-dependent platelet activation (in infants with PPHN).[90]
Increase risk of hemorrhage—CNS and pulmonary	No increase in IVH in preterms treated with iNO (16% grade IV IVH) versus 27% control group[332]; fewer iNO with grade II-IV IVH, but not significant.[332]
	No effect on incidence of IVH, PVL, pulmonary or GI hemorrhage (in infants with PPHN).[416]
Acute lung injury in surfactant dysfunction that increases the incidence/severity of BPD/CLD	A trend toward decrease in BPD/CLD in preterms treated with iNO. Fewer days on ventilators for iNO group and antiinflammatory effects of iNO on pulmonary tissue may be the cause of less lung injury.[332] Fewer days on ventilators for near-term but not preterm (<33 weeks) infants.[194]
	No effect on incidence of BPD/CLD (infants with PPHN)[416]; decrease in BPD/CLD in infants with PPHN versus controls.[100]
Methemoglobinemia	No increased incidence.[416,477]
Poorer neurodevelopmental outcomes	No increased incidence of adverse neurodevelopmental sequelae in infants with PPHN.[95,416,485]
	No increase in IVH[332]; increased frequency of severe (≥grade III) IVH and poor neurodevelopmental outcome in early childhood.[88]
Increased mortality	No improvement in overall survival in preterms treated with iNO (52%) compared with 47% control preterms.[332]
	In infants with PPHN:
	• Number of deaths similar in iNO group versus control group.[478]
	• No effect on mortality.[416]
	• Increased mortality treated with iNO versus placebo group.[131]
	• Decreased incidence in mortality.[182]

ADP, Adenosine 5'-diphosphate; *BPD/CLD,* bronchopulmonary dysplasia/chronic lung disease; *IVH,* intraventricular hemorrhage; *GI,* gastrointestinal; *ppm,* parts per million; *PPHN,* persistent pulmonary hypertension of the newborn; *PVL,* periventricular leukomalacia.

neonates are unresponsive to maximum conventional support.[460] ECMO/ECLS criteria include (1) gestational age 34 weeks or older, weight 2000 g or more, (2) no more than 7 to 10 days of assisted ventilation, (3) reversible lung disease, (4) no CNS or multisystem disease; no lethal congenital anomalies, (5) no intracranial hemorrhage above grade I or uncorrectable coagulopathy, (6) no cardiac disease (unless ECMO/ECLS is to be used for the preoperative/postoperative period for cardiac surgery), (7) no severe asphyxia, (8) failure of maximal medical management, and (9) a ventilatory index (MAP × Rate) of 1500 or above or an oxygenation index (MAP × Fio_2 ×100/PaO_2) of 40 or more.[316,460] **Conditions treated with ECMO/ECLS and their survival rates are listed in Table 23-9.**

In the last decade the number of neonates being treated with ECMO/ECLS has declined by 50%.[95,460] Because ECMO/ECLS is invasive, labor intensive, costly, and involves risks associated with systemic anticoagulation (e.g., intracranial hemorrhage), alternative therapies (e.g., surfactant replacement, iNO and HFV) are initially used and have reduced the need for ECMO.[95,316,460] These therapies have changed the population being treated with ECMO/ECLS, shortened length of stay, reduced costs, and raised concerns in delay of use of ECMO/ECLS.[316,460] In one study initial use of alternative therapies did not result in prolongation of bypass time, longer mechanical ventilation, or increased length of stay for ECMO/ECLS patients (transported into the ECMO/ECLS center).[316] However, this study did document a decline in overall survival (from 84% to 56%) of neonates requiring ECMO/ECLS after alternative therapies began to be used.

Considerable variability exists between centers, however, suggesting that the use of these techniques is partly dependent upon the clinical strategy and other issues in patient management.

Complications of ECMO/ECLS are dependent on initial disease process, pre-ECMO/ECLS factors (e.g., asphyxia, coagulopathy, hypo/hyperventilation) and type of ECMO/ECLS used (e.g., venoarterial versus venovenous).[460] Mortality rates in neonates treated with ECMO/ECLS are 15% to 20% and 10% to 20% developmental delay in survivors.[217,218,549,581] The most common complications are hemorrhagic (e.g., intracranial [incidence 4.6%; survival 50%]), and nonhemorrhagic (e.g., infarctions [incidence 10.7%; survival 50%]) central nervous system insults. Neonates who develop intracranial hemorrhage are at highest risk for mortality and poor neurodevelopmental outcomes. Two 5-year follow-up studies of ECMO/ECLS survivors found (1) normal range IQs, although as a group survivors IQs were lower than a control group; (2) increased risk for school failure; and (3) need for follow-up through school age.[218,461]

Partial Liquid Ventilation

Although prenatal administration of steroidal agents, use of surfactant, and HFOV therapies have improved the clinical course of sick preterm newborns with respiratory failure, the morbidity of severe RDS persists. Based on 40 years of experimental (animal) studies, **perfluorocarbon (PFC) liquids have been found to improve gaseous exchange, lung mechanics, and cardiopulmonary stability in various respiratory diseases.**[119,227] PFC liquids are suitable for liquid ventilation because of their high

Table 23-9	CONDITIONS TREATED WITH ECMO/ECLS	
TYPE/CONDITION	PERCENTAGE TREATED	PERCENTAGE SURVIVAL
Meconium aspiration syndrome	35	94
Congenital diaphragmatic hernia	21	55
Respiratory distress syndrome	0-9 (n = 98)	84
Sepsis/pneumonia	15	76
Persistent pulmonary hypertension of the newborn	14	80
Air leak syndromes	0.5	68
Others	5	68

Modified from Neonatal ECMO registry, 1999; and Rais-Bahrami K, Short B: The current status of neonatal ECMO, *Semin Perinatol* 24:406, 2000.
ECMO/ECLS, Extracorporeal membrane oxygenation/extracorporeal life support.

solubility of respiratory gases, easy elimination by evaporation from the lungs, and lack of metabolism by the body.[227] Instillation of a functional residual capacity of PFC liquid into the lungs during gaseous ventilation constitutes partial liquid ventilation (PLV). The best ventilator management during PLV has not been determined and may differ with underlying lung pathology.[227]

PLV is applicable to the surfactant and structurally deficient preterm lung because it reduces/eliminates surface tension forces, optimizes lung recruitment, and reexpands atelectasis. In a term infant, PLV is applicable to structural lung disease (e.g., diaphragmatic hernia) or lung disease associated with airway debris (e.g., aspiration syndromes or pneumonia). A nonrandomized, nonblinded clinical study of 13 preterm infants with severe RDS who failed to improve with CMV showed improved oxygenation within one hour of initiation of PLV.[351] In infants with respiratory failure, a combination of PLV, iNO, and surfactant may produce optimal response.[126] Currently the safety and efficacy of PLV is undergoing phase III trials in adults in the United States; trials are contemplated in infants and children in Europe.

Weaning From the Ventilator

When the infant's condition improves, ventilatory support is slowly removed. **Evidence of improvement includes biochemical parameters and clinical parameters:**

- Arterial blood gases are stable and physiologic.
- Spontaneous respiratory efforts occur in addition to the ventilator settings and if the infant is disconnected from the ventilator for suctioning.
- There is increased activity, muscle tone, and progressively decreasing FiO$_2$ requirement.

Weaning an infant as soon as possible from intubation and the ventilator is associated with a decrease in the complications of intubation (see Table 23-5) and the incidence of BPD/CLD resulting from barotrauma, volutrauma, and oxygen toxicity.[27,321,383] With IMV there is a gradual decrease in mechanical ventilation with a corresponding increase in spontaneous respiration. **One ventilator setting at a time is changed, and arterial blood gases and pulse oximetry values are evaluated to determine the infant's response before another adjustment is made.** Because each ventilator parameter has risks and benefits, each parameter must be evaluated before the decision is made as to which one will be lowered. Because high concentrations of

oxygen may be toxic to the lungs and hyperoxia may damage the eyes, oxygen is usually lowered first to a level below 80% in 5% to 10% increments. **PIP is lowered in 1- to 2-cm increments to a level of 16 to 18 cm of water, and respiratory rate is lowered in increments of 1 to 5 breaths/min until the infant has a rate of 15 to 20 breaths/min.**

Failure of extubation results in a reintubation rate in LBW infants of approximately 25% to 40%.[21,271,544] **Nasal CPAP is effective in preventing extubation failure and decreasing BPD/CLD by preventing atelectasis, improving oxygenation, decreasing apnea/bradycardia, and improving thoracoabdominal motion synchrony which indicates improved breathing strategy.**[29,321,322] Weaning an intubated neonate to ventilator CPAP increases the work of breathing associated with endotracheal tube resistance and dead space (e.g., breathing through a straw). A metaanalysis of three randomized controlled trials comparing use of ventilator CPAP with extubation to nasal CPAP showed a significant advantage (e.g., decreased the risk of reintubation and ventilation) for extubation to nasal CPAP especially using nasal prongs.[140]

Extubation directly to nasal CPAP has also been shown to be more effective than extubation directly to supplemental oxygen in a hood.[21,140,271,544] A metaanalysis of six randomized controlled trials comparing nasal CPAP (by any method) with use of an Oxyhood after extubation found that nasal CPAP (1) decreases adverse clinical events (e.g., apnea, bradycardia, respiratory acidosis, and hypoxia), (2) decreases the incidence of BPD/CLD, and (3) decreases the incidence of reintubation.[139,141] These positive effects increase when nasal-prong CPAP is used, compared with nasopharyngeal CPAP, and the benefits are consistent across ranges of weight and gestational age.[139,141]

For weaning preterm infants from mechanical ventilation, prophylactic use of nasal CPAP (with nasal prongs) has been defined as the standard of care.[29] However, variations in therapeutic methods and devices are associated with variations in outcomes. Although RCTs demonstrate a clear advantage of nasal prongs over nasopharyngeal administration, differences in design of nasal prongs may alter effectiveness.[29] Use of binasal prongs is more effective than a single nasal prong in weaning ELBW infants from the ventilator.[142] Various clinical strategies for initiation, management, and weaning of nasal CPAP are used. Use of nasal CPAP with the Aladdin/Infant Flow System (e.g., residual gas pressure is provided by the constant flow of gas) decreases the work of breathing by a more stable volume recruitment in the lungs[117,434] and has been shown to facilitate extubation in VLBW infants compared with nasal pharyngeal CPAP.[434,489,490] Other studies show equal efficacy (e.g., no differences in apnea, bradycardia, or desaturation) when nasal prong CPAP is compared with nasal synchronized IMV[489] or nasal CPAP on a ventilator compared with the Infant Flow System.[547]

If nasal CPAP fails, the nasal route may also be used to administer mechanical ventilation. At extubation of VLBW infants, nasal IMV was more effective than nasal CPAP in reducing apnea and bradycardia.[358,359,399] In two recent studies, both preterm infants (34 weeks' gestational age) and VLBW preterm infants extubated to synchronized nasal intermittent positive-pressure ventilation (SNIPPV) had a significantly higher success rate at 72 hours after extubation when compared with an NCPAP group.[41,321] Another study, in which a single nasopharyngeal tube and high-frequency ventilation were used, showed a decrease in PCO_2 in preterm infants with moderate respiratory insufficiency who deteriorated (e.g., increased respiratory acidosis, increased PCO_2, and hypoxia) with nasal CPAP.[562] A group of VLBW infants, extubated to nasopharyngeal SIMV, were compared with VLBW infants extubated to nasopharyngeal CPAP. The VLBW infants extubated to NPSIMV had a failure rate of 5%, compared with 37% in VLBW infants on nasopharyngeal CPAP. In the SIMV infants respiratory failure requiring reintubation was one and a half times less likely to occur than in the VLBW infants receiving nasopharyngeal CPAP.[199]

Once adequate oxygenation and ventilation on CPAP alone have been maintained, the infant may be extubated and placed in an oxygen hood. Oxygen should be adjusted with the use of pulse oximetry.

During the recovery phase of RDS (approximately 72 hours), changes in lung compliance occur rapidly. Hyperoxia, air leaks, increased intracranial pressure, and decreased cardiac output easily occur if high pressures and high oxygen concentrations are not decreased as rapidly as the lung is recovering.

Infants who are difficult or impossible to wean from the ventilator may have BPD/CLD, PDA, or CNS damage that affects the respiratory control center.

GENERAL COMPLICATIONS

Acute Complications

Acute and chronic complications are the result of the disease process, treatment, or both. Beginning with the least invasive therapy and progressing to more complicated ones only as needed accomplishes two goals: individualizes therapy and minimizes risk of complications. Continuous monitoring of the individual infant's progress is vital to decrease complications from the disease and from the interventions used to support the infant or to treat the primary condition. **Complications of respiratory diseases are listed in Box 23-5.**

Sudden deterioration of the infant's condition is an emergency, and the cause must be found and corrected as soon as possible to minimize further damage. **Causes of sudden deterioration are listed in Box 23-6.**

Respiratory

Management of an infant who has suddenly deteriorated begins with a visual inspection. The oxygen hood, CPAP, or ventilator must be properly connected and free of water. If all connections are intact, the infant must be disconnected from assisted

---

Box 23-5	COMPLICATIONS OF RESPIRATORY DISEASE

I. Acute
  A. Sudden deterioration of condition
  B. Air leaks
  C. Central nervous system
    1. Hypoxic-ischemic injury
    2. Increased intracranial pressure
    3. Hemorrhage
  D. Cardiac
    1. Patent ductus arteriosus
    2. Decreased cardiac output
  E. Infection
  F. Bleeding diathesis
  G. Tube
  H. Pulmonary hemorrhage
II. Chronic
  A. Oxygen toxicity and barotrauma (BPD)
  B. Hyperoxia (retinopathy of prematurity)
  C. Hypoxia
  D. Tube

BPD, Bronchopulmonary dysplasia.

Box 23-6	CAUSES OF SUDDEN DETERIORATION

I. Tube
   A. Accidental extubation
   B. Accidental disconnection
   C. Plug
II. Machine malfunction
   A. Ventilator or CPAP device
   B. Oxygen blender
   C. Tubing and connections
III. Alarm system "off"
IV. Severe hypoxia
V. Metabolic factors
VI. Air leak
VII. Intraventricular hemorrhage

CPAP, Continuous positive airway pressure.

Table 23-10	FINDINGS AND CAUSES OF INFANT'S CONDITION WITH CHEST AUSCULTATION

FINDING	POSSIBLE CAUSE
No air entry bilaterally	Air leak
	Plugged endotracheal tube
Diminished air entry	Air leak
	Endotracheal tube too high
Air entry over stomach	Accidental extubation
Air entry unequal	Air leak
	Endotracheal tube too low
Cardiac point of maximum intensity shifted	Air leak with tension

ventilation and connected to a resuscitation bag (that is connected to an oxygen source and kept at the bedside). Manual ventilation matching pressure, rates, and FiO_2 to ventilator settings must be maintained. If the infant improves with these interventions, mechanical failure of the ventilator should be suspected. Assistance should be summoned to find the mechanical problem or replace the system. The infant's respiratory effort must be manually assisted until the problem is solved.

If the infant does not improve with manual ventilation, there is probably a problem with the tube. **The infant's condition can be assessed by auscultating the chest for quality of breath sounds. Findings and what they suggest are listed in Table 23-10.**

The endotracheal tube should be suctioned quickly. If there is no improvement in clinical condition or air entry, the tube should be replaced while supporting the infant with bag and mask ventilation. If the tube is too low, it can be repositioned by pulling it back 0.5 to 1 cm. If air entry and clinical condition improve with auscultation, the tube must be secured in the new position and a chest x-ray examination done for tube placement. If assessment of the chest leads to suspicion of accidental extubation, the tube must be removed, ventilation with bag and mask administered, and reintubation performed. If the infant does not improve with manual ventilation and the tube is in place, an air leak or IVH could be the cause.

Monitors and ventilators are equipped with alarm systems to warn care providers of sudden changes in the infant's condition or in supportive systems. It is imperative that all alarm systems be maintained in the "on" position. Turning the alarms "off" during care for such procedures as suctioning and weighing creates the risk of forgetting to turn them on again. In a busy NICU the compromised infant may not be visually noticed until the hypoxia is so severe that resuscitation is more difficult or impossible. Monitor parameters (both high and low alarm settings) must be individualized for each infant and recorded (see Chapter 7).

A sick neonate may experience a severe hypoxic insult when oxygen is too rapidly altered during caregiving procedures. Feeding, weighing, or turning without an alternative oxygen source may cause a sudden decrease in PaO_2, pulmonary vasoconstriction, hypoperfusion, and an iatrogenic worsening of the condition. Prolonged endotracheal tube suctioning (15 to 20 seconds) causes hypoxia and atelectasis. Care must be organized to conserve energy, minimize hypoxic insults, and maintain the infant in physiologic homeostasis.[127,175,368] Alternative oxygen sources must be provided when the usual method of oxygen delivery is disrupted for giving care. **Small alterations in FiO_2 prevent rapid increases or decreases in oxygen tension.**

Metabolic Factors
Hypoglycemia must never be overlooked as the cause of sudden collapse. Undetected infiltration or disconnection of IV fluids may cause a precipitous drop in blood glucose, with respiratory irregularity, apnea, or seizures. Quickly checking the blood glucose with a glucometer is always warranted. If low blood glucose is not the cause of the sudden deterioration, it may be a complication of the asphyxial episode. After the infant is stabilized, screening for hypoglycemia and providing adequate fluids and glucose are appropriate (see Chapter 15).

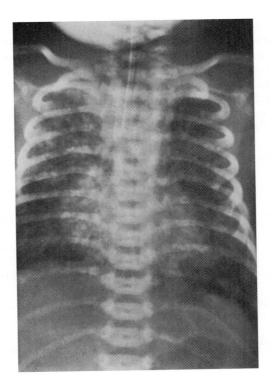

FIGURE 23-2 Pulmonary interstitial emphysema (PIE).

Hypothermia and overwhelming sepsis with their associated metabolic derangements may be the cause of sudden deterioration. Muted response to cold stress is a sequela of asphyxial insult, and cold stress must be avoided after the acute episode. **A high level of suspicion for infection should accompany sudden deterioration** (see Chapters 6 and 22).

Air Leaks
Physiology. When air dissects from an alveolus, it follows the tracheobronchial tree and may accumulate in the mediastinum (pneumomediastinum), in the pleural space (pneumothorax), in the space surrounding the heart (pneumopericardium), or in the peritoneal cavity (pneumoperitoneum) or subcutaneously (subcutaneous emphysema). **Air leaks are complications of respiratory diseases and treatment strategies.** When air continues to accumulate, pressure builds in the pleural space, compresses the lung, and pushes the mediastinum toward the unaffected side; a tension pneumothorax results.

The free air released from ruptured alveoli may lead to pulmonary interstitial emphysema (PIE) (Figure 23-2). This free air intravasates into interstitial tissue and can compromise pulmonary vascular circulation and ventilation. Localized pulmonary interstitial emphysema sometimes resolves spontaneously. Frequently it can continue for weeks or even months. Use of HFV has improved the outcome of these infants.

Etiologic Factors. **Infants at increased risk for the development of air leaks fall into three specific categories: healthy term neonates, neonates with pulmonary diseases, and neonates receiving positive-pressure support (CPAP and IMV).**

Healthy term neonates generate pressures of 40 to 80 cm of water for their first breath of life. Therefore a spontaneous air leak is more common in the neonatal period (2% to 10%) than at any other time of life.

Pulmonary diseases such as RDS result in stiff, noncompliant lungs requiring higher pressures for alveolar ventilation. Aspiration syndromes cause a ball-valve obstruction of debris with distal air trapping (meconium, milk, amniotic fluid, blood, and mucus). Hypoplastic lungs create a risk for air leaks because lung growth and development are abnormal and the lungs are stiff and noncompliant (diaphragmatic hernia and oligohydramnios syndrome). In either congenital lobar or pulmonary interstitial emphysema, alveolar rupture is associated with positive-pressure ventilation.

Positive-pressure ventilation, especially with excessive pressure, results in overdistention with alveolar rupture and air dissection. Air leaks occur in 16% to 36% of infants who are ventilated by CPAP or IMV, or resuscitated with a bag and mask or with an endotracheal tube and bag. **Administration of surfactant lowers the levels of ventilatory support necessary to adequately ventilate the preterm infant's lungs and results in a reduced incidence of pneumothorax.**[242,482,521,572]

Prevention. Using the least amount of positive pressure to obtain physiologic results decreases the chances of air leaks. The incidence of pneumothorax is reduced in surfactant-treated prematures and with the use of HFV.[92,242,482,521,572] Scrupulously clearing the airway before resuscitation and using pressure gauges on resuscitation equipment may prevent aspiration and the possibility of inadvertently using pressure that is too high. Because air leaks alter systemic hemodynamics they are associated with the development of IVH (see Chapter 26). Rapid recognition of at-risk infants, recognition of clinical manifestations and diagnosis, and rapid emergency treatment improve survival and decrease the long-term sequelae of hypoxia and ischemia.

Data Collection

History. Pneumothorax or other air leaks should be suspected when any one of the following infants takes a sudden turn for the worse:

- A preterm infant with RDS either with or without positive-pressure support
- A term or postterm infant with meconium-stained amniotic fluid
- An infant with an x-ray film of interstitial or lobar emphysema
- An infant requiring resuscitation at birth
- An infant receiving CPAP or positive-pressure ventilation

Signs and Symptoms. Asymptomatic air leaks occur in term neonates; these frequently require no treatment and resolve spontaneously in 24 to 48 hours. Gradual onset of symptoms is characterized by increasing difficulty in ventilation, oxygenation, and perfusion. Early clinical manifestations may include restlessness and irritability; lethargy; tachypnea; and use of accessory muscles including grunting, flaring, and retractions. These subtle clinical changes may be unnoticed until the infant progresses to a sudden, profound collapse.

Sudden and severe deterioration in clinical course is characterized by:

- Profound generalized cyanosis
- Bradycardia
- Decrease in the height of the QRS complex on the monitor
- Air hunger including gasping and anxious facies
- Diminished or shifted breath sounds
- Chest asymmetry
- Diminished, shifted, or muffled cardiac sounds and point of maximal intensity (PMI)
- Severe hypotension and poor peripheral perfusion
- Easily palpable liver and spleen
- Subcutaneous emphysema
- Cardiorespiratory arrest

Laboratory Data. Arterial blood gas determinations reveal increasing hypoxemia ($\downarrow Pao_2$), increasing hypercapnia ($\uparrow Paco_2$), and a persistent metabolic acidosis with gradual onset of symptoms. Transillumination of the chest with a fiberoptic probe may reveal hyperlucency of the affected side

when compared with the other side.[345] A chest x-ray examination is the definitive diagnostic technique in air leaks. **Because clinical manifestations of many other diseases may be similar to air leaks, the only way to be sure of the diagnosis is to obtain a chest x-ray examination. Anteroposterior and lateral films must be obtained. Occasionally a decubitus lateral x-ray film may be of value.** X-ray findings in pneumothorax, the most common air leak, include the following:

- Increased lucency, overall increase in size, and flattened diaphragm on the affected side
- Widened intercostal spaces
- Decreased or absent pulmonary vascular markings
- Sharp contrast of the cardiac border and diaphragm (sharp edge sign)

Tension pneumothorax results in mediastinal shifts with decreased volume, increased opacity of opposite lung, and deviation of heart and trachea to the other side.[76]

Treatment. **An air leak is a surgical emergency of the chest.** Tension within the chest cavity compromises lung excursion and cardiac output; without prompt treatment the infant will not survive. Trained care providers must be immediately available to provide emergency management in any institution that provides positive-pressure ventilatory support.

Evacuation of trapped air to decrease tension and allow proper organ function is the goal of treatment. Pneumomediastinum rarely needs to be treated, but pneumopericardium often results in cardiac tamponade and requires needle aspiration and/or tube drainage. Pneumoperitoneum must be differentiated from a perforated viscus.

A suggested conservative treatment is endotracheal intubation of the unaffected lung. The tube is advanced 1 to 2 cm beyond the carina to occlude the involved lung. This procedure is difficult to perform if the left lung is involved. If the pulmonary interstitial emphysema is localized to one lung or lobe of the lung, differential ventilation or surgical removal of the lobe may be curative. **Pneumothorax may be treated with needle aspiration of air. Tube thoracotomy with suction drainage is frequently required.**

Immediate Supportive Care. **The head of the bed is elevated 30 to 40 degrees.** This decreases the work of breathing by using gravity to localize the air in the upper chest and to push the abdominal organs downward away from the diaphragm.

Oxygen at 100% concentration is administered. The two goals for using 100% oxygen for immediate care are to attempt to improve oxygenation in a severely compromised infant and to use a nitrogen washout technique to increase by as much as sixfold the rate of absorption of the trapped air.[335]

CAUTION: Prolonged administration of 100% oxygen to treat an air leak in term infants has been used. However, exclusive use of 100% oxygen to treat trapped air is not recommended in preterm infants because of the risk of developing retinopathy of prematurity and the length of time necessary to obtain complete resolution.

A severely compromised infant requires immediate emergency procedures. A diagnostic and therapeutic thoracentesis may be necessary in life-threatening situations where there is not time to wait for x-ray examination.

Needle Aspiration. A scalp vein needle (23 to 25 gauge) or an Angiocath (24 gauge), a three-way stopcock, and a 10- to 20-ml syringe may be used for needle aspiration. The equipment is connected (syringe-stopcock-needle/Angiocath), the chest is asceptically prepared, and the needle inserted into the third intercostal space in the anterior axillary line. A slight pop may be felt when the pleura is entered. Air is withdrawn into the syringe and evacuated into the room by turning the stopcock. This procedure is repeated until no more air can be aspirated or until a chest tube can be placed.

Chest Tube. Chest tube thoracotomy is the definitive treatment for pneumothorax. The insertion of a chest tube is an invasive procedure that requires strict surgical technique, with each operator wearing a gown, gloves, mask, and cap. The infant should be appropriately positioned, restrained, and monitored before the chest is prepared for asepsis. Ideally, the anterior chest wall should be prepared with a scrub solution for a minimum of 3 minutes. If a special tray is not available, a minor suture tray will usually contain the necessary instruments. Necessary equipment is as follows:

- Chest tube (8 to 12 Fr Argyle)
- Iodine or povidone-iodine (Betadine) scrub solution
- Gloves, gown, mask, hat
- Sterile drapes
- Syringes
- Sterile sponges (gauze)
- Medicine cups
- Lidocaine 1% without epinephrine
- Scalpel blades (No. 11 or 15)
- Hemostat (mosquito and Kelly)
- Scissors
- Needle holder
- Sterile suture
- Sterile connectors (straight)
- Tubing
- Infant disposable underwater seal drainage system (two- or three-bottle or Pleurevac system)
- Wall suction
- Sterile saline solution
- Tape, Tegaderm, or OpSite
- Chest tube clamp for emergency disconnection

The insertion site depends on the clinician's preference. **In the lateral approach, the site is the fourth to sixth intercostal space on or lateral to the anterior axillary line. In the superior approach, the site is the second or third intercostal space on or just lateral to the midclavicular line (Figure 23-3).**

After infiltration of the area with 1% lidocaine, a small incision is made. A pursestring suture should be placed around the incision with ends left loose. A curved hemostat is inserted into the incision and opened. The catheter is advanced through the interspace and into the pleural space. The most frequent error by an inexperienced operator is applying too little force to enter the pleural cavity. The pursestring is tightened and tied, then tied to the chest tube. The tube is connected to the underwater drainage system, which may then be connected to a continuous suction (10 to 20 cm of water is most commonly recommended) device. The tube should be secured with tape. An x-ray examination is used to confirm placement of the tube and to evaluate the effectiveness of the therapy.

Complications. In some instances complications have arisen from the placement of chest tubes in neonates. These include hemorrhage, lung perforation, infarction, and phrenic nerve injury with eventration of the diaphragm. Clinical signs of eventration (elevation of the diaphragm into the thoracic cavity) include a shift of the umbilicus upward and toward the affected side.[381]

Care of Chest Tube and Drainage System. The chest tube drainage system removes air and fluid material from the pleural space to restore

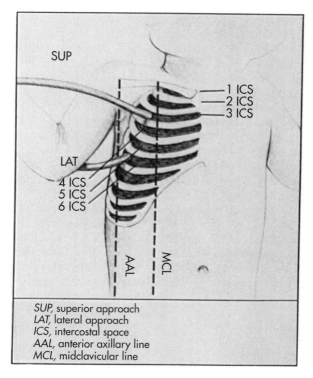

SUP

1 ICS
2 ICS
3 ICS

LAT

4 ICS
5 ICS
6 ICS

AAL   MCL

SUP, superior approach
LAT, lateral approach
ICS, intercostal space
AAL, anterior axillary line
MCL, midclavicular line

FIGURE 23-3   Chest tube insertion site. (From Oellrich RG: Pneumothorax; chest tubes and the neonate, *Matern Child Nurs J* 10:31, 1985.)

negative pressure and expand the lung. Care providers must be familiar with the operation of the drainage system used in the nursery. The single-bottle water seal system drains air and fluid by gravity and blocks atmospheric air from being drawn into the pleural space. In addition to the water seal, the multiple-bottle systems allow suction to be applied to facilitate drainage and expansion. The Pleurevac system is a single plastic unit divided into three chambers: the collection, water seal, and suction chambers.

Oscillation of fluid in the tube demonstrates effective communication between the pleural space and the drainage bottle. In the small, sick infant, intrapleural pressure may only cause fluctuation in the tube at the chest wall. Fluctuation in either the tube or bottle should be observed. Fluctuation may cease as a result of fibrin or blood clots obstructing the tube, kinked or compressed tubing, or the suction apparatus not working properly. Milking and stripping the chest tube is generally unnecessary if only air is being removed. Presence of clots or debris may require gentle kneading of the tube.[80] Milking and stripping generate tremendously high pressures that may entrap and damage the lung in the chest tube eyelets.[165]

Bubbling in the drainage bottle indicates that air is being removed from the pleural space. Continuous bubbling may indicate an air leak in the system. To locate the source of the leak, the tube is momentarily clamped (beginning close to the chest and working toward the bottle) with a rubber-tipped hemostat. When the clamp is placed between the air leak and the water seal, the bubbling will stop. Patency of the tube, fluctuation, and bubbling should be observed and charted hourly.

Excessive or insufficient fluid in the drainage bottles may interfere with proper function of the drainage system. The bottle may need to be changed, or sterile saline may need to be added.

Frequent turning is important for maximum drainage and lung expansion. Proper stabilizing and positioning of the chest tube is necessary for function, comfort, and prevention of accidental removal.

The tubing may be secured by encircling it with an adhesive tab, placing a safety pin through the tape (not the tube), and securing it to the bed. If the tube becomes dislodged, the opening should be covered with sterile gauze and pressure applied until the tube can be replaced.

When the infant is moved for such procedures as x-ray examination and weighing, the tube must be stabilized by holding it close to the chest. If the closed system is disturbed (e.g., a broken bottle), the tube should be clamped with a rubber-tipped hemostat that should always be kept at the bedside. The chest tube should be clamped for as short a time as possible. After necessary clamping, vital signs and clinical conditions should be closely monitored.

Bottles should be stabilized by being taped to an incubator or warmer so that they are not accidentally broken or picked up. The bottles must always be below the level of the infant's chest to prevent water from being pulled into the pleural space.

Removal of Chest Tubes. When bubbling has ceased for at least 24 hours, and the chest x-ray films show no free air for 12 to 24 hours, the chest tube may be removed. Rapid, sterile removal of the tube is followed by application of a petrolatum gauze pressure dressing.

CNS Insult
Acute insult to the CNS may result in increased intracranial pressure, hemorrhage, or hypoxic ischemic brain injury (see Chapter 26).

Cardiac Complications
CDP or IMV may exert sufficient pressure on the pulmonary capillary bed to raise pulmonary artery pressure and interfere with cardiac output.[277] The effect of CDP or IMV on the pulmonary vascular bed and cardiac output may be alleviated by lowering the PIP, or PEEP, or both. At times a fluid infusion to increase the intravascular volume may overcome the resistance to the pulmonary blood flow. The effect of MAP on cardiac output is difficult to monitor in most NICUs, because pulmonary artery or pulmonary wedge pressures are not routinely obtained. Until such time as these measurements are routinely obtained, the best CPAP is determined only on clinical grounds.

PDA is the most common cardiac complication in neonates with respiratory disease. Most often it is manifested by an increasing oxygen requirement or increased dependency on ventilatory support (see Chapter 24).

Infection and Bleeding
Procedures such as intubation expose the neonate to the risk of acquired (nosocomial) infection.* Scrupulous attention to technique when caring for respiratory equipment[225] and performing procedures such as sterile suctioning of the endotracheal tube minimizes the risks of infection. Handwashing before and after every contact with the neonate is the best method of preventing hospital-acquired infection in an already compromised, sick neonate. Neonates who are severely ill with respiratory disease may exhibit bleeding diathesis at birth or during the acute phase of their disease. Early recognition and treatment is important (see Chapter 20).

Chronic Complications
Bronchopulmonary Dysplasia/Chronic Lung Disease
Bronchopulmonary dysplasia/chronic lung disease (BPD/CLD) was first described by Northway and Rosan[421] as serial roentgenographic changes occurring in the lungs of premature infants who survived hyaline membrane disease (HMD). BPD/CLD also occurs in a variety of conditions, including esophageal atresia, aspiration pneumonia, congenital heart disease, PDA, and meconium aspiration. The clinical course of BPD/CLD is one of increasing respiratory distress and often is described as the chronic phase of RDS.

Recent changes in neonatal care have modified the classic stages of BPD as first described by Northway and Rosan.[421] In comparison with the infants in earlier studies, today neonates with chronic lung disease are far more premature and have lower birth weights[274,522] and generally lack many of the radiographic changes of cystic lung disease. **The "new BPD" is characterized by arrestive lung development resulting from interference with alveolarization and vascularization.[293] VLBW neonates who require supplemental oxygen at 28 to 30 days of life, or at 36 weeks' postmenstrual age have chronic lung disease.[152]** Despite these changes, the incidence of chronic lung disease in infants after NICU care remains a significant clinical problem, with an incidence approaching 17% to 54% in VLBW infants.[383]

The incidence of BPD/CLD varies among NICUs[74,96,563,565] because of variations in respiratory management associated with oxygen toxicity and

---

*References 113, 177, 230, 383, 483, 554.

baro/volutrauma.[278,563] Although use of nasal CPAP is associated with lower BPD/CLD rates,* increased use of intubation, mechanical ventilation, and high pressures (PIP and MAP) is associated with increased BPD/CLD rates.[456,563] When mechanical ventilation is used, the shorter the duration, the less BPD/CLD occurs.[78,563]

Pathophysiology. BPD/CLD is a disorder of premature infants that is characterized by respiratory distress and impaired gas exchange. **The pathogenesis of BPD is one of chronic and constant and recurring lung injury, with ongoing repair and healing of the injury.** Chronic injury and repair may in itself prolong the need for the very factors that contribute to the development of BPD: oxygen therapy and mechanical ventilation. In RDS there is injury to the alveolar mucosa, airway mucosa, serum exudation membranes, and fibrin coagulation–forming hyaline membranes. If sufficient hypoxia occurs with resultant damage, the alveolar and airway epithelium and its basement membrane will hemorrhage, and round cell infiltration will begin. Cellular and noncellular debris fill the alveoli and small airways. The obstruction causes microatelectasis, and nonobstructed airways become hyperexpanded and emphysematous.

In the healing and repair process, type II alveolar cells or their precursors multiply and differentiate into type I pneumocytes, which provide alveolar epithelium. Cells of the basal layer of the pseudo-stratified, ciliated, columnar epithelium lining the airways multiply and migrate to cover the injured airway and rejuvenate the epithelium. During this healing phase the rapidly multiplying and differentiating transitional cells are squamous or cuboidal and therefore appear "metaplastic." Epithelial metaplasia is one of the characteristics of BPD.

As healing occurs, increased inspired oxygen tensions, barotrauma, and infection continue to injure the cells that are taking part in the healing process.

Etiology. **BPD/CLD is an iatrogenic disease caused by oxygen toxicity and barotrauma resulting from pressure ventilation.** Even preterm infants with mild respiratory distress in the first week of life may develop BPD/CLD.[483] BPD/CLD is multifactorial so that lung immaturity, fluid overload, infection, PDA, and familial predisposition to asthma also contribute to its development.†

Oxygen Toxicity. **BPD/CLD has been documented in both long- and short-term exposure to oxygen at both low and high levels (greater than 60% to 80%), as well as in infants treated with mechanical ventilation without supplemental oxygen.**[106,455] As a result of these findings, many units have instituted guidelines for oxygen use and monitoring of levels with pulse oximetry. Avoidance of excessive oxygen exposure, careful attention to oxygen saturations, and arterial PaO_2 may help reduce lung injury due to oxygen exposure.[105]

Barotrauma/Volutrauma. **BPD/CLD has also been related to barotrauma and volutrauma.** BPD has been described in infants who have received high peak inspiratory pressures (PIP) and high PEEP[32,60,230,555] and in neonates with pneumothorax and PIE. A decrease in the incidence of BPD has been noted when lower peak inspiratory pressures are used.[106,164,295] Although peak inspiratory pressures should be limited whenever possible, some infants with very noncompliant lungs require the use of high pressure for survival. Volutrauma (e.g., increased lung volume [stretch]), results in regional overdistention of lung units or airways which may promote lung injury more than pressure itself.[96,230] Using the smallest possible tidal volumes to inflate the lung avoids overdistention and volutrauma that causes BPD/CLD.[106]

Use of surfactant therapy and newer ventilatory techniques[106,367,380,474,500] has decreased the pressures necessary to adequately oxygenate and ventilate the neonate's lungs as well as resultant air leaks. A recent study showed that more aggressive ventilator management was not associated with an increase in BPD/CLD, but that ventilator therapy greater than 24 hours was associated with BPD/CLD.[383,610] A ventilator strategy of low tidal volume and adequate PEEP minimizes lung injury.[106,164,295] **A gentler ventilator strategy has been used to decrease exposure of preterm lungs to barotraumas/volutrauma necessary to maintain PCO_2 in the normal range.** A strategy of "permissive hypercapnia" (e.g., accepting a $PaCO_2$ of 45 to 55 mm Hg)[204] using lower PIP, MAP, and ventilator rate reduces the duration of assisted ventilation, supplemental oxygen (at 28 days of life and total days) and rate of reintubation.[380] Although alterations in $PaCO_2$ are associated with fluctuations in cerebral blood flow,[204] there was no difference in IVH and PVL compared with the control group.[380] There was also no difference in mortality, air leaks, ROP, or PDA.[380]

Hypocarbia has been associated with the occurrence of PVL.[226,426,600] A recent study examining the

---

*References 27, 216, 305, 373, 383, 563, 570.
†References 27, 60, 106, 177, 312, 419, 483, 555, 564, 565.

relationship between ventilator setting and hypocarbia found that although the ventilator settings were similar (to the group with PVL), hypocarbia and an increased respiratory rate (of 5 breaths/min) did exist in the infants with PVL on the third day. Rather than being the cause of PVL, these authors speculated that hypocarbia may be the result of or part of the sequence of PVL.[426] Another recent study showed conflicting results: hypercarbia, not hypocarbia, is associated with the development of BPD/CLD.[536] Clearly, further studies are needed to clarify the relationship between hypocarbia/hypercarbia and PVL.

The goal of HFV—adequate gaseous exchange with less lung injury—is accomplished by the use of smaller tidal volumes, uniform lung inflation, more constant MAP, and avoidance of pressure swings.[106] **Combining HFOV with surfactant has been shown to lead to less lung injury than HFOV alone or CMV with surfactant.**[286]

Conflicting results in the use of HFV and reduction in BPD/CLD in published trials are the result of a multitude of factors.[94] Use of "high-volume" technique has been associated with less BPD/CLD and no increase in IVH.[59,111] A recent study showed that using HFOV immediately after intubation, along with early lung volume optimization, resulted in fewer ventilator days, fewer days on oxygen, and a significant decrease (0% versus 34%) in BPD/CLD in VLBW infants.[474] Although the use of HFV reduces BPD/CLD and neurologic injury, if used improperly, HFV worsens neurodevelopmental outcomes.[319] In the future, computer-controlled ventilators may stabilize physiologic parameters, decrease barotraumas/volutrauma, and expedite weaning.[500] However, these new devices are yet to be proven and require further RCTs.

Patent Ductus Arteriosus. There is a high incidence of BPD among infants with PDA[230,383,455,537] and congestive heart failure.[483,564] **The amount of oxygen and peak inspiratory pressure required to support a neonate through the pulmonary complications of PDA may result in damage from oxygen toxicity and barotrauma.** The increased pulmonary blood flow that occurs may also contribute to pulmonary damage. Because of these findings, medical closure of the ductus with indomethacin or surgical ligation is advocated (see Chapter 24) but has not affected the incidence of BPD.[32]

Nutrition. SGA infants who were undernourished in utero have been shown to have an in-

creased risk of BPD/CLD.[223] **Inadequate nutrition caused by poor intake and/or increased nutritional requirements resulting in catabolism may potentiate the effects of oxygen and barotrauma on the neonatal lung.**[525] Inadequate intake of antioxidants, trace elements, vitamins, and polyunsaturated fatty acids may also predispose the lung to injury.[525] Among VLBW infants two studies show an increased rate of esophageal reflux in infants with chronic lung disease,[201,281] and one study shows no association between gastroesophageal reflux and BPD/CLD.[302]

Fluids. BPD has also been detected in infants who have developed symptoms of fluid overload within the first few days of life.[383,537,564,565] Fluid balance in a VLBW infant is complicated by huge insensible water loss and often an intolerance for enteral feedings. Intake, output, and changes in weight must be closely monitored to calculate the fluid needs.

Family History of Asthma. Infants who develop BPD may have relatives with asthma who require hospitalization.[419] The lungs of these infants may be less tolerant of the insults of pulmonary disease, oxygen, pressure, and fluids.

Prematurity. Developmental immaturity is of principal importance in the etiologic picture of BPD/CLD.[563] Premature births alone may have a significant effect on pulmonary development, because prematurity results in differences in the development of small airways. As a result, premature infants are more susceptible to additional damage to the small airways from oxygen, ventilator pressure, fluids, and circulatory overload. As the survival rate of VLBW infants of less than 28 weeks' gestation increases, the occurrence of BPD/CLD is increasing (e.g., the lower the gestational age, the higher the risk).[33,383] However, the current form of BPD/CLD is less severe, with fewer infants requiring tracheostomies and long-term ventilation therapy (6 months or more).[293]

Oxygen and Antioxidants. Oxygen accepts free electrons generated by oxidative metabolism within the cell and produces free radicals, molecules that are toxic to living cells and/or tissues.[487] Normally, antioxidants protect cells against free radicals, but this balance may be upset by increased free radical production or decreased antioxidant defense. **A preterm neonate may be deficient in antioxidants**

and thus more susceptible to lung damage from free radicals.

Inflammation. Oxygen radicals, barotrauma, infection, and other factors initiate the inflammatory process, resulting in the infiltration of leukocytes, with release of other inflammatory mediators, resulting in pulmonary damage (e.g., decrease in capillary endothelial integrity, albumin leakage in the alveoli resulting in pulmonary edema). Neonates whose lungs are mechanically ventilated have increased pulmonary cytokine levels.* Activated neutrophils release enzymes that directly destroy the elastin and collagen of the lung. **Lung inflammation and injury predisposes the lung to increased susceptibility to volutrauma and oxidant-induced lung injury.**[293,295] This inflammatory cycle produces significant pulmonary injury during a critical period of rapid lung growth and development (24 to 40 weeks) (see Table 23-1). Preterm infants exposed to antenatal inflammation and infection are at increased risk of developing BPD/CLD.[527,585,609] Postnatal nosocomial infection is associated with an increased risk of BPD/CLD.† Variation in nosocomial infection rates may be a factor in the variation in inter-NICU BPD/CLD rates.[106,278]

Preterm infants with increased lung inflammation who subsequently develop BPD/CLD have been shown to have early adrenal insufficiency.[584,586,587] Even very early preterm infants (24 to 25 weeks) have been shown to have an increase in cortisol levels after birth, reaching maximal levels at 24 hours, with a gradual decrease of 14 to 28 days.[33] Low cortisol levels may be associated with an increased risk for developing BPD/CLD.[584,587] In one recent study, low cortisol levels at 3 to 7 days (but not 14 to 28 days) of life minimally increased the risk of BPD/CLD.[33] However, use of early low-dose hydrocortisone therapy (to achieve cortisol levels in the physiologic range) was found in one study to increase survival without BPD/CLD and without side effects.[586] Further studies are needed.

Prevention. **Widespread use of antenatal steroids and surfactant administration have not reduced the rate of BPD/CLD nor the NICU disparities in BPD/CLD rates.**[434,452,563,610] Use of surfactant does reduce the severity of BPD/CLD.[293,295] A sin-

gle course of antenatal steroid therapy decreases the incidence and severity of BPD/CLD.[411,412,455,589] Widespread use of both antenatal and postnatal steroid therapy has not improved the outcome in ELBW infants.[236,238] Premature and full-term infants (with pneumonia, MAS) treated with surfactant replacement have a lower incidence of BPD/CLD because of (1) better ventilation and pressure distribution in the alveoli, (2) stabilization of the alveoli, (3) prevention of overdistention, and (4) decreased cytokines and inflammatory response.[25,369,408]

Use of nasal CPAP may reduce or eliminate the need for intubation and mechanical ventilation, as well as assist in successful extubation.* In an attempt to prevent reinjury and allow healing, inspired oxygen tensions should be kept as low as is reasonable to provide adequate arterial oxygen tension. Pressures on the ventilator should be reduced when possible to prevent barotrauma. Although the collaborative HFV trial did not demonstrate a difference in the incidence of BPD between HFV and conventional ventilation,[215,269] early use of HFV and/or use of HFV with surfactant may decrease lung damage and resultant BPD/CLD.[319,474] In a recent RCT, inhaled nitric oxide, with its antioxidant and antiinflammatory effects on lung tissue[330] and its potentially protective effects on surfactant function,[378] decreased the incidence of BPD/CLD in preterm infants.[332] For infants older than 36 weeks' gestational age who are unresponsive to conventional ventilation, ECMO is used in selected cases. Scrupulous care of respiratory equipment[225] and sterile procedure for ETT suctioning is imperative. Infections should be treated with appropriate antibiotic agents and PDA vigorously treated medically and/or surgically.

In a recent multicenter trial, administration of vitamin A (e.g., 5000 IU IM three times a week for 4 weeks) to VLBW infants reduced the risk of BPD/CLD.[560] Monitoring of serum levels (the desired range of plasma vitamin A concentrations is 30 to 60 μg/dl; the desired plasma RBP concentration is above 25 mg/dl)[510] and assessment for manifestations of toxicity (e.g., lesions on skin/mucous membranes, bone and joint abnormalities, jaundice, hepatomegaly, and increased ICP) should accompany vitamin A administration.[106,510] In a more recent study oral supplementation of vitamin

*References 30, 293, 296, 303, 343, 527, 548, 614.
†References 113, 177, 230, 383, 483, 555.

*References 27, 29, 139, 140, 271, 383.

A (e.g., 5000 IU/day for 28 days) in ELBW infants did not significantly alter the incidence of BPD/CLD.[583]

Prevention of oxygen free radical injury to the pulmonary and central nervous systems (e.g., BPD/CLD and IVH/PVL)[496] occurs with intratracheal injection of recombinant human CuZn superoxide dismutase (rhSOD).[135,487] A significant decrease in markers of pulmonary inflammation occurred in rhSOD-treated preterm infants without short- or long-term abnormalities.[135,137,487] A multicenter, placebo-controlled trial of rhSOD in 301 VLBW infants showed that treated infants had a 60% decrease in the incidence of severe IVH (grades 3 and 4) and PVL.[135,487,496] Further study of rhSOD effects on preventing pulmonary and neurologic injury await multicenter RCTs of larger numbers of infants.[137]

Data Collection

History. A history of prematurity, moderate to severe RDS, intubation with oxygen and positive-pressure ventilation in the first week of life, inability to be weaned from the ventilator, and increasing oxygen requirement at the end of the first week of life are associated with BPD. Long-term features include tachypnea, rales, retractions, abnormal chest x-ray examination results, and the need for supplemental oxygen for more than 28 to 30 days of life or at 36 weeks' postmenstrual age.[152]

Signs and Symptoms. Tachypnea, exercise intolerance (feeding and handling), oxygen dependence, and respiratory distress (retractions, nasal flaring, fine rales at the bases or throughout the lung fields) are associated with BPD.

Laboratory Data. X-ray findings (Figure 23-4) correlate with the stage of disease; however, the pathologic changes are often more severe than the chest x-ray findings indicate[168,421]:

Stage I   Reticulogranular pattern and air bronchogram or RDS (first 3 days of life)

Stage II   Coarse granular infiltrates that are dense enough to obscure the cardiac markings (first 3 to 10 days of life)

Stage III   Multiple small cyst formation within the opaque lungs and visible cardiac borders (first 10 to 20 days of life)

Stage IV   Irregular larger cyst formation that alternates with areas of increased density (after 28 days of life)

Mild hyperinflation as demonstrated on a chest x-ray film is a common finding in VLBW infants with BPD/CLD.[187]

Cardiovascular changes include (1) right ventricular hypertrophy on ECG, (2) elevated right ventricular systolic time intervals or left ventricular and septal wall thickening on echocardiogram, or (3) elevated pulmonary vascular pressures and resistance at cardiac catheterization.[569]

Treatment. **The therapeutic goal is to reduce those factors that produce reinjury and to allow the lung to heal so that normal function can resume.** This process may take weeks, months, or even years in severe lung injuries or in small infants under 1000 g.

Concurrent supportive therapies include (1) maintenance of adequate oxygenation and ventilation, (2) adequate nutrition and fluid restriction, (3) early PDA closure, and (4) pharmacologic management. Sufficient PIP should be used to prevent atelectasis while maintaining the lowest FiO_2 (if possible, 0.5 or lower) to maintain adequate oxygenation (i.e., PaO_2 60 to 80 mm Hg; O_2 saturation 90% to 95%). **Weaning from mechanical ventilation is done slowly and may be facilitated by (1) use of SIMV that reduces the work of breathing, (2) use of methylxanthines before extubation, and (3) use of nasal CPAP after extubation.*** **Usually in BPD/CLD the infant's ability to maintain ventilation develops before the ability to maintain adequate oxygenation.** Often infants are discharged from the NICU on home oxygen therapy. **Infants with BPD/CLD who require oxygen at a rate of 20 ml/kg/min or less and those who are able to maintain oxygen saturations of 92% or above after 40 minutes of breathing room air are ready to begin successful weaning from supplemental oxygen.**[515]

Neonates with BPD have an increased resting metabolic expenditure as the major reason for growth failure, especially in the smallest, sickest infants.[347] These infants may require 150 to 200 kcal/kg/day to support adequate growth (i.e., 10 to 30 g/day weight gain).[206] Without adequate protein and/or caloric intake, damaged pulmonary tissue cannot heal,[170,525] and provision of appropriate nutrition to the neonate with BPD is essential (see Chapters 14 to 19).

---

*References 27, 29, 139, 140, 271, 383.

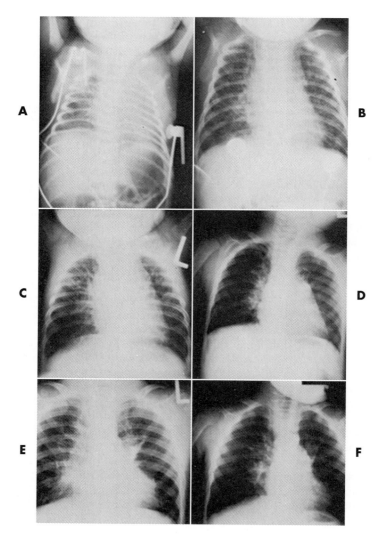

FIGURE 23-4   Serial chest x-ray films of premature infant with BPD over 2-year period. **A,** Newborn. **B,** 2 months. **C,** 3 months. **D,** 1 year. **E,** 2 years. Infant's disease process was characterized by multiple hospitalizations for reactive airway disease and pulmonary hypertension. Note progressive lung disease characterized by hyperinflation and eventual clearing of infiltrate by 2 years of age **(F).**

Pharmacologic management of BPD/CLD includes the use of bronchodilators, steroids, and diuretics (Table 23-11).[2] Inhaled and systemic bronchodilators improve lung mechanics and gaseous exchange by relaxation of bronchial smooth muscle.[136,196,308] However, bronchodilators may fail to relieve airway obstruction because of relatively poor development of bronchial smooth muscle in preterm infants. Use of inhaled nitric oxide in preterm infants with BPD/CLD improves oxygenation without adverse outcomes in a phase II trial.[101]

Methylxanthine therapy promotes weaning of infants with RDS from low rates of ventilatory sup-port.[253] Diuretics and diuretics combined with methylxanthines improve lung mechanics, clinical respiratory status, and ability to wean from mechanical ventilation.[307,308]

Use of antenatal[122,411,412,455] **and postnatal steroid therapy is associated with improved survival,**[243-246,248,369] **more rapid ventilator weaning, and decreased need for supplemental oxygen in at-risk neonates.**[243-246,248,314,607] Steroids reduce lung inflammation and improve pulmonary function in severe RDS.[390,437] Antenatally, steroidal agents are administered to 50% of mothers and postnatally to 50% of VLBW infants.[573] Even the choice of

Table 23-11 PHARMACOLOGIC AGENTS USED IN TREATMENT OF BPD

DRUG	DOSAGE	COMMENTS
I. Bronchodilators		
A. Inhaled		
1. Beta₂-agonists		
a. Albuterol (Proventil, Ventolin)	0.1 mg/kg up to 5 mg in 2 ml of normal saline solution q 4-6 hr Max dose: 0.5 ml or 2.5 mg/treatment; up to six treatments/24 hr	Drug of choice for bronchospasm—improves pulmonary resistance and lung compliance by bronchial smooth muscle relaxation; tachycardia, tremors, nausea and vomiting; can cause paradoxical bronchoconstriction: irritability; onset 5-15 min; peak action in 30 min to 2 hr; duration 3-4 hr; MDI dosage improves lung function as well as nebulization and is faster and more cost-effective[320]
b. Terbutaline (Brethine)	0.03-0.3 mg/kg/day	Same as for albuterol above; onset 5-30 min; duration 3-4 hr
2. Histamine inhibitor (Cromolyn: 20 mg/2 ml solution for nebulizer)	10-20 mg tid	Prevents release of inflammatory mediators and reduces airway hypersensitivity; urticaria, rash, and throat irritation; dosage may need adjusting in patients with hepatic and/or renal dysfunction
B. Systemic		
1. Methylxanthines		
a. Caffeine citrate	Loading: 20 mg/kg Maintenance: 5 mg/kg/day IV or PO	Promotes weaning from low rates of ventilatory support by reduction of pulmonary resistance, improved lung compliance, and improved skeletal muscle and diaphragmatic contractility; has diuretic effect; half-life as long as 100 hr; excreted unchanged in urine; safer drug with fewer side effects than theophylline; side effects rare but include tachycardia, diuresis, dysrhythmias, glucosuria, seizures, ketonuria, vomiting, hyperglycemia, jitteriness, hemorrhagic gastritis
b. Theophylline (PO)	4-6 mg/kg of active theophylline, which should produce a serum level of 10-20 μg/ml; maintenance calculated by rate of plasma clearance, usually 3-7 mg/kg/day q 12 hr	Half-life is 30-40 hr, metabolized to caffeine in the liver and excreted in urine; multisystem effect: CNS stimulant; increases respiratory rate, inspiratory drive and surfactant production; increases GFR; increases heart rate, contractility, and output; decreases GI motility and increases GI secretions; increases glucose levels, ketonuria, and glycosuria; increases muscle contractility; increases catecholamine and insulin levels; side effects: same as for caffeine citrate
2. Beta₂-agonists		
a. Terbutaline	5 μg/kg SC q 4-6 hr	Improves pulmonary mechanics; side effects same as for albuterol above; adjunct to methylxanthines
b. Albuterol	0.15 mg/kg/dose PO q 8 hr	Reduces pulmonary resistance; adjunct to methylxanthines; side effects same as for albuterol above
II. Steroids		
A. Inhaled		
1. Corticosteroids (Dexamethasone [Decadron])	100 μg/inhalation from MDI	30%-60% systemic bioavailability versus 53%-78% from oral intake; majority removed from lung within 20 min after administration; anatomic, physiologic, and pathophysiologic variations in the neonate, coupled with the aerosol delivery system and its use influence the amount of drug administered and the aerosol's efficacy[105]; side effects: oral candidiasis, bronchospasm, and pituitary-adrenal suppression[108]; tongue hypertrophy[360]

BPD, Bronchopulmonary dysplasia; *BUN,* blood urea nitrogen; *CNS,* central nervous system; *GFR,* glomerular filtration rate; *GI,* gastrointestinal; *KCl,* potassium chloride; *MDI,* metered dose inhaler.

Continued

Table 23-11	PHARMACOLOGIC AGENTS USED IN TREATMENT OF BPD—cont'd	
DRUG	DOSAGE	COMMENTS

2. Glucocorticosteroids
  a. Flunisolide (Nasalide)
  b. Beclomethasone (Beconase; Vancenase)
	250 µg/inhalation
	42 µg/inhalation
		Unknown stability—do not mix with other drugs; bronchospasm may result from buffers and/or preservatives; side effects: same as for dexamethasone above

B. Systemic (Corticosteroids—dexamethasone [Decadron])	0.5 mg/kg/day IV or PO q 12 hr for 3 days; decrease to 0.3 mg/kg/day for 3 days Taper 10%-20% q 3 days	Hyperglycemia; hypothalamic-pituitary-adrenal axis suppression; renal calcification; protein depletion and/or tissue catabolism (increase BUN; failure to gain weight); gastric irritation, perforation, bleeding; restlessness and/or irritability; myocardial hypertrophy; hypertension; increased risk for infection (see Long-Term Adverse Effects of Steroid Use, Box 23-7)
III. Diuretics A. Furosemide (Lasix)	1-2 mg/kg/dose IV bid or 2-4 mg/kg/dose PO bid	Treatment of choice for fluid overload in BPD— decrease interstitial edema and pulmonary vascular resistance; daily or alternate-day administration improves pulmonary mechanics and facilitates weaning from ventilator; side effects: metabolic alkalosis, hypokalemia, hypocalcemia; hypochloremia, hyponatremia, renal calcifications, gallstones, ototoxicity; KCl supplementation; onset 5 min IV; 1 hr PO; duration 2-4 hr
B. Thiazides 1. Chlorthiazide (Diuril)	5-20 mg/kg/dose IV or PO bid	Less potent than furosemide; promotes potassium and bicarbonate excretion with sodium and chloride; spares calcium; given with spironolactone; combination of thiazide and spironolactone results in improved lung mechanics and increased urine output; side effects: electrolyte imbalance, hypercalcemia, hyperglycemia, decreased magnesium level, hypersensitivity, GI upset, glycosuria
2. Hydrochlorothiazide (Hydro Diuril)	1-2 mg/kg/dose PO bid	Side effects: electrolyte imbalance, hypercalcemia, hyperglycemia, metabolic alkalosis; increased urinary losses of sodium, potassium, magnesium, chloride, phosphorus, and bicarbonate; spares calcium; onset 1-2 hr; duration 6-12 hr
3. Spironolactone (Aldactone)	1.5 mg/kg/dose PO bid	Weak diuretic; causes increased sodium chloride and water loss; spares potassium; side effects: irritability, lethargy, vomiting, diarrhea, rash; onset 2-3 days
4. Bumetanide (Bumax)	0.015 mg/kg/day up to 0.1 mg/kg/day PO	40 times the potency of Lasix; used in neonates and infants who are refractory to Lasix therapy; side effects same as for furosemide, above, plus hypophosphatemia

BPD, Bronchopulmonary dysplasia; *BUN,* blood urea nitrogen; *CNS,* central nervous system; *GFR,* glomerular filtration rate; *GI,* gastrointestinal; *KCl,* potassium chloride; *MDI,* metered dose inhaler.

which glucocorticoid to use antenatally may be significant: antenatal dexamethasone increases PVL compared with antenatal betamethasone.[44] An NIH consensus statement[412] discourages multiple courses of antenatal steroids because of (1) impaired head growth,[198] (2) impaired brain development and behavior,[197,236,238,590] (3) increased mortality and lung disease,[33,355] (4) gastroesophageal reflux,[58] and (5) an increased severity of ROP.[148]

Postnatal steroid use became widespread in the 1990s without properly conducted RCTs for safety and efficacy,[184] despite warnings from re-

Box 23-7	LONG-TERM ADVERSE EFFECTS OF STEROID USE

Slower growth—*References 51, 406, 407, 417, 436, 530, 531, 590*
- Somatic and head growth
- Arrested lung development caused by interference in pulmonary alveolarization and vascularization[293]

"Neurotoxic" substances—*References 39, 42, 576*
- Further reduces size of premature brain—*References 406, 407*
- Increased rate of cerebral palsy—*References 44, 160, 161, 431, 512, 606*
- Increased cognitive deficits—*References 236, 512, 531, 576*
- Increased severity of ROP—*References 244-246, 576*

Contributes to long-term
- Cardiovascular disease—*References 160, 427*
- Immune system disorders/autoimmune diseases—*Reference 31*
- Renal calcifications—*References 33, 304*
- Neurologic and behavioral deficits—*References 51, 236, 306, 407, 576, 590*

ROP, Retinopathy of prematurity.

searchers in the 1970s about serious potential dangers.[195,543,588] Steroid use has been enthusiastically accepted because of the dramatic, short-term improvements in respiratory status, although long-term effects were unknown. Two large RCTs of postnatal steroid use were halted because of serious short-term complications—intestinal perforation, growth retardation, PVL, hyperglycemia, hypertension, and infection.* **Adverse long-term outcomes are listed in Box 23-7. Adverse developmental outcomes are the result of the effects of steroids on the developing nervous system.**[294] The choice of postnatal glucocorticoid therapy may also be significant.[548] Use of methylprednisolone is as effective as dexamethasone with fewer side effects, including a decreased incidence of PVL.[20]

The efficacy of inhaled steroids in decreasing pulmonary inflammation and BPD/CLD while decreasing the incidence and severity of complications of systemic steroid usage is being studied with conflicting results.[348] An RCT of beclomethasone found no reduction of BPD/CLD but a decrease in (1) usage of subsequent systemic steroid, (2) bronchodilator therapy, (3) the proportion of infants re-

quiring ventilatory therapy at 1 month of age, and (4) tracheal inflammation markers and mucosal injury.[1,107] Another study in which inhaled fluticasone was used showed that more treated babies were extubated at 14 days, with no significant differences in the mortality rate, BPD/CLD, or subsequent systemic steroid therapy.[191] A recent review of trials of inhaled steroidal agents concluded that although there are short-term benefits (e.g., improved lung function and decreased need for later systemic steroids), there are no apparent long-term benefits and no effect on mortality rates or risk of BPD/CLD.[243] When early treatment with dexamethasone was compared with delayed treatment with inhaled steroids, preterm infants receiving early dexamethasone had (1) improved survival without BPD/CLD, (2) increased weight loss at the beginning of treatment, (3) decreased incidence of PDA, (4) increased risk of complications (e.g., hyperglycemia, hypertension, gastrointestinal problems, and major cerebral abnormalities), and (5) increased rate of death before discharge.[248] Neither this study[248] nor a recent review of inhaled steroids[508] showed that inhaled steroids are more effective than systemic steroids. Dosing of inhaled steroids with MDI remains a problem, because the desired amount may not be the dose delivered.[105]

Currently steroids are in common use, with widely varying practices about dosage as well as when and how they are used.* In a recent survey, less than 10% of the physician respondents reported involving parents in informed consent regarding steroid use.[546] Parents (in addition to health care providers)[407,548] must be honestly informed about the experimental nature of steroid use and its short- and long-term complications, so that they are able to participate in giving or withholding their fully informed consent.[254] After reviewing the short-term and long-term effects of systemic and inhaled corticosteroid use for the prevention and treatment of BPD/CLD in the VLBW infant, the AAP and Canadian Pediatric Society have published joint recommendations, as follows[17a]:
- Routine use of systemic dexamethasone to prevent or treat BPD/CLD in VLBW infants is **not** recommended.
- Postnatal use of systemic dexamethasone should be limited to carefully designed RCTs.
- Long-term neurodevelopmental assessment is strongly encouraged.

---

*References 209, 222, 243, 248, 354, 393, 437, 484, 529, 530, 533.

*References 17a, 184, 207, 243, 246, 342, 431, 436, 484, 504, 512, 519, 546, 586, 606.

Box 23-8	COMPLICATIONS OF BPD*

Increased Mortality

Pulmonary

Acute: PIE, air leaks, pulmonary hypertension, cyst formation
Chronic: altered pulmonary function, respiratory infections, rehospitalizations, and home oxygen

Cardiac

Cor pulmonale and right-sided heart failure

Growth Restriction

Somatic growth (weight)
Head growth

Orthopedic

Fractures, rickets

Neurodevelopmental Delay

Cognitive impairment
Cerebral palsy
Behavior problems
Cerebral ventriculomegaly

Sensory Deficits

Sensorineural hearing loss
Increased severity (stage 3) ROP

Long-Term Effects of Steroid Use (see Box 23-7)

---

*References 2, 11, 35, 98, 152, 172, 188, 236-239, 287, 288, 299, 377, 392, 430, 433, 480, 516, 520, 569, 576.
BPD/CLD, Bronchopulmonary dysplasia/chronic lung disease; *PIE,* pulmonary interstitial emphysema; *ROP,* retinopathy of prematurity.

Box 23-9	RISK FACTORS FOR RSV[16,231,297]

- Preterm infant ≤32 wk gestation without BPD/CLD
- Preterm infant with BPD/CLD ≤2 yr old requiring medical treatment within 6 mo before RSV season
- Preterm infant of 32-35–wk gestational age with additional risk factors:
  Neurologic disorders
  Number of young siblings
  Childcare attendance
  Exposure to second handsmoke
  Anticipated heart surgery
  Distance and availability of hospital care for severe respiratory viral illness
- History of RSV illness
- Infants with congenital heart disease, multiple congenital anomalies, and immunodeficiencies
- Male gender

BPD/CLD, Bronchopulmonary dysplasia/chronic lung disease; *RSV,* respiratory syncytial virus.

- The use of alternative antiinflammatory corticosteroids, both systemic and inhaled, awaits RCTs before additional recommendations.
- Outside of RCTs, use of corticosteroids should be limited to exceptional clinical circumstances and willfully informed parental consent.

Complications. **Complications of BPD are most common in the smallest, sickest infants (Box 23-8).**

Respiratory Syncytial Virus

More than 50% of infants with BPD/CLD are rehospitalized within the first 2 years of life, usually with viral respiratory infections. Respiratory syncytial virus (RSV) is the major cause of pneumonia, bronchiolitis, and otitis media in young children.[16] There is increased morbidity and mortality in preterm infants less than 6 months of age and in young children (2 years of age or younger) with BPD/CLD or congenital heart disease.[16] **RSV risk factors are found in Box 23-9.** RSV is a seasonal infection that occurs from winter (October to December) to early spring (March to May).

RSV may be prevented by educating parents and pharmacologic prophylaxis. Parents should be taught these principles of infection control: (1) practice good handwashing technique; (2) restrict contacts with the infant—no one with a cold; (3) avoid crowds—daycare, shopping areas, church nurseries, children's parties; (4) reduce or eliminate daycare or use daycare with fewer than two or three children; and (5) eliminate exposure to secondhand smoke.[16]

Palivizumab (Synagis), a humanized monoclonal antibody, reduces hospitalization for RSV by 55%; for infants with BPD/CLD by 39%; and for preterm infants without BPD/CLD by 78%.[550] Infants treated with Synagis have fewer hospitalizations, fewer days on higher oxygen levels, less severe infection, and fewer ICU admissions.[550] Respiratory syncytial virus immune globulin (RSV-IVIG; RespiGam), a polyclonal antibody, is intravenously administered monthly through RSV season. RSV-IVIG prevents serious RSV infection in high-risk infants, reduces hospitalization by 41%, and reduces the incidence of otitis media.[110,231] When at-risk infants are about to be discharged during RSV season, RSV-IVIG may be given for the first month of prophylaxis.[16] **RSV prophylaxis (Table 23-12) should be initiated at the begin-**

Table 23-12	PHARMACOLOGIC PROPHYLAXIS FOR RSV INFECTION	
DRUG	DOSAGE	COMMENTS
Palivizumab (Synagis)	15 mg/kg IM once a month during RSV season First dose administered before onset of RSV season Use open vial within 6 hr	Does not interfere with MMR/varicella vaccine; not recommended for infants with cyanotic CHD[16] Adverse effects: mild/transient erythema at the injection site; pain; induration and swelling; bruising; fever; rash; URI; otitis media; rhinitis; hernia; increased SGOT[550] Monitor vital signs, blood pressures, and oxygen saturation before and after administration
RSV-IVIG (RespiGam)	750 mg/kg IV over 3-4 hr once a month during RSV season Total fluid volume of 15 ml/kg	Must defer MMR and varicella vaccines for 9 mo after last dose Protects against other respiratory viruses, decreases frequency of otitis media May be preferred for high-risk infants receiving IV immune globulin for HIV or immunodeficiency syndromes Blood product with potential risk of transmission of bloodborne pathogens Contraindications: infants with CHD[16] Adverse effects: fever; vomiting; respiratory distress; wheezing; and rashes Monitor vital signs, oxygen saturations, and blood pressure before and after administration

CHD, Congenital heart disease; *HIV,* human immunodeficiency virus; *MMR,* measles, mumps, rubella; *RSV,* respiratory syncytial virus; *SGOT,* serum glutamate oxaloacetate transaminase; *URI,* urinary tract infection.

ning and terminated at the end of RSV season, taking into account regional differences.[16] Palivizumab is preferred to RSV-IVIG because of its ease of administration (IM rather than IV), no interference with other immunizations, and lack of the complications associated with IV administration.[16] Both Palivizumab and RSV-IVIG are costly, and studies report conflicting cost effectiveness of treatment.*

Retinopathy of Prematurity

Since the 1950s researchers have recognized the association between oxygen administration, prematurity, and subsequent retinal changes often resulting in blindness.[333] Severe restriction in the use of oxygen with premature infants resulted in less retinopathy of prematurity (ROP), but also in increased morbidity and mortality rates.[26,389] ROP develops in 84% of preterm survivors of less than 28 weeks' gestational age.[551] **Incidence rates and severity of ROP vary among NICUs. In 80% of cases, ROP spontaneously regresses without visual loss.**[551] Some centers report unchanged or decreased incidence and severity of ROP despite increasing survival of ELBW infants,[156,283,465] whereas others report an increased incidence in severity of ROP with decreased gestational age, decreased birth weight, and decreased number of days fed breast milk.[440]

Physiology. The pathophysiologic process in the development of ROP is not completely understood. **Many factors, not just oxygen, are involved in the pathogenesis of ROP (Box 23-10).** Abnormal growth and development of retinal vessels that results in ROP is dependent on the immaturity of retinal vasculature and exposure of these immature retinal vessels to injury and/or an abnormal environment. **The degree of retinal vascularization at birth determines the individual's susceptibility to the insults listed in Box 23-10.** The majority of retinal vascularization is complete by 32 weeks' gestation. However, even at 40 weeks the temporal periphery of the retina may still not be completely vascularized.

In response to hyperoxia, the retinal vessels constrict. They may permanently constrict and become necrotic (vasoobliteration). The vessels that have not been obliterated may proliferate in an attempt to reestablish retinal circulation. Proliferating vessels may extend into the vitreous, causing fluid leakage and/or hemorrhage, with retinal scar formation, traction on the retina, detachment, and blindness.

Early changes may first be evident at the temporal periphery, because this area is the last to be

Box 23-10	FACTORS ASSOCIATED WITH ROP

Pregnancy Complications

- Primary hypertension—pregnancy-induced hypertension, diabetes, bleeding, smoking.

Prematurity—LBW and Low Gestational Age

- Babies with the lowest birth weights (<1000 g) and lowest gestational ages (<29 weeks) have the highest risk for the development of ROP and blindness.[13,156,283,440,465]
- Multiple gestation

Supplemental Oxygen

- Hypoxia causes increase in vascular endothelial growth factor and protein in the retina within 30 min-2 hr after hypoxic insult. When retinal cells are exposed to normooxic environment there is a gradual decrease in vascular endothelial growth factor but not in protein levels.[375] Desaturations of oxygen (decreased pulse oximeter readings) are associated with increased severity of ROP.[311,441,494]
- Hyperoxia causes oxidant stress-induced vasoobliteration of ROP.[386] Risk of ROP from increased oxygen saturations (e.g., 96%-99%) is a concern in preterms in the earlier postnatal period (before 34 weeks' postmenstrual age). This earlier postnatal use of high oxygen saturations (hyperoxia) may make ROP worse.[259]

Ventilator Support

- Increased risk of ROP with more complex medical problems, prolonged oxygen requirements, lower overall arterial oxygen levels, and more episodes of fluctuating blood levels.[235,311] Prolonged ventilatory support with episodes of hypoxia, hyperoxia, hypocapnia/hypercapnia.

Surfactant Therapy

- Administration of surfactant may be associated with hypoxemia as a result of obstruction of the ETT.[414]

Surfactant Therapy—cont'd

- Significant improvements in supplemental oxygen needs and ventilator requirements occur within 10-15 min as a result of a change in lung compliance that may result in hypocarbia and/or hyperoxia.[14]

Apnea/Bradycardia

- Causes repeated cycles of hypoxia/hyperoxia and hypocapnia/hypercapnia with stimulation to breathe and increasing oxygen concentrations and need for cardio-pulmonary resuscitation, exposing retinal vessels to alternating ischemia and hyperoxic toxicity.[212]

Hypercapnia/Hypocapnia

Asphyxia/Acidosis/Shock

Blood Transfusion/Anemia

- Anemia, a decrease in oxygen carrying capacity, results in increased FiO_2 to maintain adequate oxygenation, thus exposing the lung/retina to more oxygen/oxygen toxicity.[70]
- Blood transfusions in preterms of lower gestational ages are associated with increased risk of ROP.[128,129,481]

Sepsis

- Associated with increased risk of severe ROP and need for laser surgery.[310,439]
- Cytokines that are released during sepsis may be involved in neovascularization of the retina.

Steroids

Antenatal

Conflicting study results:
- Significant increased risk of ROP[148]
- No effect of antenatal steroids on increased risk of ROP[144,439]

ETT, Endotracheal tube; *IVH,* intraventricular hemorrhage; *LBW,* low birth weight; *NEC,* necrotizing enterocolitis; *RCTs,* randomized controlled trials; *ROP,* retinopathy of prematurity; *VLBW,* very low birth weight.

---

completely vascularized. Proliferation of new vessels may remain localized and spontaneously resolve or may progress to cause total retinal detachment.

ROP is classified by location of disease in the retina (zone), by degree (stage) of vascular abnormality, and by extent of developing vasculature (clock hour)[12,19] (**Figure 23-5 and Table 23-13**). Changes are first readily seen between 6 and 8 weeks of life. When reabsorption of excessive vessels and normal vascularization is re-established, the central retinal regression of ROP occurs.

Etiology. **ROP is considered primarily a disease of prematurity,** because once vascularization is complete the retinal vessels are no longer susceptible to injury. **The incidence is inversely proportional to birth weight and gestational age.** Damage may occur in any preterm infant and has its highest incidence in infants younger than 28 weeks' gestation. Infants weighing less than 1500 g (appropriate weight for gestational age) have the highest incidence of disease and the highest incidence of blindness.[13,156,283,440,465]

Box 23-10	FACTORS ASSOCIATED WITH ROP—cont'd

Steroids—cont'd

Postnatal

Conflicting study results:

- Increased risk of stage 3 ROP with decreasing gestational age and increased number of courses of steroids.[144]
- Increased risk of ROP as a result of increased vascular tortuosity; steroids have an angiogenic effect on retinal vascular development.[23]
- Increased risk of ROP—15% without versus 48% with postnatal steroid use.[71]
- Use of postnatal steroids associated with increased risk of severe ROP requiring cryotherapy.[43]
- Increased risk of ROP—8% without versus 32% with steroid use.[464]
- No significant association with severe ROP.[338]

IVH/Seizures

- Infants with severe IVH and PVL are at increased risk for development of ROP and prethreshold disease.[47]
- Severe IVH in the first 72 hr of life is associated with severe ROP at 5-7 wk. Grades III and IV IVH at birth are a marker for the development of severe (≥stage 3) ROP.[151]
- Preterm infants with ROP requiring laser surgery are at significantly increased risk of nonvision neurodevelopmental impairments.[591]

Nutritional Deficiency (e.g., antioxidants)

- Preterms have low antioxidant (vitamin E)[85] reserves and are vulnerable to tissue damage as a result of required supplemental oxygen. Plasma vitamin E levels are positively correlated with vitamin E intakes; early nutrient intervention may decrease susceptibility to tissue damage from oxygen exposure.[200]

Nutritional Deficiency—cont'd

- Vitamin E supplementation has been associated with toxic levels, increased incidence of sepsis, and late-onset NEC.[268]

Ethnicity

- Caucasian infants develop severe ROP and require laser therapy more often than African-American infants,[439] whose fundal pigmentation may modify the risk of ROP.
- African-American infants are less likely to develop ROP[123] and have a significant protective effect in slowing the progression to threshold ROP.[551]

Exposure to Bright Light

- May contribute to free radical–induced oxidative retinal vascular damage and ROP.[212]
- Multicenter study of light reduction not associated with decrease in ROP or morbidity for VLBW infants.[317,472]

Photopic Adaptation

- Exposure of the eye to room light decreases oxygen consumption of the retina, thus decreasing retinal ischemia; retinal oxygen consumption increases in the dark, rather than in light exposure.[120] Perhaps preterms should be exposed to low light levels until prethreshold, stage 2+ or 3+ disease develops; then exposing the infant to room light may assist photopic adaptation to decrease retinal ischemia.[211] The role of light in the development of ROP is confusing—RCTs are necessary.[211]

Bilirubin/Phototherapy

- Retrospective study of 128 infants (≤800 g; ≤27 wk gestational age)—severe visual loss as a result of ROP significantly associated with low peak serum bilirubin concentrations (≤9.4 mg/dl), low gestational age, and longer duration of phototherapy.[608]

Prevention. **Preventing prematurity is the best way to prevent ROP.** Because multiple gestation is associated with birth of LBW and low gestational age babies, higher order multiples should be avoided.

Decreasing light levels and the vulnerable preterm infant's exposure to bright light has not been shown to decrease the incidence of ROP.[472] However, in this study the eye protection (goggles) was placed within the first 24 hours of life, after the infant had already been exposed to the bright lights at birth, during NICU admission, and to the ophthalmoscopic examination.

The usefulness and safety of vitamin E is still unclear. Its use is considered experimental, and its routine administration for the prevention of ROP is not recommended. Vitamin E supplementation to achieve serum levels as high as 4 to 5 mg/dl may be used in combination with cryotherapy to decrease the sequelae of ROP.[301]

Because an infant who is hyperoxic (Pao₂ greater than 100 mm Hg) will clinically look no

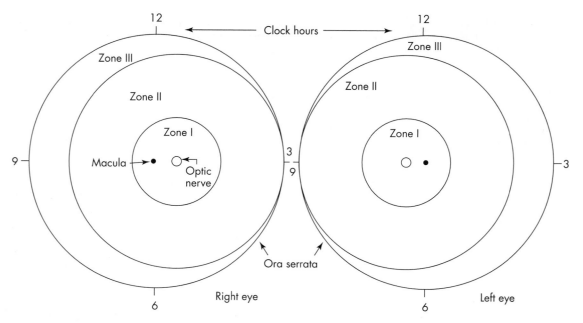

FIGURE 23-5 International classification of retinopathy of prematurity (ROP). (From AMA: *Arch Ophthalmol* 102:1131, 1984. Courtesy Ross Laboratories, Columbus, Ohio.)

Table 23-13	STAGES OF RETINOPATHY OF PREMATURITY (ROP)
STAGES	**DESCRIPTION**
Stage 1: Demarcation line	A thin white line separates the avascular retina anteriorly from the vascularized retina posteriorly. Abnormal branching vessels lead to the demarcation line, which is flat and lies in the plane of the retina.
Stage 2: Ridge	The ridge has a definite height and width, occupies a volume, and extends up out of the plane of the retina. Its color may change from white to pink. Small, isolated tufts of new vessels may appear posterior to the structure.
Stage 3: Ridge with extraretinal fibrovascular proliferations	To the ridge of stage 2 is added the presence of extraretinal fibrovascular proliferative tissue. Characteristic locations: 1. Continuous with the posterior aspect of the ridge (ragged ridge) 2. Immediately posterior to the ridge but not always appearing to be connected to it 3. Into the vitreous perpendicular to the retinal plane
Stage 4: Retinal detachment	To stage 3 is added unequivocal detachment of the retina caused by exudative effusion of fluid, traction, or both.
Stage 4A	Detachment of the retina does not include the macula; vision may be good.
Stage 4B	Macula is detached: visual potential markedly reduced.
Threshold disease	Occurs with stage 3 ROP, the presence of "plus" disease and includes 5 or more consecutive or 8 or more accumulated clock hours.
Rush disease	A rapid progression (in days rather than weeks) to severe ROP and retinal detachment. ROP in zone 1 with "plus" disease: poorer prognosis for sight.
Stage 5: Total detachment	Complete retinal detachment: the retina is pulled into a funnel-shaped configuration by the fibrovascular scar tissue. Complete blindness in affected eye.

ROP, Retinopathy of prematurity.

different from an infant whose PaO$_2$ is normal, monitoring of oxygen saturations and partial pressure of oxygen with arterial blood gases is mandatory whenever oxygen is administered. In a national survey of noninvasive monitoring of oxygen therapy in infants who weighed less than 1500 g, 76% of respondent NICUs used pulse oximetry exclusively and 26% combined pulse oximetry with TcO$_2$ monitoring.[574] For detection of hyperoxemia during use of pulse oximetry, the recommendation for high alarm setting is 96% or below.[457] In this survey only 31% used the recommended high setting, whereas 69% set the high alarm in the 97% to 100% range.[574] Setting the pulse oximetry alarm at 100% or accepting an oxygen saturation of more than 98% exposes vulnerable preterm infants to the risk of hyperoxemia and subsequent oxygen toxicity to their eyes (ROP) and lungs (BPD/CLD).

Based on the clinical observation that some infants progress to threshold ROP when their clinical courses improved and they were being weaned from supplemental oxygen, a nonrandomized case series suggests that moderate supplemental oxygen (e.g., oxygen saturations of 99% with PaO$_2$ no higher than 100 mm Hg) is associated with a decrease in the number of infants with prethreshold ROP who progress to threshold ROP.[212] **A moderate increase in the administered oxygen to achieve a higher oxygen saturation in infants with prethreshold ROP may decrease the progression of ROP by decreasing retinal hypoxia and ischemia so that developing retinal vessels are able to mature.**[212] By decreasing retinal hypoxia and retraining neovascularization by decreasing angiogenic drive, oxygen limits the scarring traction, retinal detachment, and blindness.[212,259]

The STOP-ROP trial, a randomized, multicenter controlled study to test the safety and efficacy of administering supplemental oxygen (to keep pulse oximetry saturations at 96% to 99%) to infants with prethreshold ROP to decrease progression to ROP, reported that ROP progression rates were decreased with supplemental oxygen (48.5% to 40.9% [not statistically significant]).[551] In a subset analysis in infants without "plus" disease, the progression to threshold ROP was 32% in the supplemented group versus 46% in the conventional use group (saturations 89% to 94%). The progression to ROP took longer in the supplemental group (2.5 weeks) than in the conventional (2.4 weeks) group. Diagnosis of threshold ROP was at 37.3 weeks' postmenstrual age in the supplemented group and 36.8 weeks' post-

menstrual age in the conventional group. **Administering oxygen to keep saturations at 96% to 99% does not increase the severity of ROP in infants with prethreshold ROP.**[551] Infants in the oxygen-supplemented group did not gain weight faster, and those infants with the worst lung disease had more pulmonary complications than infants on conventional oxygen supplementation.[551]

However, these studies do not mean that increased saturation is safe for immature eyes that do not yet have established ROP. The data of the STOP-ROP trial apply to infants well beyond the initial weeks after birth and *do not* show the safety of supplemental oxygen levels (saturations 96% to 99%) at younger ages.[259,551] **The risk of developing ROP from increased oxygen exposure (saturations of 96% to 99%) is of concern only in the earlier postnatal period, before 32 weeks' postmenstrual age.**[259]

Data Collection. **Because treatment with laser/ cryotherapy is associated with a 50% decrease in retinal detachment,**[123] **screening examinations of preterm infants for ROP are essential (Box 23-11).** Although AAP guidelines recommend screening at birth weights of 1500 g or below or gestational age of 28 weeks or less, some centers

---

Box 23-11 SCREENING EXAMINATION OF PREMATURE INFANTS FOR ROP[13]

Target population:
Infants with birth weight ≤1500 g or gestational age ≤28 wk
Infants >1500 g with unstable clinical courses felt to be at increased risk
  Dilated (cyclomydril drops—1 drop in each eye q 15 min ×3) indirect ophthalmoscopic examination
  Ophthalmologist with experience in examining preterm infants
Initial examination: between 4-6 wk chronologic age or between 31-32 wk postconceptual age (PCA)
  (PCA = gestational age at birth + chronologic age)
Follow-up examinations: Determined by finding on first examination (follow-up 2-4 wk until vascularization proceeds to zone 3)
With ROP or immature vessels in zone 1: Follow-up at least every 1-2 wk until normal vascularization proceeds to zone 3 or risk of attaining threshold condition has passed
Threshold disease: Consider a candidate for ablative therapy of at least one eye within 72 hr of diagnosis

recommend birth weights below 1250 g[352,391] or gestational age at 32 weeks or less.[465] Timing of first screening for ROP examinations correlates with the timing of the events of ROP. The median postmenstrual age when prethreshold ROP (without "plus" disease) was first confirmed was 34.6 weeks; the first examination to detect prethreshold ROP (without "plus" disease) may have to be as early as 31 to 32 weeks postmenstrual age[449] or 4 to 6 weeks chronologic age.[535] The median postmenstrual age when prethreshold ROP (with "plus" disease) was first confirmed was 36 weeks. The first eye examination to detect threshold ROP for possible ablative surgery can be later at 31 to 33 weeks' postmenstrual age, consistent with AAP guidelines.[449] Healthier infants with prethreshold ROP have a much lower risk of progression to threshold ROP than infants with prethreshold ROP who have greater lung dysfunction.[388]

Eye examinations are stressful for an infant. Swaddling and providing an external heat source to prevent cold stress are useful. The infant should be positioned supine, swaddled with the head immobilized. The infant may have apnea, bradycardia, increased blood pressure, and bronchospasm as a result of the use of mydriatic (Cyclomydril) eye drops and ocular stimulation during the examination. Provide monitoring with pulse oximetry and cardiorespiratory monitoring, an oxygen source, CPR equipment, and rest periods as needed. Topical anesthesia for pain control may be used (see Chapter 12).

Treatment. **The best treatment is prevention. NOTE: Even strict adherence to all principles of good care may still not prevent ROP in VLBW infants.**

Peripheral retinal ablation (with laser or cryotherapy) is effective for threshold ROP in reducing visual loss.[72,551] Use of laser therapy has become the standard treatment for advanced (e.g., threshold ROP, stages 4 and 5) ROP.[551] The laser is directed through the infant's pupil where the light photocoagulates retinal tissue, stops abnormal vessel growth, and halts the progression of ROP.[153] Laser surgery is less invasive, requires no anesthesia, and enables deeper tissue penetration and more predictable tissue interaction. In addition, it is less painful postoperatively than cryosurgery.[458,497]

Cryotherapy freezes the abnormal retinal tissue when the probe is inserted through an incision in the conjunctiva. Freezing of the tissue stops leakage of blood vessels and halts the progression of ROP.

Cryotherapy is more expensive, more painful, requires general anesthesia, and is associated with more systemic effects (e.g., apnea, bradycardia, dysrhythmias, hypotension, cyanosis) than laser surgery.[72,153] When retinal detachment has occurred, surgical procedures known as scleral buckling and vitrectomy may be performed; the visual results after these surgeries are poor.

Complications. Long-term visual consequences of laser surgery for ROP are unknown.[259,551] Complications of laser surgery include choroidal hemorrhage, scarring, increased risk of cataracts, burns of the cornea, iris or lens, and (rarely) pain.[153] Complications of cryotherapy include pain, infection, periorbital edema, retinal scarring, and detachment. In a follow-up study at 5 years (of children who had been 1000-g preterm infants of less than 28 weeks' gestation), 43% of the survivors had some ocular disorder, indicating a significant relationship between ocular disorders and ROP, and there was a 31% incidence of ocular disorders in preterm children without ROP.[260] Disorders included decreased visual acuity (27%), myopia (12%), hypermyopia (8%), astigmatism (11%), and strabismus (14%).[260] Severe myopia may develop as early as 6 months of age. Early detection and correction with lenses is essential to save the child's remaining sight. When the eyes are not used, microphthalmia (small sunken eyes) results. Glaucoma, strabismus, amblyopia, and late retinal detachment (in teens or early twenties) may develop.

Parent Teaching. Blindness is defined by many in our society as one of the worst handicaps. Parents will experience grief over this devastating loss and will need help to cope before they will be able to bond to their blind child. Parents must be taught to care for their blind or visually impaired child.[396]

Blind infants are unable to communicate with care providers through the signs and signals of facial expressions.[193] Because of the absence of eye language, no cues to infant needs and no feedback of preference, recognition, and delight can be given. Absence of a smile from the blind infant connotes a negative response to the care provider. When care providers understand these behavioral differences, they can assist parents to understand the lack of facial expression. Instead of facial expression, parents are taught to read the special hand language of their infants as an expression of emotions, intentions, preference, and recognition.[193] Appropriate referrals to occupational therapy, physical therapy, and community agencies that are resources for the blind and their families may help avoid developmental delays from insufficient or inappropriate stimulation.

Chronic CNS Sequelae
The highest incidence of abnormal findings occurs in infants with intracranial hemorrhage, the lowest birth weights (less than 1500 g), and BPD/CLD.* For a review of sequelae and outcomes of prematurity, see Chapter 13 (Tables 13-17 and 13-18 and Box 13-9) and Chapter 32 for follow-up care.

ACUTE RESPIRATORY DISEASES

Respiratory Distress Syndrome
Pathophysiology. RDS is a disease of immature lung anatomy and physiology. Anatomically the preterm lung is unable to support oxygenation and ventilation, because alveolar saccules are insufficiently developed, causing a deficient surface area for gas exchange. Also, the pulmonary capillary bed is deficient and the interstitial mesenchyme is present to a greater extent, increasing the distance between the alveolar and the endothelial cell membranes.

Physiologically the volume of surfactant is insufficient to prevent collapse of unstable alveoli. Because the alveoli collapse with each breath, normal functional residual capacity (FRC) is not established. Because of alveolar collapse, oxygenation and ventilation are insufficient, and each breath requires increased energy output.

Compliance is related to the volume achieved during a given application of pressure. Compliance of the lung is equal to the ratio of the change in volume to the change in pressure. The lung in RDS has low compliance (i.e., little change in volume is achieved with a relatively great application of pressure), thereby contributing to increased work of breathing. However, the chest wall of the neonate is unfortunately very compliant; a slight application of pressure results in a large change in volume. The infant may not be able to create enough inspiratory pressure to open the alveoli as the chest wall retracts and collapses about the relatively stiff lung. Thus in RDS the diaphragm contracts, creating an inspiratory pressure that moves less volume into

the lung than expected and simultaneously causes large sternal and intercostal retractions of the chest wall.

The increased effort of these opposing forces usually results in hypoxemia and acidemia that cause constriction of the pulmonary vascular (arterial) musculature, severely limiting pulmonary capillary blood flow. The integrity of pulmonary capillary blood flow is critical for the integrity of the alveolar epithelial membrane and the production of surfactant. Without adequate pulmonary capillary blood flow, the type II pneumocytes become deficient in the precursor material required for production of surfactant. Lack of surfactant production compounds the deficiency and leads to low compliance. These physiologic factors (surfactant deficiency and decreased lung compliance) promote increased work of breathing (WOB), fatigue, atelectasis, reduced FRC, and ventilation/perfusion (V/Q) mismatch.

In the fetus, pulmonary vascular resistance is high, and pulmonary artery blood pressure is greater than systemic blood pressure, causing blood flow from the main pulmonary artery to travel through the open ductus arteriosus to the descending aorta. A second right-to-left shunt occurs across the foramen ovale in the fetus. The high pulmonary vascular resistance is "reactive" to the normal fetal "hypoxemia," because the pulmonary vascular resistance and the pulmonary artery blood pressure decrease as the PaO_2 of the neonate increases. At birth the ductus arteriosus actively constricts in response to the increase in PaO_2 (PaO_2 greater than 50 mm Hg), eliminating blood flow across the ductus and completing the transition to neonatal circulation.

The fetal circulatory pattern may persist from birth or be initiated by a transient hypoxemic episode. In the instance of neonatal hypoxemia, the pulmonary vasculature "reacts" by vasoconstriction, raising pulmonary vascular resistance, and the ductus arteriosus "reacts" by relaxing, once again allowing blood flow from the pulmonary artery to the descending aorta, as normally occurs in the fetus. Pulmonary vascular resistance is increased with shunting through the ductus arteriosus. Fetal circulatory patterns are perpetuated by hypoxemia and acidemia and produce systemic hypoxemia that aggravates and perpetuates the condition.

Endothelial damage and alveolar necrosis aggravate the already existing surfactant deficiency. A cyclic deterioration is established, and hypoxia and acidosis persist unless treatment is initiated.

*References 9, 152, 188, 221, 228, 236, 239, 299, 377, 392, 402, 433, 493, 516, 520, 540, 541, 576.

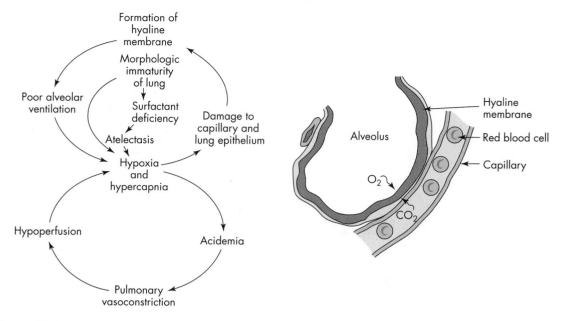

FIGURE 23-6 Interdependent relationship of factors involved in pathology of RDS. (From Pierog SH, Ferrara A: *Medical care of the sick newborn,* ed 2, St Louis, 1976, Mosby.)

Microscopically, the events that occur in the lung include injury to and death of the alveolar epithelial cells and airway epithelial cells. This injury and death are followed by sloughing of the cells from the respiratory basement membrane, leaving the basement membrane denuded followed by exudation of serum. Fibrin in the serum clots, and hyaline membranes are formed, covering the denuded basement membranes in the airways and alveolar spaces. If there is sufficient hypoxic damage to the cells and basement membranes, frank hemorrhage may fill the alveolar spaces. These factors decrease the total surface area of the gas exchange membrane. The end result is hypoxemia, acidemia, and increasing respiratory distress.

The entire sequence of events in RDS is related to the inability to maintain lung expansion and alveolar stability as a result of surfactant deficiency. RDS evolves from two interrelated problems: atelectasis and persistence of or reversion to the fetal levels of pulmonary hypertension (Figures 23-6 and 23-7).

Etiology. RDS occurs in infants born prematurely and is a consequence of immature lung anatomy and physiology. In premature or stressed infants, atelectasis from the collapse of the terminal alveoli because of lack of surfactant appears after the first few hours

of life. In a premature infant surfactant production is limited, and stores are quickly depleted. Surfactant production may be further diminished by other unfavorable conditions such as high oxygen concentration, poor pulmonary drainage, excessive pulmonary hygiene, or effects of respirator management.

Data Collection

History. A history of prematurity, cesarean section, and/or asphyxial episodes may be seen in infants with RDS.

Physical Examination. Infants with RDS are often tachypneic, and they grunt, flare, and retract within the first few minutes to hours of life. Pallor or cyanosis may also be present. The trachea is midline, and there is a normal apical pulse. **Auscultation of the chest reveals decreased breath sounds and often rales. Many of these infants may be hypotensive with prolonged capillary refill.**

Laboratory Data. Chest x-ray examinations in RDS include (1) reduced lung volume, (2) air bronchograms, (3) reticulogranularity, and (4) lung opacification.[558] Surfactant deficiency results in diffuse atelectasis, a reduction in lung volume, and decreased lung expansion as demonstrated on

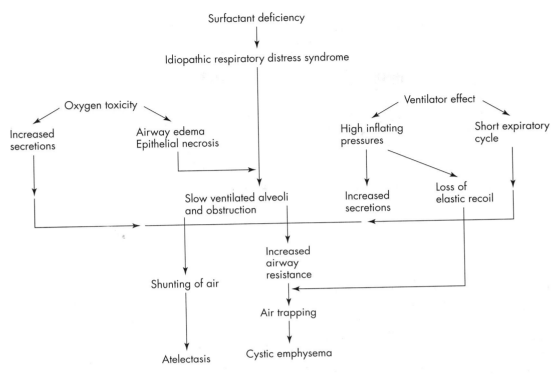

FIGURE 23-7   Schematic representation of pathogenesis of RDS.

x-ray examination. Atelectasis increases lung density and results in visible outlines of air-filled bronchi (e.g., air bronchograms) against opaque lung tissue. Chest x-ray examination also reveals a ground-glass appearance that represents areas of atelectatic respiratory alveoli adjacent to expanded or even hyperexpanded respiratory units. **This bilateral reticulogranular pattern is uniformly distributed throughout the lung fields and may also contain air bronchograms (Figure 23-8).** Diffuse opacification caused by (1) nonexpanded alveoli with little or no terminal airway aeration, (2) pulmonary edema, or (3) pulmonary hemorrhage results in loss of visible heart borders, with a **"white out" appearance on chest x-ray films (Figure 23-9).**

Arterial blood gases reveal hypoxemia and often acidemia that may be metabolic, respiratory, or a combination of both (see Chapter 11).

Prevention. A single course of antenatal steroids has decreased the incidence and severity of RDS, comorbidities (e.g., NEC, ICH, CLD) and mortality in infants of less than 32 weeks' gestation. Even a partial course appears to be beneficial.[411,412]

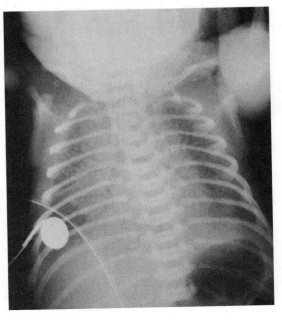

FIGURE 23-8   Chest x-ray film of 27-week premature infant with RDS. Note characteristic infiltrate pattern with air bronchograms.

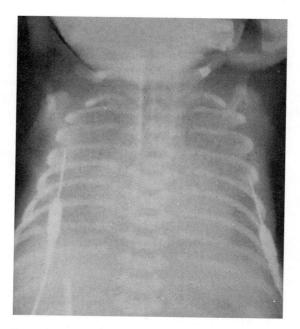

FIGURE 23-9 Chest x-ray film of 28-week preterm infant with severe RDS. Note "white out" appearance.

Prophylactic use of surfactant in animal studies is associated with more uniform and homogenous distribution when administered to a fluid-filled lung.[296,506] Administration of surfactant to a previously unventilated lung precludes exposure to causes of BPD/CLD (e.g., oxygen and barotrauma) and to cytokine release secondary to inflammatory response.[408] **Delayed surfactant administration (even by 15 minutes after the onset of assisted ventilation) may offset the benefits of surfactant.**[506] **Studies comparing timing of administration found increased survival, decreased mortality, and less pneumothorax (especially in infants of less than 26 weeks' gestation) associated with prophylactic versus rescue usage.*** **Because 30% to 40% of preterm infants of less than 30 weeks' gestational age will not have RDS, prophylactic use is associated with overtreatment so that it is reserved for the smallest, most immature infants at increased risk for RDS (e.g., 29 weeks' gestation or below).** There is no benefit of surfactant administration to preterm infants (32 weeks' gestation or below) with mild RDS who require 40% or less of Fio_2.[255]

Treatment

Surfactant Replacement Therapy. Because surfactant deficiency is the primary abnormality of RDS, the development of an effective clinical strategy for administering exogenous surface-active material to premature infants has been the focus of research efforts for many years. In addition to replacing deficient surfactant in the lungs of preterm infants, surfactant has been shown to modulate levels of inflammatory cytokines involved in the pulmonary inflammatory process.[408,527] **Administration of surfactant leads to (1) dramatic and rapid improvement in gas exchange, (2) decreases the need for high levels of supplemental oxygen and ventilatory support, (3) leads to less barotrauma, and (4) improves chest x-ray findings by improving lung compliance and lung volume.**[14,154,220,397] The use of lower levels of ventilatory support decreases the mortality rate* and the incidence of pneumothorax.[242,482,521,572] However, surfactant administration does not fully correct lung abnormalities of the VLBW infant with RDS.[313]

Coexistant morbidities (e.g., NEC, nosocomial infections, PDA, IVH, and BPD/CLD) of VLBW have not been affected by surfactant therapy.[14,255,397] The increased survival of VLBW as a result of surfactant use may contribute to the increased incidence of NEC.[365] Optimal clinical strategies—the type of surfactant to use, the timing and method of administration, and the number of doses—affect surfactant safety and efficacy.[126,479] Numerous studies comparing surfactants have documented more rapid improvement in respiratory status, decreased incidence of pneumothorax, lower mortality rates, improved survival, and less ROP and BPD/CLD with natural versus synthetic surfactant.†

Various methods of surfactant administration have been studied, with bolus injection improving the homogenous distribution of surfactant in lungs when compared with slow injection or ultrasonic nebulization.[265] A recent study of aerosolized surfactant therapy, in infants receiving CPAP, showed no beneficial effects.[53] In some studies there has been an increased incidence of IVH with surfactant administration[279] while others cite no decrease in

*References 169, 275, 315, 353, 401, 524.

*References 242, 274, 280, 503, 522, 572.
†References 242, 280, 282, 521, 522, 572.

IVH with surfactant therapy.[292] Rapid bolus injection has been associated with alteration in CBF (that may increase the risk of IVH).[118,498] A recent study of bolus administration showed no alteration in CBF (with careful attention to FiO_2 and pressures); however, alterations in CBF were related to changes in mean systolic blood pressure.[422] Studies of the number of doses document (1) decreased severity of RDS, but no improvement of survival with a single dose, and (2) increased survival, decreased mortality, and decreased incidence of pneumothorax with multiple doses.[275,353,615]

Surfactant administration has not reduced the rate of BPD/CLD nor the NICU disparity of BPD/CLD rates.* Because smaller and more immature infants survive after surfactant therapy, there is no decrease in BPD/CLD, especially in VLBW infants weighing less than 750 g.[274,432,503,522] In addition to type, timing, method, and number of doses of surfactant,[126,273] the methods of resuscitation, types of ventilators (CMV versus HFOV),[286] and ventilation style[285] (e.g., as few as six large tidal volume breaths in a surfactant-deficient lung causes lung injury)[61] contribute to lung injury resulting in BPD/CLD.

Studies have documented an increased incidence of significant PDA after birth among surfactant-treated preterm infants.[275,462] One study reports an association between PDA and pulmonary hemorrhage,[207] whereas another found no relationship.[462] However, this study did find a 50% increase in pulmonary hemorrhage after surfactant treatment especially in LBW preterm infants and when synthetic surfactant had been administered.[462]

Long-term outcome studies of preterm infants who have received surfactant therapy show no benefits, no significant effects on overall rates of handicap, and no adverse long-term effects on growth or neurodevelopmental outcome.[14,116,179] Among the smallest preterm neonates (ELBW infants) given surfactant, there is no improvement in survival rate or multiple neurosensory impairments.[361] For preterm infants of less than 28 weeks' gestational age, surfactant administration has not changed long-term pulmonary outcomes.[232]

Surfactant therapy in premature infants with RDS constitutes a major historical milestone in neonatal care[126] (see Chapter 1). There has been a marked decrease in RDS-related mortality since surfactant use

---

*References 179, 237, 435, 452, 563, 573, 610.

| Box 23-12 | RECOMMENDATIONS FOR SURFACTANT REPLACEMENT THERAPY[14] |

Target population: High risk, LBW infants, with multisystem disorders

Directed by physicians qualified and trained in use/administration, including management of mechanical ventilation of LBW infants.

Nursing and respiratory therapy experienced in management of LBW infants, including mechanical ventilation available at the bedside during administration.

Equipment available to manage/monitor LBW infants being mechanically ventilated; support services (e.g., radiology and laboratory) available.

Used only in institutions with facilities and personnel experienced in and available for the management of multisystem disorders of LBW infants.

Existence of an institutionally approved surfactant therapy protocol.

In situations in which timely transfer cannot be achieved, surfactant may be administered by a physician skilled in endotracheal intubation, after consultation with tertiary center and transfer to tertiary center arranged as soon as possible.

LBW, Low birth weight.

---

began in the 1990s. **In the postsurfactant era (1990 to 1995), the adjusted average annual decline in RDS mortality has been reported to be 11.5%.**[379] The mortality rate from RDS has decreased for both whites (59%) and African-Americans (45%) and for males (58.7%) and females (51.8%).[379] However, changes in RDS mortality vary considerably when birth weight and gestational age categories are considered: (1) less than 500 g and less than 24 weeks' gestational age—little or no effect, (2) 500 to 749 g—minimal effect reported until after 1991, (3) 750 to 1999 g—the most change was noted temporarily related to surfactant introduction, and (4) 2000 to 2499 g and 33 to 36 weeks' gestational age—the largest average annual decline in mortality rate.[379]

Recommendations for surfactant replacement therapy for RDS are outlined in Box 23-12. Surfactant preparations are commercially available as (1) organic solvent extract of minced bovine lung, (2) artificial or synthetic surfactant, (3) modified porcine-derived minced lung extract, and (4) natural surfactant extracted from calf lung lavage. **Table 23-14 summarizes the commercially available products for surfactant replacement. Other**

Table 23-14	SURFACTANT REPLACEMENT THERAPY		
DRUG/SOURCE	**INDICATIONS**	**ADMINISTRATION AND DOSAGE**	**ADVERSE EFFECTS**
Beractant (Survanta) exogenous surfactant from bovine lung extract	Prevention and treatment ("rescue") of RDS in premature infants; significantly reduces the incidence of RDS, mortality caused by RDS, and air leak complications Prevention: In premature infants <1250 g birth weight or with evidence of surfactant deficiency, give as soon as possible, preferably within 15 min of birth Rescue: To treat infants with RDS confirmed by x-ray examination and requiring mechanical ventilation, give as soon as possible, preferably by 8 hr of age	Administration: For *intratracheal* administration only; instillation through a 5 Fr end-hole catheter inserted into the infant's endotracheal tube with the tip of the catheter just beyond the end of the endotracheal tube and above the infant's carina; each dose is 100 mg of phospholipids/kg birth weight (4 ml/kg); four doses can be administered in the first 48 hr of life; give doses no more frequently than every 6 hr; repeat doses are based on the infant's birth weight	The most commonly reported adverse experiences are associated with the dosage procedure: transient bradycardia and oxygen desaturation
Colfosceril (Exosurf) artificial surfactant	Prevention and treatment ("rescue") of RDS in premature infants	Administration: Suction the infant before administration, but do not suction for 2 hr after administration, except when clinically necessary; administer via the sideport on the special endotracheal tube adapter without interrupting mechanical ventilation Dosage: Each dose is administered in two 2.5 ml/kg half-doses; each half-dose is instilled slowly over 1 to 2 min in small bursts	See above
Poractant alfa (Curosurf) Modified porcine derived minced lung extract	Prevention and treatment ("rescue") of RDS in premature infants	For *intratracheal* administration see above procedure Dosage: Initial dose: 2.5 ml/kg divided into two aliquots Subsequent dose: up to two doses of 1.25 ml/kg/dose given 12 hr apart, if needed	See above
Calfactant (Infasurf) Natural surfactant extracted from calf lung lavage	Prevention and treatment ("rescue") of RDS in premature infants	Administration: For *intratracheal* administration see above Dosage: Initial dose: 3 ml/kg divided into two aliquots Subsequent dose: Up to three doses of 3 ml/kg/dose given 12 hr apart, if needed	See above

RDS, Respiratory distress syndrome.

treatment is directed toward the indications in Box 23-13.

Transient Tachypnea of the Newborn (TTN) (RDS Type 2)

Pathophysiology. Transient tachypnea of the newborn (TTN) is the result of delayed reabsorption of normal lung fluid, and thus an alternative name is *wet lung syndrome,* or RDS type 2. Lung fluid accumulates in the peribronchiolar lymphatics and the bronchovascular spaces. Thus TTN is an "obstructive" lung disease, whereas RDS is a "restrictive" lung disease. Lung function of neonates with TTN includes: high total ventilation, high breathing frequency, low tidal volume, high dead space, prolonged nitrogen clearance, and low dynamic compliance.[495] Reabsorption of lung fluid occurs by (1) slowing of lung liquid production, (2) pulmonary epithelial changes from chloride-secreting to sodium-absorbing barrier, (3) air intake at birth shifts fluid from alveoli to interstitium and perivascular spaces, and (4) a higher protein content and

osmotic pressure of blood/lymph facilitates flow of lung fluid.[77]

Etiology. **TTN generally occurs in term or near-term infants with a history of cesarean section,[344] low Apgar scores,[247] pulmonary artery hypertension, poor left ventricular function,[247] and precipitous delivery.** In these situations there is a lack of the gradual compression of the chest that eliminates some fluid during a normal vaginal delivery. Accumulation of interstitial fluid interferes with the forces that hold the bronchioli open, causing collapse and air trapping.

Data Collection

History. Term or near-term infants with a history of cesarean section, precipitous delivery, or other abnormalities of labor/transition are predisposed to TTN. Onset is usually 2 to 6 hours after birth.

Physical Examination. Respiratory distress, including tachypnea, mild retractions, grunting, and flaring, may be seen. Cyanosis in room air may also be present.

Laboratory Data. Mild hypoxemia (requiring less than 40% oxygen) and mild acidemia are usually present. A significant degree of hypoxemia or acidemia will tend to constrict the pulmonary vasculature and aggravate the problem. Chest x-ray examination reveals hyperexpansion with streaky infiltrates radiating from the hilum. These infiltrates are thought to represent interstitial fluid along the bronchovascular spaces. Air trapping causes the appearance of mild to moderate hyperaeration/inflation on the chest x-ray film.[77] Visible fluid in the pulmonary fissures and cardiomegaly may also be seen on chest x-ray film.[77]

Treatment. In general, support of the patient with TTN requires only provision of sufficient supplemental oxygen to maintain an arterial oxygen tension of more than 70 to 80 mm Hg and maintenance of usual supportive neonatal care. Although diuretic agents have been advocated, usually little more than general support is necessary while the normal absorption of lung fluid through the lymphatics takes place. As the lung fluid clears, both the x-ray findings and clinical presentation resolve within 72 hours.

Box 23-13   TREATMENT FOR RDS

I. Reducing hypoxemia (see section on general treatment strategies in this chapter and in Chapter 11)
  A. Maintain in neutral thermal environment (see Chapter 6)
  B. Maintain blood pressure and hematocrit (see Chapters 5 and 20)
  C. Decrease stimuli from the NICU environment (see Chapter 13)
  D. Recognize and relieve pain and/or agitation (see Chapter 12)
II. Correcting acidemia (see Chapter 11)
III. Increasing the functional residual capacity (see section on general treatment strategies)
  A. Maintaining appropriate temperature (see Chapter 6)
  B. Monitoring vital signs and arterial blood gases (see Chapters 7 and 11)
  C. Providing appropriate fluid, electrolytes, glucose, and calories (see Part III)
  D. Observing for complications of disease and treatments (see section on general complications)
IV. Monitor for complications (see section on general complications, acute and chronic)

NICU, Neonatal intensive care unit; *RDS,* respiratory distress syndrome.

Meconium Aspiration Syndrome (MAS)

Pathophysiology. Before meconium aspiration can occur, meconium must find its way into the amniotic fluid. This condition occurs more often in term or postterm infants when a hypoxic episode is experienced in utero.[10,410] With fetal asphyxia the anal sphincter relaxes and colonic peristalsis ensues, expelling meconium into the amniotic fluid. Subsequently a second episode of asphyxia occurs, during which the infant makes gasping respiratory movements. These movements open the glottis so that meconium flows into the oropharynx and on into the lung. Thus the pathophysiology of lung disease in MAS is related to the mechanisms causing fetal stress as well as the direct adverse effects of meconium in the lung.

Etiology. Meconium aspiration produces disease by several mechanisms: (1) meconium physically obstructs the glottis, trachea, or any number of smaller airways, resulting in atelectasis, air trapping, alveolar collapse, and ventilation/perfusion mismatching, (2) promotes an inflammatory response known as *chemical pneumonitis*,[559] (3) inhibits surfactant function,[404] and (4) increased pulmonary vascular resistance, caused by asphyxial episodes, results in increased right-to-left shunting and the development of persistent pulmonary hypertension of the newborn (PPHN) (Figure 23-10). **Of the 8% to 19% of infants born through meconium-stained amniotic fluid, 2% to 33% will develop meconium aspiration syndrome.**[201] Of those with meconium aspiration syndrome (1) 30% to 50% will require mechan-

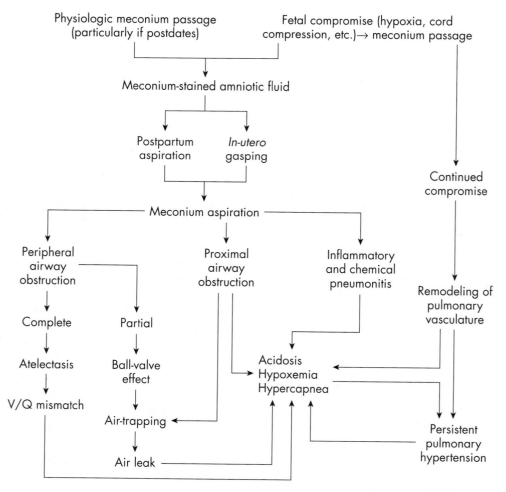

FIGURE 23-10   Pathophysiology of meconium passage and the meconium aspiration syndrome. (From Wiswell T, Bent R: *Pediatr Clin North Am* 4:957, 1993.)

ical ventilation of the lungs, (2) 15% to 33% will develop pneumothorax, (3) 33% will have accompanying PPHN, and (4) 4% to 19% will die.[103,201]

Prevention. Before an infant is born, meconium aspiration may be prevented by early recognition of the compromised fetus and appropriate intervention. Amnioinfusion, to dilute meconium in amniotic fluid, is considered experimental until its efficacy is confirmed by large randomized control trials.[201]

At birth, suction of the infant's oropharynx on the perineum before the first breath is preventive. Universal suctioning at birth of infants born through meconium-stained amniotic fluid is responsible for the significant decline in the development of MAS and mortality from it.[598] On delivery of the head and before delivery of the rest of the body of an infant with meconium-stained fluid, removing meconium, blood, and mucus from the infant's nose, mouth, and pharynx with a wall suction apparatus is essential. This prevents aspiration of the contents into the bronchi with the first gasp of respiration.[79] Oropharyngeal suction at the perineum is associated with better Apgar scores, fewer abnormal chest x-ray findings, and less need for mechanical ventilation in infants born through meconium-stained amniotic fluid.[596]

After birth, intubation and tracheal suction have been shown in a retrospective study to decrease the risk of developing MAS by 70%.[554] **A selective intubation study recommended intubation only for depressed infants born through meconium-stained amniotic fluid.**[125] Only 20% to 30% of meconium-stained infants are depressed at birth, but depressed infants and those born through the thickest consistency of meconium have an increased incidence of respiratory problems (e.g., thin meconium 2.3%; moderate meconium 6.3%; and thick meconium 15.4%).[363,488,597,599] **Based on these data, routine tracheal suction is recommended only for depressed infants and those with respiratory symptoms.**[201,599]

Data Collection

History. A history of asphyxia, IUGR, postterm delivery, and meconium-stained amniotic fluid may be present. There is a positive association between chorioamnionitis/infection and the passage of meconium at term gestation.[467]

Physical Examination. Tachypnea, rales, and cyanosis are seen in mild cases. In moderately severe cases, grunting, retractions, and nasal flaring may also be seen. In severe cases the infant is asphyxiated and severely depressed at birth. There is profound cyanosis and pallor, irregular gasping respirations, and an increased anteroposterior diameter of the chest (a barrel chest) as a result of gas trapping and alveolar overdistention.

Laboratory Data. The chest x-ray examination shows marked air trapping, hyperexpansion, and hyperinflation. There are bilateral, diffuse, coarse, patchy infiltrates (Figure 23-11). Complete occlusion by debris results in atelectatic areas.[77] Air leaks are frequently seen. Pleural effusion may occur as a result of the inflammatory process in the lung. Cardiomegaly may be present; this results from intrauterine asphyxia and/or cardiac hypoxia.[77]

Severe hypoxemia and hypercapnia as a result of ventilation perfusion mismatching and right-to-left shunting caused by pulmonary hypertension is present. Severe acidosis is usually a combined respiratory and metabolic acidosis. Infants with meconium aspiration syndrome may exhibit an increase in absolute nucleated RBC count (ANRBC) as a result of intrauterine hypoxia that was of a duration to evoke an increase in ANRBC counts.[155]

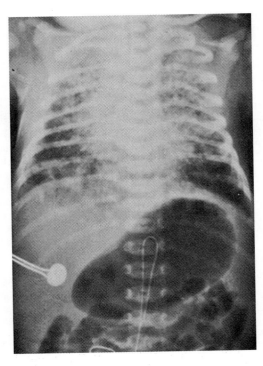

FIGURE 23-11   Chest x-ray film of infant with meconium aspiration. Note diffuse infiltrates.

Treatment. **Because the major problem in meconium aspiration is hypoxemia, treatment should be directed at improving oxygenation.** Mildly affected infants will frequently require only warmed, humidified oxygen by hood. Increasing severity of meconium aspiration will require increased levels of intervention. Some infants will respond to CPAP (4 to 6 cm of water), but others will require full ventilator support. A recent study of 62 infants with MAS showed that the majority (77%) of infants were adequately oxygenated on 5 cm of CPAP with no air leaks and no ventilator support; 23% of infants required mechanical ventilation.[418] **Because these infants are usually term or postterm, they resist assisted ventilation and may require paralyzation (Table 23-15), sedation, and/or analgesia (see Chapter 12) to ventilate and oxygenate the lungs adequately.** With paralysis, these infants may require rapid rates, high peak inspiratory pressure, and PEEP for adequate oxygenation and ventilation.

Because meconium inhibits surfactant function in a dose-dependent manner,[126,538] surfactant replacement to infants with MAS is being studied.[180] Improved oxygenation/ventilation, decreased air leaks, and use of ECMO have been observed in some studies[25,138] while inconsistent results are found in other studies.[249] Variable study results of surfactant use in MAS may be the result of (1) timing, (2) type, (3) amount, and (4) method of surfactant administration.[201] Surfactant lavage has been shown to improve oxygenation/ventilation and pulmonary function measurements in several small studies.[350,425,542] Currently, surfactant lavage versus routine management of infants with moderate to severe MAS is being studied; surfactant lavage is an experimental therapy.[201] Studies suggest that surfactant replacement therapy improves oxygenation in some patients with severe respiratory failure and MAS.[25,370]

Mucosal irritation and increased mucosal secretion hamper respiratory and mucociliary clearance efforts. Frequent pulmonary hygiene (every 2 to 3 hours) may help alleviate this problem.

As with any sick infant, close attention must be given to physiologic support and homeostasis. (See the section on general treatment strategies, Chapters, 6, 7, and 11, and Part III.)

Complications. **Persistent pulmonary hypertension frequently complicates MAS, potentiates the difficulties in oxygenation, and contributes to a large portion of the mortality associated with MAS.**[201] Air leaks are complications of both the disease (ball-valve obstruction causing air trapping) and the treatment. Being born through thick meconium-stained amniotic fluid is associated with an increased risk for seizures, mental retardation, and CP.[54,357,413] Infants with MAS are at increased risk for adverse neurologic outcomes (e.g., seizures and

Table 23-15	DRUGS USED FOR PARALYZATION	
DRUG	**DOSAGE**	**COMMENTS**
Pancuronium (Pavulon)	0.1 mg/kg IV push (0.04-0.15 mg/kg) every 1-2 hr based on duration of paralysis Onset: 1-2 min	Indications: Paralysis for mechanical ventilation to improve oxygenation/ventilation; reduce barotrauma and alteration in cerebral blood flow Although paralyzed, neonate still feels pain—analgesia necessary for painful procedures (see Chapter 12) Adverse effects: corneal drying (lubricate eyes); tachycardia; increased salivation; blood pressure changes (hypotension and hypertension) Reversed by: Neostigmine: 0.04-0.08 mg/kg IV Atropine: 0.02 mg/kg
Vecuronium	0.1 mg/kg IV push (0.03-0.15 mg/kg) every 1-2 hr based on duration of paralysis Onset: 1-2 min	Indications: same as above Adverse effects: corneal drying (lubricate eyes); decreases in heart rate and blood pressure when used with narcotics; special sensitivity by preterms (that diminishes with age); duration of effect prolonged in preterm infants Reversed by: same as above

Modified from Young T, Magnum B: *Neonfax 2000,* Raleigh, NC, 2000, Acorn Publishing.

CP)[189,387,511] and long-term pulmonary problems (e.g., increased airway reactivity, abnormal pulmonary function tests).[374,539,611] A recent study of term and near-term newborns with moderate to severe respiratory failure (resulting from MAS or pneumonia) treated with surfactant recovered completely without long-term pulmonary problems, normal neurodevelopmental outcome, and school performance.[24]

Neonatal Pneumonia

Neonatal pneumonia occurs perinatally or postnatally in about 1% of term neonates and 10% of preterm neonates.[77] Neonates requiring prolonged hospitalization in the NICU are at risk for developing pneumonia from nosocomially acquired organisms. The organisms most often causing neonatal pneumonia are mainly Group B *Streptococcus* and gram-negative organisms (e.g., *Escherichia coli, Klebsiella, Pseudomonas,* and *Serratia marcescens*) but also include *Staphylococcus aureus, Staphylococcus epidermidis,* and *Candida.* Less commonly acquired viral infections include herpes, cytomegalovirus, varicella-zoster, and syphilis. Community-acquired viral infections also occur in the NICU setting and include respiratory syncytial virus, enterovirus, adenovirus, and parainfluenza virus (Table 23-16).

Physiology. In bacterial pneumonia, alveoli are often more edematous and inflamed than in viral infections. Protein-rich fluid may partially or completely fill the alveoli. This is often followed by an influx of

Table 23-16	ETIOLOGIC FACTORS AND CHEST X-RAY FINDINGS IN NEONATAL PNEUMONIA	
CAUSATIVE AGENT	**CHEST X-RAY FINDINGS**
Bacterial	
Group B beta-hemolytic Streptococcus (GBS)	Diffuse reticulogranular pattern, opacity ("white out"), patchy infiltrates, and pleural effusion
Streptococcus pneumonia	Patchy infiltrates (lobar), pleural effusion
Staphylococcus aureus	Diffuse infiltrates; pneumatocele (nodular or miliary)
Staphylococcus epidermidis	Hazy lung fields; infiltrates
Listeria monocytogenes	Bilateral patchy infiltrates
Escherichia coli	Lobular consolidation; pneumatocele
Klebsiella	Bilateral consolidation, lung abscess, pneumatocele
Pseudomonas and *Serratia*	Parenchymal consolidation (patchy or basilar); pneumatocele
Hemophilus influenza	Nonspecific; x-ray findings similar to those of GBS (above) or RDS
Viral	
Herpes	Perihilar infiltrates; streaky, lobar consolidation, pleural effusion (late onset)
Cytomegalovirus	Nonspecific, perihilar streaking; hazy lung fields; infiltrates; opacification
Rubella	Interstitial infiltrates; hazy lung fields
Respiratory syncytial virus	Hyperexpansion; patchy consolidation
Adenovirus, enterovirus	Hyperexpansion; patchy consolidation
Fungal	
Candida albicans	Diffuse granularity; coarse infiltrates; opacification
Mycoplasma	
Ureaplasma urealyticum	Fine reticular pattern progressing to opacification and consolidation
Mycoplasma hominis	Diffuse reticular pattern, opacity, and pleural effusion
Other	
Treponema pallidum (syphilis)	Diffuse opacification; consolidation
Chlamydia trachomatis	Hyperinflation; streaky infiltrates
Pneumocystis carinii	Diffuse haziness; granularity; opacity

Modified from Carey B, Trotter C: *Neonatal Netw* 19(4):46, 2000.
GBS, Guillain-Barré syndrome; *RDS,* respiratory distress syndrome.

polymorphonuclear leukocytes and RBCs. Macrophages enter the alveoli and remove intraalveolar debris, restoring normal lung functioning.[77,167] *S. aureus* and *Klebsiella* organisms often cause severe damage to alveoli and often destroy lung tissue by causing necrosis of the septum between the alveoli. In some cases abscess formation occurs.[77]

Viruses and *Mycoplasma* organisms may also be acquired transplacentally, during the delivery, or postnatally. Viral and mycoplasmal pneumonias commonly involve the bronchi and peribronchial interstitium more often than the alveoli. Viral and mycoplasmal organisms cause loss of epithelial ciliary appendages and sloughing into the airways. This results in stasis of mucus and secretions and bronchial obstruction with atelectasis. A secondary inflammatory response is characterized by mononuclear infiltration into the submucosa and perivascular areas causing narrowing of the airway lumen. Another response to this inflammatory process is smooth muscle constriction that leads to increased airway obstruction and bronchospasm. In severe cases of viral and mycoplasmal infection, the inflammatory process involves the alveoli.[84]

Fungal infections, the most common being *Candida*, may be acquired in utero, during the birth process, or in the postnatal period. Congenitally acquired pneumonia can be diffuse resulting from the inflammatory process at birth. *Candida* often invades the pharynx and larynx and may produce a thick layer of hyphae that lines the upper and lower respiratory tract. Ulceration of the pharynx, larynx, and the lower respiratory tract can occur.

Etiology. Predisposing factors that lead to the development of neonatal infections and pneumonia include, in part, the immaturity of the immune system, colonization of the mothers' genital and vaginal tracts with pathogens, amnionitis, prolonged rupture of membranes, prematurity, and nosocomial infections acquired in the NICU. Bacterial pneumonia can occur secondary to the spread of pathogens from the mother to the baby in utero. Pneumonia acquired in utero often leads to stillbirth and premature delivery. **Neonates who require NICU care are at particularly high risk of colonization of their upper respiratory tract with pathogenic organisms and the passage of pathogens from caregivers or contaminated equipment.**

Prevention. Prevention begins by identifying mothers at risk for infection (e.g., GBS, herpes, chlamydia, syphilis, and gonorrhea); early management of infections with antibiotic therapy, meticulous equipment disinfection and handwashing practices by health care providers in the NICU; and restricting the entry of anyone with respiratory infections in the NICU (see Chapter 22).

Data Collection

History. The clinical presentation of neonatal pneumonia varies, depending on the infecting organism and the incidence of acquisition. Acute respiratory distress is frequently seen in intrauterine and intrapartally acquired secondary infections. Neonates with pneumonia often have a history of low Apgar scores, temperature instability, and poor tone and activity. **The clinical signs and symptoms of pneumonia are similar to those of respiratory distress, TTN/retained lung fluid, or sepsis.** Late-acquired pneumonia may have a gradual or abrupt onset, depending on the organism. Infants with chlamydial pneumonia frequently present with a cough.

Physical Examination. The infant with pneumonia often presents with respiratory distress (e.g., tachypnea, low pulse oximetry readings, respiratory deterioration, apnea, and temperature instability). The signs and symptoms of pneumonia often are difficult to differentiate from other neonatal respiratory problems without the aid of chest x-ray evaluation.

Laboratory Data. The appearance of pneumonia varies depending on the duration of infection, cause of the pneumonia, and presence of respiratory disease (e.g., RDS or BPD). **Serial x-ray films are more valuable than one isolated x-ray examination in making the diagnosis and following the course of the disease. Infiltration patterns on chest x-ray films include lobar consolidation, patchy alveolar infiltrates, hilar and peribronchial infiltrates, reticulogranular, nodular, or miliary infiltrates, and hazy or opaque lungs**[77] (see Table 23-16).

Tracheal aspirates and blood cultures are also useful tools in identifying the organisms of pneumonia. A workup for sepsis is often part of the diagnostic evaluation for these neonates (see Chapter 22).

Treatment. **Treatment of neonatal pneumonia includes supportive care (e.g., thermoregulation, nutrition, oxygenation, ventilation if necessary, and parental support). If the causative agent is bacterial, antibiotic therapy must be instituted after a sepsis workup; if viral, an antiviral agent** is considered; if fungal, an antifungal agent is used (see Chapter 22).

Complications. The mortality rate for perinatally acquired pneumonia is variable but has been estimated at 20%, with a higher mortality rate, 50%, for cases of postnatally acquired pneumonia.[77,150] In a recent review of perinatally acquired neonatal infections, the overall mortality rate for pneumonia was 10%.[77,450] The decline in mortality is the result of perinatal antibiotic use.

Persistent Pulmonary Hypertension of the Newborn (PPHN)

PPHN presents as severe pulmonary hypertension with pulmonary artery pressure elevation to levels equal to or higher than systemic pressure and large right-to-left shunts through the foramen ovale and the ductus arteriosus. PPHN presents early in life: 77% diagnosed in the first 24 hours of life, 93% in the first 48 hours, and 97% by 72 hours of age.[326,581]

Physiology. Once the placental blood source is severed, adequate oxygenation of the newborn depends on inflation of the lungs, closure of the fetal shunts, a decrease in pulmonary vascular resistance, and an increase in pulmonary blood flow (an eightfold to tenfold increase at the first breath). Normally, pulmonary vascular resistance decreases with the first breath of life. When it remains high, successful transition from fetal to neonatal circulation is impaired. In an infant manifesting PPHN, high pulmonary vascular resistance and pulmonary hypertension impede pulmonary blood flow. **Factors that increase and decrease pulmonary vascular resistance are listed in Table 23-17.** Increased PVR leads to hypoxemia, acidemia, hypercarbia, and eventually lactic acidosis. The pulmonary arterioles respond to this process with further constriction, promoting an additional decrease in blood flow; thus a cyclic pattern is established. Pulmonary vascular resistance also maintains higher right-sided pressures in the heart that equal or exceed systemic pressures resulting in right-to-left shunting that is characteristic of PPHN. PPHN also produces direct and indirect effects on myocardial function. A combination of pressure alterations, hypoxia, and acidemia leads to a cyclic pattern of decreased cardiac output, decreased pulmonary blood flow, and further vasoconstriction (Figure 23-12).

Etiology. **PVR remains high after birth because of underdevelopment, maldevelopment, or maladap-**

Table 23-17	FACTORS THAT INCREASE AND DECREASE PULMONARY VASCULAR RESISTANCE
LOWERS PVR	**INCREASES PVR**
Endogenous mediators and mechanisms	Endogenous mediators and mechanisms
Oxygen	Hypoxia
Nitric oxide	Acidosis
PGI_2, E_2, D_2	Endothelin-1
Adenosine, ATP, magnesium	Leukotrienes
Bradykinin	Thromboxanes
Atrial natriuretic factor	Platelet activating factor
Alkalosis	Ca^{++} channel activation
K^+ channel activation	Alpha-adrenergic stimulation
Histamine	PGF_{2a}
Vagal nerve stimulation	Mechanical factors
Acetylcholine	Overinflation or underinflation
Beta-adrenergic stimulation	Excessive muscularization, vascular remodeling
Mechanical factors	Altered mechanical properties of smooth muscle
Lung infection	Pulmonary hypoplasia
Vascular cell structural changes	Alveolar capillary dysplasia
Interstitial fluid and pressure changes	Pulmonary thromboemboli
Shear stress	Main pulmonary artery distention
	Ventricular dysfunction, venous hypertension

From Kinsella J, Abman S: Recent developments in the pathophysiology and treatment of PPHN, *J Pediatr* 126:855, 1995.
ATP, Adenosine triphosphate; *PGF$_{2a}$,* prostaglandin F$_{2a}$; *PGI$_2$, E$_2$, D$_2$,* prostaglandins I2, E2, and D2; *PVR,* pulmonary vascular resistance.

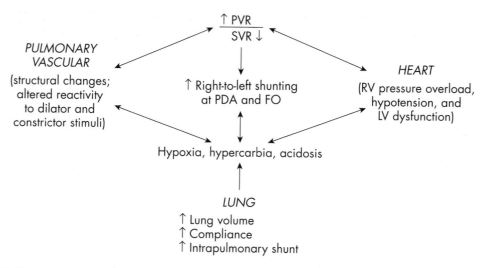

FIGURE 23-12 Cardiopulmonary interactions in PPHN. (*FO,* Foramen ovale; *LV,* left ventricle; *PDA,* patent ductus arteriosus; *PVR,* pulmonary vascular resistance; *RV,* right ventricle; *SVR,* systemic vascular resistance.) (From Kinsella J, Abman S: Recent developments in the pathophysiology and treatment of PPHN, *J Pediatr* 126:855, 1995.)

tation of pulmonary vasculature (Table 23-18). In utero, development of increased vascular smooth muscle or perinatal factors that cause or contribute to vasospasm are thought to be prime mechanisms of PPHN.

Prevention. Prevention of PPHN includes minimizing intrauterine and perinatal risk factors when possible, maintaining postnatal physiologic homeostasis, and detecting and correcting any underlying abnormality.

Data Collection

History. In addition to the risk factors listed in Table 23-18, maternal tobacco use and premature rupture of membranes[405] and maternal lack of or public insurance[581] are associated with an increased risk of PPHN.

There are two major considerations in the history of these infants: (1) the recognition of major disease processes or syndromes that are highly associated with pulmonary hypertension and (2) the timing of the onset of cyanosis and the deterioration of the infant.

Physical Examination. The initial clinical presentation is usually a near-term (34 weeks' or greater gestational age), term, or postterm infant

with worsening cyanosis within the first 24 hours of life. Tachypnea is a common finding and when accompanied by retractions is indicative of decreased pulmonary compliance. Cyanosis may either be intense at birth or progressively worsen in association with increased right-to-left shunting. Despite increasing FiO_2 the infant continues to have low PaO_2 (hypoxemia) as a result of right-to-left shunting. Milder cases of PPHN have minimal tachypnea and cyanosis, frequently associated with stress from crying or feeding. Severe cases are characterized by marked cyanosis, tachypnea, low systemic blood pressure, and decreased peripheral perfusion.

Increased pulmonary artery pressure results in the following symptoms[264]:
- Pulmonic systolic ejection clicks
- A second heart sound that is single, loud, or narrowly split with a loud pulmonary component
- A prominent right ventricular impulse that is visible or palpable at the lower left sternal border
- A soft systolic murmur in the pulmonary area

Laboratory Data. The laboratory evaluation of an infant with potential PPHN should include a CBC with differential, platelet count, chest x-ray examination, and serum glucose, calcium, electrolytes and arterial blood gas de-

Table 23-18	ETIOLOGIC FACTORS IN PPHN	
DEVELOPMENTAL PROCESS	**PATHOPHYSIOLOGY**	**ASSOCIATED CONDITIONS**
Underdevelopment, a decreased number of pulmonary vessels	Interruption in lung development, resulting in shunting of blood because of fewer pulmonary vessels and less area for gaseous exchange	Pulmonary hypoplasia (e.g., diaphragmatic hernia, aligohydramnios, Potter syndrome) Pulmonary masses (e.g., diaphragmatic hernia, cysts) Congenital heart disease (e.g., pulmonary or tricuspid atresia)
Maldevelopment, abnormally developed pulmonary vessels	Hypertrophy of musculature and extension into nonmuscularized arteries resulting in smaller lumen size, which increases PVR	Intrauterine asphyxia/hypoxia,[349] MAS Intrauterine fetal ductus arteriosus closure increases pulmonary blood flow Congenital heart defects that result in abnormal pulmonary vessel formation
Maladaptation (from intra-uterine to extrauterine life) as a result of transient or persistent vasoconstriction	Results in remodeling and abnormal muscularization of small pulmonary arteries Results in pulmonary vasospasm and vascular remodeling Pulmonary vasospasm and decreased cardiac output resulting from release of endotoxins and reaction to systemic inflammatory response	Hypoxia/acidosis/asphyxia Acute asphyxia may result in persistent vasospasm Pulmonary parenchymal disease[581] Bacterial sepsis[509] Prenatal pulmonary hypertension (e.g., fetal systemic hypertension or premature closure of ductus arteriosus) associated with maternal ingestion of NSAIDs (e.g., ibuprofen, Naproxyn, indomethacin), salicylates, phenytoin, lithium, prostaglandin inhibitors[8,186,349,444,581]
	Prevents normal circulatory transition at delivery	Delayed or ineffective resuscitation, narcosis, other CNS depression, hypothermia, hypotension
	Potentiation of vasoconstriction	Hypothermia,[613] hypoglycemia, hypocalcemia, acidosis, hypoxia, myocardial dysfunction, and ischemia[214]
	Functional obstruction of pulmonary vascular bed	Polycythemia, hyperviscosity

Modified from VanMarter L: Persistent pulmonary hypertension of the newborn. In Cloherty J, Stark A, eds: *Manual of neonatal care*, ed 4, Philadelphia, 1998, Lippincott-Raven; and Weardon M, Hansen T: Persistent pulmonary hypertension of the newborn. In Hansen T, Cooper T, Weisman L, eds: *Contemporary diagnosis and management of neonatal respiratory diseases*, ed 2, Newton, Pa, 1998, Handbook of Health Care.
CNS, Central nervous system; *MAS*, meconium aspiration syndrome; *NSAIDs*, nonsteroidal antiinflammatory drugs; *PVR*, pulmonary vascular resistance.

terminations. The CBC is used to detect anemia that could contribute to systemic hypertension, to detect polycythemia that could lead to increased pulmonary vascular resistance, and to detect an infectious process such as group B streptococcal sepsis or pneumonia.

Arterial blood gases demonstrate acidosis, hypoxia, and increased $PaCO_2$. If a blood gas is obtained simultaneously in the right radial artery (preductal) and in the descending aorta (postductal), the right-to-left shunt can be documented (preductal PaO_2 greater than postductal). Simultaneous preductal and postductal pulse oximetry and/or trans-cutaneous oxygen measurements may also be useful in the diagnosis. **Other diagnostic tests are outlined in Table 23-19.**

The most common chest x-ray findings associated with PPHN include the following[264]**:**
- Prominent main pulmonary artery segment
- Mild-to-moderate cardiomegaly
- Variable pulmonary vasculature (increased, decreased, or normal)
- Signs of left ventricular dysfunction that include pulmonary venous congestion and cardiomegaly

The electrocardiogram is usually normal but may demonstrate right ventricular hypertrophy, evidence

Table 23-19	DIAGNOSTIC TESTS FOR PPHN
TEST	**USE**
Hyperoxia test	If PO_2 does not increase in 100% oxygen, a right-to-left shunt is demonstrated (may be secondary to either PPHN or congenital heart disease)
Comparison of preductal and postductal arterial PO_2	Demonstrates ductal shunting; if negative, it does not rule out PPHN; most congenital heart disease has no ductal shunting
Contrast echocardiography "bubble echo"	Demonstrates foramen ovale shunting but should be present in most PPHN
Hyperoxia-hyperventilation	Most definitive test; if PO_2 <50 mm Hg prehyperventilation and rises to above 100 mm Hg, is almost always PPHN

From Duara S, Gewitz MH, Fox WW: *Clin Perinatol* 11:641, 1984.
PPHN, Persistent pulmonary hypertension of the newborn.

of pulmonary hypertension, and signs of myocardial ischemia. Echocardiography is used to evaluate cardiac structures and rule out cyanotic cardiac lesions, as well as diagnose right-to-left shunting at the foramen ovale and ductus arteriosus.

Treatment. **The optimal approach to treatment of PPHN is controversial[581] and has undergone major changes in the last 5 years[132] with the use of iNO, HFV, and surfactant administration.** In a recent multicenter (12 level III NICUs) observational study, the incidence of PPHN was 1.9/1000 live births. The time from admission to diagnosis was a mean of 12 hours of age; a wide variety and use of treatments occurred (Table 23-20), and there was no significant difference in mortality rates (range, 4% to 33%) among centers.[581]

Although the treatments listed in Table 23-20 are widely used, no RCTs to test safety and efficacy have been conducted,[15,581] and none of these treatments has improved survival in infants with PPHN.[182] In the study to evaluate whether therapies were equivalent, neonates treated with hyperventilation were compared with those treated with alkali infusion. Use of hyperventilation reduced the neonate's risk of needing ECMO/ECLS without increasing pulmonary morbidity (e.g., BPD/CLD). Neonates treated with hyperventilation were 2.8 times more likely to receive alkali infusions than those not undergoing hyperventilation therapy. However, the use of alkali infusion was associated with an increased use of ECMO/ECLS and BPD/CLD. This study recommended a reevaluation of hyperventilation, alkali infusion, and paralysis by randomized controlled trials.[581]

Treatment of PPHN focuses on preventing and/or

Table 23-20	TREATMENTS FOR PPHN IN TWELVE LEVEL III NICUs[581]	
TYPE OF TREATMENT	**OVERALL USE (%)**	**RANGE (%)**
Sedation	94	77-100
Inotrope IV administration	84	46-100
Continuous IV infusion of alkali	75	27-93
Paralysis*	73	33-98
Hyperventilation	65	33-92
Vasodilator drugs IV administration	39	13-81
HFV*	39	0-76
HFOV	72	
HFJV	26	
Surfactant administration	36	12-71
ECMO/ECLS*	34	0-85

*Associated with increased mortality risk, which disappeared when neonates with congenital diaphragmatic hernia were removed from analysis.
ECMO, Extracorporeal membrane oxygenation; *ECLS,* extracorporeal life support; *HFJV,* high-frequency jet ventilation; *HFOV,* high-frequency oscillator ventilation; *HFV,* high-frequency ventilation.

intervening in the development of the cyclic pattern illustrated in Figure 23-12. Pulmonary blood flow should increase if PVR is decreased or if SVR is increased. The goals of treatment include pulmonary vasodilation by improving pulmonary blood flow[182] and impeding right-to-left shunting by decreasing PVR and/or increasing SVR.[145]

Maintaining adequate oxygenation is a prime goal of care of infants with PPHN, alterations in "routine" care and handling are essential. Because handling a sick newborn for any reason causes a fall in PaO_2, the benefits of handling for

Table 23-21	**VASOPRESSOR RESPONSE IN THE NEONATE**
DRUG DOSE	**DISADVANTAGES**
Dopamine	
<4 µg/kg/min: renal vasodilation, mesenteric and cerebral vasodilation (effects unknown) plus increase in cardiac output	May decrease systemic arterial pressure
5-20 µg/kg/min: increase in cardiac output depending on myocardial norepinephrine	Loss of renal and mesenteric perfusion
>20 µg/kg/min: systemic arterial pressure increases more than pulmonary artery pressure	Cardiac output may decrease Myocardial oxygen consumption increases Marked increase in left ventricular afterload Dysrhythmias noted
Dobutamine	
10 µg/kg/min: increases cardiac contractility directly; cardiac output increases depending on myocardial catecholamine stores	No selective renal or mesenteric vasodilation Tends to increase skeletal blood flow at the expense of viscera Increase in pulmonary artery pressure
Isoproterenol	
0.05-1.0 µg/kg/min: lowers pulmonary vascular resistance in pulmonary hypertensive and vascular disease in child and adult; lowers hypoxemia-induced pulmonary vascular resistance in animal models	Dysrhythmias No specific vasodilation effects
Nitroprusside	
0.4-5.0 µg/kg/min: cardiac output increases because of decreased left ventricular afterload; systemic vascular resistance (indicated by blood pressure) decreases because of decrease in left ventricular afterload	Systemic vascular resistance remains constant if CO_2 increases

Modified from Drummond W: *Clin Perinatol* 11:715, 1984.

routine care such as changing linens, weighing, suctioning, and taking vital signs must be balanced against the risk of iatrogenic hypoxia. Pao_2 variations in the newborn are as follows[127,175]:

At rest	±15 mm Hg variation
While crying	↓Pao_2 by as much as 50 mm Hg
With routine care	↓Pao_2 by as much as 30 mm Hg

Maintaining organized, coordinated care and minimizing disturbances are therefore very important. Keeping the infant calm is important because severe hypoxia accompanies crying. Using pacifiers and decreasing noxious stimuli (e.g., invasive procedures) keeps struggling and crying to a minimum. Continuously monitoring vital signs, blood pressure, and pulse oximetry decreases the need for physical manipulation and disturbance. **These large, vigorous infants require sedation (see Chapter 12) and/or paralysis (see Table 23-15) to promote effective oxygenation and ventilation and decrease air leaks.**

Use of inotropic support (e.g., vasopressors) (Table 23-21) increases systemic vascular resis-

tance that decreases right-to-left shunting through the foramen ovale and ductus arteriosus. Cardiac output, cardiac contractility, and systemic blood pressure are all increased.[145]

Continuous (or bolus) infusion of alkali solution aids in achieving the desired pH (e.g., metabolic alkalosis) to counteract the vasoconstriction of acidosis.[145,316]

Conventional mechanical ventilation uses hyperventilation to produce hypocarbia (↓$Paco_2$) and respiratory alkalosis. Both metabolic and respiratory alkalosis have a direct vasodilatory effect on pulmonary vasculature that decreases PVR and improves oxygenation.[145] The neonate's lungs should be ventilated with whatever combination of rate, pressure, and oxygen is needed to lower $Paco_2$ and raise pH.

In addition to mechanical ventilation the use of pharmacologic vasodilators (e.g., tolazoline, sodium nitroprusside, and prostaglandin E_1) have been used to decrease PVR. These medications have resulted in variable and unpredictable results and are associated with systemic hypotension,[316] the need for volume expansion, fluid resuscitation,[376] and an inability to achieve and maintain pulmonary vasodilation.[326] When vasodilators are infused in dosages sufficient to decrease pulmonary hypertension, there is increased venous admixture as a result of right-to-left shunting of venous blood and pulmonary ventilation/perfusion mismatch.[476]

Surfactant replacement therapy is used when significant parenchymal lung disease is the cause of PPHN. Secondary surfactant deficiency may also exist in PPHN.[126] One study shows that surfactant replacement in the early phase of PPHN significantly decreases the need for ECMO/ECLS in term newborns without increasing the risk of complications.[371] In the ECMO/ECLS population, surfactant use has increased from 0% to 36%.[95]

HFV, both oscillator and jet, are used in treating PPHN. Use of HFOV optimizes lung inflation and oxygenation, improves ventilation, and achieves respiratory alkalosis.[316] HFOV is an effective rescue treatment for some neonates meeting ECMO/ECLS criteria who were unresponsive to CMV.[97,566] In the only prospective randomized controlled trial comparing HFJV with CMV, HFJV acutely improved oxygenation and ventilation without a significant increase in mortality and morbidity.[173] Because of the small samples, a multicenter RCT is needed.[173]

Endogenous nitric oxide (NO) production dilates the fetal pulmonary vascular bed. **Since endogenous production of NO in the pulmonary vasculature of neonates with PPHN is reduced,**[476] **treatment with iNO is beneficial because iNO is a selective pulmonary vasodilator (e.g., decreases pulmonary hypertension and increases oxygenation without reducing systemic blood pressure).**[131,327,476,477] Early clinical studies of iNO demonstrated brief exposure actually improved oxygenation and lowered pulmonary artery pressure.[327,329,477] RCTs for multicenters[182,326] have confirmed that prolonged iNO treatment for PPHN (1) results in sustained improvement of oxygenation,* (2) decreases the need for ECMO/ECLS treatment,† (3) is an adjunct to CMV,[194,326,331,416] and (4) combined therapy (e.g., iNO and HFOV) is more effective than either therapy alone.[331] The Neonatal Inhaled Nitric Oxide Study Group[416]

found that iNO had no effect on mortality, length of stay, number of days of ventilatory support, incidence of air leak, BPD/CLD, IVH/PVL, seizures, and pulmonary and GI hemorrhages. The effectiveness of iNO depends on (1) the initial degree of pulmonary vasoconstriction and hypoxemia, (2) the severity of parenchymal lung disease, and (3) recruitment of adequate lung volume/inflation that decreases intrapulmonary shunting and improves iNO delivery to the pulmonary system.[325,331,478] In the ECMO/ECLS population, iNO use has increased from 0% to 24%.[95]

Inhaled NO is an effective treatment for PPHN but "should be considered a part of the overall clinical strategy that cautiously manages parenchymal lung disease, cardiac performance, and systemic hemodynamics."[326] **Inhaled NO has been approved by FDA for treatment of near-term (more than 34 weeks' gestational age) and term neonates with PPHN. Recommendations for use of iNO are listed in Table 23-22.**

Use of HFOV and iNO to treat PPHN has decreased the number of neonates meeting ECMO/ECLS criteria who subsequently require ECMO/ECLS treatment, has shortened length of hospital stay, and has decreased costs.[316] There is increased survival and a decrease in short-term morbidity in neonates (34 weeks' gestational age or older) with PPHN who are treated with ECMO/ECLS versus conventional therapies.[561]

Complications. In the study evaluating the myriad of treatments of PPHN,[581] overall survival of PPHN (88%) varied according to centers and diagnostic categories: (1) MAS 94%, (2) RDS/pneumonia 91%, and (3) congenital diaphragmatic hernia 61%. **Despite the diversity of treatment within level III centers, there was no statistically significant difference in survival rates among centers (67% to 96%).**[581]

In a study of conservative management (e.g., no paralysis or hyperventilation) of PPHN, outcomes included (1) 100% survival, (2) no sensorineural hearing loss, and (3) better neurodevelopmental outcomes (e.g., average IQ in the normal range).[382] In a recent retrospective study of 14 near-term and term neonates treated with surfactant for moderate-to-severe PPHN, only one survivor showed significant cognitive impairment and abnormal school performance.[24]

A follow-up of term neonates with PPHN treated with iNO found an 11.8% (at 1 year) and 12.1% (at 2 years) rate of severe neurodevelop-

---

*References 115, 131, 181, 194, 326, 331, 332, 416, 476, 478.
†References 100, 131, 182, 326, 332, 416, 476.

Table 23-22   RECOMMENDATIONS FOR USE OF INHALED NITRIC OXIDE (iNO)

RECOMMENDATION	RESEARCH BASIS
Gestational Age	
≥34 weeks' gestation	Clinical trials[15,100,416] and FDA approval support use of iNO in near-term/term newborns
Postnatal Age	
0-14 days of age	Clinical trials support iNO use within first week of life; may also be used as adjunct therapy after ECMO/ECLS treatment
Severity of Illness	
Oxygenation index (OI) = (MAP × FiO_2 × 100 ÷ PaO_2) >25 with echocardiographic evidence of extrapulmonary right-to-left shunting	Mean OI in multicenter trials was 40; earlier use of iNO at lower OI have not resulted in reduction of ECMO/ECLS use[22,131,438]
Dose	
Initial: 20 ppm in term newborns with PPHN	Increasing dose to 40-80 ppm does not improve oxygenation if there was no response to 20 ppm*
Brief exposure to 40-80 ppm is safe	
Sustained treatment with 80 ppm increases risk of methemoglobinemia[131]	Initial treatment with subtherapeutic dose may decrease the clinical response to 20 ppm of iNO[115]
Duration	
Typically <5 days	Longer usage may be necessary in pulmonary hypoplasia; for therapy >5 days, other causes of pulmonary hypertension should be investigated
Weaning and Discontinuation	
After 4 hr at 20 ppm iNO reduced to 6 ppm without change in oxygenation[325,331]	Withdrawal of iNO can be associated with life-threatening elevations in PVR, profound oxygen desaturation, and systemic hypotension as a result of decreased cardiac output[132]
iNO decreased by 20% increments in stepwise fashion to dose of 1 ppm before discontinuation[132]	Dose-response relationship between iNO given and a drop in PaO_2. A decrease in iNO to 1 ppm before discontinuation minimizes the decrease in PaO_2, and compensatory changes in FiO_2 and ventilator parameters are unnecessary[132]
Ventilator Management	
High-frequency oscillatory ventilation (HFOV)	Inadequate lung inflation results in less response to iNO therapy[326]
• With significant parenchymal lung disease	Combination of HFOV and iNO results in best improvement in oxygenation[331] because of improved lung inflation during HFOV that augments response to iNO by reducing intrapulmonary shunting and improving iNO delivery to pulmonary circulation[325]
• Without significant parenchymal lung disease	Combination of HFOV and iNO and iNO alone are more effective than HFOV alone

Modified from Kinsella, J, Abman, S: Inhaled nitric oxide: current and future uses in neonates, *Semin Perinatol* 24:387, 2000; and American Academy of Pediatrics: Use of inhaled nitric oxide, *Pediatrics,* 106:344, 2000.

AAP, American Academy of Pediatrics; *BPD/CLD,* bronchopulmonary dysplasia/chronic lung disease; *IVH,* intraventricular hemorrhage; *ECMO/ECLS,* extracorporeal membrane oxygenation/extracorporeal life support; *PPHN,* persistent pulmonary hypertension of the newborn; *PVR,* pulmonary vascular resistance; *RCT,* randomized controlled trial; *VLBW,* very low birth weight.

*References 131, 329, 330, 416, 477, 478.

Continued

Table 23-22	RECOMMENDATIONS FOR USE OF INHALED NITRIC OXIDE (iNO)—cont'd
RECOMMENDATION	**RESEARCH BASIS**

Use in ECOM/ECLS Centers

Recommendations of AAP[15]

- Center must have expertise and experience in multiple modes of rescue and ventilator therapy or be transferred in a timely manner to such a center
- Inhaled NO therapy should be given according to product label. Center will develop criteria for treatment failure so that timely consideration for treatment alternatives is possible
- Therapies should be directed by qualified physicians (e.g., educated and experienced in the use of iNO); offered only at centers qualified and able to provide multisystem support, including on-site ECMO/ECLS capability

Initial use of iNO, HFOV, and surfactant in one ECMO/ECLS resulted in a decline in overall survival (from 84% to 56%) of neonates requiring ECMO/ECLS[316]

Use in Non-ECMO/ECLS Centers and Transport With iNO

Recommendations of AAP[15]

- Centers without capability to provide experience and expertise in multiple modes of rescue and ventilator therapy for PPHN must be able to transfer in a timely manner to such a center
- Centers without capability for ECMO/ECLS who give iNO for geographic or other compelling reasons must prospectively and mutually establish treatment failure criteria and mechanisms for timely transfer to a collaborating ECMO/ECLS center; iNO must *not* be interrupted during transport

Concerns regarding use of iNO in non-ECMO/ECLS centers[316,326]

- Undue delay in initiation of transport to ECMO/ECLS center
- Increases risks of transport
- Significant delay in use of ECMO/ECLS that results in poorer outcomes for neonates requiring ECMO/ECLS

Uses in ECMO/ECLS and Non-ECMO/ECLS Centers

Recommendations of AAP[15]

- Centers providing iNO should provide comprehensive long-term medical and neurodevelopment follow-up care
- Centers providing iNO should collect prospective data regarding timing of treatment, toxic effects, treatment failure, use of alternative therapies, and outcomes

Use in Preterm Infants (<34 weeks' Gestation)

Potential for increased toxicity of iNO and poorer outcomes in preterms (see Table 23-8)
Recommendations of AAP[15]

- Use in populations not approved by FDA is experimental use and requires formalized FDA and institutional review board approved protocol and informed parental consent

- RCT of low-dose (5 ppm) iNO in preterm infants with severe hypoxemic respiratory failure found improved oxygenation after 60 min of iNO, decreased need for mechanical ventilation, improved survival without increase in IVH or BPD/CLD[332]; iNO may decrease BPD/CLD because of its antiinflammatory and antioxidant effects[332]
- High mortality rate despite improved systemic oxygenation in VLBW (≤1500 g) rescued with iNO; survivors: increased frequency of severe (≥grade III) IVH and poor neurodevelopmental outcome in early childhood[88]

Modified from Kinsella, J, Abman, S: Inhaled nitric oxide: current and future uses in neonates, *Semin Perinatol* 24:387, 2000; and American Academy of Pediatrics: Use of inhaled nitric oxide, *Pediatrics,* 106:344, 2000.
AAP, American Academy of Pediatrics; *BPD/CLD,* bronchopulmonary dysplasia/chronic lung disease; *IVH,* intraventricular hemorrhage; *ECMO/ECLS,* extracorporeal membrane oxygenation/extracorporeal life support; *PPHN,* persistent pulmonary hypertension of the newborn; *PVR,* pulmonary vascular resistance; *RCT,* randomized controlled trial; *VLBW,* very low birth weight.

mental disability, similar to the neurodevelopmental disability of ECMO/ECLS survivors.[485,581] The mortality rate of these infants was 29%.[485] Follow-up at 18 to 24 months of age of the neonates in the NINOSG trial found no increase in neurodevelopmental, behavioral, or medical abnormality.[181]

The survival rate of neonates treated with ECMO/ECLS is 80% to 91%; 10% to 21% of the survivors have substantial developmental delays that include cognitive and motor delays, behavioral problems, and school failure.* Risk factors for higher abnormal neurodevelopmental outcome include infants requiring prolonged (15 days or more) assisted ventilation, supplemental oxygen (22 days or more), and black race.[346] Survivors of PPHN have significant pulmonary and neurodevelopmental impairment whether treated with conventional methods (listed in Table 23-20) or with ECMO/ECLS.[485,581] In one study ECMO/ECLS treated neonates had neurodevelopmental outcomes (e.g., hearing loss, blindness, cognitive delay) (26% at 20 months of age) similar to conventionally treated neonates (24%).[581] The same ECMO/ECLS treated infants had less BPD/CLD, better pulmonary outcomes, and an increased rate of macrocephaly.[581] **Survivors of PPHN are at increased risk for impaired function at school age, regardless of the treatment modality used, and should have long-term follow-up.**[485,581]

Apnea

Physiology. The two major control mechanisms that regulate pulmonary ventilation are the neural and chemical systems. The cerebral cortex and brainstem are the governing agents for the neural control system, which regulates respiratory rate and rhythm. The peripheral components of this system are found in the upper airway and lung. The chemical control center is found in the medulla and is sensitive to changes in $PaCO_2$. The peripheral portion of the chemical system lies in the carotid and aortic vessels and is sensitive to changes in $PaCO_2$.[385] Alveolar ventilation is controlled by the chemical system, and this system is the principal defense against hypoxia. Neonates have a unique response to hypoxemia and carbon dioxide retention. Unlike adults, who have sustained increase in ventilation, infants have a brief period of increased ventilation followed by respiratory depression.

Carbon dioxide responsiveness is less developed in the preterm infant and may be the result of decreased sensitivity in the chemical center or mechanical factors that prevent an increase in ventilation.[385] Apnea of prematurity or primary apnea is not associated with other specific disease entities. **The younger the gestational age, the greater the incidence of apnea.** In infants born at 27 weeks' gestation or earlier, 58% to 60% have persistent apnea at 36 weeks' postconceptual age.[171] Apnea may be associated with hypoxemia, neuronal immaturity, sleep, catecholamine deficiency, and respiratory muscle fatigue.

Etiology. **Causes of apnea in the premature are characterized as central apnea (absence of breathing effort), obstructive apnea (breathing efforts occur but the airway is blocked), or most commonly mixed apnea (an initial central apnea followed by obstruction of the airway).**[291] **Clinically, various conditions may cause apnea in the premature infant by producing hypoxia and/or altering the sensitivity of peripheral or central chemoreceptors**[385] **(Table 23-23).** Neuronal immaturity seems a plausible cause for apnea. Respiratory efforts are more unstable at a younger gestational age. The decreased response appears to be the result of a general lack of dendritic formation and limited synaptic connections, therefore decreasing the excitatory drive. Another postulation is that apneic episodes are manifestations of synaptic disorders that occur without a motor component. Such phenomena have been confirmed on electroencephalogram. Infants depend on alternating excitation and inhibition to establish rhythmic breathing, and therefore imbalances (e.g., hypoxia, hypoglycemia, and hypocalcemia) may cause respiratory arrest.

Apnea has been noted to appear with greater frequency during sleep and especially during REM or active sleep in both term and preterm infants. Apnea is uncommon in non-REM sleep, but periodic breathing may be observed. The effects of REM sleep are inhibition of spinal motor neurons, increase in brain activity causing increasing eye movements and muscular twitching, and changes in brain temperature and cerebral blood flow and CNS arousal, shown by EEG changes.

Decreased amounts of peripheral catecholamines in a premature infant have also been postulated as a cause of apnea. This would become critical if hemorrhage or infection was also present in the premature infant and stores were depleted.

---

*References 55, 217, 218, 346, 382, 549, 567, 581.

Table 23-23	CAUSES OF APNEA IN THE PREMATURE INFANT
CAUSES	**SPECIFICS**
Infection	Pneumonia, sepsis, meningitis
Respiratory distress	RDS, airway obstruction, CPAP application, postextubation, congenital anomalies of the upper airways
Cardiovascular disorders	Patent ductus arteriosus, congestive heart failure
Gastrointestinal disorders	Gastroesophageal reflux, necrotizing enterocolitis, deglutition, syncope[257]
CNS disorders	Depressant drugs, intraventricular hemorrhage, seizure, kernicterus, infection, tumors
Metabolic disorders	Hypoglycemia, hypocalcemia, hyponatremia
Environmental	Rapid increase of environmental temperature, hypothermia, vigorous suctioning, feeding, stooling, stretching, fatigue/stress
Hematopoietic	Polycythemia, anemia

CPAP, Continuous positive airway pressure; *RDS,* respiratory distress syndrome.

A premature infant has a more compliant chest cage and less compliant lungs; this situation results in a greater workload. Respiratory muscle fatigue occurs easily in the absence of fatigue-resistant fibers.

Apnea associated with the sleep state becomes more significant in that premature infants, particularly those of less than 32 weeks' gestation, spend 80% of their time asleep. Equally significant is the time spent in REM sleep, the predominant sleep state of premature infants. The percentage of quiet sleep or non-REM sleep will increase from 20% to 60% of the total sleep period by the time an infant is 3 months old.

Secondary apnea may be associated with a particular disease entity or in response to special procedures. Many disorders leading to secondary apnea may exert their influence through hypoxemia and subsequent respiratory center depression.

The majority of cases of secondary apnea arise from four conditions. In RDS, apnea is related to the degree of parenchymal disease and may result from muscle fatigue. With CNS hemorrhage and seizures, apnea arises from asphyxia with subsequent hypoxemia and respiratory center depression or actual brain injury. Apnea is related to central depression in sepsis. In addition, carbon dioxide retention and hypoxemia associated with the left-to-right shunting of a PDA may cause apnea.

Iatrogenic causes of apnea include increased environmental temperature, sudden increases in environmental temperature, vagal response to suctioning of the nasopharynx or to a gavage tube, gastroesophageal reflux, and obstruction of the airway. Reflex apnea occurs when foreign material (milk or secretions) is present in the oropharynx. This laryngeal chemoreflex is protective in that it prevents inhalation of the substance into the airway and has been documented in preterm and hospitalized infants.[133,443,453,454] Obstruction may occur from improper neck positioning or aspiration.

Cerebral blood flow (CBF) velocity decreases with apnea and bradycardia,[446] is directly correlated with the severity of bradycardia,[463] and an increase in CBF may occur on recovery.[291,364] Decreased oxygen saturation also correlates with the duration of apnea, regardless of type.[291] Obstructive apnea is associated with significantly greater maximum fall in cerebral blood volume than central or mixed apneic episodes.[291] Because alteration of CBF may cause or exacerbate IVH, obstruction of upper airways with resultant apneic episodes should be prevented.[291]

Prevention. **All infants assessed as high risk for apneic spells should be carefully monitored for a period of at least 10 to 12 days.** Impedance apnea monitors do not distinguish normal respiratory efforts from gasping movements associated with obstruction. Both heart rate and respiratory rates should be monitored. Alarm systems should be used at all times. A qualified observer is essential.

Apneic episodes are frequently associated with alterations in heart rate and oxygen saturation— the degree of these changes is related to the duration of apnea. Apnea generally precedes a drop in heart rate and oxygen desaturation. Changes in oxygen saturation are distinct from heart rate changes so that the desaturation cannot be predicted from changes in heart rate patterns. Because episodes of apnea and bradycardia are associated with a decrease in CBF[446] and oxygen desaturation (as little as 5% to 10%) is associated with alteration of cerebral circulation,[364,372] **oxygen saturation monitoring should accompany cardiorespiratory monitoring (both in-hospital and home monitoring).**[75]

Pulse oximetry monitors may detect hypoxemic conditions that may lead to apneic spells. In a premature infant younger than 32 weeks' gestation this type of apnea is common. Care should be organized to decrease stressful, hypoxic episodes.

Apneic episodes may be prevented or decreased by several means. Reducing environmental stress by providing adequate rest has resulted in a faster rate of decline in apneic episodes.[556] Gentle tactile stimulation alone has been shown to be effective in decreasing and preventing apneic spells in most premature infants. Noxious stimuli such as shaking or banging on the incubator should be avoided. If tactile stimulus is ineffective and temporary bag and mask ventilation is required, attention should be paid to preventing undue pressure on the lower chin and neck so that the airway remains open. Bagging that is too vigorous may also stimulate pulmonary stretch receptors and induce apnea; therefore it should be avoided. Waterbed flotation may decrease the frequency of apnea but generally does not completely eliminate it. **Apneic episodes are decreased when twins are co-bedded, either because of a change in sleep patterns (e.g., more frequent arousal by the co-bedded twin) or a more regular breathing pattern, reflecting a positive physiologic response to skin-to-skin contact between the twins.**[557]

Because increased environmental temperature and sudden changes in temperature have resulted in apneic episodes, prevention includes maintaining the environmental temperature at the lower end of the normal spectrum, particularly if an apneic episode has already occurred. Incubator temperature may require a 0.5° to 1.0° C (1° to 2° F) decrease to counter the problem. Phototherapy may provide sufficient radiant energy to increase an infant's temperature and contribute to the incidence of apnea. **Care should be taken to avoid sudden changes in temperature.** An infant should not be placed on a cold scale; he or she should be placed in a prewarmed incubator or bed. Oxygen should be warmed and humidified before administration.

Careful attention must be paid to prevent airway obstruction. Small neck rolls under the neck and shoulders have been used to decrease neck flexion and prevent airway obstruction when in the supine position. Close monitoring should be done during procedures such as lumbar puncture where accidental airway obstruction may occur.

Data Collection. Evaluation of apnea should include studies to rule out treatable causes.

History. Evaluation of the prenatal and birth history may give a clue to the causes and also provide a basis for further study.

Physical Examination. A thorough physical and neurologic examination rules out grossly apparent abnormalities. **Observation and documentation of apneic and bradycardic episodes and any relationship to precipitating factors help differentiate primary from secondary apnea.**

Laboratory Data. A CBC and CRP assess for infection and anemia as causes of apnea. Measurements of serum glucose, calcium, phosphate, magnesium, sodium, potassium, and chloride levels assess metabolic causes. Arterial blood gas measurements assess hypoxemia and metabolic and respiratory contributions to apnea. Blood, urine, and CSF cultures rule out sepsis as the cause of apnea. The CSF culture is usually performed only when other signs and symptoms of infection are present. Chest x-ray examinations assess cardiac and respiratory causes. The examinations may also rule out aspiration of abdominal contents caused by gastroesophageal reflux. Ultrasonographic examination of the head and an EEG may be used to rule out IVH or other neurologic causes of apnea.

Treatment. **Treatment of secondary apnea is aimed at the diagnosis and management of the specific causes. In the treatment of primary apnea (apnea of prematurity), initial efforts should begin with the least invasive intervention possible.** Gentle tactile stimulation is frequently successful, especially with early recognition and intervention. When infants do not immediately respond to external stimuli, bag and mask ventilation must be initiated. Generally, an FiO_2 approximating that used before the spell but not exceeding a 10% increase will alleviate hypoxemia and avoid marked elevations in the arterial PaO_2. The use of pulse oximetry monitoring will allow closer evaluation of PaO_2 fluctuation and helps prevent complications of oxygen toxicity. Elevation in ambient oxygen concentrations, although decreasing the frequency of apnea, causes prolongation of apnea spells.

Apnea will respond to low pressure (3 to 5 cm of water) nasal CPAP. Mechanical ventilation may be required if the infant fails to respond to lesser measures and continues to have repeated and prolonged apneic episodes. It may also be required in extremely immature, unstable, or debilitated infants. **Mechanical ventilation for apnea may be administered with nasal prongs or nasotracheal tube to avoid intubation.**[358,547]

Methylxanthines (caffeine, theophylline, and aminophylline) are used to treat apnea of prematurity (Table 23-24). They are used only in primary apnea (i.e., when pathologic causes have been eliminated). Methylxanthines are potent cardiac, respiratory, and CNS stimulants and smooth muscle relaxers. Their effect on decreasing the frequency of apnea is related to central stimulation[203] rather than to changes in pulmonary function. Caffeine citrate is considered the drug of choice because (1) dosing is once a day, (2) there is an earlier onset of action, (3) it has a wide therapeutic range, requiring fewer serum blood level evaluations, and (4) there are fewer side effects than with theophylline.[203] Although methylxanthines reduce the frequency of apnea and are associated with a decrease in the use of mechanical ventilation, there is no evidence that they decrease hypoxemia.[73,261-263,428,499] Because use of methylxanthines may worsen hypoxic tissue damage in preterms, a large RCT with long-term follow-up has been launched to study their use in preterm infants.[499]

Although gastroesophageal reflux is frequent in preterm infants because of lower esophageal sphincter relaxation,[38] recent studies do not find an association between predischarge apnea and reflux.[42,323] Reflux events are unrelated to apneic events; apneic events are not a frequent marker of reflux.[82] Because antireflux medications (some of which are unsafe, e.g., cisapride) have not been found to decrease the incidence of apnea and bradycardia in preterms, their efficacy requires randomized controlled trial testing.[324]

Complications. **Side effects of xanthines include gastric irritation, hyperactivity (restlessness, irritability, and wakefulness), myocardial stimulation (tachycardia and hypotension), and increased urinary output.** Medications to improve gastric emptying (e.g., metoclopramide) have been used to treat reflux and decrease apnea secondary to reflux, although a relationship between gastric emp-

Table 23-24	METHYLXANTHINES USED TO TREAT APNEA OF PREMATURITY		
DRUG	**DOSAGE**	**THERAPEUTIC LEVELS**	**SIDE EFFECTS**
Caffeine citrate	Route: PO Loading: 20-40 mg/kg Maintenance: 5-8 mg/kg/day administered 24 hr after loading dose Route: IV Cafcit 20 mg/ml Administer IV over 15 to 30 min to avoid cardiac dysrhythmias	Afterload: 8-14 μg/ml Maintenance: 5-25 μg/ml Toxic: >40-50 μg/ml	Administer orally with feedings: administer in morning so the infant's sleep pattern is less disrupted than with PM administration Tachycardia (withhold dose if >180/min), dysrhythmias, diuresis, glucosuria, ketonuria, hyperglycemia, jitteriness, seizures, vomiting, hemorrhagic gastritis, NEC
Theophylline	Route: PO Loading: 4-6 mg/kg Maintenance: 1.5 mg/kg q 8 hr to 3 mg/kg q 12 hr IV: Aminophylline 4-6 mg/kg over 30 min	5-15 μg/ml, although levels of 3-4 μg/ml have been shown to be effective in decreasing apnea	See above

Modified from Young T, Magnum B: *Neofax 2000,* Raleigh, NC, 2000, Acorn Publishing; and Gannon B: Theophylline or caffeine: which is best for apnea of prematurity? *Neonatal Netw* 19:33, 2000.
NEC, Necrotizing enterocolitis.

tying and reflux in preterm infants has not been supported by research.[37] Metoclopramide is associated with significant adverse neurologic effects (e.g., seizure, extrapyramidal symptoms [dystonic posturing], and tardive dyskinesia.) Cisapride has been associated with prolonged QT interval when administered alone or with other drugs to preterm infants.[48,356,582] The manufacturer and the U.S. Food and Drug Administration (FDA) have taken cisapride off the US market.[582] Because a large proportion of preterm infants have abnormally high degrees of esophageal acid, administration of acid-reducing agents (e.g., ranitidine and omeprazole) may be beneficial, and these will have fewer side effects and drug interactions.

The prognosis for apnea arising from an underlying cause depends on the outcome of the disease process itself. The prognosis for apnea is generally good in infants who are otherwise well and healthy and for whom the apnea is not prolonged. In one study no significant difference in cognitive outcome was reported for infants with apnea of prematurity compared with the control group. However, there were a greater percentage with persistent apnea that had mild motor delays compared with the control group.[341] The prognosis becomes increasingly less favorable with an increased frequency and duration of episodes. There is an association between the frequency and degree of oximetry desaturations during predischarge apnea and neurodevelopmental outcome in early childhood. Apnea associated with severe oxygen desaturations is a marker for subsequent adverse neurodevelopmental outcomes (e.g., CP, cognitive delay, blindness, hearing loss, and seizures).[89,372] Prompt recognition and intervention decrease the possibility of severe complications from hypoxia.

PARENT TEACHING

Parental attachment to an infant with respiratory disease is especially difficult. It is made more difficult if the infant is also premature. Normal interaction is curtailed by the infant's condition and appearance, the environment, and the parent's reaction to these factors. **An infant who is in an oxygen hood or receiving ventilation therapy to the lungs may give inadequate cues to arouse parental attachment and instead may arouse feelings of grief and loss (see Part VI).**

The goal of discharge planning is the best possible outcome with the least family disruption. **Evaluation of parental readiness to care for their infant is essential to effective teaching and learning.** Physical surroundings and preparations for the infant are assessed when possible by a home visit. Parental concerns at bringing home an infant with special care needs must be assessed and discussed. The parents learn to be comfortable in handling and caring for their infant gradually throughout hospitalization. A specially designated or decorated room is used for family visiting and caretaking. Before discharge, the mother and/or father spend the night caring for the infant. Positive reinforcement and praise from the professional staff should be freely given to parents who attend classes and successfully master the tasks of caregiving for their infant.

Special equipment such as oxygen tanks, nasal cannulas, a ventilator, and suction equipment for home use must be acquired before discharge. Sources, mode of delivery, and use of equipment must all be taught to parents before discharge. Pulmonary hygiene for infants with prolonged difficulty in handling secretions must also be taught. Written protocols and instructions should be provided to parents whenever possible. **Parents must be informed of dosage, route of administration, side effects, and planned duration of use of all medications.**

Because fluid and nutritional status is so important to any infant with a chronic condition, nutritional information for parents is required. Infants with tachypnea (BPD/CLD) often have difficulty with coordinating suck and swallow. Often smaller, more frequent feedings are necessary when using supplemental oxygen. Alternative feeding methods such as gavage feeding may be necessary to safely provide enough calories with a minimum of work.

Apnea is especially distressing to parents because of their fears of recurrence once the child goes home. If apnea is related to an underlying disease, treatment of the cause should result in resolution of the apneic episodes. Parents can be reliably assured that recurrence is unlikely unless the disease recurs. With apnea of prematurity assurance can be offered that infants do grow into a regular ventilatory pattern as their respiratory center matures and that all means to protect the infant will be used until that time. Also, the parents can be assured that the infant will not go home until he or she is ready and the parents are adequately prepared to handle situations that may arise.

Before an infant needing a home monitoring system is discharged from the hospital, the parents must be given adequate support and instruction. Classes on the use of the apnea monitors must include demonstration of the equipment and return demonstrations. Minor equipment checks and repairs should be mastered before discharge.

Support by the primary care providers after discharge is essential. Parents must have telephone numbers of the medical facility and personnel they can call 24 hours a day in case of problems or equipment failure.

Anticipatory support includes discussion of potential stress factors related to having an infant on a monitor and oxygen at home: sibling rivalries, marital stresses, scheduling problems, potential problems with baby-sitters, and the parent's own fears of the situation.[612] An apnea monitor in the home may provoke anxiety despite discussion and instruction. **When infants are discharged with apnea monitors, there is a marked increase in maternal fatigue one month after discharge when compared with a similar group discharged without monitors.**[592] Increased fatigue interferes with activities of daily living, ability to parent, and increases caregiver stress.[451,592] Interventions to alleviate fatigue after discharge may include spousal support, household help, child care for siblings, and opportunities for increasing sleep.[205]

The parents of every infant who has apneic episodes or serious respiratory disease must be taught cardiopulmonary resuscitation (CPR). This is a set of skills that is learned over the course of time by reading written materials and seeing and returning the demonstration. Learning CPR cannot be done on the day of discharge but must be a staged process of individual and class instruction. Supplying instructional pamphlets written just for parents aids in initial learning and provides a quick reference. If other family members or baby-sitters will provide child care during work or evening hours, they too must be able to resuscitate the infant.

Other emergency actions for which parents must be prepared include clearing the infant's airway, calling for help (having emergency phone numbers easily accessible), planning for an alternative communication source (i.e., neighbor's phone), and notifying the community rescue squad of the infant's presence in the home.

Parents must be taught how to recognize signs of illness or significant deterioration in the condition of their infant. In addition to information about special care needs, parents need informa-tion about normal newborn care. Developing realistic expectations and positive parenting skills is as important to these parents as to all new parents.

For the parents of an infant with special respiratory problems, the importance of continuous follow-up care must be emphasized. Follow-up visits should coincide with developmental stages, the natural course of the disease, and expected complications of the disease.

The parents whose child has special respiratory needs must learn a myriad of involved technical information. The primary care provider (frequently the primary nurse) is responsible for organizing, teaching, coordinating, and documenting the information. This nurse is also responsible for ensuring that the parents have not only been taught but in fact understand these concepts.

REFERENCES

1. Abbasi S, Cole C, Frantz I et al: Effect of early inhaled glucocorticoid therapy on tracheobronchial lesions in mechanically ventilated preterm infants, *Pediatr Res* 45:179A, 1999.
2. Abman SH, Groothuis JR: Pathophysiology and treatment of bronchopulmonary dysplasia, *Pediatr Clin North Am* 41:277, 1994.
3. Abman SH, Kinsella JP: Inhaled nitric oxide therapy of pulmonary hypertension and respiratory failure in premature and term neonates, *Adv Pharmacol* 34:457, 1995.
4. Abrams C, Johnson B: Endotracheal tube suctioning of the neonate: an informal procedural study, *Neonatal Netw* 3:18, 1984.
5. Ackerman MH, Ecklund MM, Abu-Jumah M: A review of normal saline instillation: implications for practice, *Dimens Crit Care Nurs* 15:31, 1996.
6. Ahmed N, Parvez B, LaGamma E: Does high frequency oscillatory ventilation cause more IVH in ELBW? *Pediatr Res* 45:180A, 1999.
7. Al-Alaiyan S, Dyer D, Khan B: Chest physiotherapy and post-extubation atelectasis in infants, *Pediatric Pulmonol* 21:227, 1996.
8. Alano M, Ngougmna E, Ostrea E et al: Analysis of non-steroidal anti-inflammatory drugs in meconium and its relation to PPHN, *Pediatrics* 107:519, 2001.
9. Allen MC, Donohue PK, Dusman AE: The limit of viability: neonatal outcome of infants born at 22 to 25 weeks' gestation, *N Engl J Med* 329:1597, 1993.
10. Alexander GR, Hulsey TC, Robillard PY et al: Determinants of meconium-stained amniotic fluid in term pregnancies, *J Perinatol* 14:259, 1994.
11. Ambalavanan N, Nelson KG, Alexander G et al: Prediction of neurologic morbidity in ELBW infants, *J Perinatol* 20:496, 2000.

12. American Academy of Pediatrics: An international classification of retinopathy of prematurity, *Pediatrics* 74:127, 1984.

13. American Academy of Pediatrics: Policy statement: screening examination of premature infants for ROP, *Pediatrics* 100:273, 1997.

14. American Academy of Pediatrics, Committee on Fetus and Newborn: Surfactant replacement therapy for RDS, *Pediatrics* 103:684, 1999.

15. American Academy of Pediatrics, Committee on Fetus and Newborn: Use of inhaled nitric oxide, *Pediatrics* 106:344, 2000.

16. American Academy of Pediatrics, Committee on Infectious Diseases and Committee on Fetus and Newborn: Prevention of respiratory syncytial virus infections: indications for the use of palivizumab and update on the use of RSV-IVIG, *Pediatrics* 102:1211, 1998.

17. American Academy of Pediatrics and American College of Obstetricians and Gynecologists: *Guidelines for perinatal care,* ed 5, Evanston, Ill, 2002, American Academy of Pediatrics.

17a. American Academy of Pediatrics, Canadian Pediatric Society: Postnatal corticosteroids to treat or prevent chronic lung disease in preterm infants, *Pediatrics* 109:330, 2002.

18. American Association of Respiratory Care, Clinical Practice Guideline: Application of continuous positive airway pressure to neonates via nasal prongs or nasopharyngeal tube, *Respir Care* 39:817, 1994.

19. American Medical Association: International classification of retinopathy of prematurity, *Arch Ophthalmol* 102:1130, 1984.

20. Andre P, Thebaud B, Odievre MH et al: Methylprednisolone, an alternative to dexamethasone in very premature infants at risk for CLD, *Intensive Care Med* 26:1496, 2000.

21. Annibale DJ, Hulsey TC, Engstrom PC et al: Randomized, controlled trial of nasopharyngeal continuous positive airway pressure in the extubation of very low birth weight infants, *J Pediatr* 124:455, 1994.

22. Antunes M, Paul D, Leef K et al: RCT of early vs. late inhaled nitric oxide in term infants with respiratory failure, *Pediatr Res* 47:386A, 2000.

23. Aubert L, Schmitt A, Fresson J et al: Impact of postnatal dexamethasone on the incidence and severity of ROP in the surfactant era, *Pediatr Res* 45:183A, 1999.

24. Auten RL, Merzbach J, Myers G et al: Neurodevelopmental and health outcomes in term infants treated with surfactant for severe respiratory failure, *J Perinatol* 20:291, 2000.

25. Auten RL, Notter RH, Kendig JW et al: Surfactant treatment of full-term newborns with respiratory failure, *Pediatrics* 87:101, 1991.

26. Avery M, Oppenheimer E: Recent increases in mortality from hyaline membrane disease, *J Pediatr* 57:553, 1960.

27. Avery ME, Tooley, WH, Keller et al: Is chronic lung disease in low birth weight infants preventable? A survey of eight centers, *Pediatrics* 79:26, 1987.

28. Aziz H, Martin J, Moore J: The pediatric disposable end-tidal carbon dioxide detector role in endotracheal intubation in newborns, *J Perinatol* 19:110, 1999.

29. Bachman TE: Evidence based medicine: NCPAP in weaning preterm infants from ventilators, *Neonatal Intensive Care* 13:15, 2000.

30. Bagghi A, Viscardi R, Taciak V et al: Increased activity of interleukin-6 but not tumor necrosis factor-alpha in lung lavage of premature infants is associated with the development of BPD, *Pediatr Res* 36:244, 1994.

31. Bakker JM, Kavelaars A, Kamphuis PJ et al: Neonatal dexamethasone treatment increases susceptibility to experimental autoimmune disease in adult rats, *J Immunol* 165:5932, 2000.

32. Bancalari E, Sosenko J: Pathogenesis and prevention of chronic lung disease: recent developments, *Pediatr Pulmonol* 8:109, 1990.

33. Banks B et al: Multiple courses of antenatal corticosteroids (ANCS): association with increased mortality and early severe lung disease (ESLD) in preterm neonates, *Pediatrics* 104 (part 3):739, 1999.

34. Banks BA, Stouffer N, Cnaan A et al: Association of plasma cortisol and chronic lung disease in preterm infants, *Pediatrics* 107:494, 2001.

35. Bardin C, Zelkowitz P, Papageorgiou A: Outcome of small-for-gestational age and appropriate-for-gestational age infants born before 27 weeks of gestation, *Pediatrics* 100:E4, 1997.

36. Barnes C, Asonye U, Vidyasager D: The effects of bronchopulmonary hygiene in PtCO$_2$ values in critically ill neonates, *Crit Care Med* 9:819, 1981.

37. Barnett C, Haslam R, Davidson G et al: Gastric emptying in preterm infants with pH probe positive gastroesophageal reflux, *Pediatr Res* 45:277A, 1999(b).

38. Barnett C, Omari T, Benninga M et al: Esophageal motor function and mechanisms of gastrosophageal reflux in the extremely premature neonate, *Pediatr Res* 45:277A, 1999a.

39. Barrington K: Postnatal steroids and neurodevelopmental outcomes: a problem in the making, *Pediatrics* 107:1425, 2001.

40. Barrington K: The adverse neuro-developmental effects of postnatal steroids in the preterm infant: a systematic review of RCTs, *BMC Pediatr* 1:1, 2001.

41. Barrington K, Bull D, Finer N: Randomized trial of nasal synchronized intermittent mandatory ventilation compared with continuous positive airway pressure after extubation of very low birth weight infants, *Pediatrics* 107:638, 2001.

42. Barrington K, Tan K, Rich W: Lack of association between pre-discharge apnea and acid GE reflux in formerly preterm infants, *Pediatr Res* 45:184A, 1999.

43. Batton D, Roberts C, Trese M et al: Severe retinopathy of prematurity and steroid exposure, *Pediatrics* 90:534, 1992.

44. Baud O, Foix-L'Helias L, Kaminski M, et al: Antenatal glucocorticoid treatment and cystic periventricular leukomalacia in very premature infants, *N Engl J Med* 341:1190, 1999.

45. Bauer J, Maier K, Linderkamp O et al: Effect of caffeine on oxygen consumption and metabolic rate in very low birth weight infants with idiopathic apnea, *Pediatrics* 107:660, 2001.

46. Baumer J: International randomized controlled trial of patient triggered ventilation in neonatal respiratory distress syndrome, *Arch Dis Child Fetal Neonatal Educ* 82:F5, 2000.

47. Baumgart S, Saunders T, Desai S et al: Maternal antenatal magnesium does not prevent ROP or severe head ultrasound abnormalities in VLBW premature infants: severe HUS abnormalities and ROP significantly related, *Pediatr Res* 45:185A, 1999.

48. Bedu A, Lupoglazoff JM, Faure C et al: Cisapride high dosage and long QT interval, *J Pediatr* 130:164, 1997.

49. Beeram M, Dhanireddy R: Effects of saline instillation during tracheal suction on lung mechanics in newborn infants, *J Perinatol* 7:120, 1992.

50. Bell P, Ellerbee S: Impaired cerebral vascular flow in the premature infant, *J Perinatol Neonatol Nurs* 7:49, 1993.

51. Benesova O, Pavlik A: Perinatal treatment with glucocorticoids and the risk of maldevelopment of the brain, *Neuropharmacology* 28:89, 1989.

52. Beresford MW, Shaw NJ, Manning D: Randomised controlled trial of patient triggered and conventional fast rate ventilation in neonatal respiratory distress syndrome, *Arch Dis Child Fetal Neonatal Educ* 82:F14, 2000.

53. Berggren E, Liljedahl M, Winbladh B et al: Pilot study of nebulized surfactant therapy for neonatal respiratory distress syndrome, *Acta Paediatr* 89:460, 2000.

54. Berkus MD, Langer O, Samueloff A et al: Meconium-stained amniotic fluid: increased risk for adverse neonatal outcomes, *Obstet Gynecol* 84:115, 1994.

55. Bernbaum J, Schwartz IP, Gerdes M et al: Survivors of extracorporeal membrane oxygenation at one year of age: the relationship of primary diagnosis with health and neurodevelopmental sequelae, *Pediatrics* 96:907, 1995.

56. Bernert G, von Siebenthal K, Seidl R et al: The effect of behavioural states on cerebral oxygenation during endotracheal suctioning of preterm babies, *Neuropediatrics* 28:111, 1997.

57. Bernstein G, Mannino F, Heldt G et al: Randomized multicenter trial comparing synchronized and conventional intermittent mandatory ventilation (SIMV vs. IMV) in neonates, *J Pediatr* 128:4, 1996.

58. Bhandari V, Brodsky N: Repetitive doses of antenatal steroids (ANS) are associated with increased gastroesophageal reflux (GER), *Pediatr Res* 45:186A, 1999.

59. Bhuta T, Henderson-Smart D: Elective high-frequency oscillatory ventilation versus conventional ventilation in preterm infants with pulmonary dysfunction: systematic review and meta-analysis, *Pediatrics* 100:E6, 1997.

60. Bhutani V, Abbasi S: Relative likelihood of bronchopulmonary dysplasia based on pulmonary mechanics measured in preterm neonates during the first week of life, *J Pediatr* 120:605, 1992.

61. Bjorklund L, Ingimarsson J, Curstedt T et al: Manual ventilation with a few large breaths at birth compromises the therapeutic effect of subsequent surfactant replacement in immature lambs, *Pediatr Res* 42:348, 1997.

62. Blauer T, Gerstmann D: A simultaneous comparison of three neonatal pain scales during common NICU procedures, *Clin J Pain* 14:39, 1998.

63. Bloomfield FH, Teele RL, Voss M et al: The role of neonatal chest physiotherapy in preventing post-extubation atelectasis, *J Pediatr* 133:269, 1998.

64. Boros SJ, Matalon SV, Ewald R et al: The effect of independent variations in inspiratory-expiratory ratio and end expiratory pressure during mechanical ventilation in hyaline membrane disease: the significance of mean airway pressure, *J Pediatr* 91:114, 1977.

65. Bos AF, Martijn A, van Asperen RM et al: Qualitative assessment of general movements in high-risk preterm infants with chronic lung disease requiring dexamethasone therapy, *J Pediatr* 132:300, 1998.

66. Bostick J, Wendelgass ST: Normal saline instillations as part of the suctioning procedure: effects on Pao_2 and amount of secretions, *Heart Lung* 16:532, 1987.

67. Bragonier R, Imong S: Oscillatory ventilation for infants with respiratory distress syndrome: survey of current practice in the UK, *J Perinat Med* 26:201, 1998.

68. Briet J, Van Wassenaer A, Dekker F et al: Risk factors of behavior problems at two years of age in children born <30 wks g.a., *Pediatr Res* 45:238A, 1999.

69. Brodsky L, Reidy M, Stanievich J: The effects of suctioning techniques on the distal tracheal mucosa in intubated low birth weight infants, *Int J Pediatr Otorhinolaryngol* 14:1, 1987.

70. Brooks S, Marcus DM, Gillis D et al: The effect of blood transfusion protocol in retinopathy of prematurity: a prospective, randomized study, *Pediatrics* 104:514, 1999.

71. Brown D, Cohen M, Myers M et al: Dexamethasone use is associated with an increased risk of ROP in neonates with birthweight <1001 gm, *Pediatr Res* 45:187A, 1999.

72. Brown GC, Brown MM, Sharma S et al: Cost-effectiveness of treatment for threshold retinopathy of prematurity, *Pediatrics* 104:955, 1999.

73. Bucher H, Duc G: Does caffeine prevent hypoxemic episodes in premature infants? A randomized controlled trial, *Eur J Pediatr* 147:288, 1988.

74. Byrne B, Mellen B, Lindstrom D et al: The BPD epidemic is diminishing, *Pediatr Res* 45:239A, 1999.

75. Carbone T, Marrero LC, Weiss J et al: Heart rate and oxygen saturation correlates of infant apnea, *J Perinatol* 19:44, 1999.

76. Carey B: Neonatal air leaks: pneumothorax, pneumomediastinum, PIE, pneumopericardium, *Neonatal Netw* 18:81, 1999.

77. Carey B, Trotter C: Radiology basics, Part III: TTN, MAS and neonatal pneumonia, *Neonatal Netw* 19:37, 2000.

78. Carlo WA, Stark A, Bauer C et al: Effects of minimal ventilation in a multicenter randomized controlled trial of ventilator support and early corticosteroid therapy in ELBW infants, *Pediatr Res* 47:391A, 2000.

79. Carson BS, Losey RW, Bowes WA Jr et al: Combined obstetric and pediatric approach to prevent meconium aspiration syndrome, *Am J Obstet Gynecol* 126:712, 1976.

80. Carroll P: Pneumothorax in the newborn, *Neonatal Netw* 10:27, 1991.

81. Carter J, Gerstmann D, Clark R et al: HFOV and ECMO for the treatment of acute neonatal respiratory failure, *Pediatrics* 124:661, 1994.

82. Cashore C, Haslam R, Davidson G et al: Gastric emptying in preterm infants with ph probe positive gastroesophageal reflux, *Pediatr Res* 45:277A, 1999.

83. Cassani V: Hypoxemia secondary to suctioning in the neonate, *Neonatal Netw* 2:8, 1984.

84. Cassel G, Waites K, Crouse D: Perinatal mycoplasmal infections, *Clin Perinatol* 18:263, 1991.

85. Chan D, Lim M, Choo S et al: Vitamin E status of infants at birth, *J Perinat Med* 27:395, 1999.

86. Chang M, Williams PD: Oxygenation during CPT of VLBW infants: relations among fraction of inspired oxygen units, number of hand ventilations and transcutaneous oxygen pressure, *J Pediatr Nurs* 4:411, 1989.

87. Cheema I, Ahluwalia J: Feasability of tidal volume-guided ventilation in newborn infants: a randomized, crossover trial using the volume guarantee modality, *Pediatrics* 107:1323, 2001.

88. Cheung PY, Peliowski A, Robertson CM: The outcome of very low birth weight neonates, *J Pediatr* 133:735, 1998.

89. Cheung PY, Barrington KJ, Finer NN et al: Early childhood neurodevelopment in very low birth weight infants with predischarge apnea, *Pediatr Pulmonol* 27:14, 1999.

90. Christou H, Adaxia I, Van Marter L et al: Inhaled nitric oxide does not affect adenosine 5'-diphosphate-dependent platelet activation in infants with PPNN, *Pediatrics* 102:1390, 1998.

91. Chulay M: Why do we keep putting saline down ETT? Is it time for a change in the way we suction! *Capsules & Comments in Crit Care Nurs* 2:7, 1994.

92. Clark R: High frequency ventilation, *J Pediatr* 124:661, 1994.

93. Clark R: How do we safely use inhaled nitric oxide? *Pediatrics* 103:296, 1999.

94. Clark R, Gerstmann D: Controversies in high-frequency ventilation, *Clin Perinatol* 25:113, 1998.

95. Clark R, Rycus P, Conrad S: How the practice of neonatal ECMO has changed, *Pediatr Res* 45:298A, 1999.

96. Clark R, Slutsky A, Gerstmann D: Lung protective strategies of ventilation in the neonate: what are they? *Pediatrics* 105:112, 2000.

97. Clark R, Yoder B, Sell M: Prospective, randomized comparison of high-frequency oscillation and conventional ventilation in candidates for extracorporeal membrane oxygenation, *J Pediatr* 124:447, 1994.

98. Clark S, Draper E, Field D et al: Chronic lung disease and survival in four tertiary neonatal units, *J Perinat Med* 27:490, 1999.

99. Clark R, Gerstmann D, Null D et al: Prospective randomized comparison of high-frequency oscillatory and conventional ventilation in respiratory distress syndrome, *Pediatrics* 89:5, 1992.

100. Clark RH, Kueser TJ, Walker MW et al: Low-dose nitric oxide therapy for persistent pulmonary hypertension of the newborn, *N Engl J Med* 342:469, 2000.

101. Clark P, Castor C, Kaytan H et al: A phase II trial of inhaled nitric oxide in neonatal CLD, *Pediatr Res* 45:190A, 1999.

102. Claure N, Gerhardt T, Everett R et al: Closed-loop controlled inspired oxygen concentration for mechanically ventilated very low birth weight infants with frequent episodes of hypoxemia, *Pediatrics* 107:1120, 2001.

103. Cleary G, Wiswell T: Meconium-stained amniotic fluid and the meconium aspiration syndrome: an update, *Pediatr Clin North Am* 45:511, 1998.

104. Cobley M, Atkins M, Jones P: Environmental contamination during tracheal suction, *Anaesthesia* 46:957, 1991.

105. Cole C: Special problems in aerosol delivery: neonatal and pediatric considerations, *Respir Care* 45:646, 2000.

106. Cole C, Fiascone J: Strategies for prevention of neonatal chronic lung disease, *Semin Perinatol* 24:445, 2000.

107. Cole CH, Colton T, Shah BL et al: Early inhaled glucocorticoid therapy to prevent bronchopulmonary dysplasia, *N Engl J Med* 340:1005, 1999b.

108. Cole CH, Shah B, Abbasi S et al: Adrenal function in premature infants during inhaled beclomethasone therapy, *J Pediatr* 135:65, 1999.

109. Coney S: Physiotherapy technique banned in Auckland, *Lancet* 345:510, 1995.

110. Conner E, PREVENT Study Group: Reduction of RSV hospitalization among premature infants and infants with BPD using RSV immune globulin prophylaxis, *Pediatrics* 99:93, 1997.

111. Cools F, Offringa M: Meta-analysis of elective high frequency ventilation in preterm infants with respiratory distress syndrome, *Arch Dis Child Fetal Neonatal Educ* 80:15F, 1999.

112. Copnell B, Fergusson D: Endotracheal suctioning: time-worn tradition or timely intervention? *Am J Crit Care* 4:100, 1995.

113. Cordero L, Ayers L, Davis K: Neonatal airway colonization with gram-negative bacilli association with severity of bronchopulmonary dysplasia, *Pediatr Infect Dis J* 16:18, 1997.

114. Cordero L, Sananes M, Ayers L: Comparison of a closed (Trach Care MAC) with an open endotracheal suction system in small premature infants, *J Perinatol* 3:151, 2000.

115. Cornfield D: Randomized, controlled trial of low-dose inhaled nitric oxide in the treatment of term and near-term infants with respiratory failure and pulmonary hypertension, *Pediatrics* 104:1089, 1999.

116. Courtney SE, Long W, McMillan D et al: Double-blind 1-year follow-up of 1540 infants with respiratory distress syndrome randomized to rescue treatment with two doses of synthetic surfactant or air in four clinical trials: American and Canadian Exosurf Neonatal Study Groups, *J Pediatr* 126:543, 1995.

117. Courtney SE, Pyon KH, Saslow JG et al: Lung recruitment and breathing pattern during variable versus continuous flow nasal positive airway pressure in premature infants: an evaluation of three devices, *Pediatrics* 107:304, 2001.

118. Cowan F, Whitelaw A, Wertheim D et al: Cerebral blood flow velocity changes after rapid administration of surfactant, *Arch Dis Child* 66:1105, 1991.

119. Cox C, Wolfson M, Shafer T: Liquid ventilation: a comprehensive overview, *Neonatal Netw* 15:31, 1996.

120. Cringle SJ, Yu DY, Alder V, et al: Light and choroidal PO_2 modulation of intraretinal oxygen levels in an avascular retina, *Invest Ophthalmol Vis Sci* 40:2307, 1999.

121. Cross JH, Harrison CJ, Preston PR et al: Postnatal encephaloclastic porencephaly—a new lesion? *Arch Dis Child* 67:307, 1992.

122. Crowley P: Prophylactic corticosteroids for preterm birth. In The Cochrane Library, Issue 4, Oxford, England: Update Software, 1999.

123. CRYO-ROP Cooperative Group: Multicenter trial of cryotherapy for ROP, *Arch Ophthalmol* 106:471, 1988.

124. CRYO-ROP Cooperative Group: The natural ocular outcome of premature birth and retinopathy: status at one year, *Arch Ophthalmol* 112:903, 1994.

125. Cunningham AS, Lawson EE, Martin RJ et al: Tracheal suction and meconium: a proposed standard of care, *J Pediatr* 116:153, 1990.

126. Curley A, Halliday H: The present status of exogenous surfactant for the newborn, *Early Hum Dev* 61:67, 2001.

127. Dangeman BC et al: The variability of PaO_2 in newborn infants in response to routine care, *Pediatr Res* 10:149, 1976.

128. Dani C, Bertini G, Piva D et al: Retinopathy of prematurity in infants with birth weight lower than 1250 gms: role of blood transfusion, iron and erythropoietin treatment, *Pediatr Res* 45:193A, 1999.

129. Dani C, Reali MG, Bertini G et al: The role of blood transfusions and iron intake on retinopathy of prematurity, *Early Hum Dev* 62:57, 2001.

130. Darlow BA, Sluis KB, Inder TE et al: Endotracheal suctioning of the neonate: comparison of two methods as a source of mucous material for research, *Pediatr Pulmonol* 23:217, 1997.

131. Davidson D, Barefield ES, Kattwinkel J et al: Inhaled nitric oxide for the early treatment of persistent pulmonary hypertension of the term newborn: a randomized, double-masked, placebo-controlled, dose-response, multicenter study, *Pediatrics* 101:325, 1998.

132. Davidson D, Barefield ES, Kattwinkel J et al: Safety of withdrawing inhaled nitric oxide therapy in persistent pulmonary hypertension of the newborn, *Pediatrics* 104:231, 1999.

133. Davies A, Koenig J, Thach B: Upper airway chemoreflex responses to saline and water in preterm infants, *J Appl Physiol* 64:1412, 1988.

134. Davis J et al: Safety and pharmacokinetics of multiple doses of recombinant human CuZn superoxide dismutase administered intratracheally to premature neonates with respiratory distress syndrome, *Pediatrics* 100:24, 1997.

135. Davis J, Rosenfeld W, Richter S et al: The effects of multiple doses of recombinant human superoxide dismutase in premature infants with RDS, *Pediatr Res* 45:193A, 1999.

136. Davis JM, Bhutani VK, Stefano JL et al: Changes in pulmonary mechanics following caffeine administration in infants with bronchopulmonary dysplasia, *Pediatr Pulmonol* 6:49, 1989.

137. Davis JM, Richter SE, Biswas S et al: Long-term follow-up of premature infants treated with prophylactic, intratracheal recombinant human CuZn superoxide dismutase, *J Perinatol* 4:213, 2000.

138. Davis JM, Richter SE, Kendig JW et al: High frequency jet ventilation and surfactant treatment of newborns with severe respiratory failure, *Pediatr Pulmonol* 13:108, 1992.

139. Davis P, Henderson-Smart D: Prophylactic postextubation nasal CPAP in preterm infants, Cochrane Collaboration Library: Neonatal Group, November, 1996.

140. Davis P, Henderson-Smart D: Extubation of premature infants from low rate IPPV vs. extubation after a trial of endotracheal CPAP, Cochrane Collaboration Library: Neonatal Group, May, 1998.

141. Davis P, Henderson-Smart D: Post-extubation prophylactic nasal continuous positive airway pressure in preterm infants: systemic review and meta-analysis, *J Paediatr Child Health* 35:367, 1999.

142. Davis P, Davies M, Faber B: A randomized controlled trial of two methods of delivery post-extubation nasal CPAP to infants <1000 g: binasal versus single nasal prongs, *Pediatr Res* 47:395A, 2000.

143. Dean E: Effect of body position on pulmonary function, *Phys Ther* 65:613, 1985.

144. deBethmann O, Relier J, Delivoria-Papadapoulous M: Corticosteroid therapy and retinopathy of the newborn, *Pediatr Res* 45:193A, 1999.

145. DeBoer S, Stephens D: PPHN: case study and pathophysiology review, *Neonatal Netw* 16:7, 1997.

146. DeGrazie M, Guthrie E, Richardson D: Survey of chest physiotherapy practices during extrauterine transition of newborns, *Pediatr Res* 47:395A, 2000.

147. Delgado M, Friedland D, Rothschild M et al: Bacterial colonization of the subglottis in neonates, *Pediatr Res* 45:193A, 1999.

148. delMoral T, Claure N, Van Buskirk S et al: Antenatal steroids and incidence of ROP in ELBW infants, *Pediatr Res* 47:395A, 2000.

149. Demers R, Saklad M: Minimizing the harmful effects of mechanical aspiration, *Heart Lung* 2:542, 1973.

150. Dennehy P: Respiratory infections in the newborn, *Clin Perinatol* 14:667, 1987.

151. DePaz J, Aghai Z, Konduri G: Severe IVH, a marker of severe ROP, *Pediatr Res* 45:194A, 1999.

152. DeRegnier RA, Roberts D, Ramsey D et al: Association between the severity of chronic lung disease and first-year outcomes of very low birth weight infants, *J Perinatol* 17:375, 1997.

153. DeRoo-Merritt L: Lasers in medicine: treatment of ROP, *Neonatal Netw* 19:21, 2000.

154. Dimitriou G, Greenough A, Kavvadia V: Change in lung volume, compliance and oxygenation in the first 48 hours of life in infants given surfactant, *J Perinat Med* 25:49, 1997.

155. Dollberg S, Livni S, Mordeclayer N et al: Increased nucleated RBC counts in MAS, *Pediatr Res* 47:396A, 2000.

156. Donn S, Becker M: Mandatory minute ventilation: a neonatal mode of the future, *Neonatal Intensive Care* 11:22, 1998.

157. Donn S, Sinha S: Management of BPD using pressure support ventilation, *Pediatr Res* 39:331A, 1996.

158. Donn S, Sinha S: Controversies in patient-triggered ventilation, *Clin Perinatol* 25:49, 1998.

159. Doray B, Orquin J: A low rate of ROP over 11 years in spite of increasing survival of small prematures, *Pediatr Res* 45:242A, 1999.

160. Doyle L: Antenatal corticosteroid therapy and blood pressure at 14 years of age in preterm children, *Clin Sci* 98:137, 2000.

161. Doyle L, Davis P: Postnatal corticosteroids in preterm infants: effects on mortality and cerebral palsy, *Pediatr Res* 45:194A, 1999.

162. Doyle L, Davis P: Postnatal corticosteroids in preterm infants: systematic review of effects on mortality and motor function, *J Paediatr Child Health* 36:101, 2000.

163. Dulock HL: Chest physiotherapy in neonates: a review, *AACN Clin Issues Crit Care Nurs* 2:446, 1991.

164. Dreyfuss D, Saumon G: Ventilator-induced lung injury: lessons from experimental studies, *Am J Respir Crit Care Med* 157:294, 1998.

165. Duncan C, Erikson R: Pressures associated with chest tube stripping, *Heart Lung* 11:166, 1982.

166. Durand M, Sangha B, Cabal L et al: Cardiopulmonary and intracranial pressure changes related to endotracheal suctioning in preterm infants, *Crit Care Med* 17:506, 1989.

167. Edwards D: The newborn infant with respiratory distress. In vonWaldenburg H, Edwards D, eds: *Practical pediatric radiology,* Philadelphia, 1994, WB Saunders.

168. Edwards DK, Colby TV, Northway W: Radiologic pathologic correlations in bronchopulmonary dysplasia, *J Pediatr* 85:834, 1979.

169. Egberts J, Brand R, Walti H et al: Mortality, severe respiratory distress syndrome and chronic lung disease of the newborn are reduced more after prophylactic than after therapeutic administration of the surfactant Curosurf, *Pediatrics* 100:E4, 1997.

170. Ehrenkranz RA, Younes N, Lemons JA et al: Longitudinal growth of hospitalized very low birth weight infants, *Pediatrics* 104:280, 1999.

171. Eichenwald E, Abimbola A, Stark A: Apnea frequently persists beyond term gestation in infants delivered at 24-28 weeks, *Pediatrics* 100:354, 1997.

172. El-Metwally D, Vohr B, Tucker R: Intraventricular hemorrhage (IVH) in the 90's: prevalence, risk factors and neurodevelopmental outcome, *Pediatr Res* 45:242A, 1999.

173. Engel W, Yoder M, Andreali S et al: Controlled prospective randomized comparison of HFJV and conventional ventilation in neonates with respiratory failure and PPHN, *J Perinatol* 17:3, 1997.

174. Etches P, Scott B: Chest physiotherapy in the newborn: effect on secretions removed, *Pediatrics* 62:713, 1978.

175. Evans J: Incidence of hypoxia associated with caregiving in premature infants, *Neonatal Netw* 10:17, 1991.

176. Evans J: Reducing the hypoxemia, bradycardia and apnea associated with suctioning in low birthweight infants, *J Perinatol* 7:137, 1992.

177. Fanaroff AA, Korones SB, Wright LL et al: Incidence, presenting features, risk factors and significance of late onset septicemia in very low birth weight infants, *Pediatr Infect Dis J* 17:593, 1998.

178. Fanconi S, Duc G: Intratracheal suction in the sick preterm infant: prevention of intracranial hypertension and cerebral hypoperfusion by muscle paralysis, *Pediatrics* 79:538, 1987.

179. Ferrara TB, Hoekstra RE, Couser RJ et al: Survival and follow-up of infants born at 23 to 26 weeks of gestational age: effects of surfactant therapy, *J Pediatr* 124:119, 1994.

180. Findlay R, Taeusch H, Walther F: Surfactant replacement therapy for meconium aspiration syndrome, *Pediatrics* 97:48, 1996.

181. Finer N, Vohr B, Robertson C et al: Inhaled nitric oxide and hypoxic respiratory failure in term infants: neurodevelopmental follow-up, *Pediatr Res* 45:196A, 1999.

182. Finer NN, Barrington KJ: Nitric oxide therapy for the newborn infant, *Semin Perinatol* 24:59, 2000.

183. Finer NN, Boyd J: Chest physiotherapy in the neonate: a controlled study, *Pediatrics* 61:282, 1978.

184. Finer NN, Craft A, Vaucher YE et al: Postnatal steroids: short-term gain, long term pain? *J Pediatr* 137:9, 2000.

185. Firme S, McEvoy C, Alconcel C et al: Episodes of hypoxemia during SIMV in VLBW infants: a randomized study, *Pediatr Res* 47:398A, 2000.

186. Fittenberg J: Persistent pulmonary hypertension after lithium intoxication in the newborn, *Eur J Pediatr* 138:321, 1982.

187. Fitzgerald D, Van Asperen P, Lam A et al: Radiologic abnormalities in survivors of chronic neonatal lung disease, *J Paediatr Child Health* 32:491, 1996.

188. Fitzgerald D, Mesiano G, Brasseau L, et al: Pulmonary outcome in extremely low birth weight infants, *Pediatrics* 105:1209, 2000.

189. Fleisher A, Anyaeqbunam A, Guidetti D et al: A persistent clinical problem: profile of the term infant with significant respiratory complications, *Obstet Gynecol* 79:185, 1992.

190. Flenady V, Gray P: Chest physiotherapy for babies extubated from mechanical ventilation (Cochrane Review). In The Cochrane Library, Issue 3, Oxford, England: Update Software, 1998.

191. Fok TF, Lam K, Dolovich M et al: Randomized controlled study of early uses of inhaled corticosteroid in preterm infants with respiratory distress syndrome, *Arch Dis Child Fetal Neonatal Educ* 80:F203, 1999.

192. Fox W, Schwartz J, Shaffer T: Pulmonary physiotherapy in neonates: physiologic changes and respiratory management, *J Pediatr* 92:977, 1978.

193. Fraiberg S: Blind infants and their mothers: an examination of the sign system. In Lewis M, Rosenblum L, eds: *The effect of the infant on its caregiver,* New York, 1974, John Wiley & Sons.

194. Franco-Belgium Collaborative NO Trial Group: Early compared with delayed inhaled nitric oxide in moderately hypoxaemic neonates with respiratory failure: a randomised controlled trial, *Lancet* 354: 1066, 1999.

195. Frank L: The use of dexamethasone in premature infants at risk for bronchopulmonary dysplasia or who already have developed chronic lung disease: a cautionary note, *Pediatrics* 88:413, 1991.

196. Frank M: Theophylline: a closer look, *Neonatal Netw* 6:7, 1987.

197. French N, Hagan R, Evans S et al: Repeated antenatal corticosteroids (CS): behavior at outcomes in a regional population of very preterm (VP, <33 W) infants, *Pediatr Res* 43:214A, 1998.

198. French NP, Hagan R, Evans SF et al: Repeated antenatal corticosteroids: size at birth and subsequent development, *Am J Obstet Gynecol* 180:114, 1999.

199. Friedlich P, Lecart C, Posen R et al: A randomized trial of nasopharyngeal: synchronized intermittent mandatory ventilation versus nasopharyngeal continuous positive airway pressure in very low birth weight infants after extubation, *J Perinatol* 19:413, 1999.

200. Friel J, Ziegler E, Widness J et al: Antioxidant status and oxidant stress in VLBW infants during the first month of life, *Pediatr Res* 45:197A, 1999.

201. Fuloria M, Wiswell T: Resuscitation of the meconium-stained infant and prevention of meconium aspiration syndrome, *J Perinatol* 19:234, 1999.

202. Fuloria M, Hiatt D, Dillard R et al: Gastroesophageal reflux in very low birth weight infants: association with chronic lung disease and outcomes through 1 year of age, *J Perinatol* 4:235, 2000.

203. Gannon B: Theophylline or caffeine: which is best for apnea of prematurity?, *Neonatal Netw* 19:33, 2000.

204. Gannon C, Wiswell T, Spitzer A: Volutrauma, $PaCO_2$ levels, and neurodevelopmental sequelae following assisted ventilation, *Clin Perinatol* 25: 159, 1998.

205. Gardner J: Fatigue in postpartum women, *Appl Nurs Res* 4:57, 1991.

206. Gardner S, Hagedorn M: Physiologic sequelae of prematurity: the nurse practitioner's role. Part V. Feeding difficulties and growth failure (pathophysiology, cause and data collection), *J Pediatr Health Care* 5:122, 1991.

207. Garland J, Buck R, Weinberg M: Pulmonary hemorrhage risk in infants with a clinically diagnosed PDA: a retrospective cohort study, *Pediatrics* 94:719, 1994.

208. Garland J, Nelson D, Rice T et al: Increased risk of gastrointestinal perforations in neonates mechanically ventilated with either face mask or nasal prongs, *Pediatrics* 76:406, 1985.

209. Garland JS, Alex CP, Pauly TH et al: A three-day course of dexamethasone therapy to prevent chronic lung disease in ventilated neonates: a randomized trial, *Pediatrics* 104:91, 1999.

210. Gaston B, Keith J: Nitric oxide and bleeding time, *Pediatrics* 94:134, 1994.

211. Gaynon MW, Stevenson DK: What can we learn from STOP-ROP and earlier studies, *Pediatrics* 105:420, 2000.

212. Gaynon MW, Stevenson DK, Sunshine P et al: Supplemental oxygen may decrease progression of prethreshold disease to threshold retinopathy of prematurity, *J Perinatol* 17:434, 1997.

213. George T, Johnson K, Bates J et al: The effect of inhaled nitric oxide therapy on bleeding time and platelet aggregation in neonates, *J Pediatr* 132:721, 1998.

214. Gersony W: Neonatal pulmonary hypertension: pathophysiology, classification, etiology, *Clin Perinatol* 11:517, 1984.

215. Gerstman DR, Minton SD, Stoddard RA et al: The Provo multicenter early high-frequency oscillatory ventilation trial: improved pulmonary and clinical outcomes in respiratory distress syndrome, *Pediatrics* 98:1044, 1996.

216. Gittermann M, Fusch C, Gittermann A et al: Early nasal continuous positive airway pressure treatment reduces the need for intubation in very low birth weight infants, *Eur J Pediatr* 156:384, 1997.

217. Glass P, Bulas DI, Wagner AE et al: Severity of brain injury following neonatal extracorporeal membrane oxygenation and outcome at age 5 years, *Dev Med Child Neurol* 39:441, 1997.

218. Glass P, Wagner AE, Papero PH et al: Neurodevelopmental status at age five years of neonates treated with extracorporeal membrane oxygenation, *J Pediatr* 127:447, 1995.

219. Gluck L, Kulovich M: Fetal lung development, *Pediatr Clin North Am* 20:367, 1973.

220. Goldsmith LS, Greenspan JS, Rubenstein SD et al: Immediate improvement in lung volume after exogenous surfactant: alveolar recruitment after distension, *J Pediatr* 119:424, 1991.

221. Goldson E: The micropremie: infants with birth weight less than 800 gms, *Infants Young Child* 8:1, 1996.

222. Gordon P, Rutledge J, Sawin R t al: Early postnatal dexamethasone increases the risk of focal small bowel perforation in extremely low birth weight infants, *J Perinatol* 19:573, 1999.

223. Gortner L, Wauer RR, Stock GJ et al: Neonatal outcome in small for gestational age infants: do they really do better? *J Perinat Med* 27:484, 1999.

224. Graff M, France J, Hiatt IM et al: Prevention of hypoxia and hyperoxia during endotracheal suctioning, *Crit Care Med* 15:1133, 1987.

225. Gray J, George RH, Durbin GM et al: An outbreak of *Bacillus cereus* respiratory tract infections on a neonatal unit due to contaminated ventilator circuits, *J Hosp Infect* 41:19, 1999.

226. Graziani LJ, Spitzer AR, Mitchell DG et al: Mechanical ventilation in preterm infants: neurosonographic and developmental studies, *Pediatrics* 90:515, 1992.

227. Greenspan J, Wolfson M, Shaffer T: Liquid ventilation, *Semin Perinatol* 24:396, 2000.

228. Gregoire M, LeFebvre F, Glorieux J: Health and developmental outcomes at 18 months in very preterm infants with BPD, *Pediatrics* 101:856, 1998.

229. Gregory G: Respiratory care of newborn infants, *Pediatr Clin North Am* 19:311, 1972.

230. Gribar S, Byun A, Parimi P et al: Ventilatory indices and *Ureaplasma ureolyticus* during the first week of life are very strongly associated with severe BPD in VLBW infants, *Pediatr Res* 45:199A, 1999.

231. Groothuis J, Simoes E, Levin M et al: Prophylactic administration of RSV-immune globulin to high-risk infants and young children, *N Engl J Med* 329:1524, 1993.

232. Gross S, Anbar R, Kueselis D: Pulmonary function at age 8 years in children born <28 wks g.a. in the pre (1985) and post (1990) surfactant era, *Pediatr Res* 47:400A, 2000.

233. Grylack L, Anderson K: Diagnosis and treatment of traumatic granuloma in tracheobronchial tree of newborn with history of chronic intubation, *J Pediatr Surg* 19:200, 1984.

234. Gunderson L, McPhee A, Donovan E: Partially ventilated endotracheal suction, *Am J Dis Child* 140:462, 1986.

235. Gunn T: Risk factors in retrolental fibroplasia, *Pediatrics* 65:1096, 1980.

236. Hack M, Fanaroff A: Outcomes of children of extremely low birthweight and gestational age in the 1990's, *Early Hum Dev* 53:193, 1999.

237. Hack M, Friedman H, Fanaroff A: Outcomes of extremely low birth weight infants, *Pediatrics* 98:931, 1996.

238. Hack M, Friedman H, Minich N et al: Antenatal steroids have not improved the outcomes of surviving ELBW infants (<750 gm), *Pediatr Res* 43:216A, 1998.

239. Hack M, Taylor HG, Klein N et al: School-age outcomes in children with birth weights under 750 g, *N Engl J Med* 331:753, 1994.

240. Hacking D, Watkins A, Fraser S et al: Respiratory distress syndrome and birth order in premature twins, *Arch Dis Child Fetal Neonatal Educ* 84:F117, 2001.

241. Hagler D, Travner G: ET saline and suction catheters: sources of lower airway contamination, *Am J Crit Care* 3:444, 1994.

242. Halliday H: Synthetic or natural surfactants, *Acta Paediatr* 86:233, 1997.

243. Halliday H: Clinical trials of postnatal corticosteroids: inhaled and systemic, *Biol Neonate* 76;29, 1999.

244. Halliday H, Ehrenkranz R: Delayed (>3 weeks) postnatal corticosteroids for CLD in preterm infants, *Cochrane Database Syst Rev* 2:CD001145, 2000.

245. Halliday H, Ekrenkranz R: Early postnatal (<96 hours) corticosteroids for preventing CLD in preterm infants, *Cochrane Database Syst Rev* 2:CD001146, 2000.

246. Halliday H, Ekrenkranz R: Moderately early (7-14 days) postnatal corticosteroids for preventing CLD in preterm infants, *Cochrane Database Syst Rev* 2:CD001144, 2000.

247. Halliday HL, McClure G, Reid MM: Transient tachypnoea of the newborn: two distinct clinical entities, *Arch Dis Child* 56:322, 1981.

248. Halliday HL, Patterson CC, Halahakoon CW: A multicenter, randomized open study of early corticosteroid treatment (OSECT) in preterm infants with respiratory illness: comparison of early and late treatment and of dexamethasone and inhaled budesonide, *Pediatrics* 107:232, 2001.

249. Halliday HL, Speer CP, Robertson B: Treatment of severe meconium aspiration syndrome with porcine surfactant, *Eur J Pediatr* 155:1047, 1996.

250. Han H, Shackelford G, Hamvas A: Infants undergoing long-term high frequency ventilation develop hydrocephalus, *Pediatr Res* 45:200A, 1999.

251. Hanley M, Rudd T, Butler J: What happens to intratracheal saline instillations? *Am J Resp Dis* 117(suppl):S124, 1978.

252. Harding JE, Miles FK, Becroft DM et al: Chest physiotherapy may be associated with brain damage in extremely premature infants, *J Pediatr* 132:440, 1998.

253. Harris MC, Baumgart S, Rooklin AR et al: Successful extubation of infants with respiratory distress syndrome using aminophylline, *J Pediatr* 103:303, 1983.

254. Harrison H: Preemies on steroids: a new iatrogenic disaster? *Birth* 28:57, 2001.

255. Harrison J, Mangat R, Singh A et al: Preterm infants requiring <40% Fio_2 do not benefit from surfactant therapy, *Pediatr Res* 47:402A, 2000.

256. Harrison VC, Heese H, Klein M: The significance of grunting in hyaline membrane disease, *Pediatrics* 41:549, 1968.

257. Hartfield D, Sankaran K: Deglutition syncope in a preterm infant, *Neonatal Intensive Care* 13:50, 2000.

258. Hay J, Ernst R, Meissner H: Respiratory syncytial virus immune globulin a cost-effectiveness analysis, *Am J Manag Care* 2:851, 1996.

259. Hay W, Bell E: Oxygen therapy, oxygen toxicity and the STOP-ROP trial, *Pediatrics* 105:424, 2000.

260. Hebbandi SB, Bowen JR, Hipwell GC et al: Ocular sequelae in extremely premature infants at 5 years of age, *J Paediatr Child Health* 33:339, 1997.

261. Henderson-Smart D, Subramanian P, Davis P: CPAP vs. theophylline for apnea in preterm infants (Cochrane Review). In The Cochrane Library, Issue Dec 16, 1997, Oxford, England: Update software: 1997.

262. Henderson-Smart D, Steer P: Prophylactic caffeine to prevent postoperative apnea in preterm infants (Cochrane Review). In The Cochrane Library, Issue May 28, 1997, Oxford, England: Update software, 1997.

263. Henderson-Smart D, Steer P: Methylxanthine treatment for apnea in preterm infants (Cochrane Review). In The Cochrane Library, Issue 4, 1998, Oxford, England: Update Software: 1998.

264. Henry G: Noninvasive assessment of cardiac function and pulmonary hypertension in persistent pulmonary hypertension, *Clin Perinatal* 11:626, 1984.

265. Henry MD, Rebello CM, Ikegami M et al: Ultrasonic nebulized in comparison with instilled surfactant treatment of preterm lambs, *Am J Respir Crit Care Med* 154:366, 1996.

266. Herrera C, Everett R, Gerhardt T et al: Randomized, crossover study of volume guarantee vs SIMV in VLBW infants recovering from respiratory failure, *Pediatr Res* 45:304A, 1999.

267. Herrera C, Everett R, Gerhardt T et al: Volume guarantee ventilation with two different tidal volumes vs SIMV in VLBW infants: a randomized crossover study, *Pediatr Res* 47:361A, 2000.

268. Hittner HM, Godia L, Rudolph A et al: Retrolental fibroplasia: efficacy of Vitamin E in a double-blind clinical study of preterm infants, *New Engl J Med* 305:1365, 1981.

269. HiFi Study Group: High-frequency oscillatory ventilation compared with conventional mechanical ventilation in the treatment of respiratory failure in preterm infants, *N Engl J Med* 320:88, 1989.

270. HiFi Study Group: High-frequency oscillatory ventilation compared with conventional mechanical ventilation in the treatment of respiratory failure in preterm infants: assessment of pulmonary function at 9 months of corrected age, *J Pediatr* 116:933, 1990.

271. Higgins RD, Richter SE, Davis JM: Nasal CPAP facilitates extubation of VLBW infants, *Pediatrics* 88:999, 1991.

272. Hird MF, Greenough A: Patient triggered ventilation using a flow triggered system, *Arch Dis Child* 66:1140, 1991.

273. Hoekstra R: Surfactant in the treatment and prevention of RDS, *Associates in Medical Marketing Co* 9:1, 1999.

274. Hoekstra R, Ferrara T, Payne N: Effects of surfactant therapy on outcome of extremely premature infants, *Eur J Pediatr* 153:S12, 1994.

275. Hoekstra RE, Jackson JC, Myers TF et al: Improved neonatal survival following multiple doses of bovine surfactant in very premature neonates at risk for respiratory distress syndrome, *Pediatrics* 88:10, 1991.

276. Hoelin T, Krause M, Buhrer C: Inhaled nitric oxide in preterm infants: a meta-analysis, *J Perinatol Med* 28:7, 2000.

278. Horbar JD, Rogowski J, Plsek PE et al: Collaborative quality improvement for neonatal intensive care, *Pediatrics* 107:14, 2001.

277. Holzman BH, Scarpelli EM: Cardiopulmonary consequences of positive end expiratory pressure, *Pediatr Res* 13:1112, 1979.

279. Horbar JD, Soll RF, Schachinger H et al: A European multicenter randomized controlled trial of single dose surfactant therapy for idiopathic respiratory distress syndrome, *Eur J Pediatr* 149:416, 1990.

280. Horbar JD, Wright LL, Soll RF et al: A multicenter randomized trial comparing two surfactants for the treatment of neonatal respiratory distress syndrome, *J Pediatr* 123:757, 1993.

281. Hrabovsky E, Mullett M: Gastroesophageal reflux and the premature infant, *J Pediatr Surg* 21:583, 1986.

282. Hudak ML, Farrell EE, Rosenberg AA et al: A multicenter randomized, masked comparison trial of natural vs. synthetic surfactant for the treatment of respiratory distress syndrome, *J Pediatr* 128:396, 1996.

283. Hussain N, Cline J, Bhandari V: Current incidence of ROP, 1989-1997, *Pediatrics* 104:e26, 1999.

284. Ignarro LJ, Buga GM, Wood KS et al: Endothelium-derived relaxing factor produced and released from artery and vein is nitric oxide, *Proc Natl Acad Sci USA* 84:9265, 1987.

285. Ikegami M, Wada K, Emerson GA et al: Effects of ventilation style on surfactant metabolism and treatment response in preterm lambs, *Am J Respir Crit Care Med* 157:638, 1998.

286. Jackson JC, Truog WE, Standaert TA et al: Reduction in lung injury after combined surfactant and high-frequency ventilation, *Am J Respir Crit Care Med* 150:534, 1994.

287. Jacobs S et al: Long term pulmonary outcome of severe BPD, *Am J Respir Crit Care Med* 151:A664, 1995.

288. Jacobs S et al: Exercise ability in severe BPD, *Am J Respir Crit Care Med* 151:A664, 1995.

289. Jacobsen T, Gronvall J, Peterson S et al: Minitouch treatment of the VLBW infant, *Acta Paediatrics* 83:934, 1993.

290. Jaille J, Levin T, Wung J et al: Benign gaseous distension of the bowel in premature infants treated with NCPAP, *Am J Rheumatol* 158:125, 1992.

291. Jenni OG, Wolf M, Hengartner M et al: Impact of central, obstructive and mixed apnea on cerebral hemodynamics in preterm infants, *Biol Neonate* 70:91, 1996.

292. Jobe A: Pulmonary surfactant therapy, *N Engl J Med* 326:861, 1993.

293. Jobe A: The new BPD: an arrest of lung development, *Pediatr Res* 46:641, 1999.

294. Jobe A: Glucocorticoids in perinatal care: misguided rockets? *J Pediatr* 137:1, 2000.

295. Jobe A, Ikegami M: Mechanisms initiating lung injury in the preterm, *Early Hum Dev* 53:81, 1998.

296. Jobe A, Ikegami M, Jacobs H et al: Surfactant and pulmonary blood flow distributions following treatment of premature lambs with natural surfactant, *J Clin Invest* 73:848, 1984.

297. Joffe S, Escobar GJ, Black SB et al: Rehospitalization for respiratory syncytial virus among premature infants, *Pediatrics* 104:894, 1999.

298. Joffe S, Ray GT, Escobar GJ et al: Cost-effectiveness of respiratory syncytial virus prophylaxis among preterm infants, *Pediatrics* 104:419, 1999.

299. Johnson A, Townshend P, Yudkin P et al: Functional abilities at age 4 years of children born before 29 weeks of gestation, *Br Med J* 306:1715, 1993.

300. Johnson KL, Kearney PA, Johnson SB et al: Closed versus open endotracheal suctioning: costs and physiologic consequences, *Crit Care Med* 22:658, 1994.

301. Johnson L, Quinn GE, Abbasi S et al: Severe retinopathy of prematurity in infants with birth weights less than 1250 grams: incidence and outcome treatment with pharmacologic serum levels of vitamin E in addition to cryotherapy from 1985 to 1991, *J Pediatr* 127:632, 1995.

302. Jolley S, Halpern C, Sterling C, et al: The relationship of respiratory complications from gastroesophageal reflux to prematurity in infants, *J Pediatr Surg* 25:755, 1990.

303. Kakkera D, Parton L: Elevation of the proinflammatory cytokine interleukin 1 in tracheal aspirates from preterm infants who progress to BPD, *Pediatr Res* 45:203A, 1999.

304. Kamisuka M, Williams M, Nyberg D et al: Renal calcification: a complication of dexamethasone therapy in preterm infants with BPD, *J Perinatol* 15: 359, 1995.

305. Kamper J, Wulff K, Larsen C et al: Early treatment with NCPAP in VLBW infants, *Acta Paediatr* 82: 193, 1993.

306. Kamphuis P, Coiset G, Bakker J et al: Neonatal treatment with dexamethasone selectively reduces pituitary-adrenal responsiveness of rats to novelty stress in adulthood, *Pediatr Res* 47:71A, 2000.

307. Kao LC, Durand DJ, McCrea RC et al: Randomized trial of long-term diuretic therapy for infants with oxygen-dependent bronchopulmonary dysplasia, *J Pediatr* 124:772, 1994.

308. Kao LC, Durand DJ, Phillips BL et al: Oral theophylline and diuretics improve pulmonary mechanics in infants with bronchopulmonary dysplasia, *J Pediatr* 111:439, 1987.

309. Kaplan-Machlis B, Beane J: Healthcare resource utilization and costs of RSV-related hospitalizations, *Neonatal Intensive Care* 13:17, 2000.

310. Karlowicz M et al: Does candidemia predict threshold retinopathy of prematurity in extremely low birth weight (<1000 gm) neonates? *Pediatrics* 105:1036, 2000.

311. Katzman G, Satish M, Krishnan V: Hypoxemia and retinopathy of prematurity, *Pediatrics* 80:972, 1987.

312. Kavvadia V, Greenough A, Dimitriou G et al: Early prediction of chronic oxygen dependency by lung function test results, *Pediatr Pulmonol* 29:19, 2000.

313. Kavvadia V, Greenough A, Itakura Y et al: Neonatal lung function in very immature infants with and without RDS, *J Perinat Med* 27:382, 1999.

314. Kazzi N, Brans Y, Poland R: Dexamethasone effects on the hospital course of infants with BPD who are dependent on artificial ventilation, *Pediatrics* 86: 722, 1990.

315. Kendig JW, Ryan RM, Sinkin RA et al: Comparison of two strategies for surfactant prophylaxis in very premature infants: a multicenter randomized trial, *Pediatrics* 101:1006, 1998.

316. Kennaugh JM, Kinsella JP, Abman SH et al: Impact of new treatments for neonatal pulmonary hypertension on extracorporeal membrane oxygenation use and outcome, *J Perinatol* 17:366, 1997.

317. Kennedy K, Fielder A, Hardy R et al: Medical outcomes in a multi-center randomized trial of light reduction for prevention of ROP in VLBW infants, *Pediatr Res* 47:407A, 2000.

318. Kerem E, Yatsiv I, Goitein KJ: Effect of endotracheal suctioning on arterial blood gases in children, *Intensive Care Med* 16:95, 1990.

319. Keszler M, Modanlou HD, Brudno DS et al: Multicenter controlled clinical trial of high-frequency jet ventilation in preterm infants with uncomplicated respiratory distress syndrome, *Pediatrics* 100:593, 1997.

320. Khalof M, Hurley J, Bhandari V: A prospective controlled trial of albuterol aerosol via metered dose inhaler-spacer device (MDI) vs. jet nebulizer in ventilated preterm infants, *Pediatr Res* 47:407A, 2000.

321. Khalof N, Brodsky N, Hurley J et al: A prospective randomized, controlled trial comparing synchronized nasal intermittent positive pressure ventilation vs. nasal continuous positive airway pressure as modes of extubation, *Pediatrics* 108:13, 2001.

322. Kiciman NM, Andreasson B, Bernstein G et al: Thoracoabdominal motion in newborns during ventilation delivered by endotracheal tube or nasal prongs, *Pediatr Pulmonol* 25:175, 1998.

323. Kikkert M, Conrad C, Mirmiran M et al: Apnea and gastroesophageal reflux in preterm and term infants: a retrospective study, *Pediatr Res* 47:407A, 2000.

324. Kimball AL, Carlton DP: Gastroesophageal reflux medications in the treatment of apnea and bradycardia in premature infants, *Pediatr Res* 47:408A, 2000.

325. Kinsella J, Abman S: Recent development in the pathophysiology and treatment of persistent pulmonary hypertension of the newborn, *J Pediatr* 126:853, 1995.

326. Kinsella J, Abman S: Inhaled nitric oxide: current and future uses in neonates, *Semin Perinatol* 24:387, 2000.

327. Kinsella JP, McQueston JA, Rosenberg AA et al: Hemodynamic effects of exogenous nitric oxide in ovine transitional pulmonary circulation, *Am J Physiol* 263:H875, 1992.

328. Kinsella JP, Neish SR, Ivy DD et al: Clinical responses to prolonged treatment of persistent pulmonary hypertension of the newborn with low doses of nitric oxide, *J Pediatr* 123:103, 1993.

329. Kinsella JP, Neish SR, Shaffer E et al: Low-dose inhalation nitric oxide in persistent pulmonary hypertension of the newborn, *Lancet* 340:819, 1992.

330. Kinsella JP, Parker TA, Galan H et al: Effects of inhaled nitric oxide on pulmonary edema and lung neutrophil accumulation in severe experimental hyaline membrane disease, *Pediatr Res* 41:457, 1997.

331. Kinsella JP, Truog WE, Walsh WF et al: Randomized, multicenter trial of inhaled nitric oxide and high-frequency oscillatory ventilation in severe, persistent pulmonary hypertension of the newborn, *J Pediatr* 131:55, 1997.

332. Kinsella JP, Walsh WF, Bose CL et al: Inhaled nitric oxide in premature neonates with severe hypoxaemic respiratory failure: a randomised controlled trial, *Lancet* 354:1061, 1999.

333. Kinsey VE: RLF: Cooperative study of retrolental fibroplasia and use of oxygen, *Arch Ophthalmol* 56:481, 1956.

334. Klaus M, Fanaroff A: *Care of the high-risk neonate,* ed 3, Philadelphia, 1986, WB Saunders.

335. Klaus M, Meyer BP: Oxygen therapy for the newborn, *Pediatr Clin North Am* 13:725, 1966.

336. Kleiber C: Clinical implications of deep and shallow suctioning in neonatal patients, *Focus Crit Care* 13:36, 1986.

337. Kleiber C, Krutzfield N, Rose EF: Acute histologic changes in the tracheobronchial tree associated with different suction catheter insertion techniques, *Heart Lung* 17:10, 1988.

338. Klein K, Cuculich P, Mellen B et al: Effect of dexamethasone on ROP in preterm infants, *Pediatr Res* 45:205A, 1999.

339. Kling P: Nursing intervention to decrease the risk of periventricular-intraventricular hemorrhage, *J Obstet Gynecol Neonatal Nurs,* Nov/Dec 1989, p. 457.

340. Knox AM: Performing endotracheal suction on children: a literature review and implications for nursing practice, *Intensive Crit Care Nurs* 9:48, 1993.

341. Koons AH, Mojica N, Jadeja N et al: Neurodevelopmental outcome of infants with apnea of infancy, *Am J Perinatol* 10:208, 1993.

342. Kothadia JM, O'Shea TM, Roberts D et al: Randomized placebo-controlled trial of a 42-day tapering course of dexamethasone to reduce the duration of ventilator dependency in very low birth weight infants, *Pediatrics* 104:22, 1999.

343. Kotecha S, Wilson L, Wangoo A et al: Increase in interleukin (IL)-1 beta and IL-6 in bronchoalveolar lavage fluid obtained from infants with chronic lung disease of prematurity, *Pediatr Res* 40:250, 1996.

344. Krantz ME, Wennergren M, Bengtson LG et al: Epidemiological analysis of the increased risk of disturbed neonatal adaptation after cesarean section, *Acta Paediatr Scand* 75:832, 1986.

345. Kuhns LR, Bednarek FJ, Wyman ML et al: Diagnosis of pneumothorax and pneumomediastinum in the neonate by transillumination, *Pediatrics* 56:355, 1975.

346. Kumar P, Shankaran S, Bedard MP et al: Identifying at risk infants following neonatal extracorporeal membrane oxygenation, *J Perinatol* 19:367, 1999.

347. Kurzner SI, Garg M, Bautista DB et al: Growth failure in infants with bronchopulmonary dysplasia: nutrition and elevated resting metabolic expenditure, *Pediatrics* 81:379, 1988.

348. Laforce W, Bruno D: Controlled trial of beclomethasone dipropionate by nebulization in oxygen and ventilator-dependent infants, *J Pediatr* 122:285, 1993.

349. Lakshminrusimha S, Steinhorn R: Pulmonary vascular biology during neonatal transition, *Clin in Perinatol* 26:601, 1999.

350. Lam B, Yeung C: Surfactant lavage for the management of severe meconium aspiration syndrome, *Biol Neonate* 76:10, 1999.

351. Leach CL, Greenspan JS, Rubenstein SD et al: Partial liquid ventilation with perflubron in premature infants with severe respiratory distress syndrome, *N Engl J Med* 335:761, 1996.

352. Lee S, Normand C, McMillan D, et al: Cost-effectiveness of screening for ROP: evidence from Canada, *Pediatr Res* 45:248A, 1999.

353. Liechty E, Donovan G, Purohit D et al: Reduction of neonatal mortality after multiple doses of bovine surfactant in LBW neonates with RDS, *Pediatrics* 88:19, 1991.

354. Leitch C, Ahlrichs J, Karn C et al: Energy expenditure and energy intake during dexamethasone therapy for CLD, *Pediatr Res* 46:109, 1999.

355. Leung E, Kenney S, O'Riordan M et al: The effect of antenatal corticosteroids on the clinical course and complications of RDS in extremely premature infants, *Pediatr Res* 47:410, 2000.

356. Lewin MB, Bryant RM, Fenrich AL et al: Cisapride-induced long QT interval, *J Pediatr* 128:279, 1996.

357. Lien JM, Towers CV, Quilligan EJ et al: Term early-onset neonatal seizures: obstetric characteristics, etiologic classifications and perinatal care, *Obstet Gynecol* 85:163, 1995.

358. Lin C, Tsai T, Lin Y et al: Efficacy of nasal intermittent positive pressure (NIPPV) in treating apnea of prematurity, *Pediatr Res* 39:338A, 1996.

359. Lin CH, Wang ST, Lin YJ et al: Efficacy of nasal intermittent positive pressure ventilation in treating apnea of prematurity, *Pediatr Pulmonol* 26:349, 1998.

360. Linder N, Kuint J, German B et al: Hypertrophy of the tongue associated with inhaled corticosteroid therapy in premature infants, *J Pediatr* 127:651, 1995.

361. Ling E, Battin M, Whitfield M: Has the 18 month outcome of extremely low gestational age infants of 23-25 weeks gestation improved? *Pediatr Res* 46:271A, 1997.

362. Lista G, Maragione P, Azzoli A et al: Volume guarantee during SIMV reduces the risk of barovolutrauma in preterm infants with RDS, *Pediatr Res* 47:367A, 2000.

363. Liu W, Borden D, Harrington T: Delivery room risk factors for development of meconium-related respiratory distress, *Pediatr Res* 47:413A, 2000.

364. Livera LN, Spencer SA, Thorniley MS et al: Effects of hypoxaemia and bradycardia on neonatal cerebral haemodynamics, *Arch Dis Child* 66:376, 1991.

365. Llano A, Moss M, Pinzon M et al: Epidemiology of neonatal NEC in the post-surfactant era: a population-based study, *Pediatr Res* 45:249A, 1999.

366. Locke RG, Wolfson MR, Shaffer TH et al: Inadvertent administration of positive end-distending pressure during nasal cannula flow, *Pediatrics* 91:135, 1993.

367. Lockridge T: Following the learning curve: the evolution of kinder, gentler neonatal respiratory technology, *J Obstet Gynecol Neonatal Nurs* 28:443, 1999.

368. Long JG, Phillip AGS, Lucey JF, Excessive handling as a cause of hypoxemia, *Pediatrics* 65:203, 1980.

369. Long W, Thompson T, Sundell H et al: Effects of two rescue doses of a synthetic surfactant on mortality rate without bronchopulmonary dysplasia in 700- to 1350-gram infants with respiratory distress syndrome, *J Pediatr* 118:595, 1991.

369a. Lorenz J: Survival of the extremely preterm infant in North America in the 1990's, *Clin Perinatol* 27:255, 2000.

370. Lotze A, Knight GR, Martin GR et al: Improved pulmonary outcome after exogenous surfactant therapy for respiratory failure in term infants requiring extracorporeal membrane oxygenation, *J Pediatr* 122:261, 1993.

371. Lotze A, Mitchell lBR, Bulas DI et al: Multicenter study of surfactant use in the treatment of term infants with severe respiratory failure, *J Pediatr* 132:40, 1998.

372. Lou H: Etiology and pathogenesis of attention-deficit hyperactivity disorder (ADHD): significance of prematurity and perinatal hypoxic-haemodynamic encephalopathy, *Acta Paediatr* 85:1266, 1996.

373. Lundstrom K: Initial treatment of premature infants: CPAP or ventilation? *Eur J Pediatr* 155:525, 1996.

374. MacFarlane P, Heaf D: Pulmonary function in children after neonatal MAS, *Arch Dis Child* 63:368, 1988.

375. Madan A, Varma S, Cohen H: Hypoxic induction of vascular endothelial growth factor (VEGF) and HIF-1 protein in retinal pigment epithelial cells, *Pediatr Res* 45:209A, 1999.

376. Mahmood B, Varma A, Devaskar U: Massive fluid resuscitation is required in neonates with primary pulmonary hypertension, *Pediatr Res* 45:209A, 1999.

377. Majnemer A, Riley P, Shevell M et al: Severe bronchopulmonary dysplasia increases risk for late neurological and motor sequelae in preterm survivors, *Dev Med Child Neurol* 42:53, 2000.

378. Mallman M: Molecular interactions between nitric oxide and lung surfactant, *Biol Neonate* 71:44, 1997.

379. Malloy M, Freeman D: Respiratory distress syndrome mortality in the United States, 1987-1995, *J Perinatol* 20:414, 2000.

380. Mariani G, Cifuentes J, Carlo W: Randomized trial of permissive hypercapnia in preterm infants, *Pediatrics* 104:1082, 1999.

381. Marinelli PV, Ortiz A, Alden ER: Acquired eventration of the diaphragm: a complication of chest tube placement in neonatal pneumothorax, *Pediatrics* 67:552, 1981.

382. Marron MJ, Crisafi MA, Driscoll JM Jr et al: Hearing and neurodevelopmental outcome in survivors of persistent pulmonary hypertension of the newborn, *Pediatrics* 90:392, 1992.

383. Marshall DD, Kotelchuck M, Young TE et al: Risk factors for chronic lung disease in the surfactant era: a North Carolina population-based study of very low birth weight infants, *Pediatrics* 104:1345, 1999.

384. Martin RJ, Miller MB, Carlo WA: Pathogenesis of apnea in preterm infants, *J Pediatr* 109:733, 1986.

385. Martin RJ, Herrell N, Rubin D et al: Effect of supine and prone positions on arterial oxygen tension in the preterm infant, *Pediatrics* 63:528, 1979.

386. Martinez-Bermudez K, Almazan G, Lachapelle P et al: Isoprostanes induce retinal obliteration, a key feature of ROP, *Pediatr Res* 45:210A, 1999

387. Mazor M, Furman B, Wiznitzer A et al: Maternal and perinatal outcome of patients with preterm labor and meconium-stained amniotic fluid, *Obstet Gynecol* 86:830, 1995.

388. McClead R, McGregor M, Bremer D et al: HOPE-ROP (high oxygen percentage in ROP) study: ROP outcome in infants with prethreshold ROP and SpO_2 >94% in room air, *Pediatr Res* 47:415A, 2000.

389. McDonald AD: Cerebral palsy in children of very low birth weight, *Arch Dis Child* 38:579, 1963.

390. McEvoy C, Bowling S, Williamson K et al: Measurements of FRC one week after treatment with a seven day tapering course of dexamethasone in VLBW infants, *Pediatr Res* 47:416A, 2000.

391. McMillan D, Vincer M, Ohlsson A et al: Retinopathy of prematurity in Canada, *Pediatr Res* 45:250A, 1999.

392. Ment LR, Vohr B, Allan W et al: The etiology and outcome of cerebral ventriculomegaly at term in very low birth weight preterm infants, *Pediatrics* 104:243, 1999.

393. Merz U: Early versus late dexamethasone treatment in preterm infants at risk for CLD: a randomized pilot study, *Eur J Pediatr* 158:318, 1999.

394. Miller KE, Edwards DK, Hilton S et al: Acquired lobar emphysema in preterm infants with BPD: an iatrogenic disease? *Radiology* 138:589, 1981.

395. Mitchell A, Greenough A, Hird M: Limitations of patient triggered ventilation in neonates, *Arch Dis Child* 64:924, 1989.

396. Mitchell S: Caring for the visually impaired infant, *Neonatal Netw* 18:41, 1999.

397. Modanlou HD, Beharry K, Padilla G et al: Comparative efficacy of Exosurf and Survanta surfactants on early clinical course of RDS and complications of prematurity, *J Perinatol* 17:455, 1997.

398. Moler F, Brown R, Faix R, Gilsdorf J: Comments on Palivizumab, *Pediatrics* 103:495, 1999.

399. Moretti C, Gizzi C, Papoff P et al: Comparing the effects of nasal synchronized intermittent positive pressure ventilation (nSIPPV) and nasal continuous positive airway pressure (nCPAP) after extubation in VLBW infants, *Early Hum Dev* 56:167, 1999.

400. Moriette G, Paris-Llado J, Walti H et al: Prospective randomized multicenter comparison of high-frequency oscillatory ventilation and conventional ventilation in preterm infants of less than 30 weeks with RDS, *Pediatrics* 107:363, 2001.

401. Morley C: Systematic review of prophylactic vs. rescue surfactant, *Arch Dis Child* 77:F70, 1997.

402. Morris BH, Miller-Loncar CL, Landry SH et al: Feeding, medical factors and developmental outcome in premature infants, *Clin Pediatr (Phila)* 38:451, 1999.

403. Mosca FA, Colnaghi M, Lattanzio M et al: Closed versus open endotracheal suctioning in preterm infants: effects on cerebral oxygenation and blood volume, *Biol Neonate* 72:9, 1997.

404. Moses D, Holm BA, Spitale P et al: Inhibition of pulmonary surfactant function by meconium, *Am J Obstet Gynecol* 164:477, 1991.

405. Muraskas J, Weiss M, Juretschke L: Perinatal risk factors for the development of PPHN of the newborn in premature newborns, *Pediatr Res* 47:419A, 2000.

406. Murphy B, Inder T, Huppi P et al: Quantitative brain growth following treatment with dexamethasone for neonatal CLD, *Pediatr Res* 47:419A, 2000.

407. Murphy BP, Inder TE, Huppi PS et al: Impaired cerebral corticol gray matter growth after treatment with dexamethasone for neonatal chronic lung disease, *Pediatrics* 107:217, 2001.

408. Nadya S, Kazzi J, Romero R et al: Surfactant therapy modulates levels of interleukin-6 and interleukin-1B in tracheal aspirates of premature infants with RDS, *Pediatr Res* 45:204A, 1999.

409. Nagaraj HS, Shott, R, Fellows R et al: Recurrent lobar atelectasis due to acquired bronchial stenosis in neonates, *J Pediatr Surg* 15:411, 1980.

410. Nathan L, Leveno KJ, Carmody TJ III et al: Meconium: a 1990s perspective on an old obstetric hazard, *Obstet Gynecol* 83:329, 1994.

411. National Institutes of Health: Effect of corticosteroids for fetal maturation on perinatal outcomes, *JAMA* 273:413, 1995.

412. National Institutes of Health: Antenatal corticosteroids revisited: repeat courses, *NIH Consensus Statement* 2000 17:1, 2000.

413. Nelson K, Ellenberg J: Obstetrics complications as risk factors for CP or seizure disorders, *JAMA* 251:1843, 1984.

414. Nelson M, Nicks JJ, Becker MA et al: Comparison of two methods of surfactant administration and the effect on dosing-associated hypoxemia, *J Perinatol* 17:450, 1997.

415. Neonatal ECMO registry of the extracorporeal life support organization (ELSO), Ann Arbor, Mich, July 1999.

416. Neonatal Inhaled Nitric Oxide Study Group: Inhaled nitric oxide in full-term and nearly full-term infants with hypoxic respiratory failure, *N Engl J Med* 336:597, 1997.

417. Ng P: The effectiveness and side effects of dexamethasone in preterm infants with BPD, *Arch Dis Child* 68:330, 1993.

418. Ng S, Gomez J: Safety profile and therapeutic usefulness of CPAP/PEEP in MAS, *Pediatr Res* 45:214A, 1999.

419. Nickerson B, Taussig L: Family history of asthma in infants with BPD, *Pediatrics* 65:1140, 1980.

420. Norris S, Campbell A, Brenkert S: Nursing procedures and alterations in transcutaneous oxygen tension in newborns, *Nurs Res* 31:330, 1982.

421. Northway W, Rosan R: Radiographic features of pulmonary oxygen toxicity in the newborn: bronchopulmonary dysplasia, *Radiology* 91:49, 1968.

422. Nuntnarumit P, Bada H, Yang W et al: Cerebral blood flow velocity changes after bovine natural surfactant instillation, *J Perinatol* 4:240, 2000.

423. Odita J, Kayyali M, Ammari A: Post-extubation atelectasis in ventilated newborn infants, *Pediatr Radiol* 23:183, 1993.

424. Ogawa Y, Miyasaka K, Kawano T et al: A multicenter randomized trial of high frequency oscillatory ventilation as compared with conventional mechanical ventilation in preterm infants with respiratory failure, *Early Hum Dev* 32:1, 1993.

425. Ogawa Y, Omaha Y, Itakura Y et al: Bronchial lavage with surfactant solution for the treatment of MAS, *J Jpn Med Soc Biol Interface* 26:179, 1996.

426. Okumura A, Hayakawa F, Kato T et al: Hypocarbia in preterm infants with periventricular leukomalacia: the relation between hypocarbia and mechanical ventilation, *Pediatrics* 107:469, 2001.

427. Ortiz L, Quan A, Weinberg A et al: Prenatal dexamethasone causes reduced glomerular number and hypertension in adult rats, *Pediatr Res* 47:450A, 2000.

428. Osborn D, Henderson-Smart D: Kinesthetic stimulation vs. theophylline for apnea in preterm infants (Cochrane Review). In The Cochrane Library, Issue Feb. 19, 1998, Oxford, England: Update Software, 1998.

429. O'Shea TM, Sevick MA, Givner LB: Costs and benefits of RSV immunoglobulin to prevent hospitalization for lower respiratory tract illness in VLBW infants, *Pediatr Infect Dis J* 17:587, 1998.

430. O'Shea TM, Goldstein DJ, deRegnier RA et al: Outcome at 4 to 5 years of age in children recovered from neonatal CLD, *Dev Med Child Neurol* 38:830, 1996.

431. O'Shea TM, Kothadia JM, Klinepeter KL et al: Randomized placebo-controlled trial of a 42-day tapering course of dexamethasone to reduce the duration of ventilator dependency in very low birth weight infants: outcome of study participants at 1-year adjusted age, *Pediatrics* 104:15, 1999.

432. Palta M, Weinstein M, McGuinness G et al: Mortality and morbidity after availability of surfactant therapy, *Arch Pediatr Adolesc Med* 148:1295, 1994.

433. Palta M, Sadek-Badawi M, Evans M et al: Functional assessment of a multicenter very-low-birthweight cohort at age 5 years, *Arch Pediatr Adolesc Med* 154:23, 2000.

434. Pandit P, Pyon K, Courtney S et al: Inspiratory work of breathing with a demand flow vs. constant flow nasal continuous positive airway pressure (NCPAP) device in preterm neonates, *Pediatr Res* 45:314A, 1999.

435. Pandit PB, Dunn MS, Kelly EN et al: Surfactant replacement in neonates with early chronic lung disease, *Pediatrics* 95:851, 1995.

436. Papile LA, Tyson JE, Stoll BJ et al: A multicenter trial of two dexamethasone regimens in ventilator-dependent premature infants, *N Engl J Med* 338:1112, 1998.

437. Parimi PS, Birnkrant DJ, Rao LV et al: Effect of dexamethasone on lymphocyte subpopulations in premature infants with BPD, *J Perinatol* 19:347, 1999.

438. Parker TA, Kinsella JP, Abman SH: Response to inhaled nitric oxide in persistent pulmonary hypertension of the newborn: relationship to baseline oxygenation, *J Perinatol* 18:221, 1998.

439. Parupia M, Dhanireddy R: Association of sepsis and race in the development of severe ROP and progression to laser therapy in ELBW infants, *Pediatr Res* 47:423A, 2000.

440. Pena I, Barton L: Which very low birthweight (VLBW) infants are proven to develop severe ROP? *Pediatr Res* 45:218A, 1999.

441. Penn J, Henry M, Wall P et al: The range of P_aO_2 variation determines the severity of oxygen-induced retinopathy in newborn rats, *Invest Ophthalmol Vis Sci* 36:2063, 1995.

442. Pepke-Zaba J, Higenbottam TW, Dinh-Xuan AT et al: Inhaled nitric oxide as a cause of selective pulmonary vasodilation in pulmonary hypertension, *Lancet* 338:1173, 1991.

443. Perkett E, Vaughan R: Evidence for a laryngeal chemoreflex in some human preterm infants, *Acta Paediatr Scand* 71:969, 1982.

444. Perkin R, Levin D, Clark R: Serum salicylate levels and right to left ductus shunts in newborn infants with persistent pulmonary hypertension of the newborn, *J Pediatr* 96:721, 1980.

445. Perlman J, Volpe J: Suctioning in the preterm infant: effects on cerebral blood flow velocity, intracranial pressure and arterial blood pressure, *Pediatrics* 72:329, 1983.

446. Pearlman J, Volpe J: Episodes of apnea and bradycardia in the preterm newborn: impact on cerebral circulation, *Pediatrics* 76:33, 1985.

447. Peters K: The physiologic responses of the respiratory distressed neonate to two different forms of chest physiotherapy, PhD dissertation, University of Alberta, Edmonton, 1983.

448. Peters K: Infant handling in the NICU: does developmental care make a difference? An evaluative review of the literature, *J Perinat Neonat Nurs* 13:83, 1999.

449. Phelps D, Oden N, Cole C et al: Timing of ROP events: screening implications, *Pediatr Res* 47:425A, 2000.

450. Philip A: The changing face of neonatal infection: experience at a regional medical center, *Pediatr Infect Dis J* 13:1098, 1994.

451. Phipps S, Drotar D: Determinants of parenting stress in home apnea monitoring, *J Pediatr Psychol* 15:385, 1990.

452. Phyu P, Tin W, Sinha S: Effect of surfactant treatment on trends in BPD, *Pediatr Res* 45:314A, 1999.

453. Pickens DL: Pharyngeal fluid clearance and aspiration preventive mechanisms in sleeping infants, *J Appl Physiol* 66:1164, 1989.

454. Pickens DL, Schefft G, Thach BT: Prolonged apnea associated with upper airway protective reflexes in apnea of prematurity, *Am Rev Respir Dis* 137:113, 1988.

455. Piuze G, Usher R, Barrington K: Etiologic factors for the development of CLD in infants <30 weeks gestation, *Pediatr Res* 47:426A, 2000.

456. Poets C, Sens B: Change in intubation rates and outcomes of very low birth weight infants: a population-based study, *Pediatrics* 98:24, 1996.

457. Poets CF, Southall DP: Noninvasive monitoring of oxygenation in infants and children: practical considerations and areas of concern, *Pediatrics* 93:737, 1994.

458. Preslan M: Laser therapy for retinopathy of prematurity, *J Pediatr Ophthalmol Strabismus* 30:80, 1993.

459. Purohit DM, Caldwell C, Levkoff AH: Multiple fractures due to physiotherapy in a neonate with hyaline membrane disease, *Am J Dis Child* 129:1103, 1975.

460. Rais-Bahrami K, Short B: The current status of neonatal ECMO, *Semin Perinatol* 24:406, 2000.

461. Rais-Bahrami K, Wagner AE, Coffman C et al: Neurodevelopmental outcome in ECMO vs near-miss ECMO patients at 5 years of age, *Clin Pediatr (Phila)* 39:145, 2000.

462. Raju T, Langenberg P: Pulmonary hemorrhage and exogenous surfactant therapy: a meta analysis, *J Pediatr* 123:603, 1993.

463. Ramaekers V, Casaer P, Daniels H: Cerebral hyperperfusion following episodes of bradycardia in the preterm infant, *Early Hum Dev* 34:199, 1993.

464. Ramanathan R, Siassi B, deLemos RA: Severe retinopathy of prematurity in extremely low birth weight infants with short-term dexamethasone therapy, *J Perinatol* 15:178, 1995.

465. Ramanathan R, Siassi B, Sardesai S: Current incidence of > Stage III ROP and need for retinal surgery for ROP in VLBW infants, 1993-1998, *Pediatr Res* 47:428A, 2000.

466. Ramsay S: The Birmingham experience, *Lancet* 345:510, 1995.

467. Rao S, Pavlova Z, Incerpi M et al: Incidence of meconium-stained amniotic fluid in term pregnancies with histologic evidence of acute chorioamnionitis and/or acute funisitis, *Pediatr Res* 47:428A, 2000.

468. Raval D, Cuevas A, Mora A et al: The efficacy of chest physiotherapy (CPT) in the first postnatal day in infants with RDS (abstract), *Pediatr Res* 19(suppl):359A, 1985.

469. Raval D, Yeh T, Mora A et al: Changes in transcutaneous PO_2 during tracheobronchial hygiene in neonates, *Perinatology-Neonatology* 4:41, 1980.

470. Raval D, Yeh T, Mora A et al: Chest physiotherapy in preterm infants with RDS in the first 24 hours of life, *J Perinatol* 7:301, 1987.

471. Rettwitz-Volk W, Veldman A, Roth B et al: A prospective, randomized, multicenter trial of high-frequency oscillatory ventilation compared with conventional ventilation in preterm infants with respiratory distress syndrome receiving surfactant, *J Pediatr* 132:249, 1998.

472. Reynolds JD, Hardy RJ, Kennedy KA et al: Lack of efficacy of light reduction in preventing retinopathy of prematurity, *N Engl J Med* 338:1572, 1998.

473. Riegel B, Forshee T: A review and critique of the literature on preoxygenation for endotracheal suctioning, *Heart Lung* 14:507, 1985.

474. Rimensberger P, Beghetti M, Hanquinet S et al: First intention high-frequency oscillation with early lung volume optimization improves pulmonary outcome in VLBW infants with RDS, *Pediatrics* 105:1202, 2000.

475. Robbins JM, Tilford JM, Jacobs RF et al: A number-needed-to-treat analysis of the use of respiratory syncytial virus immune globulin to prevent hospitalization, *Arch Pediatr Adolesc Med* 152:358, 1998.

476. Roberts J, Zapol W: Inhaled nitric oxide, *Semin Perinatol* 24:55, 2000.

477. Roberts JD, Polaner DM, Lang P et al: Inhaled nitric oxide in persistent pulmonary hypertension of the newborn, *Lancet* 340:818, 1992.

478. Roberts JD Jr, Fineman JR, Morin FC III et al: Inhaled nitric oxide and persistent pulmonary hypertension of the newborn, *N Engl J Med* 336:605, 1997.

479. Robertson B, Halliday H: Principles of surfactant replacement, *Biochem Biophys Acta* 1408:346, 1998.

480. Robertson C, Etches P, Goldson E et al: Eight-year school performance, neurodevelopmental and growth outcome of neonates with BPD: a comparative study, *Pediatrics* 89:365, 1992.

481. Rodrigues F, Berezin A, Paulo P: Times of oxygen therapy and mechanical ventilation and number of blood transfusions in premature babies with and without BPD and ROP, *Pediatr Res* 47:429A, 2000.

482. Rodriguez R, Martin R: Exogenous surfactant therapy in newborns, *Resp Clin North Am* 5:595, 1999.

483. Rojas MA, Gonzalez A, Bancalari E et al: Changing trends in the epidemiology and pathogenesis of neonatal chronic lung disease, *J Pediatr* 126:603, 1995.

484. Romagnoli C, Zecca E, Vento G et al: Effect on growth of two different dexamethasone courses for preterm infants at risk of—chronic lung disease: a randomized trial, *Pharmacology* 59:266, 1999.

485. Rosenberg AA, Kennaugh JM, Moreland SG et al: Longitudinal follow-up of a cohort of newborn infants treated with inhaled nitric oxide for persistent pulmonary hypertension, *J Pediatr* 131:70, 1997.

486. Rosenfeld W, Davis J: Prevention of oxygen radical disease in the newborn: possible therapeutic approaches, *Semin Neonatal* 3:239, 1998.

487. Rosenfeld WN, Davis JM, Parton L et al: Safety and pharmacokinetics of recombinant human superoxide dismutase administered intratracheally to premature infants with respiratory distress syndrome, *Pediatrics* 97:811, 1996.

488. Rossi C, Almeida F, Guinsburg R et al: Delivery room management of meconium-stained neonates: risk factors for MAS, *Pediatr Res* 47:430A, 2000.

489. Roukema H, O'Brien K, Nesbitt K et al: A crossover trial of infant flow (IF) CPAP vs. nasopharyngeal (NP) CPAP in the extubation of babies <1250 gms birthweight, *Pediatr Res* 45:317A, 1999.

490. Roukema H, O'Brien K, Nesbitt K et al: A randomized controlled trial of infant flow (CPAP) vs. nasopharyngeal CPAP in the extubation of babies <1250 gms, *Pediatr Res* 45:318A, 1999.

491. Rudy E, Baun M, Stone K, et al: The relationship between endotracheal suctioning and changes in intracranial pressure: a review of the literature, *Heart Lung* 15:488, 1986.

492. Ruof H, Fahwenstich H: Closed versus open ET suctioning in ventilated preterm infants, *Pediatr Res* 47:430A, 2000.

493. Saigal S, Rosenbaum P, Stoskopf B et al: Comprehensive assessment of the health status in extremely low birth weight children at 8 years of age: comparison with a reference group, *J Pediatr* 125:411, 1994.

494. Saito Y, Omoto T, Cho Y et al: The progression of retinopathy of prematurity and fluctuation in blood gas tension, *Graefes Arch Clin Exp Ophthalmol* 231:151, 1993.

495. Sandberg K, Sjoqvist BA, Hjalmarson O et al: Lung function in newborn infants with tachypnea of unknown cause, *Pediatr Res* 22:581, 1987.

496. Saugstad O: Oxygen radical disease in neonatology, *Semin Neonatal* 3:231, 1998.

497. Schecter R: Laser treatment of ROP, *Arch Ophthalmol* 111:730, 1993.

498. Schipper JA, Mohammad GI, van Straaten HL et al: The impact of surfactant replacement therapy on cerebral and systemic circulation and lung function, *Eur J Pediatr* 156:224, 1997.

499. Schmidt B: Methylxanthine therapy in premature infants: sound practice, disaster or fruitless byway? *J Pediatr* 135:526, 1999.

500. Schulze A: Enhancement of mechanical ventilation of neonates by computer technology, *Semin Perinatol* 24:429, 2000.

501. Schulze A, Gerhardt T, Musante G et al: Proportional assist ventilation in low birth weight infants with acute respiratory disease: a comparison to assist/control and conventional mechanical ventilation, *J Pediatr* 135:339, 1999.

502. Schwartz R: Effect of position on oxygenation, heart rate, and behavioral state in the transitional newborn infant, *Neonatal Netw* 12:73, 1993.

503. Schwartz R, Luby A, Scanlon J et al: Effect of surfactant on morbidity, mortality and resource use in newborn infants weighing 500-1500 gm, *N Eng J Med* 330:1476, 1994.

504. Scott S, Backstrom C, Bessman S: Effect of 5 days of dexamethasone therapy in ventilatory dependence and adrenocorticotropic hormone-stimulated cortisol concentrations, *J Perinatol* 17:24, 1997.

505. Segar J, Merrill D, Chapleau M et al: Hemodynamic changes during endotracheal suctioning are mediated by increased autonomic activity, *Pediatr Res* 33:649, 1993.

506. Seidner SR, Ikegami M, Yamada T et al: Decreased surfactant dose-response after delayed administration to preterm rabbits, *Am J Respir Crit Care Med* 152:113, 1995.

507. Shah AR, Kurth CD, Gwiazdowski SG et al: Fluctuations in cerebral oxygenation and blood volume during endotracheal suctioning in premature infants, *J Pediatr* 120:769, 1992.

508. Shah V, Ohlsson A, Halliday H et al: Early administration of inhaled corticosteroids for preventing CLD in ventilated VLBW preterm neonates. In The Cochrane Library, I. Oxford, England: Update Software, 2000.

509. Shankaran S, Farooki Z, Desai R: Beta hemolytic streptococcal infection appearing as persistent fetal circulation, *Am J Dis Child* 136:725, 1982.

510. Shenai J: Vitamin A supplementation in VLBW neonates: rationale and evidence, *Pediatrics* 104:1369, 1999.

511. Shields J, Schifrin B: Perinatal antecedents of CP, *Obstet Gynecol* 71:899, 1988.

512. Shinwell ES, Karplus M, Reich D et al: Early postnatal dexamethasone treatment and increased incidence of cerebral palsy, *Arch Dis Child Fetal Neonatal Educ* 83:F177, 2000.

513. Shorten D, Byrne P, Jones R: Infant responses to saline instillations and endotracheal suctioning, *J Obstet Gynecol Neonatal Nurs* 20:464, 1991.

514. Simbruner G, Coradello H, Fodor M et al: Effect of tracheal suction on oxygenation, circulation and lung mechanics in newborn infants, *Arch Dis Child* 56:326, 1981.

515. Simoes E, Rosenberg A, King S et al: Room air challenge: prediction for successful weaning of oxygen-dependent infants, *J Perinatol* 17:125, 1997.

516. Singer L, Yamashita T, Lilien L et al: A longitudinal study of developmental outcome of infants with bronchopulmonary dysplasia and very low birth weight, *Pediatrics* 100:987, 1997.

517. Sinha S, Donn S: Advances in neonatal conventional ventilation, *Arch Dis Child* 75:F135, 1996.

518. Sinha S, Donn S, Gavey J et al: A randomized trial of volume-controlled vs. time-cycled, pressure-limited ventilation in preterm infants with RDS, *Arch Dis Child* 77:F202, 1997.

519. Sinkin RA, Sweck HS, Horgan MJ et al: Early dexamethasone: attempting to prevent chronic lung disease, *Pediatrics* 105:542, 2000.

520. Skidmore MD, Rivers A, Hack M: Increased risk of cerebral palsy among very low-birthweight infants with chronic lung disease, *Dev Med Child Neurol* 32:325, 1990.

521. Soll R: Surfactant therapy in the USA: trials and current routines, *Biol Neonate* 71:1, 1997.

522. Soll R: Surfactant therapy of the very preterm infant, *Biol Neonate* 74:35, 1998.

523. Soll R: Early postnatal dexamethasone therapy for the prevention of chronic lung disease, *Pediatr Res* 45:226A, 1999.

524. Soll R, Morley C: Prophylactic vs selective use of surfactant for preventing morbidity and mortality in preterm infants. In The Cochrane Library, Issue 1, 2000, Oxford, Update Software.

525. Sosenko I: Nutrients and the respiratory status of the preterm neonate: strategies to optimize outcome, *Perspect Neonatol* 1:4, 2000.

526. Sottile FD, Marrie TJ, Prouth DS: Nosocomial pulmonary infection: possible etiological significance of bacterial adhesion to ETT, *Crit Care Med* 14:265, 1986.

527. Speer C, Groneck B: Oxygen radicals, cytokines, adhesion molecules and lung injury in neonates, *Semin Neonatol* 3:712, 1998.

528. Sreenan C, Lemke R, Hudson-Mason A et al: High-flow nasal cannulae in the management of apnea of prematurity: a comparison with conventional nasal continuous positive airway pressure, *Pediatrics* 107:1081, 2001.

529. Stark A, Carlo W, Bauer C et al: Complications of early steroid therapy in a randomized controlled trial, *Pediatr Suppl* 104:739A, 1999.

530. Stark AR, Carlo WA, Tyson JE et al: Adverse effects of early dexamethasone treatment in extremely-low-birth-weight infants, *N Eng J Med* 344:95, 2001.

531. Stathis SL, O'Callaghan M, Harvey J et al: Head circumference in ELBW babies is associated with learning difficulties and cognition but not ADHD in the school aged child, *Dev Med Child Neurol* 41:375, 1999.

532. Stern L: Therapy of the respiratory distress syndrome, *Pediatr Clin North Am* 19:221, 1972.

533. Stoll BJ, Temprosa M, Tyson JE et al: Dexamethasone therapy increases infection in very low birth weight infants, *Pediatrics* 104:1121, 1999.

534. Storm W: Transient bacteremia following ET suctioning in ventilated newborns, *Pediatrics* 65:487, 1980.

535. Subhani M, Combs A, Weber P et al: Screening guidelines for retinopathy of prematurity: the need for revision in extremely low birth weight infants, *Pediatrics* 107:656, 2001.

536. Subramanian K, Dhanireddy R, El-Mohandes A et al: Hypercarbia and not hypocarbia is associated with the risk of BPD in VLBW infants: a multicenter study, *Pediatr Res* 45:320A, 1999.

537. Subramanian K, Dhanireddy R, El-Mohandes A et al: Interrelationship of PDA and fluid intake during the first 6 days of life and development of BPD in VLBW infants: a multicenter study, *Pediatr Res* 45:320A, 1999.

538. Sun B, Curstedt T, Robertson B: Surfactant inhibition in experimental meconium aspiration, *Acta Paediatr* 82:182, 1993.

539. Swaminathan S, Quinn J, Stabile MW et al: Long-term pulmonary sequelae of meconium aspiration syndrome, *J Pediatr* 114:356, 1989.

540. Sweet D, Halliday H: A risk-benefit assessment of drugs used for neonatal chronic lung disease, *Drug Saf* 22:389, 2000.

541. Synnes AR, Ling EW, Whitfield MF et al: Perinatal outcomes of a large cohort of extremely low gestational age infants (twenty-three to twenty-eight completed weeks of gestation), *J Pediatr* 125:952, 1994.

542. Szymankiewicz M, Kowalski K, Gadzinowski J et al: Pulmonary function measurements after surfactant lavage in MAS, *Pediatr Res* 47:435A, 2000.

543. Taeusch H: Glucocorticoid prophylaxis for respiratory distress syndrome: a review of potential toxicity, *J Pediatr* 87:617, 1975.

544. Tapia J, Bancalari A, Gonzalez A et al: Does continuous positive airway pressure (CPAP) during weaning from intermittent mandatory ventilation in very low birth weight infants have risks or benefits? A controlled trial, *Pediatr Pulmonol* 19:269, 1995.

545. Taquino L, Blackburn S: The effects of containment during suction and heelstick on physiological and behavioral responses of preterm infants, *Neonatal Netw* 13:55, 1994.

546. Taylor R: Postnatal steroid use among neonatologists: survey results December 2000. http://www.cheo.on.ca/rtaylor/PNSteroid-r.htm.

547. Telenko T, Peliowski A, Hudson-Mason A: CPAP in the treatment of apnea of prematurity: a comparison of two CPAP delivery systems, *Pediatr Res* 45:228A, 1999.

548. Thebaud B, Watterberg K: Postnatal glucocorticoids in very preterm infants: "the good, the bad, and the ugly"? *Pediatrics* 107:413, 2001.

549. The Collaborative UKECMO trial: follow-up to 1 year of age, *Pediatrics* 101:690, 1998.

550. The Impact-RSV Study Group: Palivizumab, a humanized respiratory syncytial virus monoclonal antibody, reduces hospitalization from respiratory syncytial virus infection in high-risk infants, *Pediatrics* 102:531, 1998.

551. The STOP-ROP Multicenter Study Group: Supplemental therapeutic oxygen for prethreshold retinopathy of prematurity (STOP-ROP), a randomized controlled trial I: primary outcomes, *Pediatrics* 105:295, 2000.

552. Thome U, Kossel H, Lipowsky G et al: Randomized comparison of high-frequency ventilation with high-rate intermittent positive pressure ventilation in preterm infants with respiratory failure, *J Pediatr* 135:39, 1999.

553. Thompson C, O'Neil P, Kendra M: Patient fatigue and mucus removal with and without saline during suction, *Crit Care Med* 23(1 suppl):A46, 1995.

554. Ting P, Brady J: Tracheal suction in meconium aspiration, *Am J Obstet Gynecol* 122:767, 1975.

555. Todd D, Jana A, John E: Chronic oxygen dependency in infants born at 24-32 weeks gestation: the role of antenatal and neonatal factors, *J Pediatr Child Health* 33:402, 1997.

556. Torres C, Holditch-Davis D, O'Hale A et al: Effect of standard rest periods on apnea and weight gain in preterm infants, *Neonatal Netw* 16:35, 1997.

557. Touch S, Epstein M, Pohl C et al: Impact on sleep patterns of co-bedding multiple gestation infants, *Pediatr Res* 47:436A, 2000.

558. Trotter C, Carey B: Radiology basics, Part II: RDS and BPD, *Neonatal Netw* 19:37, 2000.

559. Tyler D, Murphy J, Cheney F: Mechanical and chemical damage to lung tissue caused by meconium aspiration, *Pediatrics* 62:454, 1978.

560. Tyson JE, Wright LL, Oh W et al: Vitamin A supplementation for extremely-low-birth-weight infants, *New Engl J Med* 340:1962, 1999.

561. United Kingdom Collaborative ECMO Trial Group: UK collaborative randomized trial of neonatal ECMO, *Lancet* 348:75, 1996.

562. Vander Hoeven M, Brouwer E, Blanco C: Nasal high frequency ventilation in neonates with moderate respiratory insufficiency, *Arch Dis Child Fetal Network Educ* 79:F61, 1998.

563. Van Marter LJ, Allred EN, Pagano M et al: Do clinical markers of barotrauma and oxygen toxicity explain interhospital variation in rates of chronic lung disease? *Pediatrics* 105:1194, 2000.

564. Van Marter LJ, Leviton A, Allred EN et al: Hydration during the first days of life and the risk of bronchopulmonary dysplasia in low birth weight infants, *J Pediatr* 116:942, 1990.

565. Van Marter LJ, Pagano M, Allred EN et al: Rate of bronchopulmonary dysplasia as a function of neonatal intensive care practices, *J Pediatr* 120:938, 1992.

566. Varnholt V, Lasch P, Suske G et al: High frequency oscillatory ventilation and extracorporeal membrane oxygenation in severe persistent pulmonary hypertension of the newborn, *Eur J Pediatr* 151:769, 1992.

567. Vaucher Y, Dudell G, Bejar R et al: Predictors of early childhood outcome in candidates for ECMO, *Pediatrics* 128:109, 1996.

568. Velasco-Whetsell M, Evans J, Wang M: Do postsuctioning transcutaneous PO_2 values change when a neonate's movements are restrained? *J Perinatol* 12:333, 1992.

569. Verclan M: BPD: its effects upon the heart and lungs, *Neonatal Netw* 16:5, 1997.

570. Verder H, Albertsen P, Ebbesen F et al: Nasal continuous positive airway pressure and early surfactant therapy for respiratory distress syndrome in newborns of less than 30 weeks' gestation, *Pediatrics* 103:E241, 1999.

571. Vermont Oxford Network: 1998 Database Summary, Burlington, VT: Vermont Oxford Network, 1999.

572. Vermont-Oxford Neonatal Network: A multicenter, randomized trial comparing synthetic surfactant with modified bovine surfactant extract in the treatment of neonatal RDS, *Pediatrics* 97:1, 1996.

573. Vermont-Oxford Trials Network Database Project: The Vermont-Oxford Trials Network: very low birth weight outcomes for 1990, *Pediatrics* 9:540, 1993.

574. Vijayakumar E, Ward G, Bullock C et al: Pulse oximetry in infants <1500 gm birth weight on supplemental oxygen: a national survey, *J Perinatol* 17:341, 1997.

575. Visveshwara N et al: Patient triggered synchronized assisted ventilation of newborns: report of a preliminary study and three years experience, *J Perinatol* XI:347, 1991.

576. Vohr BR, Wright LL, Dusick AM et al: Neurodevelopmental and functional outcomes of extremely low birth weight infants in the National Institute of Child Health and Human Development Neonatal Research Network, 1993-1994, *Pediatrics* 105:1216, 2000.

577. Voyles JB: Bronchopulmonary dysplasia, *Am J Nurs* 81:51, 1981.

578. Wagaman MJ, Shutack JG, Moornjian AS et al: Improved oxygenation and lung compliance with prone positioning of neonates, *J Pediatr* 94:787, 1979.

579. Walsh CM, Bada HS, Korones SB et al: Controlled supplemental oxygenation during tracheobronchial hygiene, *Nurs Res* 36:211, 1987.

580. Walsh-Sukys MC, Bauer RE, Cornell DJ et al: Severe respiratory failure in neonates: mortality and morbidity rates and neurodevelopmental outcomes, *J Pediatr* 125:104, 1994.

581. Walsh-Sukys MC, Tyson JE, Wright LL et al: Persistent pulmonary hypertension of the newborn in the era before nitric oxide: practice variation and outcomes, *Pediatrics* 105:14, 2000.

582. Ward R, Lemons J, Molteni R: Cisapride: a survey of frequency of use and adverse events in premature newborns, *Pediatrics* 103:469, 1999.

583. Wardle S, Hughes A, Chen S et al: Randomized controlled trial of oral vitamin A supplementation in preterm infants to prevent chronic lung disease, *Arch Dis Child Fetal Neonatal Educ* 84:F9, 2001.

584. Watterberg K, Scott S: Evidence of early adrenal insufficiency in babies who develop BPD, *Pediatrics* 95:120, 1995.

585. Watterberg K, Demers L, Scott S et al: Chorioamnionitis and early lung inflammation in infants in whom bronchopulmonary dysplasia develops, *Pediatrics* 97:210, 1996.

586. Watterberg K, Gerdes J, Gifford K et al: Prophylaxis against early adrenal insufficiency to prevent CLD in preterm infants, *Pediatrics* 104:1258, 1999.

587. Watterberg KL, Scott SM, Backstrom C et al: Links between early adrenal function and respiratory outcome in preterm infants: airway inflammation and patent ductus arteriosus, *Pediatrics* 105:320, 2000.

588. Weichsel M: The therapeutic use of glucocorticoid hormones in the neonatal period: potential neurological hazards, *Ann Neurol* 2:364, 1977.

589. Wells LR, Papile LA, Gardner MO et al: Impact of antenatal corticosteroid therapy in very low birth weight infants on chronic lung disease and other morbidities of prematurity, *J Perinatol* 19:578, 1999.

590. Whitelaw A, Thorensen M: Antenatal steroids and the developing brain, *Arch Dis Child Fetal Neonatal Educ* 83:154, 2000.

591. Whitfield M, Rogers M, Grunau R et al: Neurodevelopmental outcome at 18 mo. following photocoagulation for severe ROP compared to controls, *Pediatr Res* 47:440A, 2000.

592. Williams PD, Press A, Williams AR et al: Fatigue in mothers of infants discharged to the home on apnea monitors, *Appl Nurs Res* 12:69, 1999.

593. Wilson B, Donn S, Sinha A et al: Does spontaneous minute ventilation predict readiness for extubation in mechanically ventilated preterm infants? *Pediatr Res* 43:303A, 1998.

594. Wilson G et al: Evaluation of two endotracheal suction regimes in babies ventilated for respiratory distress syndrome, *Early Hum Dev* 25:87, 1991.

595. Wilson J, Arnold C, Connor R et al: Evaluation of oxygen delivery with use of nasopharyngeal catheters and nasal cannulas, *Neonatal Netww* 15:15, 1996.

596. Wiswell T, Bent R: Meconium staining and the meconium aspiration syndrome, *Pediatr Clin North Am* 40: 955, 1993.

597. Wiswell T, Fuloria M: Management of meconium-stained amniotic fluid, *Clin Perinatol* 26:659, 1999.

598. Wiswell T, Henley M: Intratracheal suctioning, systemic infection and the MAS, *Pediatrics* 89:203, 1992.

599. Wiswell T, Gannon CM, Jacob J: Delivery room management of the apparently vigorous meconium-stained neonate: results of the multicenter collaborative trial, *Pediatrics* 105:1, 2000.

600. Wiswell T, Graziani LJ, Kornhauser MS et al: Effects of hypocarbia on the development of cystic periventricular leukomalacia in premature infants treated with high-frequency jet ventilation, *Pediatrics* 98:918, 1996.

601. Wittmer MT, Hess D, Simmons M: An evaluation of the effectiveness of secretion removal with the Ballard closed-circuit catheter, *Respir Care* 36:844, 1991.

602. Wood B: Infant ribs: generalized periosteal reaction resulting from vibrator chest physiotherapy, *Radiology* 162:811, 1987.

603. Wright J: Closed-suctioning procedure in neonates, *Neonatal Netw* 15:87, 1996.

604. Wrightson D: Suctioning smarter: answers to eight common questions about endotracheal suctioning in neonates, *Neonatal Netw* 18:51, 1999.

605. Yamada Y, Sugai M, Woo M et al: Acquired subglottic stenosis caused by methicillin resistant *Staphylococcus aureus* that produce epidermal cell differentiation inhibitor, *Arch Dis Child Fetal Neonatal Educ* 84:F38, 2001.

606. Yeh TF, Torre JA, Rastoqi A et al: Early postnatal dexamethasone therapy in premature infants with severe respiratory distress syndrome: a double-blind controlled study, *J Pediatr* 117:273, 1990.

607. Yeh TF, Lin YJ, Huang CC et al: Early dexamethasone therapy in preterm infants: a follow-up study, *Pediatrics* 101:E71, 1998.

608. Yeo KL, Perlman M, Hao Y et al: Outcomes of extremely preterm infants related to their peak serum bilirubin concentrations and exposure to phototherapy, *Pediatrics* 102:1426, 1998.

609. Yoon BH, Romero R, Jun JK et al: Amniotic fluid cytokines (interleukin-6, tumor necrosis factor-alpha, interleukin-1 beta, and interleukin-8) and the risk for the development of bronchopulmonary dysplasia, *Am J Obstet Gynecol* 177:825, 1997.

610. Young TE, Kruyer LS, Marshall DD et al: Population-based study of chronic lung disease in very low birth weight infants in North Carolina in 1994 with comparisons with 1984, *Pediatrics* 104:292, 1999.

611. Yuksel B, Greenough A, Gamsu H: Neonatal MAS and respiratory morbidity during infancy, *Pediatr Pulmonol* 16:358, 1993.

612. Zanardo V, Ronconi M, Magarotto M et al: Maternal anxiety level during home oxygen therapy of infants with CLD, *Pediatr Res* 47:442A, 2000.

613. Zayek M, Hamm C, O'Donnell K et al: Induced moderate hypothermia markedly exacerbates pulmonary hypertension and dysfunction of neonatal piglet model of elevated pulmonary vascular resistance, *Pediatr Res* 47:442A, 2000.

614. Zimmerman J: Bronchoalveolar inflammatory pathophysiology of BPD, *Clin Perinatol* 22:429, 1995.

615. Zola Me, Gunkel JH, Chan RK et al: Comparison of three dosing procedures for administration of bovine surfactant to neonates with respiratory distress syndrome, *J Pediatr* 122:453, 1993.

24 Cardiovascular Diseases and Surgical Interventions

Kimberly D. Montoya, Reginald L. Washington

Approximately one of every 100 infants has a congenital heart defect. Some infants have life-threatening defects requiring immediate action within the first few hours or days of life.[7] Others require no intervention until later in life, or possibly not at all. It is important for the practitioner to recognize the presence of congenital heart disease, differentiate it from other conditions, and institute appropriate treatment. This chapter is designed to give the reader a clear understanding of neonatal circulation, signs and symptoms of congenital heart disease, and current management practices.

CONGENITAL HEART DISEASE OVERVIEW

Physiology

Profound hemodynamic changes occur with the delivery of the newborn. Sancoucie and Cavaliere[16] provide an excellent detailed review of this topic. However, because a basic understanding of these physiologic principles is mandatory to understanding congenital heart disease, these principles are briefly presented here.

Fetal Circulation

Three shunts affect fetal circulation: the ductus venosus, the ductus arteriosus, and the foramen ovale. These three shunts allow mixing of the fetal blood and are important in the development of a normal heart.

The blood with the highest oxygen saturation in the fetus is in the umbilical veins and is shunted directly to the heart, bypassing the liver through the ductus venosus. Once in the heart, most of this highly saturated blood is shunted directly through the foramen ovale to the left atrium, left ventricle, and aorta. Therefore the blood with the highest oxygen saturation is directed to the tissues with the highest oxygen demand—the myocardium and the

brain. The desaturated blood returning to the superior vena cava is primarily directed into the right ventricle, main pulmonary artery, ductus arteriosus, and descending aorta. where it ultimately enters the placental circulation and is resaturated. Only a small percentage of blood flow is directed to the fetal lungs, where oxygen is delivered to the lung tissue rather than extracted from it.

Changes That Occur in the Fetal Circulation With Birth. In utero the systemic vascular resistance is low, primarily because of the low resistance in the placenta. The pulmonary arterioles, which are constricted and hypertrophied, are relatively resistant to blood flow. At birth the placenta is removed from the circulation, thereby greatly increasing the systemic vascular resistance. Initiation of respirations produces increased oxygen tension, which decreases pulmonary vascular resistance and increases pulmonary blood flow. In addition, the left atrial pressure increases, closing the foramen ovale and eliminating the right-to-left shunt through the foramen ovale (Figure 4-1).

The ductus arteriosus is extremely sensitive to the oxygen content of the blood. The neonatal PaO_2 increases after birth and initiates the constriction of the ductus arteriosus.

Once these changes take place, the newborn's circulation resembles that of an adult. Desaturated blood returns to the heart by the inferior and superior venae cavae and enters the right atrium, right ventricle, pulmonary artery, and pulmonary circulation where oxygen and carbon dioxide are exchanged. The saturated blood then returns to the heart through the pulmonary venous system and enters the left atrium, left ventricle, and ultimately the aorta and systemic arterial system. However, pulmonary vascular resistance and pressures in the right ventricle and pulmonary system remain elevated in the neonate because of the hypertrophy of the pulmonary vessels. This hypertrophy slowly resolves, and the pulmonary vascular resistance and right heart pressures decrease to normal low levels between 1 and 2 months of age.

Etiology

Traditionally, the etiologic picture for congenital heart defects has been viewed as multifactorial, involving a complex interaction between genetic and environmental factors.[15] Population-based studies have revealed data challenging these views. One study, the Baltimore-Washington Infant Study, identified all liveborn infants with a heart defect in the mid-Atlantic region and compared environmental and genetic characteristics.[14] The single greatest risk factor was genetic, defined as a history of congenital cardiovascular disease in the family. Additionally, familial congenital heart defects were often concordant by phenotype and developmental mechanism. Table 24-1 lists the most common environmental risk factors and Box 24-1 lists other risk factors associated with an increased likelihood of congenital heart defects.[14] These studies, plus the recent advances toward identification of specific genes responsible for certain cardiovascular defects, suggest that genetic factors play a far more prevalent role than previously thought.[4]

Table 24-1	MOST COMMON ENVIRONMENTAL TRIGGERS AND SPECIFIC DEFECTS ASSOCIATED WITH EACH		
POTENTIAL TERATOGENS	FREQUENCY OF CARDIOVASCULAR DISEASE (%)	MOST COMMON MALFORMATIONS	
Drugs			
Alcohol	25-30	Ventricular septal defect, patent ductus arteriosus, atrial septal defect	
Amphetamines	5-10	Ventricular septal defect, patent ductus arteriosus, atrial septal defect, transposition of great arteries	
Anticonvulsants	2-3	Pulmonary stenosis, aortic stenosis, coarctation of aorta, patent ductus arteriosus	
Trimethadione	15-30	Transposition of great arteries, tetralogy of Fallot, hypoplastic left heart syndrome	
Lithium	10	Ebstein's anomaly, tricuspid atresia, atrial septal defect	
Sex hormones	2-4	Ventricular septal defect, transposition of great arteries, tetralogy of Fallot	
Infections			
Rubella	35	Peripheral pulmonary artery stenosis, ventricular septal defect, patent ductus arteriosus, atrial septal defect	
Maternal Conditions			
Diabetes	3-5	Transposition of great arteries, ventricular septal defect, coarctation of aorta	
	30-50	Cardiomegaly, myopathy	
Lupus erythematosus	?	Heart block	

Box 24-1	OTHER RISK FACTORS ASSOCIATED WITH CONGENITAL HEART DEFECTS

Exposure to Environmental Agents During Work and/or Hobby

- Paternal exposure to cold temperature
- Maternal exposure to various solvents, hairdyes, autobody repair work

Drug Exposure

- Diazepam, phenothiazines
- Corticosteroids
- Gastrointestinal drugs
- Paternal exposure to cocaine

Maternal Reproductive History

- Genetic risk factor (family history of congenital heart disease), >3 prior pregnancies and an increased number of miscarriages
- Without genetic risk but with premature births and previous induced abortion

Syndromic Associations

- 27.7% of all cases had either chromosomal anomalies, heritable syndromes, or an additional major organ system defect (see Table 24-2)

About 8% of congenital heart defects are associated with specific syndromes (e.g., trisomy 21 syndrome and Turner's syndrome) (Table 24-2). An additional 2% of congenital heart defects predominantly originate because of known environmental factors (rubella, maternal anticonvulsant therapy, or maternal alcohol consumption). Approximately 1% of infants in North America have congenital heart disease. Approximately 50% of these have a ventricular septal defect (VSD) alone or in combination with other cardiac abnormalities. Table 24-3 shows the most common congenital heart defects and their time of presentation.

Data Collection

History

A family history of congenital heart disease, a prenatal history of maternal viral infections (rubella and CMV) or drug or toxic substance ingestion, asphyxia or dysrhythmias before or at birth, a history of hydrops fetalis, or Rh incompatibility give clues about the possible presence of congenital heart dis-

Table 24-2	CHROMOSOMAL ABERRATIONS EVIDENT IN NEONATAL PERIOD THAT ARE ASSOCIATED WITH CONGENITAL HEART DISEASE			
POPULATION	**INCIDENCE OF CONGENITAL HEART DISEASE (%)**	**MOST COMMON LESIONS**		
		1	**2**	**3**
Trisomy 21 syndrome	50	Ventricular septal defect, endocardial cushion defect	Atrial septal defect	Patent ductus arteriosus
Trisomy 18 syndrome	99+	Ventricular septal defect	Patent ductus arteriosus	Pulmonary stenosis
Trisomy 13 syndrome	90	Ventricular septal defect	Patent ductus arteriosus	Dextrocardia
Turner's syndrome	35	Coarctation of aorta	Aortic stenosis	Atrial septal defect
DiGeorge Deletion 22q[10]	50	Truncus	Tetrology of Fallot	Interrupted aortic arch

Table 24-3	DIAGNOSIS OF INFANTS AT SELECTED AGES*				
0-6 DAYS (%)		**7-13 DAYS (%)**		**13-20 DAYS (%)**	
Transposition of great arteries	(17)	Coarctation of aorta	(19)	Ventricular septal defect	(20)
Hypoplastic left ventricle	(12)	Ventricular septal defect	(15)	Transposition of great arteries	(17)
Lung disease	(10)	Hypoplastic left ventricle	(11)	Coarctation of aorta	(16)
Tetralogy of Fallot	(9)	Transpostion of great arteries	(9)	Tetralogy of Fallot	(8)
Coarctation of aorta	(7)	Tetralogy of Fallot	(6)	Endocardial cushion defect	(6)
Ventricular septal defect	(7)	Heterotaxia	(4)	Heterotaxia	(6)
Pulmonary atresia (with intact ventricular septum)	(7)	Truncus arteriosus	(4)	Patent ductus arteriosus	(4)
Heterotaxia	(6)	Single ventricle	(4)	Total anomalous pulmonary venous return	(3)
Other	(25)	Other	(28)	Other	(20)
Total 896	(100)	Total 210	(100)	Total 116	(100)

From Fyler D et al: Report of the New England Regional Infant Cardiac Program, *Pediatrics* 65:391, 1980.
*These numbers are intended as a rough guideline because there is considerable overlap. Infants with congenital heart disease are often active initially and appear well for several hours or days after birth. In contrast, infants with respiratory distress often have characteristic symptoms within the first several hours after birth.

ease. **The timing of the onset of symptoms may indicate the type of anomaly (see Table 24-3).**

Clinical Presentation of Infants With Severe Cardiac Disease

Newborns with severe congenital heart disease usually have one or more of the following signs or symptoms: (1) cyanosis, (2) respiratory distress, (3) congestive heart failure and diminished cardiac output, (4) abnormal cardiac rhythm, and (5) cardiac murmurs. Although cardiac murmurs in the neonatal period do not necessarily indicate severe cardiac disease, they must be carefully evaluated. Absence of a murmur does not exclude cardiac disease. **Infants with severe life-threatening congenital anomalies of the cardiovascular system may not have a murmur.**

Each of these previously mentioned categories is considered on an individual basis. The differential diagnosis of any individual sign or symptom is important, especially in the neonatal period, when there is considerable overlap and several disease entities have identical symptoms. In this section we will discuss each sign or symptom and briefly detail the laboratory evaluation of each.

Cyanosis. **Cyanosis is a bluish discoloration of the skin, nail beds, and mucous membranes resulting from the presence of 3 mg/dl or more of reduced hemoglobin in the arterial blood or 4 to 5 mg/dl or more of reduced hemoglobin in the peripheral capillary blood.** Cyanosis therefore depends on the total hemoglobin concentration and the arterial oxygen saturation and requires immediate assessment.

When the causes of cyanosis are being considered, the six components of oxygen delivery must be considered individually. These are the CNS, musculoskeletal system, airways, gas exchange interface in the lungs, hemoglobin, and cardiovascular system. Each of these is briefly reviewed here. The reader is referred to other sections of this book for a more complete discussion of the individual lesions.

Several disorders of the CNS and neuromuscular system cause poor oxygenation as a result of the abnormal rate or rhythm of respiration. Iatrogenic depression of the cardiovascular system may result from the anesthetic administered to the mother before delivery. Birth trauma can cause either asphyxia or diaphragmatic paralysis and result in generalized cyanosis. Metabolic abnormalities that

cause neuroencephalopathy and resultant cyanosis are hypoglycemia and hypocalcemia.

Several disorders of the lung result in poor oxygenation from alveolar hypoventilation. These include hypoplastic lung, bronchiogenic cysts, pulmonary arteriovenous malformation, atelectasis with resultant lobar emphysema, pneumothorax, aspiration pneumonia, RDS, and shock lung. Differentiating between these disorders and primary cardiac disease is often difficult.

Because the cyanosis depends on the amount of reduced hemoglobin present, any abnormality of the blood that alters either the hemoglobin structure or content may result in cyanosis. Disorders such as polycythemia, hypovolemia, methemoglobinemia, and other hemoglobinopathies may account for cyanosis and must always be considered.

Finally, several disorders of the cardiovascular-pulmonary system may cause cyanosis, even though they do not involve actual structural defects. These include persistent pulmonary hypertension, pulmonary edema, dysrhythmias, and low cardiac output from any cause.

Respiratory Distress. Respiratory distress may occur from pulmonary venous congestion as a result of a defect in the cardiovascular system, pulmonary disease, or both. This differentiation is often difficult, and newborns may have both primary pulmonary disease and cardiac defects.

Most infants with cyanosis from congenital heart disease do not have respiratory distress. When respiratory distress is present, the cyanosis is not proportional to the amount of respiratory distress evaluated from the physical and chest x-ray examinations. **If cyanosis is present and is caused by a fixed right-to-left shunt (cardiac lesion) increasing inspired oxygen will have little effect on the arterial blood gases.** However, if the cyanosis is caused by a diffusion defect in the lungs (pulmonary disorder), the degree of cyanosis often decreases with increasing inspired oxygen.

The shunt study is beneficial in differentiating respiratory disease from cyanotic heart disease. Shunt studies are performed by obtaining arterial blood gas measurements (preferably from the right radial artery) when the infant is in room air and then after the infant has been in 100% oxygen for 5 to 10 minutes. If the PaO_2 is greater than 150 mm Hg, the presence of a right-to-left shunt and cyanotic congenital heart disease as the cause of cyanosis is unlikely.

Congestive Heart Failure. Congestive heart failure is a clinical syndrome reflecting the inability of the myocardium to meet the metabolic requirements of the body. Therefore the signs and symptoms of congestive heart failure reflect the decreased cardiac output and decreased tissue perfusion.

Congestive heart failure may be caused by (1) volume overload, (2) pressure overload, (3) cardiomyopathy, or (4) dysrhythmias. However, in the newborn, asphyxia and anemia must also be considered as causes of congestive heart failure.

The common symptoms associated with congestive heart failure can be explained using the physiologic principles previously outlined.

Tachycardia. The heart attempts to compensate for the decrease in cardiac output by increasing either the heart rate or the stroke volume (CO = HR × SV). The newborn has a reduced capacity to increase stroke volume, primarily because the fetal myocardium has relatively few contractile elements and is poorly innervated by the sympathetic nervous system. **Therefore the newborn increases cardiac output mainly by increasing the heart rate, resulting in tachycardia.**

Cardiac Enlargement. Dilation and/or hypertrophy of the heart occurs in response to the volume or pressure overload, or the dysfunction associated with cardiomyopathies and dysrhythmias. Dilation of the cardiac chambers is evident on chest x-ray examination, with enlargement of the cardiac silhouette.

Tachypnea. Inefficient emptying or overloading of the lungs results in interstitial pulmonary edema. Tachypnea is the first clinical manifestation of pulmonary edema. As pulmonary edema progresses, however, alveolar and bronchiolar edema occur, resulting in intercostal retractions, grunting, nasal flaring, dyspnea, rales, and possibly cyanosis.

Gallop Rhythm. The gallop rhythm is an abnormal filling sound caused by the dilation of the ventricles. It is heard as a triple rhythm on auscultation.

Decreased Peripheral Pulses and Mottling of the Extremities. Decreased cardiac output results in a compensatory redistribuiton of blood flow to vital tissues. Peripheral tissue perfusion is therefore decreased, resulting in mottling of the skin and a grayish or pale skin color, as well as decreased pulses.

Decreased Urine Output and Edema. Decreased renal perfusion results in decreased glomerular filtration. This is interpreted by the body as a decrease in intravascular volume, initiating compensatory mechanisms such as vasoconstriction and fluid and sodium retention. **Infants normally manifest this as weight gain or may have periorbital edema.**

Diaphoresis. Diaphoresis represents the increased metabolic rate with congestive heart failure and most likely increased activity of the autonomic nervous system. The increased metabolic rate is in response to the increased workload of the heart in failure.

Hepatomegaly. The right ventricle in congestive heart failure is less compliant and may not adequately empty, leading to elevated pressures in the right atrium, central venous system, and hepatic system. **Hepatomegaly results from hepatic congestion caused by the elevated central venous pressure.**

Decreased Exercise Activity. The decreased perfusion to peripheral tissues and the increased energy required by the heart in failure leave little energy reserve for activities such as feeding and crying. The infant may sleep a majority of the time, fall asleep during feedings, and have a weak cry.

Failure to Thrive and Feeding Problems. Multiple factors contribute to the infant's failure to thrive and feeding difficulties. **Tachypnea compromises the infant's ability to feed. The basal metabolic rate increases in infants with congestive heart failure, necessitating a higher caloric intake (150 kcal or more).** The infant must expend more energy to consume the calories but lacks the energy to do so.

Diminished Cardiac Output. An infant with poor peripheral pulses and skin mottling often has a profound decrease in cardiac output. This is commonly found in infants with coarctation of the aorta or hypoplastic left heart syndrome but may also be noted in asphyxia, metabolic disease, and sepsis.

Abnormalities of the cardiac rhythm and murmurs are discussed individually later.

Cardiac Examination

See the section on specific cardiac lesions.

Laboratory Data

Arterial Blood Gases. The $PaCO_2$ in cardiac disease is often normal or increased if a primary pulmonary disease is present. Frequent monitoring of blood gases is unnecessary, but the acid-base balance should be monitored closely. The $PaCO_2$ may be normal or decreased, depending on the cardiac lesion and pulmonary status of the infant.

Chest X-ray Examination. The chest x-ray examination may be normal even if life-threatening congenital heart disease is present. However, the degree of pulmonary vascularity helps define the type of congenital heart disease present and is characterized as being increased, normal, or decreased. Likewise, the heart size should be evaluated and is described as being increased, normal, or decreased.

Electrocardiogram. See the section on specific cardiac lesions.

Echocardiogram. Echocardiograms are used to define cardiac anatomy, estimate pressures, measure gradients, and evaluate cardiac function. The transthoracic echocardiogram is the most commonly used approach. It is noninvasive and performed with the transducer on the infant's chest. The transesophageal echocardiogram (TEE) is used for intraoperative and postoperative evaluations, as well as in patients in whom it is not possible to obtain adequate views of the cardiac anatomy or evaluation of function by transthoracic echo. TEE requires general anesthesia for control of the airway and patient comfort. TEE can be performed on infants as small as 2500 g.

MRI offers three-dimensional reconstruction and high-resolution images of the heart and great vessels. The MRI is of particular use in evaluation of extracardiac vascularity, such as arch anomalies, vascular rings, and pulmonary arterial venous anomalies. The MRI provides high spatial resolution, excellent soft-tissue definition, a large field of view, and unrestricted demonstration of cardiovascular morphology. It does require sedation and a stable patient, and it is expensive.

General Treatment Strategy

Optimal management of infants with heart disease requires specialized expertise. Infants are monitored closely for hypoxia, hypoglycemia, acidosis, and congestive heart failure.

The infant must be kept in an incubator or warmer in which body temperature is maintained while color changes (pallor and increased cyanosis) may be observed. A cardiorespiratory monitor for continuous cardiac monitoring detects bradycardia, tachycardia, and dysrhythmias. Monitoring of oxygen saturations is helpful in determining adequacy of pulmonary blood flow and/or increased need for oxygen. The respiratory effort is assessed for tachypnea, shallow breathing, apnea, retractions, grunting, and nasal flaring. Observe and document activity level such as muscle tone, spontaneous movement, and seizure activity.

Management of Congestive Heart Failure[6]

The medical management of congestive heart failure attempts to reverse the process outlined previously and helps the heart compensate with increased cardiac output.

Digoxin acts primarily as a positive inotropic (improves contractility) agent but decreases the heart rate and increases urine output (Box 24-2). This drug should be used with caution if acidosis, myocarditis, or obstructive lesions (e.g., tetralogy of Fallot, subvalvular pulmonary stenosis, and asymmetric septal hypertrophy) are present.

Diuretics such as furosemide (Table 24-4) help decrease total body water (which is increased as a result of congestive heart failure). In general, chronic fluid restriction and low-salt diets are not commonly used in newborns or infants with congestive heart failure.

Infants with congestive heart failure may be difficult to feed, and the process is often frustrating. They may have trouble sucking, swallowing, and breathing simultaneously. They may need to rest frequently during a feeding, thus prolonging feeding times, and they may fall asleep exhausted before adequate caloric intake is achieved. **Because caloric requirements are higher in infants with congenital heart disease, adequate nutrition must be assured by (1) observing the infant's ability to nipple feed (a soft free-flowing [premature] nipple offers the least resistance to sucking and helps the infant conserve energy), (2) providing adequate calories for growth and if necessary using alternative feeding methods (i.e., gavage or continuous nasogastric drip) if the infant is sucking poorly, (3) anticipating the infant's hunger and offering feedings before the infant uses energy by crying, (4) positioning the infant in a semierect position for feeding, (5) burping the infant after every half ounce to help minimize vomiting, and (6) weighing the infant daily and checking for appropriate weight**

Table 24-4 CARDIAC DRUGS

DRUG	ROUTE	DOSE	ONSET OF ACTION	COMMENTS
Atropine	IV	0.01-0.03 mg/kg/dose PRN (max 0.4 mg)	Seconds	May cause tachycardia, urinary retention, or hyperthermia
	PO	0.01-0.03 mg/kg/dose q 4-6 hr (max 0.4 mg)	Minutes	May cause tachycardia
Calcium chloride (10% solution)	IV	0.2-0.3 ml (20-30 mg)/kg/dose q 10 min PRN (max 500 mg)	Minutes	Slow infusion; must be IV; potentiates digoxin; bradycardia
Diazoxide (Hyperstat)*	IV	5 mg/kg/dose q 30 min PRN	1-2 min	May cause hypotension or hyperglycemia
Dobutamine (Dobutrex)†	IV	2-10 µg/kg/min	Minutes	Do not use in IHSS or tetralogy of Fallot; may cause ventricular ectopy, tachycardia, or hypertension Incompatible with alkaline solutions
Dopamine (Intropin)*	IV	5-30 µg/kg/min	Minutes	Often combined with a vasodilator when used at higher doses to counteract alpha vessel constriction; inactivated in alkaline solution
Epinephrine (1:10,000)	IV	0.1 ml/kg/dose (max 5 ml/dose) q 3-5 min PRN (0.01 mg/kg/dose)	Seconds	May cause tachycardia, dysrhythmias, or hypertension; not effective if acidosis is present
Furosemide (Lasix)	IV	1-2 mg/kg/dose	5-15 min	May cause metabolic alkalosis + hypokalemia
	PO	1-4 mg/kg/dose	30-60 min	Follow electrolytes; may need KCl supplementation; renal calcification
Hydralazine (Apresoline)	IV	0.1-0.5 mg/kg/dose q 3-6 hr	15-30 min	May cause lupuslike syndrome, tachycardia, or hypotension
	PO	0.1-0.5 mg/kg q 6 hr; may increase to max of 2 mg/kg q 6 hr	Often days until titrated effect achieved	Same as above
Hydrochlorothiazide (HydroDiuril)	PO	1-2 mg/kg q 12 hr	1-2 hr	May cause electrolyte imbalance; may need KCl supplementation

*Safety and efficacy of these agents in children have not been established.
†Mix: 6 × weight (kg) = milligrams to be added to 100 ml D₅W. Yields: 1 ml/hr = 1 µg/kg/min.
  Example: 6 × 3 kg = 18 mg (dopamine, dobutamine, or Nipride) to be added to 100 ml D₅W.

Table 24-4   CARDIAC DRUGS—cont'd

DRUG	ROUTE	DOSE	ONSET OF ACTION	COMMENTS
Indomethacin	IV	0.1-0.2 μg/kg/dose; may be repeated q 8 hr for total of 3 doses		Less effective if administered after 7 days of age; probably will have no effect after 14 days of age
Isoproterenol (Isuprel)‡	IV	0.1-0.4 μg/kg/min	30-60 sec	May cause tachycardia/ventricular tachy-dysrhythias; may also cause subendo-cardial ischemia
Lidocaine (Xylocaine)	IV	IV bolus 1-3 mg/kg; IV drip 30-50 μg/kg/min		May cause dysrhythmia, CNS agitation, or depression
Nitroprusside (Nipride)†	IV	1-10 μg/kg/min over 10 min to control blood pressure; chronic infusion—2 μg/kg/min (protect from light; change solution q 4 hr)	Seconds	May cause hypotension and reflex tachycardia; may cause thiocyanate toxicity, especially if decreased renal function is present
Phentolamine (Regitine)	IV	1-20 μg/kg/min	5-10 min	May cause hypotension; commonly used with an inotropic agent
	PO	5 mg/kg/day qid	N/A	May cause hypotension
Phenytoin (Dilantin)	IV	Load: 10-15 mg/kg over 5 min slow infusion Maintenance: 3-5 mg/kg/day bid	5-10 min	May cause cardiac depression
	PO	3-5 mg/kg/day bid	2-4 hr	Therapeutic blood levels (5-20 μg/ml)
Procainamide (Pronestyl)	IV	Load: 10-15 mg/kg/dose (max 1000 mg) over 5 min Maintenance: IV 30-80 μg/kg/min	1-5 min	May cause hypotension or lupuslike syndrome
	IM	5-8 mg/kg q 6 hr	15-30 min	Same as above
Propranolol (Inderal)	IV	Dysrhythmias: 0.01-0.15 mg/kg/dose slow IV q 6-8 hr PRN (max single dose, 10 mg); hypercyanotic spell: 0.15-0.25 mg/kg/dose slow IV push q 15 min (max dose 10 mg)	2-5 min	May severely decrease cardiac output
	PO	Dysrhythmias: 0.5-1.0 mg/kg/dose tid-qid (max daily dose 60 mg); hypercyanotic spells: 1-2 mg/kg/dose qid	30-60 min	Same as above
Prostaglandin E₁ (Prostin VR)	IV	0.01-0.1 μg/kg/min	Minutes	May cause apnea, fever, or hypotension
Quinidine gluconate (Duraquin)	PO	5-10 mg/kg q 6 hr	4-8 hr	May cause gastrointestinal symptoms, hypotension, or blood dyscrasia
Spironolactone (Aldactone)	PO	1-2 mg/kg/day	3-5 days	Hyperkalemia, gastrointestinal upset, drowsiness
Tolazoline	IV	Test: 1-2 mg/kg slow IV push Maintenance: 1-2 mg/kg/hr	Minutes	May cause hypotension; gastrointestinal or pulmonary hemorrhage
Adenosine	IV	30-250 μg/kg		Slows the spontaneous heart rate and prolongs the PR interval, may cause transient complete heart block and hypotension, half-life is only 9.3 seconds so its effects quickly dissipate

‡Mix: 0.6 × weight (kg) = milligrams to be added to 100 ml D_5W. Yields: 1 ml/hr = 0.1 μg/kg/min.

Example: 0.6 × 3 kg = 1.8 mg (Isuprel) to be added to 100 ml D_5W.

†,‡From Pediatric Life Support, Children's Hospital and Medical Center, Seattle, Washington, 1987.

gain. **Before discharge from the nursery, the infant should be in stable condition (e.g., feeding well and gaining weight appropriately).**

An important fact for families to understand is that many infants will gain weight very slowly because of their cardiac defects, regardless of the method of feeding that is used. The family of an infant in congestive heart failure needs support and teaching. **Explanation of the term** *congestive heart failure* **should be given early, because it is a frightening term for parents. The words "heart failure" are often interpreted as "heart attack." It is important that parents understand that saying an infant is in heart failure does not imply that the infant's heart will stop.** A simple explanation describing heart failure as a condition in which the heart shows signs of being less able to pump sufficient blood to meet all the needs of the body is helpful in decreasing anxiety for the family.

SPECIFIC CONDITIONS[1,5,9,17-20]

Patent Ductus Arteriosus
Physiology
The ductus arteriosus is a normal pathway in the fetal circulatory system and allows blood from the right ventricle and pulmonary arterial system to flow into the descending aorta for ultimate delivery to the placenta (Figure 24-1). **Functionally, the PDA closes**

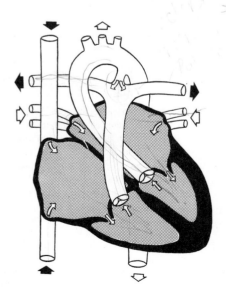

FIGURE 24-1 Patent ductus arteriosus. (Courtesy Ross Laboratories, Columbus, Ohio.)

within a few hours to several days after birth, but this closure is often delayed in premature infants. After birth, as a result of a decrease in the pressure of the pulmonary circulation and an increase in the pressure of the aorta, the blood flow through a PDA is predominantly from the aorta to the pulmonary artery (left-to-right shunt). The hemodynamic changes and the resultant clinical manifestations of a PDA depend on the magnitude of the pulmonary vascular resistance and the size of the ductal lumen.

Approximately 15% of infants with PDAs have additional cardiac defects (VSD, coarctation of the aorta, aortic stenosis, or pulmonary stenosis). PDA can be associated with known syndromes, most commonly rubella.

Data Collection
History. Asphyxial insult or RDS, inability to wean from a respirator, and an increasing Fio_2 demand usually accompany PDA.

Physical Findings. Increased flow to the pulmonary circulation and volume overload of the left ventricle are the two major physiologic abnormalities in a PDA.

Cyanosis. Generally, cyanosis is not present in an isolated PDA, because the predominant shunt is from left to right.

Heart Sounds. Infants with a PDA may have audible murmurs as a result of the left-to-right shunting through the ductus during systole. A grade I through III systolic murmur is best heard at the upper left sternal border with radiation to the left axilla and faintly to the back. Although this murmur may occasionally flow into diastole, the classical continuous machinery-like murmur is an unusual occurrence in the newborn period. It is often helpful to briefly disconnect the newborn from the ventilator before auscultating. There are cases of large PDAs in which no murmur is audible.

Pulses. Because of the rapid upstroke and wide pulse pressure, the peripheral pulses are bounding. Pulses are hyperdynamic and easily palpated. **Assessment of the pulses should include palpation of palmar, plantar, and calf pulses. The calf pulses are not usually palpable in infants.** The presence of an easily palpated pulse in these areas suggests the presence of an aortic run-off lesion, which is most commonly a PDA.

Congestive Heart Failure. Because of the volume overload of the left ventricle, the infant may show signs of congestive heart failure and pulmonary edema (see discussion of congestive heart failure).

Laboratory Data
Arterial Blood Gases. Arterial blood gas values are normal.

Chest X-ray Examination. Chest x-ray examination is normal in small shunts. Cardiomegaly is present with increased pulmonary vascularity in large shunts.

Electrocardiogram. The ECG may be normal, demonstrate left ventricular hypertrophy, or demonstrate combined ventricular hypertrophy. Ischemia is rarely seen.

Echocardiogram. An increased left atrial/aortic ratio suggests a moderate to large left-to-right shunt (i.e., PDA, VSD). **An echocardiogram should be performed before medical or surgical closure of the PDA to rule out a ductal-dependent lesion or other associated anomalies.** Color flow mapping allows for visualization of the PDA, as well as determination of the direction of blood flow across the PDA (i.e., left to right, right to left, or bidirectional).

Cardiac Catheterization. If the echocardiogram has eliminated a ductal-dependent lesion, cardiac catheterization is usually not required before treatment.

Treatment
Medical Management. Asymptomatic infants with PDAs generally do not require medical management or surgical ligation. These infants should be monitored for evidence of congestive heart failure, failure to thrive, increasing oxygen requirement, or other complications.

Symptomatic infants require ductal closure by either ductal ligation or indomethacin therapy. Medical management such as fluid restriction is rarely successful. Indomethacin is administered orally (PO) or intravenously (IV) at a dose of 0.1 to 0.2 mg/kg/dose and may be repeated every 8 hours for a total of three doses. It is much less effective if administered after 7 days of age and probably will have no effect after 14 days of age. Urine output should be continuously monitored, and if there is a dramatic decrease, the drug should be discontinued.

Surgical Treatment. **Surgical ligation or clipping the ductus arteriosus through a lateral thoracotomy incision is a low-risk procedure when performed by an experienced surgical team.** Coil closure of a PDA in the cardiac catheterization laboratory or video-assisted transthoracic endoscopic closure of a PDA is usually not done in infants less than 3 to 6 months of age.

Complications and Residual Effects
Complications and residual effects, although rare, include **(1) recannulization, (2) recurrent laryngeal or phrenic nerve palsies, or (3) false aneurysms. The surgical mortality in the neonatal period is generally less than 1%.**

Prognosis and Follow-up
Asymptomatic infants have an excellent prognosis, although close follow-up is necessary because if the ductus remains patent until 9 to 12 months of age, ligation is recommended.

Symptomatic infants with a persistent ductus arteriosus generally experience failure to thrive, continued congestive heart failure, increased oxygen requirements with resultant BPD, or pulmonary infections.

Ventricular Septal Defect
Physiology
VSDs may involve various portions of the ventricular septum and are classified according to the anatomic position that they occupy when viewed from the right ventricle (Figure 24-2).

A VSD may occur as an isolated anomaly or may be part of a more complex cardiac lesion. Only isolated VSDs are discussed in this section. The effect of the VSD on the circulation depends on both the size of the VSD and the relative pulmonary vascular resistance. Pulmonary vascular resistance is nearly systemic immediately after birth but rapidly falls to one-fourth to one-third systemic in the first several days of life.

In a small VSD the left-to-right shunting at the ventricular level is minimal and the infants are asymptomatic.

Larger VSDs may have a mild to moderate left-to-right shunt, resulting in congestive heart failure and pulmonary edema. Premature infants tend to have lower pulmonary vascular resistance at birth,

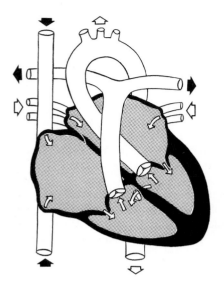

FIGURE 24-2 Ventricular septal defects. (Courtesy Ross Laboratories, Columbus, Ohio.)

allowing greater left-to-right shunting, and therefore may be symptomatic. Infants with severe lung disease (RDS, BPD, or pneumonia) may have elevated pulmonary vascular resistance and therefore minimal left-to-right shunting.

Data Collection

See Table 24-1 for infants at increased risk.

Physical Findings

Cyanosis. Infants with isolated VSDs are rarely cyanotic in the neonatal period.

Heart Sounds. Most infants with VSDs have a heart murmur. The time when this murmur is first audible depends on the pulmonary vascular resistance and the size of the defect. The murmur is typically a grade II to III/VI systolic murmur heard best at the lower left sternal border. A diastolic flow rumble at the apex indicates a large left-to-right shunt.

Congestive Heart Failure. Congestive heart failure is unusual in the newborn with an isolated VSD. When it occurs, however, it is a result of the volume overload of the left ventricle (see the section on congestive heart failure).

Laboratory Data

Arterial Blood Gases. Arterial blood gas values are normal.

Chest X-ray Examination. A chest x-ray examination shows a normal to increased heart size with an increased pulmonary vascular flow.

Electrocardiogram. The ECG in an infant with a VSD is usually normal but may demonstrate ventricular hypertrophy.

Echocardiogram. A two-dimensional echocardiogram is able to demonstrate the VSD in 90% of the cases. Doppler interrogation of the ventricular septum and/or color flow mapping have greatly increased the accuracy of diagnosing a VSD noninvasively. The use of color flow is particularly advantageous in identifying the presence of multiple VSDs and the direction of blood flow across the VSD.

Cardiac Catheterization. A cardiac catheterization is diagnostic but not required in the neonatal period unless there is some question regarding the diagnosis or if surgery is being considered.

Treatment

Medical Management. **If the patient demonstrates failure to thrive or intractable congestive heart failure with maximum medical management, surgical intervention at any age is necessary** (see the section on general treatment strategy).

Surgical Treatment. **Surgical treatment of a VSD consists of either suture closure or patching (using most commonly a synthetic material such as Dacron).** The surgical approach is through a median sternotomy incision. The defect is approached through the right atrium and tricuspid valve, thereby avoiding a right or left ventriculotomy.

If the infant is small (less than 2 kg) or single or multiple muscular VSDs are present, it may be necessary to perform a palliative procedure of pulmonary artery banding to decrease pulmonary blood flow until the infant is older and can undergo debanding and closure of the VSDs.

Complications and Residual Effects

Complications and/or residual effects may include (1) a persistent shunt (residual VSD), (2) conduction abnormalities (right bundle-branch block and third-degree heart block), and (3) aortic or tricuspid insufficiency (<1%).

The mortality in infants is less than 5%, with higher mortality found in the neonatal period.

Contraindications to primary VSD closure include the diagnosis of double-outlet right ventricle and multiple muscular VSDs. The combined risk of pulmonary banding plus later debanding and VSD closure is about 10%.

Prognosis and Follow-up

Approximately 50% to 75% of small VSDs will spontaneously close.

If a large left-to-right shunt is persistent after 9 to 24 months of age, the infant is susceptible to pulmonary vascular disease.

Coarctation of the Aorta

Physiology

Coarctation of the aorta is a localized constriction of the aorta that usually occurs at the junction of the transverse aortic arch and the descending aorta in the vicinity of the ductus arteriosus (Figure 24-3). However, coarctation can occur anywhere in the aorta from above the aortic valve to the abdominal aorta. The precise location of the coarctation and the presence or absence of associated anomalies affect the clinical presentation. **Associated anomalies include PDA, VSD, and bicuspid aortic valve (50%).** Coarctation is frequently observed in infants with Turner's syndrome.

Data Collection

Physical Findings. Newborns with critical coarctation of the aorta usually have signs and symptoms of congestive heart failure and low cardiac output. **Coarctation of the aorta is a medical and surgical emergency.**

Cyanosis. Generally, cyanosis in the newborn is not present in the isolated coarctation of the aorta.

Heart Sounds. Cardiac murmurs are generally not found in an isolated, severe coarctation of the aorta. If other associated cardiac defects are present, however, a murmur may be heard. A soft grade I to II/VI systolic murmur may be present at the left sternal border, radiating to the left axilla and to the back. A gallop rhythm is usually present. The murmurs of associated anomalies, however, are usually dominant.

Pulses and Blood Pressure. The blood pressure proximal to the area of obstruction is higher than the blood pressure distal to the area of obstruction. **The most consistent physical finding in infants with critical coarctation of the aorta is a higher**

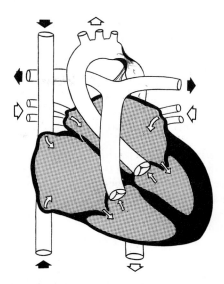

FIGURE 24-3 Coarctation of aorta. (Courtesy Ross Laboratories, Columbus, Ohio.)

systolic blood pressure (above 15 mm Hg) in the upper extremities than in the lower extremities. This blood pressure must be measured with the appropriate-size cuff. In addition, pulses are easily palpable in one or both upper extremities but are difficult to palpate or are absent in the lower extremities. **Pulses should be carefully evaluated in all extremities and blood pressures obtained in both arms and either leg.** The coarctation may occur between the subclavian arteries, or the right or left subclavian artery may arise aberrantly distal to the coarctation, resulting in a differential pulse and blood pressure between the right and left arms.

Congestive Heart Failure. Congestive heart failure is a common finding in infants with severe coarctation as a result of a pressure overload on the left ventricle (see the section on congestive heart failure).

Laboratory Data

Arterial Blood Gases. Arterial blood gas values are normal.

Chest X-ray Examination. Cardiomegaly may be seen on the x-ray film. Pulmonary vascularity is normal unless associated anomalies are present.

Electrocardiogram. Right ventricular hypertrophy is frequently present. Left ventricular hypertrophy or combined ventricular hypertrophy is rarely seen in the newborn period. The ECG may be normal.

Echocardiogram. The area of coarctation can often be visualized using two-dimensional techniques and color flow mapping. Abnormal Doppler blood flow is diagnostic. However, cautious interpretation of the findings is suggested, if a PDA is suspected.

Cardiac Catheterization. Cardiac catheterization is diagnostic and is commonly performed before any surgical procedure is undertaken to evaluate other associated anomalies.

Treatment

Medical Management. **Congestive heart failure should be treated aggressively. Intractable congestive heart failure, acidosis, oliguria, and hypertension are indications for corrective surgery as soon as possible.** (See the section on general treatment strategy of congenital heart disease.) Balloon dilation of the coarcted site has been performed in the catheterization laboratory at some institutions with variable success. A significant incidence of aortic wall aneurysm formation has been identified 6 to 12 months later.

Surgical Treatment. **The two most common surgical procedures are resection of the coarctation with end-to-end anastomosis or the subclavian flap aortoplasty.** With the former, the coarcted segment is resected and the ends of the aorta reanastomosed together. With the latter, a longitudinal incision is made in the aorta across the coarctated site and continued to the end of the distally divided left subclavian artery. The left subclavian artery is used as a patch or flap to increase the diameter of the aorta. Both procedures are performed through a lateral thoracotomy incision and have been highly successful in relieving coarctation and providing for future growth of the aorta. Absorbable suture material is often used with the intention of decreasing the incidence of recoarctation from rigid suture lines.

Complications and Residual Effects

Complications and residual effects include (1) diminished or absent pulses in the left arm, (2) persistent hypertension, (3) Horner's syndrome, (4) paraplegia (less than 0.5%), (5) mesenteric vasculitis, and (6) residual coarctation.

The overall operative mortality is <20% in infancy. However, the high mortality is usually related to preoperative status and associated lesions. Early detection and referral in addition to the use of prostaglandin E1 may dramatically reduce this mortality in the future.

Prognosis and Follow-up

Infants with mild coarctation require minimal care until later in life. If these patients are medically managed, close follow-up is mandatory, with cardiac catheterization and surgery expected at a later date.

Infants with severe coarctation require prompt medical and surgical treatment. If this therapy is instituted early, the prognosis is generally favorable. Untreated infants with severe coarctation often have a rapidly deteriorating clinical course with left ventricular failure, severe hypertension, or intractable congestive heart failure, and the prognosis is guarded. After surgical repair, frequent follow-up is required to ensure adequate coarctation repair. Cardiac catheterization may be required several months to years after the surgical procedure is completed if recoarctation is suspected (20%).

Critical Aortic Stenosis

Physiology

Obstruction of the left ventricular outlet may occur below the aortic valve, at the aortic valve, or above the aortic valve (subvalvular, valvular, or supravalvular aortic stenosis) (Figure 24-4).

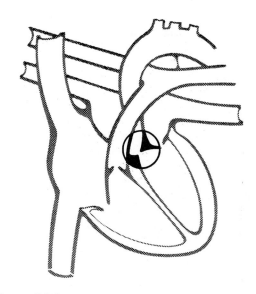

FIGURE 24-4 Aortic stenosis. (Courtesy Ross Laboratories, Columbus, Ohio.)

Valvular aortic stenosis is the most common type and is discussed here. A pressure gradient (the pressure difference from the left ventricle to the ascending aorta) of 50 mm Hg or more is indicative of significant aortic stenosis in the newborn.

Data Collection

Physical Findings. Although most infants with aortic stenosis are asymptomatic in the neonatal period, **an infant who is symptomatic from critical or severe aortic stenosis needs medical and surgical emergency treatment. The infant with critical aortic stenosis will have pale, gray, cool skin with decreased perfusion and peripheral pulses.**

Cyanosis. Cyanosis is generally not present in isolated valvular aortic stenosis.

Heart Sounds. A grade II to IV/VI harsh systolic murmur is typically heard in the upper right sternal border, radiating to the upper left sternal border and faintly to the neck. **The intensity of the murmur is unrelated to the severity of the obstruction.** An ejection click may be heard at the apex, radiating to the lower left sternal border. A suprasternal notch thrill is often palpable.

Congestive Heart Failure. Infants with critical aortic stenosis have congestive heart failure caused by a pressure overload of the left ventricle (see the section on congestive heart failure).

Laboratory Data

Arterial Blood Gases. Arterial blood gas values are generally normal.

Chest X-ray Examination. A chest x-ray examination shows cardiomegaly with normal pulmonary vascularity.

Electrocardiogram. The ECG may be normal or demonstrate left ventricular hypertrophy. **It is important to remember that there is poor correlation between an electrocardiographic abnormality and the degree of aortic stenosis present.**

Echocardiogram. The aortic valve is usually thickened and appears to close abnormally on an echocardiogram. Doppler interrogation can accurately estimate the systolic pressure gradient from the left ventricle to the ascending aorta and identify the level or levels of obstruction.

Cardiac Catheterization. Cardiac catheterization is diagnostic and may or may not be performed in cases of critical aortic stenosis. Some centers are performing balloon dilation of the aortic valve during the cardiac catheterization.

Treatment

Medical Management. Medical management is usually unsatisfactory, and **surgical intervention is necessary for critical aortic stenosis in the newborn** (see the section on general treatment strategies). However, balloon dilatation of aortic valve stenosis in the cardiac catheterization laboratory has been a successful alternative to surgical intervention in selected newborns.

Surgical Treatment. **Aortic valvulotomy through a median sternotomy incision is the surgical procedure for correcting critical aortic stenosis in infants.** This procedure can usually be accomplished in the newborn with inflow occlusion and circulatory arrest for 1 to 2 minutes. In older infants, cardiopulmonary bypass should be performed. The fused commissures of the valve are incised, permitting the leaflets to open freely during systole.

Complications and Residual Effects

Complications and residual effects include aortic insufficiency and residual aortic stenosis. **The mortality in infancy ranges from 5% to 50%, with the highest risk involving the newborn with critical obstruction.** It is hoped that avoidance of a cardiopulmonary bypass operation will reduce the mortality in this group.

Prognosis and Follow-up

Surgery for critical aortic stenosis in the neonatal period is considered a palliative measure for relief of the obstruction. Repeated catheterization and further surgical repair of the valve should be expected in the next several months to years.

Critical Pulmonary Stenosis With Intact Ventricular Septum

Physiology

In critical pulmonary stenosis with intact ventricular septum, the flow to the pulmonary artery from the right ventricle is obstructed. The obstruction may occur below the valve in the infundibular area, above the valve, or at the valve (subvalvular, supravalvular, or valvular). In valvular stenosis the orifice of the pulmonary valve is markedly narrowed, and the valvular tissue may assume the shape of a cone (Figure 24-5). The pulmonary artery distal to this area of stenosis may be dilated. Because the ventricular septum is intact, the right ventricle is subjected to a marked increase in pressure and becomes hypertrophied. A pressure gradient from the right ventricle to the pulmonary artery of 50 mm Hg or more is indicative of significant pulmonary stenosis in the newborn.

Data Collection
Physical Findings
Cyanosis. Cyanosis is generally not present in an isolated lesion but may occur in the presence of a right-to-left atrial shunt.

Heart Sounds. A harsh, grade II to III/VI systolic murmur is heard in the upper left sternal border, radiating to both axillae and faintly to the back. Diastole is quiet. A murmur of tricuspid insufficiency (grade I/VI, soft, systolic murmur at the lower left sternal border) may be heard. An ejection click may also be heard at the left sternal border.

Congestive Heart Failure. The infant with critical pulmonary stenosis typically has signs and symptoms of right-sided congestive heart failure re-

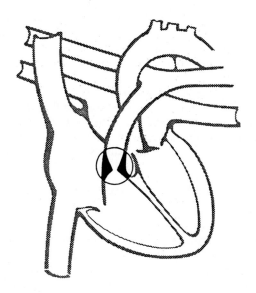

FIGURE 24-5 Pulmonary stenosis. (Courtesy Ross Laboratories, Columbus, Ohio.)

sulting from excessive pressure overload (see the section on congestive heart failure).

Laboratory Data
Arterial Blood Gases. Arterial blood gas values are generally normal.

Chest X-ray Examination. The chest x-ray examination may be normal but usually demonstrates cardiomegaly with normal or decreased pulmonary vascularity.

Electrocardiogram. The ECG may be normal or demonstrate right ventricular hypertrophy.

Echocardiogram. An abnormal pulmonary valve pattern on a two-dimensional echocardiogram is diagnostic. Doppler interrogation and color flow mapping can accurately estimate the systolic pressure gradient from the right ventricle to the pulmonary artery and identify the level or levels of obstruction.

Cardiac Catheterization. Infants suspected of having critical pulmonary stenosis with an intact ventricular septum usually undergo cardiac catheterization as soon as possible. Balloon dilation of the pulmonic valve during catheterization has been successfully performed in many institutions.

Treatment
Medical Management. Prostaglandin E₁ has been used successfully to maintain the patency of the ductus arteriosus, thereby allowing adequate pulmonary blood flow until surgery or balloon dilation is performed. If balloon dilation has been successful, surgical intervention may be postponed or may not be necessary at all.

Surgical Treatment. The degree of pulmonary stenosis and the size of the pulmonary arteries determine surgical approach. If the right ventricle and pulmonary arteries are of adequate size, then pulmonary valvulotomy through a median sternotomy incision is the preferable procedure. This involves incising the pulmonary valve commissures, allowing the leaflets to open freely during systole. Like aortic valvulotomy, this procedure can often be performed under inflow occlusion.

Complications and Residual Effects
Complications and residual effects include pulmonary insufficiency and residual pulmonary

stenosis. **The mortality of pulmonary valvulotomy is 17% in newborns.**

If the right ventricle and pulmonary arteries are too small to allow antegrade flow, then a palliative procedure such as the Blalock-Taussig operation is performed. This procedure consists of bringing down the subclavian artery opposite the aortic arch and anastomosing it to the ipsilateral pulmonary artery or placing a Gore-Tex or Dacron tube graft (conduit) between the subclavian artery and the pulmonary artery.

Complications and residual side effects of Blalock-Taussig shunts include (1) diminished or absent pulses in the affected arm, (2) congestive heart failure from an overlarge shunt, and (3) inadequacy of the shunt. The mortality in this group is higher than in infants with adequately sized right ventricles and pulmonary arteries.

Prognosis and Follow-up

If a palliative shunt has been used, follow-up catheterization and surgical procedures should be anticipated either when the shunt becomes nonfunctional or when total repair is expected. If the lesion has been primarily corrected surgically in the neonatal period, repeated catheterization may be performed several months later to evaluate the residual obstruction if it is suspected. However, evaluation by echocardiogram may be sufficient without catheterization.

Atrioventricular Septal Defect, Endocardial Cushion Defect (AV Canal)
Physiology
The complete type of endocardial cushion defect is characterized by a large central hole in the endocardial cushion of the heart with free communication among all four chambers. The anterior leaflet of the mitral valve and the septal leaflet of the tricuspid valve both have clefts and are continuous with each other through the defect. Thus the atrioventricular (AV) valves are represented by a valve common to both sides of the heart.

These infants usually have a left-to-right shunt at both the atrial and ventricular levels. If the cleft in the mitral valve is substantial, mitral insufficiency may also be present. The symptomatology depends on the degree of shunting at the atrial and ventricular levels and the amount of mitral insufficiency present. There is an association between endocardial cushion defects and Down syndrome.

Data Collection
Physical Findings
Cyanosis. Generally, cyanosis is not present with an isolated endocardial cushion defect.

Heart Sounds. If mitral insufficiency is present, a blowing, systolic, apical murmur with radiation to the left axilla and/or a VSD murmur is heard.

Congestive Heart Failure. Congestive heart failure may be present because of volume overload of the ventricles as a result of mitral insufficiency and left-to-right shunting at either the atrial or ventricular level (see the section on congestive heart failure).

Laboratory Data
Arterial Blood Gases. The $PaCO_2$ may be elevated if there is severe mitral insufficiency and pulmonary edema. The pH is usually normal. The PaO_2 is also usually normal.

Chest X-ray Examination. The heart size may be normal or increased. The pulmonary vascularity is generally increased.

Electrocardiogram. An ECG with a left axis deviation, counterclockwise loop in the frontal plane, and superior axis suggests AV septal defect.

Echocardiogram. A two-dimensional echocardiogram with Doppler and color flow mapping demonstrates the atrial septal defect (ASD), VSD, and common AV valves, and the degree of AV valve insufficiency. This technique is diagnostic.

Cardiac Catheterization. Cardiac catheterization is diagnostic but generally not performed in the neonatal period in a typical AV septal defect. An echocardiographic diagnosis may be sufficient without cardiac catheterization.

Treatment
Medical Management. See general section on medical therapy.

Surgical Treatment. If the infant does not respond to medical treatment and exhibits congestive heart failure, severe mitral regurgitation, or pulmonary hypertension, surgical repair is necessary. The surgical procedure through a median sternotomy incision involves closing the ASD and

VSD, separating the common leaflets of the mitral and tricuspid valves, and reconstructing the mitral valve.

Complications and Residual Effects
Complications and residual effects include (1) persistent shunt (residual ASD or VSD); (2) conduction abnormalities (dysrhythmias and third-degree heart block), (3) mitral regurgitation, and (4) tricuspid regurgitation. The mortality in infancy is 10% to 25%.

The alternative to total repair is pulmonary artery banding. This is, however, contraindicated when mitral regurgitation or atrial shunting is severe. The cumulative risk of banding and debanding may approach the risk of total repair.

Prognosis and Follow-up
In the complete AV septal defect, congestive heart failure is a frequent problem and early surgical intervention is generally required. The prognosis of surgical repair in the neonatal period is guarded, with a generally favorable outcome if the surgery can be postponed until the infant is older than 6 months of age. The prognosis is guarded if pulmonary hypertension develops before surgical intervention.

Ebstein's Anomaly
Physiology
Ebstein's anomaly consists of an abnormally low insertion of the tricuspid valve, incorporating a portion of the right ventricle into the right atrium. The resultant right ventricular cavity is small, and because the elevated pulmonary artery pressure is normally present in the newborn period, the cardiac output from the right ventricle to the pulmonary artery is decreased. This cardiac output generally increases as the pulmonary artery pressure decreases after birth. Tricuspid insufficiency is present in varying degrees in the infant.

Data Collection
Physical Findings
Cyanosis. Varying degrees of cyanosis are present and depend on (1) the amount of right-to-left shunting at the foramen ovale and (2) the amount of blood that enters the pulmonary circulation by the right ventricle. In severe cases, the amount of pulmonary blood flow is markedly decreased, and these infants may be deeply cyanotic.

Heart Sounds. The second heart sound, S_2, is normal in the mildly affected infant, but the pulmonary component of S_2 may be diminished or inaudible in severely affected patients. **A nonspecific systolic murmur is usually present and varies from a grade I/VI to a grade V/VI, representing tricuspid insufficiency.** Diastolic murmurs, ejection clicks, and triple or quadruple rhythms are frequently heard.

Congestive Heart Failure. Newborns who are symptomatic usually have congestive heart failure resulting from volume overload of the left ventricle (see the section on congestive heart failure).

Arterial Blood Gases. The PaO_2 may be normal to very low, depending on the amount of antegrade blood flow through the pulmonary valve. PaO_2 in the low 20s is not uncommon.

Chest X-ray Examination. The chest x-ray examination shows cardiomegaly with decreased pulmonary vascularity. Massive cardiomegaly generally indicates severe tricuspid insufficiency.

Electrocardiogram. An ECG shows abnormal P waves and various degrees of heart block. The QRS generally demonstrates a right bundle-branch block pattern. **Wolff-Parkinson-White (preexcitation) syndrome is frequently present, and dysrhythmias are common.**

Echocardiogram. An echocardiogram with abnormal tricuspid valve patterns on an M mode suggests Ebstein's anomaly. A two-dimensional echocardiogram is diagnostic. Doppler interrogation and color flow mapping are very useful in evaluating the amount of antegrade blood flow through the pulmonary valve and the degree of tricuspid insufficiency present.

Cardiac Catheterization. There is an increased risk of dysrhythmias during catheterization. This procedure is not generally performed in the neonatal period unless a question regarding the differential diagnosis exists (to rule out pulmonary atresia).

Treatment
Medical Management. **Dysrhythmias, especially supraventricular tachycardia, should be anticipated and appropriately managed (see the section on general treatment strategies).**

Surgical Treatment. Surgical treatment for Ebstein's anomaly is rarely indicated in infancy. The procedure through a median sternotomy incision involves repositioning the tricuspid valve and an anuloplasty to improve the competency of the valve. In addition, plication of the atrialized ventricle is performed. Replacing the tricuspid valve may be required.

Complications and Residual Effects
Complications and residual effects include tricuspid insufficiency and dysrhythmias. The mortality in infancy is unknown because of insufficient data.

Prognosis and Follow-up
The prognosis of mild Ebstein's anomaly is generally favorable. Infants with severe Ebstein's anomaly generally improve as the right ventricular output increases. Although surgery has been used successfully in the more severe forms of Ebstein's anomaly, the prognosis is less favorable in patients requiring surgical intervention.

Persistent Pulmonary Hypertension in the Newborn (PPHN)
Physiology
Infants with abnormally elevated pulmonary vascular resistance have PPHN or persistent fetal circulation. These infants are generally hypoxic and acidotic but usually do not have severe pulmonary parenchymal disease or underlying cardiac disease. **These infants have a right-to-left shunt at the ductal or atrial level.**

Data Collection
History. PPHN is usually associated with severe antepartum or peripartum conditions that involve hypoxia reflected by low Apgar scores. These infants are generally term or near term and are symptomatic within the first hours after birth. Associated findings include hyperviscosity, hypoglycemia, or a congenital diaphragmatic hernia.

Physical Findings
Cyanosis. The milder cases of PPHN have minimal transient tachypnea and cyanosis associated with stress (crying or feeding). **Severe cases have marked cyanosis, tachypnea, acidosis, and decreased peripheral perfusion.**

Heart Sounds. A loud pulmonary component of S_2 and occasionally a nonspecific systolic ejection murmur are heard.

Congestive Heart Failure. Infants with PPHN usually have congestive heart failure because of pressure overload of the right ventricle (see the section on congestive heart failure).

Laboratory Data
Arterial Blood Gases. Arterial blood gas values demonstrate acidosis, hypoxia, and increased $Paco_2$. **If a blood gas measurement is obtained simultaneously in the right radial artery (preductal) and in the descending aorta with a UAC (postductal), the right-to-left shunt at the ductal level can be documented.** If blood gas measurements are repeated after intubation and pharmacologic intervention (see the section on treatment), the amount of hypoxia is often reduced. Simultaneous preductal and postductal transcutaneous oxygen measurement may also be used.

Chest X-ray Examination. The chest x-ray examination demonstrates mild to moderate cardiomegaly with normal pulmonary vascular markings. The lung fields may be clear.

Electrocardiogram. The ECG frequently is normal but may demonstrate right ventricular hypertrophy and signs of myocardial ischemia.

Echocardiogram. An echocardiogram helps to evaluate cardiac structures and rule out cyanotic lesions. Evaluating the right ventricular and pulmonary artery pressures by Doppler and the degree of right-to-left shunting at the atrial and ductal levels is helpful.

Cardiac Catheterization. Cardiac catheterization is usually not performed.

Treatment
Medical Management. See Chapter 23.

Complete D-Transposition of the Great Arteries
Physiology
Complete D-transposition of the great arteries (Figure 24-6) is one of the most common forms of serious heart disease. The aorta arises from the right ventricle, receives unoxygenated systemic venous blood, and returns this blood to the systemic arterial circulation. The pulmonary artery arises from the left ventricle, receives oxygenated pulmonary venous blood, and returns this blood to the

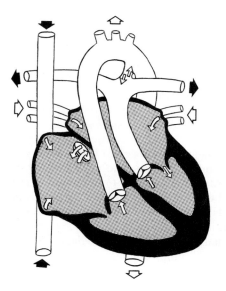

FIGURE 24-6   Complete transposition of the great arteries. (Courtesy Ross Laboratories, Columbus, Ohio.)

pulmonary circulation. D-transposition can occur by itself or can be associated with other defects (PDA, ASD, VSD, or pulmonary stenosis).

Data Collection

History. Transposition of the great arteries is more prevalent in males and is typically found in infants who are full term.

Physical Findings. The major physiologic abnormalities in D-transposition of the great arteries are an oxygen deficiency in the tissues and excessive work load of the right and left ventricles. **The only mixing of oxygenated and unoxygenated blood occurs in the presence of associated lesions (patent foramen ovale, ASD, VSD, PDA, or collateral circulation).** The extent of the mixing depends on the number, size, and position of the anatomic communications, the pressure differential between the two systems, and changes in the systemic and pulmonary vascular resistance.

Cyanosis. Cyanosis is present in varying degrees, depending on the amount of intercirculatory mixing present. Cyanosis may be mild if the mixing occurs through a significant VSD or PDA. **Cyanosis is profound with intact ventricular septum or a closing PDA. Oxygen therapy will be of limited benefit. Only a certain amount of oxygenated blood is able to reach the systemic**

circulation, **and administration of additional oxygen does not improve this situation.** Enlargement of the interatrial communication by balloon septostomy (Rashkind procedure) during cardiac catheterization is commonly performed to establish adequate intercirculatory mixing for these infants. Additional management may include surgical removal of the atrial septum (Blalock-Hanlon operation).

After these palliative procedures, the infant will continue to be cyanotic, especially in times of stress (crying, feeding, or exposure to cold temperatures). **If the Pao$_2$ at rest in room air is not greater than 35 mm mm Hg or if persistent metabolic acidosis is present, inadequate intercardiac mixing should be suspected.**

Heart Sounds. The aorta arises from the anterior (right) ventricle, and the closure of the aortic valve is easily heard. The S$_2$ is single with an increased intensity. Murmurs if present are usually those of associated lesions (see the section on individual lesions).

Congestive Heart Failure. As a result of the volume and pressure overload experienced by both ventricles, the infant may show signs of congestive heart failure. This is especially true if there is a large VSD or PDA present (see the section on congestive heart failure). Digoxin should be used with caution if subvalvular pulmonary stenosis is present.

Laboratory Data

Arterial Blood Gases. The pH and Paco$_2$ values are normal. The Pao$_2$ is typically low (20 to 40 mm Hg), but if a large VSD or PDA is present, the Pao$_2$ may approach normal levels.

Chest X-ray Examination. The chest x-ray examination may be normal or demonstrate either decreased or increased pulmonary vascularity. The cardiac silhouette may assume the shape of an egg lying on a string. However, this finding is not diagnostic.

Electrocardiogram. The ECG may be normal or demonstrate right ventricular hypertrophy. Left ventricular hypertrophy and combined ventricular hypertrophy are uncommon.

Echocardiogram. The echocardiogram is extremely useful in establishing the diagnosis and evaluating associated lesions in infants with transposition of the great arteries.

Cardiac Catheterization. Cardiac catheterization is diagnostic. **A balloon septostomy is commonly performed to improve interatrial mixing.**

Treatment

Medical Management. **Serial venous and arterial pH measurements should be obtained to rule out the presence of a persistent metabolic acidosis that would suggest inadequate intercardiac mixing.** In addition, congestive heart failure should be continually anticipated and treated appropriately if it occurs (see the section on general treatment strategies).

Surgical Treatment. **The arterial switch procedure in most centers is the treatment of choice for D-transposition of the great arteries.** This procedure through a median sternotomy incision involves amputation of the main pulmonary artery and the aorta above the respective valves. The pulmonary artery is anastomosed to the right ventricle, and the aorta is anastomosed to the left ventricle (the aortic valve becomes a functional pulmonary valve, and the pulmonary valve becomes a functional aortic valve). The coronary arteries are resected with a button of surrounding tissue and reanastomosed to the supravalvular area of the ascending aorta.

It is essential in performing this procedure that the left ventricular pressure is systemic. In infants with a VSD, the pressure tends to remain elevated; therefore this procedure may be postponed for several days or even months. However, once the left ventricular pressure decreases below that of the right ventricle, the morbidity and mortality increase dramatically. Therefore, infants with an intact ventricular septum require surgery within the first few days of life.

If the arterial switch procedure is not performed and the infant becomes refractory to medical management and exhibits congestive heart failure, failure to thrive, pulmonary hypertension, or severe hypoxia, an alternative surgical procedure is necessary. **The most common procedures other than the arterial switch for repair of D-transposition with an intact ventricular septum are the Mustard and the Senning procedures.** Both of these procedures performed through a median sternotomy incision involve intraatrial redirection of blood flow. The oxygenated blood returning from the lungs through the pulmonary veins is redirected to the tricuspid valve and right ventricle, while the systemic venous return from inferior and superior venae cavae is redirected to the mitral valve and left ventricle.

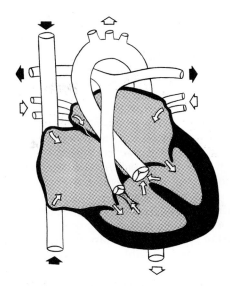

FIGURE 24-7 Tetralogy of Fallot. (Courtesy Ross Laboratories, Columbus, Ohio.)

Complications and Residual Effects

Complications and residual effects of the arterial switch procedure include (1) dysrhythmias, (2) myocardial ischemia and infarction, and (3) aortic and/or pulmonary supravalvular stenosis.

Complications and residual effects of the Mustard and Senning procedures include (1) dysrhythmias, (2) superior vena cava or inferior vena cava obstruction, (3) tricuspid regurgitation, and (4) pulmonary venous obstruction. The latter is a severe complication warranting early detection and immediate correction. The mortality to infants is 8% and is even higher in the neonatal period.

Prognosis and Follow-up

Without treatment, 30% of these infants die within the first week of life, 50% die within the first month, 70% die within the first 6 months, and 90% die within the first year. With treatment, the mortality rate is reduced to approximately 5% or less.

Tetralogy of Fallot

Physiology

Tetralogy of Fallot is the most common form of cyanotic congenital heart disease. The four components of tetralogy of Fallot are (1) VSD, (2) overriding of the ascending aorta, (3) obstruction to the right ventricular outflow tract, and (4) right ventricular hypertrophy (Figure 24-7).

Data Collection

Physical Findings. The degree of symptomatology in these infants depends on the degree of right ventricular outflow tract obstruction. Newborns who are symptomatic usually have severe right ventricular outflow tract obstruction.

Cyanosis. The predominant intercardiac shunt is right to left; therefore most infants with tetralogy of Fallot are cyanotic. However, if the right ventricular outflow obstruction is only mild or moderate, the intercardiac shunt is left to right and the infant initially will be acyanotic.

Infants with tetralogy of Fallot occasionally have a *TET,* or hypercyanotic spell. These spells consist of cyanosis, irritability, pallor, tachypnea, flaccidity, and possible loss of consciousness. TETs may be the result of a transient increase in the obstruction of the right ventricular outflow tract (usually the muscular infundibular area) and usually respond to knee-chest positioning, oxygen, propranolol, or morphine.

Heart Sounds. A grade II to IV/VI harsh systolic murmur at the mid to upper left sternal border is usually present but is diminished or absent during a TET. The S_2 is usually loud and single (representing aortic closure).

Congestive Heart Failure. Congestive heart failure is uncommon in tetralogy of Fallot.

Laboratory Data

Arterial Blood Gases. The $Paco_2$ and pH are normal. The Pao_2 is normal if the pulmonary stenosis is mild and there is little right-to-left shunting at the ventricular level. If the pulmonary stenosis, however, is more severe, the amount of right-to-left shunting increases and the Pao_2 falls.

Chest X-ray Examination. The classic chest x-ray examination of tetralogy of Fallot resembles the shape of a boot with a normal-sized heart. However, the classic chest x-ray pattern described is not common in the newborn. Pulmonary vascularity is either normal or decreased.

Electrocardiogram. The ECG demonstrates right ventricular hypertrophy.

Echocardiogram. The echocardiogram is suggestive when the overriding aorta can be demonstrated. Echocardiograms help identify the pulmonary valve to rule out pulmonary atresia. Doppler interrogation helps to define the degree and level of pulmonary stenosis. Color flow mapping identifies the VSD as well as the direction of blood flow across the VSD.

Cardiac Catheterization. Cardiac catheterization is diagnostic and performed in the newborn when there is a question regarding the differential diagnosis (pulmonary atresia).

Treatment

Medical Management. Digoxin is not routinely used because it may increase the amount of infundibular obstruction present. **Propranolol is the preferable drug for treating hypercyanotic infants,** although morphine has been used successfully (see the section on general treatment strategies).

Surgical Treatment. Total repair of tetralogy of Fallot involves patch closure of the large VSD and relief of the right ventricular outflow obstruction performed through a median sternotomy incision. Often a pericardial patch across the pulmonary valve annulus is required. The use of homograft conduits for relief of right-sided obstruction is also common. Contraindications include small size of the child, anomalous left anterior descending coronary artery, and hypoplastic pulmonary arteries.

Total surgical repair of tetralogy of Fallot is not usually recommended in the neonatal period. If surgical intervention is warranted (i.e., the infant is severely hypoxic because of inadequate pulmonary blood flow), a systemic-to-pulmonary shunt is performed. The Blalock-Taussig operation is usually preferred (see previous description of the Blalock-Taussig operation).

Complications and Residual Effects

Complications and residual effects include (1) diminished or absent pulses in the affected arm, (2) congestive heart failure from an overlarge shunt, and (3) inadequate shunt. Mortality in infancy is 10%.

Prognosis and Follow-up

Early cardiac catheterization with subsequent surgery is recommended if the child is symptomatic or refractory to medical care. Tetralogy of Fallot without surgery has a grave prognosis.

Parent Teaching
Parents should be instructed to place the infant in a knee-chest position during a TET spell and to notify the physician immediately.

Pulmonary Atresia With Intact Ventricular Septum

Physiology

Pulmonary atresia is characterized by complete agenesis of the pulmonary valve. This lesion produces severe signs or symptoms soon after birth and is not compatible with life unless there is an associated interatrial communication and an additional pathway of entry for blood into the pulmonary circulation (through a PDA and/or collateral blood flow). Because flow to the lungs may depend on a PDA, death may occur when this structure closes. The right ventricle is usually hypoplastic but may be normal or dilated, depending on the degree of tricuspid insufficiency present.

Data Collection
Physical Findings

Cyanosis. Cyanosis is always present in varying degrees, depending on the amount of pulmonary blood flow from the PDA and/or collateral blood flow.

Heart Sounds. The S_2 is single, and a soft systolic murmur is heard as a result of either the PDA or tricuspid insufficiency in about one half of the infants with pulmonary atresia.

Congestive Heart Failure. Congestive heart failure is usually present with moderate to severe tricuspid insufficiency (see the section on congestive heart failure).

Laboratory Data

Arterial Blood Gases. The pH and $PaCO_2$ are usually within normal range. The PaO_2, however, is usually very low (20 to 30 mm Hg), unless there is a large shunt at the ductal or bronchial collateral level. In some cases the amount of pulmonary blood flow is insufficient, and the pH may be low, reflecting metabolic acidosis.

Chest X-ray Examination. The heart appears enlarged on x-ray examination if tricuspid insufficiency is present. Pulmonary vascularity is either decreased or normal, depending on the amount of shunting through the PDA and/or collateral blood flow.

Electrocardiogram. The ECG is usually normal but may demonstrate left ventricular hypertrophy. It is important to differentiate this lesion from tricuspid atresia that shows a counterclockwise loop in the frontal planes with a superior axis.

Echocardiogram. The two-dimensional echocardiogram with Doppler and color flow mapping can identify absence of blood flow across the pulmonary valve and is diagnostic.

Cardiac Catheterization. Cardiac catheterization is diagnostic and may be performed if the diagnosis is suspected. A balloon atrial septostomy may be performed at the time of catheterization.

Treatment
Medical Management. Prostaglandin E_1 is used to maintain patency of the ductus arteriosus until surgical intervention (see the section on general treatment strategy).

Surgical Treatment. In most medical centers a systemic-to-pulmonary shunt such as the Blalock-Taussig operation is performed through a lateral thoracotomy incision. However, some institutions are performing a pulmonary valvulotomy or a pulmonary outflow patch procedure in addition to a shunt. This establishes an open pathway through the atretic valve area between the pulmonary artery and the right ventricle. Antegrade blood flow through the right ventricle and pulmonary artery will then promote growth of these areas. The pulmonary valvotomy and pulmonary outflow patch procedures are performed through a median sternotomy incision.

Complications and Residual Effects

Complications and residual effects of the Blalock-Taussig operation include (1) diminished or absent pulses in the affected arm, (2) congestive heart failure from an overlarge shunt, and (3) inadequate shunt. **The mortality rate in infants is 25% or higher.**

Prognosis and Follow-up

Pulmonary atresia is fatal without surgical intervention. If a palliative shunt is performed, catheterization and further surgical procedures should be anticipated when the shunt becomes nonfunctional. If primary surgical correction is undertaken in the newborn period, catheterization should be anticipated to evaluate residual obstruction. Despite the development of newer surgical techniques, the prognosis in these infants is guarded.

Total Anomalous Pulmonary Venous Return

Physiology

Total anomalous pulmonary venous return (TAPVR) is characterized by all the pulmonary veins returning directly or indirectly into the right atrium rather than the left atrium. The presence of an ASD is necessary to sustain life (Figure 24-8). The four main varieties of TAPVR are (1) supercardiac (most common), in which the drainage is to the superior vena cava through the innominate vein; (2) cardiac, in which the pulmonary veins drain into the coronary, sinus or directly into the right atrium; (3) infracardiac, in which the four veins join behind the heart, flow through the diaphragm, and connect to the portal venous system; and (4) mixed. Each of the various types of anomalous drainage can occur with or without obstruction along the pulmonary venous pathway. The presence or absence of obstruction profoundly affects the clinical course.

Data Collection

Physical Findings

Cyanosis. Infants with obstructed or unobstructed TAPVR are typically cyanotic. **Because all pulmonary venous return (oxygenated blood) ultimately enters the right atrium (as opposed to the left atrium), a right-to-left shunt at the atrial level is required to sustain life.**

Heart Sounds. Murmurs are rarely heard in infants with TAPVR and when present are nonspecific.

Congestive Heart Failure. Infants with unobstructed TAPVR usually show signs of congestive heart failure resulting from volume overload of the right ventricle. Infants with obstructed TAPVR generally do not demonstrate evidence of congestive heart failure but typically demonstrate pulmonary venous congestion (see the section on congestive heart failure).

Laboratory Data

Arterial Blood Gases. The pH and PaCO2 are usually normal. The PaO2 may be within the normal range if there is a large amount of pulmonary blood

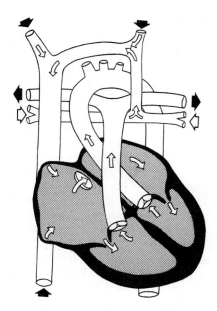

FIGURE 24-8   Anomalous venous return. (Courtesy Ross Laboratories, Columbus, Ohio.)

flow (always associated with severe congestive heart failure). If the pulmonary blood flow is limited, secondary to obstruction of blood flow, the PaO2 may be low.

Chest X-ray Examination. If the TAPVR is obstructed, the chest x-ray examination will demonstrate pulmonary venous congestion without cardiomegaly. If the TAPVR is unobstructed, the chest x-ray examination will demonstrate a marked increase in pulmonary vascularity and cardiomegaly.

Electrocardiogram. An ECG may demonstrate right axis deviation, right ventricular hypertrophy, and right atrial enlargement.

Echocardiogram. An echocardiogram is diagnostic; however, it is sometimes difficult to visualize the pulmonary veins by this method. The diagnosis of TAPVR is strongly suggested when an extra cavity is seen behind the small left atrium. With color flow mapping, the right-to-left shunting across the atrial septum, as well as the anomalous venous return as it enters through the atrium, superior vena cava, or coronary sinus, can be visualized.

Cardiac Catheterization. Infants suspected of having TAPVR may undergo cardiac catheterization to define the type of TAPVR and presence or absence of obstruction. A Rashkind balloon septostomy may be performed at that time to improve intraatrial mixing.

Treatment
Medical Management. **Obstructed TAPVR is a surgical emergency.** Nonobstructed TAPVR may be medically treated temporarily, although early surgery is generally recommended (see the section on general treatment strategy).

Surgical Treatment. Surgical correction of TAPVR depends on the variety. Supracardiac and infracardiac varieties require surgical reimplantation of the common vein into the left atrium. Intracardiac TAPVR can usually be surgically repaired by realigning the atrial septum during closure of the ASD and directing the anomalous veins to the left atrial side. All repairs are performed through a median sternotomy incision.

Complications and Residual Effects
Complications and residual effects include pulmonary venous obstruction and dysrhythmias. The mortality varies from 5% to 25% in infancy, depending on the anatomic type.

Prognosis and Follow-up
Infants with nonobstructed TAPVR generally do well if the lesion is recognized early and early corrective surgery is performed. The prognosis for obstructed TAPVR is less favorable despite early surgical intervention.

Tricuspid Atresia
Physiology
In tricuspid atresia there is complete agenesis of the tricuspid valve with no direct communication between the right atrium and right ventricle. Systemic venous blood entering the right atrium is shunted through a patent foramen ovale or ASD into the left atrium. A VSD may be present, and the right ventricle and pulmonary arteries may be normal in size. If the ventricular septum is intact but a large PDA is present, the right ventricular cavity may be hypoplastic and the pulmonary arteries are usually slightly decreased or normal in size (Figure 24-9). About 30% of these infants will have transposition of the great arteries.

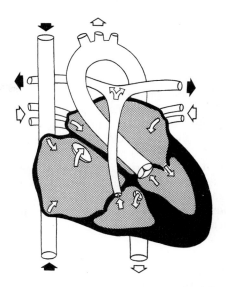

FIGURE 24-9 Tricuspid atresia. (Courtesy Ross Laboratories, Columbus, Ohio.)

Data Collection
Physical Findings
Cyanosis. The degree of cyanosis present varies. Newborns will have marked cyanosis if the pulmonary blood flow is compromised.

Heart Sounds. A single S_2 is present in infants with tricuspid atresia. Murmurs of associated shunts (VSD and PDA) are typically present.

Congestive Heart Failure. Congestive heart failure may be present with a large shunt (PDA or VSD) (see the section on congestive heart failure).

Laboratory Data
Arterial Blood Gases. The pH and $Paco_2$ are usually normal. The Pao_2 may vary from near normal if there is a large VSD or PDA to extremely low if there is limited shunting into the pulmonary system.

Chest X-ray Examination. A chest x-ray examination is nondiagnostic and may show a normal heart size or cardiomegaly. Pulmonary vascularity may be normal, decreased, or increased, depending on the degree of pulmonary blood flow.

Electrocardiogram. An ECG is highly suggestive and usually demonstrates left axis deviation with a counterclockwise loop, a superior axis in the frontal plane, and left ventricular hypertrophy.

Echocardiogram. Absence of the tricuspid valve and presence of a small hypoplastic right ventricle echocardiographically is highly suggestive of tricuspid atresia. Color flow mapping can identify the right-to-left shunt at the atrial level and the presence of a VSD and/or PDA.

Cardiac Catheterization. An infant suspected of having tricuspid atresia usually undergoes cardiac catheterization and a balloon septostomy. **A balloon septostomy is performed to improve intraatrial mixing.**

Treatment
Medical Management. See the section on general treatment strategy.

Surgical Treatment. When surgery is indicated, the preferred procedure in the neonatal period is a systemic-to-pulmonary shunt such as the Blalock-Taussig operation performed through a lateral thoracotomy incision.

Definitive repair of tricuspid atresia is accomplished with a single operation (Fontan procedure) or a staged procedure (Glenn followed by a Fontan). These operations involve the creation of a communication between the right atrium and pulmonary artery or right ventricular outflow chamber by direct anastomosis or conduit. Closure of the ASD and any VSDs present is also performed. Definitive repair is performed through a median sternotomy incision.

Complications and Residual Effects
Complications and residual effects include (1) heart failure, (2) pleural effusions, (3) renal or liver failure, (4) persistent shunts, (5) conduit obstruction, and (6) dysrhythmia. The mortality rate in infancy is unknown, but in older children it is approximately 10% to 25%.

Prognosis and Follow-up
The prognosis of tricuspid atresia is guarded. The Fontan procedure may improve this prognosis.

Truncus Arteriosus
Physiology
Truncus arteriosus is characterized by one great artery arising from the left and right ventricles, overriding a VSD. This common artery has one

valve and gives rise to the pulmonary, coronary, and systemic arteries (Figure 24-10). **Truncus arteriosus is classified into three types, depending on the origin of the pulmonary arteries:**

1. **Type I—A short, main pulmonary artery arises from the common trunk that bifurcates into the right and left pulmonary arteries.**
2. **Type II—The right and left pulmonary arteries arise directly from the posterior surface of the common trunk.**
3. **Type III—The right and left pulmonary arteries arise directly from the lateral walls of the common trunk.**

The ductus arteriosus is absent in approximately 50% of infants with truncus arteriosus. Between 30% and 35% have a right aortic arch.

Data Collection
Physical Findings. In truncus arteriosus the common trunk receives a mixture of unoxygenated blood from the right ventricle and oxygenated blood from the left ventricle. Blood flow to the lungs varies with the type of truncus but is usually increased and at systemic level pressure.

Cyanosis. Cyanosis is present at birth but varies in intensity according to the amount of pulmonary blood flow. Minimal cyanosis indicates adequate pulmonary blood flow.

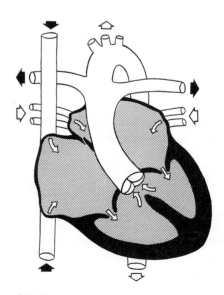

FIGURE 24-10 Truncus arteriosus. (Courtesy Ross Laboratories, Columbus, Ohio.)

Heart Sounds. The first heart sound, S_1, will be normal, but the S_2 will be single and loud because of the single valve of the common trunk. A loud systolic ejection click is frequently heard. A loud pansystolic murmur maximal at the lower left sternal border that radiates to the entire precordium is commonly heard. A middiastolic rumble may be present. If the truncal valve is insufficient, a blowing diastolic murmur may be heard. A wide pulse pressure may also be present.

Congestive Heart Failure. Congestive heart failure may be present shortly after birth or appear between 2 and 3 weeks of age. The presence of congestive heart failure depends on the amount of pulmonary blood flow. Persistent high pulmonary arteriolar resistance in the first few weeks of life will decrease pulmonary blood flow, and congestive heart failure may not be present. However, if the truncal valve is severely damaged, congestive heart failure will be present shortly after birth (see the section on congestive heart failure).

Laboratory Data
Arterial Blood Gases. The pH and $PaCO_2$ are usually normal. If there is no obstruction to pulmonary blood flow, the PaO_2 may be near normal (usually associated with severe congestive heart failure). If the pulmonary blood flow is restricted, the PaO_2 may be extremely low.

Chest X-ray Examination. Cardiomegaly, displayed pulmonary arteries, and increased vascular markings are typical findings on the chest x-ray examination.

Electrocardiogram. Combined ventricular hypertrophy is most often seen in an ECG. Left atrial enlargement is also commonly found.

Echocardiogram. A two-dimensional echocardiogram is helpful in establishing the diagnosis and in differentiating tetralogy of Fallot from truncus arteriosus. In addition, the echocardiogram is used to identify the number of truncal valve leaflets, the presence of truncal valve insufficiency, and the presence of pulmonary stenosis.

Cardiac Catheterization. A cardiac catheterization is diagnostic and is usually performed on an infant suspected of having truncus arteriosus.

Treatment
Medical Management. Medical management of these infants consists of stabilizing and treating congestive heart failure when present. **Calcium should be closely monitored because of the possibility of DiGeorge syndrome.**

Surgical Treatment. Totally repairing truncus arteriosus is rare in the newborn period. It consists of separating the pulmonary artery from the common trunk, closing the VSD with a patch, and inserting a right ventricular-to-pulmonary artery valved conduit. The use of homograft conduits for repair of truncus arteriosus has become more common. Total repair of truncus arteriosus is performed through a median sternotomy incision.

Complications and Residual Effects
Complications and side effects include (1) pulmonary vascular disease, (2) residual shunts, (3) truncal valve incompetence, and (4) conduit obstruction. The mortality is 40% to 50% in infancy.

Prognosis and Follow-up
The natural history depends on the amount of pulmonary blood flow and the competency of the truncal valve. Without treatment, more than half of these infants die before 3 months of age. Survival past 1 year of age ranges from 15% to 30%. Truncus arteriosus is often associated with DiGeorge syndrome, which has a guarded prognosis.

Hypoplastic Left Heart Syndrome
Physiology
Hypoplastic left heart syndrome represents a clinical spectrum that includes severe coarctation of the aorta, severe aortic valve stenosis or atresia, and severe mitral valve stenosis or atresia. The left ventricle and ascending aorta are hypoplastic. Coronary blood flow occurs in a retrograde fashion into the small ascending aorta through the PDA. The resultant poor myocardial perfusion leads to rapid decompensation.

Data Collection
Physical Findings
Cyanosis. These infants are usually not truly cyanotic but rather have severe pallor and a grayish skin color as a result of marked vasoconstriction and congestive heart failure.

Heart Sounds. A nonspecific systolic murmur is heard in approximately two thirds of infants with hypoplastic left heart syndrome.

Congestive Heart Failure. Congestive heart failure is present in all cases as a result of right ventricular volume and pressure overload (see the section on congestive heart failure).

Laboratory Data

Arterial Blood Gases. The arterial blood gas values are typically normal until the infant begins to deteriorate, at which time the baby will become acidotic.

Chest X-ray Examination. Cardiomegaly with increased pulmonary vascularity and pulmonary edema is seen on the x-ray examination.

Electrocardiogram. An ECG frequently demonstrates right axis deviation and right ventricular hypertrophy. However, the electrocardiogram may be normal.

Echocardiogram. An echocardiogram is usually diagnostic with a small left ventricular cavity and ascending aorta with an abnormal aortic valve pattern.

Cardiac Catheterization. Cardiac catheterization is diagnostic. In some cases only an aortic root contrast study using a UAC is required to demonstrate the typical small ascending aorta. If there is a question regarding the differential diagnosis, a heart catheterization is indicated.

Treatment

Medical Management. Hypoplastic left heart syndrome is a lethal lesion, and currently no medical therapy is effective. Surgical intervention offers the only chance of survival. Patency of the ductus arteriosus is maintained with infusion of prostaglandin E_1 (PGE) until surgical intervention (see Table 24-4). (See the section on general treatment strategy.)

Surgical Treatment. Recent advances in surgical treatment have made it possible to treat this lesion with a multistaged approach. The Norwood procedure is performed initially, consisting of enlargement of the atrial septal defect, ligation of the PDA, anastomosis of the pulmonary artery to the ascending aorta and the aortic arch, and creation of an aortopulmonary shunt (Blalock-Taussig shunt) to maintain pulmonary blood flow. In the second stage the aortopulmonary shunt is removed and an anastomosis is made between the superior vena cava and the pulmonary artery, which is called the bidirectional Glenn shunt and is performed at 6 to 12 months of age. The final stage is the Fontan procedure connecting the inferior vena cava to the pulmonary artery at 18 to 36 months of age. Cardiac transplantation is an alternative surgical option. In some centers the Norwood procedure is performed as a bridge to transplant, allowing the infant to survive until a donor heart is available.

Heart Transplantation in Infants[3]

Approximately 10% of infants born with congenital heart disease have severe, complex lesions that preclude corrective surgery. For some of these infants, heart transplantation may offer a chance of long-term survival. Hypoplastic left heart syndrome is the most common of these defects and is the most common indication for heart transplantation in early infancy. Cardiomyopathies are another indication.

Heart transplantation in infancy is severely limited by donor availability. There is a scarcity of donor hearts in this age and size group, and 31% of infants less than 6 months of age on transplant lists die waiting for donors.[3]

Contraindications for donor hearts are cardiac dysfunction and congenital heart disease (screened by echocardiogram), infection, systemic illness, and prolonged cardiac arrest. Acceptable hearts are matched with recipients by ABO blood group and approximate body weight and heart size. Specific human leukocyte antigen (HLA) matching is not done. Contraindications for recipients include major CNS abnormalities, irreversible failure of other organ systems, uncontrolled infections, and severe dysmorphism. Relative contraindications include marked prematurity (less than 36 weeks' gestational age), low birth weight (less than 2000 g), positive drug screen, and a family structure that is unable to support the long-term medical needs of the patient.[3] Abnormal structural relationships (i.e., situs inversus, dextrocardia, and abnormalities of systemic and pulmonary veins) are not contraindications to heart transplantation.[3]

Pretransplant care involves the support of the infant to maintain systemic perfusion, adequate oxygenation, and control of congestive heart fail-

ure. Great caution is used to avoid infection and maintain optimal nutritional status. If blood transfusions are necessary, washed, leukocyte-filtered red blood cells and blood products negative for CMV are used.

In performing the transplant, the donor heart atria are anastomosed to the posterior walls of the recipient atria, thus leaving the infant with two sinoatrial (SA) nodes, the native recipient SA node and the donor SA node. This will give a characteristic ECG postoperatively, with both the recipient and donor P waves present. The donor SA node controls the rhythm of the transplanted heart; therefore donor P waves will be related to the QRS complex.

Postoperative management of these infants involves isolation for prevention of infection, inotropic support as needed, immunosuppression, and surveillance for rejection. Rejection is closely monitored by clinical examination, ECG, echocardiogram, and myocardial biopsy. Rejections are treated with pulsed corticosteroids and other agents.

Immunosuppression is achieved through the administration of a variety of drugs, including cyclosporine, OKT3, FK-506, azathioprine, and corticosteroids. Each institution performing transplants uses some variation of combination of the above drugs for both immediate and long-term immunosuppression. **The highest incidence of rejection occurs in the first 6 months after transplant. Death in the perioperative period can be from graft failure, rejection, or infection.**

Long-term complications include rejection, infection, impairment of renal function, hypertension, growth restriction, neurologic sequelae, lymphoproliferative disease, and graft atherosclerosis. Most of these complications are secondary to chronic immunosuppression.

Prognosis and Follow-up

The prognosis is grim. Without surgical intervention, all infants die within several days or months of birth. Even with surgical intervention, the mortality rate is still high.

Dysrhythmias[10,13,18]
Physiology

The development of the cardiac conduction system continues after birth with a steady increase in the sympathetic innervation of the heart. This accounts for the observed heart rate variability and the high frequency of benign dysrhythmias in the newborn. Premature ventricular beats (Figure 24-11), brief episodes of ectopic atrial rhythms, wandering atrial pacemakers (Figure 24-12), and even brief episodes of sinus arrest are all frequently seen in the newborn period. The majority of these dysrhythmias do not require immediate treatment; however, if they persist, the presence of congenital heart disease, sepsis, drug toxicity, persistent hypoxia, adrenal insufficiency, disorders of electrolyte and acid-base balance, hypoglycemia, and hypocalcemia should be considered.

All cardiac tissue is capable of generating a spontaneous depolarization. However, the SA node, AV node, and His-Purkinje system consist of specialized conductive tissue with rapid spontaneous depolarization. The SA node is the normal pacemaker of the heart because it has the fastest rate of spontaneous depolarization. If, however, the spontaneous depolarization of the SA node is delayed or slower than normal, an escape rhythm (see Figure 24-12) is generated by either the AV node or His-Purkinje system (these rhythms are called *nodal escape* or *ventricular escape,* respectively). Dysrhythmias can also originate from an automatic

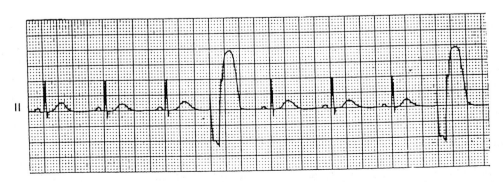

FIGURE 24-11 Premature ventricular beats.

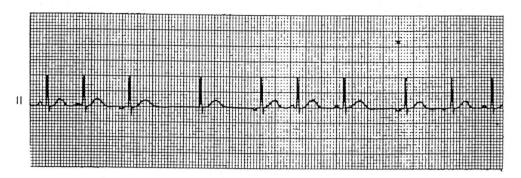

FIGURE 24-12   Wandering atrial pacemaker with junctional escape (fourth complex).

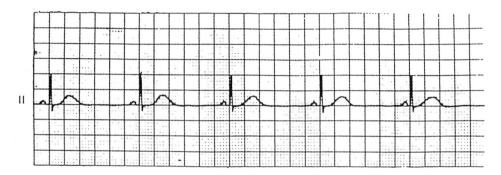

FIGURE 24-13   Sinus bradycardia.

"ectopic" pacemaker located anywhere in the heart. These ectopic pacemakers become more active in the presence of hypoxia, acidosis, digoxin toxicity, abnormal sympathetic nervous system stimulation, increased wall tension (congestive heart failure), or altered electrolyte balance. Drug therapy for dysrhythmias is based on the ability of certain medications to alter the electrophysiologic properties of cardiac tissue. One class of antidysrhythmic drugs directly increases the automaticity of certain cardiac fibers. Examples of such drugs include quinidine, procainamide, lidocaine, and phenytoin (see Table 24-4). Other drugs directly or indirectly affect the autonomic nervous system activity. Propranolol is a beta-adrenergic blocker and works in this fashion. Digoxin exerts its chronotropic activity by altering the sympathetic and parasympathetic nervous system response within the heart.

Benign Dysrhythmias: Sinus Bradycardia, Sinus Tachycardia, and Sinus Dysrhythmia
Of normal premature infants, 35% to 40% have brief episodes of sinus bradycardia (Figure 24-13), sinus tachycardia, or sinus dysrhythmia (Figure 24-14) that are benign and require no treatment. Healthy premature and term infants may have heart rates that range from 90 to 200 beats/min. Sustained heart rates (greater than 15 seconds) above or below this range should be evaluated with a 12-lead electrocardiogram and rhythm strip. These are important, because artifact created by the bedside monitors often makes accurate interpretations of dysrhythmias impossible.

Supraventricular Tachycardia
Supraventricular tachycardia (SVT) (Figure 24-15) is the most common tachydysrhythmia in the newborn period. It is the result of dual AV nodal pathways, rapid conduction through an accessory bundle (Wolff-Parkinson-White syndrome), or the existence of an ectopic atrial pacemaker. SVT is commonly associated with Ebstein's anomaly of the tricuspid valve, D-transposition of the great vessels, cardiomyopathy, or myocarditis. These lesions are present in 10% to 25% of infants with SVT and should be excluded with the appropriate evaluation.

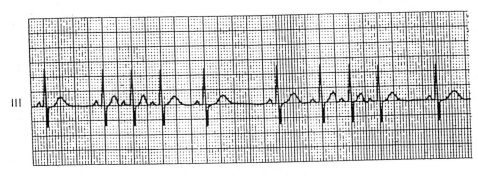

FIGURE 24-14 Sinus dysrhythmia.

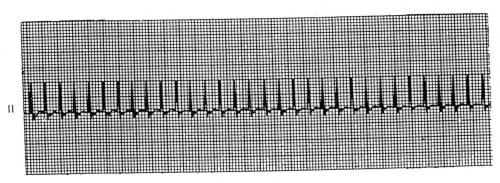

FIGURE 24-15 Supraventricular tachycardia.

Newborns with SVT will have a history of gradually developing congestive heart failure with findings of anxiousness, restlessness, tachypnea, and poor feeding. These symptoms develop after 12 to 24 hours of SVT. SVT often starts and ceases abruptly.

Criteria for SVT include (1) persistent ventricular rate over 200 beats/min, (2) a fixed and regular R-R interval, and (3) little change in heart rate with various activities (crying, feeding, or apnea).

Treatment. Various maneuvers may be used to attempt to convert the infant to normal sinus rhythm (NSR). Vagal maneuvers (unilateral carotid pressure, gagging, rectal stimulation) may be attempted but rarely work. **Ocular compression should never be used.** Stimulation of the diving reflex using an ice bag applied to the infant's face may be attempted. (Caution must be used in this procedure to ensure adequate ventilation for the infant.) **Adenosine, a purinergic agonist, is an especially effective antidysrhythmic drug for treatment of SVT. Adenosine slows the sinus rate and produces transient AV block, interrupting the SVT.** Overdrive atrial

pacing has been successful in converting SVT to NSR. However, direct-current (DC) cardioversion (1 to 2 watt-seconds/kg) is the most effective mode of treatment. The defibrillator must always be in the synchronous mode. If cardioversion is successful, maintenance drug therapy should be initiated. Other antidysrhythmic drugs such as digoxin have been used to treat this disorder. Recently, however, **it has been suggested that digoxin not be used in Wolff-Parkinson-White syndrome and that this disorder be ruled out before digoxin is used.** If not contraindicated, digoxin should be administered using standard doses (see Box 24-2).

Propranolol administered IV may be used if the patient is not in congestive heart failure. Beta-blocking agents may inhibit circulating catecholamines, which are needed for the maintenance of adequate cardiac output in the face of congestive heart failure.

Verapamil is a calcium channel blocker and when first introduced was thought to be the drug of choice in SVT. However, **this drug should not be used in children under 1 year of age and should never be used in a patient in congestive heart failure.**

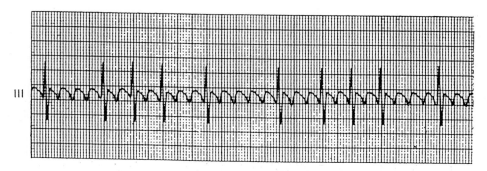

FIGURE 24-16 Atrial flutter.

If the SVT fails to convert using the methods outlined above, other drugs such as amiodarone, flecanide, or procainamide may be required. After conversion to NSR, maintenance drug therapy should be continued for 12 months or longer. **Relapses during the first 48 hours are common (70%) and should be anticipated.**

Fetal SVT is uncommon, but when present can be associated with severe congestive heart failure and hydrops fetalis. Fetal SVT requires aggressive management, including conversion with maternally administered propranolol and digoxin.

Atrial Flutter and Fibrillation
The presence of atrial flutter (Figure 24-16) usually indicates severe organic heart disease (endocardial fibroelastosis, Ebstein's anomaly of the tricuspid valve, or complex heart defects). **Atrial flutter is diagnosed when (1) the atrial rate is greater than 220 beats/min; (2) the P waves are very regular; and (3) there is a characteristic sawtooth pattern, indicating a flutter wave.** The ventricular rate will vary depending on the degree of AV block present. Atrial fibrillation is extremely rare and almost always indicates a serious organic heart disease.

Treatment. The treatment of atrial flutter or fibrillation is DC cardioversion or overdrive atrial pacing followed by maintenance therapy with digoxin.

Ventricular Tachycardia
Ventricular tachycardia is frequently associated with severe organic heart disease.

Treatment. Ventricular tachycardia is best treated with immediate DC cardioversion. Lidocaine may be used as a bolus (1 to 2 mg/kg IV) or as a continuous IV infusion of 20 to 30 μg/min. After conversion, maintenance therapy should be initiated using phenytoin, Inderal, lidocaine, procainamide, or amiodarone.

Complete Atrioventricular Block
In complete heart block, the ventricular rate is slower than the atrial rate and there is no association between the ventricular and atrial rates. Complete heart block can be seen in infants with myocarditis or endocardial fibroelastosis. There is a strong association between congenital heart block and maternal collagen diseases such as SLE. Often these mothers have no signs or symptoms of lupus, but laboratory confirmation is often possible.

Treatment. No treatment is required unless the ventricular rate falls below 55 beats/min or the infant becomes symptomatic, in which case a pacemaker is required. Isoproterenol may increase the ventricular rate until a pacemaker is placed.

PARENT TEACHING[2,4,5,12,14]

The diagnosis of congenital heart disease in their child is a frightening experience for parents. Depending on the family background, educational level, and emotional state, parents may think their infant will die regardless of the severity of the heart defect. In addition, parents may have an overwhelming sense of guilt at having borne a child with a heart defect. Frequently they ask, "What did I do wrong to cause this?" **Therefore comprehensive teaching, reassurance, and support are essential for the well-being of both the infant and the family.**[8,11,21] Understanding the heart defect aids in decreasing anxiety. Parents should also have a basic understanding of their child's heart defect to provide good care after discharge.

Explain the infant's heart defect to the parents. Draw or show a picture of the heart defect, explaining briefly and simply the normal circulation of the heart and how the circulation of their child's heart differs from normal. This explanation should be repeated often for parental understanding and retention. Careful explanation of all tubes, monitors, equipment, and procedures in the nursery also helps decrease parental anxiety.

Heart defects are not visible lesions. Most of these infants will appear quite normal and healthy. Thus it may be difficult for some parents to accept that anything is wrong with their infant. In addition, parents are under great emotional and sometimes physical stress (from labor and delivery), which decreases their ability to hear and retain explanations about the defect. Repetition of explanations is important.

Health care providers should facilitate bonding and decrease the parents' fear of holding or caring for their infant by encouraging interaction with the infant and enabling parents to participate in their infant's care. The parents' confidence in caring for their infant at home is established in the nursery. Parents must feel comfortable caring for their infant and have the opportunity to demonstrate their ability to do so before discharge from the hospital.

Teaching home care of the infant before discharge should be detailed and include medications, signs and symptoms to observe, and guidelines for care. Ideally these should be written instructions. The parents should telephone the physician if the infant demonstrates (1) poor feeding for 1 to 2 days or sweating with feeds, (2) vomiting most of feedings for a 12- to 24-hour period, (3) fast or labored breathing for several hours, (4) decreased activity level, (5) weight loss or failure to gain weight, and (6) frequent respiratory illnesses.

All medications should be explained in detail, including their purpose, action, and administration. Parents should be made aware of the potential adverse effects (side effects) of all of their infant's medications. Parents should be observed giving medications in the nursery before the infant is discharged.

Cyanotic heart disease is particularly disturbing to parents because their infant's skin color is "blue." Parents should be cautioned that their infant will appear blue, especially around the mouth, mucous membranes, hands, and feet, and the blueness will increase with activity such as crying, feeding, and bowel movements. Parents should notify the physician about any of the previously listed symptoms in addition to (1) greatly increased cyanosis, especially if associated with fast or labored breathing, (2) decreased movement in any or all of the extremities, (3) decreased responsiveness or eyes deviating to one side, and (4) seizure activity such as jerking motions or stiffness followed by the infant becoming floppy or limp.

It is important to emphasize to parents that their infant should be treated as normally as possible. **There is no activity restriction for infants with heart disease, because infants will "self-limit" themselves according to their capacities.** It is difficult for parents with a firstborn child with heart disease to differentiate "normal baby problems" from cardiac-related problems. For these parents, as well as other parents of children with cardiac defects, it is particularly important to have open communication between the family, the primary care provider, and the cardiologist. Parents should be encouraged to call these medical personnel as needed for support, answers to questions, and reassurance. Support groups of parents whose children have heart defects provide information, empathy, and practical tips to parents dealing with medical and/or surgical interventions for their child's heart defect.

ACKNOWLEDGMENT

We would like to thank David Clark, M.D., F.A.C.S., F.A.C.C., for his contribution to the sections on surgical management.

REFERENCES

1. Allen HD et al, eds: *Moss and Adams heart disease in infants, children, and adolescents,* ed 6, vol 1, Philadelphia, 2001, Williams & Wilkins.
2. American Heart Association: *If your child has a congenital heart disease: a guide for parents,* Dallas, 2001, American Heart Association.
3. Boucek MM, Shady RE: Pediatric heart transplantation. In Allen HD, Emmanouilides G, Riemenschneider T et al, eds: *Moss and Adams heart disease in infants, children, and adolescents,* Philadelphia, 2001, Williams & Wilkins.
4. Clark EB: Etiology of congenital cardiovascular malformations: epidemiology and genetics. In Allen et al, eds: *Moss and Adams heart disease in infants, children and adolescents,* Philadelphia, 2001, Williams & Wilkins.
5. Freedom RM, Benson LN, Smallhorn JF, eds: *Neonatal heart disease,* London, 1992, Springer-Verlag.
6. Furdon SA: Recognizing congestive heart failure in the neonatal period, *Neonatal Netw* 16:5, 1997.
7. Fyler DC: Report of the New England Regional Infant Cardiac Program, *Pediatrics* 65(Suppl):375, 1980.

8. Garson A Jr, Benson RS, Ivler L et al: Parental reactions to children with congenital heart disease, *Child Psych Hum Dev* 9:86, 1978.

9. Garson A, Bricker JT, Fisher DJ, et al, eds: *The science and practice of pediatric cardiology,* ed 2, vol 1, Baltimore, 1998, Williams & Wilkins.

10. Gillette PC, Garson A: *Pediatric arrhythmias: electrophysiology and pacing,* Philadelphia, 1990, WB Saunders.

11. Gottesfeld IB: Congenial heart disease: the family of the child with congenital heart disease, *MCN Am J Matern Child Nurs* 4:101, 1979.

12. Hinoki KW: Congenital heart disease: effects on the family, *Neonatal Netw* 17:7, 1998.

13. Page J, Hosking M: An approach to the neonate with sudden dysrhythmia: diagnosis, mechanisms, and management, *Neonatal Netw* 16:7, 1997.

14. Perry LW, Neill C, Ferencz C et al: Infants with congenital heart disease: the case. In Fernandez C, Rubin J, Loffredo C et al, eds: *Epidemiology of congenital heart disease: the Baltimore-Washington infant heart study 1981-1989,* Mount Kisco, NY, 1993, Futura.

15. Rose V, Clark E: Etiology of congenital heart disease. In Freedom RM, Benson LN, Smallhorn JF, eds: *Neonatal heart disease,* London, 1992, Springer-Verlag.

16. Sansoucie DA, Cavaliere TA: Transition from fetal to extrauterine circulation, *Neonatal Netw* 16:5, 1997.

17. Spilman LJ, Furdon SA: Recognition, understanding, and current management of cardiac lesions with decreased pulmonary blood flow, *Neonatal Netw* 17:7, 1998.

18. Witt C: Cyanotic heart lesions with increased pulmonary blood flow, *Neonatal Netw* 17:7, 1998.

19. Wood MK: Acyanotic lesions with increased pulmonary blood flow, *Neonatal Netw* 16:17, 1997.

20. Wood MK: Acyanotic cardiac lesions with normal pulmonary blood flow, *Neonatal Netw* 17:5, 1998.

21. Wolterman M, Miller M: Caring for parents in crises, *Nurs Forum* 22:34, 1985.

Neonatal Nephrology

Rita D. Swinford, Melvin Bonilla-Felix, Ruby D. Cerda, Ronald J. Portman

In utero the fetal kidney is not required for toxin removal or fluid and electrolyte homeostasis; that is primarily the placenta's function. Rather, by generating amniotic fluid the fetal kidney has an essential role in the normal development of the fetus. Postnatally, as the infant adapts to the external milieu, the kidney gradually assumes its role as the regulator of fluid and electrolyte homeostasis. At birth there is a dramatic change in renal function that is clinically difficult to assess. This is especially true in a premature infant, whose kidneys must perform a role for which they are not ready. In fact, **nephrogenesis continues to progress until 36 weeks' postconceptional age.**

The more complicated an organ in its development, the more subject it is to maldevelopment, and in this aspect the kidney outranks most other organs. **The genitourinary system has the highest percentage of anomalies, congenital or genetic, of all of the organ systems (10%). In some series the genitourinary system represents 22% to 50% of all abnormalities found on in utero ultrasonographic examinations.**[97] These anomalies frequently present during the neonatal period, but many may be diagnosed later in childhood. Predicting the response of the neonatal kidney to an injury can be quite complicated, because such factors as postconceptual age, presence or absence of a renal anomaly, intrinsic kidney function, and maturation can differentially affect outcome.

There is enormous clinical importance to the developmental disorders of the kidney: renal dysplasias, renal obstruction, and cystic diseases account for a majority of the patients with end-stage renal failure. Similarly, inherited metabolic disorders can cause significant renal diseases. Although as in oxalosis, the defect does not lie within the kidney, or in other conditions, such as cystinuria and renal tubular acidosis, tubular disorders are directly caused by molecular defects. Recently it has been suggested that essential hypertension, which manifests in adolescence and adulthood, can be the sequela of neonatal events.

In this section we will discuss the anatomic and physiologic development of the kidney and its clinical assessment, presenting prenatal and postnatal indicators of renal disease and the most common and important clinical conditions involving the genitourinary system in the neonatal period.[30,50,88,121]

GENERAL PHYSIOLOGY

Normal Development of the Kidney

The mammalian embryo develops three sets of organs, all of which might be called the *embryonic kidneys*.[30,56,88,121,129] The pronephros and the mesonephros regress in the human but induce the metanephros, the direct precursor of the adult kidney (Figure 25-1). The pronephros, a solid mass of cells along the nephrogenic cord, is located at the cervical level at approximately 3 weeks' gestation. Degeneration of the pronephros begins soon after its formation, and no excretory function occurs. Infection or other insults at this stage in development may result in agenesis or abnormal development of the kidney. The primitive ureter of the pronephros forms the Wolffian, or mesonephric duct, which induces the formation of the second kidney, the mesonephros.

At approximately 4 weeks' gestation the mesonephros originates more caudally. It develops from the nephrogenic cord and forms 40 pairs of thin-walled tubules and glomeruli with excretory function. At the end of the fourth month these degenerate as the metanephric kidney develops. Portions of the mesonephric duct system are retained in the male fetus and form the ducts of the epididymis, the ductus deferens, and the ejaculatory duct. In the female, near-complete degeneration occurs.

The metanephros appears at 4½ to 5 weeks' gestation. The metanephric kidney is the product of a series of inductive interactions between the metanephric mesenchyme and the epithelial ureteric bud. Initially, the ureteric bud grows from the Wolffian duct into the mesenchymal portion of the urogenital ridge. Concomitantly, the metanephric mesenchyme changes,

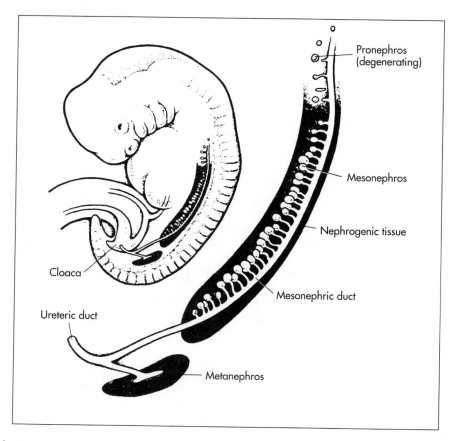

FIGURE 25-1 Schematic representation of overlapping stages in embryogenesis of human kidney. See text for a detailed description. (From Holliday MA: Developmental abnormalities of the kidney in children, *Hosp Pract* 13:101, 1978.)

becoming histologically distinct from the surrounding tissue. When the metanephric mesenchyme and the ureteric bud make contact, a condensation of cells begins along the surface of the bud, and the beginnings of pretubular aggregates develop and undergo mesenchymal-to-epithelial transformation to become the segmented nephron. In addition to the pretubular aggregates, the condensed mesenchyme is thought to produce a number of stem cells, which remain undifferentiated and proliferative. These cells maintain a supply of precursor cells until the generation of completion of nephron development. The epithelial portion of the adult kidney is therefore derived from both stem cells, which give rise to the individual nephron units and the ureteric bud, which gives rise to the collecting ducts and ureter. The ureteric bud migrates to the most caudal end of the nephrogenic cord and finally to the lumbar region and rotates medially along the longitudinal axis.

Cephalic migration of the kidney to its normal position results from straightening of the fetus from the curled position. Abnormalities in the ascent or rotation can lead to pelvic kidneys, horseshoe kidneys, or crossed fused ectopia. Nephrogenesis begins in the renal cortex closest to the medulla (juxtamedullary nephrons). The process continues in a dichotomous branching centrifugal pattern, with the outermost (superficial cortical) nephrons forming last. Finally, cells from the surrounding major vessels and spinal ganglia grow into the metanephros to complete the remaining cell types.

PHYSIOLOGIC DEVELOPMENT AND CLINICAL ASSESSMENT

Kidney function can be broadly classified into the following three categories[129]:

1. Glomerular filtration
2. Tubular reabsorption and secretion
3. The endocrine function of the kidney

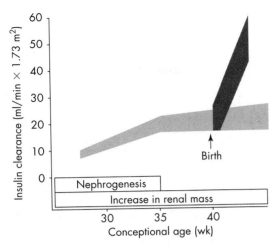

FIGURE 25-2 Correlation of glomular filtration rate (GFR) as measured by insulin clearance and postconceptional age. Note marked increase in GFR postnatally. However, this increase in GFR does not occur after 40 weeks unless birth occurs. If birth occurs before nephrogenesis is complete (usually at 35 weeks), this increase will not occur until 34 to 36 weeks' postconceptional age. (From Guignard JP: Neonatal nephrology. In Holliday MA, Barratt TM, Vernier RL, eds: *Pediatric nephrology*, ed 2, Baltimore, 1987, Williams & Wilkins.)

As early as the mesonephric phase of kidney development, glomerular filtration and tubular function occur. However, the verification or testing of this function has proved difficult in utero; therefore most data are focused on the physiologic changes that occur in the neonatal period.

The process of forming the lifelong complement of approximately 600,000 nephrons in each kidney is complete by 34 to 36 weeks after conception. The kidneys will continue their development at approximately the same rate, whether in utero or ex utero. For example, a premature infant of 28 weeks' gestation will not complete nephrogenesis for 6 to 8 more weeks (Figure 25-2). How insults such as hypoxia, asphyxia, and various toxins affect this development is not yet clear. The newborn kidney may be relatively protected from these insults, because the superficial cortical nephrons are not fully developed and the juxtamedullary nephrons are more resistant to hypoxic damage.

Glomerular Filtration Rate*

For the fetus the placenta serves as the major organ for maintenance of body fluid, electrolyte compo-

sition, and clearance of metabolic wastes in utero. It is not surprising that the percentage of cardiac output to the kidneys is low (2.2% to 3.7%) compared with 25% observed in an adult. In the immature kidney, the total renal plasma flow, directed to the more developed juxtamedullary nephrons, is only approximately 50% of adult values and total renal vascular resistance exceeds adult values, where both afferent and efferent glomerular arterioles appear to be constricted.

After birth there is a dramatic decrease in renal vascular resistance and increase in glomerular filtration rate (GFR). The GFR doubles in the first weeks of life to 30 to 40 ml/min/1.73 m² (Figures 25-2 and 25-3) and then further increases to the adult normal of 100 to 120 ml/min/1.73 m² between 1 and 2 years of life. During this period the GFR is increasing at a rate greater than the growth in body mass. Factors responsible for the striking rise in GFR are an expansion in filtration surface area caused by a greater perfusion of the superficial cortical nephrons and a decrease in renal vascular resistance. The cause of this fall in renal vascular resistance is not known but may be partly explained by a decreasing ratio of alpha-adrenergic (constrictor) to beta-adrenergic (vasodilator) receptors, fall of high levels of circulating renin and angiotensin II activity. **Premature infants of less than 34 weeks' postconceptional age have little increase in creatinine clearance before about 34 weeks' gestation, even though renal weight rises during that period; after this time glomerular filtration rate rises rapidly, increasing threefold to fivefold** (see Figure 25-2).

In term neonates, plasma creatinine falls over the first few days, from a maternal creatinine of 0.8 to 1.2 mg/dl to neonatal levels of 0.2 to 0.3 mg/dl. The rate of this decrease can be quite variable, depending on the infant's level of hydration and clinical status. This lack of steady state makes accurate measurement of creatinine clearance troublesome. Also, laboratory measurement of creatinine has a very low sensitivity for any changes in GFR. A true increase in creatinine from 0.4 to 0.5 mg/dl could reflect a decrease in GFR of as much as 25%. However, **a rising serum creatinine level is never normal. A plasma creatinine level exceeding 0.5 mg/dl in a 1-week or older infant may be an important early clinical indication of the presence of congenital disease (Figure 25-3).**

In an effort to enhance the sensitivity of serum creatinine, Schwartz[105] developed a formula correlating

*References 6, 7, 32, 40, 48, 105, 107, 113.

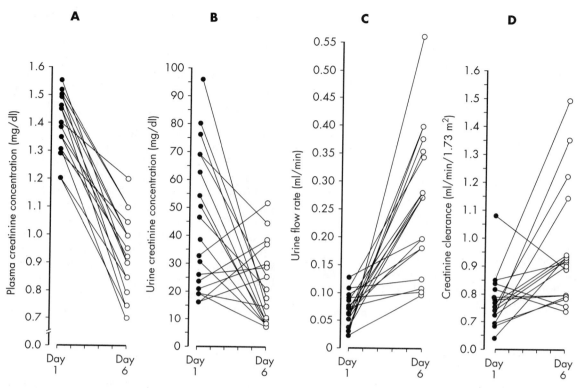

FIGURE 25-3   A, Change in plasma creatinine concentrations on day 1 *(solid circle)* and day 6 *(open circle)* of life. *Solid line con-nects* values of individual infant. **B,** Urinary creatinine concentrations. **C,** Urinary flow rate. **D,** GFR as measured by creatinine clearance. Note that increase in GFR is accompanied by decrease in creatinine concentrations as infant excretes maternal creatinine and by increase in urine flow rate. (From Sertel H, Scopes J: Rates of creatinine clearance in babies less than one week of age, *Arch Dis Child* 48:717, 1973.)

creatinine clearance to body length and plasma creatinine values:

GFR (ml/min/1.73 m²) =

$$\text{Length [cm]} \times \frac{\textbf{k [proportionality constant]}}{\textbf{plasma creatinine (mg/dl)}}$$

The proportionality constant, k, is a function of urine creatinine excretion per unit of body size. For an infant less than 2500 g at birth, the mean value of k is 0.33 throughout the first year of life. For a full-term infant during the same period, k is 0.45. Other k values are available for older children.

Determining GFR in a preterm infant is much more complicated. As mentioned previously, the GFR generally does not increase until nephrogenesis is complete. Until this time the infant's creatinine reflects the mother's creatinine. The only reasonable assessment of renal function in the premature infant

is a relative change in creatinine as measured in serial determinations. Values in excess of maternal creatinine or greater than 1.5 mg/dl may be considered abnormal.

If measurement of creatinine clearance is desired, it is best performed by placing an indwelling urinary catheter for a discrete interval of approximately 2 to 3 hours. The bladder should be drained before the start of urine collection. The clearance formula is as follows:

$$\textbf{Clearance (ml/min/1.73)} = (U \times \frac{V}{P}) \times \frac{1.73}{BSA}$$

where U is the urine creatinine concentration (milligrams per deciliter), P is the plasma concentration, also in milligrams per deciliter, V is the volume of urine divided by the time of collection in minutes, and BSA is the body surface area in square meters.

However, such maneuvers are rarely indicated, because a precise determination of GFR during the newborn period is usually not necessary.

Tubular Function*

Urine flow in utero is important for its contribution to amniotic fluid and for the development of the urinary tract. Sufficient amniotic fluid volume is critical for fetal development; low or no amniotic fluid can lead to fetal *akinesia syndrome,* also called *Potter's syndrome,* in which there is deformation of facial features and limbs and the lungs fail to develop in size, resulting in fetal demise or difficult respiratory management and a need for neonatal dialysis.

The fetal kidney excretes a hypotonic urine (10 ml/ kg/hr) with a large sodium content. After birth the urine flow rate increases in the first week of life (see Figure 25-3). Quite often infants will void unnoticed in the delivery room. **Fifty percent of infants void in the first 12 hours, 92% in the first 24 hours, and 99% in the first 48 hours of life. Causes for failure to void by this time must be carefully evaluated, including abnormalities in volume status or renal function, or anatomic abnormalities such as obstruction.** A diuresis occurs in the first 5 days of life as the expanded extracellular fluid volume of the neonate is excreted. A 10% loss of body weight can be normally seen in those first few days of life. Stimuli for this diuresis are unknown but may be related to the rise in renal blood flow and GFR, and possibly to atrial natriuretic factor release.

Oliguria is generally defined as urine output of less than 1 ml/kg/hr. This definition should not be used for the first 48 hours of life, however, because an infant with poor oral intake may not develop the appropriate signal for diuresis, so that oliguria may not imply a renal abnormality.

Urine flow depends on fluid intake and solute load, as noted in Chapter 14. The neonatal kidney can dilute urine to the same degree as an adult kidney (i.e., 50 mOsm/L); however, the neonate can have difficulty excreting a large volume of water, as acute increases in GFR are not possible. The ability of the neonate to dilute urine coincides with its nutrition, which is a calorically dilute solution (breast milk) and thus there is a need to be able to freely excrete water. The term neonatal kidney, however,

cannot maximally concentrate the urine for several reasons: a low medullary urea content, low peritubular capillary oncotic pressure, resistance to antidiuretic hormone, decreased expression of water channels, and a short loop of Henle are all postulated mechanisms. The kidneys of most infants can fully concentrate urine by 1 year of age.

Sodium*

Apart from the clearance of nitrogenous waste products; the regulation of sodium balance is the most important function of the kidney as this determines the extracellular fluid volume. Early sodium loss accounts for the 10% of extracellular volume loss seen postnatally. In a term neonate the fractional excretion of sodium—which is urinary sodium clearance factored for glomerular filtration rate—is approximately 1% to 3%. However, in preterm infants less than 30 weeks' gestation the fractional excretion rate of sodium (FENa) may be greater than 5% to 6% and in utero greater than 15% (Figure 25-4). The FENa is calculated as follows:

$$FENa = \frac{U_{Na} \times P_{Na}}{U_{Cr} \times P_{Cr}} \times 100$$

Fractional Excretion of Sodium. The extracellular fluid volume is expanded in newborns, and the aforementioned diuresis is accompanied by natriuresis. The ability of the neonatal kidney to handle rapid challenges in sodium balance is relatively fixed. The immature proximal tubule cannot reabsorb adequate amounts of sodium, and thus the distal nephron must compensate with an increase in sodium reabsorption. This is mediated by the increase in the renin, angiotensin, and aldosterone (RAA) levels seen in newborns. This mechanism cannot completely compensate for the increased distal sodium delivery; thus the "salt wasting" of the newborn is observed. Conversely, the neonatal kidney cannot increase the FENa rapidly and thus cannot handle a large sodium load. Such a load would lead to edema and volume overload. Urinary prostaglandin levels are also quite high and may also account for the increase in RAA levels. With tubular maturity and increased proximal sodium reabsorption, the RAA and prostaglandin levels gradually fall. Abnormalities in sodium concentration are discussed in Chapter 14 and are primarily problems

---

*References 6, 7, 32, 40, 49, 94, 107, 113.

*References 7, 32, 48, 53, 94, 110, 114.

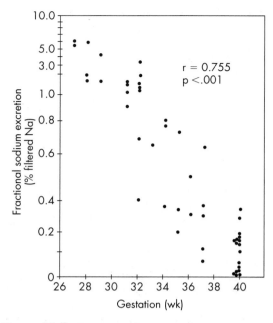

FIGURE 25-4 Decrease in fractional excretion of sodium occurs with increasing postconceptional age. (From Siegel S, Oh W: Renal function as a marker of human fetal maturation, *Acta Paediatr Scand* 65:481, 1976.)

with water balance. Sodium losses are also increased in a stressed, hypoxic infant as the major oxygen consumption of the kidney is used for sodium reabsorption.

Proximal Tubular Function

The proximal tubule appears to be less well developed anatomically than the glomerulus at birth.[7,32,113] The neonatal increase in urinary glucose and amino acid excretion has led investigators to consider the possibility of an imbalance of function between the glomeruli and tubules. In fact, there is a balance in each individual nephron for glomerular and tubular function. The tremendous heterogenicity in nephron development, however, can lead to an enhanced delivery of these substrates to certain nephrons. This filtered load overwhelms the transport systems, and thus glucose and amino acids are spilled into the urine. This is called an increase in *splay*. Neonatal expansion of extracellular fluid volume may also lead to a decrease in proximal tubular absorption of these compounds in the first days of life.

Low-molecular-weight proteins such as beta-2-microglobulin (β2M) are also absorbed exclusively in the proximal tubule. β2M is the small subunit of the HLA class I antigen. As cells die, β2M is released into the circulation and is excreted solely by the kidney. After being freely filtered by the glomerulus, β2M is 99.9% reabsorbed by the proximal tubule and metabolized to amino acids. Any increase in urinary β2M levels is suggestive of proximal tubular dysfunction.[119] Whether an increased excretion in more premature infants is a marker of tubular immaturity is a matter of some debate. β2M is, however, a very sensitive marker of damage to the proximal tubule by hypoxia or toxins and has been used clinically for this purpose.[89]

Potassium

The plasma potassium concentration of neonates tends to be higher (e.g., 5.5 to 6.0 mEq/L) than the values in children and adults.[7,102,113] It appears that the connecting tubule and cortical collecting ducts of the immature kidney are less able to excrete a potassium load as a result most likely to a resistance to aldosterone (9% vs 15%) compared with the mature organ even when the lower glomerular filtration rate is taken into account. This elevated level is rarely of pathologic significance.

Acid-Base Balance[7,22,32,48,113]

With regard to hydrogen ion homeostasis by the kidney, **the plasma bicarbonate level is lower in a newborn (19 to 21 mEq/L) than in an adult.** This is a result of increased endogenous acid production, decreased bicarbonate reabsorption in the proximal tubule, and decreased proton secretion in the collecting duct. Another contributing factor is the neonate's expanded extracellular fluid volume, which leads to a reduction in sodium and bicarbonate reabsorption in the proximal tubule. Carbonic anhydrase activity in the second trimester human kidney is not impaired, and neonates are able to excrete acid urine, frequently with a pH greater than 6. The tubular maximum gradually increases to near-adult levels by the first year of life so that serum bicarbonate increases from 21 to 24 mEq/L. Moreover, the capacity to excrete ammonium and titratable acids increases to adult values, when factored for glomerular filtration rate, by the first month post-term.[118]

A nonanion gap metabolic acidosis secondary to either diarrhea or a renal tubular acidosis can be seen transiently in neonates. Renal tubular acidosis with normal anion gap acidosis in the newborn can also be seen as the tubule recovers from acute renal failure, renal vein thrombosis, nephrocalcinosis (tubular deposition of calcium oxalate), rapid expansion of extracellular fluid, addition of acid (most commonly seen with parenteral nutrition), and urinary diversions into an ileal.

Uric Acid

Serum uric acid levels are elevated in the newborn because of an increase in production.[48,115] Infants who are stressed have particularly high levels from nucleotide breakdown. There is also a fivefold to sevenfold increase in uric acid excretion in newborns compared with excretion in adults. The fractional excretion of uric acid is 30% at 30 weeks' gestation and 18% at 40 weeks' gestation, as opposed to 5% in adults. Newborns are relatively protected from this excessive uric acid excretion by the normal alkalinity of the urine improving the solubility of uric acid. **Uric acid crystals can appear reddish in the diaper and can be mistaken for blood.**

CONGENITAL AND ACQUIRED RENAL ABNORMALITIES

Chromosomal Disorders

Although lower urinary tract and renal anomalies are seldom the presenting features of chromosomal disorders, they frequently form part of a multisystem malformation syndrome caused by chromosomal anomalies.[22,36,73,120,129] Renal disorders seen with chromosomal disturbance include fused kidneys, duplication defects, renal agenesis or hypoplasia, hydronephrosis and hydroureter, renal dysplasia or cystic disease, hypospadias, micropenis, and cryptorchidism.

The overall pattern of malformation seen with individual chromosomal disorders is usually sufficient for diagnosis; however, variation can be seen from one individual to another, even for patients with complete monosomies or trisomies. Although certain renal anomalies are characteristic of many of the more common chromosomal disorders, the picture is otherwise characteristically nonspecific, that is no one renal malformation is unique to any particular chromosomal disorder.

There appears to be two distinct processes involved in the generation of renal defects in chromosomal disorders. On one hand, there may be a developmental error or failure of growth, which occurs during embryogenesis (e.g., horseshoe kidney or duplication defects). Or, there may be obstruction in the urinary tract, either unilateral (e.g., pelviureteric or ureterovesical obstruction) or bilateral (e.g., posterior urethral valves). Consequences to the obstructed developing nephron unit can be hydronephrosis, hydroureter and cortical cysts as seen in trisomy 13 and other chromosomal anomalies or renal agenesis and dysplasia. Renal agenesis and dysplasia may also be secondary to developmental growth failure and also be unilateral or bilateral. In the case of the multicystic dysplastic kidney there may be no evidence of obstruction while in prune belly syndrome the dysplastic kidney may be secondary to bilateral dilation of ureters and obstruction. Typically, when followed longitudinally, the dysplastic kidney does not keep up with patient growth and gradually shrinks, eventually disappearing.

ACQUIRED DISORDERS*

Neonatal renal involvement should be considered with the use of three drugs—loop diuretics, aminoglycosides, and nonsteroidal antiinflammatory drugs (NSAIDs)—because the neonate's immature and lower GFR may be adversely affected in a concentration-dependent fashion. Complicating the issue of dosage is the rapid maturation of the neonate's GFR.

Although furosemide, a loop diuretic, is used in the neonatal population, it is associated with significant side effects. Furosemide is freely filtered by the glomerulus but primarily secreted in the proximal tubule where an increased dose is required in the newborn with a lower GFR. A common side effect of furosemide is electrolyte disturbance including, hyponatremia, hypochloremia, hypokalemia, and metabolic alkalosis that can be treated with electrolyte supplementation and adjustment of diuretic agents. Furosemide also increases the excretion of urine calcium and therefore is associated with renal calcifications, including commonly interstitial calcifications or nephrocalcinosis, less commonly renal stones or nephrolithiasis, secondary hyperparathyroidism, and osteopenia. In neonates, high

---

*References 5, 14-18, 21, 23, 31, 35, 46, 58, 59, 61, 79, 103, 108.

urinary calcium excretion and an alkaline urinary pH is thought to promote calcium salt crystallization, although the cause of nephrocalcinosis in preterm neonates has not been fully elucidated.

More recently it has been proposed that the higher dietary intake of calcium, phosphate, ascorbic acid, low urinary citrate to creatinine ratio, high urine calcium to creatinine ratio, immaturity, and prevalent use of diuretics enhancing urinary calcium excretion elevates the incidence of nephrocalcinosis in neonates, especially those with lower birth weight and lower gestational age. Nephrocalcinosis develops secondary to an imbalance between stone-favorable versus stone-inhibiting factors. The more mature medullary nephrons within a premature infant's kidney are thought to have relatively longer loops of Henle and lower urine velocity, which would favor crystal formation and aggregation. **Paradoxically, the higher concentration of calcium and phosphate needed to ensure bone development are not beneficial for the kidney. Hypercalciuria is defined as a urinary calcium loss greater than 0.15 mmol/kg/24 hr. Interestingly, neonates receiving only short-term therapy of about a week of furosemide can develop this abnormality and develop short-term complications including nephrolithiasis with ureter obstruction and urinary tract infection. Although nephrocalcinosis occurs in premature infants without the use of furosemide, it is the single major risk factor in this form of renal damage; the incidence varies between 17% and 64% depending on different patient populations and ultrasonographic criteria and equipment.**

With the development of nephrocalcinosis, one may also see a renal tubular acidosis requiring treatment with oral bicarbonate for maintenance of linear growth. This type of calcification and renal tubular acidosis may be halted or reversed by the addition of a thiazide diuretic that promotes the reabsorption of calcium and potassium citrate, which increases the favorability of crystal solubility. The long-term outcome of nephrocalcinosis in preterm infants has not been defined, but small-scale studies suggest a possible decline in renal function.

Furosemide is used in neonates and infants to treat the pulmonary congestion associated with acute respiratory distress syndrome, bronchopulmonary dysplasia, and transient tachypnea of the newborn. In preterm infants who are greater than 3 weeks of age with chronic lung disease (CLD) acute and long-term administration of furosemide improves lung compliance and oxygenation. However, data are lacking to support routine use of this agent with developing CLD. Indeed, there are no current data to support the routine diuretic use in preterm infants with respiratory distress syndrome as the risk of hypovolemia, hemodynamic instability, and symptomatic patent ductus is increased. The potential for furosemide ototoxicity is also a significant complication, especially when used in combination with aminoglycosides. Interestingly, the incidence of sensorineural hearing loss in preterm NICU graduates is approximately 20%, where risk factors of hyponatremia (secondary to diuretic use or inappropriate antidiuretic hormone secretion) seem to enhance the development of adverse sequelae.

Aminoglycosides have long been one of the commonest causes of drug-induced nephrotoxicity. **Pharmacokinetic analysis of gentamicin therapy in the newborn can achieve desired concentrations (peak 6 to 8 μg/ml and trough less than 2 μg/ml) and minimize overall dosing.** The recognition of patient- and treatment-related risk factors have improved the safety of aminoglycosides to that of the other main wide-spectrum antibiotics. The neonatal kidney may be at less risk for nephrotoxicity from aminoglycosides than is the mature kidney. However, gentamicin-induced renal toxicity was recently confirmed in the neonatal kidney without any relationship to peak and trough serum levels. In fact, the long-term effects of neonatal aminoglycoside exposure on renal development have yet to be adequately evaluated. Ototoxicity, which is the second main adverse effect of aminoglycosides and which, in contrast to nephrotoxicity, is irreversible.

The nephrotoxicity induced by aminoglycosides manifests clinically as nonoliguric renal failure, with a slow rise in serum creatinine and a hypoosmolar urine developing after several days of treatment. The nephrotoxicity of the aminoglycosides is believed to be secondary to a small percentage of retained drug within the kidney's proximal epithelial cells, where at low or appropriate doses, tubular alterations can generate proteinuria, hypoosmotic urine, and increases in blood BUN and creatinine, reflecting a decrease in GFR. At higher doses of aminoglycosides, tubular wasting of potassium, magnesium, and calcium, decreased reabsorption of water, bicarbonate, and glucose occurring concomitantly with tubular necrosis can be seen.

Since the 1970s, premature infants with symptomatic patent ductus arteriosus (PDA) have been treated with indomethacin, a nonspecific prostaglandin inhibitor. Indomethacin, as well as other NSAIDs, has been shown to have various side effects including hemodynamic changes in cerebral, mesenteric and renal circulations. The renal side effects seen with indomethacin appear to be related to the following three phenomena:

1. Intrauterine cyclooxygenase (COX) inhibition may induce renal dysplasia, dysgenesis and alter renal maturation by slowing glomerular maturation.
2. Oligohydramnios may be the end result of fetal indomethacin exposure with concomitant decline in renal blood flow and glomerular filtration.
3. Indomethacin given in three divided doses of 0.2 mg/kg every 12 hours for closure of PDA may induce and exacerbate renal failure by changing the balance of cortical juxtamedullary nephron perfusion. The fragile balance of vasoconstrictor (mediated by angiotensin II and endothelin) and vasodilatory (atrial natriuretic peptide, nitric oxide, prostaglandins, kallikrein-kinin) forces is now altered in favor of vasoconstriction, and further reduction of the already low GFR.

For preterm infants and newborns, the administration of NSAIDs should be done with care and frequent monitoring of renal function, even though these changes are often reversible. When a change or decline in GFR is noted, such as a plasma creatinine increase, administration of the NSAID should be halted. Indomethacin has been shown to have clinically important renal side effects, including proteinuria, oliguria, renal failure, hyperkalemia, and hyponatremia. Patients at higher risk include infants with persistent patent ductus, dehydration, and simultaneous administration of other nephrotoxic drugs. In a randomized controlled study of furosemide versus a distal diuretic chlorothiazide in preterm infants, furosemide was shown to increase the incidence of PDA mediated by prostaglandin. Unfortunately, the combined use of furosemide and indomethacin does not improve outcome. At this time, in the absence of large randomized and controlled trials, guidelines for NSAID administration must rely on animal studies. Additionally, there are no studies on the effect of selective COX inhibitors on PDA closure.

GENERAL DATA COLLECTION

History

Obtaining a complete family history of renal diseases or syndromes involving the kidneys can aid in the ultimate diagnosis of a preterm infant (e.g., a history of prenatal maternal infections, drugs, toxin, or medication intake as risk factors for the development of fetal nephropathy).[13,48,74,92] Paternal smoking and advanced age can also be associated with an increased risk of urinary tract anomalies.

The quantity of amniotic fluid is the only reliable indicator of renal function in the fetus. A clinical change in volume and its subsequent correlation to impaired renal function may be assessed in utero in selected abnormalities. Fetal swallowing, breathing, and urination are thought to regulate amniotic fluid volume beginning in the second trimester. Abnormalities in these regulatory mechanisms result in alteration of amniotic fluid volume. Normally, amniotic fluid volume increases during gestation, peaking at 34 weeks' gestation. Decreased volume, or oligohydramnios, is caused by fetal genitourinary abnormalities (Table 25-1). Polyhydramnios, or excessive amniotic fluid, occurs in varying degrees with moderate (2000 ml) to extreme (15,000 ml) increases in fluid volume. A correlation between perinatal outcome and the degree of hydramnios has been reported. Gastrointestinal abnormalities that inhibit fetal swallowing are implicated as a major etiological factor in polyhydramnios. Conditions characterized by a severe urinary concentrating defect (e.g., diabetes insipidus and Bartter's syndrome) have been associated with polyhydramnios.

A perinatal asphyxia scoring system that uses fetal heart rate monitoring, Apgar scores, and metabolic acidosis has been developed. A high score is an excellent predictor of renal damage.

Signs and Symptoms

Physical findings that are indicators of genitourinary tract abnormalities are outlined in Table 25-1. The table points out the importance of a careful physical examination as a first step in a nephrologic evaluation.

Laboratory Data

Ultrasonography

Ultrasonography may identify urinary tract dilation beginning at the seventeenth and twenty-fourth weeks of gestation.[8] Fetal ultrasonography for the

Table 25-1	PERINATAL INDICATORS OF ABNORMALITIES OF THE GENITOURINARY TRACT
FINDING	**SUSPECTED ABNORMALITY**
Oligohydramnios	Bilateral renal agenesis, PKD, or dysplasia
	Amnion nodosum
Polyhydramnios	Nephrogenic diabetes insipidus, trisomy 18 or 21, anencephaly, esophageal or duodenal obstruction, Klippel-Feil syndrome, Bartter's syndrome
Enlarged placenta (>25% of infant birth weight)	Congenital nephrotic syndrome
Velamentous insertion of umbilical cord	Increased congenital anomalies
Asphyxia neonatorum	Renal failure
Physical Examination	
Hypertension	See text
Skin	
Hemangioma	Hemangioma of kidney or bladder
Edema	Congenital nephrotic syndrome, hydrops fetalis
Adenoma sebaceum	Tuberous sclerosis—cystic kidneys
Head	
Encephalocele	Meckel's or Meckel-Gruber syndrome—polycystic kidney disease
Cleft lip and palate	Urinary tract anomalies
Macroglossia	Beckwith-Wiedemann syndrome—renal dysplasia
	Johanson-Blizzard syndrome—hydronephrosis, orofaciodigital syndrome—renal microcystic disease
Eyes	
Phakoma (tubular sclerosis)	Angiomyolipoma of the kidney
Retinitis pigmentosa	Medullary cystic disease of the kidney
Cataracts	Cystic diseases, Lowe's syndrome, Wilms' tumor, congenital rubella
Aniridia	Wilms' tumor
Ears	
Low set or malformed	Increased risk of renal abnormalities, Potter's syndrome
Ear tags	Brancho-oto-renal (BOR) syndrome
Preauricular pits	
Skeleton	
Hemihypertrophy	Wilms' tumor
Spina bifida	Neurogenic bladder
Arthrogryposis	Oligohydramnios, Potter's syndrome

Modified from Retik AB: Genitourinary problems in children, *Hosp Pract* 11:133, 1976.

assessment of renal function can provide (1) estimation of amniotic fluid volume, (2) information on the appearance and echogenicity of kidneys on ultrasonography, (3) degree of upper urinary tract dilation, and (4) provide guidance for amniocentesis to analyze fetal urine electrolytes. Prenatal ultrasonography can define the structure and anatomy of renal tract abnormalities but does not predict neonatal and postnatal urinary tract function. The term *dilation* does not always imply urinary tract obstruction and must be used in conjunction with the amount of amniotic fluid in estimating kidney function. The most common finding on ultrasonography in the fetal urinary system is a dilated renal pelvis or hydronephrosis. Often this is physiologic and nonobstructing, although an etiology relating to obstruction must be considered. Although the definition of hydronephrosis in the fetus is not definitive, the following have been observed:

1. The more severe the dilation (greater than 9 mm in the second trimester), the more likely that the infant will either need conservative

Table 25-1	PERINATAL INDICATORS OF ABNORMALITIES OF THE GENITOURINARY TRACT—cont'd
FINDING	**SUSPECTED ABNORMALITY**
Skeleton—cont'd	
Dysplastic nails	Nail patella syndrome
Vertebral anomalies	VATER syndrome—renal dysplasia
Polydactyly	Meckel's or Meckel-Gruber syndrome—polycystic kidneys
Abdomen	
Absence of abdominal musculature	Prune-belly syndrome
Single umbilical artery	Increased congenital anomalies of the urinary tract
Umbilical discharge	Patent urachus
Abdominal mass	See Table 25-5
Hepatomegaly	Storage diseases—renal tubular dysfunction, Beckwith-Wiedemann syndrome, Zellweger's syndrome
Pulmonary	
Spontaneous pneumothorax	Increase in renal abnormalities
Pulmonary hypoplasia	Oligohydramnios
Genitourinary—Male	
Undescended testes	Prune-belly syndrome, Noonan's syndrome, Lawrence-Moon-Biedel syndrome
Congenital absence of vas deferens	Renal agenesis or ectopia
Hypospadias	Increase in renal abnormalities
Abnormal urinary stream	Bladder dysfunction or urethral outlet obstruction
Genitourinary—Female	
Enlarged clitoris	Adrenogenital syndrome
Cystic mass in urethral region	Ectopic ureterocele, paraurethral cyst
	Sarcoma botryoides
Bulging in vagina	Hydrometrocolpos
Abnormal urinary stream or dribbling	Bladder dysfunction, urethral obstruction
Common cloaca	Urinary tract abnormalities
Rectal	
Deficient anal sphincter tone	Neurogenic bladder dysfunction
Dilated prostatic urethra	Posterior urethral valves, prune-belly syndrome
Masses	Tumor
Anal atresia	VATER syndrome—renal dysplasia
Urinalysis	See text

long-term follow-up care or surgical intervention in the first year of life.

2. The later in pregnancy the sonogram is performed, the more likely the diagnosis of hydronephrosis will be confirmed postnatally.

Other Imaging Studies

The resolution of neonatal nuclear scans may be inadequate for diagnosing all but the most glaring abnormalities (e.g., lack of renal perfusion). A voiding cystourethrogram is an invasive procedure used to evaluate the lower urinary tract and is typically reserved for the more mature infant.

Amniocentesis

Amniocentesis, performed during the second trimester, involves the aspiration of amniotic fluid with a needle transabdominally under ultrasound guidance for safety of the fetus and to increase the likelihood of a successful tap.[11,52] Amniocentesis reveals information on fetal lung maturity, presence of fetal chromosomal abnormalities, Rh isoimmunization, and prenatal diagnosis of many inherited disorders. The determination of alpha-fetoprotein, the major serum protein present in early gestation, yields important data from amniocentesis. Produced initially by the yolk sac, levels of AFP peak between 14 and 18 weeks' gestation. High concentrations of AFP are associated with open neural tube defects and other conditions such as congenital nephrosis, hydrocele, esophageal atresia, and Meckel's syndrome (Meckel-Gruber syndrome). Cystinosis can be diagnosed by measuring the cystine content of cells obtained by amniocentesis.

Urinalysis

Urinalysis is frequently overlooked but can be an important adjunct for diagnosis of renal disease in preterm infants.[118] Sampling can be accomplished by thorough cleansing of the perineum and placement of a urine bag; the subsequent sample can be sent for urine dipstick and analysis including pH, specific gravity, protein, glucose, heme, nitrate, leukocyte esterase, and cell count.

Specific Gravity. **A newborn's urine specific gravity reflects the immature kidney's ability to concentrate and dilute the urine. Initially, the specific gravity will be low (1.001 to 1.005) in the term neonate and maximally 1.015 to 1.020.** Other components of the urine, such as glucose, protein, and dyes, can alter the specific gravity. Urine osmolality measurements should be obtained and correlated to serum osmolality if issues of inappropriate water or salt losses are being considered.

Glucosuria. Glucose may be found only in trace quantities in a term infant's urine but more frequently is noted in a premature infant's urine. Even minor elevations of plasma glucose concentrations may cause significant glucosuria in this population. Large glucose loads given during parenteral alimentation may lead to an osmotic diuresis.

Urinary pH. **Urinary pH is typically relatively acidotic at 6.0. Most neonates can acidify the urine to a pH below 6.0 and if challenged to 5.0.**

Hematuria. **Hematuria, defined as greater than five to six red blood cells per high-powered field (HPF) is abnormal in a neonate, indeed, any individual.**[28,69,113] A positive dipstick for heme occurs with hemoglobinuria, during hemolytic states, and with myoglobinuria from severe asphyxia. Hema-

turia may occur after the trauma of delivery, especially with an enlarged kidney (e.g., cystic disease or obstruction). Hematuria is most commonly seen in perinatal asphyxia. Other common conditions associated with hematuria include renal vein thrombosis, urinary tract infections, sepsis, embolization to the renal artery (especially from UACs), renal necrosis, hypercalciuria, coagulopathies and, rarely, congenital glomerulonephritis or nephrosis. Hematuria may also be observed from blood outside of the genitourinary tract that is mixed with urine. This includes blood from a circumcision, blood from perineal irritation, and uterine bleeding caused by withdrawal from the effects of maternal hormones. If the hematuria is persistent, it should be evaluated with urine culture, assessment of proteinuria and urine calcium excretion, measurement of GFR, and an anatomic evaluation of the kidneys, such as renal ultrasound.

Pyuria. **Pyuria is frequently noted in the newborn, especially females.**[48] **As many as 25 to 50 white blood cells/HPF may be observed in the first days of life. Pyuria may be a marker of infection, and a urine culture should be obtained where clinically indicated with fever or signs and symptoms of sepsis. However, pyuria may also be seen with stress and other injuries to the kidney.**

Proteinuria.[33,48,63] The urine dipstick test for protein is based on a color change that occurs when the tetrabromophenol present on the strip reacts with the amino groups of proteins. Both albumin and low-molecular-weight proteins will give positive results; therefore a dipstick test cannot be used to distinguish between glomerular and tubular proteinuria. Protein detection by dipstick is also pH dependent; thus alkaline urine (approximately 8.0) may give false-positive results. Other factors that can confound the detection of protein include prolonged immersion of the strip and the presence of detergents and urine white cells or bacteria. The dipstick measures protein concentration, where 1+ is approximately 30 mg/dl, 2+ is approximately 100 mg/dl, and so on. If a urine specimen is very concentrated, even very small amounts of protein can give a falsely elevated reading. Conversely, if the urine is quite dilute (e.g., a specific gravity of 1.002), significant amounts of protein will go undetected.

For accurate measurement of protein excretion rates, timed urine collections are necessary. In children the rate of protein excretion rates varies with age and size, with minimal discrepancy if normalized to body surface area (BSA). Proteinuria (greater than or equal to 1+ on the urine dipstick) is frequently seen in newborns. Protein excretion that is considered "acceptable" can range from 182 (88 to 377) mg/24 hr/m² in preterm infants to 145 (68 to 309) mg/24 hr/m² in full-term infants. At 2 months to 1 year the protein excretion is seen to vary between 48 and 244 mg/24 hr/m². As a point of reference an adult may have a 24-hour protein value of 63 (22 to 81) mg/24 hr/m². Proteinuria is highest in the first day of life but then rapidly decreases; this is thought to be secondary to a low tubular reabsorptive capacity. Typically (although not for newborns), a protein excretion rate of less than 4 mg/m²/hr is considered normal; 4 to 40 mg/m²/hr is elevated; and greater than 40 mg/m²/hr is considered nephritic-range proteinuria. Proteinuria is seen in many renal parenchymal diseases and should be evaluated if persistent. Spot urine protein/creatinine ratios are a reasonable substitute in assessing proteinuria in most clinical situations, as a timed urine collection can be quite difficult if the infant is not catheterized. Values of less than 0.5 are considered normal for a child less than 6 months of age; for children from 6 months to 2 years of age, 0.2 to 0.25 is acceptable.

ACUTE RENAL FAILURE*

Pathophysiology

Acute renal failure (ARF) is defined as the sudden deterioration of the kidneys' baseline function, resulting in an inability to maintain the body's fluid and electrolyte homeostasis.[62,123] Steady-state creatinine equilibrium is not achieved until the preterm and term infant is approximately 1 year of age; therefore the detection of acute and chronic renal failure can be difficult (see Figure 25-3). Preterm and term newborns will have a serum creatinine clearance in the first few days of life reflective of the mother's creatinine clearance at delivery (e.g., 0.8 to 1.2 mg/dl). As mentioned earlier, a preterm infant will continue nephrogenesis until about week 36 of life, with serum creatinine clearance ranging from 0.5 to 1.2 mg/dl. As a general rule, the more premature the infant, the higher the serum creatinine. **Any rising serum creatinine from initial baseline or a serum creatinine greater than 1.5 mg/dl with normal mater-**

nal function should be investigated. Recall that a 1-week-old term infant can have a serum creatinine level of approximately 0.2 to 0.4 mg/dl.

Etiology*

Both preterm and term infants are born with significantly low renal function, tenuously balanced between vasoconstrictor and vasodilatory intrarenal factors. **The preponderance of factors causing acute renal failure in a newborn is prerenal (e.g., hypoxia, hypovolemia, hypotension and positive pressure ventilation) in nature, because primary renal and postrenal factors (e.g., autosomal polycystic kidney disease, posterior urethral valves with obstruction) are much less common.**

Acute renal failure has been reported to occur in up to 8% of neonates admitted to an NICU. This is probably an underestimate because of the difficulty in making the diagnosis, especially in nonoliguric acute renal failure. A scoring system for diagnosing the severity of perinatal asphyxia suggests that up to 60% of patients with severe asphyxia may have acute renal failure, predominantly nonoliguric in nature. In fact, asphyxia is the most common cause of acute tubular necrosis in the term neonate (65%); sepsis is the most common in the preterm infant (35%). Patients with congenital heart disease appear to be especially vulnerable to tubular necrosis after cardiac catheterization and cardiac surgery.

Urinary/blood indices have been used to separate these entities and are based on the appropriateness of the renal response to a challenge and gestational age. By example, the FENa should be very low in a prerenal patient as reabsorption of all fluid would be physiologic (e.g., less than 1%); an inappropriate response suggesting tubular damage would be an increased FENa (e.g., greater than 3%). Similarly, a urine creatinine to serum creatinine ratio of greater than 40 implies water conservation and a prerenal cause, whereas a ratio of less than 20 suggests intrinsic renal damage. But it is important to note that urinary/blood indices not only vary according to gestational age and maturity in preterm infants but also in term infants, thereby undermining the usefulness of spot urine samples in the early neonatal period. Although we have categorized these groups into pretubular, tubular, and posttubular causes of acute renal failure, the use of these indices is ineffective in

---

*References 34, 45, 48, 76, 87, 116.

*References 62, 75, 87, 116, 120,127.

Table 25-2	ETIOLOGY OF ACUTE RENAL FAILURE IN THE NEONATE				
	URINARY INDEXES OF ACUTE RENAL FAILURE				
	U_{Na} (mEq/L)	FENa (%)	RFI	U/P_{CRE}	U/P_{OSM}
Pretubular	31.4 ± 19.5	0.95 ± 0.55	1.29 ± 0.82	29.2 ± 15.6	>1.3
Renal parenchymal (tubular) obstruction	63.4 ± 34.7	4.25 ± 2.2	11.6 ± 9.6	9.6 ± 3.6	>1.0

Modified from Matthew OP, Jones AS, James E et al: Neonatal renal failure: usefulness of diagnostic indices, *Pediatrics* 65:57, 1980.

Pretubular: hypotension-sepsis, shock, hypovolemia-dehydration, hemorrhage, hypoproteinemia, cardiac failure, renal artery stenosis, hypoxemia, asphyxia, glomerulonephritis, mechanical ventilation, pressor agents.

Renal parenchymal (tubular): acute tubular necrosis, corticomedullary necrosis, asphyxia neonatorum, pyelonephritis, interstitial nephritis, polycystic kidney disease, renal parenchymal/aplasia/hypoplasia, intrauterine infection, endogenous toxins (uric acid, hemoglobinuria, myoglobinuria), exogenous toxins (aminoglycosides, indomethacin, contrast media), renal vein thrombosis, disseminated intravascular coagulation, congenital nephrotic syndrome.

Obstruction: ureteral obstruction, urethral obstruction.

U, Urine concentration; *P,* plasma concentration; *FENa,* fractional excretion of sodium; *Cre,* creatinine (mg/dl); *Osm,* osmolarity (mOsm/L); *RFI,* renal failure index ($U_{Na} \times$ P/U creatinine).

infants and premature infants causing problems with interpretation (Table 25-2).

Prevention

The prevention of acute renal failure in preterm and term infants is a complicated discussion[62]; nonetheless, some recommendations include the following: minimization of perinatal asphyxia; avoidance of maternal and infant ACE-inhibitor use; aggressive management of hypoxemia, hypovolemia, hypotension, acidosis, and hypothermia, and early detection and treatment of infections and with careful attention to agents with vasoactive or nephrotoxic properties that can exacerbate renal injury (e.g., diuretics, aminoglycosides, and NSAIDs).

Laboratory Data

Renal ultrasonography should be performed in all neonates with suspected ARF to assess possible urinary tract obstruction, renal vein thrombosis, and congenital renal abnormalities such as dysplasia, polycystic disease, or aplasia.

Treatment*

When the diagnosis of acute renal failure secondary to prenatal causes is made, treatment should begin e.g., rapid volume challenge without waiting for urine studies etc. and removal, if possible, of the precipitating agent or agents. Prenatal causes require increasing perfusion of the kidney by fluid

therapy and restoring cardiac output and blood pressure to normal. Any obstruction or thrombosis needs immediate attention.

A fluid challenge of 5 to 10 ml/kg of body weight of crystalloid for small preterm infants and up to 20 ml/kg of body weight for term infants should be attempted. With no signs of congestive heart failure and continuing oliguria or anuria, fluid administration continues with the administration now of colloid, 5% albumin, in a similar amount. If heart failure is present, inotropic agents should be considered (see Chapter 24).

Central venous pressure (CVP) is an important, underutilized parameter in measuring the appropriateness of fluid therapy. Use of CVP is especially important in infants with capillary leak syndrome or with third spacing of fluids postoperatively. These infants appear fluid overloaded but may be intravascularly depleted. Therapeutically, diuretic administration removes fluid, but it does not help diagnostically because an increase in urine output does not differentiate between renal involvement and prerenal causes. Diuretics may in fact cause dehydration and further exacerbation of ARF. Mannitol should be avoided because of its hyperosmolarity and increased risk for IVH.

The indications for the acute application of renal replacement therapy include fluid overload with/without limitation of nutritional therapy, severe acidosis, hyperkalemia with EKG changes, symptomatic uremia, hyperuricemia, hyperammonemia, and drug overdose (e.g., theophylline, gentamicin, vancomycin, carbamazepine). Current modalities of renal replacement therapy available for preterm in-

*References 24, 26, 27, 34, 37, 44, 47, 48, 52, 60, 62, 64, 66, 72, 116, 125.

fants are quite limited as the degree of vascular access and abdominal musculature prevent placement of dialysis catheters. However, for a term infant hemodialysis, continuous venovenous hemodialysis (CVVHD), and peritoneal dialysis (PD) are feasible and should be offered as a standard of care.

Continuous Venovenous Hemodialysis

Although there is clear support for the use of CVVHD in infants who are critically ill with acute renal failure, there are other illnesses without renal involvement per se for which CVVHD can be of value.[43,71,95,96] These include sepsis and inflammatory syndromes, such as acute respiratory distress syndrome; postcardiopulmonary bypass, in which removal of inflammatory mediators by membrane adsorption may improve outcome in addition to regulation of volume status; inborn errors of metabolism; and severe lactic acidosis. The goal of CVVHD is to maintain normal electrolyte balance with ongoing slow fluid removal until the infant has recovered from the initiating insult. CVVHD is only feasible in the critical care setting and is not an alternative to chronic care.

For the last few years CVVHD has been our first choice for dialysis of small infants with ARF. Although there is the potential for complications related to the characteristic need for patient anticoagulation to prevent filter clotting, the current availability of CVVHD equipment adapted for the small patient, the availability of small double lumen vascular catheters, experienced intensive care nursing, and wide publication of successful pediatric experiences are all factors which have contributed the acceptance and availability of this technique (Figure 25-5). Because the extracorporeal blood volume will be in most cases more than 10% to 20% of the patient's blood volume, we routinely prime the lines with whole blood or packed red blood cells. In our experience, all infants, including those weighing 2 kg, have tolerated the procedure well. Maintenance of normal electrolyte balance is achieved often by adjustment of dialysate electrolyte solutions as hypophosphatemia, hypokalemia, and hyponatremia is fairly frequent. Heparinization may not be necessary if a preexistent coagulopathy exists; if necessary regional anticoagulation therapy using citrate can be done as an alternative. CVVHD offers a great alternative for acute dialysis, especially in an infant with labile hemodynamic status in whom hemodialysis and peritoneal dialysis are not feasible.

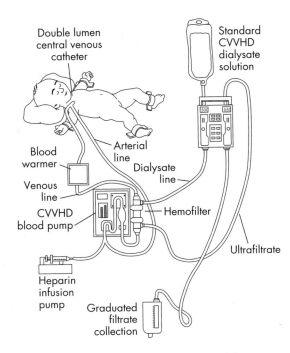

FIGURE 25-5 Continuous venovenous hemodialysis (CVVHD) in newborn. Blood access is provided by a central venous line. Blood is pumped through the system by a hemofiltration pump at a blood flow of 5 to 8 ml/kg/min (minimum 30 ml/min). A constant heparin infusion is maintained to keep an activated clotting time between 180 and 220 seconds. The amount of ultrafiltrate is regulated (according to the individualized needs) by using an infusion pump at filter outflow. A standard CVVHD dialysate solution is used unless severe metabolic acidosis develops. Before the blood is returned to the patient, it is passed through a blood warmer to prevent hypothermia.

Peritoneal Dialysis*

As a renal replacement therapy, PD is useful for both the acute and chronic care setting; therefore it remains the intervention of choice for the neonate with end stage renal disease. The goal of long-term PD is ideally to permit normal growth and development up to the time of transplantation, if needed. The ability of PD to perform ultrafiltration and removal of solute through the process of diffusion is mediated by the peritoneal membrane, a dialysis catheter and a method for filling the abdomen with fluid/dialysate and for removal of such fluid after a

---

*References 19, 26, 44, 47, 52, 57, 64, 66, 70, 98, 100, 109, 128.

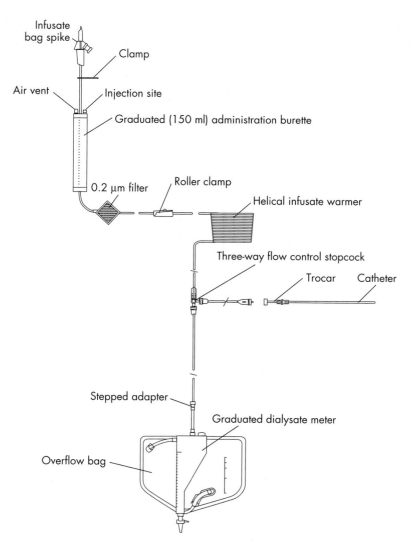

FIGURE 25-6 An example of a commercially available dialysis set for neonatal peritoneal dialysis. The graduated burette in this closed system allows for easily varying the amount of dialysate delivered. The helical coils allow dialysate to be warmed in the same manner as in exchange transfusion. A graduated meter allows accurate measurement of outflow. (Courtesy Gesco International, San Antonio, Texas, 1987.)

specified amount of time (Figures 25-4 through 25-6 and Table 25-3).

Long-term dialysis, as provided by PD, has become the standard of care for even very small infants with clinical conditions requiring renal replacement therapy. Many newborns who require peritoneal dialysis do not have primary renal failure, but require dialysis because of prenatal, perinatal, and/or postnatal conditions that have resulted in poor renal perfusion. As this statement implies, it can be difficult to judge before initiation of dialysis which infant will benefit and which will not. Therefore **it would seem reasonable to *initially* present acute dialysis as a temporary adjunct to care within a limited time frame, such as 1 or 2 weeks, as agreed on by the family and medical team.** With the available infant-specific equipment and expertise, dedicated support of the renal team and family, aggressive nutritional

Table 25-3	NURSING CARE PLAN FOR PERITONEAL DIALYSIS IN THE NEONATE
PROBLEMS	**NURSING ACTIONS**

Potential peritonitis	1. Sterile technique to be used at all tubing connections and bag spikes; all connections clamped and taped.
	2. Assess PD effluent with each drain for color, turbidity, and the presence of fibrin.
	3. Should turbidity exist:
	   a. Obtain cell count, differential, gram stain, and culture of PD fluid.
	   b. Administer antibiotics as ordered.
	4. Occlusive dressing at catheter site.

Potential fluid overload and/or dehydration	1. Measure and record the exact amount of inflow and outflow of dialysate with each exchange.
	2. Weigh neonate at regular intervals during drain to determine real weight of infant.
	3. Assess for fluid reabsorption:
	   a Peripheral and dependent edema
	   b. Weight gain
	   c. Failure to drain out all of dwell volume
	4. Assess for dehydration:
	   a. Weight loss
	   b. Poor skin turgor and sunken eyes
	   c. Hypotension
	5. Notify physician of weight discrepancies or other symptoms.

Potential temperature maintenance problems	1. Warm all PD fluid to body temperature by blood warmer or heating pad immediately before inflow.
Inflow and/or outflow obstruction	1. Check for kinks in line. 2. Reposition patient, inflow and/or drain bags. 3. Plain radiograph of the abdomen to check position of catheter—should be toward pelvis. 4. Add heparin to dialysate if fibrin is present.
Potential respiratory compromise	1. Use smaller exchange volumes. 2. Position patient with HOB elevated to reduce pressure on the abdomen. 3. If distress exists after drain, obtain chest x-ray to rule out pneumonia or hydrothorax.

HOB, Head of bed; *PD,* peritoneal dialysis.

supplementation, maintenance of hemoglobin with erythropoietin and growth with vitamin D and recombinant growth hormone, survival with an improved quality of life and development has been achieved.

Although there has been a clear improvement in the availability of infant catheters and dialysis tubing, it remains a real challenge for the parents of an infant on PD when they recognize that ultimately this is a home-based therapy they must implement. Even when they surmount this hurdle, feeding issues remain paramount. The recommendation is for early placement of nasogastric tubes or gastrostomy buttons. These patients require truly devoted families who can focus on detail for the better part of each 24 hours, day in and day out.

Although renal replacement therapy for infants has become a standard-of-care therapy, the careful final decision to begin long-term dialysis remains in the hands of both the multidisciplinary team and the parents. An infant cannot speak for himself or herself; therefore the guiding principle should remain "to do what is best" for the infant. As difficult as this decision process may seem (and we often wish we could see into the future), there are data and experience to draw from, because chronic infant dialysis has been offered successfully since the mid-1980s. On one hand, infants with concomitant extrarenal organ dysfunction, particularly pulmonary disease and/or hypoplasia and oliguria and anuria, have great mortality risk within the first year of life (approximately 80%), compared with infants without those complications (approximately 25%). Nevertheless, the ethics of individualized decisions to withhold, continue, or discontinue treatment involve clinical, theoretic, legal, and economic considerations. Thus the multidisciplinary team and family must make the "ideal" decision, together, with compassion, and with complete awareness of the facts and feelings, and eventually plan for a transplant as appropriate.

HYPERTENSION

In the past decade it has become apparent that hypertension is a significant clinical problem in the neonate cared for in a NICU setting.[2,4,29,38,48] The incidence of hypertension in healthy term infants appears to be quite low, and the majority of hypertensive infants have a definable cause. Nearly universal blood pressure monitoring in nurseries with established normal blood pressure ranges enables more frequent diagnosis. A hypertensive infant may be quite ill, with symptoms similar to those of an infant with sepsis or heart or lung disease. If the infant is properly diagnosed and treated, the outcome may be quite favorable.

Blood pressures (BPs) vary by gestational age, body weight, cuff size, and state of alertness. Normal values have been developed by body weight and by postnatal age, but no criteria combining these variables are available. BP begins low and postnatally increases by 1 to 2 mm Hg/day for the first 3 to 8 days and 1 mm Hg/week for 5 to 7 weeks, and reaches a steady value for the first year of life by 2 months of age. Whether the percentile for an infant's BP will track into later childhood or adulthood is still controversial at this point. Normal values for BPs in infants are listed in Figure 25-7.

Etiology

The causes of hypertension[2,38] can be seen in Box 25-1. All infants with hypertension must be assumed to have a specific secondary etiology. The most common cause may be a complication of umbilical artery catheterization (UAC).

Prevention

Obtaining accurate, reliable measurements of BP is necessary to prevent falsely elevated (or depressed) values.[29,122] Under study conditions, the best determinant of BP is the direct arterial measurement, usually through a UAC. Older techniques such as auscultation, palpation, and flush blood pressure measurements have been replaced by Doppler measurements and oscillometry. These latter two techniques have correlated very well with direct arterial measurements for systolic BP but not as well with diastolic BP. **Cuff selection is also important, because small cuffs give falsely high values. The**

Box 25-1	ETIOLOGIC FACTORS IN HYPERTENSION IN THE NEONATE

Vascular

Renal artery stenosis
Renal artery thrombosis
Coarctation of the aorta
Hypoplastic abdominal aorta
Renal vein thrombosis
Idiopathic arterial calcification

Renal

Renal dysplasia and/or hypoplasia
Polycystic kidney disease (autosomal dominant or recessive)
Renal failure
Obstructive uropathy
Reflux nephropathy
Pyelonephritis
Glomerulonephritis
Tumors
    Wilms'
    Neuroblastoma

Endocrine

Adrenogenital syndrome
Cushing's disease
Hyperaldosteronism
Thyrotoxicosis

Other

Closure of abdominal wall defects
Fluid overload
Genitourinary surgery
Hypercalcemia
Increased intracranial pressure
Medications
    Phenylephrine
    Corticosteroids
    Theophylline
    Deoxycorticosterone
Seizures
Bronchopulmonary dysplasia

Modified from Adelman RD: Neonatal hypertension. In Loggie JMH, et al, eds: *NHLBI workshop on juvenile hypertension*, New York, 1983, Biomedical Information; and Gulgnard JP: Neonatal nephrology. In Holliday MA, Barratt TM, Vernier RL, eds: *Pediatric nephrology*, ed 2, Baltimore, 1987, Williams & Wilkins.

---

cuff should completely encircle the extremity and be the largest cuff possible without impinging on the joints of the upper arm or leg. In this way, BP in the arms and legs should be equal. Frequently the same cuff is used for the arm and the leg, with the result that the leg pressures appear to be higher,

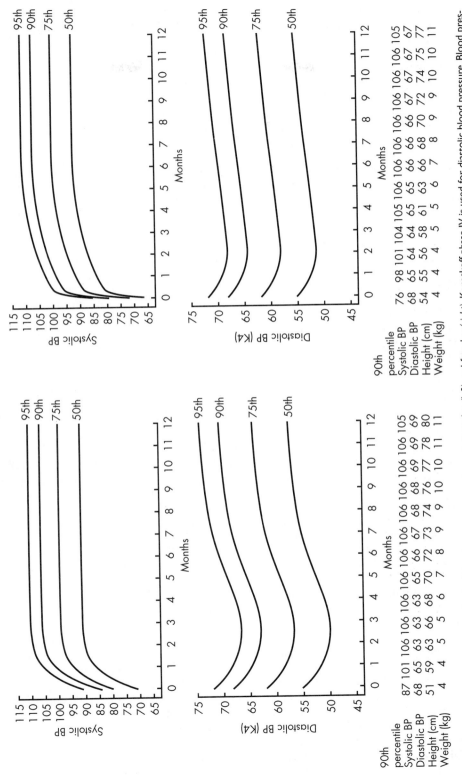

FIGURE 25-7 Age-specific percentiles of blood pressure measurements in males (*left*) and females (*right*). Korotkoff phase IV is used for diastolic blood pressure. Blood pressures exceeding the 90th percentile are considered hypertensive unless the infant's height and weight exceeds the 90th percentile. Blood pressures exceeding the 90th percentile are always considered hypertensive. (From Report on the Second Task Force on Blood Pressure Control in Children: *Pediatrics* 79:1, 1987.)

because the cuff is too small. The size of the cuff and extremity used for measurement should be documented so that serial measurements will be consistent. The position for measuring BP is always supine. BPs taken on extremities elevated above the level of the heart may give erroneously low values; the converse is true of pressures taken on extremities lower than the level of the heart. BP can vary greatly with the state of alertness and with crying. Frequently a sick infant will have a BP measured directly through a UAC as well as by oscillometric techniques. Significant discrepancies between these measurements may be seen, and it is often difficult to discern which one is the "true" BP. Aside from equipment malfunction, discrepancies can be caused by a UAC with a caliber too small for the infant's size, a thrombus at the tip of the catheter, or poor peripheral perfusion.

Data Collection

History

Nearly all hypertensive infants (88%) have had a UAC.[2,38] The incidence of renal artery thrombosis in neonates with indwelling UACs is 3% to 20%; however, only 13% of these infants were clinically diagnosed. Of patients with UACs, 3% develop hypertension.

Signs and Symptoms

Any infant exceeding the 95th percentile for BP is considered to be hypertensive. Thus 5% of the population on initial screening would be hypertensive.[2,3,29,48] **For the term infant, any BP exceeding 95 mm Hg systolic or 75 mm Hg diastolic is considered hypertensive. In premature infants the definition is less clear but is considered to be 80 mm Hg systolic and 50 mm Hg diastolic.** Hypertension usually occurs during the first week of life in the full-term infant and in the second week in preterm infants. However, new data suggest that hypertension can occur much later in the course of a sick infant and even after discharge.

BP measurements should be taken in all extremities to seek evidence for coarctation of the aorta.

The symptoms of hypertension may be severe but very nonspecific. Hypertension presents with respiratory distress in 50% of infants; PDA in 50%; neurologic symptoms such as seizures, tremor, and abnormalities in tone in 30%; and congestive heart failure in 40%. Intracranial hemorrhage, hemiparesis, hepatosplenomegaly, and cyanosis may also occur. Approximately 50% of infants, however, are asymptomatic. Fundoscopic examination revealed typical changes of hypertensive retinopathy in 11 of 21 hypertensive infants studied. The true incidence of hypertension in the newborn has been reported to be 1.2% to 5% of NICU admissions.

Laboratory Data

Hypertension in a neonate demands a full evaluation to determine the cause.[2,38,114] In one study of 17 hypertensive infants, five had a definable cause, two had UACs, and 10 had no definable cause. Evaluation should consist of a study of renal anatomy by ultrasonography. If this fails to reveal a cause, a renal scan or angiography should be performed, depending on the degree of elevation and the infant's response to therapy. Serum creatinine clearance is usually normal or may be only slightly elevated. Urinalysis may be normal, but hematuria and proteinuria may also be noted (either as a sign of a cause of hypertension or as a result of the hypertension). Peripheral renin activities are generally elevated but must be compared with age-matched normal values—references that can be difficult to locate. The effects of hypertension should also be evaluated, including a fundoscopic examination by an ophthalmologist and a cardiologist's evaluation for evidence of hypertensive damage if the hypertension has been long-standing or severe.

Treatment*

Hypertension should be treated in a neonate, particularly if it exceeds the definition of severe hypertension (greater than 110 mm Hg systolic). However, an overly rapid normalization of BP should not be sought, because an excessive lowering of BP may also be detrimental. Rather, an initial 30% decrease is preferable. A definable cause, such as a urinary tract obstruction, abdominal tumor, or coarctation, should be treated surgically. Nephrectomy of the involved kidney may be recommended in cases of medically unmanageable severe hypertension.

Drugs and dosages commonly used in neonates for controlling BP are found in Table 25-4. Captopril should be used with caution if it is possible that bilateral renal artery stenosis is present, because renal failure has been reported in this situation. Generally, ACE-inhibition is not recommended as a first-line therapy, because its adverse effect on over-

---

*References 2, 38, 51, 86, 93, 126

Table 25-4	ANTIHYPERTENSIVE MEDICATIONS FOR USE IN THE NEONATAL PERIOD*			
MEDICATIONS	DOSE	SCHEDULE	ROUTE	COMMENTS
Propranolol	1-4 mg/kg/dose	bid-tid	PO	Contraindicated in heart failure, possibly in BPD, sedation
Hydralazine	0.025-1 mg/kg/dose	bid	IV	
	0.25-1.5 mg/kg/dose (max 4.5 mg/kg/day)	bid-qid	PO	Tachycardia, sodium retention
	0.1-0.5 mg/kg/dose with beta blocker	q6h	IV	
	0.4-0.8 mg/kg/dose (sole agent)			
Captopril	0.1-2.0 mg/kg/dose	tid	PO	Leukopenia, rash, proteinuria, hyperkalemia, acute renal failure, seizures
Enalapril	0.1-0.3 mg/kg/dose	qd-q12h	PO	Hypotension
Enalaprilat	0.005-0.05 mg/kg/dose	qd-q12h	IV	Hypotension
Diazoxide	1-5 mg/kg/dose	q4-24h	IV	Hyperglycemia, fluid retention, hyperuricemia
Sodium nitroprusside	0.5-10 µg/kg/min	Continuous infusion	IV	Keep covered in foil, careful observation for infiltration of IV or varying rate of administration

*No reported experience in the newborn with nifedipine, clonidine, labetalol, or verapamil. Furosemide and thiazides are not antihypertensive medications but are used for volume overload.
BPD, Bronchopulmonary dysplasia.

all nephron development has not been adequately ruled out. For an acute hypertensive crisis, an oral challenge with nifedipine, hydralazine, or clonidine can be tried. If there is no success, intravenous hydralazine, labetolol, nicardipine, or nitroprusside would be the drug of choice. Calcium channel blockers have great potential for the treatment of neonatal hypertension. Typically they do not, within recommended dosing, cause fluid retention or reflex tachycardia. Some pharmacies are able to make a liquid preparation of nifedipine and amlodipine.

Complications

The prognosis for hypertensive infants is excellent if BP is well controlled medically or cured surgically.[3,4,38] These infants have normal somatic growth and development, and in most their antihypertensive medications may be discontinued after 1 to 2 years of follow-up. Poor renal growth is noted on the side of renal artery pathology, and renal scans tend to be persistently abnormal. Creatinine clearances appear to be normal for most infants.

ABDOMINAL MASS

Slightly more than 50% of abdominal masses present during the newborn period are of renal origin.[48,67,68,69,78] The literature offers no consistent

data on the frequency of abdominal masses in infants, but there is general agreement that these patients must be evaluated quickly and thoroughly before planning intervention. The differential diagnosis in an infant with an abdominal mass is shown in Table 25-5.

Physical Examination

Visualization of the abdomen before manual exploration enables the examiner to note a mass that may be missed on a tense abdomen. Bimanual palpation using the flat surface of the fingers while supporting the infant's flank with the other hand permits exploration of the abdomen during deep palpation. Renal masses are usually smooth to palpation and move with respirations. The size of the mass is not helpful in determining its cause.

Percussion may be used to outline the suspected area, and transillumination is sometimes helpful in identifying hydronephrosis and multicystic kidneys, which are both positive when transilluminated. Some renal masses are quite soft, so excessive pressure during the examination will frequently cause the mass to be missed.

Laboratory Data

Ultrasonography is the most desirable diagnostic tool for initial evaluation of an abdominal

Table 25-5	NEONATAL ABDOMINAL MASSES
TYPE OF MASS	**PERCENT OF TOTAL**
Renal Masses	55
Hydronephrosis	
Multicystic dysplastic kidney	
Polycystic kidney disease	
Mesoblastic nephroma	
Renal ectopia	
Renal vein thrombosis	
Nephroblastomatosis	
Wilms' tumor	
Genital Masses	15
Hydrometrocolpos	
Ovarian cyst	
Gastrointestinal Masses	15
Duplication	
Volvulus	
Complicated meconium ileus	
Mesenteric-omental cyst	
"Pseudocyst" proximal to atresia	
Nonrenal Retroperitoneal Masses	10
Adrenal hemorrhage	
Neuroblastoma	
Teratoma	
Hepatosplenobiliar Masses	5
Hemangioendothelioma	
Hepatoblastoma	
Hepatic cyst	
Splenic hematoma	
Choledochal cyst	
Hydrops of gallbladder	

From Kirks DR, Merten DF, Grossman H et al: Diagnostic imaging of pediatric abdominal masses: an overview, *Radiol Clin North Am* 19:527, 1981.

mass in a newborn. The advantages of this technology include its noninvasive nature, accessibility for bedside studies, improved resolution, and relatively low cost. Ultrasonography reveals a kidney with communicating cystic masses in hydronephrosis. Renal dysplasia most often is seen as noncommunicating cyst formations on the sonogram. When this diagnostic tool is incapable of differentiating dysplasia and hydronephrosis, renal scintigraphy is indicated. With this modality, dysplasia is noted as having no functional activity on nuclear scan. A hydronephrotic kidney demonstrates "rim" activity, with delayed accumulation of the radionuclide in the pelvis and calyces. Selected isotopes (gluco-

heptonate) used in renal scintigraphy will reveal fine anatomic detail, making this modality a useful tool in assessing renal function. Rarely, a percutaneous nephrostogram is performed to determine whether cysts are caused by obstruction or dysplasia. A voiding cystourethrogram is the method of choice to diagnose vesicoureteral reflux. CT scans can be helpful, especially for differentiating renal masses.

INTRINSIC RENAL PARENCHYMAL ABNORMALITIES

Renal abnormalities can be classified by the amount of tissue, the differentiation of tissue, and the position of the kidneys.[68,78,88,122] Ronco et al[95,96] present a thorough summary of renal involvement with various syndromes.

A congenital absence or agenesis of renal tissue can occur unilaterally or bilaterally. Unilateral renal agenesis is seen more frequently (1:1000 live births) and may present as a solitary kidney on examination with enlargement caused by compensatory hypertrophy. Unilateral agenesis has been associated with Turner syndrome, Poland syndrome, and VATER syndrome. Bilateral agenesis, or Potter's disease, is seen rarely, with an incidence of 1:4000 births.

Hypoplasia is a deficiency in the amount of renal tissue expressed as an abnormally small kidney. Morphologically, the kidney is normal, and renal function is unaffected in the neonatal period. Later in life patients can sometimes "outgrow" their renal function.

Signs and Symptoms

In unilateral agenesis, patients are often asymptomatic and are diagnosed inadvertently by ultrasonography or based on the significant association with malformations of the lower genitourinary tract. There is no need for long-term follow-up if only a solitary kidney without additional involvement is found.

In bilateral agenesis the majority of affected infants are male and small for gestational age, with a history of maternal oligohydramnios. The characteristic facial features accompanying Potter's syndrome include wide-set eyes, parrot-beak nose, receding chin, and large, low-set ears with little cartilage. Other associated malformations include pulmonary hypoplasia, hydrocephalus, meningocele, multiple skeletal anomalies, and imperforate anus. Death usually occurs within hours to several days.

Differentiation of Tissue

Abnormalities in renal tissue differentiation are most commonly expressed as dysplastic kidneys.[84,91,106] Renal dysplasia is a failure of the metanephric tissue to mature appropriately, frequently because of obstruction of the urinary tract early in gestation. The result is a persistence of immature structures and very little normal-functioning renal tissue.

Renal dysplasia may be seen in one or both kidneys and may involve the entire kidney, segments of the kidney, or microscopic areas (foci) of a kidney. Dysplasia is most commonly expressed as cyst formation. Bilateral multicystic dysplastic kidneys (MCDK) are nonfunctional and not compatible with life. Unilateral MCDK involvement is both the most common cystic lesion of the neonatal kidney and one of the most frequently palpated abdominal masses in newborns. Unilateral MCDK shows no predilection for males or females or for involvement of right or left kidney. Usually the ureter is absent, atretic, or stenotic. No orifice is found in the bladder. Renal function and structure may be normal in the remaining kidney of infants with unilateral dysplasia; however, frequently vesicoureteral reflux or ureteropelvic (UPJ) obstruction is present in the contralateral kidney. Therefore a voiding cystourethrogram should be performed on every patient suspected of having this condition. Additionally, hypertension is a potential complication (estimates of 20% have been made) of MCDK and requires treatment and/or long-term follow-up.

Renal dysplasia is usually sporadic, but some familial cases have been reported. A lack of blood flow, as demonstrated on a ^{99}mTc DPTA nuclear renal scan, confirms the diagnosis.

Treatment

Generally, in an infant with this condition, the kidneys involute with time; therefore a conservative approach rather than a surgical correction is recommended. The association between renal dysplasia and neoplasia has not been confirmed. However, removal of the kidney is sometimes indicated if its size prevents adequate nutrition.

POLYCYSTIC KIDNEY DISEASE

Pathophysiology

Polycystic kidney disease (PKD)[11,25,88] may present as one of two types in the infant: (1) autosomal recessive polycystic kidney disease (ARPKD) and (2) autosomal dominant polycystic kidney disease (ADPKD). Traditionally, ADPKD has not been associated with onset during the first year of life, but recent studies have confirmed both presentations in the infant, and conversely, ARPKD has been reported in the old child.

ARPKD presents with varied severity, but it is always bilateral. The kidneys become enlarged with a proliferation of renal tubules and dilated collecting tubules. These are not true "cysts," and the kidney has a renoform shape. Autosomal dominant disease involves cyst formations in any portion of the nephron, Bowman's space, and liver. Rarely, cyst formation in the pancreas and spleen is present. There is a strong association with autosomal dominant PKD and cerebral artery aneurysms.

Data Collection

History

Criteria for making a definitive diagnosis for both diseases have been developed.[25] Autosomal recessive disease includes infants with the following: (1) congenital hepatic fibrosis as demonstrated on liver biopsy or through evidence of portal hypertension, (2) renal histologic studies consistent with collecting tubule ectasis, and/or (3) a sibling with the disease. Infants diagnosed with ARPKD have a positive parental history or known liver cysts or Berry aneurysm.

Signs and Symptoms

Both types of PKD can present initially with an abdominal mass. The infant may present with bilateral flank masses, hepatic enlargement, Potter's facies caused by oligohydramnios, oliguria, acute renal failure, hypoplastic lungs, respiratory distress, and spontaneous pneumothorax. Hypertension is common in both types of the disease.

Laboratory Data

Differentiation of ADPKD from ARPKD may be difficult, even with ultrasonography, because radiographic studies are not consistently accurate in discerning differences. Indeed, retrospectively, it is not uncommon to find infants who have been misclassified. Nevertheless, there are ultrasonographic criteria that can be relied on.

Treatment

Management consists of serial monitoring of blood pressure, renal function, and urine cultures. Neonates with either form of PKD need aggressive treatment of BP with captopril as the drug of choice, treatment of any urinary tract infection, and aggressive nutritional management.

HYDRONEPHROSIS*

Physiology

The collecting system of the kidney is composed of the ureter, pelvis, and calyces, all of which function as a system for removing urine from the kidneys. Hydronephrosis, one of the most common abdominal masses in the newborn, involves a dilation of the pelvis and calyces, most often as a result of congenital obstruction. The impaired movement of urine as a result of severe or chronic obstruction may lead to dysplastic and cystic changes that further impair kidney function if the obstruction occurs early in gestation.

The most common ureteral site of obstruction is the ureteropelvic junction. The infant presents with a ballooning of the renal pelvis. Obstruction at the ureterovesical junction, also known as *congenital megaureter* in its primary form, occurs more often in male infants and more frequently affects the left ureter. Posterior urethral valves (PUV) in males are the major cause of urethral obstruction. This distal obstruction may result in bladder hypertrophy, hydroureter, and hydronephrosis if severe. Dysplastic changes can be seen if the obstruction occurs early in gestation. The neonate with PUV is at risk for developing an ascending infection and subsequent renal damage. *Prune-belly syndrome,* also known at *Eagle-Barrett syndrome,* is a less common cause of obstruction and dilation of the pelvis and calyces; there is a strong male predominance. This triad of anomalies includes (1) absence or hypoplasia of the abdominal wall muscles, (2) bilateral cryptorchidism, and (3) urinary tract abnormality. The loose, shriveled abdomen is responsible for the prune-belly appearance, which diminishes with age and does not require surgical correction. Renal dysplasia is usually seen in prune-belly syndrome and may range from mild to severe involvement. The enlarged bladder may be seen in conjunction with a patent urachus draining urine. The prostatic urethra is usually hypoplastic.

Etiology

The cause of most types of hydronephrosis remains unclear. Primary prune-belly syndrome may be a re-

sult of a mesenchymal developmental arrest. A variant of the syndrome can also be seen as a sequela of an intrauterine distention of the abdomen by an obstructed urinary system. The existence of this secondary cause of prune-belly syndrome is controversial. Another cause of calyceal dilation not associated with obstruction is vesicoureteral reflux, as discussed further under urinary tract infections.

Infants may have few if any symptoms, and there are usually no physical findings unless a bladder or kidney is palpated on routine examination. These infants can present with a poor urinary stream and frequently with failure to thrive.

Treatment

Mild to moderate unilateral obstruction does not require immediate treatment.[41,42] Close follow-up is indicated for monitoring of kidney growth and obstruction as surgery may be a postnatal consideration; bilateral dilation with normal amounts of amniotic fluid is treated with close observation. **Treatment of bilateral dilation with decreased amniotic fluid depends on the gestational age of the fetus.**

A viable fetus with dilated collecting systems, initial normal amount of amniotic fluid, and evidence of decreasing amniotic fluid should be delivered early. Other conditions such as bilateral vesicoureteral reflux, prune-belly syndrome, and primary megaureter may present with dilated collecting systems and are not amenable to in utero surgery. Surgical intervention in utero is very controversial, center dependent, and the morbidity of this therapy is very high.

Complete obstruction at the uteropelvic and/or uterovesical junctions is surgically corrected. For uterovesical obstructions, surgical correction involves excising the stenotic segment in the obstructed megaureter as well as ureteric reimplantation and is successful in the large majority of infants. Management of obstruction secondary to posterior urethral valves (PUV) depends on the age at presentation and infant's condition. After initial stabilization, relief of obstruction with a catheter provides quick decompression. Permanent repair consists of removal of the obstructing valves. The use of a vesicostomy versus a higher diversion is controversial.

RENAL VEIN THROMBOSIS

Renal vein thrombosis (RVT), can be an acute life-threatening condition or insidious with the develop-

---

*References 9, 13, 77, 83, 85, 117.

ment of microhematuria and hypertesnion.[81,89,104] RVT is associated with conditions that cause circulatory collapse and decreased oxygenation within the kidney.

Etiology

Perinatal causes of neonatal RVT include maternal diabetes, toxemia, maternal thiazide therapy, polycythemia, placental insufficiency, birth asphyxia, prematurity, RDS, and sepsis. Angiography has also been associated with RVT. Thrombosis most often occurs in the smaller renal veins rather than the main renal vein.

Data Collection

Signs and Symptoms

The involved kidney may enlarge secondary to obstruction to blood flow and forms a palpable flank mass. Other clinical symptoms may include hematuria (60% of cases), anemia, oliguria, and thrombocytopenia (less than 75,000 platelets).

Laboratory Data

A urine dipstick test that is positive for blood, urine output of less than 1 ml/kg/hr, and a low platelet count may indicate RVT.

Treatment

Management includes treatment of the underlying illness, treatment of sepsis if suspected, fluid therapy, and possibly dialysis in select cases. Heparin therapy remains controversial for RVT. Surgical excision of the thrombus is not usually indicated during the acute phase but may be appropriate at a later time. Rarely, nephrectomy is required. Renal tubular dysfunction is often observed after recovery from RVT.[65]

MISCELLANEOUS CAUSES OF ABDOMINAL MASS

Wilms' tumor, also known as *nephroblastoma,* **is the most common intraabdominal tumor seen in children, occurring at a rate of 8 to 9/100,000/yr in the United States. Two thirds of patients present in the first 3 to 6 months of life.** The tumor is described as firm, smooth, and confluent with the kidney or attached to the organ. In 10% of cases both kidneys are involved. This condition has an excellent prognosis with treatment. Surgical removal of the tumor is followed by irradiation for most patients and chemotherapy.

Neuroblastoma, on the other hand, is the most common malignant tumor in infancy. The primary site of the tumor may be any area of neural crest tissue, with the most common site identified in the adrenal gland. Presenting in the neonate as a palpable abdominal mass, this tumor may also cause urinary obstruction. Prognosis is related to the site of the primary tumor, histologic appearance of the tumor, staging of the disease, and age of the patient.

RENAL TUBULAR DISORDERS

Although most of the renal tubular disorders are congenital, they rarely manifest clinically during the newborn period.[10] However, in sick infants admitted to the intensive care unit, these tubular abnormalities can lead to severe, and frequently life-threatening, electrolyte disorders.

Etiology

With the advent of routine prenatal ultrasonographic examination, a number of newborns referred for evaluation of polyhydramnios and polyuria have been diagnosed with diabetes insipidus (central or nephrogenic) and Bartter's syndrome. In addition, obstruction of the urinary tract, which is frequently diagnosed prenatally, is commonly associated with RTA, particularly the hyperkalemic type (type IV).

Data Collection

History and Signs and Symptoms

Infants with Fanconi syndrome and distal RTA most commonly present after the neonatal period with the complaint of failure to thrive. Frequently there is a history of previous admissions to the hospital for evaluation of sepsis and/or dehydration.

Laboratory Data

The diagnosis of Fanconi syndrome is confirmed by demonstration of a generalized dysfunction in the proximal tubule, evidenced by the presence of glycosuria, proteinuria (low-molecular-weight proteins), bicarbonaturia, phosphaturia, and uricosuria. Distal RTA is diagnosed by demonstrating a decreased urinary excretion of ammonium. Because the measurement of urinary ammonium is cumbersome, calculation of the urine net charge may be done by the following formula:

$$([Na^+] + [K^+]) - [Cl^-]$$

Where $[Na^+]$, $[K^+]$, and $[Cl^-]$ represent the concentration of the respective electrolytes in a random urine sample (in milliequivalents per liter). This formula has been proposed as a bedside tool for screening for distal RTA. If the result of this calculation is a negative number (less than zero), then distal RTA is ruled out. A positive urine net charge (higher than zero) is consistent with RTA. However, because of the presence of other organic anions in the urine during the first 2 weeks of life, the validity of this test during the neonatal period has been questioned. Disorders of vitamin D metabolism and/or phosphate reabsorption (rickets) usually present by the end of the first year of life, after the child starts walking. Infants with diabetes insipidus typically present during the first 2 months of life with dehydration and a sepsis-like picture.

Complications

Thus, although most of the tubular disorders are not clinically evident at birth, it is important for the clinician to keep a high index of suspicion in those infants with prenatal diagnosis of urologic abnormalities or serious abnormalities in water and electrolyte metabolism. Early evaluation and treatment of renal tubular disorders may prevent catastrophic complications such as life-threatening episodes of dehydration and delayed growth and development.

URINARY TRACT INFECTIONS

Urinary tract infections (UTIs) affect approximately 1% of full-term infants and 3% of premature infants.[3,48,55] Male infants are affected five times more frequently than females. Vesicoureteral reflux is a common radiographic finding in infants. Primary reflux is seen in abnormalities of the vesicoureteral junction, ureteral duplication, and ureterocele. Secondary reflux is associated with infection, PUV, and neurogenic diseases.

Etiology

Abnormalities of the urinary tract are responsible for a large number of UTIs in the neonate. Whether the infection is ascending from the bladder or hemotogenously spread is a matter of debate. The high association of reflux with UTI makes determining the etiology of reflux a priority for planning appropriate treatment. Reflux is graded on a four-point scale, with grade IV denoting massive hydronephrosis and hydroureter.

Maternal urinary infections have also been associated with neonatal UTIs. Symptomatic manifestations include abnormal weight loss during the first days of life, decreased feeding, dehydration, irritability, lethargy, cyanosis, jaundice, and septicemia. In some cases the affected kidneys are palpable. Infected infants may also be asymptomatic.

Data Collection

Laboratory Data

Evaluation of a neonate with suspected UTI includes an immediate ultrasound to rule out upper tract abnormalities. Urine should be obtained for culture, blood cultures, and a CBC. The optimal method of obtaining urine for culture is suprapubic aspiration of the bladder. Successful results depend on a full bladder. Catheterization may not be recommended in a neonate because of possible urethral stricture formation in the male and frequent culture contamination in the female. Urine obtained in a urine bag should not be used for cultures. Skin contamination frequently yields false-positive cultures; conversely, one drop of povidone-iodine solution (Betadine) in a bag of urine can prevent in vitro bacterial growth. Grades of reflux are diagnosed by voiding cystourethrogram (VCUG). Sterile urine is necessary before a VCUG is undertaken.

Treatment

Pyuria (10 to 15 WBC/hpf) can be observed in the neonate normally. Treatment for UTI is indicated when an organism is cultured from the urine. Any growth in a urine specimen obtained by suprapubic aspiration should be considered an infection if the procedure was cleanly done. Any aspiration of bowel contents must affect the interpretation of culture results. Traditional antibiotic coverage consists of both ampicillin and an aminoglycoside. The advent of third-generation cephalosporins has allowed for excellent gram-negative coverage without the nephrotoxicity of the aminoglycosides. *Escherichia coli* is the organism most often implicated in neonatal UTIs, followed by *Klebsiella*. Sulfonamides are contraindicated in the neonate because of their potential to complicate hyperbilirubinemia.

Antibiotic therapy should continue for 14 days, with a follow-up urine culture 3 days after therapy is discontinued.

Complications

After urine is sterile, a VCUG is used to assess any lower urinary tract abnormalities, specifically reflux. A normal study result indicates that

antibiotic therapy may be discontinued. These patients should be followed with monthly urine cultures. Patients who demonstrate reflux should be maintained on suppressive antibiotic therapy. VCUG should be repeated in 12 months if reflux was initially present.

NEUROGENIC BLADDER

Neurogenic bladder is an anatomic interruption of the micturition reflex normally triggered by a full bladder.[1,12,99] The bladder may be flaccid and unable to empty urine or spastic and hyperreflexive and unable to store urine. Infants with lumbosacral spinal malformations commonly have a urinary tract dysfunction known as neurogenic bladder. Lower motor neuron deficit causes bladder atony, and upper motor neuron deficit can cause spasticity.

Data Collection
Signs and Symptoms
Often there is a mixed presentation of symptoms. It is the flaccid bladder that requires aggressive intervention in the neonate. Diagnosis begins immediately at the bedside when the newborn has no apparent voiding stream or the urine flow rate falls below expectations without other explanations. Further clarification of the diagnosis can be made by VCUG and by cystometric studies.

Treatment
Surgical intervention is indicated in the neonate with neurogenic bladder when there is severe reflux with renal damage present or recurrent UTI. The urologist creates a vesicostomy to allow the free flow of urine into diapers.

Complications
Early diagnosis and intervention for infants with neurogenic bladder can decrease the risks of the complications associated with this problem. Long-term complications of neurogenic bladder include UTI and vesicoureteral reflux leading to hydronephrosis, electrolyte imbalances, and permanent damage to the kidney.

NEONATAL CHRONOBIOLOGY*

The human time structure consists of a spectrum of rhythms of different frequencies, which are super-imposed on trends such as development and aging. These rhythms are genetically determined and are adjusted in time (synchronized) by environmental factors, which adapt the organism to its periodic surroundings. The genetic environmental interactions in the establishment and maintenance of these rhythms begins in early intrauterine life and continues during infancy and childhood with the establishment of mature time structure similar to adults by 2 years of age. The rhythms reach their peak in amplitude in adolescence, before stabilization during adult life and return to a more infantlike pattern in old age. These rhythms are often defined as *circadian* (*circa,* "about"; *dian,* "day") for 24-hour rhythms (e.g., heart rate and blood pressure), *ultradian* for rhythms of less than 24 hours (e.g., various cycles of sleep), and *infradian* for rhythms of greater than 24 hours (e.g., menstrual cycles). Hundreds of studies have defined the human time structure in health. Examples include body temperature, the circadian variations of gastrointestinal motility and blood flow, gastric acid secretion, hepatic enzyme activity, peripheral blood lymphocyte helper/suppressor ratios, adrenergic receptor activity, and many cardiovascular parameters.[82]

Disease states have very specific periodic rhythms as well. Examples include exacerbation of asthma at night, arthritis in the morning, and ulcer disease in the evening. The peak incidence of myocardial ischemia, migraine headache, angina pectoris, and thrombotic stroke occurs in the early morning hours when blood coagulation is at a peak and early morning rises in heart rate, blood pressure, sympathetic tone, and adrenergic receptor activity are observed. Diagnostic tests are also time dependent, with significant diurnal variations noted (e.g., in casual BP measurements, pulmonary function testing, glucose tolerance, and cutaneous antigen testing). *Chronokinetics* refers to rhythm effects on the rate and extent of drug absorption, distribution, and elimination. Circadian changes in gastric hydrogen ion excretion, gastric emptying, intestinal transit time, hepatic enzyme activity, and renal function lead to administration time differences in pharmacokinetic studies. The effects may also depend on the chemical nature of the medication or the attributes of new drug delivery systems. Chronokinetic data are known for many classes of medications, including beta-adrenergic receptor agonists and antagonists, nonsteroidal antiinflammatory drugs (NSAIDs), and antihypertensive medications. There also exists a rhythm dependency in the body's response to medications, termed *chronesthesy.* Chronestheses may result

*References 20, 39, 53, 80, 82, 90, 91, 101, 111, 112, 124, 130.

from many factors, including rhythms in cell receptor number, rate limiting steps in metabolic pathways, and cell turnover. Variations in response to medications have been described for analgesics, IV heparin, beta-adrenergic receptor antagonists, and cancer chemotherapy. The knowledge of these rhythms is important for the understanding of disease states and their development as well as administration of appropriate therapies. It is important to understand how these principles may be applied in neonatology.

The development of the time structure has two distinct phenomena: the spontaneous maturation within the framework of genetic makeup and the accumulation of experience by the child. It is now established that a biologic clock, the suprachiasmatic nucleus, is oscillating in the mammalian fetus and reflects the endocrine, metabolic, cardiovascular, and nutritional functions of the mother. The fetal clock is entrained by redundant circadian signals from the mother, which include feeding times, breathing movements, heart rate, and sleep-wake patterns. Although this maternal-fetal communication of circadian phase is apparent, the potential for direct perception of light by the fetus in utero also exists. An entrainable circadian clock during fetal life allows the developing mammal to prepare more readily for life outside the womb and confers a significant survival advantage for those species whose rhythms are fully developed at birth.

At the time of birth the transplacental maternal influences cease and direct environmental stimuli become operative. During the first week of life, some of the infant's rhythmicity may represent maternal influences. Ultradian rhythms predominate in the newborn at the time of birth and shortly thereafter. The development of recognizable circadian periodicity in the infant occurs gradually during the first month and may extend over the first 2 years of life by maturation of the infant and by environmental synchronization of the genetically determined circadian oscillators. After birth the child is exposed to new stimuli, which show marked circadian periodicity. These stimuli act as synchronizers of endogenous oscillators. The strongest of these stimuli are the alternation of light and dark, noise and silence, heat and cold, and hunger and satiety, and the relations of the neonate to its human environment. *Circaseptan* (weekly) rhythms based on the day of birth have also been found. The effect of external stimuli for sick infants in an intensive care nursery on the development of rhythms is not well defined. During the first 2 years of life a variance transposition takes place with the circadian rhythms gaining in importance and development of a time structure more and more similar to that seen in the adult.

The classic cross-sectional studies by Helbrugge[53] circadian rhythms in infants still provide the best information on the development of rhythms in human infants. Conclusions from this study of 297 children from the first week of life to 15 years of age include six important points: (1) physiologic functions develop circadian rhythms independently of each other; (2) rhythms develop at different times after birth; (3) increased range of oscillation occurs in all physiologic functions with age; (4) increase in oscillation can occur from increase of upper width of oscillation during light (activity) or increases in lower oscillation during dark hours (sleep); (5) in humans monophasic rhythms or circadian rhythms originate out of polyphasic or ultradian ones; and (6) maturation of the infant at birth is essential to rhythm development. The details of the study can be seen in Figure 25-8.[53]

More recent studies confirm Hellbruegge's findings. Mirmiran and Kok,[80] in a group of 12 premature infants 29 to 35 weeks of gestational age, found a circadian pattern of heart rate in about half of the subjects by 1 to 2 weeks of age. Gemelli et al[39] studied BP and heart rate patterns in 21 term newborns at 4 days of age. Single cosinor analysis reveals few significant rhythms. None of the subjects had rhythms of heart rate, but males had greater BP variability than did females. Sitka et al[111] examined circadian patterns in 17 infants on day 2 and at 4 weeks of age. Almost all subjects had rhythms in body temperature unrelated to activity, and greater than 50% had rhythms for systolic blood pressure. None demonstrated a circadian rhythm in diastolic blood pressure.[111] In all of these studies, activity, environment, and feeding times played a significant role in pattern development. However, the infant rhythm was distinct and could be separated from maternal rhythms.

The suprachiasmatic nucleus is felt to be the master biologic clock. The pineal gland is felt to be the effector of this clock through the production of the hormone melatonin. During intrauterine development, the fetus does not produce noteworthy amounts of melatonin. However, because of melatonin's excellent placental permeability, maternal

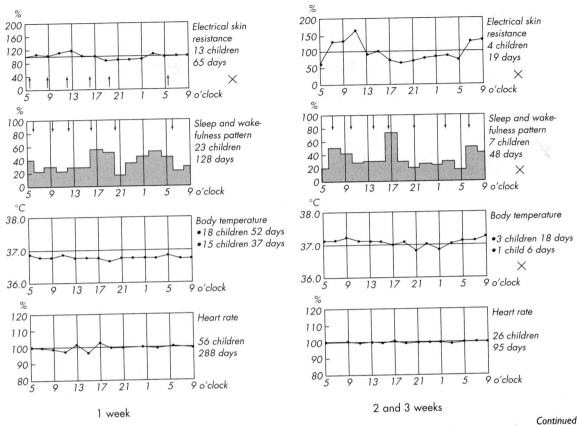

FIGURE 25-8   Development of circadian rhythms in children. Presented are six sets of graphs of 297 patients at different ages, with hours of the day along the x axis. Arrows along this axis represent feeding times. The X at the right of each graph represents the statistical significance of the circadian rhythm detected by cosinor analysis. During the first week of life, only electrical skin resistance demonstrates a circadian rhythm. Other variables such as sleep, body temperature, and heart rate (as well as urine output and sodium and potassium excretion, not shown) demonstrate no discernible circadian pattern. By 2 to 3 weeks of life, circadian patterns are demonstrated with skin resistance, sleep, and temperature. By 4 to 20 weeks of age, and certainly by 5 to 9 months, infants continue to have significant patterns for all variables with the same acrophase as earlier in life, but with deeper amplitude. The MESOR (24-hour mean) increases with increasing age. The 1- to 7- and 7- to 15-year-old children continue to have significant rhythms now similar to an adult pattern.

melatonin crosses the placenta freely in rhythmic fashion and thus the fetus is exposed to the same environmental stimuli as the mother. Melatonin levels are slightly higher as pregnancy progresses. Labor and delivery do not alter the maternal circadian rhythm of melatonin. Shortly after birth, all maternal melatonin is cleared and there is a virtual lack of melatonin for a period of 2 to 3 months. Melatonin production then increases and becomes circadian with a steadily rising melatonin level and increased amplitude. The period of melatonin deficiency is

longer for premature infants, suggesting the onset of melatonin production occurs approximately 10 to 12 months after conception and may be the result of a genetically determined maturation process. Melatonin is stimulated by darkness but not by sleep. Peak lifetime levels occur in the first 3 to 7 years of life (250 pg/ml). There is a gradual decline in melatonin levels (120 pg/ml) until a marked decrease in melatonin levels occurs at the time of puberty (50 pg/ml). There is speculation that this marked melatonin decline not only marks the onset of puberty, but as in

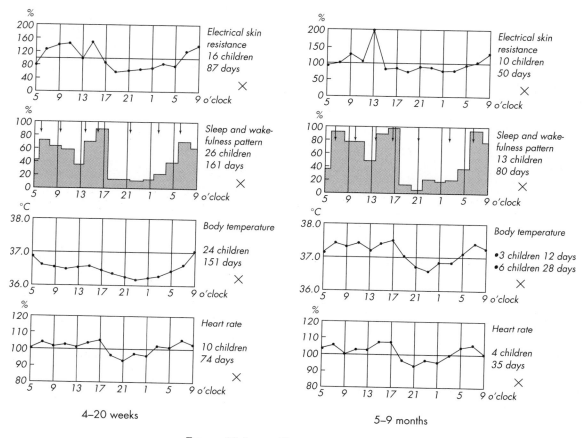

FIGURE 25-8, cont'd For legend see p. 637.

lower mammals may stimulate the onset of puberty. Delayed puberty has been noted with melatonin-producing tumors. Tumor removal normalizes melatonin levels and puberty then proceeds normally. The common calcification of the pineal gland has no known functional effect. During adult life, nocturnal melatonin levels average 20 pg/ml and fall to much lower levels in the aged.

In adults, diurnal rhythms of hormones lead to as much as 70% variation in blood levels. In the newborn, many hormones do not have the same rhythms as later in life. It has been shown that a circadian rhythm in cortisol excretion is absent in the newborn. Variations do occur but are related more to stress than a specific circadian rhythm. Further, the rhythm of this vital hormone does not achieve a mature rhythm until 2 years of age. Growth hormone does not have a normal circadian pattern until approximately 10

weeks of age, but neonates have a very definable ultradian rhythm, and newborns, with their eyes covered for phototherapy, have a marked increase in growth hormone levels. Certain enzymes such as glucose phosphate isomerase and hexosaminidase are circadian in the newborn at birth and synchronous with the mother. Sankaran, Hindmarsh, and Tan[101] showed, in 17 infants with a mean gestational age of 32 weeks and birth weight of 1790 ± 898 g at a mean of day 3 of life, a significant circadian variation in plasma concentrations of beta-endorphins. Various other physiologic parameters rapidly become circadian, as noted in Helbrugge's work,[53] even in the absence of melatonin.

In summary, the mother entrains the fetal biologic clock. The effects of maternal rhythms quickly abate after birth. Although infants of lower mammals have well-defined and mature rhythms at birth,

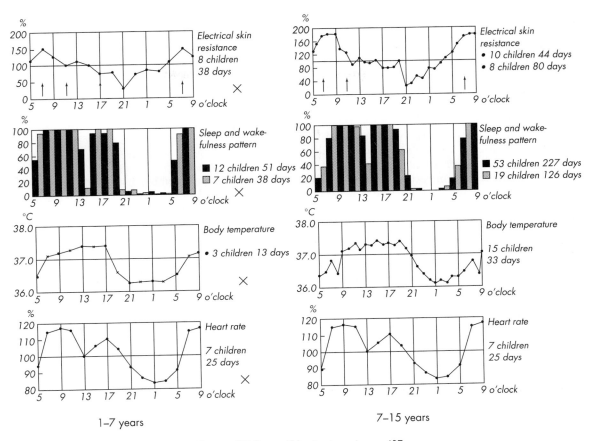

1–7 years   7–15 years

FIGURE 25-8, cont'd   For legend see p. 637.

the human newborn's patterns are low in amplitude and ultradian in pattern with the virtual absence of melatonin. Statistically, significant circadian rhythms are often absent at birth, especially with increasing prematurity, and rhythms observed are most likely a reflection of activity. With age the rhythms become more organized, less ultradian and more circadian, less variable in acrophase and higher in amplitude. The circadian rhythms in children have the same pattern as seen in adults but with a lower 24-hour mean level and occasionally with the circadian peaks (acrophases) shifted because of earlier sleep or awake times. Because there are marked variations in body size, there are also marked individual variations in biologic time structure. Whether these genetically based rhythms track throughout development is not established. The field of chronobiology itself is in its infancy and requires a great deal

of investigation before neonatal rhythms are fully understood so that chronotherapeutics can be applied.

PARENT TEACHING

Because many renal problems are secondary to abnormalities, parents need the information that nothing they have done or did not do caused the anomaly. Grief work over the loss of the perfect infant is necessary before attachment and caregiving is possible (see Chapters 29 and 30). Genetic counseling enables parents to make informed choices about subsequent pregnancies (see Chapter 27).

Most infants with renal problems require accurate intake and output measurement. The importance and necessity of measuring intake and not overfeeding must be stressed to parents, as well as the necessity of saving and weighing diapers. Infants who are fluid restricted may be "difficult" for care providers and parents because they are fussy and irritable. Adherence to the prescribed formula and/or breast milk is very important to regulate sodium intake and fluid retention.

Long-term complications that parents may have to recognize and/or manage must be explained and instructions given in writing. Because abnormalities in renal function and anatomy may be sequelae of renal diseases, follow-up by a pediatric nephrologist and/or urologist for urinalysis, cultures, and other diagnostic tests is important. General health maintenance is also important, because growth failure may be a manifestation of ongoing or recurring renal problems.

The importance of administering antihypertensive medications must be stressed to parents. Because hypertension is often a silent condition, the need for continuation of medications must be thoroughly explained. Side effects of hypertensive medications such as sedation, tachycardia, and excessive weight gain, as well as the necessity of medical follow-up, must also be emphasized.

REFERENCES

1. Action Committee on Myelodysplasia: Current approaches to the evaluation and management of children with myelomeningocele, *Pediatrics* 63:663, 1979.
2. Adelman RD: Neonatal hypertension. In Loggie JMH et al, eds: *NHLBI workshop on juvenile hypertension,* New York, 1983, Biomedical Information.
3. Adelman RD: Urinary tract infections in children. In Brenner BM, Stein JH, eds: *Contemporary issues in nephrology,* New York, 1984, Churchill-Livingstone.
4. Adelman RD: Long-term follow-up of neonatal renovascular hypertension, *Pediatr Nephrol* 1:35, 1987.
5. Adelman RD, Wirth F, Rubio T: A controlled study of the nephrotoxicity of mezlocillin and gentamicin plus ampicillin in the neonate, *J Pediatr* 111:888, 1987.
6. Arant BS: Renal disorders of the newborn infant. In Brenner BM, Stein JH, eds: *Contemporary issues in nephrology,* New York, 1984, Churchill-Livingstone.
7. Arant BS: Postnatal development of renal function during the first year of life, *Pediatr Nephrol* 1:308, 1987.
8. Aviram R, Pomeran A, Sharony R et al: The increase in renal pelvis dilatation in the fetus and its significance. *Ultrasound Obstet Gynecol* 16:60, 2000.
9. Barrat TM, Manzoni GA: The dilated urinary tract. In Holliday MA, Vermier RL, eds: *Pediatric nephrology,* ed 2, Baltimore, 1987, Williams & Wilkins.
10. Battle DC, Hizon M, Cohen E et al: The use of the urinary anion gap in the diagnosis of hyperchloremic metabolic acidosis, *N Engl J Med* 318:594, 1988.
11. Blyth H, Ockenden BG: Polycystic disease of the kidneys and liver presenting in childhood, *J Med Genet* 8:257, 1971.
12. Borzyskowski M, Mundy AR: Management of the neuropathic bladder in childhood, *Pediatr Nephrol* 2:56, 1988.
13. Boylan P, Parisi V: An overview of hydramnios, *Semin Perinatol* 10:136, 1986.
14. Brion LP, Campbell DE: Furosemide in indomethacin-treated infants: systematic review and meta-analysis, *Pediatr Nephrol* 13:212, 1999.
15. Brion LP, Campbell DE: Furosemide for symptomatic patent ductus arteriosus in indomethacin-treated infants, *Cochrane Database Syst Rev* 3:CD001148, 2001.
16. Brion LP, Primhak RA: Intravenous or enteral loop diuretics for preterm infants with (or developing) chronic lung disease, *Cochrane Database Syst Rev* 4:CD001453, 2000.
17. Brion, LP, Soll RF: Diuretics for respiratory distress syndrome in preterm infants, *Cochrane Database Sys Rev* 2:CD001454, 2001.
18. Brion LP, Primhak RA, Ambrosio-Perez I: Diuretics acting on the distal renal tubule for preterm infants with (or developing) chronic lung disease, *Cochrane Database Syst Rev* 3:CD001817, 2000.
19. Bunchman TE: Infant dialysis: the future is now, *J Pediatr* 136:1, 2000.
20. Cavallo A: The pineal gland in human beings: relevance to pediatrics, *J Pediatr* 123:843, 1993.
21. Chamaa, NS, Mosig D, Drukker A et al: The renal hemodynamic effects of ibuprofen in the newborn rabbit, *Pediatr Res* 48:600, 2000.
22. Chan JCM: Renal tubular acidosis, *J Pediatr* 102:327, 1983.
23. Chavez GF, Mulinare J, Codero JF: Maternal cocaine use during early pregnancy as a risk factor for congenital urogenital anomalies, *JAMA* 262:795, 1989.
24. Cohen C: Ethical and legal considerations in the care of the infant with end-stage renal disease whose parents elect conservative therapy, *Pediatr Nephrol* 1:166, 1987.
25. Cole BR, Conley SB, Stapleton FB: Polycystic kidney disease in the first year of life, *J Pediatr* 111:693, 1987.
26. Conley SB: Supplemental nasogastric feedings in infants undergoing continuous peritoneal dialysis. In Fine R, ed: *Chronic ambulatory peritoneal dialysis and chronic cycling peritoneal dialysis in children,* Boston, 1987, Martinus-Nyhoff.
27. Conley SB, Portman RJ, Lemire JM et al: Five years' experience with cyclosporine in children, *Transplant Proc* 20(suppl 3):280, 1988.

28. Cruz C, Spitzer A: When you find protein or blood in the urine, *Contemp Pediatr*, Sept, 1998.
29. DeSwiet M, Fayers P, Shinebourne EA: Systolic blood pressure in a population of infants in the first year of life: the Brompton study, *Pediatrics* 65: 1028, 1980.
30. Donovan MJ, Natoli TA, Sainio K et al: Initial differentiation of the metanephric mesenchyme is independent of WT1 and the ureteric bud, *Dev Genet* 24:252, 1999.
31. Drukker A, Mosig D, Guignard J-P: The renal hemodynamic effect of Aspirin in newborn and young adult rabbits, *Pediatr Nephrol* 16:113, 2001.
32. Edelmann CM Jr: Developmental renal physiology. In Gruskin AB, Norman ME, eds: *Pediatric nephrology*, Boston, 1980, Martinus-Nyhoff.
33. Elinder G, Aperia A: Development of glomerular filtration rate in excretion of beta 2-microglobulin in the neonate during gentamicin treatment, *Acta Paediatr Scand* 72:219, 1983.
34. Engle WD: Evaluation of renal function in acute renal failure in the neonate, *Pediatr Clin North Am* 33:129, 1986.
35. Ertl T, Hadzsiev K Vincze O et al: Hyponatremia and sensorineural hearing loss in preterm infants, *Biol Neonate* 79:109, 2001.
36. Ferris M et al: Is in utero cocaine exposure a risk factor for urinary tract anomalies? *J Am Soc Nephrol* 2:307A, 1991.
37. Fine RN, Gruskin AB, eds: *End stage renal diseases in children*, Philadelphia, 1984, WB Saunders.
38. Friedman AL, Hustead VA: Hypertension in babies following discharge from a neonatal intensive care unit, *Pediatr Nephrol* 1:30, 1987.
39. Gemelli M, Manganaro R, Marni C et al: Circadian blood pressure pattern in full-term newborn infants, *Biol Neonate* 56:315, 1989.
40. Gallini F, Maggio L, Romagnoli C et al: Progression of renal function in preterm neonates with gestation age less than or equal to 32 wks, *Pediatr Nephrol* 15:119, 2000.
41. Glick PL, Harrison MR, Golbus MS et al: Management of the fetus with congenital hydronephrosis. II. Prognostic criteria and selection for treatment, *J Pediatr Surg* 20:376, 1985.
42. Golbus MS, Filly RA, Callen PW et al: Fetal urinary tract obstruction: management and selection for treatment, *Semin Perinatol* 9:91, 1985.
43. Goldstein SL, Currier H, Graf CD et al: Outcome in children receiving continuous venovenous hemofiltration. *Pediatrics* 107:1309, 2001.
44. Gong N-K et al: Eighteen years in pediatric acute dialysis: analysis of predicted outcome, *Pediatr Res* 16:212, 2001.
45. Gordon I, Barratt TM: Imaging the kidneys and urinary tract in the neonate with acute renal failure, *Pediatr Nephrol* 1:321, 1987.
46. Green TP, Thompson TR, Johnson DE et al: Furosemide promotes patent ductus arteriosus in premature infants with the respiratory-distress syndrome, *N Engl J Med* 308:743, 1983.
47. Gruskin AB: Developmental aspects of peritoneal dialysis kinetics. In Fine R, ed: *Chronic ambulatory peritoneal dialysis and chronic cycling peritoneal dialysis in children,* Boston, 1987, Martinus-Nyhoff.
48. Guignard J-P: Neonatal nephrology. In Holliday MA, Barratt TM, Vernier RL, eds: *Pediatric nephrology,* ed 2, Baltimore, 1987, Williams & Wilkins.
49. Guignard J-P. Renal function in preterm neonates, *Pediatr Res* 36:572, 1994.
50. Guignard J-P, Gouyan J-B: Adverse effects of drugs on the immature kidney, *Biol Neonate* 53:243, 1988.
51. Hanssens M, Keirse MJ, Vankelecom F et al: Fetal and neonatal effects of treatment with angiotensin-converting enzyme inhibitors in pregnancy, *Obstet Gynecol* 78:128, 1991.
52. Harmon WE: Treatment of children with chronic renal failure, *Kidney Int* 47:951, 1995.
53. Helbrugge T et al: Circadian periodicity of physiological function in different stages of infancy and children, *NY Acad Sci* 117:361, 1964.
54. Helin I, Persson P-H: Prenatal diagnosis of urinary tract abnormalities by ultrasound, *Pediatrics* 78: 879, 1986.
55. Hellstrom M, Jacobsson B, Jodal U et al: Renal growth after neonatal urinary tract infection, *Pediatr Nephrol* 1:269, 1987.
56. Holliday MA: Developmental abnormalities of the kidney in children, *Hosp Pract* 13:101, 1978.
57. Holtfa T, Ronnholm K, Jalanko H et al: Clinical outcomes of pediatric patients on peritoneal dialysis under adequacy control, *Pediatr Nephrol* 14:889, 2000.
58. Hufnagle KG, Khan SN, Penn D et al: Renal calcifications: a complication of long-term furosemide therapy in preterm infants, *Pediatrics* 70:360, 1982.
59. Jacinto JS, Modanlou HD, Crade M et al: Renal calcification incidence in very low birth weight infants, *Pediatrics* 81:31, 1988.
60. Kalia A, Brouhard BH, Travis LB et al: Renal transplantation in the infant and young child, *Am J Dis Child* 143:47, 1988.
61. Kao, Warburton D, Cheng MH et al: Use of diuretics in bronchopulmonary dysplasia, *Pediatrics* 74:37, 1984.
62. Karlowicz MG, Adelman RD: Nonoliguric and oliguric acute renal failure in asphyxiated neonates, *Pediatr Nephrol* 9:718, 1995.
63. Karlsson FA, Hardell L-I, Hellsing K: A prospective study of urinary proteins in early infancy, *Acta Paediatr Scand* 68:663, 1979.
64. Katz A, Bock GH, Mauer M: Improved growth velocity with intensive dialysis: consequence or coincidence, *Pediatr Nephrol* 14:710, 2000.

65. Keidan I, Lotan D, Gazit G et al: Early neonatal renal venous thrombosis: long-term outcome, *Acta Paediatr* 83:1225, 1994.

66. Kohaut EC, Alexander S: Ultrafiltration in the young patient on CAPD. In Moncrief J, Popovich R, eds: *CAPD update,* New York, 1981, Masson.

67. Kirks DR, Merten DF, Grossman H et al: Diagnostic imaging of pediatric abdominal masses: an overview, *Radiol Clin North Am* 19:527, 1981.

68. Kissane JM: Congenital malformations of the kidney. In Hamburger J, Crosnier T, Gruenfeld J-P, eds: *Nephrology,* 1979, Wiley-Flammarion.

69. Kleinman LI, Stewart CL, Kaskel FJ: Renal disease in the newborn. In Edelmann CM, ed: *Pediatric nephrology,* ed 2, Boston, 1992, Little, Brown.

70. Ledermann SE, Scanes ME, Fernando ON et al: Long-term outcome of perinatal dialysis in infants. *J Pediatr* 136:24, 2000.

71. Lieberman K: Continuous arteriovenous hemofiltration in children, *Pediatr Nephrol* 1:330, 1987.

72. Lieberman K, Nardi L, Bosch JP: Treatment of acute renal failure in an infant using continuous arteriovenous hemofiltration, *J Pediatr* 106:646, 1985.

73. Lindemann R: Congenital renal tubular dysfunction associated with maternal sniffing of organic solvents, *Acta Paediatr Scand* 80:882, 1991.

74. Manning FA: Ultrasound in perinatal medicine. In Creasy RF, Resnik R, eds: *Maternal and fetal medicine principles and practice,* Philadelphia, 1984, WB Saunders.

75. Matos V, Drukker A, Guignard J-P: Spot urine samples for evaluating solute excretion in the first week of life, *Arch Dis Child Fetal Neonatal Educ* 80: F240, 1999.

76. Matthew OP, Jones AS, James E et al: Neonatal renal failure: usefulness of diagnostic indices, *Pediatrics* 65:57, 1980.

77. McLean RH, Gearhart JP, Jeffs R: Neonatal obstructive uropathy, *Pediatr Nephrol* 2:48, 1988.

78. McVicar M, Margouleff D, Chandra M: Diagnosis and imaging of the fetal and neonatal abdominal mass: an integrated approach, *Adv Pediatr* 38:135, 1991.

79. Mingeot-Leclercq M-P, Tulkens PM: Aminoglycosides: nephrotoxicity, *Antimicrob Agents Chemother* 43:1003, 1999.

80. Mirmiran M, Kok JHL: Circadian rhythms in early human development, *Early Hum Dev* 26:121, 1991.

81. Mocan H, Beattie TJ, Murphy AV: Renal vein thrombosis in infancy: long term follow-up, *Pediatr Nephrol* 5:45, 1991.

82. Muehlendahl KE, Ballowitz L: Growth hormone and cortisol in neonates during phototherapy, *Z Kinderheilk* 119:53, 1975.

83. Murphy JL, Kaplan GW, Packer MG et al: Prenatal diagnosis of severe urinary tract anomalies improves renal function and growth, *Child Nephrol Urol* 9:290, 1988.

84. Murugasu B, Cole BR, Hawkins EP et al: Familial renal adysplasia, *Am J Kid Dis* 18:490, 1991.

85. Parkhouse H, Barrett JM: Investigation of the dilated urinary tract, *Pediatr Nephrol* 2:43, 1988.

86. Perlman JM, Volpe JJ: Neurologic complications of captopril treatment of neonatal hypertension, *Pediatrics* 83:48, 1989.

87. Portman RJ, Carter BS, Gaylord MS et al: Predicting neonatal morbidity after perinatal asphyxia: a scoring system, *Am J Obstet Gynecol* 162:174, 1990.

88. Potter EL: Normal and abnormal development of the kidney, St. Louis, 1972, Mosby.

89. Rasoulpour M, McLean RH: Renal venous thrombosis in neonates, *Am J Dis Child* 134:276, 1980.

90. Reppert S, Weaver D: A biological clock is oscillating in the fetal suprchiasmatic nucleus. In Klein DC, Moore RY, Reppert SM, eds: *Suprachiasmatic nucleus: the mind's clock,* New York, 1991, Oxford University Press.

91. Reppert SM, Weaver DR, Rivkees SA et al: Putative melatonin receptors in a human biological clock, *Science* 242:78, 1988.

92. Retik AB: Genitourinary problems in children, *Hosp Pract* 11:133, 1976.

93. Reznik VM, Kaplan GW, Murphy JL et al: Follow-up of infants with bilateral renal disease detected in utero, *Am J Dis Child* 142:453, 1988.

94. Robillar JE, Smith FG et al: Mechanisms regulating renal sodium excretion during development, *Pediatr Nephrol* 6:205, 1992.

95. Ronco C, Bragantini L, Brendolan A et al: Arteriovenous hemodiafiltration (AVHDF) combined with continuous arteriovenous hemofiltration (CAVH), *Trans Am Soc Prof Artif Organs* 31:349, 1985.

96. Ronco C, Brendolan A, Bragantini L et al: Treatment of acute renal failure in newborns by continuous arterio-venous hemofiltration, *Kidney Int* 29: 908, 1986.

97. Rosendahl H: Ultrasound screening for fetal urinary tract malformations: a prospective study in general population, *Eur J Obstet Gynecol Reprod Biol* 36:27, 1990.

98. Rotundo A, Nevins TE, Lipton M et al: Progressive encephalopathy in children with chronic renal insufficiency in infancy, *Kidney Int* 21:489, 1982.

99. Roussan MS: Neurogenic bladder dysfunction, *Med Times* 109:43, 1981.

100. Salusky IB, von Lilien T, Anchondo M et al: Experience with continuous cycling peritoneal dialysis during the first year of life, *Pediatr Nephrol* 1:172, 1987.

101. Sankaran K, Hindmarsh KW, Tan L: Diurnal rhythm of J-endorphin in neonates, *Dev Pharmacol Ther* 12:1, 1989.

102. Satlin LM: Maturation of renal potassium transport, *Pediatr Nephrol* 5:260, 1991.

103. Schell-Feith EA: Etiology of nephrocalcinosis in preterm neonates: association of nutritional intake and urinary parameters, *Kidney Int* 58:2102, 2000.

104. Schmidt B, Andrew M: Neonatal thrombosis: report of a prospective Canadian and international registry, *Pediatrics* 96:939, 1995.

105. Schwartz GJ, Brion LP, Spitzer A: The use of plasma creatinine concentration for estimating glomerular filtration rate in infants, children, and adolescents, *Pediatr Clin North Am* 34:571, 1987.

106. Seeman T, John U, Blahova K et al: Ambulatory blood pressure monitoring in children with unilateral multicystic dysplastic kidney, *Eur J Pediatr* 160:78, 2001.

107. Sertel H, Scopes J: Rates of creatinine clearance in babies less than one week of age, *Arch Dis Child* 48:717, 1973.

108. Shankaran S, Liang KC, Ilagan N et al: Mineral excretion following furosemide compared with bumetanide therapy in premature infants, *Pediatr Nephrol* 9:159, 1995.

109. Shooter M, Watson M: The ethics of withholding and withdrawing dialysis therapy in infants, *Pediatr Nephrol* 14:347, 2000.

110. Siegel S, Oh W: Renal function as a marker of human fetal maturation, *Acta Paediatr Scand* 65:481, 1976.

111. Sitka U, Weinert D, Berle K et al: Investigations of the rhythmic function of heart rate, blood pressure, and temperature in neonates, *Eur J Pediatr* 153:117, 1994.

112. Smolensky MH, D'Alonzo GE: Medical chronobiology concepts and applications, *Am Rev Respir Dis* 147:S2, 1993.

113. Springate JE, Fildes RD, Feld LG: Assessment of renal function in newborn infants, *Pediatr Rev* 9:51, 1987.

114. Stalker HP, Holland NH, Kotchen JM et al: Plasma renin activity in healthy children, *J Pediatr* 89:256, 1976.

115. Stapleton FB: Renal uric acid clearance in human neonates, *J Pediatr* 103:290, 1983.

116. Stapleton FB, Jones DP, Green RS: Acute renal failure in neonates: incidence, etiology and outcome, *Pediatr Nephrol* 1:314, 1987.

117. Straub E, Spranger J: Etiology and pathogenesis of the prune belly syndrome, *Kidney Int* 20:695, 1981.

118. Sulyok E, Guigard J-P: Relationship of urinary anion gap to urinary ammonium excretion in the neonate, *Biol Neonate* 57:98, 1990.

119. Tack ED, Perlman JM, Robson AM: Renal injury in sick newborn infants: a prospective evaluation using urinary beta 2 microglobulin concentrations, *Pediatrics* 81.432, 1988.

120. Task Force on Blood Pressure Control in Children: Report of the Second Task Force on Blood Pressure Control in Children—1987, *Pediatrics* 79:1, 1987.

121. Temple JK, Shapira E: Genetic determinants of renal disease in neonates, *Clin Perinatol* 8:361, 1981.

122. Toth-Heyn P, Drukker A, Guignard J-P: The stressed neonatal kidney: from pathophysiology to clinical management of neonatal vasomotor nephropathy, *Pediatr Nephrol* 14:227, 2000.

123. Vainio SJ, Uusitalo MS: A road to kidney tubules in the Wnt pathway, *Pediatr Nephrol* 15:151, 2000.

124. Walhauser F, Weiszebacher G, Tatzer E et al: Alterations in nocturnal serum melatonin levels in humans with growing and aging, *J Clin Endo Metab* 66:648, 1988.

125. Warady BA, Bunchman T: Dialysis therapy for children with acute renal failure: survey results, *Pediatr Nephrol* 15:61, 2000.

126. Wells JG, Bunchman TE, Kearns GL: Treatment of neonatal hypertension with enalapril, *J Pediatr* 117:664, 1990.

127. Wilkins IA, Chitkara U, Lynch L et al: The nonpredictive value of fetal urinary electrolyte: preliminary report of outcomes and correlates with pathologic diagnosis, *Am J Obstet Gynecol* 157:694, 1987.

128. Wood EG, Hand M, Briscoe DM: Risk factors for mortality in infants and children on dialysis, *Am J Kidney Dis* 37:573, 2001.

129. Woolf AS: Developmental anatomy and physiology. In Morgan SH, Grunfeld J-P. *Inherited disorders of the kidney,* Oxford, England, 1998, Oxford University Press.

130. Wu J et al: Circaseptan and circannual modulation of circadian rhythms in neonatal blood pressure and heart rate. In Hayes D, Pauly J, Reiter R, eds: *Chronobiology: its role in clinical medicine, general biology and agriculture,* 1990, Wiley-Liss.

26 Neurologic Disorders

Patti L. Paige, Paul R. Carney

The developing nervous system provides an ongoing challenge for researchers and clinicians alike. Investigation continues in a wide variety of areas, yet basic mechanisms for a pathophysiologic understanding of common events such as neonatal seizures and intraventricular hemorrhages (IVHs) remain unclear.

Improved neonatal care in recent years has not significantly reduced neurologic residua. How much of this is a reflection of sicker and more immature infants being salvaged is difficult to assess. Primary neurologic disease and secondary neurologic complications from such common conditions as cardiopulmonary disease, metabolic derangements, shock, infection, and coagulopathy still represent major problems encountered in every intensive care nursery. Serious anomalies still appear with regularity, albeit in small numbers.

In this chapter we deal with selected topics in neonatal neurology, including congenital malformations, trauma, seizures, hypoxic-ischemic encephalopathy, and IVH.

CONGENITAL MALFORMATIONS

Physiology, Etiologic Factors, and Clinical Features

Congenital malformations of the nervous system occur when the usual sequence of maturation and development is interrupted[81] (Table 26-1). By definition, the malformation is present at birth. Causes are multiple and largely unknown. Although strictly destructive lesions (such as hydranencephaly resulting from bilateral carotid artery occlusion) are separate from primary failures of morphogenesis, both may be included in the broad category of congenital malformations. The distinction between the two types lies in an understanding of the causes.

Understanding congenital malformations requires an appreciation of the normal embryologic sequence.[82] The clinical and pathologic identification of normal and abnormal structures makes it possible to determine the timing of the insult or development failure. Once timing is established, an appropriate search for the cause can be made.

Neural Tube Defects

The incidence in the United States of neural tube defects (NTDs) is approximately 1:1000 births. NTDs represent one of the most common birth defects contributing to mortality and morbidity of infants.[69] **NTDs include three of the most serious birth defects: anencephaly, encephalocele, and spina bifida.** Folic acid supplements before and during pregnancy have been cited as substantially lowering the incidence of these NTDs. **As many as 50% or more of NTDs are preventable.** The U.S. Public Health Service issued a recommendation that women of childbearing years consume 400 µg of folic acid each day to prevent NTDs. The American Academy of Pediatrics also supports this recommendation.[16,75]

Although the incidence of NTDs is decreasing, it is important to note that prenatal diagnosis and elective termination of pregnancies may have skewed these statistics. Nor should we expect total prevention of NTDs with improved consumption of folic acid, because NTDs result from environmental as well as genetic factors. Other environmental factors include maternal consumption of certain anticonvulsants, maternal obesity, and diabetes.[47]

At the end of the first embryonic week the *primitive streak* is present on the rostral surface of the embryo. A second streak, the *notochordal process,* develops alongside the primitive streak. The notochord is responsible for the induction of both the *neural plate* and the *neurenteric canal.* Cells proliferate along the lateral margin of the neural plate to form the neural folds around the central *neural groove.*[47,85]

Cells at the apex of the neural folds make up the *neural crest.* Schwann cells, piarachnoid cells, sensory ganglia, melanocytes, and various secretory cells arise from the neural crest. The neural folds meet and fuse with the rostral (anterior) and caudal (posterior) ends (neuropore), closing approximately by the end of the fourth embryonic week.[85]

Table 26-1	CENTRAL NERVOUS SYSTEM DEVELOPMENT AND RELATED DEFECTS	
MATURATIONAL PROCESS	TIME	ASSOCIATED DEFECTS
Neural tube defects (dorsal induction, neurulation)	3-4 wk	Craniorrhachischisis Anencephaly Myeloschisis Encephalocele Myelomeningocele Arnold-Chiari malformation
Prosencephalic development[18]	2-3 mo	Cyclopia Holoprosencephaly Arhinencephaly Septooptic dysplasia Agenesis of corpus collosum Agenesis of septum pellucidum
Proliferation	2-4 mo	Microcephaly Megalencephaly Neurocutaneous syndromes (?)
Migration[1,2]	3-5+ mo	Schizencephaly Lissencephaly Pachygyria (macrogyria) Microgyria (polymicrogyria) Neuronal heterotopias
Neuronal organization and functional organization	6 mo	Down syndrome (?) Mental retardation (?) Genetic epilepsy (?)
Myelination[5]	8 mo	Anoxic/ischemic damage

Failure of development at this stage results in the defects of neurulation (or dorsal induction). The most severe of these defects is craniorachischisis, in which there is significant malformation of the brain (as in anencephaly), absence of the posterior skull, and an open spine the full length of the spinal cord. Only a few survive to early fetal stages.[85]

Anencephaly is similar to craniorachischisis without the spinal defect. There is essentially no normal brain tissue above the brainstem and thalami, and parts of those structures are malformed. Onset is thought to occur before 24 days' gestation. About one fourth of these infants survive to the neonatal period, but three fourths are stillborn. The majority of anencephalic infants die within the first week of life without intensive care.[85]

Myeloschisis involves the failure of the posterior neural tube to close. No skull defect is present.

Encephaloceles are caused by a limited failure of closure at the rostral (head) end of the neural tube. Extensions of meninges or brain tissue through the skull may occur on the ventral or rostral surface.[85]

Myelomeningoceles (or even the more limited meningoceles) are a limited form of myeloschisis with failure of closure at the caudal (tail) end of the neural tube. The Arnold-Chiari deformities are usually included here. These malformations, often seen with myelomeningoceles, involve structures of the brainstem and cerebellum. Generally, the cerebellar tonsils are pulled down through the foramen magnum, and the brainstem is elongated in later life. Hydrocephalus is common. Dilatation of ventricles often occurs without increased head circumference or clinical symptoms of increased intracranial pressure in this group of infants; therefore, it is important to perform serial CT or ultrasonographic scans. Symptoms of brainstem involvement may occur. Open myelomeningoceles and anencephaly (any defect in which the spinal or cranial contents are "open" to the outside) will cause an elevation of AFP in the amniotic fluid. This is important in prenatal diagnosis.[85]

Segmentation Defects

After formation and closure of the neural tube, the development of the different regions of the brain begins to occur. Suprasegmental structures are formed. The division of the brain into hemispheres, formation of the ventricular system, and formation of the major gyral patterns are all part of this period of development. Major areas of the brain, including the cerebellum, basal ganglia, brainstem nuclei, thalamus, and hypothalamus, form at this time.[45,85] Defects of segmentation and cleavage occur during this phase of neural development. For unknown reasons, defects of segmentation and cleavage are far less common than defects of neurulation. Because these malformations involve abnormalities of ventral induction rather than dorsal induction (such as neurulation), the face, eyes, nose, mouth, and hair are also involved in the malformation. These features should always be investigated carefully for specific anomalies.

Holoprosencephaly is characterized by a single midline lateral ventricle; incomplete or absent interhemispheric fissure; absent olfactory system; midfacial clefts; and hypotelorism. The most severe form of holoprosencephaly is cyclopia (a single fused midline eye) and supraorbital nasal structure. At times, the nasal structure and eye are absent. An intermediate form is cebocephaly, which includes ocular hypotelorism (abnormally decreased space between the eyes) and a flat nose with single nostril.[85]

When any of these malformations are suspected or when features suggestive of them are seen, careful examination of the hair, eyes, ears, mouth, and nose may reveal other related anomalies.

Migration and Cortical Organizational Defects

A critical aspect of brain development has yet to be described. The remaining development of the brain takes over twice as long as the previously described development and includes cellular proliferation, migration, organization, and myelination. The cells that later form the cerebral cortex begin in the germinal matrix (near the caudate nucleus around the lateral ventricles). These cells then migrate in a radial fashion to their final positions near the surface of the brain. Abnormalities of cellular migration result in collections of gray matter in unusual places (heterotopias), abnormal gyri and sulci, abnormal spaces in the brain, and frequent clinical signs of gray matter dysfunction. Frequently, these clinical problems are not apparent in the newborn period. The malformations in this grouping show no characteristic cranial or somatic features, because the timing of the malformations is after the formation of large brain structures, divisions, and connections.[43]

Microcephaly means "small brain" and is manifested by a head circumference measuring greater than two standard deviations below average for infants at that gestational age. Microcephaly may be (1) genetic (dominant, recessive, sex-linked) or chromosomal (translocation [see Chapter 27]), (2) caused by teratogens (cocaine, alcohol), (3) caused by infection (rubella, cytomegalovirus), or (4) of unknown cause. Occasionally there is a paucity of germinal matrix cells, or they fail to adequately migrate, resulting in a brain cortex with lessened neuronal cells.[85]

Schizencephaly is a malformation in which atypical clefts, most often in the region of the sylvian and rolandic fissures, are present within the brain substance. Schizencephaly is unilateral in over half of the cases. A portion of the germinative zones and cerebral wall is believed to fail to develop. If the cleft lips become widely separated, it may result in dilation of the lateral ventricles and hydrocephalus.[85]

In contrast to schizencephaly, **porencephaly** (not a malformation) is most often thought to be the result of destruction of previously normal tissue. Porencephaly is the occurrence of a cavity within the brain.[85] This theory of porencephaly is confirmed by the identification of porencephalic cysts after strokes or meningitis.

In **lissencephaly** the brain is smooth in appearance, having little or no gyri (convolutions). Although not generally present at birth, microcephaly usually occurs within the first year in type I lissencephaly. Appearance is marked by hollowing at both temples, a small jaw, and hypotonia. Neonatal seizures may be present but seizures more commonly present at 6 to 12 months of age. Another form of type I lissencephaly is Miller-Dieker syndrome, in which craniofacial deviations occur. In type II lissencephaly, macrocephaly is generally present is birth or develops soon afterward. Retinal, cerebellar, and muscular abnormalities are always present.[85]

Macrogyria (pachgria) may be a localized hemispheric malformation or a diffuse malformation. The involved gyri show large, abnormal neurons and dense gliosis. Unusually wide gyri with compressed sulci can be seen.

Microgyria or **polymicrogyria** occurs as a response to an arrest in neuronal maturation before the fifth gestational month. CMV and maternal carbon monoxide poisoning (at 20 to 24 weeks' gestation) have been shown in some instances to produce this malformation, but most often the cause is unknown. Anatomically, areas of very small gyri are present in the involved area.

Agenesis of the corpus callosum most likely represents a midline anomaly and is often seen as a part of a more extensive malformation such as Aicardi's syndrome, in which agenesis of the corpus callosum is accompanied by a chorioretinal lacuna and infantile spasms.

Schizencephaly and other malformations often have associated agenesis of the corpus calosum. In this malformation, there is a large subarachnoid space between the two hemispheres, and the lateral ventricles are displaced laterally (a commonly looked-for sign on a CT scan). The third ventricle is often dilated. An X-linked form has been reported, but most cases are sporadic. Clinically the X-linked cases generally show multiple neurologic problems, whereas the isolated malformations of the corpus callosum have been found incidentally at autopsy in patients in whom it was not at all suspected.

Migrational anomalies easily lead to problems of gray matter dysfunction. These problems include seizures, mental retardation, motor dysfunction (cerebral palsy), and sensory dysfunction (blindness or deafness). Common manifestations in the newborn period are seizures, microcephaly, SGA, abnormal cry, and abnormal transillumination. Findings that are present later in life and probably not seen in neonates are mental retardation and spasticity.

Clinical features of schizencephaly include seizures, retardation, spastic quadriparesis, or minimal findings.

Clinical features of porencephaly include seizures, motor problems, increased intracranial pressure if the cyst is enlarging, and abnormal transillumination if the cyst is superficial. On occasion, no symptoms are perceptible.

Clinical features of lissencephaly include seizures, microcephaly, abnormal cry, SGA, polyhydramnios, micrognathia, downward-slanted palpebral fissures, anteverted nares, and prominent forehead and occiput. Later, severe spasticity, hypsarrhythmia, and severe mental retardation may develop.

Clinical features of macrogyria include spastic hemiplegia or diplegia (depending on the site of involvement). If the area of involvement is very limited, there may be a paucity of findings. Clinical features of microgyria include absence of findings in the newborn period. Later, spasticity and mental retardation are observable.

Signs and symptoms of absence of the corpus callosum are most often a result of associated malformations and anomalies.[23] These include seizures, mental retardation, hydrocephalus, motor abnormalities, and asynchrony as demonstrated on an EEG.

Additional Defects

Cerebellar malformations are quite varied. Most often, at least a portion of the cerebellum is preserved, but total absence occurs. Hemispheric aplasia or vermal aplasia are seen, and familial forms have been reported. The **Dandy-Walker cyst** is another complex malformation involving the cerebellum. In it the fourth ventricle is dilated into a cystic structure. The foramena of Magendie and Lushka are atretic, and hydrocephalus results. The cerebellum is small and displaced upward. Associated anomalies include heterotopias, microgyria, agenesis of the corpus callosum, aqueductal stenosis, and syringomyelia. No specific causes are known. The differential diagnosis includes an arachnoid cyst of the posterior fossa. In the case of an arachnoid cyst, the fourth ventricle is not part of the malformation and is normal, although it may be displaced.

Clinical features of cerebellar malformations include absence of symptoms in the newborn period, cerebellar findings in family members, and the proband (hypotonia, incoordination, and nystagmus), especially in vermal aplasia, or total absence of symptoms throughout life.

Clinical features of the Dandy-Walker cyst include frequent progressive hydrocephalus, associated malformations that cause additional specific symptoms, possible absence of symptoms in the newborn period, enlargement of the occipital shelf and posterior part of the skull, positive transillumination in a triangular shape, nystagmus, lateral gaze palsy, abnormalities of respiratory control, and, later in life, ataxia.

Craniosynostosis is the abnormal fusion of the bones of the skull. The causes of this malformation are unknown. The premature closure of sutures may involve one or many sutures, with resulting deformity of the skull. Numerous terms are used to describe the shapes the skull assumes when craniosynostosis is present. Among these terms are plagiocephaly, scaphocephaly, dolichocephaly, keel-shaped deformity, and clover-leaf skull. Any of the atlases of human malformations give striking examples of these deformities.

Craniosynostosis should be suspected in the presence of microcephaly or a misshapen head. Appropriate evaluation requires x-ray films of the skull and a CT scan to define which if any of the sutures are stenosed and what problems might exist with brain structure (pressure or malformation).

Hydrocephalus may occur in many different situations from many separate causes. An inherited X-linked form exists. Intrauterine infections are another cause. Hydrocephalus may be associated with many of the malformations listed above. Hydrocephalus results when the normal flow of ventriculospinal fluid is obstructed. This may be the result of an atretic portion of the ventricular system, blockage from the outside, inflammation within the ventricular system causing a permanent blockage, or (very rarely) overproduction of ventriculospinal fluid.[85] Therefore, if the cause is an inflammatory process that caused degeneration and destruction of part of the ventricular pathway, hydrocephalus may at times be more appropriately categorized with the destructive lesions. These infectious processes may also be responsible for some of the cases of congenital porencephaly. Vascular occlusion is the other cause thought to be responsible for some malformations in the "destructive lesion" category, including cases of porencephaly and hydranencephaly.

Data Collection

The diagnosis of malformations of the CNS may be quite obvious (as in anencephaly) or totally unrecognized during life (as in some cases of agenesis of the corpus callosum).[23] Careful examination of all newborns will result in the identification of most malformations. At times the diagnosis will be suspected not on the basis of findings on examination but because of an accompanying sign, such as seizures.

When a congenital malformation is suspected, whether or not somatic signs are present, careful evaluation of the status of the CNS is in order. **CT scanning is important for a better understanding of the intracranial structures, and electrophysiologic studies (EEG and evoked potentials) will help assess the functional aspects of the malformations.** Clearly, there is no need for these studies in a seriously malformed infant who is not expected to survive.

Two very important tests have become available in recent years that allow prenatal diagnosis of certain congenital malformations of the nervous system. **Ultrasonographic examination (an abdominal ultrasound scan of the mother) provides an opportunity to identify certain malformations by viewing the fetus during development.** Hydrocephalus, encephaloceles, myelomeningoceles, and anencephaly may be identified prenatally. **Determination of alpha-fetoprotein (AFP) in the amniotic fluid allows for the identification of anencephaly and open myelomeningoceles. A nonenclosed nervous system will cause a significant rise in AFP in the amniotic fluid.** Amniocentesis provides the amniotic fluid necessary for this determination. Testing of maternal serum for AFP is less specific and more controversial. At present, the combination of ultrasonographic examination and amniocentesis provides the most helpful information.

Clinical signs and symptoms have been described for each individual nervous system malformation presented earlier in this chapter.

Treatment

Very limited treatment is available for congenital malformations of the nervous system. A variety of strategies are available for reducing secondary complications or providing earlier management to handle these complications more efficiently.

The greatest efforts and accomplishments have been made for infants with congenital malformations who might be expected to live productive lives. When secondary complications are managed appropriately, children with myelomeningoceles often become well-adjusted, productive adults. This is not possible when the malformation causes severe retardation.

Some of the malformations are lethal in a short period of time (anencephaly and hydranencephaly), making intervention unnecessary and inappropriate. When intervention results only in increased time of survival without any improvement in profound physical and mental handicaps, the desirability of intervention should be questioned.

Treatment of many of the malformations of the brain is limited to the management of the manifestations of the malformation. These would include seizures, hearing impairment, spasticity, and secondary orthopedic problems. Because the primary defect cannot be changed, it is important to recognize that for many of the conditions, one cannot hope for substantial improvement.

In certain malformations, some specific treatment is indicated. **If the encephalocele is small and a large amount of the brain is not contained in the sac, the defect should be closed. Associated neurologic problems such as seizures should be treated.**

When treatment is thought to be appropriate, closure of the myelomeningocele should be performed as soon as possible. In this way the risk of meningitis and ventriculitis can be reduced. Untreated infants often die within the first year of life. Soon after closure of the primary defect, many infants develop hydrocephalus or experience a more severe case of antecedent hydrocephalus. Shunting then becomes necessary (Boxes 26-1 and 26-2 and Figures 26-1 and 26-2).[32]

The only situation in which microcephaly could be considered surgically treatable is total craniosynostosis. Generally, skull deformity is also present in infants with craniosynostosis, but it is always wise to consider the possibility of craniosynostosis in any infant with a small head. If present, total craniosynostosis should be treated surgically.

The management of congenital hydrocephalus consists primarily of early shunting as soon after

Box 26-1	POSTOPERATIVE VENTRICULOPERITONEAL SHUNT CARE

I. Positioning
- A. Place on unaffected side (may position on shunt side with "dough" over operative site once incision has healed). Keep head of bed flat (15 to 30 degrees) to prevent too-rapid fluid loss.
- B. Support head carefully when moving infant.
- C. Turn q 2 hr from unaffected side of head to back.

II. Shunt site
- A. Use strict aseptic technique when changing dressing.
- B. Pump shunt if and only as directed by neurosurgeon.
- C. Observe for fluid leakage around pump.

III. Observe and document all intake and output. Watch for symptoms of excessive drainage of CSF:
- A. Sunken fontanel
- B. Increased urine output
- C. Increased sodium loss

IV. Observe, document, and report any seizure activity or paresis.

V. Observe for signs of ileus:
- A. Abdominal distention (serially measure abdominal girth)
- B. Absence of bowel sounds
- C. Loss of gastric content by emesis or through oro-gastric tube

VI. Perform range-of-motion exercises on all extremities.

VII. Observe and assess for symptoms of increased intracranial pressure (shunt failure):
- A. Increasing head circumference (measure head daily)
- B. Full and/or tense fontanel
- C. Sutures palpably more separated
- D. High-pitched, shrill cry
- E. Irritability and/or sleeplessness
- F. Vomiting
- G. Poor feeding
- H. Nystagmus
- I. Sunset sign of eyes
- J. Shiny scalp with distended vessels
- K. Hypotonia and/or hypertonia

VIII. Observe and assess for signs of infection:
- A. Redness or drainage at shunt site
- B. Hypothermia and/or hyperthermia
- C. Lethargy and/or irritability
- D. Poor feeding and/or weight gain
- E. Pallor

IX. Parent teaching (see Figure 26-1)
- A. Demonstrate and receive return demonstration of drug administration.
- B. Teach parents side effects of medications.
- C. Document on NICU's routine discharge teaching checklist with routine care.

Box 26-2	WOLFSON CHILDREN'S HOSPITAL PARENT HANDOUT NEWBORN VENTRICULOPERITONEAL (VP) SHUNT (FOR USE WITH VP SHUNT TEACHING CHECKLIST)

Purpose of VP Shunt. Ventricles are compartment-like spaces that are located in the normal brain. Spinal fluid forms daily in these ventricles. This clear fluid flows out over the brain and down around the spinal cord. Spinal fluid helps cushion the brain from injury, keeps the brain moist, and carries away waste products.

Hydrocephalus is a condition in which an abnormally large amount of spinal fluid builds up in your baby's ventricles and is usually caused by a blockage in the spinal fluid path. Because the ventricles continue to make spinal fluid daily, a build-up of fluid occurs when it can't escape. This excess fluid can cause pressure on the brain and result in permanent damage to the brain unless it is properly treated.

The purpose and function of your baby's VP shunt is to allow the excess spinal fluid to drain through a tube from the ventricle into the abdomen, where it is absorbed.

Pathway of the VP Shunt. A small incision is made on the scalp and the tube is passed through the skull and into the ventricle. Located under the skin, the tube passes behind the ear, down the side of the neck, and continues to the abdomen where a second incision is made to put the end of the tube

into the abdominal cavity. A third incision is sometimes needed in the neck area with some babies.

The scalp incision will be hidden as your baby's hair grows. You'll see and feel the shunt tubing (like a large vein under the skin), but it is barely noticeable after the baby gains weight.

Signs and Symptoms of Shunt Infection. The shunt is at risk for infection because it is a foreign object located inside the body. You will need to watch for these signs of shunt infection and report them **immediately** to your doctor:
- Temperature of 101° F or higher
- Swelling, redness, and/or drainage along the pathway of the shunt tube
- Lethargy or irritability (change in behavior)
- Loss of appetite or poor feeding

Signs and Symptoms of Shunt Failure/Increased Intracranial Pressure (ICP). The spinal fluid contains proteins and chemicals that may build up and block off the shunt. It is also possible for tissue within the brain or abdomen to block the shunt or for the shunt device itself to fail. This shunt failure (malfunction) means that the spinal fluid will once again build up and result in pressure on the brain and possible irreversible

Courtesy Baptist Medical Center, Wolfson Children's Hospital Jacksonville, Fla.

Continued

Box 26-2	WOLFSON CHILDREN'S HOSPITAL PARENT HANDOUT NEWBORN VENTRICULOPERITONEAL (VP) SHUNT (FOR USE WITH VP SHUNT TEACHING CHECKLIST)—cont'd

damage. It is therefore very important for you to watch for the signs of increased pressure in the brain that occurs with shunt failure and report them immediately to your doctor.

- Lethargy or sleepiness
- Unusual irritability, fussiness, or excessive crying
- Repeated vomiting
- Poor feeding
- Bulging soft spot when baby is sitting up quietly
- Shrill, high-pitched cry
- Eyes that look downward
- Increase in spaces between the bones of the skull
- Seizures/posturing

Reason and Importance of Prompt Treatment of Health Problems. Prompt treatment of your baby's health problems (ear infections, skin infections, etc.) is important to pre-

vent infections spreading to the shunt. It is also vital to seek medical care for signs of shunt infection or failure as noted above.

Importance of Close Medical Follow-up. Your baby will need to be followed up by a neurosurgeon and your pediatrician after being discharged. It is important for you to bring the baby to every follow-up appointment so that your baby's head can be measured and physical condition can be evaluated. Your baby will also go to the Developmental Evaluation Clinic where a specialist in baby development can examine him or her. If development problems occur, this will ensure early diagnosis and treatment.

Care of the Shunt. You can handle, cuddle, and play with your baby like any baby. Your baby can also sleep in any position after the initial postoperative period.

Courtesy Baptist Medical Center, Wolfson Children's Hospital Jacksonville, Fla.

birth as possible. Fetal surgery for placement of a ventriculoamniotic shunt has been proposed, but an improvement in outcomes when compared with surgery after birth is uncertain. Additionally, hydrocephalus in the fetus is often associated with serious developmental abnormalities that have an impact on morbidity and mortality.[85]

In Volpe's series, outcome was variable, and the procedures were not as reliable as hoped. It was not always possible to distinguish true hydrocephalus from ventriculomegaly without increased pressure. **Shunting soon after birth often produces a far better outcome than would be assumed, with minimal motor deficit and only a mild to moderate deficit in intellect.**[85]

Monitoring of pregnancies with fetal ultrasound allows for the detection of congenital hydrocephalus. Induction of lung maturation with steroids has been suggested to allow a preterm delivery (with a smaller head) without excessive pulmonary complications. In this way, a permanent shunt can be placed sooner than with term delivery.[18]

Complications

Many of the expected complications were dealt with previously in the sections describing the malformations and their associated problems. It is difficult to separate true complications from problems occurring by the nature of the malformation. For example, hydrocephalus after closure of a myelomeningocele is not truly a complication of the procedure or the

disease, but merely a condition brought out by the procedure.

Malformations carry with them disturbed anatomy and physiology that are reflected in abnormal function. General problems commonly encountered are seizures, retardation, sensorimotor abnormalities, disturbances in primary sensory function such as vision and hearing, orthopedic problems, and vegetative functions.

The problems encountered are ordinarily explainable on the basis of the malformation. Midline defects in the brain (particularly at the base of the brain) will often have clinical problems involving the hypothalamus. Diabetes insipidus may be present.

To some extent, the anatomy predicts the kinds of problems encountered. Involvement of the cortex causes seizures, retardation, and sensorimotor problems. White matter damage can cause spasticity. If the brainstem participates in the malformation, apnea, deafness, sleep disturbance, oculomotor disturbances, and problems with sucking and swallowing may be seen. Spinal cord lesions cause quadriplegia or paraplegia. Genitourinary problems, and to a lesser extent gastrointestinal problems, are also seen.

Apnea and other brainstem findings may occur when the malformation involves the brainstem, as in Arnold-Chiari deformities, Dandy-Walker cysts, occipital encephaloceles, and arachnoid cysts.

Pituitary-hypothalamic dysfunction may manifest itself in impaired temperature regulation,

BAPTIST MEDICAL CENTER
WOLFSON CHILDREN'S HOSPITAL
JACKSONVILLE, FLORIDA

VENTRICULOPERITONEAL (VP) SHUNT TEACHING CHECKLIST

GOAL/SKILL	NURSING (Date and Initials)	CARE GIVER #1	CARE GIVER #2	CARE GIVER #3
1. Verbalizes understanding of reason for VP shunt.	H - "An Introduction to Hydrocephalus" ☐			
2. Identifies the pathway of the VP shunt and the shunt's function.	H - "Ventriculoperitoneal Shunt" (Newborn) ☐ H - "Hydrocephalus and Shunts" (For infants with Cordis Shunts) ☐ H - "Your Valve System for Hydrocephalus" (For Cordis Valve System Shunts) ☐ H - "Just Like Any Other Little Beagle" ☐ V - "Just Like Any Other Little Beagle" ☐			
3. Lists signs and symptoms of shunt infection and emergent need to notify MD.				
4. Lists signs and symptoms of shunt failure and emergent need to notify MD.				
5. Discuss the reason and importance of prompt treatment of health problems.				
6. Verbalizes understanding of importance of close medical follow-up.				

SIGNATURE/INITIAL	TEACHING CODES	PARENT SIGNATURE(S)
	L - Lecture/Discussion	
	D - Demonstration (or return demo)	
	U - Verbalizes Understanding	
	R - Reinforced Teaching	PATIENT LABEL
	V - Video	
	H - Handout	
	E - Equipment	

20-207 Rev 5/96

FIGURE 26-1   Ventriculoperinatal (VP) shunt teaching checklist. (Courtesy Wolfson Children's Hospital, Jacksonville, Fla, 1996.)

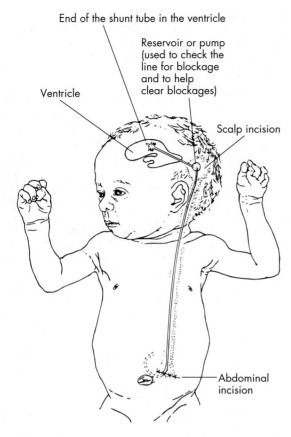

End of the shunt tube in the ventricle

Reservoir or pump (used to check the line for blockage and to help clear blockages)

Ventricle

Scalp incision

Abdominal incision

FIGURE 26-2   Ventricular peritoneal shunt. (From Harrison H, Kositsky A: *The premature baby book,* New York, 1983, St Martin's Press.)

thyroid abnormalities, diabetes insipidus, and adrenal insufficiency.

Most of the complications occur after the newborn period, although the causes are already present at birth. These include seizures, retardation, spasticity, genitourinary problems, and orthopedic problems. In many of these circumstances the problem is already present, but the functional expression, such as impaired ambulation, retardation, and deafness, is lacking. In the infant's follow-up examinations, careful attention must be given to those problems likely to develop or intensify with age. When a specific malformation is identified, it is necessary to become familiar with the expected problems, not only to anticipate them as they appear, but also to lessen any secondary damage that might occur if they go unrecognized.

Parent Teaching

Parents of an infant born with congenital malformations are faced with a stressful event that may develop into a major life transition. **Parents (especially mothers) report feelings of guilt and self-blame, although they may not initially share these feelings with hospital staff. After the birth of a malformed child, they go through stages of grief (see Chapters 29 and 30): shock and/or denial, anger, bargaining, depression, and acceptance.** Some authors question whether full acceptance occurs for the family of the handicapped child because of return of grief and sorrow each time a developmental milestone is missed or the child experiences illness.[36,50]

Social support received from hospital personnel, family, and friends can help parents feel less stressed and more able to cope with the illness of their infant. The ability of the staff to accurately anticipate and assess parental feelings and concerns can be invaluable when assisting families through this difficult time. **Parents should be encouraged to verbalize their feelings and fears in a supportive environment.** Reassurances, when appropriate, should be provided (e.g., parents were not responsible for the congenital malformation; it is normal for the mother to experience [or at least report] more fears than her husband, etc.). **The ultimate goal of intervention is to reduce stress, assist families to confront fears, improve coping, and facilitate the bonding process.**[26,50]

Infants with congenital malformations present such a complex variety of problems that parent teaching and emotional support needs to begin as early as possible. Often parents will know from the time of birth or earlier that a major problem exists. In other circumstances the anomaly will be detected only after appropriate studies are performed.

When the infant is not viable, care should be directed to meeting the emotional needs of the family. Every effort should be made to give family members positive experiences and memories by encouraging early parental holding of the infant and, whenever possible, participation with care (see Chapter 30). Anticipatory counseling from social services and chaplain staff can help the family during grieving and with funeral arrangements. **There will also be questions about etiologic factors and genetics, and these questions should be dealt with according to the family's wishes.**

If serious handicaps are anticipated and the infant is expected to survive, the parents should

be encouraged to participate in the care of the infant from the beginning. Not only will the adjustment occur more easily, but also the important aspects of care in special circumstances will be learned more effectively. A multidisciplinary team approach to parent education and support will allow hospital resources to be individualized to the specific needs of the patient and family. In addition to medical, nursing, social service, and chaplain involvement, team members can be drawn from psychologic, developmental, PT/OT, and other services based on specific needs and circumstances. Parent teaching and support must be individualized according to the anomaly. When available, support groups and specialized clinics can help with postdischarge care and parent education.

Parent teaching for the mothers and fathers of infants with congenital anomalies should be started early, involve the parents in the care of the infant, use the resources of the hospital for specialized help, and continue after the infant has gone home from the hospital.[46]

BIRTH INJURIES

Physiology and Etiology

Birth injuries (birth traumas) are the direct result of difficulties encountered during the delivery process. They may be minor injuries without expected sequelae or may be the direct cause of death in the neonatal period. Classification of birth injuries is usually etiologic (predisposing factors or mechanisms of injury) or anatomic. An anatomic classification is used in this discussion to illustrate the commonly encountered problems (Table 26-2).

The timing of birth injuries can be used to describe causes. Etiologic classification of birth injuries includes uterine injury (antenatal), fetal monitoring procedures, abnormal or difficult presentations or methods of delivery, and multifactorial injuries. It should be recognized that the same injury might be caused in several ways. Thus a cephalhematoma could be the result of forceps delivery or vacuum extraction. A variety of specific predisposing factors increase the risk for birth injury:

- Macrosomia
- Cephalopelvic disproportion
- Dystocia
- Prematurity
- Prolonged or precipitous labor
- Breech presentation

Table 26-2	ANATOMIC CLASSIFICATION OF BIRTH INJURIES	
SITE OF INJURY	**TYPE OF INJURY**	
Scalp	Caput succedaneum	
	Subgaleal hemorrhage	
	Cephalhematoma	
Skull	Linear fracture	
	Depressed fracture	
	Occipital osteodiastasis	
Intracranial	Epidural hematoma	
	Subdural hematoma (laceration of falx, tentorium, or superficial veins)	
	Subarachnoid hemorrhage	
	Cerebral contusion	
	Cerebellar contusion	
	Intracerebellar hematoma	
Spinal cord (cervical)	Vertebral artery injury	
	Intraspinal hemorrhage	
	Spinal cord transection or injury	
Plexus injuries	Erb's palsy	
	Klumpke's paralysis	
	Total (mixed) brachial plexus injury	
	Horner's syndrome	
	Diaphragmatic paralysis	
	Lumbosacral plexus injury	
Cranial and peripheral nerve injuries	Radial nerve palsy	
	Medial nerve palsy	
	Sciatic nerve palsy	
	Laryngeal nerve palsy	
	Diaphragmatic paralysis	
	Facial nerve palsy	

- Forceps usage
- Rotation of fetus
- Version and extraction
- Handling after delivery

Multiple factors are often present. When multiple predisposing factors are present, a single underlying maternal disease often causes them. A common example would be a premature, macrosomic fetus with a diabetic mother in whom labor is not progressing properly.

The common factors that are present in deliveries complicated by birth injuries are as follows:
- Unusual progress of labor
- Unusual size or shape to the fetus (large for gestational age and hydrocephalus)
- Problems encountered during delivery (dystocia and forceps application)

- **Unusual or unexpected presentations (breech or unexpected twin)**

The maternal history must always be studied for the underlying disease process or conditions that might increase the risk for a birth injury.

Prevention

Most birth injuries may be preventable, at least in theory. Careful attention to risk factors and the appropriate planning of delivery should reduce the incidence of birth injuries to a minimum. Transabdominal ultrasonography facilitates predelivery awareness of macrosomia, hydrocephalus, and unusual presentations. Particular pregnancies may then be delivered by controlled elective cesarean section to avoid significant birth injury. Care must be taken to avoid substituting a procedure of greater risk. Often a small percentage of significant birth injuries cannot be anticipated until the specific circumstances are encountered during delivery. Emergency cesarean section may provide last-minute salvage, but in these circumstances the injury may truly be unavoidable.

Specific Birth Injuries

Injuries to the Scalp

The three commonly encountered forms of extracranial hemorrhage (caput succedaneum, subgaleal hemorrhage, and cephalhematoma) are distinguished not only in clinical manifestations, but also in pathophysiology.[85] These three extracranial scalp injuries are included with neurologic birth injuries not because they have associated neurologic problems, but because the family or health care providers often raise the question of possible neurologic involvement.

Physiology and Etiology. **Caput succedaneum is caused by trauma to the scalp, usually during a routine vertex vaginal delivery.** The caput is the result of hemorrhagic edema superficial to the aponeurosis of the scalp. Spread of the edema is therefore not restricted to suture lines and is soft and pitting because of its superficial location.[85]

Forces that compress and then drag the head through the pelvic outlet cause subgaleal hemorrhage. Significant acute blood loss can occur with shock as the presenting symptom. Bleeding may continue after birth with enlargement of the accumulated blood and dissection of the blood along tissue planes into the neck. Such a hemorrhage carries

the greatest potential for complications, but fortunately it is the least common form of birth injury to the scalp.[85]

Cephalhematoma is a subperiosteal collection of blood that is confined by the sutures. The incidence is 1% to 2% of all live births. The cause is nearly always mechanical trauma and its occurrence is more common in primiparous women and in forceps delivery. Males are generally more likely to be affected than females. The firm, tense collection of blood may increase in size after birth, but significant blood loss does not occur.[85]

Data Collection. **With caput succedaneum, physical examination reveals soft, pitting edema that is diffuse and crosses suture lines. There is no need for laboratory tests.**[85]

Since the subgaleal collection of blood is under the aponeurosis connecting the occipitofrontalis muscle and superficial to the periosteum, **subgaleal hemorrhage crosses suture lines. It is firm but fluctuant to palpation. Vital signs should be carefully monitored for symptoms of shock. The hematocrit should be serially followed, and bilirubin levels should be determined during recovery.**[85]

Cephalhematoma may occur anywhere but is most commonly found in the parietal area on one side. Because the location of the blood is subperiosteal, the blood is confined by suture lines. Symptoms are normally absent. **A skull fracture underlying the cephalhematoma is present in 10% to 25% of affected infants. X-ray examination of the skull defines the fracture.** Rare complications include infection, osteomyelitis, hyperbilirubinemia, meningitis, and late-onset anemia.[85]

Treatment. **No treatment is required for any of these three lesions. In subgaleal hemorrhage, treatment of blood loss and shock may be necessary.** During resolution the breakdown of the blood may cause hyperbilirubinemia requiring treatment (see Chapter 21).

Parent Teaching. Careful preparation of the parents for the acute side effects of subgaleal hemorrhage is important. **Parents should be warned of the possibility of swelling and discoloration of the face, head, and neck.** Parents of an infant with a cephalhematoma can remain unconcerned unless localized changes occur, suggesting secondary infection (erythema, induration, or drainage). **Cephal-**

hematoma may be evident for 6 to 8 weeks. Outpatient evaluation of bilirubin levels may be needed in some cases.

Skull Fractures

Three forms of skull fracture should be identified and differentiated: linear fractures, depressed fractures, and occipital osteodiastasis.[85]

Physiology and Etiology. Linear skull fracture (a nondepressed fracture) is the most common type of skull fracture. **The result of compression of the skull during delivery, a linear skull fracture most often has no associated injuries and causes no symptoms.** Bleeding may be seen extracranially (common) or intracranially (rare). Intracranial bleeding causes symptoms referable to the bleeding rather than to the fracture itself.[85]

The typical depressed skull fracture is of the "ping-pong" type, an indentation without loss of bony continuity. Forceps are usually the direct cause of injury, which most often is without complication or sequelae. **When neurologic signs are present, direct cerebral injury, intracranial bleeding, or free bone fragments should be suspected.**[85]

Data Collection. A linear skull fracture usually has no signs or symptoms unless intracranial bleeding has occurred. **Skull x-ray films** most frequently demonstrate a parietal fracture. A depressed skull fracture is usually a palpable "ping-pong" fracture in the parietal area. No other signs and symptoms are present unless intracranial bleeding or focal irritation of the cortex causes them. **Evaluation with a skull x-ray examination or CT scan is necessary to delineate the fracture and to identify complications.**

Treatment. **No treatment is necessary for a linear skull fracture.** The controversy over treatment of a depressed skull fracture centers on the mode of treatment and the necessity for treatment. **If free bone fragments or clots are identified, neurosurgical intervention is required.** More conservative approaches are indicated when no complications are present. Vacuum extractors and breast pumps have been used with success.[85]

Complications. **With a linear skull fracture the single complication to be aware of is a "growing" skull fracture.** A dural tear may allow leptome-

ninges to extrude into the fracture site, setting up the possibility of a leptomeningeal cyst. As the cyst enlarges, the edges of the fracture may fail to fuse and even spread apart, giving the appearance of a "growing" fracture. Palpation and x-ray examination demonstrate the lesion. Surgical correction may be required to ensure healing and prevent further complications. With a depressed skull fracture, intracranial bleeding and direct cerebral injury with seizures or residual neurologic deficit are rare.

Parent Teaching. Parents should be instructed to have the fracture site checked for several months to ensure that reunion of the bone has taken place. Patients will have no other aftercare unless neurosurgical intervention was necessary or complications developed.

Intracranial Birth Injuries

Three major forms of bleeding occur intracranially: epidural hematoma, subdural hemorrhage, and subarachnoid hemorrhage. Added to these are cerebellar hemorrhages, cerebellar contusions, and cerebral contusions. Each has its own particular set of symptoms and signs, and complications and sequelae. IVH is usually not related to trauma and is covered separately in this chapter.

Physiology and Etiology. Epidural hematoma is pathophysiologically difficult to form in newborns because of a relatively thick dura. When present, it is almost always accompanied by a linear skull fracture across the middle meningeal artery.

Subdural hemorrhage is more common in term infants than in preterm infants and occurs from trauma tearing veins and venous sinuses. Four major pathologic entities are defined: laceration of the tentorium, laceration of the falx, laceration of the superficial cerebral vein, and occipital osteodiastasis. Tentorial laceration causes a posterior fossa clot with compression of the brainstem. The straight sinus, Galen's vein, lateral sinus, and infratentorial veins may be involved. Laceration of the falx is caused by rupture of the inferior sagittal sinus. The laceration usually occurs at the junction of the tentorium and the falx, and the clot appears in the longitudinal cerebral fissure over the corpus callosum. Laceration of superficial cerebral veins causes subdural bleeding over the convexity of the brain. Subarachnoid bleeding or contusion of the brain may also be present.

Subarachnoid hemorrhage is the most common type of neonatal intracranial hemorrhage. In term infants, trauma is the most common cause, whereas in preterm infants hypoxia is more often the cause. Small hemorrhages are more common than massive ones and usually result from venous bleeding. Underlying contusion may occur.

Cerebral contusion is uncommon as an isolated event. Focal blunt trauma is necessary to produce a contusion. Pathologically, focal areas of hemorrhage and necrosis are seen. Shearing forces may cause slitlike tears in the white matter.

Cerebellar contusion and intracerebellar hemorrhage are uncommon events usually seen in association with occipital osteodiastasis and infratentorial subdural hemorrhage. These are catastrophic events, as described previously, and most often result in the death of the patient.

Data Collection. **For epidural hemorrhage the signs and symptoms may be diffuse (increased intracranial pressure with a bulging fontanel) or focal or lateralizing seizures, eye deviation, and hemisyndromes. Laboratory tests should include x-ray examination to look for fractures and CT scanning to identify bleeding.**

Infants with subdural hemorrhage are neurologically abnormal at birth. Tentorial lacerations and laceration of the falx tend to produce signs by pressure on the brainstem. These signs include skew deviation of the eyes, apnea, coma, or unequal pupils. Nuchal rigidity and opisthotonos are signs of progressive herniation. Signs and symptoms of subdural hemorrhage from laceration of the superficial cerebral veins are variable. Small clots may produce no identifiable dysfunction. Typical symptoms are those of focal or lateralized cerebral dysfunction, although increased intracranial pressure may occur. CT scans including views of the posterior fossa should be obtained immediately when a subdural hemorrhage is suspected.

With subarachnoid hemorrhage, underlying contusions may cause focal neurologic signs. Often no significant increase in intracranial pressure is found acutely. Irritability and a depressed level of consciousness may persist. Seizures are frequent in term infants, whereas apnea is common in preterm infants. Useful laboratory data include lumbar puncture and CT scan results. Focal signs predominate in cerebral contusions.

Treatment. **Surgical evacuation of epidural and subdural clots may be necessary as emergency procedures. Subdural taps may be useful in the symptomatic infant with subdural bleeding from laceration of superficial cerebral veins. Many infants with intracranial bleeding may require treatment of seizures.**

Complications. The complications of epidural hemorrhage range from none to permanent neurologic deficits with or without seizure. Sequelae of subdural hemorrhage occur in 20% to 25% of affected infants. The most common sequelae are focal neurologic signs. Seizures and hydrocephalus are seen less often. Hydrocephalus is the major potential complication of subarachnoid hemorrhage and directly alters outcome. When hydrocephalus is not present, as many as 90% of affected infants are normal at follow-up. Only 35% to 50% of children in whom hydrocephalus develops will be normal.

Parent Teaching. Because the long-term outcome is variable and may be abnormal even in infants who appear normal at discharge from the nursery, parent teaching must be individualized. It is important to emphasize the need for appropriate follow-up and intervention. Referral to available support groups is usually beneficial.

Spinal Cord Injuries
Physiology and Etiology. Injuries to the spinal cord (usually the cervical portion) are most often seen in complicated breech deliveries. Before cesarean sections were performed routinely for breech delivery, fatal attempts to deliver vaginally were often associated with interspinal hemorrhage. The breech presentation in conjunction with a hyperextended head is the most dangerous situation and is worsened by a depressed fetus. Traction, rotation, and torsion cause mechanical strain on the vertebral column. Cephalic deliveries are not entirely safe, because of the difference in mechanical forces; a different clinical picture is seen with a higher lesion.[85]

Data Collection. **Clinical manifestations depend on the severity and location of the injury.** Clinical syndromes include stillbirth or rapid neonatal death, respiratory failure, and spinal shock syndrome. High cervical cord injuries are more likely to cause stillbirths or rapid death of the neonate. Lower lesions cause an acute cord syndrome. **Common signs of spinal shock include flaccid extremities (may just** involve the lower extremities if the cervical cord is spared), a sensory level, diaphragmatic breathing, paralyzed abdominal movements, atonic anal sphincter, and distended bladder. Useful laboratory tests include myelography, an MRI or CT scan of the spine, and somatosensory-evoked potentials to help determine the extent and site of the lesion. The differential diagnosis includes dysraphism, neuromuscular disease, and cord tumors.[85]

Complications. After the acute phase, chronic lesions include cysts, vascular occlusions, adhesions, and necrosis of the spinal cord. Flaccid or spastic quadriplegia is expected. Some infants with spinal cord injuries will be respirator dependent. Bowel and bladder problems will continue.

Parent Teaching. Parents need to understand fully the implications of severe injury to the spinal cord. Recovery is frequently minimal to nonexistent. Continued specialized care may be required, including ventilator therapy. The overwhelming implications for the family cannot be emphasized strongly enough.

An individualized multidisciplinary team approach to discharge planning is vital to parental confidence and a timely discharge. The problems of both patient and family are complex and not limited to medical concerns. A successful discharge is unlikely unless family emotional, financial, and educational concerns are addressed early in the planning process. The timely assessment of needs and involvement of supportive agencies will allow resolution of problems well before the projected discharge date. Such assistance should include early family referral to available federal programs for financial aid (e.g., SSI) and assistance with patient transportation to their multiple outpatient follow-up appointments. Early assessment of equipment needs and home nursing requirements is also of primary importance and should include a determination of the availability of these resources in the community, parent acceptance of their use, and whether the home can accommodate them (i.e., adequate electrical system and space).

Plexus Injuries
Physiology and Etiology. Plexus injuries occur much more commonly than cord injuries and result from lateral traction on the shoulder[31] (vertex deliveries) or the head (breech deliveries).[54,70] Most often a depressed fetus or dystocia from a large infant is a contributing factor. Inappropriate augmentation of

labor is another possible additive cause. **Estimates of the incidence of brachial plexus injuries range from 0.5 to 2.0 per 1000 live births.**[85] Extremely mild cases may have undetectable findings and may remain unidentified.

Pathologic changes range from edema and hemorrhage of the nerve sheath to actual avulsion of the nerve root from the spinal cord. Of the reported cases of plexus injuries, **90% involve the C5 to C7 nerve roots and are classified as Erb's palsy.**[85] In a small minority of cases, the C4 nerve root is also affected, causing diaphragmatic problems. The site of injury in Erb's palsy is Erb's point where C5 and C6 nerve roots join to form the upper trunk. **Total brachial plexus palsy occurs in 8% to 9% of the cases and has findings referable to C5 to T1 (and possibly C4).** When T1 is involved, the sympathetic fibers become affected with an ipsilateral Horner's syndrome (ptosis, anhydrosis, and miosis) and possible delay in pigmentation of the iris. Less than 2% of the cases have Klumpke's paralysis involving only C8 to T1. In this form, the site of pathologic conditions is the point at which C8 to T1 join to form the lower trunk.

Data Collection. Signs of brachial plexus palsies vary somewhat, most often because of overlap of the pure clinical syndromes. **Shoulder and arm findings are characteristic of a true Erb's palsy. Involvement of the hand and fingers is seen in total forms or Klumpke's paralysis.** Table 26-3 lists

Table 26-3	BRACHIAL PLEXUS EXAMINATION: DISTINGUISHING FEATURES
PART EXAMINED	**SPINAL LEVEL**
Diaphragm movement (downward)	C4 (C3-5)
Deltoid muscle	C5
Spinatus muscle	C5
Biceps muscle	C5-6
Brachioradialis muscle	C5-6
Supinator of arm	C5-6
Biceps tendon reflex	C5-6
Wrist extensors	C6-7
Long extensor of the digits	C6-7
Triceps tendon reflex	C6-7
Wrist flexors	C7-8, T1
Finger flexors	C7-8, T1
Dilator of iris	T1
Eyelid elevator (full elevation)	T1
Moro reflex (shoulder abduction)	C5
Moro reflex (hand motion)	C8-T1
Palmar grasp	C8-T1

the specific cord levels involved in various functions that might be addressed.

Evaluation of diaphragmatic function by x-ray examination is at times necessary. Myelography or MRI may be required to identify nerve root avulsion, which generally should be suspected when recovery does not occur. Electromyography often shows abnormalities early in the course of the injury, suggesting that the process may actually have begun in the last weeks of pregnancy rather than at the time of delivery.

Clinical syndromes of plexus injuries include Erb's palsy, total palsy, and Klumpke's paralysis. Erb's palsy accounts for about 90% of plexus injuries.[85] It involves the upper part of the plexus, C5 to C7 and occasionally C4. The shoulder and upper arm are involved, and the biceps reflex is decreased. When C4 is involved, diaphragmatic dysfunction is present.

Total palsy occurs in 8% to 9% of the cases. Plexus involvement is diffuse (C5 to T1 and occasionally C4). The upper and lower arm and hand are involved. Horner's syndrome (ptosis, anhydrosis, and miosis) exists when T1 is involved. The diaphragm is affected when C4 is involved. Biceps and triceps reflexes are decreased.

Klumpke's paralysis is seen in less than 2% of cases. The lower part of the plexus, C8 to T1, is involved. The lower arm and hand are involved. T1 involvement is associated with Horner's syndrome. Triceps reflex is decreased.

Treatment. **Treatment may include immobilization for 1 to 5 days to prevent contractures. Finger and wrist splints may be necessary. Passive range-of-motion exercises follow, and then gradual increase of activity to the affected limb is permitted.**[85]

Complications. Associated trauma may occur and should be carefully investigated. **Common associated injuries include clavicular fracture, shoulder dislocation, cord injury, facial nerve injury, and humeral fracture. Full recovery of plexus function was seen in 88% to 92% of cases in the first year of life during the National Collaborative Perinatal Study.**[85] Children that show no signs of improvement during the first 3 months after delivery should be referred to a clinic specializing in brachial plexus injury. Rarely, graph surgery of the injured nerve root is required.

Parent Teaching. **Parents should be taught passive range-of-motion exercises to encourage mo-**bility and prevent contractures. Instructions should begin before discharge from the hospital. Most often a neonatal nurse or an occupational or physical therapist gives the instructions.

Parents may equate the presence of a brachial plexus injury with poor obstetric care. Most often this will not be the case. The awareness of early changes on electromyography should be used to help families understand that the factors causing injury to the plexus may begin long before the onset of labor.

Cranial and Peripheral Nerve Injuries

Median and sciatic nerve injuries are usually postnatal and result from brachial and radial artery punctures (median nerve) and inferior gluteal artery spasm (umbilical artery line drug instillation). Recovery is variable.

Median nerve palsy is manifested by decreased pincer grasp, decreased thumb strength, and the continuous flexed position of the fourth finger. Sciatic nerve palsy is manifested by decreased hip abduction and decreased distal joint movement. Hip adduction, flexion, and rotation are normal, because the femoral and obturator nerves control them.

Radial nerve damage is usually seen in conjunction with a humeral fracture. Prolonged labor is normally present. Congenital bands may also be causative. Recovery takes place in weeks to months.

Radial nerve palsy is manifested by wrist drop (decreased finger and wrist extension) and normal grasp.

Laryngeal nerve palsy may be seen in conjunction with facial or diaphragmatic paralysis. If the paralysis is unilateral, a hoarse cry may be heard. Bilateral involvement causes breathing to be difficult and the vocal cords to remain closed in the midline. It is important to rule out intrinsic brainstem disease. Often the presence of other brainstem findings such as oculomotor problems, apnea, or facial palsy will help clarify this. Evoked potentials, both brainstem auditory and somatosensory, may also help rule out brainstem involvement.

Laryngeal nerve palsy is manifested by difficulty in swallowing (superior branch), difficulty in breathing (bilateral), and difficulty in vocalizing (recurrent branch). Also, the head is held high and flexed laterally with slight rotation. Severe cases may require tracheotomy and feedings by gavage.[85]

Diaphragmatic paralysis is most often seen in association with plexus injuries (80% to 90% have an associated plexus injury) and has the

same cause. Some series involving unilateral paralysis have a mortality of 10% to 20%. Most patients recover fully in 6 to 12 months. Although less than 10% of patients have bilateral diaphragmatic paralysis, the mortality for these patients is higher (almost 50%). **Treatment has consisted of using rocking beds, electric pacing of the diaphragm, CPAP, respirators, or plication.** Because diaphragmatic paralysis may occur in other conditions such as a myotonic dystrophy, attention to the differential diagnosis is important, particularly when associated brachial plexus problem is not present.[85]

Diaphragmatic paralysis is demonstrated by respiratory difficulty in the first few hours of life. X-ray film shows elevation of the hemidiaphragm with paradoxic movement that may disappear on PEEP or CPAP.[85]

Facial palsy may be part of intrinsic brainstem disease (see previous discussion of laryngeal nerve palsy) or other conditions such as Möbius syndrome, myotonic dystrophy, or facial muscle agenesis. When it is traumatic in origin, facial palsy is thought to be caused by the position of the face on the sacral promontory at the exit of the nerve from the stylomastoid foramen.[85] Normally both the upper (temporofacial) and lower (cervicofacial) branches are involved. Known complications (from lack of total resolution) include contractures and synkinesis. Cosmetic surgical procedures are occasionally necessary but are often delayed for years.

Facial palsy is seen on the left side in 75% of cases. Features include a widened palpebral fissure, flat nasolabial fold, and decreased facial expression. Most infants completely recover within 3 weeks, although some infants continue to have deficits months later.[85]

Parent Teaching. **Infants with facial palsy may require the use of artificial tears if unable to completely close the eye on the involved side.** Occasionally it may be necessary to tape the eye to prevent injury to the cornea. Parents should also be taught to expect some drooling of formula from the corner of the mouth during feedings.

Although most infants with laryngeal nerve palsy recover in the first 6 to 12 months of life, their symptoms will initially require supplemental parent education and support. **Infant risk of aspiration necessitates careful feeding and appropriate response should choking occur. Additional education for gavage feedings, a tracheotomy, or an apnea monitor may be required for the parents of a few infants.** The teaching requirements of the infant with diaphragmatic paralysis must also be tailored to meet the individual needs and circumstances of the child and family involved.

NEONATAL SEIZURES

Seizures may be the most frequent, and often the only, clinical sign of central nervous system dysfunction in the neonate.[51,85] The occurrence of seizures typically prompts urgent medical attention for infants who experience them. Seizures raise immediate concerns about the underlying cause of the brain disorder, associated clinical condition, the effect seizures may have on the developing brain, the need for antiepileptic drugs (AEDs), and the effect AEDs may have on the neonate with seizures.

Although the exact incidence of neonatal seizures is difficult to ascertain, Volpe noted marked differences in incidence associated with variations in birth weight: ranging from 57.5 per 1000 infants weighing less than 1500 g to 2.8 per 1000 infants weighing 2500 to 3999 g at birth.[85]

Neonatal seizures increase the risk of impaired neurological and developmental functioning in infancy and increase the risk of death.[76] Volpe notes that multiple or extended neonatal seizure activity is associated with significantly poorer prognosis than when seizures are controlled.[85]

Recognition of neonatal seizures with identification of etiology and prompt treatment is critical. Although not a disease entity, seizures are commonly related to significant disorders, which may require specific treatment. Untreated neonatal seizures may interfere with supportive therapies such as assisted ventilation and nutrition. **Finally, there is experimental data suggesting that seizures themselves may result in brain injury.**[12,85]

Seizures result when an excessive synchronous electrical discharge of neurons within the CNS occurs (i.e., depolarization).[85] Neonatal seizures are not a specific disease entity but rather a symptom.[12,44] They may be associated with any disorder directly or indirectly affecting the CNS. **Primary intracranial processes that may result in neonatal seizures include meningitis, intracranial hemorrhage (subdural, IVH, primary subarachnoid), encephalitis, and tumor. Seizures, however, also occur secondary to systemic or metabolic disturbances including hypoglycemia, hypoxia-ischemia, hypocalcemia, hypomagnesemia, hyponatremia, and drug withdrawal.**[6,85] They have also been reported in the literature as a complication of the

usage of opiates for sedation/analgesia in the newborn period.[72]

Clinical presentation of seizures is considerably different in the newborn period when compared to the well-organized seizure activity seen in older children and adults. The incomplete neurophysiologic development of a premature infant results in even less organized seizure activity than that seen with the term infant.[85]

Seizures are signs of malfunctioning neuronal systems. It is most useful to think of a localized or generalized loss of inhibitory control as the source of the seizure activity. This inhibitory loss may be the result of damage to the developing brain or transient effects such as disturbances in blood flow, glucose availability, or hypoxia. These disturbances may cause paroxysmal electrical activity recorded as seizures on the EEG.[68] Ordinarily there are clinical signs that mimic what might, under other circumstances, be normal brain activity but in the context of the seizure, cause stereotyped, repetitive, and inappropriate activity.

Seizures may be the only manifestation of brain dysfunction, but this is extremely uncommon in the neonate. **Most often, seizures in the newborn period are the result of a very significant brain insult; the clinical signs of the insult are multiple.**

Etiology and Data Collection

Neonatal seizures may be caused by a variety of acute and chronic stresses on the brain.[7,30,34,73] **Table 26-4 lists the general groups of causes of neonatal seizures.** The search for a cause proceeds in an orderly, methodical way. Most often the known history of perinatal problems will narrow the differential diagnosis to one or two likely causes. Acute metabolic changes that are likely to cause seizures should be rapidly investigated first. **Blood glucose**

Table 26-4	COMMON CAUSES OF NEONATAL SEIZURES	
CLASSIFICATION	**CAUSES**
Acute metabolic conditions (assess blood gases, pH, HCO_3^-, Na, K, Ca, Mg, glucose, BUN)	Hypocalcemia Hypoglycemia; hyperglycemia Hypomagnesemia Pyridoxine dependency or deficiency Hyponatremia; hypernatremia
Inherited metabolic conditions (acidosis, common; assess urine amino acids, organic acids, NH_3, galactose)	Maple syrup urine disease Nonketotic hyperglycemia Hyperprolinemia Galactosemia Urea cycle abnormalities Organic acidemias
Infections (12% of cases, assess CSF; culture blood, ?CSF; PCR of CSF; imaging)	Viral encephalitis, herpes, or enterovirus Congenital infections Bacterial meningitis Sepsis Brain abscess Septic venous thrombosis
Intracranial hemorrhage (15% of cases, imaging; ?CSF exam)	Subdural hematoma Cerebral contusion Subarachnoid hemorrhage Epidural hemorrhage Intraventricular hemorrhage (premature)

Hypoxic ischemic (0-3/day) most common (60%)
Congenital malformations
Neonatal drug withdrawal (see Chapter 10) (e.g., opiates)
Local anesthetic intoxication
Kernicterus
Specific nongenetic syndromes
Benign familial neonatal seizures
Idiopathic (in only 10%, no cause is found)

should be immediately checked both in the NICU (Accucheck with glucose meter reading) and lab since hypoglycemia is a dangerous but very treatable cause of seizures.[85] See Table 26-7 for treatment of hypoglycemia.

Volpe[85] also listed lumbar puncture as the other urgent laboratory test to be completed because bacterial meningitis is another dangerous but treatable cause of seizures. Sepsis should never be overlooked as a potential cause. The infectious agent (meningitis, encephalitis, empyema, abscess, septic thrombosis, and ventriculitis) may directly affect the CNS. Systemic infection may cause seizures through the complication of shock, coagulopathy, impaired oxygenation, and multisystem organ failure. When the CSF is examined, not only will the changes associated with infection be identified, but evidence of bleeding (red blood cells) or cell destruction (protein) may also be found.[6,81,90]

Structural studies are routinely performed as part of the evaluation. Presently the most useful studies are CT scans and cranial ultrasonographic examination, which can document intracranial hemorrhage.[6,90]

The infant's history should be carefully reviewed to narrow the possible causes to the most likely ones. Physical examination may further narrow the differential diagnosis. Once these are quickly done, blood should be drawn for assessment of arterial blood gases, electrolytes, glucose, calcium, and magnesium.[6,90]

Appropriate cultures must be obtained. Usual culture sites or specimens include blood, urine, spinal fluid, and pharyngeal or tracheal aspirate. The CSF should be examined for red blood cells and white blood cells, organisms (by Gram's stain), protein, and sugar.[6,90]

Ultrasonographic examinations are particularly useful for identifying and following intraventricular bleeding and hydrocephalus. The infant is exposed to no radiation, either immediately or long-term; no complications, either immediate or long-term, have been identified. The test may be repeated as often as needed and is usually performed at the bedside.

Although it provides better resolution for identifying subtle changes in brain structure, a CT scan exposes the developing brain to significant radiation. The larger the number of "cuts" made, the greater the exposure. The exact amount of radiation varies with the type of machine and duration of the study. Short-term effects have not been detected, but the potential for long-term or cumulative effects of radiation exposure has not been determined. In addition, the use of a contrast medium is occasionally necessary for a complete study. This may be contraindicated in newborns with impaired renal function or in those with delicate fluid balance.

Although they provide interesting and helpful information in older patients with seizures, newer imaging techniques such as positron emission tomography (PET) have not been widely available and/or applied to newborns except in research. The potential hazards of isotopic scanning need further study before PET can be put to general use in newborns.

MRI produces exceptional detail and is sensitive to changes in cellular composition. Presently the studies often require transport and up to an hour's time, limiting their practicality in a sick newborn.

Clinical Seizure Types

The application of technology used in the assessment of patients with epilepsy has finally been applied to neonates having seizures.[42] Simultaneous EEG and video recording allow the accurate diagnosis of difficult-to-assess subtle behaviors, apneic and bradycardiac spells, and the jerks and twitches commonly seen in preterm newborns.[51] Many have been surprised to find no correlation between events thought to be seizures and changes on the EEG.[11,68,85]

Volpe[81] defined seizures clinically as "a paroxysmal alteration in neurologic function, i.e., behavioral, motor, or autonomic function." He included in this definition behavioral, motor, or autonomic clinical phenomena that are associated with EEG seizure activity and also clinical phenomena not consistently correlated with EEG seizure activity. He cited an increasing body of literature indicating that epileptic phenomena can be formed at subcortical levels and are therefore not detectable by surface-recorded EEG. Table 26-5 lists classification types and usual EEG findings. It has also been noted that many neonatal seizures identified by EEG are not correlated with motor and behavioral seizure activity.[68] The most immature infants are more prone to this finding.[85]

Focal clonic and multifocal clonic seizures are the most likely to have true cortical origins. Eye blinking (a clonic manifestation) may be seen, as may nystagmus. Focal clonic seizures have been seen as an important manifestation of stroke in the neonate.[14] Apnea with electrical seizure activity has been seen as an ictal manifestation but

Table 26-5	TRADITIONAL CATEGORIZATION OF NEONATAL SEIZURES	
CLASSIFICATION/TYPES	**DEFINITION/DESCRIPTION**	**CLINICAL MANIFESTATIONS**
Clonic • Focal clonic • Multifocal clonic Tonic • Focal tonic • Generalized tonic	• Rhythmic jerks (1-3/sec) • Rate slows during seizure • + EEG seizure activity • Characterized by posturing • Focal: + EEG seizure activity • Generalized: usually no EEG seizure activity seen	Focal: well-localized to a body part Multifocal: several body parts jerking simultaneously or in migrating order Focal: continued posturing of limb or a posturing (asymmetric) of trunk or neck Generalized: extension of lower limbs with either upper limb extension (looks like decerebrate posturing) or with upper limb flexion (looks like decorticate posturing)
Myoclonic • Focal myoclonic • Generalized myoclonic	• Faster jerking than clonic seizures • Flexor muscles (limbs) involved • Focal: usually no EEG seizure activity • Generalized: + EEG seizure activity	Focal: flexor jerking of upper limbs Generalized: bilateral jerking of upper extremities; sometimes lower limbs also are involved
Subtle (more common in the premature infant)	• Abnormal behavioral, autonomic, or motor activities that are not due to the other 3 seizure classifications • + EEG seizure activity only with some of the seizure activities	**Ocular:** nystagmus, horizontal or vertical deviation of eyes, staring episodes, eyelid flutter or blinking **Facial:** repetitive sucking, mouth movements, tongue protrusion, chewing, drooling **Limb:** bicycling, swimming movements, "boxing" or "hooking" motions, stepping **Apnea:** only 2% result from seizures **Autonomic or vasomotor changes**

is more commonly seen in a full-term infant. The majority of apneic episodes in the premature population "are not epileptic in origin."[85]

The lack of ongoing monitoring of brain activity in most neonatal units makes accurate identification of seizures extremely difficult. The best correlation can be made by obtaining an EEG during periods of suspected seizure activity. The EEG can confirm clinical manifestations as true epileptic seizure activity. As previously discussed, however, there is "evidence that epileptic discharges" may be present without EEG detection.[85]

The traditional categorization of neonatal seizures is presented in Table 26-5. The classification does not have the same significance as the International Classification of Seizures in older individuals. Some general observations may pertain, even with the confusion surrounding the accurate diagnosis of neonatal seizures. **However, seizures continue to be more difficult to recognize in neonates. Newborn jitteriness compounds this difficulty, so care must be taken to avoid mistaking this jitteriness for seizure activity**[14,85] (Table 26-6).

Episodes characterized as tonic and subtle are most likely to be seen in premature infants. Tonic episodes are quite commonly associated with IVH. Clonic and multifocal clonic seizures are more common in term infants. Myoclonic seizures often include a metabolic cause, such as nonketotic hyperglycemia or urea cycle disorder. For a review of neonatal clinical manifestations, see Table 26-5. The article by Mizrahi and Kellaway[51] is suggested for a more extensive review.

Prevention

Many neonatal seizures can be successfully prevented through careful attention to possible metabolic changes expected on the basis of the infant's condition. Hypoglycemia, hypocalcemia, hypomagnesemia, and often hypoxia can be anticipated and controlled.

Seizures resulting from intracranial malformations, infections, or prenatal injury most often cannot be prevented. Inherited metabolic disorders may not be identified until after initial symptoms (often including seizures) appear.

Whether neonatal seizures can be prevented by pretreatment of the mother (in high-risk situations thought likely to result in neonatal seizures) has not been adequately investigated. As progress in ante-

Table 26-6	SEIZURES VS JITTERINESS	
CLINICAL OBSERVATIONS	SEIZURE	JITTERINESS
Ocular abnormalities (eye deviations or staring)	Yes	No
Gentle restraint of the involved body part halts the activity	No	Yes
Activity is easily elicited with stimulation (voice, motion, etc.)	No	Yes
Dominant movement is a slower clonic jerking having both a fast and slow element	Tremor in which the amplitude and rate of the alternating movements is equal	Yes
Autonomic changes are present: apnea, tachycardia, elevated BP, pupil changes, increased salivation, etc.	Yes	No

natal treatment of the fetus continues, this may become an area for further investigation.[85]

Treatment

The rational treatment of neonatal seizures involves a vigorous attempt to achieve four specific goals: acute treatment, correction, prevention, and minimization.

Acute Treatment

The first goal is acute treatment of prolonged or multiple seizures and status epilepticus.[51] Prolonged seizures and frequent, multiple seizures may result in metabolic changes and cardiorespiratory difficulties. Whether seizures themselves may cause brain damage is an unanswered question. It seems appropriate to make vigorous efforts to control seizures completely, although this may not always be possible. When the administration of a single drug does not result in lasting control, a second or third should be tried.[29,30,55,66]

The most commonly used drugs for the control of acute seizures and status epilepticus in the newborn are phenobarbital and phenytoin (Table 26-7). In a randomized, controlled study, these two drugs performed almost exactly equally in controlling electroencephalography-confirmed seizures; combined therapy was needed in over half of the infants, regardless of which drug was received first.[56] Both are given in loading doses of 20 mg/kg. In most infants this load achieves a blood level within the therapeutic range. Because both drugs are always given intravenously (IV) for this indication, the blood level is promptly achieved.[4,85,91] **When these antiepileptic drugs are unsuccessful in bringing the seizure(s) under control, alternative drugs such as lorazepam or midazolam may be used.[51] More recently, fosphenytoin (Cerebyx) was approved by the U.S. Food and Drug Administration (FDA) for use as a parenteral AED in adults. Its efficacy and safety in neonates is currently under investigation.[51]** However, some important features of fosphenytoin differentiate it from phenytoin and should be appreciated if fosphenytoin is eventually approved for use in the newborn. **With fosphenytoin there is less potential for local toxicity such as abscess formation. An additional potential advantage of the use of fosphenytoin over phenytoin is the ability to administer fosphenytoin intramuscularly if no intravenous sites are available. A considerable advantage of fosphenytoin is that it can be infused safely at a much faster rate than phenytoin.** In adults, fosphenytoin can be infused at a rate of 225 mg/min (equivalent to 150 mg/min of phenytoin), whereas phenytoin itself can only be infused safely at a rate not to exceed 50 mg/min.[60]

Correction

The second goal is correction of underlying remediable causes. This goal is often more important than the first goal, because some seizures induced by metabolic abnormalities cannot be controlled with antiepileptic drugs until the metabolic derangement is corrected. It is especially inappropriate to treat a newborn with antiepileptic drugs before correctable causes have been excluded.

After blood has been drawn for glucose, calcium, magnesium, electrolytes, and blood gas determination, therapy may begin. It is always proper to administer glucose. Inspired oxygen concentration may be raised temporarily if hypoxia is suspected. The IV administration of 50 to 100 mg pyridoxine should ideally be performed under simultaneous EEG monitoring so that the true causes of pyridoxine dependency or deficiency can be detected.[85]

Table 26-7 DRUG THERAPY FOR NEONATAL SEIZURES

DRUG	DOSE	COMMENTS
Glucose, 10% solution as indicated	2 ml/kg bolus IV if hypoglycemic[56] **Maintenance:** as high as 8 mg/kg/min IV[85] (see Chapter 15)	Treat if hypoglycemic with glucose meter (e.g., Accucheck; One Touch II)
Phenobarbital (drug of choice for neonatal seizures)	**Loading:** 20 mg/kg IV given slowly over 10-15 min; additional 5 mg/kg can be given to a maximum of 40 mg/kg total for refractory seizures[85,90,91] **Maintenance:** 3-4 mg/kg/24 hr in 2 divided doses beginning no earlier than 12 hr after last loading dose[85,91]	**Therapeutic level:** 15-30 μg/ml (obtain levels any time 1 hr after dose); respiratory depressant; incompatible with other drugs in solution Maintain adequate oxygenation and ventilation
Fosphenytoin (Cerebyx) preferred over phenytoin* (added if seizures not controlled by phenobarbital alone)	Fosphenytoin dose expressed in phenytoin equivalents (PE); fosphenytoin 1 mg PE = phenytoin 1 mg[91] **Fosphenytoin loading:** 15-20 mg PE/kg IM or IV† given slowly over minimum of 10 min; flush IV with NS before and after[91] **Fosphenytoin maintenance:** 4-8 mg PE/kg/24 hr IM or IV slow push (see above for dilution); infuse no faster than 1.5 mg/kg/min; NS flush IV before/after Begin maintenance 24 hr after loading dose Term infants >1 wk of age may need up to 8 mg PE/kg/dose every 8-12 hr[91]	**Fosphenytoin advantages:** high water solubility; pH value closer to neutral; faster safe rate of administration; safe to give IM; absence of tissue injury with IV infusion; easy to prepare in IV solution[85] **Therapeutic level:** measure trough serum phenytoin (not fosphenytoin) 48 hr after IV loading dose; "probably 6-15 ml μg/ml (?10-20)"[91] Monitor BP closely during the infusion; can be given with lorazepam Safety in newborns still not clearly established; use with caution in infants with hyperbilirubinemia[85,91]
If phenytoin used instead of Cerebyx to control seizures that are not controlled by phenobarbital alone	**Phenytoin Loading:** 15-20 mg/kg IV infusion over at least 30 min (no more rapidly than 0.5 mg/kg/min); flush with NS before and after giving NEVER GIVE IM!![91] **Phenytoin Maintenance:** 4-8 mg/kg/24 hr‡ IV slow push or po (no more rapidly than 0.5 mg/kg/min). Flush with NS before and after. Absorption erratic with po route. NO IM[91] Term infants >1 week of age may need up to 8 mg/kg/dose q 8-12 hr.[91]	**Phenytoin disadvantages:** incompatible with glucose and all other drugs; cannot be given IM (crystallizes in the muscle); rapid administration can result in bradycardia, dysrhythmias, hypotension The pH of IV solution is 12, which is very irritating to veins Extravasation may result in tissue necrosis[85,91] **Phenytoin therapeutic level:** measure trough level 48 hr after loading dose "probably 6-15 μg/ml (?10-20),"[91] although a therapeutic blood level of 15-20 μg/ml is cited by Volpe[85]
Pyridoxine (Vitamin B₆) as indicated	50-100 mg IV push or IM[85] Monitor EEG while giving Protect from light	Used to diagnose and treat seizures resulting from pyridoxine (vitamin B₆) deficiency Diagnostic when seizures cease within minutes and the EEG normalizes within minutes or hours[85]
Lorazepam (Ativan) For seizures uncontrolled by phenobarbital and fosphenytoin (or phenytoin if used)	0.05 to 0.1 mg/kg IV slow push over several min[85,91]	Enters brain rapidly; onset of action in less than 5 min Monitor for respiratory depression[85,91] Monitor IV site for phlebitis or extravasation[91] Safer to use than diazepam (Valium), which is contraindicated for use in the newborn[85]

Additional therapy as indicated:
Calcium gluconate, 5% solution
Magnesium sulfate, 50% solution
IV antibiotics (bacterial infection) (see Chapter 22)
Acyclovir (herpes) (see Chapter 22)

---

*Appears to be preferred, although safety has not been clearly established.[85]
†MUST be diluted in NS or D₅W to a concentration of 1.5-25 mg PE/ml for IV use.
‡Volpe cited 3-4 mg/kg/24 hr IV in divided doses every 12 hr, starting 12 hr after loading dose.[85]

Prevention

Prevention of further seizures is the third goal (see Table 26-7). Seizure prophylaxis is a worthwhile goal for patients of all ages, but it is often not easily achieved in newborns. Often, despite the appropriate and vigorous administration of several antiepileptic drugs, seizures persist for several days, only to remit spontaneously and never return. Despite this observation, attempts to provide adequate seizure prophylaxis seem justified.

Phenobarbital remains the most studied and most used drug for seizure control in the newborn.[51,85] Because the half-life of phenobarbital is long and may vary from 40 to 200 hours, serum concentration is monitored and it may not be necessary to give routine maintenance doses on a fixed schedule.[91]

Phenytoin is also used extensively in neonatal seizures.[51,85] Although it may be very useful in acute treatment, phenytoin is often quite difficult to use as a maintenance drug. The most frequently encountered problem is the extremely variable half-life in newborns. It is not predictable, and frequent blood level determinations are necessary to estimate a useful half-life for the individual infant. Not uncommonly, repeated loading doses must be used several times a day to maintain an adequate blood level.[9] This pharmacokinetic problem is dramatically compounded by oral administration. It is reasonable to avoid the oral use of phenytoin in the newborn altogether.

A second problem is the variability in binding of phenytoin to albumin in blood. The binding is affected by the amount of albumin, concurrent drugs, and other poorly understood factors. Because changes in binding alter the amount of drug available to enter the brain, there is often little control over the true unbound "level."[85] Whenever the unbound level of phenytoin (normal 1 to 3 mg/ml) can be measured, it is more useful than the total level. Using the unbound level does not make the calculation of an appropriate dosage any simpler, but it does give information that can help avoid needless toxicity. **Maintenance doses of phenobarbital (3 to 5 mg/kg) should be given after blood level determinations indicate that the level is dropping.[22,24,91] Phenytoin and fosphenytoin maintenance doses are difficult to predict. Frequent blood level assessments may be necessary.[85]**

If unbound levels of phenytoin are available, these are often easier to use to ensure that a therapeutic range is maintained. **Because the characteristic signs of phenytoin toxicity are cerebellar,**

they are ordinarily not recognized in the newborn. One must rely on the accurate determination of blood levels to safeguard against excessive administration. Maintenance doses for phenytoin range from 4 to 8 mg/kg IV every 24 hours for the neonate.[60,91]

Other antiepileptic agents such as primidone, carbamazepine, and valproic acid are used less frequently. Fewer data about safety, effectiveness, and dosage are available than for phenobarbital, phenytoin, and lorazepam.[85]

Minimization

The fourth goal is minimization of the side effects of antiepileptic drug therapy. In the attempt to control seizures, the potential of antiepileptic drugs to produce side effects must not be ignored. Drug-induced encephalopathy may mimic the clinical changes seen in hypoxic-ischemic encephalopathy (HIE) or numerous metabolic derangements. The possibility that the pharmaceutical agent may be causing some of the findings being attributed to the underlying disorder always exists. Likewise, improvement in the underlying disorder may be masked by changes induced by the drug.

More significant side effects such as respiratory or cardiovascular depression produced by large doses of any of the drugs, hepatotoxic changes induced by valproic acid, or hyperbilirubinemia intensified by diazepam are rare but worthy of recognition.[85]

The issue of long-term side effects of the antiepileptic drugs is far from being settled. Virtually all of the drugs used have been shown in animal or tissue culture studies to have detrimental effects on the growth or development of the brain. The extent to which any of this information can be transferred to the human situation remains the subject of extensive investigation.[85]

Complications and Outcome

The evidence for long-term clinical complications that can be directly related to the presence of neonatal seizures is limited and controversial.[88] This should not be surprising, because most neonatal seizures occur in the course of significant insults to the developing brain (hypoxia, ischemia, infection, and malformation).

Studies to date have been unable to separate satisfactorily the effect of the seizures from the effect of the cause of the seizures.[86] Hypoglycemia is a good example. Infants with significant hypoglycemia are likely to have identifiable problems, whether or not they actually had neonatal hypoglycemic seizures.

Another curious example is the syndrome of benign familial neonatal seizures.[86] In this condition, infants may have 10 to 20 or more seizures daily. No neurologic sequelae occur in this condition, and seizures generally resolve within 1 to 6 months.[85]

Early hypocalcemia (often seen in stressed newborns) is another example of a relatively benign cause of neonatal seizures. These infants have an excellent chance of recovery without complications. For acute treatment, 2 ml/kg of a 10% solution of calcium gluconate (9 mg of elemental Ca/ml) should be diluted in an appropriate IV solution and infused intravenously over 10 to 30 minutes. The infant should be closely monitored by ECG during infusion of IV calcium.[51,91]

Separate from any discussion of the direct effect of seizures on the developing brain is the question of whether seizures in the newborn period predispose to later seizures. Again, cause seems to be the most important factor. Those seizures caused by transient metabolic changes that do not cause other permanent neurologic dysfunction are themselves likely to be transient and not occur outside the neonatal period. Seizures caused by congenital anomalies or those accompanied by obvious permanent brain damage are likely to persist.

Persistent seizures with structural brain damage are among those seizures that even later in life are hardest to control. Children who develop infantile spasms or the Lennox-Gastaut syndrome frequently have significant problems, including seizures in the neonatal period.

Important prognostic findings and signs can be grouped to provide a general guide to assess newborns with seizures. **Factors favoring a good prognosis include transient metabolic causes (hypocalcemia, hypomagnesemia), normal neurologic examination, normal EEG findings, and benign familial neonatal seizures.**

Factors favoring a poorer prognosis include the presence of a congenital malformation, seizures persisting for more than several days, severe birth asphyxia as the cause,[52] presence of a major IVH, severely abnormal EEG findings (burst suppression, extremely low voltage, or isoelectric), or major signs on neurologic examination (hemi-syndrome, multiple brainstem signs, and severe hypotonia with unresponsiveness).[85]

Factors not carrying any particular prognostic significance include duration of individual seizures (other than status epilepticus), total number of seizures in the first few days of life, initial response to antiepileptic drug therapy, and presence of epilepsy in the patient's family.

Parent Teaching

Lay terms such as *fit* or *spell* provide a hint of the fear that seizure activity can instill in parents. Parent teaching should focus not only on providing pertinent information but also on the correction of existing misinformation. **Parents may initially have difficulty believing that an infant is seizing, because neonatal seizure is difficult to recognize.** It is also not unusual for parents to expect staff to insert items in the mouth, perform CPR, restrain or shake the infant, or institute other measures once they understand that the infant is seizing.

Parents may express an urgent and understandable need to know the cause and the long-term outcomes of the seizure activity. It is important to supply careful explanations of tests being performed and their purpose in identification of the cause of the seizure. The long-term impact on the infant can be harder to predict for the parents, although the presence of certain factors can result in a poorer or better prognosis (see Complications and Outcome). Close follow-up after discharge by both medical and developmental services is vital.

Once the parents are home with the infant, their ability to recognize seizures and appropriately intervene is crucial. Careful documentation of teaching and parent understanding will allow the nursing staff to build on previous knowledge and skills. Parent handouts should focus on the skills and goals listed on this teaching checklist (Figure 26-3). Care should be taken to use short, easy-to-understand sentences and to explain all terminology that parents might find confusing (e.g., what an EEG is). Without parent handouts, attempting to teach the volume of information required is more stressful on both the caregiver and the family. It is even more important that handouts improve the parents' retention of what has been learned.

Providing parents with a form on which to document seizures is also helpful. It can guide the parents in the appropriate observations to make during seizure activity: date, time, duration, seizure activities observed, color changes, behavior after seizure, etc. Parents should practice using this form while the infant is in the hospital so that staff members can assist them with their

BAPTIST MEDICAL CENTER
WOLFSON CHILDREN'S HOSPITAL
JACKSONVILLE, FLORIDA

SEIZURE DISORDER FAMILY TEACHING CHECKLIST

GOAL/SKILL	PRESENTATION/ NURSE DEMONSTRATION DATE AND INITIAL	CARE GIVER/ PATIENT DEMONSTRATION DATE AND INITIAL	CARE GIVER/ PATIENT DEMONSTRATION DATE AND INITIAL	COMMENTS/ HANDOUTS DATE AND INITIAL
1. Verbalizes understanding of seizure pathophysiology.				Handouts given:
2. Describes signs that indicate a seizure.				
3. Lists important observations to make during a seizure.				"Seizure Recognition"
4. Describes care of a child during a seizure.				
5. Identifies child's a. medication, dosage and schedule b. side effects of anticonvulsants c. consequences of non-compliance d. correct administration of medication				Medication _____ Dosage _____ Schedule _____ Medication handout given _____
6. Verbalizes how to seek emergency assistance from home.				
7. Identifies resources for families with a child with a seizure disorder.				
VIDEOS FOR PARENTS (Date that care giver/ patient views)	_____ "How Medications Work" _____ "Understanding Seizure Disorders"			

FIGURE 26-3   Seizure disorder family teaching checklist. (Courtesy Wolfson Children's Hospital, Jacksonville, Fla, 1996.)

assessments and documentation until they gain confidence. **Parents should also administer the medications whenever possible during the infant's hospitalization to establish skills and to reinforce their confidence.**

With the transition to the use of neonatal nurse practitioners (NNP) and physician assistants (PA) in the NICU, collaboration has been identified as essential to the provision of effective health care.[41] Certainly this holds true for the provision of effective discharge teaching as well, because the involvement with the multidisciplinary team approach to discharge planning is crucial. **This planning and parental education must be initiated early in the hospitalization for successful outcomes. A multidisciplinary approach to follow-up after discharge is also required.**[8]

In summary, quality of life issues for patients who have experienced seizures have been almost exclusively discussed in relationship to older children and adults. **However, discharge from the hospital after the diagnosis and treatment of neonatal seizures is a period of both relief and increased anxiety for parents, other family members, and caregivers. For infants with a good prognosis, efforts should be made to help family members look past the neonatal seizures and view their newborn as "healthy" rather than as an "ill" child. For infants whose neurologic outcome will clearly not be normal, clinicians should stress the needs of the multiply handicapped child. The clinician should take the lead in providing the basis for this discussion and guidance in the normalization of the lives of these infants and children.**

HYPOXIC-ISCHEMIC ENCEPHALOPATHY

Physiology

A common identified cause of brain damage in newborns is HIE.[35,38,80,85] Hypoxemia refers to a diminished amount of oxygen in the blood, and ischemia refers to a diminished amount of blood perfused in the brain. Asphyxia refers to the impairment of the exchange of respiratory gases, implying low oxygen and high carbon dioxide in the blood.[53]

Etiology

The timing may be antepartum (i.e., before the onset of labor), with faulty placental gas exchange because of maladies such as diabetes or prediabetes in the mother or preeclampsia.[53] IUGR suggests a chronic antepartum circulatory insult.

The antepartum insult may be acute (e.g., acute hypotension in the mother or placental separation with uterine hemorrhage).

Intrapartum asphyxia may be caused by cord strangulation or placental problems, such as abruption, during labor. Difficult delivery with transverse arrest would be another example of intrapartum cause or contribution to asphyxia. More rare in term infants are postnatal causes. In premature infants RDS, prolonged apnea, severe cyanotic congenital heart disease, or enlarged patent ductus might affect gas exchange enough to result in asphyxia. Many times a combined insult (intrapartum and antepartum) may be causative.

About 1 to 2 of every 1000 newborns experience HIE; 0.3 per 1000 have permanent sequelae.

Data Collection

Prevention

Prevention and management of this entity include optimizing prenatal, parturitional, and postnatal care.[85]

History

Infants with intrapartum cause of HIE show symptoms as a newborn. These infants will have fetal distress in utero, will be depressed at birth, and will have prolonged low Apgar scores. Most have evidence of systemic organ damage: renal, cardiac, and sometimes pulmonary dysfunction will be readily apparent, accompanying the neurologic features of HIE. Diagnosis of HIE depends on careful prenatal and perinatal history-taking and a thorough postnatal neurologic examination. Severe and persistent neurologic findings suggest an unfavorable prognosis.

Signs and Symptoms

Multiple diagnostic criteria have confused the recognition of intrapartum asphyxia in term infants.[13,18,52] Diagnosis of acute perinatal asphyxia should meet one of the three sets of criteria in the Report of the Workshop on Acute Perinatal Asphyxia in Term Infants.[89] The basic requirement for making this diagnosis is a pH less than 7.0, with a 5-minute Apgar score of 3 or less. The addition of abnormal fetal heart rate patterns to these two parameters has been used to develop a scoring system that improves the predictive value of these parameters.[62,66] The American Academy of Pediatrics/American College of

Obstetricians and Gynecologists add multiple organ system failure and neurologic sequelae to their definition.[3]

The neurologic syndrome presents as stupor or coma, ventilatory problems (e.g., periodic breathing or apnea), hypotonia, and often, early onset seizures.[67] The seizures, often subtle, may be epileptic seizures (i.e., with brain electrical discharges), or the seizures may be nonepileptic release phenomenon such as decerebrate/decorticate posturing. There may be extraocular movement and pupillary irregularities (e.g., miosis or unequal pupils).

In the next few days, seizures, apnea, hypotonia, jitteriness, weakness, and even respiratory arrest may occur. In premature infants IVH may be catastrophic. Increased intracranial pressure with or without respiratory arrest may happen in the most severely involved infants. In those infants who survive, tube feedings, weak suck, and continued stupor may persist for days to weeks.

Laboratory Data
Metabolic or laboratory parameters will often be abnormal, and blood gases and pH should be assessed. Acidosis, hypoxemia, and hypercarbia are frequent findings. Other parameters possibly needing correction include a low blood sugar (hypoglycemia), hypocalcemia, hyponatremia, and more rarely, hyperammonemia. Creatine phosphokinase, especially the BB (brain fraction), correlates with parenchymal brain damage.

One should sample the spinal fluid to see whether there is bleeding and to rule out infectious possibilities. The infant[68] should be monitored with an EEG for seizures. In a term infant, a severely abnormal pattern such as burst suppression, very low amplitude, or isoelectric EEG suggest an ominous prognosis.

Accurately performed ultrasonography may show periventricular increased echodensities, later to become lucencies or even large cysts or cystic encephalomalacia.

Early CT scans may show cerebral edema, sometimes difficult to quantify and to differentiate from the normal brain in a newborn. Hemorrhagic lesions are clearly seen. The CT scan has more utility in follow-up, showing location of white matter malacia, basal ganglia lesions, etc.

An **MRI** may show cortical necrosis on a T1 weighted image and loss of the gray-white delineation on T2.

Treatment
Treatment includes the broad principles of adequate ventilation, gas exchange, and perfusion; maintenance of normal glucose and electrolyte levels; control of seizures; and prevention and control of brain swelling.

New therapies may include excitotoxic amino acid antagonists and free-radical scavengers.[57] These are the same new approaches taken for management of stroke and ischemic brain damage in adults.

Complications
A variety of sequelae may result from selective neuronal necrosis and periventricular leukomalacia.[28] The former often correlates with mental retardation, spastic quadriparesis, seizure disorder, ataxia, pseudobulbar palsy, and attention deficit hyperactivity disorder. Periventricular leukomalacia has been most commonly associated with spastic diplegia.

Prognosis, of course, depends on the severity of the insult, but in large studies, 50% of affected infants have normal outcome, 20% to 30% have abnormal sequelae, and 10% to 30% die with the more unfavorable statistics noted in premature infants.[64,85]

INTRAVENTRICULAR HEMORRHAGE

Physiology
The problem of bleeding into and around the ventricular system has received more attention in the last decade than any other neurologic problem in neonates. In large measure, this relates to the frequency with which the problem develops, generally estimated to be 15% in premature infants under 1501 g.[85] The growth of routine cranial ultrasonographic examination in premature infants has resulted directly from the need to evaluate this common problem. Recently, however, the incidence of these hemorrhages has appeared to be decreasing. With the advent of CT and ultrasonographic scanning, a large number of infants who were not otherwise suspected of having intraventricular bleeding were diagnosed on scans.

Although the bleeding is regularly spoken of as *intraventricular* and *intracranial hemorrhage,* these terms do not accurately reflect its causes. Highly vascularized areas, which have relatively fragile and poorly supported blood vessels, are the source of bleeding. In a premature infant the most common source of hemorrhage is the germinal matrix.[38,63,81] The width of the matrix is 2.5 mm at 23 to 24 weeks but decreases to 1.4 mm at 32 weeks. By 36 weeks, almost complete involution has occurred. Volpe listed principal clinical features as a premature baby requiring a ventilator secondary to respiratory distress syndrome. **Approximately 90% of bleeding events occur in the first 72 hours of life, and at least one in two affected infants will hemorrhage in the first 24 hours.**[85]

The incidence of IVH in term infants is approximately 3.5% to 5%, making IVH both an uncommon and unanticipated diagnosis. Approximately 50% of IVH in the term newborn are caused by asphyxia and/or trauma with symptoms appearing in the first 48 hours after birth. About 25% of these infants with IVH have no significant risk factors and symptoms tend to appear at a later age (approximately 1 week of age).[21]

In term infants the choroid plexus of the lateral ventricles is the most common site in which bleeding originates.[21] In premature infants the germinal matrix, in the subependymal area adjacent to the caudate nucleus, is the primary site

of bleeding.[39] Both of these are areas of high arterial and capillary blood flow; in addition, they use an anatomically awkward venous drainage system, eventually draining into the internal cerebral vein (Figure 26-4).

The extent of bleeding generally predicts the likelihood of complications and residua. Bleeding may be confined to the germinal matrix or the choroid plexus, or it may enter the ventricular system. When filled under pressure, the ventricular system may dilate. Blood may also extravasate out into the brain parenchyma (more likely with germinal matrix bleeding than with choroid plexus bleeding).

Several classification schemes have been used, each trying to assess the degree of bleeding or amount of blood present. Ideally, a classification should relate to pathophysiology, treatment, or outcome, but with present knowledge this is not possible.

Volpe listed three grades of germinal matrix-IVH using ultrasonographic scanning to identify the presence and extent of blood in the germinal

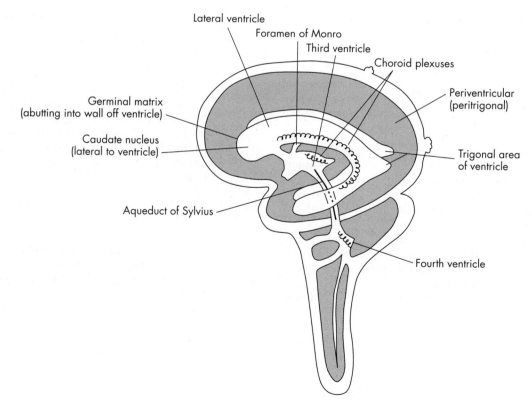

FIGURE 26-4   Central nervous system/ventricular system.

matrix and lateral ventricles (Table 26-8). A "separate notation" is made for the existence of "periventricular hemorrhage infarction or of other parenchymal lesions." He clarified the use of this separate notation by noting that these abnormalities are not usually the result of simple "extension" of matrix or IVH hemorrhage into "normal brain parenchyma."[85] Others also use this classification system.[58]

The use of an older classification system based on the extent of hemorrhage seen on the CT scan grades germinal matrix hemorrhages as follows (Figure 26-5). Since both grading systems are still cited in the literature, we have included each.*

0—No bleeding

I—Germinal matrix only

II—Germinal matrix with blood in the ventricles

III—Germinal matrix with blood in the ventricles and hydrocephalus (ventricular dilation)

IV—Intraventricular and parenchymal bleeding (other than germinal matrix)

Etiology

The factors identified in infants who have experienced IVH are multiple. **These include asphyxia, severe respiratory distress, pneumothorax, hypoglycemia, shock, acidosis, blood transfusions, seizures, and rapid volume expansion (Box 26-3).** What appears to be the common factor underlying the pathologic condition is a fluctuation in cerebral blood flow.†

At times, this may have a systemic counterpart, such as in shock. At other times, changes in brain perfusion occur without any reflection in systemic blood pressure, pulse, or respiration. The fragility of the germinal matrix and choroid plexus seem to allow for the disruption of capillary or small blood vessel integrity with resultant bleeding.[39]

Intraventricular bleeding tends to occur in the first few hours or days of life. The profound physiologic changes normally seen after birth are coupled with the multiple problems (primarily cardiorespiratory) typically experienced by the premature infant to make intraventricular bleeding common. The degree to which the aggressive management of premature newborns has a role in the development of bleeding cannot be accurately assessed. In general, although not exclusively, it is the sicker infants who both require more intervention and have a greater likelihood of bleeding. The decreased incidence of intraventricular bleeding with antenatal (but not with neonatal) phenobarbital administration suggests a role for prenatal and intrapartum events in the etiology of intraventricular bleeding.[37] **In a recent study of 3721 premature infants, the authors concluded that a significant reduction of the incidence of IVH would occur if "extremely premature infants, the vast majority of patients suffering from IVH, didn't have to be transferred postnatally to another hospital."[27]**

Data Collection

As mentioned earlier, the historical information is somewhat varied. Some infants, generally those who are at term, will have IVH associated with severe asphyxia. **Premature infants often show one or more of the following: birth weight less than 1500 g, gestational age less than 34 weeks, shock, RDS, need for blood transfusions, coagulopathy, hyperviscosity, hypoxia, and birth asphyxia.**

Because premature infants, particularly those weighing less than 1500 g, tend to have multiple

---

*References 10, 20, 21, 25, 27, 48, 49, 63, 74, 78.
†References 15, 17, 25, 81, 83, 84.

Table 26-8	GRADING OF SEVERITY OF GERMINAL MATRIX—INTRAVENTRICULAR HEMORRHAGE BY ULTRASOUND SCAN	
SEVERITY	**DESCRIPTION**	
Grade I	Germinal matrix hemorrhage with no or minimal intraventricular hemorrhage (10% of ventricular area on parasagittal view)	
Grade II	Intraventricular hemorrhage (10%-50% of ventricular area on parasagittal view)	
Grade III	Intraventricular hemorrhage (>50% of ventricular area on parasagittal view; usually distends lateral ventricle)	
Separate notation	Periventricular echodensity (location and extent)	

From: Volpe JJ: *Neurology of the newborn,* ed 4, Philadelphia, 2001, WB Saunders.

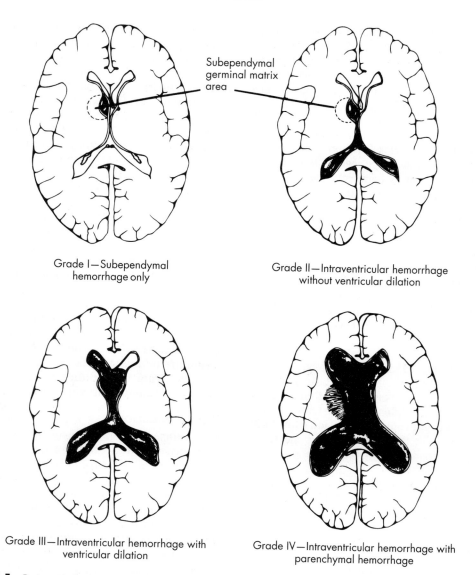

Subependymal germinal matrix area

Grade I—Subependymal
hemorrhage only

Grade II—Intraventricular hemorrhage
without ventricular dilation

Grade III—Intraventricular hemorrhage with
ventricular dilation

Grade IV—Intraventricular hemorrhage with
parenchymal hemorrhage

FIGURE 26-5   Periventricular-intraventricular hemorrhage, grades I-IV. (From Rozmus C: Periventricular-intraventricular hemorrhage in the newborn, *Matern Child Nurs* 17:79, 1992.)

Box 26-3	FACTORS THAT PREDISPOSE TO INTRAVENTRICULAR HEMORRHAGE (IVH)

Prematurity

Birth weight <1500 g
<34 wk gestation

Asphysia (see Chapters 4 and 11)

Before, during, after birth

Respiratory (see Chapters 11 and 23)

Idiopathic respiratory distress syndrome (IRDS)
Hypoxia
Positive pressure ventilation
Pneumothorax
Apnea

Cardiovascular (see Chapter 4)

Rapid volume expansion
Elevated venous pressure
Elevated or lowered arterial pressure (shock; transfusions)

Hematologic (see Chapter 20)

Hyperosmolarity
Coagulation disorders
Hyperviscosity

Metabolic (see Chapters 11, 14, and 15)

Hypoglycemia/hyperglycemia
Hypernatremia
Metabolic acidosis
Rapid pH shifts

Miscellaneous

Hypothermia (see Chapter 6)
Acetysalicyclic acid ingestion by mother
Neonatal pain (see Chapter 12)
Neonatal environmental stressors (see Chapter 13)

Modified from Gardner S, Hagedorn M: Physiologic sequelae of prematurity: the nurse practitioner's role, Part VIII. Neurologic conditions, J Pediatr Nurs 6:265, 1992.

hematocrit, flaccidity, areflexia, full fontanel, tonic posturing, and oculomotor disturbances.

When intracranial bleeding is suspected, appropriate studies of intracranial structures should be performed as soon as possible. **For periventricular-intraventricular hemorrhage both ultrasonography and CT scanning are useful tools for defining the presence of bleeding and for following its evolution.** Ultrasonographic scanning is listed by Volpe as "the procedure of choice in the diagnosis of germinal matrix-IVH."[85] Because ultrasonography is the safer procedure and uses no radiation, it should be used for follow-up.

Treatment and Intervention

The primary treatment of IVH is confined to supportive care. Ventilatory support, maintenance of oxygenation, regulation of acid-base balance, suppression of seizures, and treatment of any attendant coagulopathy are all extremely important in reducing mortality and morbidity. The role that successful management has in the amelioration or prevention of complications is unclear.

Many therapies have been proposed or used but remain unproved. These are listed here not to recommend them for general clinical use, but to suggest the ways in which the problem has been approached.

When the hemorrhage is confined to the germinal matrix, little can be done, even from a theoretic standpoint.

The removal of blood from the ventricular system has been used for many years as a treatment for IVH. Many studies have shown it to have limited effectiveness. The rationale for removing blood is twofold: (1) to remove an irritating substance from the ventricular system, at the same time reducing clot formation, and (2) to remove protein in the hope of preventing hydrocephalus. Yet, because of high spinal fluid protein levels and the potential for a block in the flow of fluid, there is a concern that repeated lumbar punctures may be ineffective in clearing blood from the ventricles. **Lumbar puncture has much less chance of morbidity and was the preferred procedure. Ventricular taps can be used but are rarely recommended.** In a review of pediatric, neurosurgical, and general medical journals back to 1976, White-law sought to ascertain whether repeated CSF tapping (via ventricular or lumbar routes) decreased morbidity and mortality in neonates at risk of or with posthemorrhagic hydrocephalus. **There was**

problems, it is not surprising that the clinical presentation of germinal matrix hemorrhage may range from subtle (or even undetectable) to catastrophic.

Deterioration in clinical condition followed by apnea, flaccid quadriparesis, unresponsiveness, and death from circulatory collapse is a recognizable syndrome. Common signs of germinal matrix hemorrhage include apnea, hypotension, drop in

no statistically significant difference between repeated CSF tapping and conservative management except for an increased risk of CSF infection when CSF tapping was used. Whitelaw's conclusion was that "early repeated CSF tapping cannot be recommended for neonates at risk of, or actually developing, post-hemorrhagic hydrocephalus."[87]

Intraventricular fibrinolytics (streptokinase/ urokinase) have been utilized to dissolve the clot and prevent hydrocephalus. After noting that intraventricular blood clots have been successfully dissolved by urokinase in the adult population with subsequent improved outcomes, several neonatal studies were completed. **Initial favorable results were followed by two studies that showed no benefit from the use of fibrinolytic therapy.**[85]

Care must be given to reduce the risk for continued bleeding, working to maintain perfusion of the brain and to reduce wide fluctuations in blood pressure, oxygenation, and pH.

Another theoretical (and unproved) objection to these methods suggests that removing blood will allow for further bleeding by reducing the pressure in the ventricles and therefore upsetting the homeostatic balance.

Medications to reduce intracranial pressure and therefore treat secondary effects of the bleeding include furosemide, acetazolamide, and steroidal agents. Mannitol and glycerol have also been used. The same unproved argument concerning upsetting the homeostatic balance may be applied here.

Helpful pharmacologic preventive agents (glucocorticoids and possibly phenobarbital administered prenatally and indomethacin, vitamin E, and phenobarbital postnatally) have had varying success.*

Apparently, the best recommendation for the treatment of IVH is to continue the management of ensuing problems without undue attention to the intracranial bleeding.

Complications

The complications from IVH relate to the underlying causes and the extent of bleeding. Massive bleeding with dilation of the ventricular system is much more likely to cause an acute change in brain function, with increased intracranial pressure, brainstem findings, and apnea. Milder degrees of hemorrhage may be asymptomatic or associated with seizurelike events, changes in muscle tone, or apnea.

When bleeding extends into the parenchyma, porencephaly may result from liquefactive necrosis or ischemia-induced encephalomalacia. Follow-up structural brain studies may show hypodense areas where blood was present; later they may show areas of porencephaly.

The most common complication is posthemorrhagic hydrocephalus. The possibility of this developing is directly related to the severity of the hemorrhage, with up to 10% of survivors of mild IVH and 65% to 100% of survivors of severe IVH showing progressive ventricular dilation. Posthemorrhagic hydrocephalus should be sought in all survivors of germinal matrix hemorrhage. CT scanning or ultrasonography to assess ventricular size should be used. Clinical signs alone are not reliable.[40]

With the hope of avoiding the necessity of placing a shunt, some attempts at control of the hydrocephalus have been attempted. Osmotic and diuretic agents, including furosemide, isosorbide, and acetazolamide, have been used to reduce the formation of CSF. Some clinicians have been enthusiastic about this approach, but it has not gained widespread acceptance. As mentioned, early, repeated lumbar and intraventricular taps are sometimes used in an attempt to avoid shunting. This approach holds questionable benefits.[86] In some small premature infants, ventricular drainage without a full shunt (to the peritoneal cavity) is used.

Outcome studies have been difficult to assess. Clearly, the sickest infants tend to do poorly. They also tend to have more complications, including CNS complications. **There is a clear correlation between the grade of bleed and the likelihood of significant neurologic residua, but the correlation is far from perfect.**[79] The influence of other factors on neurologic outcome may be more significant than the actual bleed itself. Hypoxia, hypoperfusion, and other conditions known to damage the developing nervous system cannot easily be separated as individual factors in outcome.[71] **Patients with grade I and II hemorrhages usually do as well as patients with no hemorrhage. Patients with grade III and IV hemorrhages most often have long-term morbidity.**

---

*References 19, 37, 39, 48, 49, 59, 61, 65, 77, 85.

PARENT TEACHING

Parents of an infant with IVH should be involved with their infant's care plan. The rationale for a minimal handling protocol needs to be explained. Encouraging parents to participate in setting "time out" and "touch me" times will facilitate their ability to visit and assist with care. **During visits, they should be encouraged to recognize signs of overstimulation and appropriate interventions.**[17,26,33]

The infant with IVH will have varying degrees of problems.[79] Often the acute situation resolves without ongoing problems. In these cases, parents should understand the possible complications such as hydrocephalus that may occur in the short term. **Teaching the parents to measure head circumference and alerting them to the signs of increased intracranial pressure such as poor feeding, posturing, eye movement difficulties, full fontanel, and lethargy will enable them to par-**ticipate more fully in the medical follow-up (see Box 26-2). **Up to 80% to 90% of infants with hydrocephalus need a shunt because of ventricular dilation.**[8]

Parents must understand the risk for long-term neurologic sequelae. Even though these sequelae are difficult to predict with any degree of certainty, parents should understand that mental and motor handicaps, delays in the acquisition of milestones, seizures, and problems associated with hydrocephalus and potential shunt placement may occur.[79] Specific preparation for these potential problems should begin in the nursery but will be increased during follow-up visits if the possibility for such problems seems greater. Prompt and appropriate referral to medical specialists and supportive services is important in both inpatient and outpatient settings. **Parents may also find support and information from national and state organizations such as those listed in Box 26-4.**

Box 26-4	PARENT RESOURCES FOR NEUROLOGIC DISORDERS

The Hydrocephalus Association
870 Market Street
Suite 705
San Francisco, CA 94102
Phone: (888) 598-3789 toll free
Phone: (415) 732-7040
Fax: (415) 732-7044
Web: www.hydroassoc.org
E-mail: hydroassoc@aol.com

Family Support Center of New Jersey
35 Beaverson Blvd.
Suite 8A
Brick, NJ 08723
Phone: (732) 262-8020
Fax: (732) 262-4373

National Organization for Rare Disorders (NORD)
P.O. Box 8923
New Fairfield, CT 06812-8923
Phone: (800) 999-6673—help line
Phone: (203) 746-6518
Fax: (203) 746-6927
TDD: (203) 746-6927
Web: www.rarediseases.org
E-mail: orphan@rarediseases.org

Epilepsy Foundation of America
4351 Garden City Drive
Landover, MD 20785
Phone: (800) 332-1000 toll free
Phone: (301) 459-3700
Web: www.epilepsyfoundation.org

Exceptional Parent Magazine
555 Kinderkamack Road
Oradell, NJ 07649
Phone: (800) 372-7368 toll free
Fax: (201) 634-6599
Web: www.eparent.com

National Hydrocephalus Foundation
12413 Centralia
Lakewood, CA 90715-1623
Phone: (888) 260-1789 toll-free pager
Phone: (562) 402-3523
Fax: (562) 924-6666
Web: www.nhfonline.org
E-mail: hydrobrat@earthlink.net

NOTE: The presence of a group on this list of parent resources does not constitute a recommendation by the authors for the group or the information that they may provide.

Continued

| **Box 26-4** | **PARENT RESOURCES FOR NEUROLOGIC DISORDERS—cont'd** |

Hydrocephalus Family Support of Central Florida
702 Robert Street
Kissimmee, FL 34741
Phone: (800) # is pending
Web: www.HFSG.net (under construction)
E-mail: mrssm1000@aol.com

American Self-Help Clearing House
100 East Hanover Avenue
2nd Floor
Cedar Knolls, NJ 07927-2020
Phone: (800) 367-6274 toll free
Phone: (973) 326-6789
Web: www.selfhelpgroups.org

American Epilepsy Society
342 North Main St.
West Hartford, CT 06117
Phone: (860) 586-7505
Web: www.aesnet.org

Medic Alert
2323 Colorado Ave
Turlock, CA 95382
Phone: (800) 432-5378 toll free
Web: www.medicalert.org

NOTE: The presence of a group on this list of parent resources does not constitute a recommendation by the authors for the group or the information that they may provide.

REFERENCES

1. Aicardi J: Disorders of neuronal migration: a spectrum of cortical abnormalities, *Int Pediatr* 8:162, 1993.
2. Altman N, Brunberg J, Elster A et al: Advanced MRI of disorders of neuronal migration and sulcation, *Int Pediatr* 10(suppl):16, 1995.
3. American Academy of Pediatrics and American College of Obstetricians and Gynecologists: *Guidelines for perinatal care,* ed 4, Elk Grove Village, Ill, 1997, The Academy.
4. Ballweg DD: Neonatal seizures: an overview, *Neonatal Netw* 10:15, 1991.
5. Barkovich AJ, Kjos BO, Jackson DE Jr et al: Normal maturation of neonatal and infant brain: MR imaging at 1.5 T, *Radiology* 166:173, 1988.
6. Beers MH, Berkow R, Bogin R et al: *The Merck manual,* ed 17, West Point, P, 1999, Merck.
7. Bernes SM, Kaplan AM: Evolution of neonatal seizures, *Pediatr Clin North Am* 41:1069, 1994.
8. Blackburn S: Problems of preterm infants after discharge, *J Obstet Gynecol Neonatal Nurs* 24:43, 1995.
9. Bourgeois BFD, Dodson WE: Phenytoin elimination in newborns, *Neurology* 33:173, 1983.
10. Bromberger P: Intraventricular hemorrhage (IVH) of the newborn, *Clinical Reference Systems,* Nov, 1999, p 795.
11. Camfield PR, Camfield CS: Neonatal seizures: a commentary on selected aspects, *J Child Neurol* 2:244, 1987.
12. Carlson C: Neonatal seizures, *Central Lines* 16:7, 2000.
13. Carter BS, Haverkamp, AD, Merenstein GB: The definition of acute perinatal asphyxia, *Clin Perinatol* 20:287, 1993.
14. Clancy R, Malin S, Larangue D et al: Focal motor seizures heralding stroke in full-term infants, *Am J Dis Child* 139:601, 1985.
15. Cordis Corp.: *Hydrocephalus and shunts: your valve system for hydrocephalus,* and *Just like any other beagle,* Miami, 1989, Cordis Corp.
16. Desposito F, Cunniff C, Frias J et al: Folic acid for the prevention of neural tube defects, *Pediatrics* 104:325, 1999.
17. Dietch JS: Periventricular-intraventricular hemorrhage in the very low birth weight infant, *Neonatal Netw* 12:7, 1993.
18. Edwards MSB: Fetal hydrocephalus, *Int Pediatr* 2:89, 1987.
19. Faix RG, Stowell J: Comparative efficacy and safety of indomethacin and phenobarbital for prevention of intraventricular hemorrhage, *Pediatrics* 104:A753, 1999.
20. Finer NN, Horbar JD, Carpenter JH: Cardiopulmonary resuscitation in the very low birth weight infant: The Vermont Oxford Network experience, *Pediatrics* 104:428, 1999.
21. Fink S: Intraventricular hemorrhage in the term infant, *Neonatal Netw* 19:13, 2000.
22. Fischer JH, Lockman LA, Zaske D et al: Phenobarbital maintenance dose requirements in treating neonatal seizures, *Neurology* 31:1042, 1981.
23. Fujii Y, Konishi Y, Kuriyama M et al: Corpus callosum in developmentally retarded infants, *Pediatr Neurol* 11:219, 1994.

24. Gal P, Toback J, Boer HR et al: Efficacy of phenobarbital monotherapy in treatment of neonatal seizures: relationship to blood levels, *Neurology* 32: 1401, 1982.

25. Gardner SL, Hagedorn MI: Physiologic sequelae of prematurity: the nurse practitioner's role. Part VIII. Neurologic conditions, *J Pediatr Health Care* 6:263, 1992.

26. Gennaro S: Facilitating parenting of the neonatal intensive care unit graduate, *J Perinat Neonatal Nurs* 4:55, 1991.

27. Gleissner M, Jorch G, Avenarius S: Risk factors for intraventricular hemorrhage in a birth cohort of 3721 premature infants, *J Perinat Med* 28:104, 2000.

28. Goetz MC, Gretebeck RJ, Oh KS et al: Incidence, timing, and follow-up of periventricular leukomalacia, *Am J Perinatol* 12:325, 1995.

29. Hahn JS: Controversies in treatment of neonatal seizures, *Pediatr Neurol* 9:330, 1993.

30. Halslam RAH: Neonatal seizures. In Behrman R, ed: *Nelson's textbook of pediatrics,* ed 15, Philadelphia, 1996, WB Saunders.

31. Hankins GDV, Clark SL: Brachial plexus palsy involving the posterior shoulder at spontaneous vaginal delivery, *Am J Perinatol* 12:325, 1995.

32. Harrison H, Kositsky A: *The premature baby book,* New York, 1983, St. Martin's Press.

33. Haskins R, finkelstein NW, Stedman DJ: Infant stimulation programs and their effects, *Pediatr Ann* 7:123, 1978.

34. Holmes GL: Neonatal seizures, *Acta Neuroped* 1:241, 1995.

35. Hull J, Dodd KL: Falling incidence of hypoxic-ischemic encephalopathy in term infants, *Br J Obstet Gynaecol* 99:386, 1992.

36. Hummel PA, Eastman DL: Do parents of preterm infants suffer chronic sorrow? *Neonatal Netw* 10:59, 1991.

37. Kaempf JW, Porreco R, Molina R et al: Antenatal phenobarbital for the prevention of periventricular and intraventricular hemorrhage: a double-blind, randomized placebo-controlled multihospital trial, *J Pediatr* 111:931, 1990.

38. Leviton A, Nelson KB: Problems with definitions and classifications of newborn encephalopathy, *Pediatr Neurol* 8:85, 1992.

39. Leviton A, Kuban KC, Pagano M et al: Antenatal corticosteroids appear to reduce risk of postnatal germinal matrix hemorrhage in intubated low birth weight newborns, *Pediatrics* 81:1083, 1993.

40. Lin JP, Goh W, Brown JK et al: Neurological outcome following neonatal post-haemorrhagic hydrocephalus: the effects of maximum raised intracranial pressure and ventriculo-peritoneal shunting, *Childs Nerv Syst* 8:190, 1992.

41. Little GA, Buus-Frank ME: Transition from housestaff in neonatal intensive care unit, *Am J Perinatol* 13:127, 1996.

42. Lombroso C: Neonatal seizures: historic note and present controversies, *Epilepsia* 37(suppl):5, 1996.

43. Martin-Padilla M: Review of perinatal brain damage in premature born infant, *Int Pediatr* 10(suppl):26, 1995.

44. McCance KL, Huether SE: *Pathophysiology: the biologic basis for disease in adults and children,* ed 3, St. Louis, 1998, Mosby.

45. McGrath, JM: Developmental physiology of the neurological system, *Central Lines* 16:1, 2000.

46. McLone D, Reigel D, Sommers M et al: *An introduction to hydrocephalus,* Chicago, 1982, Children's Memorial Hospital.

47. Melvin EC, George TM, Worley G et al: Genetic studies in neural tube defects, *Pediatr Neurosurg* 32:1, 2000.

48. Ment LR, Oh W, Ehrenkranz RA et al: Low-dose indomethacin and prevention of intraventricular hemorrhage: a multicenter randomized trial, *Pediatrics* 93:543, 1994.

49. Ment LR, Vohr B, Allan W et al: Outcome of children in the indomethacin intraventricular hemorrhage prevention trial, *Pediatrics* 105:485, 2000.

50. Miles MS, Carlson J, Funk SG: Sources of support reported by mothers and fathers of infants hospitalized in a neonatal intensive care unit, *Neonatal Netw* 15:45, 1996.

51. Mizrahi EM, Kellaway P: *Diagnosis and management of neonatal seizures,* ed 1, Philadelphia, 1998, Lippincott-Raven.

52. Nelson KB, Leviton A: How much of neonatal encephalopathy is due to birth asphyxia? *Am J Dis Child* 143:1325, 1991.

53. Nelson KB, Leviton A: Problems with definition and classification of newborn encephalopathy, *Pediatr Neurol* 8:85, 1992.

54. Painter MJ: Brachial plexus injuries in neonates, *Int Pediatr* 3:120, 1988.

55. Painter MJ, Gaus LM: Neonatal seizures: diagnosis and treatment, *J Child Neurol* 6:101, 1991.

56. Painter MJ, Scher MS, Stein AD et al. Phenobarbital compared with phenytoin for the treatment of neonatal seizures, *N Engl J Med* 341:485, 1999.

57. Palmer C, Vannucci RC: Potential new therapies for perinatal cerebral hypoxia-ischemia, *Clin Perinatol* 20:411, 1953.

58. Perlman JM, Rollins N: Surveillance protocol for the detection of intracranial abnormalities in premature neonates, *Arch Pediatr Adolesc Med* 154:822, 2000.

59. Perlman JM, Risser RC, Gee JB: Pregnancy-induced hypertension and reduced intraventricular hemorrhage in preterm infants, *Pediatr Neurol* 17:29, 1997.

60. *Physician's Desk Reference,* ed 55, Montvale, N.J., 2001, Medical Economics Data Production.

61. Poland SRL: Vitamin E for prevention of intracranial hemorrhage, *Pediatrics* 85:865, 1990.

62. Portman RJ, Carter BS, Gaylord MS et al: Predicting neonatal morbidity after perinatal asphyxia: a scoring system, *Am J Obstet Gynecol* 162:174, 1990.

63. Ramey J: Evaluation of periventricular-intraventricular hemorrhage in premature infants using cranial ultrasounds, *Neonatal Netw* 19:31, 2000.

64. Robertson CM, finer NM: Long-term follow-up of term neonates with perinatal asphyxia, *Clin Perinatol* 20:483, 1993.

65. Rozmus C: Periventricular-intraventricular hemorrhage in the newborn, *Maternal Child Nurs* 17:74, 1992.

66. Rust RS, Volpe JJ: Neonatal seizures. In Dodson WE, Pellock JM, eds: *Pediatric epilepsy: diagnosis and therapy,* New York, 1993, Demos Publications.

67. Sarnat HB: Disturbances of late neuronal migrations in the perinatal period, *Am J Dis Child* 141:969, 1987.

68. Scher MS, Painter MJ, Bergman I et al: EEG diagnoses of neonatal seizures: clinical correlations and outcome, *Pediatr Neurol* 5:17, 1989.

69. Schultz AW: Improving child and family health through primary prevention of neural tube defects, *Pediatr Nurs* 25:419, 1999.

70. Sellinger C: Brachial plexus injuries, *Pediatr Rev* 13:77, 1992.

71. Shinnar S, Molteni RA, Gammon K et al: Intraventricular hemorrhage in the premature infant: a changing outlook, *N Engl J Med* 306:1464, 1982.

72. da Silva O, Alexandrou D, Knoppert D et al: Seizure and electroencephalographic changes in the newborn period induced by opiates and corrected by naloxone infusion, *J Perinatol* 19:120, 1999.

73. Stafstrom CE: Neonatal seizures, *Pediatr Rev* 16:248, 1995.

74. Steinbach MT: Traumatic birth injury: intracranial hemorrhage, *Mother Baby J* 4:5, 1999.

75. Stevenson RE, Allen WP, Pai GS et al: Decline in prevalence of neural tube defects in a high-risk region of the United States, *Pediatrics* 106:677, 2000.

76. Strober JB, Bienkowski RS, Maytal J: The incidence of acute and remote seizures in children with intraventricular hemorrhage, *Clin Pediatr* 36:643, 1997.

77. Thorp JA, Parriott J, Ferrette-Smith D et al: Antepartum vitamin K and phenobarbital for preventing intraventricular hemorrhage in the premature newborn: a randomized, double-blind, placebo-controlled trial, *Obstet Gynecol* 83:70, 1994.

78. Vergani P, Patane L, Doria P et al: Risk factors for neonatal intraventricular haemorrhage in spontaneous prematurity at 32 weeks gestation or less, *Placenta* 21:402, 2000.

79. Vohr B, Ment LR: Intraventricular hemorrhage in the preterm infant, *Early Hum Dev* 45:169, 1996.

80. Volpe JJ: Brain injury in the premature infant: current concepts, *Biol Neonat* 69:165, 1956.

81. Volpe JJ: Neonatal intracranial hemorrhage: pathophysiology, neuropathology and clinical features, *Clin Perinatal* 4:77, 1977.

82. Volpe JJ: Normal and abnormal human brain development, *Clin Perinatol* 4:3, 1977.

83. Volpe JJ: Intraventricular hemorrhage and brain injury in the premature infant: diagnosis, prognosis and prevention, *Clin Perinatol* 16:387, 1989.

84. Volpe JJ: Intraventricular hemorrhage and brain injury in the premature infant: neuropathology and pathogenesis, *Clin Perinatol* 16:361, 1989.

85. Volpe JJ: *Neurology of the newborn,* ed 4, Philadelphia, 2001, WB Saunders.

86. Webb R, Bobele G: "Benign" familial neonatal convulsions, *J Child Neurol* 5:295, 1990.

87. Whitelaw A: Repeated lumbar or ventricular punctures for preventing disability or shunt dependence in newborn infants with intraventricular hemorrhage, *Cochrane Database Syst Rev,* CD000216, 2000.

88. Wiscal BS: Neonatal seizures and electrographic analysis: evaluation and outcomes, *Pediatr Neurol* 10:271, 1994.

89. Wright LL, Merenstein GB, Hirtz DG, eds: *Report of the workshop on acute perinatal asphyxia in term infants,* Bethesda, Md, 1996, National Institutes of Health.

90. Yager JY, Vannucci RC: Development and disorders of organ systems. In Fanaroff A, Martin R, eds: *Neonatal-perinatal medicine: diseases of the fetus and infant, vol. 1,* ed 6, St. Louis, 1997, Mosby.

91. Young TE, Mangum OB: *Neofax: a manual of drugs used in neonatal care,* ed 13, Raleigh, NC, 2000, Acorn Publishing.

27 | Genetic Disorders, Malformations, and Inborn Errors of Metabolism

Anne L. Matthews, Nathaniel H. Robin

A neonate born with a malformation, genetic syndrome, or an acute metabolic disorder represents a management challenge for the NICU staff. If these conditions are not suspected and diagnosed in a critically ill neonate, an appropriate course of action might not be taken. Thus a specific diagnosis becomes imperative. An accurate diagnosis provides the staff with information about the cause of the condition, points the way toward appropriate treatment, and indicates the prognosis so that the most appropriate care of the infant can be initiated. Moreover, the broader issues of providing supportive care and counseling for the affected infant's family can be addressed.

Genetic evaluation is a complex process that requires expertise in differentiating normal variations from abnormal findings and knowledge of the principles of embryology and dysmorphology to provide an accurate diagnosis. Skills in obtaining detailed information of prenatal and family histories may be equally important.

The field of genomics and genetic medicine has witnessed an explosion of new knowledge, much of which has been generated by the efforts of the Human Genome Project.[10] Our understanding of the genetic basis of development and function, as well as the interaction of genes and the environment, continues to provide new insights into human health.

This chapter is a concise overview of the major categories of genetic disorders and the appropriate techniques to establish specific diagnoses. For an excellent review and detailed explanation of concepts, terminology, and specific genetic mechanisms refer to *Thompson and Thompson Genetics in Medicine*.[32] See Box 27-1 for a comprehensive list of terms.

GENETIC PRINCIPLES

Genes

A **gene** is a segment of a DNA molecule coded for the synthesis of a single polypeptide and contains the hereditary information needed for development or function. DNA, which allows for the storing, duplicating, and processing of hereditary information, consists of two long strands twisted around each other to form a double helix. Each strand of DNA is composed of four nucleotides: guanine (G), adenine (A), thymine (T), and cytosine (C). The specific order of the nucleotides determines the precise information that will be coded at that site. Genes can (1) regulate other genes by turning them "on" or "off," (2) specify the exact structure of proteins, which then control the activities of the cells, and (3) specify RNA, which is required for protein synthesis.

Chromosomes

Genes are packed in linear order on chromosomes. **Chromosomes** are found in the nuclei of cells. In humans, normal somatic cells contain 46 chromosomes (**diploid** number), of which 44 are termed **autosomes** and 2 are **sex chromosomes.** Females have two X chromosomes (XX), and males have an X and a Y chromosome (XY). Gametes—eggs or sperm—contain 23 chromosomes (**haploid** number). In the zygote and somatic cells, chromosomes are paired (**homologs**). In each pair, one homolog is maternal and the other is paternal in origin. Each chromosomal pair has unique morphologic characteristics that allow it to be distinguished from other chromosomes, such as size, position of the centromere, and the unique banding pattern that is demonstrated by special staining techniques[11] (Figure 27-1).

To pass on the genetic information to daughter cells, the chromosomes must replicate and then

679

Box 27-1 GLOSSARY

Acrocentric chromosome Chromosomes with the centromere near the end of the chromosome.

Allele One of a series of alternate forms of a gene at the same locus.

Aneuploid Any chromosome number that is not an exact multiple of the haploid set.

Autosome A chromosome that is not a sex chromosome.

Centromere The primary constriction of a chromosome where the long and short arms meet.

Chromatid After replication of a chromosome, two subunits attached by the centromere can be seen; each is called a chromatid, and after separation each becomes a chromosome of a daughter cell.

Chromosome The microscopic structures in the cell nucleus composed of DNA and proteins that contain the genes.

Congenital Present at birth.

Dermatoglyphics The dermal ridge patterns on the digits, palms, and soles.

Diploid Two copies of all chromosomes; the number of chromosomes normally present in somatic cells. In humans, this is 46 and is sometimes symbolized as 2N.

Dominant A gene (allele) that is expressed clinically in the heterozygous state. In a dominant disorder the mutant allele overshadows the normal allele.

Dysmorphic Morphological abnormality, often a minor physical finding that may or may not have any cosmetic or functional significance and is present in less than 4% of the newborn population.

Fluorescent in situ hybridization (FISH) Molecular cytogenetic method for detection of microdeletions of chromosomes.

Gamete Mature reproductive cell, the egg or the sperm, containing the haploid number of chromosomes.

Gene The functional unit of heredity.

Genotype A person's genetic constitution.

Haploid One copy of all chromosomes; the number of chromosomes present in the gamete; in humans this is 23 and can be symbolized as N.

Hemizygous The condition in which only one copy of a gene is normally present, and so its effect is expressed because there is no counterpart gene present; e.g., the genes on the X or Y chromosome of the male.

Heterozygote An individual who has two different alleles at a given locus of two homologous chromosomes.

Homologous chromosomes Members of the same chromosome pair; normally they have the same number and arrangement of genes.

Homozygote An individual who has two identical alleles at a given locus of two homologous chromosomes.

Karyotype The standard pictorial arrangement of chromosome pairs, numbered according to centromere position and length.

Locus The position or place that a gene occupies on a chromosome.

Malformation A primary structural defect that results from a localized error of morphogenesis; abnormal development.

Metacentric chromosome Chromosomes with the centromere in the center of the chromosome.

Monosomy When one chromosome of one pair is missing.

Mosaicism Presence in the same individual of two or more different chromosomal constitutions.

Mutation A heritable alteration in the genetic material.

Nondisjunction Failure of two homologous chromosomes to separate equally during cell division into two daughter cells, resulting in abnormal chromosome numbers in gametes or somatic cells.

Phenotype The observable expression of traits either physically or biochemically.

Recessive A gene (allele) that is expressed clinically in the homozygous state. In a recessive disorder, both genes at a given locus must be abnormal to manifest the disorder.

Sex chromosomes The X and Y chromosomes.

Syndrome Recognizable pattern of multiple malformations that occur together and have the same cause.

Transcription The process by which complementary messenger RNA is synthesized from a DNA template.

Translation The process whereby the amino acids in a given polypeptide are synthesized from the messenger RNA template.

Translocation Transfer of all or part of a chromosome to another location (i.e., on the same or another chromosome) after chromosome breakage.

Trisomy The presence of three homologous chromosomes rather than the normal two.

X-linked A gene located on an X chromosome.

Zygote A fertilized egg that develops into an embryo.

---

divide correctly. Somatic cells undergo **mitosis,** in which cells replicate and then divide chromosomal material into two genetically identical daughter cells with 46 chromosomes each. In gametes, the process is known as **meiosis,** which is different from mitotic division in that daughter cells contain the haploid number of chromosomes (23) and crossing over or recombination between two homologues occurs, thus facilitating genetic variation in offspring.[32]

An individual's chromosome constitution can be determined by examining dividing body cells under certain laboratory conditions from any accessible

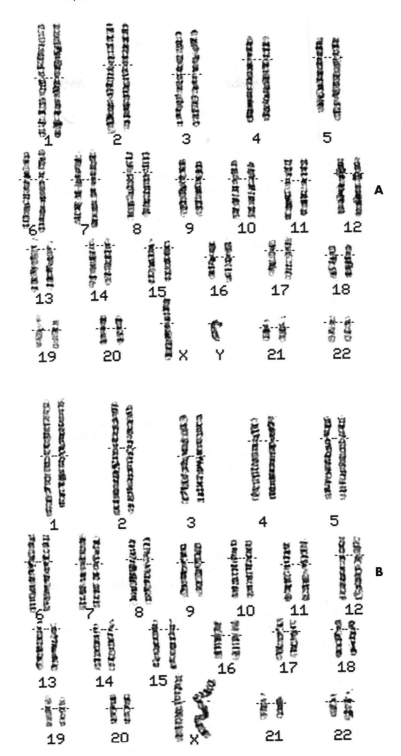

FIGURE 27-1   **A,** Normal male karyotype. **B,** Normal female karyotype. Each karyotype contains 46 chromosomes (44 autosomes and 2 sex chromosomes, XY, male; XX, female). The autosomes are numbered from 1 to 22. Note banding pattern, unique for each chromosomal pair. (Courtesy Cytogenetics, The Children's Hospital, Denver, Colo.)

tissue such as blood lymphocytes or skin fibroblasts. The resulting **karyotype** (see Figure 27-1), or pictorial arrangement, demonstrates the number and structure of that individual's chromosomes.

ETIOLOGY

Malformations and genetic disorders caused wholly or partly by genetic factors can be categorized into four major areas: (1) chromosomal disorders caused by numeric or structural abnormalities of chromosomes; (2) single-gene or mendelian disorders, which are secondary to single-gene mutations; (3) complex or multifactorial disorders resulting from interaction of genes and environmental influences; and (4) abnormalities caused by environmental exposures of the fetus during development.

More recently, better understanding of molecular processes has allowed the identification of additional genetic mechanisms contributing to genetic disorders: germline mosaicism, genomic imprinting, and uniparental disomy.

Chromosomal Disorders

Chromosomal abnormalities are relatively common. Approximately 0.5% to 0.7% of all live newborns have a chromosomal abnormality and 4% to 7% of perinatal deaths result from a chromosomal abnormality. Moreover, it is estimated that at least 50% of all recognized first-trimester miscarriages are caused by a chromosomal aberration.[15] Current cytogenetic techniques, such as high-resolution banding, fluorescence in situ hybridization, and other molecular genetic approaches, have increased the detection rate of chromosomal aberrations. Submicroscopic deletions, duplications, or other abnormal rearrangements of chromosome material that may not have been identified a few years ago are now being detected in children with congenital malformations and/or mental retardation.

Chromosomal aberrations should be suspected in any of the following situations:
- **Small for gestational age for weight, length, and/or head circumference**
- **Presence of one or more congenital malformations**
- **Presence of dysmorphic features**
- **Neurologic/neuromuscular dysfunction**
- **Family history of multiple miscarriages or siblings with mental retardation or birth defects along with one of the above**

Chromosomal abnormalities can be classified into two major categories: abnormalities of chromosome number **(aneuploidy),** in which there is an extra or missing chromosome, and abnormalities of chromosome structure that result in the loss or duplication of part of the chromosomal material. Abnormalities of autosomes usually have more significant deleterious effects on the development of the infant than those seen with sex chromosome abnormalities.

Abnormalities of Chromosome Number

Numeric chromosomal abnormalities occur as a result of nondisjunction in which aberrant segregation leads to loss or gain of one or more chromosomes. Nondisjunction can occur during either meiosis or mitosis, resulting in an abnormal gamete (egg or sperm) or abnormal somatic cell, respectively (Figure 27-2). Fertilization of an aneuploid gamete by a normal gamete produces a zygote with an extra chromosome **(trisomy)** or missing chromosome **(monosomy).** Aneuploidy in somatic cells results in chromosomal **mosaicism** (i.e., the presence of some cells with the normal number of chromosomes and other cells with an abnormal number of chromosomes) (Figure 27-3). Although nondisjunction may affect any chromosomal pair, the most commonly recognized trisomies in liveborns are trisomy 21 (Down syndrome), trisomy 18 (Edward syndrome), and trisomy 13 (Patau syndrome). On the other hand, trisomy 16 has been found exclusively in spontaneous abortions.[15] The most common monosomy is 45,X, Turner syndrome. **As a rule, numeric chromosomal abnormalities are associated with IUGR, dysmorphic features, malformations, and mental retardation. Physical abnormalities may be milder or absent in the newborn with mosaicism.**

Abnormalities of Chromosome Structure

Structural abnormalities have been described in all chromosomes. These include deletions, translocations, duplications, and inversions (Figure 27-4). A **deletion** is a loss of chromosome material and results in partial monosomy for the chromosome involved. Loss of material from the end of a chromosome is known as a **terminal deletion,** as seen in 5p–, cri du chat syndrome. An **interstitial deletion** involves a loss of chromosomal material that does not include the ends of the chromosome. A terminal deletion of both arms of a chromosome may result in reattachment of the remaining arms, leading to a

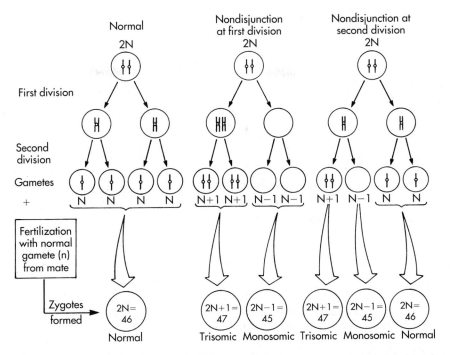

FIGURE 27-2   Nondisjunction. During formation of gametes, errors of nondisjunction can occur during either first or second meiotic division.

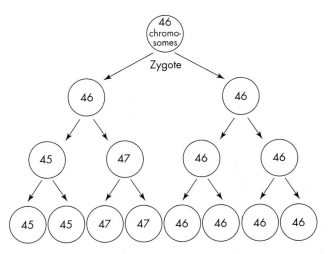

FIGURE 27-3   Mosaicism. Nondisjunction occurring after fertilization and zygote formation results in some cells containing the normal 46-chromosome complement and other cells having an abnormal number of chromosomes.

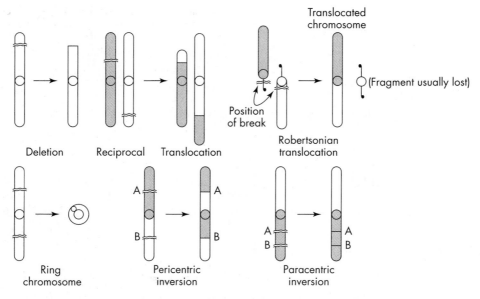

FIGURE 27-4 Schematic example of structural chromosomal abnormalities. (From Hathaway WE et al, eds: *Current pediatric diagnosis and treatment,* ed 10, Norwalk, Conn, 1991, Appleton & Lange.)

formation of a **ring** chromosome. Presence of additional chromosome material results in **duplication** or partial trisomy of a chromosome. **Translocation** is the detachment of a chromosome segment from its normal location and its attachment to another chromosome. The translocation is **balanced** if the cell contains two complete copies of all chromosomal material, although in different order. In an **unbalanced** translocation the rearrangement results in partial trisomy or monosomy.

Translocations can be reciprocal or Robertsonian. A reciprocal translocation involves exchange of segments between two chromosomes (e.g., part of the short arm of the chromosome 4 trades a place with a part of chromosome 10). Robertsonian translocations involve two acrocentric chromosomes fused at their centromeres. The most frequent Robertsonian translocation is formed between chromosomes 14 and 21.[21]

Inversions are the result of a double break in a single chromosome and reinsertion of the chromosomal material that has been inverted. Inversions are either **pericentric** (including the centromere) or **paracentric** (without the centromere). The most common inversion is a small pericentric inversion of chromosome 9, which is considered to be a normal variant, found in approximately 1% of the general population.[32] All other inversions may produce gametes that result in an individual with an unbalanced rearrangement (i.e., having both a duplication and a deletion of some chromosome material, such as that seen in recombinant 8 syndrome).

Microdeletions and Syndromes

At times, structural chromosomal abnormalities are submicroscopic and therefore cannot be detected by conventional cytogenetic techniques. **Fluorescent in situ hybridization (FISH) is a molecular cytogenetic method that facilitates the detection of microdeletions.** FISH utilizes segments of fluorescently labeled DNA called *probes,* constructed so that each probe can attach only to a specific segment of a chromosome, which then will be fluorescent during a microscopic visualization. In the case of deletion of that chromosome segment, the probe cannot attach to the chromosome; thus the fluorescent segment is missing from the deleted chromosome.[37]

Microdeletions result in phenotypic abnormalities. There are a number of well recognized microdeletion syndromes that may be suspected in the NICU. **Prader-Willi syndrome,** caused by an interstitial deletion of chromosome 15 (q11q13), usually presents in a newborn as severe hypotonia, feeding difficulties, and micropenis or hypoplastic labia.[22] **Williams syndrome** is caused by an interstitial deletion or mutation of the elastin gene (ELN) on the long arm of chromosome 7 (7q11).[31] The condition is often first seen in an affected newborn in the postterm period; the infant is small for family size. There may be a congenital heart defect, in particular, supravalvular aortic stenosis or peripheral pulmonic stenosis; hypotonia; failure to thrive with gastroesophageal reflux; poor suck and swallow; and vomiting and irritability or colic. Infantile hypercalcemia is seen in approximately 20% of these infants. There may be subtle dysmorphic facial features noted in the newborn.[31]

One of the most commonly seen microdeletion syndromes is velocardiofacial syndrome (VCFS), which is characterized by cleft palate or velopharyngeal insufficiency, hypernasal speech, learning disabilities, conotruncal heart defects, and characteristic facies. It actually represents one of a spectrum of clinical disorders all known to be caused by a deletion in chromosome 22q11 (del22q11). These include DiGeorge syndrome (DGS) (conotruncal heart defect, hypocalcemia, and thymic hypoplasia), and conotruncal anomaly face syndrome (CTAF) (conotruncal heart defects and typical facies). In addition, del22q11 has been found in 11% to 16% of nonsyndromic congenital conotruncal heart disease, and has been reported to present as apparently isolated neonatal hypocalcemia or learning problems.[12] Taken together, del22q11 has an estimated incidence of 1 in 2000 to 4000 newborns. The availability of molecular cytogenetic testing by FISH has led to appreciation of both the high incidence of the del22q11 as well as the increasing variety of clinical presentations that can be seen even within a single family.[25]

In the newborn period, the characteristic facial findings are seldom obvious. However, most affected individuals will manifest some of these findings by early childhood. Most prominent is the nose, which is described as long, with a "built up nasal bridge, squared off nasal root, and bulbous nasal tip."[25] The eyes appear narrow and slitlike, the mala (cheeks) are flat, and the jaw recessed. The ears are usually small and in some way abnormally formed. There may be an overt cleft of the secondary palate, a bifurcated uvula, a subtle submucosal cleft, or cleft lip with and without cleft palate. Other nonstructural palatal abnormalities can be seen, most commonly velopharyngeal insufficiency. In an older child or adult, this presents as hypernasal

speech; in a newborn, one sees excessive nasal regurgitation. Congenital heart disease is seen in 35% of del22q11 patients. The type of congenital heart disease (CHD) is fairly specific, and includes those lesions classified as "conotruncal heart defects" (truncus arteriosus, interrupted aortic arch, tetralogy of Fallot, left-sided aortic arch, vascular rings, and some types of ventricular septal defects [VSDs]). Furthermore, studies have shown del22q11 in 11% to 30% of nonsyndromic CHD. Perhaps the most consistent finding in patients of all age-groups is long, thin fingers and toes. Additional nonspecific findings include abundant scalp hair; hypospadias; renal abnormalities that can include renal agenesis; tortuous retinal vessels; ectopic/aberrant/unilateral absence of carotid and vertebral artery; microcephaly; and microdontia (there are 166 different findings to date).

Developmental delay, learning disabilities and/or mental retardation are common, and very variable. Behavioral and psychiatric problems are a common but underappreciated finding in VCFS. These individuals have a characteristic personality, marked by a flattened affect and abnormal social interaction, ranging from being intermittently withdrawn to socially precocious. A host of other psychiatric diagnoses have been seen in patients with VCFS.

Both DiGeorge syndrome and VCFS have been recognized as being caused by deletions in 22q11. More than 90% of cases of DGS and VCFS are deleted. DGS may also be caused by maternal diabetes, and has recently been shown to caused by deletions of 10p. There are a few cases of VCFS in which no 22q11 deletion can be detected. These are obviously the focus of intense research. Recent evidence suggests that the condition may in fact be caused by a single gene abnormality. Thus it is important to obtain family histories and examine parents for subtle features of the syndrome. In many cases the infant has inherited the abnormality from a parent.

Clinical Examples of Chromosomal Abnormalities

Down Syndrome. **Down syndrome has an incidence of approximately 1 in 600 live births. Approximately 95% of cases are caused by nondisjunction involving chromosome 21, 5% are caused by a translocation, and 1% are mosaic. Down syndrome may present with marked hypotonia; a number of major malformations, most commonly congenital heart defects, duodenal**

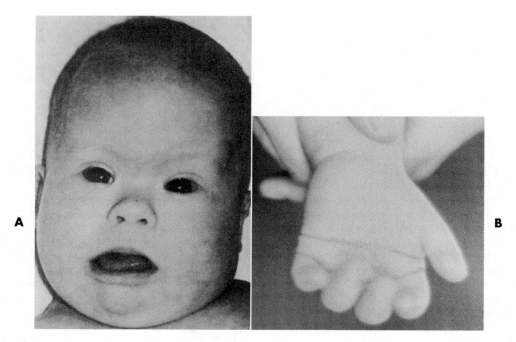

FIGURE 27-5   Infant with Down syndrome. **A,** Note midface hypoplasia, epicanthic folds, and depressed nasal bridge. **B,** Single palmar crease. (**A** from Gorlin RJ, Cohen MM, Levin LSW, eds: *Syndromes of the head and neck,* ed 3, New York, 1990, Oxford University Press; **B** courtesy Genetic Services, University of Colorado Health Sciences Center and The Children's Hospital, Denver, Colo.)

atresia, and tracheoesophageal fistula; and a characteristic pattern of dysmorphic features. The classic phenotype seen in Down syndrome includes a flattened occiput, midfacial hypoplasia, depressed nasal bridge, upward-slanting palpebral fissures, epicanthic folds, grayish speckling of the iris (Brushfield spots), micrognathia, excess nuchal skin, single palmar creases (simian creases), single flexion creases and in-curving of the fifth fingers (clinodactyly), and increased distance between the first and second toes (Figure 27-5).

In full-term infants with the classical phenotype of Down syndrome, the clinical diagnosis is not difficult. However, it is imperative that cytogenetic studies be done to confirm the diagnosis and to differentiate a nondisjunctional trisomy from a translocation. This distinction has important implications for recurrence risks (see discussion under Prevention). In premature infants the classical facial phenotype is frequently missing, making clinical diagnosis more difficult. The presence of an AV canal or duodenal atresia with minor malformations, such as abnormal dermatoglyphics, should alert the clinician to the possibility of Down syndrome.

Trisomy 18. **Trisomy 18 has an incidence of 1 in 6000 live births. The major phenotypic features include prenatal growth restriction, complex cardiac malformations, abnormal muscle tone, microcephaly, prominent occiput, low-set and malformed ears, corneal opacities, micrognathia, peculiar hand posturing with the second and fifth digits overlapping the third and fourth, hypoplasia of fingernails, abnormal dermatoglyphics, prominent calcanei, and deep plantar furrows between the first and second toes** (Figure 27-6). The prognosis is poor, and the majority of infants with trisomy 18 will die within the first few months of life. Infants who have survived into childhood are profoundly retarded.

Trisomy 13. **Trisomy 13 is seen in approximately 1 in 15,000 live births. Phenotypic features include prenatal and postnatal growth restriction, microcephaly, sloping forehead, coloboma of the iris, microphthalmia or anophthalmia, low-set or malformed ears, cleft lip and palate, postaxial polydactyly, and abnormal palmar creases and dermatoglyphics** (Figure 27-7). Internal abnormal-

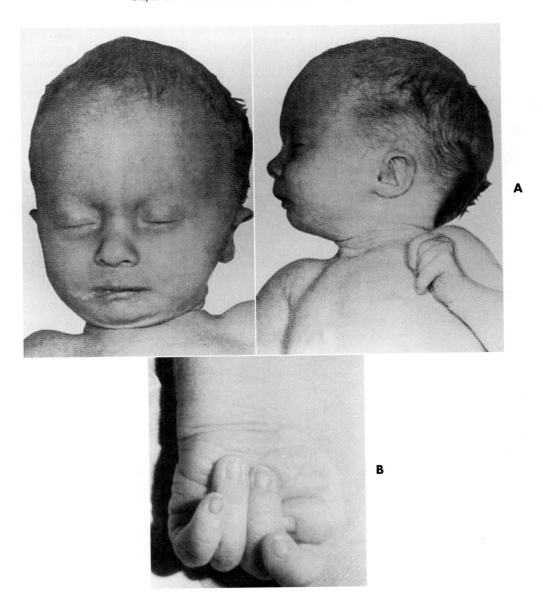

FIGURE 27-6   Infant with trisomy 18. **A,** Typical facies with small chin, abnormal pinna, and prominent occiput. **B,** Typical hand posturing with overlapping fingers. (**A** from Gorlin RJ, Cohen MM, Levin LSW, eds: *Syndromes of the head and neck,* ed 3, New York, 1990, Oxford University Press; **B** courtesy Genetic Services, University of Colorado Health Sciences Center and The Children's Hospital, Denver, Colo.)

ities may include a number of CNS malformations, such as holoprosencephaly, cardiac malformations, omphalocele, renal malformations, and urogenital abnormalities such as cryptorchidism in males and uterine malformations in females. The prognosis is extremely poor for these infants, with most dying within the first few months of life.

Turner Syndrome. **The only monosomy to be seen in live births is that of Turner syndrome—females with a 45,X karyotype.** Additionally, it is the only numeric abnormality of the sex chromosome that may be identifiable at birth. **Turner syndrome has an incidence of 1 in 5000 female births.**[34] **Clinical features that may be evident in**

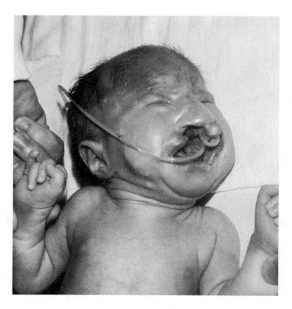

FIGURE 27-7   Infant with trisomy 13. Facial clefts and micro-cephaly; abnormal positioning of the hands. (From Hathaway WE, Groothuis J, Hay W et al, eds: *Current pediatric diagnoses and treatment,* ed 10, Norwalk, Conn, 1991, Appleton & Lange.)

the newborn period are a short, webbed neck or redundant skin on the back of the neck and marked lymphedema of the dorsum of the hands and feet (Figure 27-8). Congenital heart defects are seen in approximately half the patients, with 30% having a coarctation of the aorta. Renal anomalies may also be present.[22] Prognosis is usually excellent but depends on the presence and severity of the congenital heart defect. Intelligence is normal; however, some females with Turner syndrome have been noted to have problems with spatial perception or fine motor abilities.[34]

Cri du Chat. **Cri du chat, or cat cry syndrome, is the result of loss of the terminal end of the short arm of chromosome 5 (5p–).** The name of the syndrome reflects the unusual catlike, weak cry these infants have in the neonatal period. These infants are usually small for gestational age, hypotonic, and microcephalic, and may have ocular hypertelorism, epicanthic folds, downward slant of the palpebral fissures, low-set ears, and micrognathia. They are significantly mentally retarded.

San Luis Valley Syndrome. **Recombinant 8, or the San Luis Valley syndrome, named for the area in**

which many of these individuals were first identified, is an example of an unbalanced pericentric inversion with both a duplication and a deletion of chromosome 8 material. The pericentric inversion of chromosome 8 found in a parent and other relatives of a child with recombinant 8 syndrome has no phenotypic consequence because it is a balanced rearrangement. However, a carrier is at risk for producing unbalanced gametes during meiosis. In recombinant 8 syndrome, there is a deletion of chromosomal material of the short arm of chromosome 8 and a duplication of chromosome material of the long arm of 8. The phenotype is characterized by unusual facial features, including a wide face, depressed nasal bridge, hypertelorism, down slanting palpebral fissures, upturned nose, long philtrum, low-set and malformed ears, cleft lip and/or cleft palate, congenital heart disease, and renal abnormalities.[36]

Prevention
The identification of chromosomal abnormalities in the newborn is important not only for management issues regarding the infant, but also because of the recurrence risks the abnormality carries for the family. In general, numeric chromosomal abnormalities carry low recurrence risks (approximately 1% to 2%).[15] In the presence of structural abnormalities, recurrence risks depend on whether one of the parents carries a balanced rearrangement. If parental chromosomes are normal, the recurrence risk is minimal. However, if a parent carries a balanced chromosomal rearrangement, the recurrence risk is significantly increased. The exact risk figure will vary with the nature of the specific chromosomal rearrangement and in some cases the sex of the carrier parent. In either situation, for parents and families concerned about recurrence risk, prenatal diagnosis for chromosome analysis is available.

Single-Gene Disorders
McKusick's online catalog of mendelian inherited disorders currently lists more than 10,000 entries with approximately 6000 single-gene disorders with known patterns of inheritance.[33] Many of these disorders are singularly rare; however, collectively, they affect about 1% of the population. Single-gene disorders are the result of either a single or double dose of an abnormal gene. Single-gene disorders are classified as autosomal dominant, autosomal recessive, X-linked dominant, and X-linked recessive. Humans have two copies of each gene located at identical places (gene **loci**) on homologous chromo-

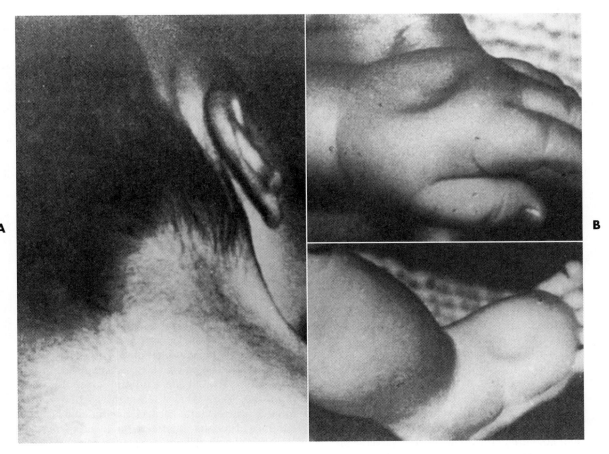

FIGURE 27-8   Female infant with Turner syndrome. **A,** Webbed neck with low posterior hairline. **B,** Lymphedema of the dorsal surfaces of the hands and feet. (From Knuppel R, Drukker JD, eds: *High risk pregnancy: a team approach,* Philadelphia, 1988, WB Saunders.)

somes. In a single-gene disorder, an abnormal or mutated **allele** (an alternate form of a gene) is found on one or both members of a pair of chromosomes.[32] Individuals with identical alleles at a particular locus are **homozygous** for the gene. Individuals with different alleles are **heterozygous** for the gene. Because males have only one X chromosome, and most genes located on the Y chromosome do not correspond to those located on the X, males are **hemizygous** for the genes on the X chromosome. Abnormal genes located on one of the 44 autosomes are the cause of **autosomal disorders:** disease-causing genes located on the X chromosome are the cause of **X-linked disorders.** Disorders are **dominant** when the phenotype is expressed in the presence of only one copy of the mutated gene. In **recessive** disorders

the phenotype is expressed only when both the chromosomes carry the mutated gene.

Autosomal Dominant Disorders

Autosomal dominant disorders are ones in which the disorder is expressed in the heterozygous state. Major characteristics include (1) multiple generations affected (i.e., an infant would have an affected parent), (2) both males and females are affected and both sexes can transmit the disorder to their offspring (i.e., male-to-male transmission can occur), (3) there is a 50% risk for each offspring to inherit the gene from an affected parent, and (4) individuals who do not have the gene cannot transmit the disorder to their offspring.

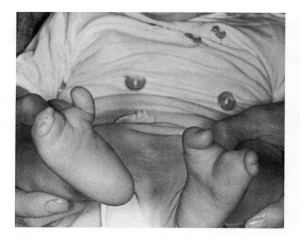

FIGURE 27-9 Ectrodactyly (lobster claw deformity) of the feet. (Courtesy Genetic Services, University of Colorado Health Sciences Center and The Children's Hospital, Denver, Colo.)

A negative family history does not rule out the presence of an autosomal dominant disorder. Possible explanations for a negative family history are (1) the infant's disorder is a result of a new mutation, (2) a parent has a very mild expression of the disorder and may not have been previously diagnosed, (3) nonpaternity, (4) decreased penetrance (i.e., not all individuals with the gene have phenotypic abnormalities [skipped generation]), and (5) germline mosaicism for the mutation (see the section on nontraditional inheritance).

Dominant disorders that may be seen in the NICU include skeletal dysplasias, such as achondroplasia (abnormality in the FGFR3 gene), osteogenesis imperfecta (abnormality in COL1A1 or COL1A2), Apert and Crouzon syndromes (abnormality in the FGFR2 gene), Treacher Collins' syndrome (abnormality in Treacle gene), and ectrodactyly (Figure 27-9).[3]

Autosomal Recessive Disorders
Autosomal recessive disorders are expressed only in the homozygous state. Thus, to be affected, an individual usually inherits an abnormal gene from each parent. The parent who is heterozygous for a disease causing gene is usually phenotypically normal and is called a carrier. **Major characteristics of autosomal recessive inheritance include (1) phenotypically normal parents, (2) affected siblings, (3) both males and females affected, (4)** offspring of two carrier parents are at a 25% risk of being affected, (5) unaffected siblings have a two-thirds chance of being carriers, and (6) there may be an increased incidence of consanguinity (mating between blood relatives). Autosomal recessive disorders that may be identified in the neonatal period include many of the metabolic disorders such as phenylketonuria (PKU), galactosemia, and isovaleric acidemia; as well as some of the multiple-malformation syndromes (such as Meckel-Gruber syndrome), cystic fibrosis presenting with meconium ileus, Zellweger (cerebrohepatorenal) syndrome (Figure 27-10), and skeletal dysplasias such as achondrogenesis. The specific gene or biochemical defect for most of these disorders is now known.

X-Linked Disorders
X-linked disorders are caused by an abnormal gene (or genes) located on the X chromosome. Most X-linked disorders are recessive. The X-linked recessive disorders are phenotypically expressed in hemizygous males; heterozygous females are generally phenotypically normal and are referred to as carriers. Affected fathers do not have affected sons (no male-to-male transmission); however, all daughters of affected males are carriers. A carrier female has a 50% chance of having an affected male offspring.

Occasionally there may be heterozygous females who are phenotypically affected, although usually less severely than males. If females are severely affected, other mechanisms, including homozygosity for the X-linked gene, may be responsible for the phenotype. X-linked recessive disorders that may be recognizable in the newborn period include factor VIII and IX deficiency (classical hemophilia A and B), X-linked hydrocephalus, and Opitz syndrome.

X-linked dominant disorders occur when the abnormal gene located on the X chromosome is expressed in both the hemizygous and heterozygous states. As in X-linked recessive conditions, there is no male-to-male transmission, because the affected male passes his Y chromosome and not his X chromosome to his sons; however, all of the daughters of an affected male will inherit his X chromosome and thus be affected. Each son and daughter of an affected female has a 50% risk of being affected; males are usually more severely affected than females. There are only a few disorders that are known to be inherited as an

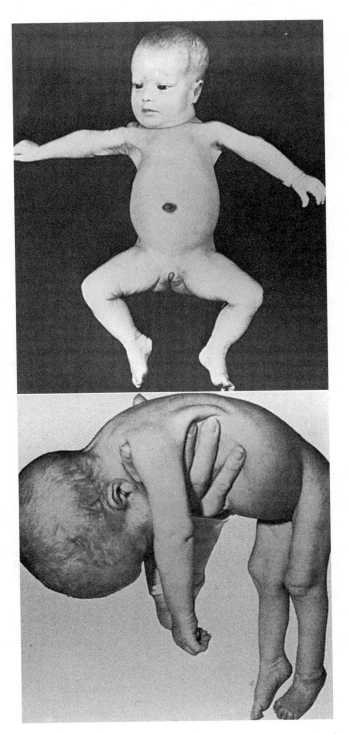

FIGURE 27-10   Infant with Zellweger syndrome, an autosomal recessive disorder. Note the high forehead, narrow facies, and extreme hypotonia. (From Gorlin RJ, Cohen MM, Levin, LS, eds: *Syndromes of the head and neck,* ed 3, New York, 1990, Oxford University Press.)

X-linked dominant, such as incontinetia pigmenti, hypophosphatemia (vitamin D–resistant rickets), and ornithine transcarbamylase (OTC) deficiency. Early diagnosis of OTC is important because, if untreated, it leads to neonatal hyperammonemia and death in affected males. In affected females the clinical picture can be variable, ranging from an asymptomatic infant to one who presents in the first week of life with lethargy, vomiting, and protein avoidance, ending in seizures and coma.

Complex/Multifactorial Disorders

Complex, common nonmendelian disorders, often called *multifactorial disorders*, are the result of both environmental and genetic factors.[20] Most isolated single malformations, including congenital heart defects, neural tube defects, cleft lip and palate, pyloric stenosis, and club feet, are inherited in this manner. Additionally, the more complex, common familial disorders, such as diabetes mellitus, coronary artery disease, affective disorders, and mild mental retardation, are the result of multifactorial inheritance. In contrast to single-gene inheritance, multifactorial disorders recur within families without a characteristic pedigree pattern, and recurrence risks are based on empiric data.[32]

Multifactorial inheritance is explained as a liability model with a threshold effect.[20] The general population as a whole has an underlying genetic predisposition for multifactorial traits and disorders that follow a normal distribution curve; only in those individuals in whom the genetic predisposition exceeds the threshold will the malformation actually be expressed (Figure 27-11).

Major characteristics of complex/multifactorial inheritance include (1) no consistent pedigree pattern between families (i.e., there may be only an isolated occurrence, or the disorder may be seen among siblings, in multiple generations, or scattered throughout the family); and (2) recurrence risks are not constant, as in single-gene disorders, but are influenced by a number of factors. These factors include (1) the number of family members affected (i.e., the more family members affected, the higher the recurrence risk becomes); (2) the degree of relatedness to those affected— first-degree relatives are at higher recurrence risk than second- or third-degree relatives; (3) the severity of the defect—the more severely affected an individual is, the higher the recurrence risk; (4) the frequency of the disorder, which may vary with eth-

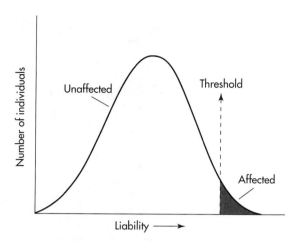

FIGURE 27-11   Multifactorial inheritance. Liability curve with a threshold beyond which the trait is expressed.

nic background (e.g., neural tube defects have a higher incidence among English and Irish populations); and (5) the sex of the individual (for disorders in which one sex is more commonly affected than the other [e.g., pyloric stenosis is more common in males]; if the less commonly affected sex has the defect, then the recurrence risk is higher).

Nontraditional Inheritance
Germline Mosaicism
Spectacular growth in the field of molecular genetics and its technologies in only the past few years has enabled the clarification of the inheritance patterns of many genetic disorders and birth defects that were previously unknown or unclear. For example, the lethal form of osteogenesis imperfecta (OI) occurring in multiple offspring of unaffected parents was thought to be the result of autosomal recessive inheritance. However, improved molecular techniques have documented it to be the result of **germline mosaicism, that is, the mutation occurs in the gonad of one of the parents, who then has some gametes with and others without the OI mutation. This distinction alters the recurrence risks and is very important for genetic counseling.[17]**

Genomic Imprinting
In the past little notice was given to whether the sex of the parent that transmitted an abnormal gene to offspring had any effect on the expression of genes. It is now recognized that **maternally and pater-**

nally derived genes may function differently, and this is called genomic imprinting.[18] For example, offspring who inherit the gene for Huntington's disease (autosomal dominant) from an affected father are more likely to have childhood onset of the disease than if they inherited the maternal gene.

Uniparental Disomy
Uniparental disomy is the result of inheriting both copies of a chromosome from one parent and none from the other.[18] It is assumed that for normal growth and development, a child must receive both maternal and paternal genes; if both copies of a gene originate only from one parent, the development is abnormal. Uniparental disomy has been seen in cystic fibrosis with short stature, and in the Prader-Willi, Angelman, and Beckwith-Wiedemann syndromes. The parental origin of a child's chromosomes can be identified only by molecular analysis; routine chromosome analysis is usually not helpful.

The possibility of a nontraditional pattern of inheritance makes genetic counseling more complex than previously thought. Thus it is imperative that health care providers be aware of such complexities and refer families to a geneticist or genetic counselor for a more detailed discussion when appropriate.

Inborn Errors of Metabolism
Genetic disorders in which defects of single genes cause clinically significant blocks in metabolic pathways are known as inborn errors of metabolism. The recognition of disorders caused by inborn errors of metabolism has increased rapidly in recent years, and they are now recognized as important causes of disease in the newborn and pediatric age-group.[16] Inborn errors of metabolism include defects of carbohydrate metabolism, amino acid metabolism, organic acid metabolism, and purine metabolism; disorders of fatty acid oxidation; lysosomal storage diseases; and disorders of peroxisomes. It is important to remember that inborn errors can present at any time and may affect almost any organ system. Specific disorders that need to be considered in symptomatic newborns include galactosemia, ornithine transcarbamylase deficiency (OTC), or carbamoyl-phosphate synthetase (CPS) deficiency, maple syrup urine disease, nonketotic hyperglycinemia, propionic and methylmalonic acidemias, isovaleric acidemia, and glutaric acidemia type II.[16]

Although the majority of infants will not be found to have an inborn error of metabolism as the etiology of their illness, early recognition is imperative and may be considered a medical emergency if appropriate treatment is to be initiated. Many of these disorders can be effectively treated and if untreated are lethal in the newborn period. Moreover, without the appropriate diagnosis, parents would not be aware of recurrence risks in future offspring.

Inborn errors of metabolism should be included in the differential diagnosis of any critically ill newborn in the following instances: (1) suspicion of neonatal sepsis; (2) recurrent vomiting and/or altered consciousness; (3) clinical findings of hypoglycemia, seizures, parenchymal liver disease, unusual odor, hyperammonemia, or unexplained acidosis; and/or (4) a family history of a sibling affected with similar symptoms, mental retardation, or SIDS.[16]

In general, laboratory analysis will depend on the presenting symptoms seen in the newborn. Laboratory studies that should be obtained before any treatment is begun are electrolytes, ammonia, glucose, urine pH, urine-reducing substances, and urine ketones. Clues to suspecting an inborn error are (1) hypoglycemia and ketonuria in the newborn, (2) acidosis with recurrent vomiting and hyperammonemia, and (3) acidosis that is difficult to correct and is out of proportion to the clinical state. If other etiologies are not readily apparent, additional laboratory tests that may be appropriate are serum and urine amino acids and urine organic acids.[39] Moreover, molecular (DNA) testing is available for several disorders.[26]

Newborn Screening
Inborn errors of metabolism, when unrecognized and untreated, may lead to severe consequences, including mental retardation and death in some instances. Thus the goal is to identify, treat, and prevent major sequelae whenever possible. Newborn screening accomplishes this goal for a small number of disorders. Screening criteria that should be met are relatively high frequency of the disorder, severity of symptomatology in untreated individuals, availability of treatment, simplicity of obtaining tissue for testing, and availability of a simple screening test with high sensitivity and specificity and reasonable cost. Screening for metabolic disorders are mandated by individual states. All states require screening for phenylketonuria (PKU) and hypothyroidism. Additional disorders screened that may be screened for include homocystinuria, maple syrup urine disease,

biotinidase deficiency, and galactosemia, hemoglobinopathies, and cystic fibrosis. Each state decides individually what will be included in the newborn screening program. **Any screening test may give both false-positive and false-negative results. Thus a positive screen must be followed by a confirmatory diagnostic test.**[1] **Moreover, if there is clinical suspicion of a particular disorder in spite of a negative screening result, further diagnostic testing is warranted.** (For an in-depth review of those disorders that may be part of the newborn screening program, refer to the American Academy of Pediatrics Newborn Screening Fact Sheets.[1])

Newborn Hearing Screening. **Newborn hearing screening tests are now available that have high sensitivity when administered properly.**[5] **Hearing loss is present in approximately 1 to 2 per 1000 infants.** Research has demonstrated that there are both genetic and nongenetic causes of deafness. **Sixty percent of prelingual deafness has a recognizable genetic etiology, and of these, the most common cause of autosomal recessively inherited nonsyndromic hearing loss is due to mutations in the connexin 26 (Cx26) gene, a member of the connexin family of gap junction proteins.**[41] **Commercial DNA-based screening tests are now available to detect common genetic forms of deafness including Cx26 and mitochondrial deafness.**[4] The American Academy of Pediatrics has recommended that all newborns be screened for hearing loss before the age of 3 months.[2] The American College of Medical Genetics has recommended, in addition to screening and subsequent confirmation of hearing loss by diagnostic tests, that protocols be developed to ensure that appropriate genetic counseling be provided if diagnostic testing includes genetic testing.[4] This would provide families with accurate information regarding causes and recurrence risks for parents, siblings, and other family members.

Environmental Causes

Environmental exposures may have adverse effects on fetal development (teratogenic effect) resulting in malformations and functional, neurodevelopmental abnormalities in infants and children. There are four major prerequisites needed for teratogenic action, as follows[19]:

1. The agent must have the potential to be teratogenic. There are few conclusive data available regarding the teratogenicity of most chemicals and drugs in humans. Animal studies provide most of the currently available data on the teratogenicity of agents; however, not all are always applicable to human situations. To prove that an agent is teratogenic, a causal relationship between the exposure and presence of a malformation must be documented; just the history of an exposure to an agent is not sufficient. **Although very few agents have been documented to be teratogenic in humans, a few stand out, such as alcohol, cocaine, anticonvulsants, and isotretinoin (Accutane) (Figure 27-12).**

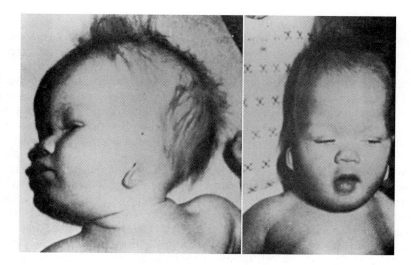

FIGURE 27-12 Infant exposed to Accutane in utero. Note dysmorphic face and auricles with atretic ear canal. (Courtesy Genetic Services, University of Colorado Health Sciences Center and The Children's Hospital, Denver, Colo.)

2. The timing of the exposure during pregnancy is of major importance. For the agent to adversely affect the fetus, it must be present during organogenesis and/or histogenesis. Exposures occurring within the first 2 weeks postconception, before cell differentiation, will cause no damage or will result in fetal wastage; exposures occurring from 2 to 12 weeks of gestation (period of organogenesis) may result in major malformations; after completion of development of the major organ systems, harmful exposures usually do not result in malformations but can be responsible for organ dysfunction. However, some agents may morphologically disrupt previously intact organs.[8] On the other hand, it has been shown that if the harmful exposure to an agent such as alcohol has been discontinued, the damage is less severe than if the exposure continues throughout the pregnancy.

3. Dosage of the teratogen is related to the severity of the teratogenic effect; the higher the dose, the more severe the effect and the higher the frequency of affected fetuses.

4. Finally, genetic makeup or genetic susceptibility of the mother and fetus may affect the metabolism as well as tissue sensitivity to the teratogen.

Teratogenic agents may be divided into four categories: (1) infectious agents, (2) chemical agents (drugs and environmental agents), (3) radiation, and (4) maternal factors. Chapter 2 provides excellent overviews of most of these exposures.

Traditionally, only maternal exposures to teratogens have been implicated in malformations. There has been a concern that some paternal exposures also may be teratogenic. Theoretically, a teratogen excreted in the semen could be introduced into the fetal environment and could be potentially teratogenic to the developing fetus.[9]

Teratogenic exposures should be considered in the differential diagnosis of congenital malformations and CNS dysfunction if one can document fetal exposure and the phenotype is compatible with the known effects of the suspected teratogen. The recognition of exposures is important for genetic counseling; if they can be avoided during subsequent pregnancies, recurrence risk is not increased. Frequently there is phenotypic overlap between the fetal abnormalities caused by specific teratogens and other syndromes. The family should be referred to a genetics clinic to rule out chromosomal, single-gene, and sporadic syndromes with overlapping phenotypes.

DATA COLLECTION

A genetic evaluation consists of the same components found in any medical evaluation; however, the emphasis may be different. Moreover, to make an accurate diagnosis and assessment, medical information regarding extended family members may need to be obtained. There is an excellent overview of the evaluation of the neonate with single or multiple congenital anomalies published by the American College of Medical Genetics and available at their website.[4]

History

Prenatal and perinatal histories, from a genetic standpoint, need to elicit information regarding potential teratogenic exposures including maternal disease and acute illness. Fetal growth and behavior (e.g., fetal movement and swallowing) provide important clues for the assessment of fetal neuromuscular function. Thus information regarding fetal position, movement, and amount of amniotic fluid should be obtained. Perinatal history should include the duration of gestation, anthropometric birth measurements, including head circumference, and information regarding perinatal adaptation. In a newborn with abnormal CNS functioning, it may be difficult to differentiate between primary maldevelopment and dysfunction caused by perinatal complications. An abnormal newborn with a genetic disorder may present with symptoms suggestive of birth asphyxia (i.e., hypoxia, acidosis, hypotonia, seizures). Moreover, **because many a priori abnormal newborns have an increased frequency of perinatal complications, a documented birth injury does not rule out the presence of a genetic cause.**

Family history may be extremely helpful in clarifying the causes and risk of recurrence. The information obtained from the parents may need to be complemented by physical examination of the parents and other family members and review of the medical records. This may be necessary because parents may not be aware that different defects in family members may be an expression of the same disorder. For example, an autosomal dominant gene may cause mild hypoplasia of thumbs in one family member and complete absence of thumb and radii in another.

Physical Examination

A physical examination should enable the examiner to detect major and minor malformations (dysmorphic features). Minor malformations are defined as structural variations found in less than 4% of the general population and having no significant medical or cosmetic effect. This is in contrast to structural variations that are found in more than 4% of the newborn population and represent a normal variation, such as a mongolian spot and capillary hemangioma on the forehead. **Minor malformations may provide important clues to the identification of a specific syndrome. None of the minor malformations as an isolated finding are clinically significant; however, a combination or pattern of minor malformations may indicate a specific disorder.** For example, dysmorphic features such as up-slanted eyes, epicanthic folds, hypertelorism (Figure 27-13), and abnormal dermatoglyphic pattern (Figure 27-14) in an infant with a congenital heart defect, are suggestive of Down syndrome. Minor malformations may also alert the clinician to the presence of major malformations. For example, preauricular ear tags are associated with an increased frequency of inner ear malformations and hearing loss. Additionally, the greater the number of minor malformations an infant has, the higher the chance of finding one or more major malformations.[28]

If minor malformations are identified, the parents of the infant should be examined. Presence of the same minor malformation in one of the parents may indicate a benign familial feature. Alternatively, finding the same dysmorphic features in other family members may represent an inherited genetic disorder. A mild syndactyly between second and third toes is frequently an isolated, inherited finding without clinical significance. However, syndactyly associated with craniosynostosis may represent an autosomal dominant disorder with variable expression and significant clinical sequelae.

If an infant looks dysmorphic, documentation of specific features should be recorded. Actual measurements compared with age-related norms should be used to measure body proportions, length of extremities, and such facial features as distance between eyes, length of eye fissures, size of ears, and length of philtrum. Description of the other features, such as the shape of the neck (webbed) or the chest size (widely spaced nipples), or a specific description of any skin lesions as to size, shape, lo-

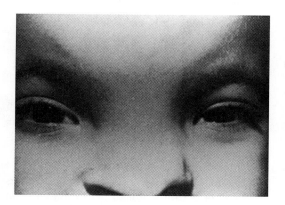

FIGURE 27-13 Dysmorphic feature of hypertelorism. Note wide-spaced eyes. (From Aase JM: *Diagnostic dysmorphology,* New York, 1991, Plenum Press.)

cation, and color (hyperpigmented or hypopigmented), may provide important clues for a specific diagnosis. Dermatoglyphic analysis, the analysis of the dermal ridges on the digits, palms, and soles, may prove useful for the timing of a fetal insult.[40] Development of ridges begins during the thirteenth week of gestation and is complete by the nineteenth week. Thus many chromosomal and genetic disorders will have disruptions of the dermal ridge patterns. For example, an infant with Down syndrome may have a single palmar crease (simian crease), a single flexion crease of the fifth digit, and an open field pattern (arch tibial) on the hallucal area of the foot.[40] Moreover, specific descriptors, or even more useful, photographs, should be used to describe dysmorphic findings. Photographs are particularly important if the infant is critically ill and the constellation of findings does not immediately suggest a specific syndrome. Thus the patient's findings may be more accurately shared with other clinicians in the future.

Smith's Recognizable Patterns of Human Malformations[22] **and other texts document a large number of syndromes, some of which are quite rare and may not be immediately recognized by neonatal staff. It may be helpful and important to consult a clinician who is familiar with dysmorphology and syndromology to help establish a diagnosis.**

Laboratory Data

When a genetic disorder is suspected, a number of diagnostic studies may be useful in delineat-

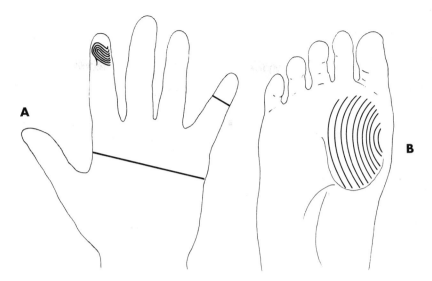

FIGURE 27-14   Dermatoglyphics commonly seen in infants with Down syndrome. **A,** Ulnar loop on the second digit, single flexion crease on the fifth digit, and single palmar crease (simian line). **B,** Arch tibial pattern in hallucal area of foot.

ing a diagnosis, including chromosome analysis, molecular DNA testing, biochemical studies to rule out inborn errors of metabolism, radiographs, organ imaging, and when appropriate, autopsy. Not all of these studies are routinely used in all patients but are based on clinical suspicion of a particular disorder.

Chromosome Analysis

Routinely, results of chromosome analysis may not be available for several weeks. However, if results of chromosome analysis are urgently needed for clinical management, chromosome analysis from bone marrow can be available within a few hours, and preliminary results from blood lymphocyte culture can be obtained in 48 hours. Indications for chromosome analysis have been listed previously. However, chromosome analysis should be obtained in all critically ill infants for whom there is no plausible explanation for their grave clinical course, before death occurs. For postmortem examination, chromosomes may also be obtained from any tissue, in particular intracardiac blood, thymus, skin, and gonad. Under sterile conditions, these tissues should be obtained as soon as possible after the infant's demise. Tissue should be transported to the laboratory in a tissue culture medium or sterile saline solution, not in formalin.

Molecular DNA Analysis

There is a growing list of disorders for which the gene has been identified and thus, molecular diagnostic tests are commercially available. Whenever the health care professional has a reasonable suspicion of a specific diagnosis based on clinical phenotype, it is reasonable to suggest molecular testing if it is available to confirm the diagnosis and provide appropriate genetic counseling. However, the clinician must remember that mutational analysis is complex, and although it can confirm a diagnosis when the test result is positive, a negative result may not determine conclusively that the neonate is *not* affected.[3] Some disorders (listed with their gene symbol and chromosomal locus) that molecular gene testing is available for and might be seen in the neonate include achondroplasia (FGFR3, 4p16), Apert syndrome (FGFR2, 10q26), cystic fibrosis (CFTR, 7q31), and congenital myotonic dystrophy (DMPK, 19q13).

Biochemical Studies

A critically ill neonate who has a condition suggestive of an inborn error of metabolism or who has no specific diagnosis should have blood and urine sent for appropriate biochemical studies (listed in the section on inborn errors of metabolism). If such studies have not been obtained, postmortem tissue such as liver should be obtained and frozen for later biochemical analysis. Care providers should request detailed instructions from a laboratory specializing in testing for inherited metabolic disorders regarding which tissue is appropriate and how it should be obtained, stored, and shipped to the laboratory.

Radiographs

X-ray examination should be obtained if a skeletal dysplasia or other skeletal abnormality is suspected or if the differential diagnosis includes a genetic syndrome that has skeletal defects as part of the phenotype. Moreover, if a localized skeletal defect is found, a skeletal survey should be obtained to identify other possible skeletal defects.

Organ Imaging

Organ imaging by ultrasonography, MRI, and CT scan should be used to rule out structural abnormalities of major organs such as the brain, heart, and kidneys. Malformations may be suspected on the basis of clinical symptoms such as anuria or on the basis of known nonrandom associations of certain birth defects, such as the vertebral/anal/T-E fistula/renal/radial (VATER) association. In addition, some dysmorphic features are associated with major malformations, and one must rule out these features. For example, there is an increased incidence of underlying midline brain defects associated with some facial dysmorphic features.

Autopsy

In the event of a neonate's death, an autopsy may provide crucial information for the establishment of a correct diagnosis. As outlined previously, chromosome analysis, biochemical studies, x-ray examination, and photographs all should be included. In the absence of a specific, confirmed diagnosis, the family should be strongly encouraged to consent to an autopsy, and a tissue sample should be frozen for further testing. Without this valuable information, subsequent genetic counseling of the parents, including clarification of the causes and recurrence risks, becomes impossible.

TREATMENT/INTERVENTION

For most genetic disorders and malformations, there are no "cures," and only symptomatic treatment is available; that is, conventional medical and surgical interventions are instituted, although the basic genetic defect is not corrected. Surgical intervention

for specific malformations will depend on the malformation, its cause, and prognosis. For example, surgical repair of a cleft lip and palate usually has an excellent outcome, although the underlying genetic cause has not been altered. In other instances, the diagnosis may provide direction and guidance to the health care professionals and family as to the appropriate course of action. An infant born with a hypoplastic left side of the heart may be considered a candidate for a heart transplant. However, if the cardiac malformation is the result of a chromosomal abnormality with an extremely poor prognosis, such as trisomy 13, the management of that infant may be palliative rather than corrective.

With the diagnosis of a metabolic disorder, treatment may be one of a nutritional or pharmacologic approach, such as the restriction of phenylalanine in an infant with PKU or the replacement of a deficient hormone, such as thyroid supplements in hypothyroidism. For some conditions, such as OI, the best approach may be educating the parents on specific techniques of holding and caring for an infant to prevent further fractures. In some disorders, organ or tissue transplantation may be appropriate. Bone marrow transplantation has been found to be effective in treating select genetic disorders, including lysosomal storage disorders[24] and beta thalassemia.[27] Because specific treatment leading to a cure is not available for most genetic disorders, the utilization of genetic counseling and available reproductive alternatives, such as prenatal diagnosis, in vitro fertilization, preimplantation diagnosis, and artificial insemination by donor, are acceptable alternatives for some families.

THE HUMAN GENOME PROJECT

The year 2000 marked the announcement that the vast majority of the human genome had been sequenced.[10] This international effort, funded in part by the National Institutes of Health (NIH), began in 1990 with the development of genetic and physical maps of the human genome and completed its initial goals in 2000 with a draft of the sequencing of the 3 billion base pairs of the human genome. Defining the sequence of the human genome is only the beginning of the application of that knowledge to current and future research opportunities that will provide avenues for innovative therapies. New powerful technologies for understanding gene expression are being applied to designing drugs that will moderate disease pathways. It is predicted that these "designer drugs" will by available within the next 20 years to treat individuals with diabetes mellitus, hypertension, and cancer. The field of genomics will also provide opportunities to predict responsiveness to drug therapies, because reactions to drugs are often based on individual genetic variations. With the identification of common gene variants involved in drug action or metabolism, health care professionals might be able to predict an infant's response—good or bad—to a particular drug regimen.[10]

With the numerous advances in molecular genetics it is predicted that many genetic disorders and malformations may be amenable to treatment in utero or after birth. In utero correction of such birth defects as urinary tract malformations, myelomeningocele, and diaphragmatic hernia have been successfully attempted.[6,13,14] In 1990 the first human trial of gene therapy was undertaken at the National Institutes of Health. The treatment was somatic gene replacement in a 4-year-old with adenosine deaminase deficiency, a rare inherited disorder that destroys the immune system.[29] Successful efforts utilizing improved gene therapy techniques continue with this disorder.[7] Since that time a number of gene therapy trials for other genetic disorders have been done. Although the arena of gene therapy in general has been somewhat disappointing, the results have led to new areas of research and experimentation with new promising techniques.[35] The development of safer and more effective vectors based on technologies spearheaded by the Human Genome Project should provide significant improvements in gene therapy, such as that seen in an application of gene therapy with hemophilia B.[23]

PARENT TEACHING

The birth of any infant with a malformation or genetic disorder is a devastating event for any family. The neonatal staff find themselves on the front lines helping families to deal with the infant's problems and provide the best environment for both the critically ill newborn and his or her family. In general, the most difficult factor for most parents and families to deal with is the unknown. Thus, once again, the need for an accurate diagnosis becomes paramount. Moreover, even when the diagnosis carries a very poor prognosis, parents would prefer having the information so they can realistically anticipate and prepare for what is to come.[38] Currently, many parents obtain information about their infant's mal-

formation or genetic disorder through prenatal diagnosis and have already begun the process of anticipatory grief by the time the infant is admitted to the NICU. Parental feelings of disbelief, shock, anger, or despair may have already been replaced with a "sense of relief" about confirmation of the abnormalities and a need to deal with the situation at hand.[30]

Chapter 29 provides an excellent review of the grief and mourning process that parents will experience when their anticipated "perfect baby" is born with a malformation or genetic disorder.

From a genetic counseling standpoint, there are a number of principles that should be incorporated into the plan of care for the neonate and his or her family. First—and it cannot be overstated—an accurate diagnosis is essential if genetic counseling is to be provided. Even with what appears to be an isolated malformation, a genetics consultation may be appropriate to rule out other causes, such as single-gene disorders or chromosomal abnormalities. After establishing the diagnosis, one can realistically address the prognosis, treatment, and other management issues with the family. Finally, at the appropriate time for the family, recurrence risks and options for future pregnancies can be addressed.

Certainly, the busy and stressful environment of the NICU is not the most conducive atmosphere for obtaining and providing detailed information. However, it is very appropriate for the geneticist to make an initial contact with the family in the NICU, where basic information regarding pregnancy and perinatal and family histories can be obtained that will aid in diagnosis and defining the cause. Diagnosis and management can then be addressed by the neonatal staff and geneticist. Later, at a time appropriate for the family, such issues as recurrence risks can be addressed. Eventually the family should receive a written summary of all the issues discussed for their own documentation.

The genetic evaluation is a complex and multifaceted process that cannot be done in isolation; it requires a team approach. The geneticist can assist the neonatal intensive care staff in determining the diagnosis, cause, and prognosis so that appropriate management of the infant can be implemented and aiding in future counseling of the families they serve. The neonatal staff should use the genetics team as a resource for consultation and assistance in providing infants and families with the most appropriate and complete health care available.

REFERENCES

1. American Academy of Pediatrics: Newborn screening fact sheets, *Pediatrics* 98:473, 1996.
2. American Academy of Pediatrics: Newborn and infant hearing loss: detection and intervention policy statement, *Pediatrics* 103:527, 1999.
3. American Academy of Pediatrics: Molecular genetic testing in pediatric practice: a subject review, *Pediatrics* 106:1494, 2000.
4. American College of Medical Genetics: Evaluation of the newborn with single or multiple congenital anomalies: executive summary. http://www.acmg.net
5. American College of Medical Genetics: Statement of the American College of Medical Genetics on Universal Newborn Hearing Screening, *Genet Med* 2: 149, 2000.
6. Bruner JP, Tulipan N, Paschall RL et al: Fetal surgery for myelomeningocele and the incidence of shunt-dependent hydrocephalus, *JAMA* 282:1819, 1999.
7. Calazzana-Calvo M, Hacein-Bey S, de Saint Basile G: Gene therapy of human severe combined immunodeficiency (SCID)-X1 disease. *Science* 288:669, 2000.
8. Clayton-Smith J, Donnai D: Human malformations. In Rimoin DL, Connor JM, Pyeritz RE, eds: *Emery and Rimoin's principles and practice of medical genetics,* ed 3, New York, 1996, Churchill Livingstone.
9. Colie CF: Male mediated teratogenesis, *Reprod Toxicol,* 7:3, 1993.
10. Collins FS, McKusick VA: Implications of the Human Genome Project for medical science, *JAMA* 285:540, 2001.
11. DeGrouchy J, Turleau C: *Clinical atlas of human chromosomes,* ed 2, New York, 1984, John Wiley & Sons.
12. Driscoll DA, Salvin J, Sellinger B et al: Prevalence of 22q11 microdeletions in DiGeorge and velocardiofacial syndromes: implications for genetic counseling and prenatal diagnosis, *J Med Genet* 30:813, 1993.
13. Flake AW: Fetal therapy: medical and surgical approaches. In Creasy RK, Resnick R, eds: *Maternal and fetal medicine,* ed 4, Philadelphia, 1998, WB Saunders.
14. Flake AW, Crombleholme TM, Johnson MP et al: Treatment of severe congenital diaphragmatic hernia by fetal tracheal occlusion: clinical experience with fifteen cases, *Am J Obstet Gynecol* 183:1059, 2000.
15. Gardner RJM, Sutherland GR: *Chromosome abnormalities and genetic counseling,* ed 2, New York, 1996, Oxford University Press.
16. Goodman SI, Greene CL: Inborn errors as causes of acute disease in infancy, *Semin Perinatol* 15(suppl): 31, 1991.
17. Hall JG: Somatic mosaicism observations related to human genetics, *Am J Hum Genet* 43:355, 1988.
18. Hall JG: Genetic imprinting: review and relevance to human disease, *Am J Hum Genet* 46:857, 1990.
19. Hanson JW: Human teratogens. In Rimoin DL, Connor JM, Pyeritz RE, eds: *Emery and Rimoin's principles and practice of medical genetics,* ed 3, New York, 1996, Churchill Livingstone.
20. Harper PS: *Practical genetic counseling,* ed 5, Oxford, England, 1998, Butterworth Heinemann.
21. Hay WW, Hayword A, Levin M: *Current pediatric diagnosis and treatment,* ed 14, Norwalk, Conn, 1999, Appleton & Lange.
22. Jones KL, ed: *Smith's recognizable patterns of human malformation,* ed 5, Philadelphia, 1997, WB Saunders.
23. Kay MA, Manno CS, Ragni MV: Evidence for gene transfer and expression of factor IX in haemophilia B patients treated with an AAV vector, *Nat Genet* 24: 257, 2000.
24. Krivit W, Whitley CB: Bone marrow transplantation for genetic diseases, *N Engl J Med* 3165:1085, 1987.
25. Leana-Cox J, Pangkanon S, Eanet KR et al: Familial DiGeorge/velocardiofacial syndrome with deletions of chromosome area 22q11.2: report of five families with a review of the literature, *Am J Med Genet* 65: 309, 1996.
26. Levy HL, Albers S: Genetic screening of newborns, *Annu Rev Genomics Hum Genet* 1:139, 2000.
27. Lucarelli G, Galimberti M, Polchi P et al: Marrow transplantation in patients with advanced thalassemia, *N Engl J Med* 316:1050, 1987.
28. Marden AM, Smith DW, McDonald MN: Congenital anomalies in the newborn infant, including minor variations, *J Pediatr* 64:357, 1964.
29. Marwick C: Two more cell infusions on schedule for gene replacement therapy patient, *JAMA* 265:2311, 1991.
30. Matthews AL: Known fetal malformations during pregnancy: a human experience of loss, *Birth Defects Orig Artic Ser* 26:168, 1990.
31. Morris CA: Williams syndrome, University of Washington. www.geneclinics.org
32. Nussbaum RL, McInnes RP, Willard HF: *Thompson and Thompson genetics in medicine,* ed 6, Philadelphia, 2001, WB Saunders.
33. McKusick VA: Online mendelian inheritance in man (OMIM), Baltimore, Johns Hopkins University, Center for Medical Genetics. http://www3.ncbi.nlm.nih.gov/omim
34. Robinson A, Bender B, Linden M et al: Sex chromosome aneuploidy: the Denver prospective study, *Birth Defects Original Article Series* 26:59, 1990.
35. Schuchman EH, Desnick RJ: Strategies for the treatment of genetic disease. In Rimoin DL, Connor JM, Pyeritz RE, eds: *Emery and Rimoin's principles and practice of medical genetics,* ed 3, New York, 1996, Churchill Livingstone.
36. Sujansky E, Smith AC, Prescott KE et al: Natural history of recombinant (8) syndrome, *Am J Med Genet* 47:512, 1993.

37. Tkachuk DC, Pinkel D, Kuo WL et al: Clinical applications of fluorescence in situ hybridization, *Genet Anal Tech Appl* 7:49, 1991.

38. Walker AP: Genetic counseling. In Rimoin DL, Connor JM, Pyeritz RE, eds: *Emery and Rimoin's principles and practice of medical genetics,* ed 3, New York, 1996, Churchill Livingstone.

39. Ward JC: Inborn errors of metabolism of acute onset in infancy, *Pediatr Rev* 11:205, 1990.

40. Wertelecy W: Dermatoglyphics. In Stevenson RE, Hall JG, Goodman RM, eds: *Human malformations and related anomalies,* ed 2, New York, 1993, Oxford University Press.

41. Zelante L, Gasparini P, Estivill X' et al: Connexin 26 mutations associated with the most common form of non-syndromic neurosensory autosomal recessive deafness (DFNB1) in Mediterraneans, *Hum Mol Genet* 6:1605, 1997.

28 | Neonatal Surgery

Denis D. Bensard, Casey M. Calkins, David Partrick, Frances N. Price

Three percent of newborns present with congenital malformations, which are an important cause of early infant death and disability. Twenty-two percent of neonatal mortality is attributed to congenital malformations, and although overall infant mortality has declined the mortality attributable to birth defects has increased.[49] In the last decade improvements in perinatology and prenatal imaging have allowed earlier diagnosis and intervention for surgically correctable malformations. Yet many surgical conditions continue to escape early detection and are diagnosed in the newborn period. The care of a neonate with a major congenital malformation is resource intensive and costly. In a study of a regional NICU, newborns with major congenital malformations accounted for 27% of the NICU referrals, 32% of total NICU days, and 40% of NICU costs. Moreover, surgery was more frequent in newborns with major malformations, and one third required ongoing medical support at the time of discharge.[30] Early diagnosis, comprehensive neonatal care, and a multidisciplinary approach are necessary to ensure an optimal outcome for both parent and child.

In this chapter we briefly discuss the clinical history, diagnostic evaluation, and therapeutic intervention of common neonatal surgical conditions.

DIAPHRAGMATIC HERNIA

Physiology and Etiology

Congenital diaphragmatic hernia (CDH) is a posteriolateral defect of the diaphragm that occurs in 1 in 4000 live births. Failure of the normal closure of the pleuropertioneal canal during the eighth week of gestation results in communication between the abdominal and thoracic cavities and is commonly referred to as the **hernia of Bochdalek.** As a result the intestine migrates into the chest as it returns from the umbilical cord. Resultant compression of the developing lung leads to a small and abnormally developed lung (or lungs). As in abdominal wall defects, because the bowel is in an abnormal location, normal rotation does not occur; thus by definition

all infants with CDH have nonrotation. Ninety percent of posterolateral diaphragmatic hernias occur on the left side, 5% on the right, and rarely, they occur on both sides. Less common defects of the diaphragm are an anteromedial **(Morgagni hernia)** defect and a central weakening of the diaphragm **(eventration).**

Data Collection

History

Ultrasonography enables antenatal diagnosis of diaphragmatic hernias, which allows early planning and intervention, as appropriate. The mother may then deliver in a high-risk perinatal center with neonatal medical and surgical support on standby. Although in utero surgical repair seemed promising initially, this has been abandoned because of a lack of demonstrable survival benefit.[53]

Signs and Symptoms

Respiratory distress commonly develops immediately after birth. If significant pulmonary hypoplasia is present, the infant becomes rapidly symptomatic, heralded by profound respiratory distress and circulatory shock. **Because the bowel is in the chest, the abdomen is scaphoid and the anteroposterior diameter of the chest may increase as the bowel distends with air. Breath sounds are diminished or absent on the affected side, and the mediastinum is displaced toward the contralateral side.** Associated anomalies include hypoplasia of the lung, malrotation of the intestine, and patent ductus arteriosus. Associated anomalies requiring evaluation include CNS malformations, genitourinary anomalies, esophageal atresia, omphalocele, cleft palate, and cardiovascular defects.[43]

Laboratory Data

A chest x-ray film is obtained and demonstrates bowel in the ipsilateral thoracic space with contralateral displacement of the heart (Figure 28-1). An echocardiogram may be necessary to assess cardiac function and exclude significant congenital cardiac anomalies.

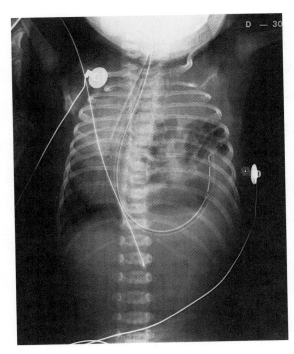

FIGURE 28-1 Diaphragmatic hernia in a newborn female with respiratory distress. Note that the nasogastric tube enters the abdomen and then curves upward into left hemithorax. Loops of bowel are visible in the left chest.

Treatment

Preoperative Care

As soon as a diaphragmatic hernia is suspected, an orogastric (OG) tube should be placed for gastric decompression to prevent further distention of the bowel and compression of the lung. The infant may require endotracheal intubation and positive pressure mechanical ventilation to maintain adequate respiration. The earlier the infant is symptomatic, the more severe the respiratory compromise and the poorer the prognosis. **Pulmonary hypertension** and **lung hypoplasia** are the major determinants of early outcome (see Chapter 23).

Operative Intervention

Surgical repair does not alter early outcome. Therefore the patient's condition should be stabilized and efforts directed to the management of the associated pulmonary dysfunction. Early repair is indicated only in infants with little or no pulmonary dysfunction. If severe respiratory insufficiency is present, medical therapies of conventional or high-frequency mechanical ventilation, inhaled nitric oxide, or extracorporeal membrane oxygenation are instituted. If this is successful, surgical repair is generally performed at 7 to 14 days of life.[54]

By a transabdominal approach, the surgeon reduces the abdominal contents from the chest to the abdominal cavity and closes the diaphragmatic defect. If the defect is large, a prosthetic patch is needed to repair the hernia. Closure of the abdomen may be difficult because of an underdeveloped abdominal cavity. If closure is not possible, a prosthetic patch or skin is closed over the top of the abdominal contents, leaving a large ventral hernia. Chest tubes are generally unnecessary, unless excessive bleeding (because of anticoagulation/ECMO therapy) or a pneumothorax is anticipated.

Postoperative Care

As in the preoperative state, the principal postoperative concern remains ventilation and oxygenation. If conventional mechanical ventilation fails, high-frequency ventilation and inhaled nitric oxide are employed.[26] **Extracorporeal membrane oxygenation (ECMO)** is reserved in this setting as a salvage therapy for infants who are believed to have a reasonable chance of survival (see Chapter 23).

Complications and Prognosis

The survival rate for infants who require mechanical ventilation in the first 18 to 24 hours of life is approximately 50%. If an infant with a diaphragmatic hernia does not present with respiratory distress in the first 24 hours of life, survival approaches 100%. With improvements in ventilator management, there has been a gradual, albeit small, increase in survival.[43] The primary **early complication** of CDH is pulmonary dysfunction. **Late complications** include recurrent diaphragmatic hernia, gastroesophageal reflux, growth restriction, and neurodevelopmental delay.[36] Bench and clinical research continue in an effort to identify improved therapies for the pulmonary dysfunction associated with congenital diaphragmatic hernia.

ESOPHAGEAL ATRESIA AND TRACHEOESOPHAGEAL FISTULA

Physiology and Etiology

Esophageal atresia (EA) is a **spectrum of anomalies** that occur early in gestation (22 to 36 days), as the trachea buds from the primitive foregut. Failure of the normal development of the esophagus and

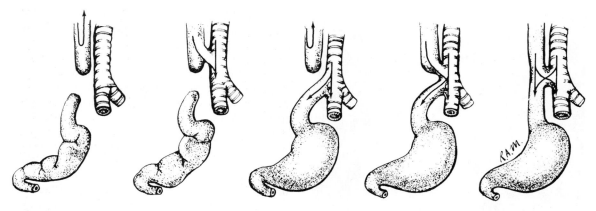

FIGURE 28-2 Most common types of esophageal atresia and tracheoesophageal fistula. (From Wong DL, Hockenberry-Eaton M, Wilson D et al: *Nursing care of infants and children,* ed 6, St Louis, 1999, Mosby.)

separation of the trachea from the esophagus results in: esophageal atresia and distal tracheoesophageal fistula (85%); isolated esophageal atresia (8%); tracheoesophageal fistula (TEF) without esophageal atresia (5%); or esophageal atresia with proximal or proximal and distal fistulas (2%) (Figure 28-2). The cause of this defect remains unclear, but it is suspected that an environmental insult occurs during this critical period of organogenesis, resulting in the malformation. Because other developing organs are vulnerable to the same insult, **associated anomalies** are common (50% to 70%), particularly vertebral, cardiac, gastrointestinal, genitourinary, and limb malformations. Although not considered a genetic disease, there is a high incidence in children with trisomy 21 and if suspected chromosomal analysis is indicated.[49]

Data Collection

History
Maternal **polyhydramnios** suggests esophageal atresia or other conditions in which the fetus does not swallow amniotic fluid normally.

Signs and Symptoms
Infants with esophageal atresia are identified soon after birth because of their excessive secretions and inability to swallow feedings. With feeding they cough and regurgitate undigested formula. If an orogastric tube is passed and meets an obstruction at 8 to 10 cm from the mouth, esophageal atresia is present. If a distal tracheoesophageal fistula is also present, air is shunted into the stomach and bowel, resulting in abdominal distention. If significant distention occurs, ventilation becomes compromised. Severe **respiratory distress**

may follow because of the combination of **pneumonitis** resulting from the reflux of gastric acid and inadequate ventilation resulting from impaired diaphragmatic excursion by the distended viscera. Symptoms of an "H"-type fistula are less obvious and require a high index of suspicion. **Coughing and choking with feedings or recurrent pneumonia over the first months of life suggests the presence of an occult tracheoesophageal fistula.**

Physical Examination
Once a TEF is diagnosed, the infant should be carefully examined to exclude the other anomalies of the VACTERL association—a combination of anomalies affecting the vertebrae, anus, heart (cardiac), trachea, esophagus, urinary tract (renal), and limbs.[6] Echocardiography permits both the identification of significant cardiac anomalies and the presence of a right or left sided aortic arch which have important implications for surgical repair.

Laboratory Data
An **x-ray film** of the chest and abdomen should be obtained after OG tube placement. The OG tube will be visible at the second or third thoracic vertebra (Figure 28-3). The stomach will contain air if there is a distal tracheoesophageal fistula. If there is no distal fistula, the abdomen will be gasless (Figure 28-4).

Treatment

Preoperative Care
Once the diagnosis is established, a suction catheter is placed in the upper pouch to prevent aspiration. While awaiting operation, the child should be kept in the head-up position to minimize gas-

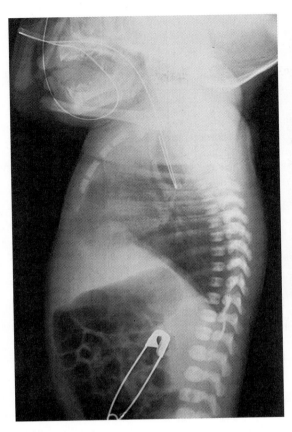

FIGURE 28-3   Esophageal atresia with tracheoesophageal fistula. Lateral x-ray film shows the gastric tube in esophageal pouch and air in the gastrointestinal tract.

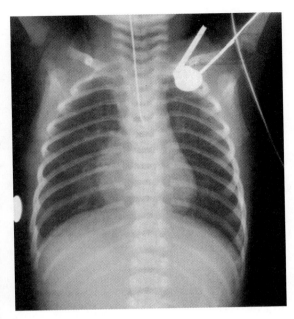

FIGURE 28-4   Esophageal atresia without tracheoesophageal fistula. Note that the nasogastric tube is in the upper esophageal pouch and the abdomen appears gasless, consistent with the absence of a distal tracheoesophageal fistula and thus air.

troesophageal reflux and the risk of pneumonitis. If a proximal fistula is present, urgent operation is indicated, because saliva will empty into the lungs despite the OG tube. In this instance, while awaiting operation the child should be kept in the head-down position to improve drainage of the upper esophagus.

Operative Intervention

The type of esophageal malformation dictates the surgical approach. Surgical repair of tracheoesophageal fistula and esophageal atresia is not an emergency but should be carried out as soon as the patient is stable. If the infant is in otherwise good health and the gap between esophageal elements is not too large, **primary anastomosis** is indicated through a right retropleural approach.

Unfortunately, in isolated esophageal atresia the gap distance is generally too great to allow early repair. If the gap length is considered too great or if the child is too ill, a **delayed or staged repair** is planned. An early gastrostomy is placed for decompression and division of the fistula to prevent soilage of the tracheobronchial tree. After a wait of several days to as long as 10 weeks to allow resolution of **pneumonitis** or maximum growth of the distal esophagus, a second operation completes the repair.

Postoperative Care

Postoperative care includes pulmonary care, IV fluids, parenteral nutrition, and antibiotics. **Tracheal and esophageal suction catheters should not come in contact with the newly repaired esophagus, because this may cause a leak or recurrent fistula.** Antibiotic therapy is continued for 3 to 5 days. A retropleural chest tube is placed for suctioning. Oral feedings may begin at 5 to 10 days after repair if an esophagram indicates no **anastomotic leak.** All of these infants have some degree of **esophageal dysmotility** and **gastroesophageal reflux (GER). Elevating the head of the bed 35 to 45 degrees, administering H_2 antagonists, and slow feeding help to control reflux symptoms.**

If delayed or staged repair is planned, secretions must be controlled. Suction catheters in their pouch are maintained to reduce the risk of aspiration. In rare cases, reconstruction using the native esophagus is not possible. In this circumstance, **esophageal replacement** using gastric or colon transposition is necessary. If the infant is not a candidate for early operation because of a lethal chromosomal defect or severe congenital heart disease, cervical esophagostomy and gastrostomy are performed to palliate the infant, and esophageal replacement is performed later if indicated.

Complications and Prognosis

Long-term complications include stricture, anastomotic leak, and esophageal dysmotility. **Anastomotic leaks** are treated conservatively with chest tube drainage, parenteral nutrition, antibiotics, and patience. The vast majority heal without operative intervention. **Strictures** are often associated with **GER** and are generally treated successfully by repeated esophageal dilation. If GER is complicated by recurrent stricture, a fundoplication procedure may be necessary.

A degree of esophageal dysmotility always exists because of the dysfunction of the distal esophagus and poor peristalsis. The child may adapt to a poorly functioning esophagus by altering his or her feeding habits. However, in infancy, gastrostomy feeding may be required to prevent vomiting and aspiration.

With modern surgical and medical techniques, long-term survival after repair of TEF/EA is very good. The **prognosis** depends on the presence of associated anomalies and their severity. A useful system to predict survival is the Spitz classification, which stratifies infant survival by birth weight and major cardiac anomaly[45]:

I: Birth weight greater than 1500 g, no major CHD, survival is greater than 97%

II: Birth weight less than 1500 g or major CHD, survival is 59%

III: Birth weight less than 1500 g and major CHD, survival is 22%

GASTROESOPHAGEAL REFLUX

Physiology and Etiology

Gastroesophageal reflux (GER) is common in the first year of life but generally improves spontaneously after this time. Gastric contents are prevented from refluxing into the esophagus by (1) a physiologic sphincter at the distal esophagus, defined manometrically as the high-pressure zone; (2) the acute angle of His of the esophagus to the stomach; and (3) maintenance of the gastroesophageal junction below the diaphragm, where intraabdominal pressure exceeds intrathoracic pressure. In infants one or more of

these elements may be absent, predisposing them to GER. Moreover, the infant's usual recumbent position, frequent increases in intraabdominal pressure because of crying, and a predominantly liquid diet may explain the predisposition to reflux during the first year of life. **Approximately 1 in 300 to 1000 infants will develop significant symptoms of GER requiring medical or surgical therapy.** In addition, certain conditions are associated with an increased risk of GER, including congenital diaphragmatic hernia, esophageal atresia, prematurity, and neurologic or pulmonary disease.

Data Collection

Signs and Symptoms

Nonbilious vomiting suggests GER. A spectrum of associated symptoms may be present, but in infants are primarily pulmonary or nutritional. Apnea, coughing, choking, wheezing (particularly when the child is recumbent), or pneumonitis suggests GER. Repeated episodes of significant emesis may lead to inadequate caloric intake and failure to thrive. Esophageal injury from repeated acid reflux is generally observed much later, but in infants with esophageal atresia, anastomotic stricture may be aggravated by uncontrolled GER.

Laboratory Data

Evaluation of suspected GER begins with an upper gastrointestinal contrast study. This study provides anatomic information (hiatal hernia, esophageal stricture, and malrotation) and may demonstrate GER. A **UGI series** will fail to demonstrate reflux in more than half of infants with pathologic GER; therefore normal findings on examination do not exclude the diagnosis. **A pH probe study is the best available test to assess GER.** Unlike UGI evaluation, a pH probe study is performed continuously over an interval of 12 to 24 hours, providing a quantitative and temporal analysis of GER. The frequency and duration of reflux (pH below 4) is quantified and scored to assess the severity of GER. A nuclear gastric scintiscan and esophagoscopy are additional modalities to assess GER, but these are rarely employed in infants.

Treatment

Preoperative Care

Treatment of GER begins with dietary and postural modification. Feedings are thickened with rice cereal and are given more frequently and in smaller volumes. Placing the infant in an upright position during and after feeding is recommended, although the use of an infant seat is dis-

couraged, because these seats increase intraab-dominal pressure. **If these conservative measures fail, then medical therapy is instituted.** An H_2 antagonist (e.g., ranitidine) or a proton pump inhibitor (e.g., omeprazole) is used to reduce gastric acid and thus also reduce the inflammatory effect on esophageal or bronchial mucosa. A prokinetic agent, such as metoclopramide, may be added in an effort to improve gastric emptying supplementing the effect of acid blockade.[50] **Together these therapies control reflux in 90% of patients** (Table 28-1).

Operative Intervention

Surgical correction of GER is intended to restore the anatomic components of the native antireflux barrier (intraabdominal GE junction, correct angle of His, closed esophageal hiatus). An **absolute indication** for surgical repair is life-threatening apnea or bradycardia or near-SIDS attributable to GER. **Relative indications** in infants include recurrent or exacerbated lung disease, failure to thrive, or refractory esophageal stricture.

A partial (270-degree) or complete (360-degree) fundoplication may be used, although a Nissen (360-degree) fundoplication is recommended most often. In addition to the fundoplication, the esophagogastric junction is restored in the abdomen and the esophageal hiatus closed. A gastrostomy is often added for feeding or gastric decompression, which may ameliorate the symptoms of gas-bloat (gagging, retching), the most common complication of a 360-degree fundoplication. The **Nissen fundoplication** can be performed either by a laparotomy incision (midline or subcostal) or laparoscopically (multiple 3- to 5-mm incisions). The results appear comparable, but the laparoscopic technique appears to allow earlier feeding, decreased postoperative pain, and earlier discharge.[12]

Postoperative Care

After an antireflux procedure **gastric decompression** should be used liberally to avoid symptoms of gas-bloat. Oral or tube feedings may be started as early as the first postoperative day and gradually advanced.

Today a **primary gastric button** (Figure 28-5) with a detachable tube is usually placed; this button

Table 28-1	MEDICATIONS FOR GASTROESOPHAGEAL REFLUX	
DRUG	**DOSAGE**	**COMMENTS**
Metoclopramide	0.1 mg/kg divided q 8 hr	GI smooth muscle stimulant May cause extrapyramidal symptoms (e.g., dystonic posturing)
Omperazole	0.3-3 mg/kg divided q 12 hr PO	Gastric acid pump inhibitor Recommended starting dose 0.7 mg/kg PO in morning
Ranitidine	1-2 mg/kg divided q 8 hr IV 3-4 mg/kg divided q 8 hr PO	H_2 antagonist

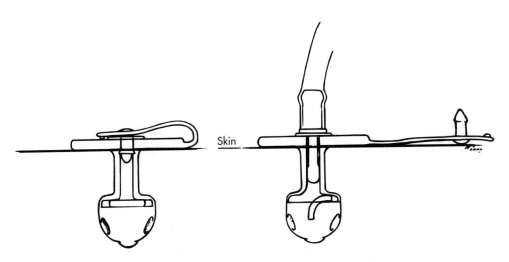

FIGURE 28-5 Gastrostomy button with a one-way valve.

reduces the incidence of wound enlargement and leakage.[18] Movement or manipulation of the button should be minimized. If a leak develops, cotton dental rolls are used to secure the button. This type of dressing serves two purposes: movement is minimized and drainage is absorbed, reducing skin breakdown. The dressing should be changed daily, and the area should be kept clean and dry. If the button is accidentally dislodged, it must be replaced quickly because the tract to the stomach shrinks in a few hours. Early displacement (less than 4 weeks) requires evaluation by the surgeon and may require operative replacement. If the gastrostomy is more than 4 weeks old, the button may be temporarily replaced with a urinary catheter until a new button is available.

Complications and Prognosis

In general, the complete or Nissen fundoplication is recommended because of its **efficacy** (more than 90%) and low **recurrence rate** (less than 10%).[15,27] Unfortunately, neurologically impaired infants have much higher failure rates (up to 30%) and complications (feeding intolerance, retching, and gagging).[14]

PYLORIC STENOSIS

Physiology and Etiology

Infantile hypertrophic pyloric stenosis is the most common cause of **gastric outlet obstruction** in children. Progressive thickening and hypertrophy of the pyloric muscle during the first month of life results in obstruction and a history of worsening nonbilious emesis. Diverse mechanisms, such as type of formula or absence of nitric oxide (smooth muscle relaxant), have been implicated, but a conclusive etiology remains elusive. Approximately 10% of children who develop pyloric stenosis are born to affected parents; affected mothers are four times more likely than affected fathers to have an affected child. Yet the mode of inheritance, like the cause, remains unknown. Males are more commonly affected than in females (4:1), in particular firstborn males.

Data Collection

History

Episodes of nonbilious emesis begin in the first weeks of life, gradually become more frequent and projectile. The infant does not appear ill and appears hungry despite the repeated emesis. Eventually the infant begins to lose weight because of inade-

quate caloric intake, and if allowed to continue will become dehydrated. Often a history of changes in formula, frequency or volume of feeds will be given, because pyloric stenosis mimics gastroesophageal reflux early in the course of the illness. **Nearly all parents observe, however, that the infant appears hungry and eager to feed after vomiting.**

Signs and Symptoms

Today the disease is often recognized early. The baby may appear normal or slightly dehydrated, but occasionally the diagnosis is considered late and the infant when initially seen is lethargic and severely dehydrated. Historically, caregivers were taught that careful examination of the abdomen revealed a palpable pyloric muscle, **"olive,"** in the majority of children. Currently, the olive is reported to be palpable in two thirds of infants.[5] One percent to 2% of infants will be jaundiced as a result of associated glucuronyl transferase deficiency.

Laboratory Data

Serum electrolytes may demonstrate low chloride and bicarbonate as a result of the repeated loss of acid (HCl) and the compensatory response of the kidney to dehydration. **If the imbalance is severe, a hypokalemic, hypochloremic, metabolic alkalosis develops and should be corrected preoperatively.** When the diagnosis is suspected but an olive is not palpable, either ultrasonography or contrast radiography (UGI) may be used. **Ultrasonography** is an excellent modality for identifying pyloric stenosis. It is noninvasive and has a diagnostic accuracy greater than 95%.[34] However, ultrasonography provides no information about GER, which is the most likely alternative diagnosis. Therefore, in the setting of early symptoms, when GER should be considered, a **UGI** is chosen, permitting examination of both possibilities without the need for further testing.

Treatment

Preoperative Care

The dehydration and electrolyte imbalance is corrected with the administration of crystalloid solution. Initially, rehydration is started with normal saline bolus. Once urine output is established, a half-normal saline solution with 20 to 30 mEq of KCl/L is infused to correct the low chloride, potassium, and elevated HCO_3^-. Because of the risk of postoperative apnea, the serum bicarbonate level should be less than 30 mEq/dl before proceeding to operation.

Operative Treatment and Postoperative Care

The Rammstedt pyloromyotomy has been the corner-stone of treatment since the turn of the twentieth century. In this simple but effective procedure the hypertrophied pyloric muscle is incised and then fractured, relieving the obstruction. The procedure may be done either through an abdominal incision or laparoscopically, using three small incisions (3 mm).[10] Both methods appear equally effective, but regardless of the technique employed, the surgeon must ensure that the mucosa has not been inadvertently injured, resulting in visceral perforation. Failure to recognize a perforation can be disastrous and even fatal.

Postoperatively, early feeding is started and advanced as tolerated. Recent studies have demonstrated that infants tolerate early and rapid advancement of feeds, although the parents should be forewarned that episodes of small volume emesis are not unexpected. In general, infants are tolerating full feeds and ready for discharge within 24 hours of operation.[3]

Complications and Prognosis

The prognosis is excellent and mortality is less than 0.1%. Some patients will demonstrate prolonged feeding intolerance due to gastric dysfunction or concomitant GER but is rarely caused by incomplete pyloromyotomy (less than 1%). However, if symptoms persist beyond 12 to 14 days, an upper GI contrast study should be obtained.[22]

MALROTATION AND VOLVULUS

Physiology and Etiology

The midgut normally herniates into the base of the umbilical cord at the beginning of the sixth week of development and returns to the abdominal cavity by the tenth to twelfth week. As it returns, the proximal midgut rotates posterior and counterclockwise to the superior mesenteric artery (SMA). Thus the duodenum comes to lie posterior to the SMA. At the transition of duodenum to jejunum the midgut is fixed by the ligament of Treitz. Concomitantly, the colon and distal small bowel rotate anterior to the SMA until the cecum lies in the right lower quadrant and is fixed by the peritoneal reflection. Failure to undergo rotation and fixation results in the clinical condition of **malrotation.** Malrotation is always present in infants who have gastroschisis, omphalocele, or congenital diaphragmatic hernia, because the bowel has herniated either through the abdominal wall or the diaphragm and does not undergo normal rotation and fixation. More often malrotation occurs in the absence of other anomalies.

The degree of malrotation covers a wide spectrum from complete nonrotation to partial malrotation or improper fixation of a segment of bowel. There may also be a reversal of rotation such that the colon lies posterior to the SMA and the duodenum lies anterior. Nonrotation or total failure of rotation is the most common. In this situation the entire small bowel is on the right side of the abdomen and the colon is mainly on the left side. Consequently, the root of the mesentery is not anchored, and the superior mesenteric artery and vein suspend the entire bowel. The lack of fixation and nonrotation predisposes the long vascular pedicle to twisting (**volvulus**). If volvulus occurs, the blood supply to the midgut becomes compromised, leading first to ischemia and finally bowel infarction.

Some individuals may never develop symptoms in their lifetime, whereas others may develop symptoms in infancy or childhood.

Data Collection

History

Malrotation may present as a mechanical bowel obstruction caused by the abnormal attachments (Ladd's bands) or as an acute abdomen due to volvulus and intestinal ischemia. In a neonate with symptomatic malrotation, the first few days of life are normal but then the infant develops bilious emesis and abdominal distention. The symptoms may progress to profound shock and distention as a result of the presence of midgut volvulus.[47]

Signs and Symptoms

The symptoms of **malrotation** mimic those of duodenal stenosis or atresia, jejunal atresia, or other conditions resulting in proximal intestinal obstruction.

Midgut volvulus presents as the sudden onset of abdominal distention, lethargy, and hypovolemic shock. The presence of bloody emesis or stools suggests intestinal ischemia with mucosal injury or necrosis. In this setting, rapid diagnosis and prompt surgical intervention is essential to avoid extensive bowel loss or death.

Laboratory Data

Abdominal radiographs may demonstrate a dilated stomach and proximal duodenum. However, the definitive study is an upper GI series, which can demonstrate both abnormal rotation of the duodenum (**malrotation**) and partial or complete obstruction of the proximal duodenum (**midgut volvulus**). A barium enema may also show abnormal rotation of the colon but provides no information regarding the presence or absence of midgut volvulus[31] (Figure 28-6). Laboratory data are generally unremarkable, unless bowel ischemia is present, as suggested by leukocytosis, anemia, and metabolic acidosis.

Treatment

Preoperative Care

Although distinguishing between volvulus in its early stages and symptomatic malrotation with obstruction may be difficult, these conditions should be treated similarly. Gastric decompression, fluid resuscitation, correction of electrolyte and acid-base abnormalities, and parenteral antibiotics are instituted in the preoperative period. Emergency abdominal exploration should be considered in any infant with suspected or confirmed volvulus, because the bowel will be irreparably damaged in as little as 4 hours. In fact, it is unwise to await correction of metabolic abnormalities or hypotension. In this setting, prompt surgical intervention with continued intraoperative resuscitation is indicated to maximize the chances for bowel salvage and survival.

Operative correction of malrotation includes division of Ladd's bands (to relieve duodenal obstruction), correction of the malrotation (by placement of the colon in the left side of the abdomen and the small bowel on the right), widening of the base of the mesentery, and appendectomy (the appendix and cecum will reside in the left upper quadrant). The procedure may be performed either via laparotomy or laparoscopy. The long-term results of the laparoscopic approach are unknown, but preliminary results suggest comparable efficacy.[2] If volvulus is present, the bowel is untwisted and allowed to reperfuse. Necrotic segments of bowel are resected and stomas created. In selected instances, substantial resection would result in short bowel syndrome. In this situation marginal intestine should be left in place rather than removed and a planned reoperation should be performed in 24 to 36 hours to reevaluate the need for additional bowel resection. With continued resuscitation the objective is to allow marginally viable intestine time to recover or become obviously necrotic and therefore minimize the amount of intestinal resection.

Complications and Prognosis

Malrotation is corrected by the Ladd's procedure, and recurrence is rare. The postoperative care consists of nasogastric decompression and IV fluid therapy until the return of gastrointestinal function (4 to 6 days).[13] Conversely, the outcome following malrotation with midgut volvulus is predicated on the degree of intestinal resection.[32] **Midgut volvulus** is a leading cause of short bowel syndrome in infants and may render the infant TPN dependent if extensive intestinal necrosis has occurred.

INTESTINAL ATRESIA

Physiology and Etiology

Any segment of the bowel may be narrowed (**stenosis**) or discontinuous (**atresia**). Duodenal atresia is the most commonly involved bowel segment, followed by ileum, jejunum, colon, and stomach.[8]

Bowel atresia results from either failure of vacuolization (fifth to sixth week of gestation) and recanalization (eighth to tenth week of gestation) of the

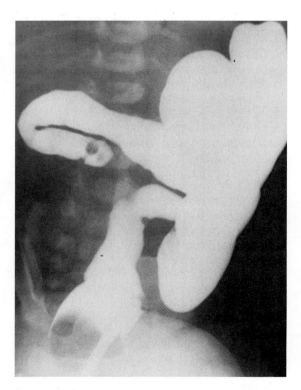

FIGURE 28-6   Malrotation in a 2-day-old male infant with bilious emesis. A barium enema shows high-lying cecum curved on itself in right upper quadrant. However, the study provides no information about the presence or absence of midgut volvulus. If volvulus is suspected, a UGI series should be performed.

duodenum or a late in utero vascular accident (jejunal, ileal, or colonic atresia). Because **duodenal atresia** results from an early in utero event, there is a high incidence of associated anomalies (30%), including trisomy 21, congenital heart disease, and VACTERL association.[19] Conversely, **intestinal atresia** is rarely associated with significant anomalies, because the insult occurs late in gestation. Atresias are classified as membranes, fibrous cords, gap defect including mesentery, and "apple-peel" atresia.[52]

Data Collection
History and Physical Examination
Typically, the affected neonate is **SGA** and there is a history of maternal **polyhydramnios.** The more proximal the site of intestinal atresia, the more likely the history of maternal polyhydramnios. **The infant presents with emesis and feeding intolerance. Bilious emesis is present when the obstruction is distal to the ampulla of Vater. However, in 15% of cases, duodenal atresia occurs proximal to the ampulla of Vater and therefore the patient will not demonstrate bilious emesis or aspirates.** The more distal the site of obstruction, the more likely that the infant will demonstrate significant abdominal distention. If the atresia occurs early in gestation, the infant fails to pass meconium, and only mucus is passed after birth.

Laboratory Data
Abdominal x-ray films demonstrate distended bowel, suggesting an intestinal obstruction. In duodenal atresia, a dilated stomach and proximal duodenum is present in a pattern called the **double bubble** (Figure 28-7). A contrast study is not indicated unless there is air present in the distal bowel and malrotation with midgut volvulus cannot be excluded. In the setting of atresia of the small intestine or colon, abdominal x-ray films demonstrate dilation of intestinal segments proximal to the site of obstruction with absence of air in the distal bowel. For intestinal atresia a barium enema is generally performed and will demonstrate a **microcolon** or **unused colon,** with no reflux of the contrast agent into the proximal bowel.

Treatment
Preoperative Care
Preoperative care includes gastric decompression, fluid resuscitation, and correction of electrolyte abnormalities. Gastric decompression is implemented to reduce the risk of vomiting and aspiration.

Operative Intervention
Intestinal atresia requires surgical correction with **restoration of intestinal continuity.** Duodenal atresia is repaired through a side-to-side anastomosis of the proximal and distal duodenum to prevent injury to the bile and pancreatic ducts. Other intestinal atresias are generally repaired by a simple end-to-end anastomosis. The size disparity between the dilated proximal loop and the decompressed distal loop may require that the proximal bowel be tapered and/or the distal bowel be cut obliquely to allow anastomosis. If these methods are not possible, then both segments may be brought out as stomas and intestinal anastomosis delayed to allow reduction of the dilation of the proximal segment and growth of the distal segment. When the caliber of the bowel becomes more comparable in size, anastomosis is performed.

Postoperative Care
Postoperatively, an OG tube is placed to decompress the bowel until bowel function begins. Stomas must be protected from desiccation by covering with petrolatum gauze or a stoma appliance. Proximal ostomies have high output because of a lack of absorptive capacity and therefore will require replacement of both fluid and electrolyte losses. The proximal output may be refed into the distal mucous fistula, but this is often technically difficult because of problems intubating the distal stoma and securing the infusion catheter to permit infusion. All infants demonstrate a significant period of **bowel dysfunction** and therefore should undergo temporary central venous access to permit nutritional support.[41] Furthermore, all infants with intestinal atresia should undergo repeat screening for **cystic fibrosis,** which may contribute to both the development of the anomaly and ongoing bowel dysfunction.

Complications and Prognosis
The overall prognosis for these patients is excellent, unless severe associated anomalies are present. **Prolonged bowel dysfunction** is the primary complication following surgical correction of intestinal atresia. In selected cases, tapering of dilated bowel segments is attempted to enhance the recovery of bowel function.[44] Some infants will fail to recover sufficient bowel function and require long-term parenteral nutritional support, either because of dysmotility or inadequate bowel length resulting from long segment atresia. Fortunately, the majority of patients have no long-term problems after postoperative recovery and return of bowel function.

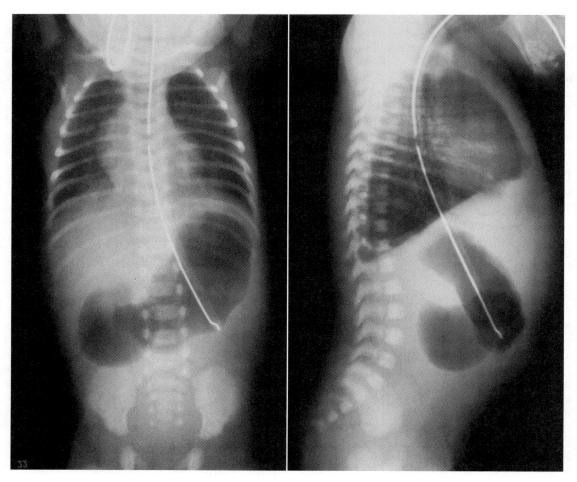

FIGURE 28-7 Duodenal atresia. The classic "double bubble" sign of gastric and duodenal dilation secondary to duodenal atresia is noted on both x-ray films. Note that no bowel gas extends beyond duodenum.

NECROTIZING ENTEROCOLITIS

Physiology and Etiology

Necrotizing enterocolitis (NEC) is an inflammatory condition of the bowel of unknown cause. NEC is primarily a disease of **premature infants,** although approximately 5% of cases involve term infants. An immature intestinal barrier, intestinal ischemia, bacterial colonization of the gut, and nutritional substrate in the gut lumen have been implicated as contributing factors present in infants developing NEC. Other conditions that result in mucosal injury have also been linked to NEC: hypoxia, polycythemia, hyperosmolar feedings, gastrointestinal infection (bacterial or viral), and se-

vere cardiopulmonary disease. Inflammation and ischemia initially involves the intestinal mucosa, but as the condition progresses the muscular layers and subserosa of the bowel become involved. The intestinal wall becomes hemorrhagic and attenuated, with evidence of gas **(pneumatosis).** Histologically, the intestine demonstrates features of acute and chronic inflammation, with areas of coagulative necrosis. NEC occurs in 1 in 1000 live births; the incidence in premature babies weighing less than 1500 g is approximately 5%. The ileocecal region is most commonly involved (50%), followed by disease limited to the colon (25%) or both large and small intestines (25%). Up to 15% of infants with NEC will have pannecrosis (more than 75%) of the bowel and significant risk of death or short bowel syndrome.[1]

Data Collection

Signs and Symptoms

The onset of NEC is heralded by the development of feeding intolerance, abdominal distention, and bloody stools in a premature infant receiving enteral feedings. A history of perinatal hypoxia, respiratory distress, congenital heart disease, or indomethacin administration for PDA closure is often elicited. As the disease progresses the infant develops signs and symptoms of septic shock (lethargy, respiratory distress, temperature instability, hypotension, and oliguria). Examination reveals a distended and tender abdomen that may demonstrate erythema and induration in severe cases.

Laboratory Data

CBC and serum electrolyte evaluations typically reveal thrombocytopenia, leukocytosis or leukopenia, and metabolic acidosis, respectively. Stool tests demonstrate occult blood and reducing substances in more than 50% of cases. The diagnostic test of choice is the **three-way abdominal series.** X-ray films are carefully reviewed for the characteristic finding of **pneumatosis intestinalis,** intramural bowel gas. The x-ray film should be assessed for free air, which would suggest visceral perforation. Other findings include dilated bowel, portal venous gas, ascites, or a fixed bowel loop that does not change on repeated studies.

Treatment

Preoperative Care

The only absolute indication for surgery is **pneumoperitoneum** and thus intestinal perforation. In a clinically stable infant with no findings of perforation, medical management consisting of bowel rest, fluid resuscitation, and broad-spectrum antibiotic therapy is indicated. The infant is monitored carefully (serial abdominal x-ray films and examination) for signs of **intestinal gangrene.** More than half of infants will respond to medical management, but up to 30% of infants treated medically will develop an **intestinal stricture** requiring surgical management.

A subset of infants will continue to deteriorate, suggesting intestinal gangrene without intestinal perforation. Intestinal gangrene should be considered in infants with persistent thrombocytopenia, leukopenia, refractory shock, erythema of the abdominal wall, or a fixed, dilated intestinal loop.[51]

Operative Intervention

The principle of surgical management is to **resect** all necrotic bowel while preserving as much of the intestinal length as possible. In cases of extensive bowel involvement, only necrotic segments of intestine are removed and reoperation at 12 to 24 hours is planned (a second look). Following bowel resection, proximal and distal ostomies are created, and the abdomen is thoroughly irrigated to reduce bacterial and fecal contamination. In severely premature infants weighing less than 1000 g, **primary peritoneal drainage (PPD)** performed in NICU is an alternative to laparotomy. PPD and laparotomy appear to have comparable survival rates, but interestingly, infants treated with PPD have substantial improvement in residual bowel length, which may be in part because up to a third of these patients will not require further operative therapy.[9]

Postoperative Care

After laparotomy, supportive care (fluids, antibiotics) and bowel rest are continued for 10 to 14 days. At 2 weeks low-osmolar elemental feedings are started and advanced as tolerated. A stoma closure procedure is planned for 6 to 8 weeks after the initial surgery. All infants must undergo a preoperative contrast study before ostomy closure to make certain there is no intestinal stricture.

Complications and Prognosis

Stomal prolapse or retraction, wound infection, intraabdominal abscess, and intestinal obstruction are **early** complications. Recurrent NEC is uncommon, but does occur in approximately 5% of infants treated medically or surgically. The most significant **late** complication is that of inadequate intestinal length (short bowel syndrome) and the need for long term parenteral nutrition. **Survival** in infants weighing more than 1000 g has improved from 50% to 80% over the last two decades. Severely premature infants weighing less than 1000 g still have a mortality rate in excess of 50%.[29]

MECONIUM ILEUS

Physiology and Etiology

Meconium ileus is an intestinal obstruction caused by **hyperviscous** secretions from the intestinal glands coupled with a lack of the pancreatic enzymes that normally help break down intestinal secretions. The result is tenacious, viscous meconium that creates a sticky plug obstructing the lumen of bowel. The obstruction generally occurs at the terminal ileum, mimicking ileal atresia. More than 90% of infants with meconium ileus have **cystic fibrosis,** a three base pair deletion on chromosome 7. This autosomal recessive genetic defect results in alteration of the chloride channel transporter and therefore fluid flux across the apical surface of epithelial cells. Meconium ileus occurs in 10% to 25% of patients with cystic fibrosis; 20% of mothers have polyhydramnios. A family history of cystic fibrosis is present in 10% to 30% of cases.

Data Collection

Signs and Symptoms

Meconium ileus is classified as **simple** (obstruction) or **complicated** (volvulus, intestinal atresia, perforation). Uncomplicated meconium ileus presents as distal ileal obstruction caused by inspissated meconium (pellets) and proximal intestinal dilation. The onset of symptoms associated with simple meconium ileus begins 24 to 48 hours after birth. Bilious emesis, progressive abdominal distention, and the failure to pass meconium suggest intestinal obstruction. The **differential diagnosis** includes ileal atresia, meconium plug, Hirschsprung's disease, and meconium ileus. Inspection demonstrates a patent anus that may express a small amount of gray meconium. Examination of the abdomen reveals moderate distention with a characteristic doughlike sensation because of the thickened meconium contained in the dilated bowel. Complicated meconium ileus often presents more abruptly and progresses more quickly. Symptoms include abdominal distention within 24 hours of birth, respiratory distress (especially if a postnatal perforation has occurred), and an edematous, erythematous abdomen.[40]

Laboratory Data

Abdominal x-ray examination demonstrates a **"soap bubble"** appearance of the bowel caused by trapped gas within the meconium, and also shows large dilated (with air) loops of bowel with few air fluid levels because of the viscous nature of the meconium. A barium enema shows a **microcolon** and pellets of inspissated meconium at the site of distal obstruction.

Treatment

Preoperative Care

After gastric decompression, IV hydration, and electrolyte replacement, a half-strength Gastrograffin enema can be attempted. NOTE: It is important that the infant be adequately hydrated be-fore the enema because of the hyperosmolarity of the Gastrograffin. Instillation of Gastrograffin draws fluid into the bowel lumen, diluting the viscous meconium and facilitating passage. If the Gastrograffin enema results in incomplete evacuation, it may be repeated over the next several days. However, if the Gastrograffin enema fails to result in passage of meconium, complicated meconium ileus or ileal atresia may be present and operative intervention is indicated.[22]

Operative Intervention

The goal of operative treatment is the **relief of intestinal obstruction.** For a simple meconium ileus, an enterotomy (appendiceal stump) is performed and the tenacious meconium is extracted and irrigated from the bowel. If complicated meconium ileus is identified, the obstructed segment is resected and ostomies are performed to permit postoperative irrigation. Ostomy closure is usually performed 4 to 6 weeks later.

Postoperative Care

Postoperatively, nasogastric tube decompression, nutritional support, and irrigation of the rectum or ostomies with saline solution or *N*-acetylcysteine (Mucomyst) are instituted. Once gastrointestinal function returns, feedings using predigested or elemental formula and pancreatic enzyme supplements are started. The diagnosis of cystic fibrosis is confirmed with genetic testing and/or sweat chloride testing.

Complications and Prognosis

One-year survival for infants with a simple or complicated meconium ileus is favorable (greater than 90%), but long-term survival is limited primarily because of the pulmonary complications of the disease.[33] **Late gastrointestinal complications** of cystic fibrosis include distal intestinal obstruction syndrome, appendicitis, intussusception, rectal prolapse, intestinal stricture, pancreatitis, and cholestatic liver disease.[16]

HIRSCHSPRUNG'S DISEASE

Physiology and Etiology

Hirschsprung's disease is a congenital intestinal disorder caused by a lack of ganglion cells in the bowel wall that prevents effective peristalsis. During development neural crest cells migrate to the intestinal musculature in a craniocaudal direction. Arrest of neural crest migration results in Hirschsprung's disease or intestinal **aganglionosis,** a common cause of neonatal intestinal obstruction. At the site of arrest a transition of normal to abnormal enervation is present and all intestine distal to this site will be aganglionic and therefore dysfunctional. The result is a functional obstruction that mimics mechanical intestinal obstruction. Rectosigmoid disease is most common (85%), with the remainder of patients developing variable lengths of more proximal colonic and rarely small intestine aganglionosis. Hirschsprung's disease occurs in 1 in 5000 live births, with a 4:1 male-to-female predominance. In general, the disease occurs sporadically, but infants with trisomy 21 appear at higher risk, and familial occurrences have been reported in 3% of reported cases. In the latter situations longer segment disease is more likely.

Data Collection

Signs and Symptoms

Ninety-eight percent of normal infants pass meconium in the first 24 to 48 hours of life. **Failure to pass meconium early, feeding intolerance, and abdominal distention suggest a diagnosis of Hirschsprung's disease.** Evacuation of stool may be noted on rectal examination and the infant may appear otherwise healthy. If **vomiting, abdominal distention, and constipation** or paradoxic diarrhea resulting from watery stool escaping around the obstipated stool continues, further investigation is indicated. Hirschsprung's disease may escape detection during the newborn period, and in **older children** a history of refractory and chronic obstipation may be the only symptom. Approximately 5% to 10% of affected infants will present with a picture of **enterocolitis,** characterized by fever, vomiting, abdominal distention/tenderness, foul-smelling diarrhea, and septic shock. The infant may rapidly deteriorate, with a 50% risk of death if an emergency colostomy is not performed. Fortunately, in most cases of Hirschsprung's disease the infant is mildly ill, allowing time for definitive diagnostic studies before surgical correction is undertaken.[7]

Laboratory Data

The diagnostic evaluation begins with a **barium enema.** The study typically demonstrates a contracted or spastic rectosigmoid, with contrast agent entering the proximal dilated bowel. The area between the contracted and dilated bowel is called the **transition zone** (Figure 28-8). If the study is equivocal, an ab-

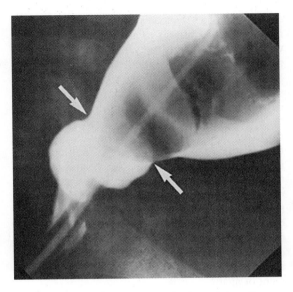

FIGURE 28-8   Hirschsprung's disease. Lateral view of a barium enema demonstrates the transition zone (arrows) of ganglionated to nonganglionated rectum.

dominal x-ray film should be repeated 24 hours after the barium study. If contrast material is retained within the distal bowel, this suggests the presence of Hirschsprung's disease. **Definitive diagnosis** is made by using a suction rectal biopsy. The biopsy demonstrates an absence of ganglion cells and hypertrophic nerve trunks within the submucosal and intermyenteric plexus. Conversely, if ganglion cells are observed on histologic examination, a diagnosis of Hirschsprung's disease is excluded.

Treatment

Preoperative Care

In infants with enterocolitis, orogastric tube decompression, IV fluid resuscitation, broad-spectrum antibiotics, and correction of acid-base deficits and electrolyte abnormalities are promptly initiated (see Chapters 4, 11, 14, and 22). In infants who are less ill with symptoms of obstruction, they are placed on NPO status and IV antibiotic therapy and orogastric decompression are instituted, permitting time to complete the diagnostic evaluation.

Operative Intervention

In the presence of enterocolitis, an emergency colostomy is indicated. In general, a colostomy is performed at a site of normal bowel (ganglion cells present), as confirmed by a frozen section histologic examination. In selected cases the infant will be too ill, so operative time is minimized by the creation of a right colon enterostomy, because most affected patients have more distal colonic involvement. If the infant presents with milder symptoms, one of several options may be selected: (1) laparoscopically assisted primary pull-through, (2) primary transanal pull-through, or (3) **staged reconstruction** (temporary colostomy, followed by a pull-through in 3 to 6 months). In all cases, multiple intestinal seromuscular biopsies are performed at the time of operation until the transition zone to normally enervated bowel is identified. A coloanal anastomosis or colostomy is performed at the site of histologically proven normal bowel. If the anastomosis or colostomy site is absent of ganglion cells, the infant will remain symptomatic—the bowel will not function normally because of a segment of aganglionosis.

Several factors influence the decision to perform a **primary pull-through procedure.** The infant should be of sufficient size (more than 3 kg), have rectosigmoid disease as demonstrated by barium enema, not have significant proximal bowel distention,

and not have evidence of enterocolitis. Infants who do not meet these criteria should be treated in a staged manner, with an immediate colostomy and a delayed pull-through procedure.[18,46]

Postoperative Care

The recovery period is generally straightforward and supportive care is provided until the return of bowel function. In children treated initially with colostomy, postoperative care includes teaching the parents about ostomy care (Box 28-1). The **pull-through procedure** entails resecting abnormal aganglionic bowel and bringing ganglionic bowel to the anus. There are several variations of the pull-through operation; each has slight advantages and disadvantages, but in general the results are equivalent.

Complications and Prognosis

Early complications of the pull-through operation include inadequate blood supply to the anastomoses, anastomotic dehiscence, and cuff abscess. The infant usually thrives postoperatively and grows normally. It is not uncommon for the infant to

---

Box 28-1	**INSTRUCTIONS FOR OSTOMY CARE**

Supplies

Skin-prep (United)*
Stoma-adhesive paste (Convatec)*
Ostomy set-up (skin wafer and bag)
Pattern for stoma

Application Instructions

1. Measure the diameter of the stoma, using the measuring guide circle enclosed in the wafer box.
2. Trace the appropriate circle onto the white paper backing of the wafer and cut out the hole. Gently bend and slightly stretch the opening with your finger. The goal is to have the hole ¹⁄₁₆ to ⅛ inch larger than the stoma. A snug but not constricting fit is needed to prevent stool from leaking onto the skin.
3. Clean and dry the skin around the stoma.
4. Apply a generous coat of Skin-prep (United) on the skin around the stoma.
5. Apply a thin border of Stoma-adhesive paste (Convatec) around the stoma.

Application Instructions—cont'd

6. Press wafer firmly to skin.
7. If using a two-piece appliance, snap on the bag and close the end of the bag with a clip or rubber band if it is open-ended. If using a one-piece appliance, the appliance may be applied directly to the skin or to a skin barrier such as Stoma-adhesive (Convatec).*

Helpful Hints

1. *Change the appliance as soon as there is any evidence of leaking!*
2. Rinsing the bags with some type of scented soap (peppermint or spice) will help cut down on the bag odor.
3. Pre-cut several wafers ahead of time.
4. When travelling, always have an extra set of clothes and a complete set of supplies as well as a new set-up with stoma holes already cut.

Courtesy Kris Altzenbeck, R.N., The Children's Hospital, Denver, Colo.
*Other products may be used in place of the brand names upon recommendation of your medical supplier, physician, or nurse.

have frequent stools during the immediate postoperative period, and later some children will experience continued **constipation** requiring some form of bowel management.[55]

IMPERFORATE ANUS

Physiology and Etiology

Imperforate anus occurs in 1 in 5000 live births, and males (58%) are more commonly affected than females (42%). **Imperforate anus is a spectrum of anomalies characterized as low, intermediate, or high.** The higher the defect, the more likely the presence of other associated malformations. Again, this relates to the concept that an insult that occurs during the critical period of organogenesis places a number of systems at risk for malformation. The development of the hindgut begins during the third week of gestation and is completed by the ninth week of gestation. The most severe anorectal malformation, cloaca, arises from an arrest in development of the hindgut during the fourth to sixth week of gestation, and thus up to 60% infants will have concomitant anomalies of other organ systems.[20] A high imperforate anus is defined as the ending of the rectum occurring above the levator ani muscles. Conversely, in low imperforate anus the rectum descends below the levator complex. A fistulous connection is uniformly present. In high lesions the rectal fistula enters the membranous urethra in the male or the vagina in the female. In low lesions the rectal fistula exits on the perineum or the posterior fourchette of the vagina.[38] Congenital VACTERL anomalies and trisomy 21 are common and require evaluation. Moreover, a high incidence of spinal dysraphism is observed with anorectal malformation; imaging of the spine is indicated.[48]

Data Collection

Signs and Symptoms

Most anorectal malformations are apparent on physical examination but may be missed if a careful inspection of the buttocks and anus is not performed. **Once the diagnosis is made, a fistula should be sought.** In low lesions there may be a thin membrane over the anal orifice, or there may be a fistula along the perineum and scrotal raphe. If meconium passes in the urine or from the vagina, a high lesion is present. If the condition remains unrecognized, the infant develops signs and symptoms of intestinal obstruction.

Laboratory Data

An **abdominal x-ray film** demonstrates bowel dilation without rectal gas, but it will not reliably show the distal extent of the rectum. **Ultrasonography** may be used to establish the level of the obstruction and to outline the fistula. A contrast study of the fistula or urethra may also delineate the degree of rectal malformation.

Treatment

Preoperative Care

The infant should be kept NPO, and an OG tube should be placed. If a fistula is present on the perineum or fourchette, it should be dilated and an early anoplasty performed. If no fistula is visualized and a high lesion or cloaca is present, a colostomy is performed and staged reconstruction is planned.

Operative Intervention

For **low imperforate anus,** early reconstruction is performed either in the newborn period (males) or in the first months of life if the infant can produce stools adequately through the fistulous tract (females). After colostomy in infants with a **high imperforate anus,** a formal repair is undertaken when the child is 3 to 6 months of age. Approached through a posterior sacral incision, the fistula is divided, the rectum is brought through the sphincter mechanism and anastomosed to the anal skin in a procedure known as a *posterior sagittal anorectoplasty* (PSARP).[39]

Postoperative Care

After an anoplasty, simple skin care is all that is necessary, and a program of anal dilation is instituted 10 to 14 days postoperatively. After a colostomy, stoma care and teaching is begun with the parents (Box 28-1).

Complications and Prognosis

Mechanical complications of the stoma (prolapse, stenosis, and skin breakdown) may arise but generally do not require revision and should be temporized until stomal closure.[37] **Urinary tract infection** (UTI) or **hyperchloremic metabolic acidosis** may result from the fistulous connection of the rectum to the urinary tract. Antibiotic prophylaxis is instituted and selected infants may require bicarbonate supplement until the fistula is divided.

Constipation is the primary long-term problem after correction of low imperforate anus. Stricture of the anoplasty should always be considered and may be treated with anal dilation or rarely revision anoplasty.

High imperforate anus is most often complicated by **incontinence** and frequent soiling. Long-term results are influenced by the degree of sphincter muscle development and enervation. Approximately 25% of infants will have good continence, 50% will have fair continence, and 25% will have poor results. Bowel programs and strategies have been developed to permit some degree of social continence so that permanent colostomy can be avoided.

BILIARY ATRESIA

Physiology and Etiology

Biliary atresia is an inflammatory condition of unknown cause that culminates in the obliteration of the bile ducts. It is thought to be an **acquired** condition: fibrosis and scarring leads to blockage of the bile ducts and obstruction of bile flow. Beginning in the newborn period, a progressive **obliteration** of the bile ducts (Figure 28-9) results in complete obstruction by 3 to 4 months of age. Both intrahepatic and extrahepatic ducts are involved, but the primary involvement of the extrahepatic (common hepatic duct and common bile duct) segment of the biliary system permits surgical palliation. Biliary atresia is the most common cause of **obstructive jaundice** in

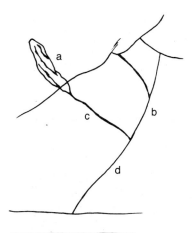

FIGURE 28-9 Extrahepatic biliary atresia is manifested as fibrosis of the gallbladder and the hepatic, cycstic, and common bile ducts.

infants, affecting females slightly more often than males.

Data Collection
History and Physical Examination
Because the gradual loss of patency of the bile ducts begins early in the neonatal period, few newborns with biliary atresia are visibly jaundiced. The infant often eats and grows normally until 1 month of age. Shortly thereafter, scleral icterus begins and the parent may note the passage of nonpigmented (clay-colored) stools and dark urine. Soon the infant appears **jaundiced,** and physical examination reveals an enlarged liver.[35]

Laboratory Data
Infantile jaundice may be caused by obstructive or nonobstructive causes (infection, hematologic, metabolic).[24] Serum liver tests (total, direct, indirect bilirubin, ALT, AST, GGT) demonstrate a pattern of **obstructive jaundice.** Ultrasonography and nuclear imaging scans are obtained. If on **ultrasound** the gallbladder is not visualized, a diagnosis of biliary atresia is suspected, although examination early after the onset of the disease may result in a false-negative study, because complete obstruction has not occurred and the gallbladder only appears to be small or contracted. A **radionuclide (HIDA) scan** demonstrates normal or delayed uptake of the marker, but secretion into the gastrointestinal tract is absent. Definitive diagnosis, however, can only be made operatively using **liver biopsy** and **cholangiography.**

Treatment
Operative Intervention
During surgical exploration, the gallbladder appears shrunken and fibrotic. An intraoperative cholangiogram demonstrates occlusion of the extrahepatic ducts and absence of flow into the duodenum. Thus an alternative conduit for bile drainage must be constructed. The fibrotic ducts are excised to the bifurcation of the major hepatic ducts and a segment of jejunum is interposed between the liver and small intestine, permitting bile flow[35] in a procedure called **Kasai portoenterostomy.** The Kasai operation results in adequate bile drainage in approximately 80% of infants under 10 weeks of age, but successful restoration of bile flow falls to less than 50% if the procedure is performed after the infant is more than 4 months of age. Thus early diagnosis and operative intervention are essential, because

successful correction appears inversely proportional to the infant's age.

Postoperative Care

Bowel rest and decompression are continued until the return of bowel function. A surgical drain placed in the area of the hepatoenteric anastomosis is monitored carefully for evidence of a leak. Feedings employing a predigested formula are started, and the stool is monitored for pigment that would suggest the return of bile flow from the liver to the intestine. Fat-soluble vitamins are started because of fat malabsorption. If bile flow appears sluggish, a steroid burst or ursodeoxycholic acid is administered. If surgery has been successful, liver function tests will normalize and jaundice will slowly resolve over the ensuing 2 to 3 months.

Complications and Prognosis

Biliary atresia is an incurable condition, but it may be palliated with the Kasai operation: one third of patients improve indefinitely, and one third improve temporarily, but one third fail to demonstrate any improvement. For the latter two thirds of patients, liver transplantation be- comes their only chance for survival.[25] Apart from the complications of progressive liver failure in those who do not respond, cholangitis is the most frequent complication affecting all patients undergoing the Kasai operation. **Cholangitis** results from bile stasis and bacterial contamination of the intestinal conduit. Characterized by fever, leukocytosis, and acholic stools, therapy consists of a 5- to 7-day course of intravenous antibiotics and a limited course of corticosteroids to promote bile flow. Repeated episodes of cholangitis accelerate the already existing liver damage and may lead to early liver failure if inadequately treated.

OMPHALOCELE AND GASTROSCHISIS

Physiology and Etiology

Omphalocele and gastroschisis are defects of the abdominal wall at or near the umbilicus. **Omphalocele is herniation of the abdominal viscera through the base of the umbilical cord and a covering of peritoneum (Figure 28-10). Omphalocele is a defect in abdominal wall development. Associated anomalies are common (30% to 35%), including trisomy 12, 18, and 21; other midline**

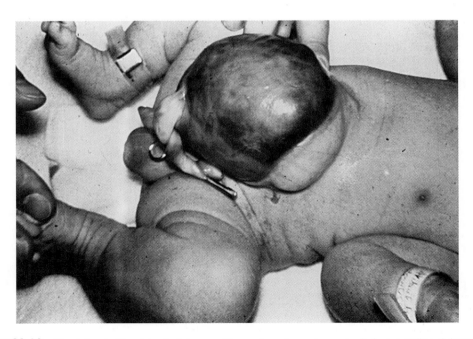

FIGURE 28-10   Omphalocele. The abdominal viscera with a peritoneal covering protrude from a midline abdominal wall.

congenital defects, including sternal and diaphragmatic defects; and congenital heart lesions. Therefore omphalocele is considered the most serious abdominal wall defect and is a potentially lethal anomaly.[4] A rare form of omphalocele is cloacal exostropy, which consists of an abdominal wall defect, hindgut defect, bladder defect, spinal abnormalities, and imperforate anus.

Gastroschisis is a defect of the abdominal wall that occurs to the right of the umbilicus and lacks a peritoneal covering (Figure 28-11). It is hypothesized that this defect results from a weakening of the abdominal wall as the right umbilical vein regresses during development. Gastroschisis occurs two to three times more frequently than does omphalocele, but this may reflect increased termination of pregnancy in infants with omphalocele because of the high incidence of associated anomalies. **Gastroschisis is typically not associated with major congenital anomalies or syndromes although 5% to 10% of affected infants will suffer intestinal atresia secondary to vascular compromise to the affected segment arising from a constricting fascial defect.**[28]

Nonrotation of the intestine is uniformly present in both conditions.

Data Collection

History

Abdominal wall defects are readily diagnosed by antenatal ultrasonography, permitting future therapy to be planned. Normal vaginal delivery may be considered, because there is a low risk of bowel injury during delivery.[21]

Severe serositis resulting from exposure of the bowel to amniotic fluid makes closure more difficult and delays the return of bowel function. Early delivery is recommended for infants with **gastroschisis** if there is sonographic evidence of progressive bowel distention and thickening suggesting bowel obstruction or severe serositis.

Signs and Symptoms

Both conditions present as a mass of abdominal contents extruding through an anterior abdominal wall defect. **Eviscerated bowel without a peritoneal covering is present in gastroschisis, whereas in omphalocele there is peritoneal covering herniated bowel and often liver as well.** Gastroschisis is herniation to the right of the midline, while omphalocele occurs through a central defect.

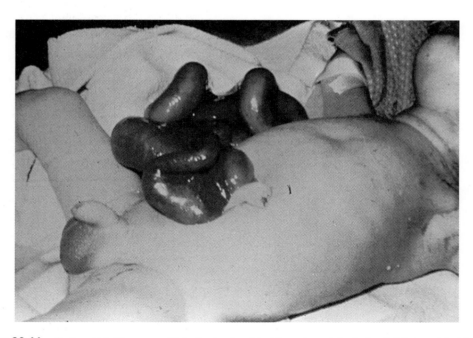

FIGURE 28-11 Gastroschisis. The exposed intestine has herniated through an abdominal wall defect to right of midline.

Laboratory Data

In a neonate with **omphalocele** a careful search for associated anomalies is performed before closure is attempted. Echocardiography and an x-ray examination of the chest and spine are performed to rule out cardiac, chest wall, diaphragmatic, and spinal anomalies.

Treatment

Preoperative Care

Initial management includes preservation of body heat and fluid, gastric decompression, protection of the intestine, and prophylaxis against infection. Covering the exposed viscera minimizes heat and fluid loss. Wrapping the intestines in warm, saline-soaked gauze covered with a plastic wrap or placing the infant into an impermeable, clear plastic bowel bag are generally employed. Both methods decrease evaporative losses; the bowel bag further allows continuous visual monitoring of the bowel. With either method, it is imperative that the bowel be positioned to prevent constriction of the blood supply at the fascial level.

Intravenous fluids and broad-spectrum antibiotics should be instituted early. To prevent bowel distention, an orogastric tube is placed on suction.

Operative Intervention

Rarely, an infant with omphalocele may be too ill to undergo operation or may have other lethal mal-formations. Under these circumstances the infant is given palliative care with a daily application of 65% alcohol or silver sulfadine to the abdominal sac. The result is eschar formation and subsequent epithelialization in 10 to 20 weeks. A large ventral hernia will remain, and if the patient survives, repair may be performed later.

Primary **surgical repair** entails reduction of the herniated abdominal contents into the abdominal cavity without increasing abdominal pressure to a point that ventilation, venous return, and intestinal blood supply are compromised. If the amount of eviscerated abdominal contents is small or moderate, primary repair is simple and safe. Before closure the surgeon searches carefully for associated atresia but makes no attempt at correction during the initial operation. The atretic bowel is returned to the abdomen, with reexploration planned in 2 to 3 weeks to allow the thickened, edematous bowel to return to normal, permitting anastomosis or enterostomy.

In selected cases the fascial defect may have to be enlarged to allow replacement of the herniated organs into the abdomen because of the small size of the abdominal cavity and the amount of intestinal herniation. The inability to perform primary closure necessitates placement of a **Silastic silo** (Figure 28-12) or patch to permit staged reduction. Over the ensuing 7 to 10 days the herniated viscera is slowly returned to the abdomen on a daily basis. Once all

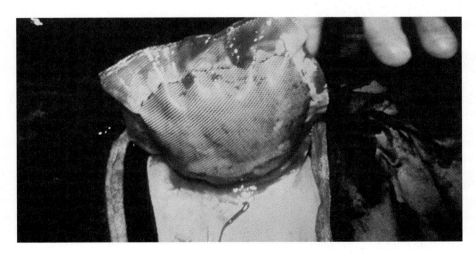

FIGURE 28-12   Silo. A silicone-coated mesh pouch has been created to accommodate the herniated intestine. Over the ensuing 5 to 7 days the abdominal contents are reduced daily until the abdominal wall can be safely reconstructed.

the contents of the silo are successfully reduced, the infant is returned to the operating room for removal of the silo and closure of the fascia.[42]

Complications and Prognosis

Bowel injury, respiratory compromise, and diminished venous return caused by increased abdominal pressure may complicate recovery. In this setting the infant is returned to the operating room for placement of a silo. Rarely, the silo may become infected, separate from the fascia, and make closure by this method impossible.

Recovery of bowel function is uniformly delayed, especially in gastroschisis caused by exposure of the bowel to amniotic fluid. A central venous catheter should be placed at the time of initial surgery for long-term nutritional support (see Chapter 17). Incisional hernia and adhesive bowel obstruction are possible short- and long-term complications. Otherwise, prognosis is good unless severe associated malformations are present.

Parent Teaching

Preoperative

The planned operative procedure and its expected results and risks of complications are discussed with the parents, ensuring that all questions and concerns are addressed. Moreover, the need for anesthesia and analgesia should be explained to parents, along with the physiologic and behavioral benefits of pain relief. **Care providers' sensitivity to the neonate's pain and advocating for pain relief is comforting for parents** (see Chapter 12).

Parents often fear what the infant will look like on return from surgery. Providing written material with simple drawings of the operative procedure helps to simply and clarify the operative procedure. **It is helpful for both the nurse and the physician to meet with the family to discuss the operation.** This is especially important for the nurse, who must answer questions, interpret information, and reassure an anxious family when the physician leaves.

Because parents' fears and fantasies about their infant's problem are frequently worse than reality, parents should see their infant before surgery (see Chapters 29 and 30). Infants who are extremely ill should have a picture taken before surgery. In the tragic situation of the neonate's death during operation, these pictures may be very valuable to the family. It may also be helpful for parents to see an infant who has had a similar procedure and has the equipment that has been described (e.g., colostomy, OG tube, and

chest tube). If this is not possible, pictures or drawings are useful in preventing postoperative surprises.

Operative

Accompanying the infant to surgery and seeing the infant as soon as possible after surgery are comforting to the parents. Progress reports of the surgery, if possible, are helpful for the anxious family members. After the operation, the pediatric surgeon should immediately see the parents to explain the procedure and any unexpected problems that occurred during the operation.

Postoperative

After surgery parents need to review the equipment and what it does to help their infant. It is important to help them focus their attention on their infant rather than the surrounding environment. Early involvement in caregiving helps the parents to feel as though they are essential to their child's recovery.

For infants with an ostomy or who will continue TPN at home, the parents should participate often and early. They may begin by cleansing the skin around the ostomy or helping to prepare the equipment. Gradually they are able to increase their responsibilities of caregiving as their infant improves. Delay until a few days before discharge does not give parents adequate time for practice and familiarity before being on their own.

The possibility of late postoperative complications should be discussed with parents. Parents should be familiar with problems that may develop and how to recognize them; for example, the ability to recognize excessive stooling in an infant with an ileostomy may lead to the family seeking early medical attention before severe dehydration develops.

The importance of follow-up care is emphasized to the parents. It may be helpful for parents to talk with a "graduate" parent who had an infant with similar problems. Available resources, such as visiting nurses, graduate parents, and physician assistants or nurses are provided with contact information. The infant's history and treatment should be easily accessible to other providers and is ideally summarized in a concise discharge plan provided to the parents.

ACKNOWLEDGMENT

We would like to thank Carol Rumack, M.D., and the Department of Radiology, University of Colorado Health Sciences Center, Denver, Colorado.

REFERENCES

1. Adzick NS, Nance ML: Pediatric surgery, *N Engl J Med* 342:1651, 2000.
2. Bax NM, van der Zee DC: Laparoscopic treatment of intestinal malrotation in children, *Surg Endosc* 12:1314, 1998.
3. Carpenter RO, Schaffer RL, Maeso CE et al: Postoperative ad lib feeding for hypertrophic pyloric stenosis, *J Pediatr Surg* 34:959, 1999.
4. Chen CP, Liu FF, Jan SW et al: Prenatal diagnosis and perinatal aspects of abdominal wall defects, *Am J Perinatol* 13:355, 1996.
5. Chen EA, Luks FI, Gilchrist BF et al: Pyloric stenosis in the age of ultrasonography: fading skills, better patients? *J Pediatr Surg* 31:829, 1996.
6. Chittmittrapap S, Spitz L, Kiely EM et al: Oesophageal atresia and associated anomalies, *Arch Dis Child* 64:364, 1989.
7. Coran AG, Teitelbaum DH: Recent advances in the management of Hirschsprung's disease, *Am J Surg* 180:382, 2000.
8. Dalla Vecchia LK, Grosfeld JL, West KW et al: Intestinal atresia and stenosis: a 25-year experience with 277 cases, *Arch Surg* 133:490, 1998.
9. Dimmitt RA, Meier AH, Skarsgard ED et al: Salvage laparotomy for failure of peritoneal drainage in necrotizing enterocolitis in infants with extremely low birth weight, *J Pediatr Surg* 35:856, 2000.
10. Downey EC Jr: Laparoscopic pyloromyotomy, *Semin Pediatr Surg* 7:220, 1998.
11. Engum SA, Grosfeld JL, West KW et al: Analysis of morbidity and mortality in 227 cases of esophageal atresia and/or tracheoesophageal fistula over two decades, *Arch Surg* 130:502, 1995.
12. Esposito C, Montupet P, Reinberg O: Laparoscopic surgery for gastroesophageal reflux disease during the first year of life, *J Pediatr Surg* 36:715, 2001.
13. Feitz R, Vos A: Malrotation: the postoperative period, *J Pediatr Surg* 32:1322, 1997.
14. Fonkalsrud EW, Ashcraft KW, Coran AG et al: Surgical treatment of gastroesophageal reflux in children: a combined hospital study of 7467 patients, *Pediatrics* 101:419, 1998.
15. Fonkalsrud EW, Bustorff-Silva J, Perez CA et al: Antireflux surgery in children under 3 months of age, *J Pediatr Surg* 34:527, 1999.
16. Fuchs JR, Langer JC: Long-term outcome after neonatal meconium obstruction, *Pediatrics* 101:E7, 1998.
17. Gauderer MW: Gastrostomy techniques and devices, *Surg Clin North Am* 72:1285, 1992.
18. Georgeson KE, Cohen RD, Hebra A et al: Primary laparoscopic-assisted endorectal colon pull-through for Hirschsprung's disease: a new gold standard, *Ann Surg* 229:678, 1999.
19. Grosfeld JL, Rescorla FJ: Duodenal atresia and stenosis: reassessment of treatment and outcome based on antenatal diagnosis, pathologic variance, and long-term follow-up, *World J Surg* 17:301, 1993.
20. Hendren WH: Cloaca, the most severe degree of imperforate anus: experience with 195 cases, *Ann Surg* 228:331, 1998.
21. How HY, Harris BJ, Pietrantoni M et al: Is vaginal delivery preferable to elective cesarean delivery in fetuses with a known ventral wall defect? *Am J Obstet Gynecol* 182:1527, 2000.
22. Hulka F, Harrison MW, Campbell TJ et al: Complications of pyloromyotomy for infantile hypertrophic pyloric stenosis, *Am J Surg* 173:450, 1997.
23. Kao SC, Franken EA Jr: Nonoperative treatment of simple meconium ileus: a survey of the Society for Pediatric Radiology, *Pediatr Radiol* 25:97, 1995.
24. Karrer FM, Bensard DD: Neonatal cholestasis, *Semin Pediatr Surg* 9:166, 2000.
25. Karrer FM, Price MR, Bensard DD et al: Long-term results with the Kasai operation for biliary atresia, *Arch Surg* 131:493, 1996.
26. Kinsella JP, Truog WE, Walsh WF et al: Randomized, multicenter trial of inhaled nitric oxide and high-frequency oscillatory ventilation in severe, persistent pulmonary hypertension of the newborn, *J Pediatr* 131:55, 1997.
27. Kubiak R, Spitz L, Kiely EM et al: Effectiveness of fundoplication in early infancy, *J Pediatr Surg* 34:295, 1999.
28. Langer JC: Gastroschisis and omphalocele, *Semin Pediatr Surg* 5:124, 1996.
29. Lemons JA, Bauer CR, Oh W et al: Very low birth weight outcomes of the National Institute of Child health and human development neonatal research network, January 1995 through December 1996, *Pediatrics* 107:E1, 2001.
30. Lindower J, Atherton H, Kotagal U: Outcomes and resource utilization for newborns with major congenital malformations: the initial NICU admission, *J Perinatol* 19:212, 1999.
31. Long FR, Kramer SS, Markowitz RI et al: Radiographic patterns of intestinal malrotation in children, *Radiographics* 16:547, 1996.
32. Messineo A, MacMillan JH, Palder SB et al: Clinical factors affecting mortality in children with malrotation of the intestine, *J Pediatr Surg* 27:1343, 1992.
33. Mushtaq I, Wright VM, Drake DP et al: Meconium ileus secondary to cystic fibrosis: the East London experience, *Pediatr Surg Int* 13:365, 1998.
34. Neilson D, Hollman AS: The ultrasonic diagnosis of infantile hypertrophic pyloric stenosis: technique and accuracy, *Clin Radiol* 49:246, 1994.
35. Nio M, Ohi R: Biliary atresia, *Semin Pediatr Surg* 9:177, 2000.
36. Nobuhara KK, Lund DP, Mitchell J et al: Long-term outlook for survivors of congenital diaphragmatic hernia, *Clin Perinatol* 23:873, 1996.
37. Patwardhan N, Kiely EM, Drake DP et al: Colostomy for anorectal anomalies: high incidence of complications, *J Pediatr Surg* 36:795, 2001.

38. Pena A: Anorectal malformations, *Semin Pediatr Surg* 4:35, 1995.

39. Pena A, Hong A: Advances in the management of anorectal malformations, *Am J Surg* 180:370, 2000.

40. Rescorla FJ, Grosfeld JL: Contemporary management of meconium ileus, *World J Surg* 17:318, 1993.

41. Sato S, Nishijima E, Muraji T et al: Jejunoileal atresia: a 27-year experience, *J Pediatr Surg* 33:1633, 1998.

42. Sauter ER, Falterman KW, Arensman RM: Is primary repair of gastroschisis and omphalocele always the best operation? *Am Surg* 57:142, 1991.

43. Skari H, Bjornland K, Haugen G et al: Congenital diaphragmatic hernia: a meta-analysis of mortality factors, *J Pediatr Surg* 35:1187, 2000.

44. Spigland N, Yazbeck S: Complications associated with surgical treatment of congenital intrinsic duodenal obstruction, *J Pediatr Surg* 25:1127, 1990.

45. Spitz L, Kiely EM, Morecroft JA et al: Oesophageal atresia: at-risk groups for the 1990s, *J Pediatr Surg* 29:723, 1994.

46. Teitelbaum DH, Cilley RE, Sherman NJ et al: A decade of experience with the primary pull-through for Hirschsprung disease in the newborn period: a multicenter analysis of outcomes, *Ann Surg* 232:372, 2000.

47. Torres AM, Ziegler MM: Malrotation of the intestine, *World J Surg* 17:326, 1993.

48. Torres R, Levitt MA, Tovilla JM et al: Anorectal malformations and Down's syndrome, *J Pediatr Surg* 33:194, 1998.

49. Trends in infant mortality attributable to birth defects: United States, 1980-1995, *MMWR Morb Mortal Wkly Rep* 47:773, 1998.

50. Vandenplas Y: Diagnosis and treatment of gastroesophageal reflux disease in infants and children, *Can J Gastroenterol* 14(suppl):26D, 2000.

51. Ververidis M, Kiely EM, Spitz L et al: The clinical significance of thrombocytopenia in neonates with necrotizing enterocolitis, *J Pediatr Surg* 36:799, 2001.

52. Waldhausen JH, Sawin RS: Improved long-term outcome for patients with jejunoileal apple peel atresia, *J Pediatr Surg* 32:1307, 1997.

53. Walsh DS, Adzick NS: Fetal surgical intervention, *Am J Perinatol* 17:277, 2000.

54. Weber TR, Kountzman B, Dillon PA et al: Improved survival in congenital diaphragmatic hernia with evolving therapeutic strategies, *Arch Surg* 133:498, 1998.

55. Yanchar NL, Soucy P: Long-term outcome after Hirschsprung's disease: patients' perspectives, *J Pediatr Surg* 34:1152, 1999.

PART VI

PSYCHOSOCIAL ASPECTS OF NEONATAL CARE

29 Families in Crisis: Theoretic and Practical Considerations

Roberta Siegel, Sandra L. Gardner, Gerald B. Merenstein

The technical advances that have characterized newborn care in the last 40 years have resulted in marked improvement in the mortality and morbidity of the high-risk infant. These developments have been accompanied by a heightened appreciation of the psychologic strain and emotional stresses encountered by the family of the sick neonate.[20,58,92,103,107,144,157] Realization of the need for a family-centered approach to perinatal care has emerged out of an enhanced understanding of individual and family functioning and their adaptation to stress.[57,71,142] It has become essential for perinatal health care teams to address the psychologic needs of families who are experiencing the painful crisis of the birth of a sick newborn. The purpose of this chapter is to discuss the complex psychosocial needs of families during this stressful period and to offer concrete suggestions for intervention.

NORMAL ATTACHMENT

Emotional investment in the child begins not at birth, but during the pregnancy. The terms *attachment* and *bonding*[81] are used to describe this process of relating between parents and their infant. Attachment behavior is characterized by the same qualities used to describe love: care, responsibility, and knowledge.[51] Attachment is an individualized process, not an automatic one.[20]

The infant's need for the parent is absolute, but the parent's need for the infant is only relative. The neonate is totally dependent, both physically and emotionally, on the caregivers. Recognition of this unique relationship is evidenced cross-culturally by immediate and prolonged contact with no evidence of separation.[75,102] In most animal species the mother engages in species-specific behaviors[81] that enable her to become acquainted with and claim the newborn. Interference during this critical period results in rejection by the animal mother and death of the young. In a recent study, adult rats whose mothers engaged in more species-specific behaviors (e.g., licking and grooming) showed significantly decreased levels of stress hormones.[97] Parental attachment and caregiving behaviors are crucial for the infant's physical, psychologic, and emotional health and survival.[20,73,97,101,132] Ultimately, this influence will affect the child's well-being as an adult and a potential parent for a subsequent generation.

Critical and Sensitive Period

In the period immediately after birth, both mother and infant are physiologically and psychologically ready for reciprocal interaction.[81] Physiologically, even though labor and birth are tiring, most mothers feel "high" and have an incredible surge of energy after birth. Psychologically, the family is ready to meet and interact with the long-awaited newcomer. Physiologically, the first hour of life is a time of alertness for the newborn. Before the sleep phase the newborn is alert, makes eye-to-eye contact, fixes and follows, begins to search, unassisted, for the maternal nipple, and begins to feed.[156] At birth all five senses are operational, and the infant is ready to cue and shape the environment (see Chapter 13).

This period of mutual readiness has been compared with the critical period in animals. This human "maternal sensitive period"[81] is the time immediately after birth in which the attachment process is initiated. Called the optimal, but not the sole, period for attachment to develop, the human critical period represents a reciprocal readiness for acquaintance. Positive effects of early and extended contact, rather than initial separation, have shown significant differences in caregiving behaviors that persist over time.

Sustained and early contact between parents and infant completes the process of labor and birth and gives the family the opportunity for interaction. The presence of the infant enables the parents to begin knowing the reality and individuality of their infant. Early parent-infant contact facilitates parent-infant attachment and contributes to the regulation of the newborn's physiology and behavior.[20,31,73,97,131] Unnecessary "routines" and procedures that interfere with initial contact should be deferred until the initial acquaintance process is completed.[20,31,73,156]

Failure to establish immediate contact because of medically indicated interventions necessary to sustain life does not promote attachment, but it also does not undermine the entire process of attachment. Unlike animals, human mothers do not automatically reject their infant if they are unable to interact immediately. Interference or failure to interact during the critical period does not condemn the resilient and adaptable human parent to rejection of or maladaptation to the infant.

Crisis Event: Pregnancy and Parenthood

Pregnancy, birth, and parenthood are almost universally defined as a life crisis.[75,90] Parenting is a major adjustment of the prepregnancy roles, lifestyle, and relationships. Because previous ideas and coping styles may not be helpful, life crisis situations challenge the individual with the potential for growth as new responses and solutions are used for problem solving. Periods of upheaval, change, and vulnerability provide a time of openness, receptiveness, and readiness for help from significant others (including professionals).

Influences on Parenting

Opportunities to experience parenting and to observe others parent within a social setting are essential learning experiences for the development of parenting behaviors. The ability to parent is influenced by a multitude of factors that occur before, during, and after the birth of the infant. Previous life events, including genetic endowment,[81] cultural practices,[75,102] being parented,[61] previous pregnancies,[76,92] and interpersonal relationships,[22,61] affect the experience of pregnancy and parenthood. The events of the current pregnancy,[32,74,81,92,147] their significance to the parent, and the availability of support and assistance influence parenting ability.[22,42,107] After birth, infant characteristics, appearance,[17,20,155] the behavior of health professionals,* separation from the infant,[16,89,97,106,131] and hospital practices† may positively or negatively influence parents. Not only the occurrence of these events, but also their meaning to the individual and the type of assistance received, influence parenting abilities.

Steps of Attachment

Klaus and Kennell[81] have proposed nine steps in the process of attachment.

Step 1: Planning the Pregnancy

This is the initial step of investment in the life-altering prospect of parenthood. Pregnancies are planned in one of two ways: consciously or unconsciously. Who planned the pregnancy and why this particular time has been chosen are important indicators of the investment of each individual in the decision and in the pregnancy.

Carrying a pregnancy is not assurance that the baby is wanted. Although it may be a legal option, abortion may not be a cultural, moral, financial, or ethical option for the individual woman. Attachment of the mother (or father) to the infant is not assured merely by the mother's remaining pregnant, giving birth, and keeping the infant.

Step 2: Confirming the Pregnancy

This occurs after the first and often subtle signs of pregnancy appear. Pregnancy confirmation begins the psychologic acceptance of the pregnancy. Delaying confirmation enables the fact of pregnancy to be denied and prevents progression to the acceptance stage.

Step 3: Accepting the Pregnancy

This usually begins early in the pregnancy and is characterized by the emotional changes of primary narcissism, introversion, and passivity. Because she is less interested in the outside world and more interested in her own inner world, the mother is able to become attuned to her own needs. Although she was previously engaged in active, extroverted be-

---

*References 41, 43, 57, 64, 81, 106, 107, 127, 134, 136.
†References 17, 20, 41-43, 52, 57, 65, 74, 82, 152.

haviors, she may, during the pregnancy, contentedly participate in quieter, more introspective activities.

At this early stage of pregnancy the fetus is not perceived by the woman as separate from herself but as an extension of her body. The psychologic changes of pregnancy have survival significance in that caring for herself assures caring for the fetus as an integral part of herself.[21]

During the early months of pregnancy, the man and woman realize that parenting will require a major adjustment of prepregnancy roles, lifestyle, and relationships. The adaptation of parenthood is characterized by upheaval and change, losses and gains. Bombarded with phenomenal lifelong changes, the future parents experience the normal feeling of ambivalence.

Step 4: Fetal Movement
Fetal movement, felt by the mother between 16 and 32 weeks of gestation, is the beginning of the acceptance of the fetus as an individual. Fetal movement is the first concrete evidence to the mother of the existence of another person within her. Hearing the baby's heartbeat, seeing the ultrasound readings, or experiencing an amniocentesis also confirms the reality of the fetus.[72] Fetal movement is such a significant event that often a pregnancy that began as unplanned and unwanted becomes wanted.

Perception of the first fetal movement is a happy event. When asked "How did you feel when the baby first moved?" most women respond in a happy tone and with a smile. A negative tone or negative words used to describe fetal movement is a concern because the individual (fetus) may already be perceived as an intruder.

Step 5: Accepting the Fetus
Accepting the fetus as an individual begins with fetal movement. The fetus asserts individuality in controlling the movement; the mother can neither start nor stop these movements. With the realization of the concrete evidence of the presence of another person, parents begin the psychologic acceptance and personification of the fetus as a separate individual. Love for the fetus as a separate individual occurs through the parents' investing a personality in the fetus and establishing a relationship with that personality. Fantasies about how the baby looks, the sex, and the wish for a perfect, healthy infant are common.

Outwardly, preparations are made for the acceptance of an infant into the home; baby clothes and furniture are purchased, and a room is prepared. The fetus may be referred to by a nickname or a term of endearment. The baby's name may be chosen. Choosing a name is a highly personal and significant event. The meaning of the name and who chooses it illustrate the power holder and decision-maker within the family. Prenatal questions such as "Do you have a nickname for the baby?" "Do you have a name picked out for the baby?" and "Who picked it out?" may be asked after the birth to elicit information.

Whether the newborn meets parental expectations for "the right sex" may be crucially important in the parents' ability to attach to the infant. "Do you have a sex preference for the baby?" may be asked before or after the birth to elicit this information. Often parents with a strong sex preference have chosen no names for a baby of the "wrong" sex.

"It doesn't matter as long as it's healthy," is often heard and may indicate no conscious sex preference. However, unconsciously the parents may have a strong sex preference as evidenced by a predominance of dreams about one sex. If dreams are equally divided between male and female children, there may indeed be no sex preference at the unconscious level.

Most parents are fearful of producing a defective child. This fear is experienced as dreams about dead, deformed, or damaged fetuses and babies, or dreams with a central theme of destruction. These unconscious contents are often experienced as frightening nightmares that may often be imbued with magical ideas such as, "If I think (or talk about) it, it will come true." Both before and after birth, it is reassuring for parents to know that this is a common and scary phenomenon, that they aren't "crazy," and that the fears are not magical.

Parental expectations of the newborn are established before birth in the personification and relationship with the unseen, unheard fetus. After birth the developmental task of parenthood is a working out of the discrepancy between the wished for and the actual infant.[146] Before attachment to the actual infant can proceed, the fantasized child must be mourned.

Step 6: Labor and Birth
Labor is a physiologic, maturational, and psychologic crisis for the family. Birth is the culmination of pregnancy and the reward for the work of labor. Parents' attitudes about the labor and birth experiences affect their reactions to the infant. Newton

and Newton[115] found mothers more likely to be pleased with their infant at first sight if the mothers were relaxed, calm, and cooperative; had rapport with the attendants; and received personalized, solicitous care.

Paternal participation in labor and birth is an important issue. In the past, health care professionals saw no benefit to the presence of the father and even wished to exclude him because of imagined "horribles" such as increased infection rate, malpractice suits, and disruption of routines.

Birth is a powerfully emotional experience, so that those who attend birth are more attached to the infant than those who do not attend.[81] Benefits attributed to a father's participation at labor and birth include use of less analgesia, a more supportive environment, and a deepened relationship[14] between parents and between parents and their infant.[125] Inclusion of the father in perinatal events may "hook" him for inclusion in parenting activities. Rather than just a financial provider, fathering may be perceived as a psychologic necessity for both fathers and children.

Parental behaviors at birth indicate involvement and investment in the infant[72a]:

- "How does the mother or father *look?*" At the sound of the infant's cry, parents smile and breathe a sigh of relief at this first breath of life. Support, joy, and happiness are positive feelings shared by couples at birth.
- "What does the mother or father *say?*" By speaking in a positive tone with words of affection and endearment, the parents relate to each other and to the new infant.
- "What does the mother or father *do?*" When offered the infant, both parents will reach out to take the infant. Spontaneously, parents engage in eye-to-eye contact and touch and explore the infant. Affectionate behaviors such as kissing, fondling, cuddling, and claiming characterize positive parental reactions.

A positive, self-affirming birth experience for the mother enhances her feelings of self-esteem, thus her self-concept as a woman and mother.[52] A birth experience that does not meet parental expectations may have a negative effect on the self-concept of the mother, her perception of her ability to parent, and her relationship with the infant.[41,52] In fact, "so intricately are mother and infant entwined in a symbiotic relationship, that what is psychically positive for the mother is positive for the infant. What is psychically negative for the mother will affect the infant."[52] Labor and delivery that have been difficult or prolonged may influence the parents' over-

protection, resentment, or antagonism toward the infant.[3,41]

So powerful is the labor and birth experience that women are unable to proceed with parenting until psychic closure of the experience has been obtained. Even women who experience a normal labor and birth process need to recount the experience to others. Maternal perception of the events is obvious in tone and content of the recounting. *Missing pieces*[3] is the term used to describe the aspects of labor and birth that are forgotten or unavailable to recall. Long labor, short labor, or medicated labor can cause missing pieces in the mother's memory of the birth. Labor that did not meet expectations because of difficulty, cesarean section, use of forceps, or episiotomy could also affect the mother.[3] To proceed with parenting, these women need to fill in their knowledge gaps by asking questions or looking at pictures or films of the birth to reconstruct the situation.

Step 7: Seeing

Seeing and touching are the species-specific ways in which humans attach to their young.[81] In a recent study, immediate attachment was facilitated by (1) positive maternal feelings toward the infant; (2) mother able to see infant immediately after birth; and (3) when there was immediate contact between mother and infant.[20] Delayed attachment may occur when the infant is premature because he does not conform to parental expectations of a full-term baby.[20]

Eye contact between parents and their infant in the initial period after birth may be a positive release of parental feelings of warmth, closeness, and caring. As parents see and inspect the newborn, they begin claiming their infant: "He has my eyes; she has your nose" and begin "letting go" of the prenatally fantasized child. Characteristics of each parent and the family are identified in the infant, and the newborn is claimed as a member of the family.

The term *en face position* is used to describe the mother's (father's) eyes and the infant's eyes positioned in the same vertical plane.[81] This positioning enables the parent and infant to look directly into each other's eyes, to focus, and to regard each other (Figure 29-1).

The newborn infant is an active participant in the acquaintance process, as he or she cues the mother with eye-to-eye contact. Even minutes old[49] newborns see and show a preference for the human face (within 7 to 12 inches from their face). The newborn is able to visually follow the parent's face and voice and to signal the parent with facial expressions, movement, and vocalization, including a dis-

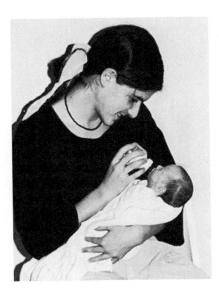

FIGURE 29-1   En face position: infant is held in close contact (mother's body touching infant's); mother is looking at infant en face; bottle is perpendicular to mouth; milk is in tip of nipple. (From Klaus MH, Kennel JH: *Parent-infant bonding*, ed 2, St Louis, 1982, Mosby.)

tress cry when separated from body contact with mother.[31]

Deterrents to the infant's full participation include removal to the nursery, medication (from analgesia), and eye prophylaxis. Unless medically indicated (necessary for physical survival), newborns should remain with their parents after birth.[131,152] Because eye prophylaxis irritates and interferes with vision, the "routine" instillation immediately after birth (in the delivery room) can be delayed until after the initial acquaintance process is completed.

Step 8: Touching
This behavior is important to the adult as a means of tactile and sensory knowledge of the infant. To the neonate the "stimulus hunger"[129] is satisfied by the parents' touch and ministrations.

In exploring the infant, parents systematically use fingertip contact with the infant's extremities. Gradually, there is progression to palm contact with the infant's trunk (Figure 29-2). With the healthy term infant, this progression occurs within minutes of the first contact. After gaining confidence and preliminary knowledge, the parent will enfold the infant close to the ventrum of the adult (a cuddling position).

With the preterm infant, this characteristic progression may take hours, days, or several visits (see

Figure 29-2). Fear of harming the small, fragile preterm infant prevents parents from feeling at ease in touching their infant. Until the parents feel confident that their actions will not harm the infant, they may be reticent to use palm contact with the trunk (vital organs).

Holding and cuddling the infant are significantly different from touching and exploring. Mothers who have only seen and touched their infant still experience "empty arms." The species-specific behavior of touch is not completely satisfied until the parent is able "to hold" the infant. Most mothers have a preference for holding their infants on the left. Explanations for this preference include hand dominance, importance of maternal heart beat, left breast sensitivity, and advantages in monitoring the infant. A more recent hypothesis proposes that maternal affective signals (both visual and auditory) are given to the infant's free left ear and processed by the more advanced right cerebral hemisphere.[143]

Step 9: Caregiving
The final step of attachment, caregiving is important for psychic closure of the task of bonding. The relationship between the primary caregiver and the infant is a reciprocal relationship. In the caregiving relationship both care provider and infant give to and receive from each other.[31,64,73] The physical and emotional needs of the helpless infant are satisfied by parental caregiving behaviors such as feeding, soothing, grooming, and playing. Based on the infant's ability to perceive and receive these ministrations, the infant responds to the care provider. Parental expectations of newborn responses include quieting, sucking, clinging and cuddling, looking, smiling, and vocalizing. The parents' capability to soothe and satisfy the infant provides emotional satisfaction and positive feedback about the parent's competency.

Personal needs for comfort, maintenance of homeostasis, and relief from painful experiences are infant expectations of the relationship with the care provider. Care-eliciting behaviors (crying, visual following, and smiling) are neonatal cues used to signal the care provider that attention is needed. Relief from discomfort enables the infant to respond positively to the care provider. The infant experiences the world through the caregiver and quickly learns that the environment is either nurturing and loving or hostile and nonresponsive. Consistent, predictable nurturing and caregiving enable the infant to develop a sense of trust in the caregiver, the world, and self (see Chapter 13).

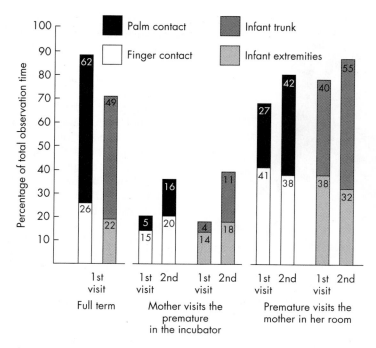

FIGURE 29-2 Fingertip and palm contact on trunk or extremities in three groups of mothers: (1) 12 mothers of term infants at their first visit, (2) 9 mothers who visited their premature infants in incubators in the NICU, and (3) 14 mothers whose premature infants were brought to their maternity rooms and placed in their beds. (From Klaus MH, Kennell JH: *Parent-infant bonding,* ed 2, St Louis, 1982, Mosby.)

Care by parents is the ideal neonatal care situation, because the infant learns and reacts to one set of cues or caregiving behaviors. Cared for by one or two people, the infant is able to regulate his physiologic behavioral processes (i.e., autonomic, neuroendocrine, behavioral, and electrophysiologic) and develop synchrony with the parents.[73] Single caregiving improves the establishment of biorhythms of the neonate[41,73] for sleep-wake cycles, feeding, and visual attentiveness. Multiple caregiving confuses the infant, increases distress with feeding, causes irritability, and upsets visual attention. Care by parents provides for mutual cuing and acquaintance and a natural setting for observation of parent-infant interaction.[32,152]

PSYCHOLOGIC ADJUSTMENTS TO A SICK NEWBORN

The birth of a sick newborn with its consequent family disruption represents to the perinatal health care team a unique crisis, a dangerous opportunity[7] within which to practice preventive health care.[111] For the involved individual and family this stressful event re-

sults in a period of psychologic disorganization during which their usual problem-solving mechanisms may not be adequate to cope with the events presented to them.[28] In addition to confronting this situational crisis, the individual or family must master the normal developmental process of parenthood.

Parental behavior and responses are determined not only by preexisting personality factors, social and cultural variables, and interactions with significant others,[22,28,43,80,92] but also by the immediate situation in which the parents are placed.* In one recent study six major sources of parental stress in the NICU were identified: (1) preexisting and concurrent personal and family factors, (2) prenatal and perinatal experiences, (3) infant illness, treatments, and appearance,[17,20] (4) concerns about the infant's outcome, (5) loss of the parental role,[17,20,107,144] and (6) health care providers.[74] Situational factors can have an important bearing on the family's ability to cope with the crisis and thus affect the overall outcome (Box 29-1).

---

*References 17, 22, 32, 43, 57, 134.

Box 29-1   SITUATIONAL FACTORS AFFECTING PARENTAL COPING*

1. The behaviors and attitudes of the hospital staff (physicians, nurses, and allied health professionals)
2. The sensitivity used in the process of separation and transfer of the infant to the intensive care unit or in some cases the referral hospital
3. The flexibility of hospital policy concerning parental and sibling involvement and visitation in the nursery
4. The instruction of parents in their infant's individual behaviors and characteristics (thus facilitating appropriate parent-child interaction and reciprocity) (see Chapter 13)
5. The staff's comprehension and appreciation of the psychosocial functioning of families and the family's responses and adaptation to stress and crisis
6. The employment of emotionally supportive intervention programs for parents within the nursery setting
7. The development of appropriate discharge planning to provide adequate follow-up care to the infant and family

*References 17, 20, 24, 39, 42, 43, 53, 57, 64, 65, 71, 74, 92, 103, 106, 107, 127, 134, 140, 142, 157.

Box 29-2   THE PRINCIPLES FOR FAMILY-CENTERED NEONATAL CARE

1. Family-centered neonatal care should be based on open and honest communication between parents and professionals on medical and ethical issues.
2. To work with professionals in making informed treatment choices, parents must have available to them the same facts and interpretation of those facts as the professionals, including medical information presented in meaningful formats, information about uncertainties surrounding treatments, information from parents whose children have been in similar medical situations, and access to the chart and rounds discussions.
3. In medical situations involving very high mortality and morbidity, great suffering, and/or significant medical controversy, fully informed parents should have the right to make decisions regarding aggressive treatment for their infants.
4. Expectant parents should be offered information about adverse pregnancy outcomes and be given the opportunity to state in advance their treatment preferences if their infant is born extremely prematurely and/or critically ill.
5. Parents and professionals must work together to acknowledge and alleviate the pain of infants in the NICU.
6. Parents and professionals must work together to ensure an appropriate environment for infants in the NICU.
7. Parents and professionals must work together to ensure the safety and efficacy of neonatal treatments.
8. Parents and professionals should work together to develop nursery policies and programs that promote parenting skills and encourage maximum involvement of families with their hospitalized infants.
9. Parents and professionals must work together to promote meaningful long-term follow-up for all high-risk NICU survivors.
10. Parents and professionals must acknowledge that critically ill newborns can be harmed by overtreatment as well as by undertreatment, and we must insist that our laws and treatment policies be based on compassion. We must work together to promote awareness of the needs of NICU survivors with disabilities to ensure adequate support for them and their families. We must work together to decrease disability through universal prenatal care.

Modified from Harrison H: The principles for family-centered neonatal care, *Pediatrics* 82:643, 1993.

Families are psychologically vulnerable after the birth of a sick infant. During this period of temporary disorganization, there is a heightened receptivity to accepting help and being responsive to change, because the family is struggling for a way to cope with the crisis. Significant potentialities exist for individual and family emotional growth and development.[20,27,28,107] The perinatal health team has an opportunity to influence how the individual and family adapt to the crisis.[20,57,107] By providing appropriate supportive interventions coupled with enlightened policies and attitudes that reflect family-centered principles (Box 29-2), the team can positively influence the family's coping, thus enhancing the likelihood for a successful resolution of the crisis and ultimately a healthy parent-child relationship.*

As discussed earlier, attachment is a complex developmental process. There are many interrelated

*References 20, 32, 39, 40, 43, 74, 92, 101, 106, 107, 110, 133, 140, 142.

factors that influence parental behavior and attachment toward the infant.[20,26,70] These include the infant, sex of the infant, social class, birth order, parental attitudes and expectations, events of the newborn period and postdischarge period, and level of family functioning.* Very important in any neonatal illness and subsequent hospitalization is the disruption and stress that is frequently created in the nuclear family system. It has been demonstrated that the family's functioning and its adaptation to stress have important effects on the family's relationship with the infant and the infant's later development. A crucial task of the perinatal health care team is to intervene in such a way as to assist families in using the unfortunate event of the birth of their sick infant to maximize their growth, adaptation, and reorganization during this period.†

To assist parents through the difficult experience of having a sick infant, it is helpful to identify the psychologic tasks and emotional reactions they experience. This section describes the six psychologic issues facing families; it discusses the clinical and behavioral indicators that parents are struggling with and then suggests interventions that the perinatal health care team can employ to help families. It is extremely important to remember that these are generalizations and that each family or person must be approached individually. Additionally, in assessing families' reactions, it is critical to look at how they cope over a period of time. Initially there may be a tremendous amount of upset, disruption, and upheaval within the individual or family system that eventually may lead to improved functioning and a sense of growth and mastery. The key is how the individuals or families reorganize, how able they are to return to a state of equilibrium, the coping strategies they are able to develop, and whether they are adaptive or maladaptive. Attachment and parenthood are complex, interactional developmental processes that must evolve and unfold over time.

Kaplan and Mason[76] describe four psychologic tasks that parents of premature infants must deal with:

1. Anticipatory grieving and withdrawal from the relationship established during pregnancy
2. Parental acknowledgment of feelings of guilt and failure

3. Resumption of the relationship with the infant that had been previously disrupted
4. Preparation to take the infant home

Two additional tasks are also significant:

1. Crisis events related to labor and delivery
2. Adaptation to the intensive care environment[39,41,57,60,123]

In general, these six psychologic tasks can be applied to any parent's reaction to a sick infant, with additional specific issues arising, depending on whether the infant was premature or born with a congenital anomaly.

Labor and Delivery

The first psychologic task involves working through the crisis events surrounding the labor and delivery. Medical problems occurring at any point during the pregnancy or delivery that threaten the health or survival of the fetus or the mother can result in the parents' delaying their planning and making an emotional investment in the fetus or infant. Parents may psychologically withdraw from the pregnancy as a way of protecting themselves. The parents of an infant born prematurely often do not have the necessary psychologic and physical time to prepare. This deprivation of time may interfere with the parents' ability to complete the final steps of attachment described earlier.[59] Parents who have been concentrating on themselves in a healthy, narcissistic way may not yet be ready to transfer their investment to the infant, because they have been prematurely thrust into the role of parents. There is an overwhelming sense of losing control of the events of the labor and delivery and their timing. Parents' wishes to retain the pregnancy can influence their attitude about the delivery and the infant.[151]

On the other hand, some parents react in the opposite way: they may wish to be rid of the pregnancy as a way of dealing with their ambivalent feelings about the infant or their fear of the unknown and the uncertainty facing them. Many mothers of premature infants feel that their infants are alien[20]; they do not feel that the infants are really theirs, making it easier to have feelings of rejection toward the infant. In addition to feeling insufficient and inadequate about their ability to deliver an infant at term, they feel empty inside, as if something is missing. This seems to occur because the mother who has been predominantly concerned about herself, her body, and the fetus growing inside is not ready to transfer that emotional investment outside of herself. With a premature birth there is usually a heightened sense

---

*References 22, 32, 43, 57, 74, 82, 92, 95, 101, 126, 134, 142, 144.
†References 20, 32, 39, 43, 57, 74, 92, 101, 103, 107, 134, 157.

of emergency and concern about the health and survival of the infant and at times the mother, who herself may have suffered complications.

In the case of a full-term infant born with a problem despite a problem-free pregnancy, there is a sense of overwhelming shock and disappointment. Parents immediately sense the problem; as their apprehension mounts, they frequently imagine and fantasize the worst. Parents of a newborn with a malformation normally experience lowered self-esteem and view this event as an affront to their reproductive capabilities. The mother specifically views it as a failure of her feminine role. Parents often feel that they have failed and that the infant symbolically represents their own defectiveness. Parents not only fear for the infant, they fear for themselves and what this child may mean to their future. The reaction of the parents is based on the specific psychologic, social, and cultural meaning of the defect to the parents and the manner in which the problem is discussed and handled with the parents by the health care team.[81]

The emotional reactions and feelings that parents have at and after the delivery of a sick infant range from shock, fright, and panic to anxiety and helplessness.[118] Parents may be so overwhelmed by the events that initially they may block any observable emotional response or affect. Staff interventions at this time are extremely important, because they lay the foundations for subsequent interactions between parents and health professionals. Early comments and influential statements during this critical time can have lasting impressions in the minds of parents. This is also an emotionally difficult time for physicians and nurses, because they too are struggling with their own feelings of inadequacy, failure, and helplessness. Unconsciously, in an attempt to deal with their own feelings, staff may withdraw from parents and not be emotionally available to help. This is a normal response, but one that needs to be guarded against, because it only perpetuates a breakdown in relationships and communication with parents that are so greatly needed at this time. Many helpful interventions can be employed that are sensitive and supportive, and that facilitate the emerging relationship between the parents and their infant.

Early Communication

In the labor and delivery phase, early communication with both parents is essential. Parents normally are apprehensive and extremely sensitive to explicit or implicit cues, such as actual statements by the staff, the atmosphere, looks, or a tone of voice that may indicate how things are progressing. Because of the emphasis on prepared childbirth, parents are extremely sophisticated in their knowledge of labor and delivery practices and immediately sense some deviation from what they expected. Prompt, direct explanations presented in a calm manner are important and reassuring to parents. This explanation of the process of what is or will be happening can be effective, because it helps to organize the parents at a time when they are extremely vulnerable and feeling out of control. Although it is normal for the staff to be guarded, members of the health care team should tell the parents the known facts and what actually is being done for their infant without giving any diagnosis, prognosis, or forecast for the future course of the infant. Avoiding or not talking to parents only accelerates parental anxiety and adds to their growing fantasies or distortions. It has been well established and documented that parents' fantasies about their infant's problems are usually worse than the reality.[81,92] Parents often report that when they actually saw their infant, they were relieved because they had imagined that the infant would appear worse.

Support of Staff

It is also important that one of the staff members stay with the parents through labor, delivery, and recovery to offer continuous support and to reassure parents that communication will continue as soon as more information is known. This is, again, an uncomfortable time for the staff, because they may feel helpless and useless and as a result may avoid parents or revert to performing more technical activities. Some parents may need someone to be with them, not only to talk to them, but more important, to listen. On the other hand, some parents may not be able to talk or verbalize their concerns or fears. Others may wish to be alone with each other or any other significant person in their life. Because of the varying responses and needs of people, it is extremely important to be sensitive to individual differences in approaching parents.

Parents have expressed their desire to be together when given "bad news."[71,87,138] As much as possible, talking to both parents at the same time is helpful when discussing the infant's condition. This decreases their distortions and misconceptions, increases the communication and support between parents, and prevents either parent from feeling excluded. The assumption is commonly made that the father is in a better emotional state to hear about the infant; this misconception leads health professionals to mistakenly exclude or "spare" the mother, which only postpones her ability to begin to cope with the reality of her infant's condition. Sparing the mother may cause the parents to be in different stages of their understanding of the infant's medical condition and in their emotional state. Because emotional support between parents is so critical, the staff should avoid sparing, because it can add to the parents' difficulty in being attuned to each other's needs and creates more opportunities for the parents to be out of synchrony with each other. Both mothers and fathers of critically ill newborns generally find each other to be the greatest source of support in the first 2 weeks of NICU hospitalization.[104,141]

Seeing the Infant

The question usually arises about the value of the parents seeing their infant, especially if the infant is very small, is not likely to survive, or is profoundly malformed. Generally, it is assumed that it is psychologically better for parents to have had the opportunity to see their infant, but this must be individualized for each family and newborn. Seeing the infant helps to facilitate attachment,[20] decrease exaggerated fantasies, decrease withdrawal from the infant, and enhance the parents' ability to grasp the reality of the situation. Because of the need to respect individual differences in people, the best approach is to give parents the opportunity to decide whether they together or individually want to see the infant. The opportunity to see and touch the infant in the delivery room or before transport may reduce stressful feelings verbalized by parents who see their infant for the first time in the NICU.[141]

This decision should be ultimately made by the parents with the support of the health care team. It is not uncommon to find a well-meaning family member, physician, nurse, or social worker advising the parents or making the decision himself or herself and concluding it would be in the parents' best interests not to see the infant. The argument is given that "It's better not to get attached," or "It would make them cry or upset them to see the anomaly," or "They could not handle it," or "They would lose control." This decision is for the parents, not the professional, to make.

Some parents may know unequivocally what they want to do; others may be ambivalent, unsure, and indecisive. It is the role of the professional to give the parents assistance (information and sup-

port) in making the decision. The parents may need time to think about it or may need to discuss their fear and ambivalence first, before being able to decide. They may need some factual information and preparation from the professional, such as the appearance of the infant and a description of the equipment. They may need assurance that someone will stay with them. Although time often is a factor and a decision must be made quickly, it is important to move at the parents' pace. The professional should still follow as much as possible the principle of facilitating the parents in seeing the infant. If for medical reasons related to the mother's condition this is not possible, a self-developing picture can be taken.[109] If it is medically possible for the parents to touch or hold the infant, the parents should be offered the opportunity. Touching or holding not only facilitates attachment[20] but can provide parents with an emotional experience that is very sustaining and reassuring, helping them proceed through a very critical time of separation.

The parents are very sensitive to the staff's attitude toward the infant as reflected by their comments and the manner in which the staff handle the infant. If the infant is regarded with respect and treated as important, the parent is given the feeling that the infant is seen as valued and worthwhile. This is especially important for parents of an infant with a congenital anomaly; the parents could wonder if their infant is viewed as "damaged goods" by society. In describing the infant to the parent, it is important to present a balanced picture of both the normal and abnormal aspects of the infant. In discussing the infant with the parents, staff should refer to the infant by name, if they have named the infant; this helps personalize to the infant and establish the infant's unique identity.

Caregiving

To reinforce the caregiving needs of parents, it is important to discuss with them their plans to feed their infant. Support and encouragement should be given whether the parents have decided on breastfeeding or bottlefeeding. In most situations, breastfeeding a sick infant may be possible. Many mothers are able to pump their breasts for milk that eventually will be given to the infant. There are many psychologic and physiologic reasons why breastfeeding or pumping may be beneficial for mothers and infants alike (see Chapter 19). The breastfeeding or pumping experience helps the mother to feel close to her infant and that she has some control over what is happening to her infant; she can uniquely contribute to her infant's care in a way no one else can. Fathers too can participate in this activity by their support and interest in the actual breastfeeding or the pumping and milk collection activities. Many mothers are able to successfully pump and eventually put the infant to breast, but others are not, because of emotional stresses, the condition of the infant, the length of time until the infant can feed, and the waning interest of the mother. Regardless of eventual success, the mother should be encouraged to try if she has an interest; then she can feel that she made an attempt to relate to her infant in this way. If a mother does not plan to breastfeed or pump, or if she tries but does not continue, she should not be made to feel guilty or that she failed in her role. She is already vulnerable to these feelings, having had an infant born with problems.

After the delivery, when the mother is taken to her room without a healthy infant, she usually experiences a void; an amputation has occurred.[81] She and those around her are beginning to grieve. The interventions of the staff should be flexible and sensitive to the individual needs of the family. Empathy, responsiveness, and an ability to listen to the parents are important at this time.

Encouraging parents to verbalize and express their feelings and concerns (at their own pace), although difficult to do at times, is useful to the parents. Listening is as important to parents as giving them information.[74] Avoiding their grief gives the mother and father the impression that they are "bad parents" for having feelings of sadness, anger, guilt, or loss; this only increases their level of guilt and isolation. Prescribing tranquilizers also gives the message that is it not permissible to talk about what has happened to them and their infant. Tranquilizers only increase the feelings of unreality that normally are experienced. This stifles the parents' coping mechanisms at a time when the parents need to begin to come to terms with what has happened.

Room assignments are a very personal matter, and the mother should be given a choice of where she will stay. Some mothers want to stay in a regular maternity unit; for others this is too painful, and they want to be in a separate area. Flexible visiting guidelines[30,39,65] for the father and other significant persons are essential so they can support one another through a very difficult, uncertain period.

In talking to parents, it is important to bear in mind that the parents do not remember much of what has been said; it is very difficult for them to assimilate all that has happened, both cognitively and emotionally. It is important for the staff to move at the parents' own pace. If the infant has been transferred or the chances for survival are limited, the mother should be discharged or given a pass to visit the infant as soon as possible. It is also important to acknowledge to the mother (and father) that they are parents and that they did give birth to a baby. They need the congratulatory cards, gifts, and attention that they would have normally received.

Anticipatory Grieving

After labor and delivery, parents are struggling with the second psychologic task of anticipatory grieving and withdrawal from the relationship established during pregnancy. This task requires that parents acknowledge that their infant's life is endangered or that the newborn might die. Events surrounding the labor, delivery, and postpartum period may have indicated to the parents that their infant's chances for survival are diminished. If this has occurred, parents can then become involved in anticipatory grieving and withdrawal from the relationship established during pregnancy. Studies have shown that the decision to transfer an infant to a NICU alone is likely to initiate an anticipatory grief reaction.[19]

Parents may also be experiencing feelings of grief and sadness over the loss of the expected, idealized child that they had wished for during the pregnancy. For some parents attaching to a critically ill or malformed infant may be too overwhelming; parents may withdraw from the infant in an attempt to protect themselves from their feelings of hurt, disappointment, and guilt.[20,60,107,111] Some parents may feel ambivalent about the infant; they may feel they could not love or cope with an infant who might die or who would have significant physical or mental problems. Feeling uncertain about whether they want the infant to survive can cause feelings of guilt that may cause the parents to withdraw from the infant as a way of avoiding confronting these difficult, painful feelings.

During this period parents may find themselves in a very stressful position; they are faced with the task of balancing the painful realities of confronting a possible loss against their hopes of the intact survival of their infant. The emotional withdrawal and grieving that parents experience is normal during the critical time that the infant's life is endangered or when parents are faced with the possibility that their infant may have a life-long problem. This withdrawal becomes pathologic only if it continues beyond the time the infant demonstrates definite signs (to the parents) of improvement and survival. In the case of a newborn with a permanent developmental or physical disability, parents who are unable to grieve their idealized infant may maintain this withdrawal, which might lead to attachment difficulties.[146]

Parental Responses

Parents exhibit many emotional responses and behaviors that indicate they are struggling with the anticipatory grieving and withdrawal. Some parents are very sad, depressed, and teary, and others may be highly anxious, at times bordering on panic states; others react by having a flat affect, being withdrawn, and appearing apathetic. Some parents may exhibit very angry, hostile, confrontational behavior as a way of dealing with their distress, others may deny the situation by optimistically feeling that "everything will be OK."

Parents who typically are verbal may ask questions reflecting their concerns about their infant's survival; this is especially true after the child has received medical attention and decisions are being made about treatment for the infant, including transfer to an NICU. The questions they ask physicians and nurses are: "Is he going to make it?" "What do you think his chances are?" "He'll be OK, won't he?" "Have you seen other babies with this problem?" "Do other babies make it?" and "How long will he be in the hospital?" Parents struggling with their fears may resist seeing, touching, or visiting the infant. If they do visit the infant in the NICU, they may remain distant by having little or no eye contact with the infant, refusing to touch, standing far from the warmer or incubator, and asking few or no questions of the staff. The parents may be reluctant to name the infant; when they do refer to the infant, they say "it," "she," "he," or "the baby." If the infant has been given a special or treasured family name, they may be reluctant to use it.

A very common phenomenon occurs when parents, being protective of each other, discourage each other's involvement with the infant. This is especially true at the time of transport, when the transport nurse may suggest to the father or family members that the infant be shown to the mother before leaving. Many fathers are afraid this will increase the emotional attachment to the infant and thus the feelings of disappointment and loss if the infant should die. The father is usually very apprehensive about how to handle the mother's feelings of grief in addition to his own. This type of behavior also is true with regard to medical information; it is not uncommon for one parent to request that all communication go through him or her. The response is: "My spouse is too upset or anxious and couldn't handle hearing any bad news." Many times it is actually the parent making the request who is most anxious and who is dealing with this anxiety by projecting it onto the other partner. Work and child care responsibilities, transportation difficulties, and financial limitations are all legitimate reasons that parents may be unable to have frequent contact with their infant.[67] However, these factors may also serve as unconscious ways to maintain distance from the infant.

It is important to keep in mind that withdrawal and grieving are part of a necessary and natural process.[20] For parents to develop an attachment to and accept the reality of their infant's condition, they must experience their feelings of grief, sadness, anger, guilt, and disappointment over the loss of the expected child.[146] This grieving serves to free the parents' emotional energy so that they can interact with and become attuned to their infant. Grieving enhances the parents' availability to the infant. This availability aids in their feeling competent to handle their infant.[151] The goal, then, of the perinatal health care team's interventions is to help the family realize that their feelings are natural and normal and will be accepted.[20] Parents need permission to have their feelings. It is essential to acknowledge to parents that it is normal to be afraid of attaching to an infant who might die or have a handicap. Giving permission diminishes the guilt that the parents may feel about their behavior being abnormal or about being bad parents because they are afraid. Simple statements such as, "Many parents tell us they are afraid of getting close to their baby," or "It's scary to attach when you think the baby may die," are helpful.

It is sometimes useful for parents to verbalize what their fears actually are. They may fear their infant's dying, being retarded, or being paralyzed. Once their fears are clarified in the minds of the parents and either confirmed or refuted by the medical staff, it is usually easier for parents to begin to accept their infant's diagnosis and prognosis and begin relating to the infant. Social workers can provide valuable emotional support to families in helping them deal with their realistic and unrealistic concerns.[116]

Communicating Medical Information

The role of the health care professionals in communicating medical information is important. There are many schools of thought about how to approach parents, ranging from being extremely cautious and pessimistic ("paint the bleakest picture") to being encouraging and optimistic ("give parents hope"). Although the approach should be individualized for each family, some professionals feel a balanced approach is the most beneficial. In a recent study, parents stated that information should be accurate, current, and comprehensive, but not unduly pessimistic.[74] Parents need a realistic assessment of the situation that is honest and direct. It is important to acknowledge the infant's condition and possible problems, but not to inundate parents with every potential problem that can arise.

Parents who hear "brain damage," "retarded," or "the baby will die" are not likely to forget these statements. These statements can linger in the minds of parents and adversely influence how the parents relate to their newborn. They may believe that some day "brain damage will show up" or that the infant is susceptible and frail and needs to be treated cautiously for fear of a life-threatening condition. These children may become victims of the *vulnerable child syndrome*,[63,124] a condition in which a child is overprotected by his or her parents and treated as if he or she had a medical problem or is in danger of death when neither is any longer the case. Parents who are told their newborn may die may have trouble attaching or becoming emotionally invested. When talking to parents, physicians and nurses should be judicious and careful in making statements of a sensitive nature. Definitive statements should be used only when appropriate and necessary. The long-term emotional implications of such statements need to be weighed.

There are several other guidelines in communicating medical information to parents.[151] As we've just discussed, parents' perceptions of their infant's condition are extremely important, remain in parents' minds, and can affect their relationship with the infant. Parents easily misperceive information given to them. They may believe that a PDA indicates open-heart surgery and therefore worry that their infant has a heart condition. Or perhaps they think a bilirubin problem means their infant has liver disease. Therefore, in beginning any discussion with parents, it is essential to determine and address their perceptions. A staff member might say, "Could you tell me what you understand about your baby's condition?" This will give the physician or nurse the opportunity to correct any misinformation or misconceptions and to hear about the parents' concerns. The perceived morbidity of the baby is a source of stress for both mothers and fathers.[141] Parents' perceptions of the severity of their infant's illness are complex, change over time, and are affected by (1) parental anxiety, (2) infant size, (3) amount and type of equipment and treatments, and (4) amount and type of information received from health care providers.[29,69,141] A team member might specifically ask about the parents' concerns or worries: "Could you tell me what concerns you have about your baby?" Asking this can make communication between the perinatal health care team and the parents more meaningful and helpful; unless the team deals with the parents' anxiety, discussions become one-sided lectures and only benefit the professional. Discussions need to be a dialog between parent and professional.

During the course of a discussion and again at the end, it is useful to determine parents' interpretations of what has been said and to modify and clarify as needed. The staff need to avoid overloading a parent with lengthy explanations that are too technical. It is more productive to move at a pace so that the parent can assimilate the information presented; it is not necessary to describe the entire course of RDS or BPD. It is always preferable to use simple language that is understandable to a layperson. For some parents the use of statistics is helpful; for some it is not. Statistics are confusing, because they do not apply to the individual case and can easily be misinterpreted. When asked about the frequency of brain damage with a grade III IVH, a team member might say, "A majority of these babies have some neurologic problem, but there are some who do not." Vivid modifiers such as "This is the worst case of sepsis we have ever had" or "Your baby is the sickest baby in the nursery" are of no real benefit to the parents and only accelerate their fantasies and anxieties. Finally, if a referring physician and the nursery team are both communicating with the parents, it is essential to coordinate the particular approach. It is very confusing to parents and decreases their trust level for one to be pessimistic and the other optimistic.

Communicating Medical Information: New Research

The principles of family-centered neonatal care clearly promote a certain approach. The first four principles concern communication, medical information, fully informed parental decision-making and parental advance directives (see Box 29-2). Recently, researchers have confirmed that information given to parents in the NICU is often communicated in euphemisms, vague statements, half-truths and shielding of parents from uncertainties and controversies of NICU care.[71] Professional attitudes that may interfere with open, honest communication include: (1) assuming that parents are too emotional to assimilate information and make a rational decision, (2) assuming that information about complications and poor outcomes may disrupt attachment to the neonate, and (3) assuming that parental guilt and psychologic harm will ensue from decision-making (despite research to the contrary[18]).[71]

Many parents desire and can handle complete, specific, honest, detailed, unbiased and meaningful information—the same facts and interpretation of those facts as the staff—delivered in a humane and respectful manner.[71] More recent research substantiates the parents' wishes. Parents express "remarkably uniform and unambiguous requests . . . to receive early, honest and detailed information in a comprehensible and sympathetic manner and to be together when given bad news."[39] Prenatal consultation has been found to be useful by 80% of mothers in one study.[122] These researchers concluded that "in our population of educated mothers, most mothers prefer to be told exact statistics, rather than generalizations, concerning major neonatal morbidities."[122] Another group of researchers uses actuarial data to counsel parents regarding infants at the limits of viability and in morbidity counseling.[113] Accuracy of prenatal and postnatal counseling of parents is of concern, because information affects practice management and influences parental decision-making.[45,85,113]

Individuals vary in their desire to be informed and involved in decision-making. Individuals also vary in the manner in which they assimilate information. Some parents may want extensive information about their situation, whereas others may not. Some parents may not wish to be decision-makers and should be able to delegate decision-making to a physician of their choice.[71] However, physicians have an ethical and legal obligation[8,9,33,45,153] to give parents the facts from which to make an informed consent regarding their neonate's condition, illnesses, outcomes, and the risks and benefits of various interventions. Proactive risk management strategies include effective communication,[68] because legal action, in the form of civil malpractice suits (60%)[149]

and criminal action,[33] may result from poor communication between parents and physicians.

Poor understanding by parents may be the result of poor communication techniques, contradictory messages, poor parental health, inexperience with medical terminology, denial, inability to ask questions, or lack of opportunity to review the information.[85] In a recent study parents claimed that they had never been spoken to by a neonatalogist, when the conversation did occur and had been recorded.[83] In this study parents were given a tape-recording of their initial conversation with the neonatalogist and any subsequent conversations of importance. The audiotape proved useful: 96% of the mothers and 68% of the fathers listened to the tape again an average of 2.5 and 1.8 times, respectively. Eight-five percent of parents who listened to the tape had forgotten elements of the conversation, and two mothers did not recall that the conversation had ever occurred. Taped conversations were found helpful by (1) 99% of parents and grandparents, (2) 76% of nurses, and (3) 36% of neonatalogists. Forty percent of the physicians were not happy about having their conversations taped—"legal implications" being the most frequent reason given. As pointed out in the study, the "legal implications" work both ways—taping encourages precise, organized, clear, and humane communication of information while providing an "alibi" if a legal complication arises. A multicenter, randomized controlled trial to evaluate the long-term effects on parenting skills and well being is in process.[83]

Research has documented that postpartum women have transient deficits in cognitive function, particularly in attention and memory function.[48,148] Because verbal communication may be poorly remembered, augmentation with written instructions is recommdned.[10,48,148] In addition to relistening to an audiotape, if parents are given written information, such as an evidence-based table of the likely outcomes of babies at different gestations, they are able to look at it again to review it. Such an evidence-based table for infants from 23 to 28 weeks' gestational age has been presented in the literature for use with parents.[85] This table contains information about mortality statistics, need for assisted ventilation, prolonged use of oxygen, length of stay, use of phototherapy, PDA needing treatment, outcomes of brain scans, and long-term neurodevelopmental outcome. A NICU staff member can create a table for parents by using their most recent data.[45,84] With the advent of computerized data bases (such as the Vermont Oxford Data Base) that compares statistics from multiple NICUs and a large cohort of infants, parents can be provided with statistical information from multiple NICUs to compare with the outcomes from the NICU in which their baby is hospitalized.[48] Parents may need assistance in interpreting statistics and making them meaningful to their individual situation. Again, some parents may want and need this type of information, whereas others may not.

Ongoing research on the *outcome of gestation table* (OGT) has documented views of parents, nurses, and physicians.[84] The majority of parents and nurses interviewed favored the table; they agreed that the information was frightening but important for parents to know. Parents wanted to keep a copy and nurses wanted a copy in the medical record. Parents also thought that the information was easy to understand, the table did not contain "too much" information, and although it was frightening, they still would rather have the information. The majority of physicians thought that the table was easy to understand, had "too much" information, and were ambivalent about using it in their practice. Parents, nurses, and physicians all agreed that the table and its information was not misleading. Twenty-one percent of doctors disagreed about including a copy of the table in the medical record so that other health care providers would know what had been said to the parents. This finding was surprising to the researchers who thought that inclusion of the table in the medical record would promote consistency in information given to the parents by different members of the perinatal team.

The principles of family-centered neonatal care (see Box 29-2) also advocate full and free access to lay and medical literature pertaining to the neonate's condition, proposed treatments, and probable outcomes.[71] Medical literature, articles, books, and videos should be available in the NICU or in the hospital library for the parents' use. A video such as *You Are Not Alone*—(see Resource Materials for Parents at the end of this chapter) is available to help parents understand the impact on the family of long-term handicaps and to support them in making informed decisions. Access to the Internet has proven to be a source of medical information (some accurate; some inaccurate) for families, as well as professionals.[46]

Acknowledgment of Guilt Feelings

The third psychologic task parents are dealing with simultaneously with anticipatory grieving and with-drawal is confronting and recognizing their feelings of failure and guilt in not delivering a healthy infant. Most parents struggling with feelings of inadequacy and guilt are likely to search for answers to the causes of their infant's situation. The mother may focus on concrete things, such as not eating well, the flu, intercourse, birth control pills, or an unwanted pregnancy. The father may also be concerned about his role in not helping his wife enough, placing too many demands on her, an argument he provoked that precipitated labor, or another family member with the same chromosomal abnormality. Parents search for reasons because they need to find a cause for such an event happening to them. It is harder for them to feel out of control and helpless than to feel guilty. Some parents place responsibility on themselves, but others shift the blame to others in their external world, such as their spouse, extended family, doctor, nurses, or God. Often both parents are concerned with the disappointment that they have caused the other. They may withdraw from each other at a time when they both need acceptance and support. Realistic answers from the medical team are helpful for some parents in diminishing guilt feelings; in other parents the guilt may be so deeply integrated in the parents' thinking that it is less easily overcome. For example, some parents may focus on irrational, unrealistic factors, such as, "This is my punishment for not being a good wife or daughter" or "This is my punishment for running away from home when I was 15." It seems that the more irrational the parent's thinking, the harder it is to assuage and resolve the guilt. Many feelings of guilt and failure are normal and expected; the feelings are a problem when the parent does not respond to the infant's progress, because the infant may continue to represent the parent's failure.

Parental Responses

Parents demonstrate many behaviors that indicate they are struggling with guilt and failure. Some parents directly verbalize these feelings and attempt to obtain helpful answers from the staff. Less obvious are the parents who are markedly depressed and remain so despite any improvement in the infant. These parents demonstrate the classic signs of depression, such as apathy, loss of interest in appearance and self, withdrawal, and loss of self-esteem. They exhibit an overwhelming sense of helplessness, because they feel responsible for causing their infant's problem and are helpless to remedy the situation. Their guilt feelings cause them to be very self-deprecating and angry themselves, a state that often results in depression. Other parents struggling with guilt are highly anxious about their ability to handle their infant; they feel they have harmed their infant and cannot tolerate facing that infant. Another manifestation of guilt is hostility and anger that is usually directed toward others, such as the spouse, the staff, or God. Instead of focusing their anger on themselves like a depressed parent, they direct it outward to rid themselves of their feelings of responsibility, projecting the guilt feelings onto others in their life. They may be angry at the physicians, nurses, or social workers for not making their infant healthy (if the child is premature) or perfect (if the child has a congenital defect). They may be hostile toward the social worker for not being able to help them with their financial problems. Unconsciously, they are trying to make the staff feel as guilty, helpless, and responsible as they do.

Facilitating Adaptation

To intervene with parents, it is useful to help the parents become aware of and acknowledge their feelings of failure and guilt.[60] By verbalizing their feelings, they can begin to identify the source of the guilt feelings, which may not always be clear to them. The staff can then intervene with appropriate information to modify and clarify the perceptions that may be the source of some of the parents' guilt feelings. Many parents directly ask about the causes of their infant's problem, and the medical team should provide them with appropriate information. Other parents are not as direct and verbal; they need to have the subject introduced. A staff member might say: "Have you wondered why this has happened?" or "Many parents find themselves feeling responsible for their baby's problem, as if they failed. Have you had these feelings?" As parents begin to talk about their feelings, they are often able to test reality and discover the irrationality in their thinking. However, some parents continue to feel guilty even though they have been told they are not to blame. Guilt feelings are very complex and may take a long time to resolve; for some they may never be completely resolved, but at least the intensity of the feelings may diminish. If a child recovers from the illness, guilt can be more easily relinquished. If the child has a chronic problem, the parent is daily confronted with feelings of responsibility. The more irrational the source of the guilt, the harder it will be to dispel. Because this persistent guilt can cause problems in the parents' relationship to the child, a

referral to a perinatal social worker or other mental health professional may be indicated.

To facilitate support between parents, it is useful to ask whether they have shared their feelings of guilt and failure with each other. Often a spouse may assume that one is angry at or disappointed with the other. Discussing this may bring a tremendous sense of relief and reassurance. However, if the parents are blaming each other and relationship problems develop, a referral to a perinatal social worker or counselor is appropriate.[117]

In some cases there may be realistic reasons (either intentional or unintentional) why the parent may feel guilty about the infant's problem. Parental drug or alcohol abuse, an accident, or an inherited genetic problem may be real reasons. In these cases the staff must acknowledge to the parent that there is a causal relationship and then give the parents support by allowing them to talk about their feelings. If causes were not intentional, it is helpful to acknowledge that fact; if they were, it is important to be nonjudgmental. A judging attitude only reinforces the feelings parents are already experiencing and further alienates them from the child and the staff. The parents need help with the problem that initially led to the impairment of the fetus. When this type of psychosocial problem arises, the involvement of a perinatal social worker or counselor is essential.

Adaptation to the Intensive Care Environment

The fourth psychologic task involves adaptation to the intensive care environment.[41,42,57,107,142] All of the reactions of guilt, anxiety, fear, anger, and disappointment become heightened when parents attempt to adapt to this unfamiliar environment. They must learn a new language, establish trust in new relationships, and adapt to their role in this setting. The intense and sometimes chaotic appearance of a high-risk nursery makes it a frightening experience that serves to increase parental feelings of helplessness and anxiety. Parents need to gain a sense of security in this environment before initiating a caregiving role with their infant. There may be cultural adaptations and geographic obstacles for families who live in small, rural communities and must travel to large, unfamiliar cities and become adapted to a large hospital. Locating the hospital and finding accommodations and meals can become overwhelming to parents who have undergone much emotional turmoil. Meeting the infant's care provider, the competent physician and nurse, can sometimes evoke a mixture of positive and negative feelings. Parents may experience reassurance and gratitude for care being given,[127] yet at the same time register a reinforcement of their feelings of uselessness, helplessness, and inadequacy can ensue. The sophistication of the highly technical care and heroic measures provided to achieve survival for their infant may be met with both awe and uncertainty. Family disruption is exaggerated by distance, especially if the infant was transported and the father must decide whether he is most needed with the infant, the infant's mother, or perhaps other children at home. Decisions must be made about work responsibilities as well as child care. The financial concerns related to providing intensive care become an added stress on families and are often compounded by the travel expenditures necessary to visit the infant.

Parental Responses

In comparing the psychosocial adjustments of parents in the NICU, both parents may experience increased levels of emotional distress.[42] In one recent study mothers were found to be more anxious, hostile, and depressed than fathers; with poorer adjustments related to work, sexual relations, social environment, and psychologic distress.[42] Mothers and fathers experience the NICU stay differently, mothers found the entire NICU experience and its aftermath more stressful than fathers.[42,105] It is important to include both mothers and fathers in assessments and interventions and to avoid overlooking the father's needs because he may be less accessible.[42]

There are a number of nonverbal and verbal signs that indicate parents are struggling to gain a sense of security in the NICU. Some parents appear frightened, overwhelmed, nervous, and withdrawn, asking few questions or being reluctant to call or visit. Others may be highly anxious and unable to focus on their infant and may instead concentrate on other activities or infants in the nursery. Some parents may ask many questions and become very interested in the technical aspects of their infant's treatment, such as respirator settings and laboratory values. Some parents, uneasy with entrusting their child to strangers, may initially feel a need to remain at their infant's side, maintaining a vigil. Some may wish to read the infant's chart or attempt to read material on their infant's particular condition. Others may become angry or upset at minor differences in the infant's care or the nursery policies,

such as a respiratory setting being off a point or discrepancies in enforcing visitation guidelines.[65]

Facilitating Adaptation

There are many interventions that can be employed to familiarize and orient families.[142] First, the obstetrician, transport team, or any other professional who has initial contact with parents can give them preparatory information and a description of intensive care. A booklet or video that includes basic information and illustrative pictures is extremely useful and should include a discussion of the type of care being provided, normal feelings and reactions parents experience, financial information, a glossary of terms, breastfeeding information, available accommodations and meals, calling and visitation policies, the discharge policy, and a city map. Both at the time of transfer and later in the nursery, a self-developing picture can be taken of the infant for the parents. If the infant is being transported, information should be given as to the approximate length of time of transport and by whom and when the parents will be contacted after the infant has been admitted and evaluated. A personal phone call from the staff with an introduction, information about the infant and unit, and an inquiry regarding parental visitation plans are useful. Parents feel less anxious when they have an orientation and a name to relate to. The staff can then be prepared to be available when the parents arrive.

Certainly, the first visit to the NICU is stressful, and members of the team should welcome the parents and stay with them to explain the equipment and procedures, answer questions, review the infant's course, give emotional support, and in general, orient the parents to this new experience. Mothers who have not previously seen their baby report more stress in seeing their baby first in the NICU.[141] Seeing the infant is stressful and may evoke shock, fear, guilt and helplessness.[105,106] It is important to be attentive to the mother's physical need; comfortable chairs or perhaps a wheelchair if the mother has had a cesarean section are helpful. The message needs to be conveyed that parents are welcome and that their visits do make a difference in that they have a useful role to play with their infant. Because many parents are uncertain about what questions to ask, it may be necessary at times to help parents construct questions ("Do you understand why we start IVs in the head?" or "Do you know what blood gases, hood oxygen, and CPAP are?") and to repeat explanations using simple, nontechnical language. Relating to the parent's affect or emotional state seems to establish a rapport with the family and helps them feel that the staff is empathetic and understanding. If parents sense the staff's genuine concern and interest in them and their infant, it is easier for them to leave their infant in the staff's care.[106,127] A team member might say, "You look frightened or scared," or "This can be an overwhelming situation," or "You look like you want to cry." Facilitating the parents' relationship with the infant is essential and can be done by offering the parents the opportunity to touch or stroke their infant, hold the infant if possible, or at least remove eye patches. Pointing out some of the unique personal characteristics of the infant is helpful. A staff member might say, "Your baby is very active," or "He responds well to touch," or "She seems to prefer lying on her side."

Families coming from out of town should be provided with a list of inexpensive housing and restaurants located near the hospital. In many cities, national and local businesses have established nearby homes run by local volunteer organizations for housing parents on a temporary basis. The homes have several sleeping rooms in addition to kitchen and laundry facilities and provide parents with a comfortable, homelike atmosphere at a nominal charge. A natural support system generally emerges among the parents using the home. A list of apartments, hotels, and boarding rooms reasonably priced and rented by the day or week can also be made available. Social workers often can secure food, parking and cab vouchers to give to families to decrease some of the financial stresses.

Parents are usually concerned with the cost of their infant's hospitalization. Some parents feel that if they are unable to pay, their child will receive less attention. Parents should be reassured that their infant's care will not depend on their ability to pay. They should, however, be referred to the appropriate funding agencies, such as the Handicapped Children's Program or Health Care Programs for Children with Special Needs, Social Security Disability, Title 19 Medicaid, and state child health insurance programs that provide financial assistance.

Because communication is so critical, regular conferences between the family and staff (physician, nurses, and social workers) should be instituted to give consistent medical information and emotional support; this is especially helpful with both extremely critical and long-term infants. Med-

ical interpreters should be made available if parents do not speak English; the same principle applies for deaf parents.[91] Parents should be given the names of the physicians and nurses taking care of their infant and the personnel's specific role in providing both care to the infant and communication to the family. If the physicians and nurses have a rotation system, this also should be explained from the beginning. At the end of a rotation the transition can be facilitated by the oncoming physician's participation in even a brief conference with the outgoing physician, primary nurse, and parents. Primary nursing, especially for long-term infants, can be very helpful in providing for continuity of care. The primary nurse has been identified by parents as the primary source and facilitator of information to parents and between parents and other health care providers and as the link between parents and infant. In a study of maternal values, mothers associated nurses with the human quality of the NICU, with a wealth of knowledge about technology and with valuing the personal characteristics of the babies.[127] In the same study, mothers identified the most desirable attributes of care providers: (1) technical skill/competency, (2) caring about or "really liking" babies, (3) communication abilities, and (4) patience.[127]

Parental access to the medical record is a legal right that cannot be denied by professionals or the hospital. Institutions, however, may have a specific policy to deal with parent requests for access to the medical record. Many institutions require the presence of a professional to answer questions and interpret medical language for parents as they read the chart.[91] The principles of family-centered neonatal care advocate not only parental access to the complete medical record, but also documentation by parents of their own observations in the medical record.[71]

For out-of-town families the telephone plays a major role in staff-to-parent communication. The establishment of a telephone calling schedule with families and the use of a toll-free number, if available, can be useful. If the family is out of town and unable to visit frequently, the local or referring physician can supplement the communication. That physician often knows the family and can talk with them in person. The physician should, of course, communicate regularly with the nursery team to obtain the current medical information and present a consistent approach to the family.

Resumption of the Relationship With the Infant

The fifth psychologic task entails the parents' reestablishment of a relationship with their infant and initiating their caregiving role, a process that usually begins when the child's improvement revives previous hopes after a disappointing experience. Certain medical events may signal to the parents that it is safe to risk a relationship with the infant. These events may be a regular weight gain, changes in feeding patterns or methods, elimination of life support equipment, the infant crying for the first time or becoming more active and responsive, or the infant's transfer from the NICU to a level II nursery. The parents may begin to read baby books or pamphlets about their infant's condition, buy clothes, set up the baby's room, send out birth announcements, or name the baby. If the infant has a congenital defect, the parents may become involved with genetic counseling and other parents whose infants have similar deficits.

Parents must begin to shift their level of involvement and activity from that of a passive participant to that of an active primary caregiver.[78,144] This shift includes the parents gaining confidence in their ability to care for their infant. The family that has been disrupted must reestablish itself and recover from the crisis in an environment that is sensitive and supportive to this essential task.* The transfer of care from staff to parent is influenced by (1) the stability or lability of the infant's condition, (2) physical health of the mother, (3) level of parental support, and (4) staff expectations.[57,135]

Involvement in caregiving lessens the parents' feelings of helplessness and frustration and facilitates their identification with their role as parents.[43,74,140] Alteration in their parental role is particularly stressful for mothers in the NICU.† When parents visit, they can help by providing skin care for their infant, learning to read and respond to infant cues, helping turn the infant even if a respirator is attached, diapering the infant, and feeding the infant if this is possible. If the parents are separated by distance, they can send family pictures that can be posted at the infant's bed; periodic pictures of the infant taken by the staff can be sent back to the family. Parents can send clothing, mobiles, simple toys, and even cassette tapes so that the infant can hear the parents' voices. Some mothers who are pumping

send frozen breast milk (see Chapter 19). All of these reminders help the nursery staff to be aware of the real family that is genuinely interested. These personal attempts made by parents that help them feel they are important to their infant's development should be encouraged. Sometimes foster grandparents or volunteers can hold, feed, and talk to infants whose parents cannot visit frequently.

Kangaroo care (see Chapter 13), skin-to-skin contact between mother and infant by placing the infant in a vertical position between the mother's breasts, has positive maternal as well as neonatal responses. Use of kangaroo care activates the maternal processes of a search for meaning and mastery of the experience of preterm birth and a recovery of self-esteem and enhancement in the parenting of a high-risk neonate.[5,6] Successive sessions of kangaroo care ease the pain and emotional suffering as mothers deal with loss and letting go and develop competence and confidence. Paternal attachment is also facilitated by fathers holding their infants and engaging in skin-to-skin contact. The first time fathers hold their babies is of special importance to the development of feelings of love, so that the earlier fathers hold their babies, the sooner they reported feelings of love and warmth.[155] In this same study fathers reported delaying attachment until they were certain of the infant's survival. The infant may become a reality to the father when he is able to hold his infant.[155]

The use of "graduate parents," parents who have had an infant in the NICU and who have successfully dealt with and resolved the crisis of the birth of their infant, can be extremely valuable.[23,71,93,96] They provide support to parents by sharing common feelings, reactions, and experiences about having a hospitalized infant. Graduate parents also visit selected infants whose parents are unable to visit. They can establish written correspondence with the parents and perhaps include a picture of the infant. Graduate parents can provide support and practical assistance for mothers interested in breastfeeding, parents who take their infant home on oxygen, or parents whose infant requires special medical care such as a shunt, tracheostomy, colostomy care, or gavage feedings. Organized graduate parent groups in large tertiary settings have become a very popular means of providing support, but locating one parent or couple to talk with parents in a small community can be just as helpful.[23]

Parent classes can also be offered on a variety of topics such as breastfeeding, infant development,

---

*References 5, 20, 53, 57, 64, 71, 144.
†References 20, 43, 57, 74, 107, 144, 155.

premature infant development, sibling and family reactions, discharge, CPR, coping with the hospitalization, and special medical needs. These classes provide specific, didactic information combined with group discussions that are mutually supportive in nature.[23] Social workers, nurses, and other related health care professionals (respiratory, occupational, and physical therapists) facilitate the group; graduate parents also participate as a resource group.

A third type of support group is counseling sessions.[134] The purpose of these sessions is to discuss and deal with common issues among parents arising from the hospitalization of their infant and the effects on their marriage and family life. This type of group has also been helpful for parents whose infant has died. The group is usually short term and is conducted by the perinatal social worker and another staff member such as a physician, nurse, or chaplain. The focus of the group is not to give specific medical information, but rather to provide parents with an opportunity to verbalize their feelings about their infant's hospitalization and to receive emotional support.

Recently telemedicine technologies have been utilized in the NICU to enhance medical, informational and emotional support for families during and after hospitalization.[25,46,62] Baby CareLink is a telemedicine program that incorporates video conferencing and Internet technologies to enhance interactions between families, NICU staff, and community health care providers. The link contains information for families about relevant issues during and after hospitalization. The video conferencing module enables distance learning by the family in their home during the NICU stay and remote monitoring after discharge. A recent survey found that families using this technology were more satisfied with the unit's physical environment and visitation policy, possibly because of the ability to facilitate visitation via teleconferencing when family members could not be present in the NICU.[62] Websites for parents of premature infants, children, and adults in the family are available so that parents can support each other, discuss common problems and share solutions (see Resource Materials for Parents).

Visiting in the NICU
Visiting Guidelines
Besides their spouse or significant other, parents identify their families and friends as the main source of support through the crisis of having a sick neo-

nate.[141] Prohibiting visiting by family and friends and/or limiting visitors to "two at a time" can isolate parents from a major source of support. NICU visiting policies should be used as guidelines, rather than rules, to facilitate visiting and caretaking by parents and families.[65,112] Care providers need to use good judgment and discretion regarding visitations while at the same time understanding and respecting the parents' need to be "in charge" of their infant (e.g., make decisions for their child).[17,74,110,127,144] Lack of perceived control by parents is associated with increased anxiety, hostility, depression, and poorer adjustment.[43,107,144] A sense of parental control in the NICU is enhanced by parental decision-making.* Parents should designate their infant's "guest list"—other family and friends who can visit and perform caretaking activities in their absence.

NICU visiting policies vary within the United States[30] and among European countries.[39] Two thirds of nurseries recently surveyed "allow" parents to visit during medical rounds, whereas visiting during nurse report was more restricted.[30] When parental visits were restricted, confidentiality was cited as the determinant of the visiting policy.[30] In this same survey 39% of parents "sometimes" or "often" complain about restricted visitation.[30] A discrepancy exists between parental requests and visitation practices in many NICUs. Parents should be permitted to visit during rounds, report, or emergencies.[65,71] Parents are interested in being included in medical rounds to actively participate in the care, discussion and decision-making about their infant.[57,65,71] Patient confidentiality can be maintained by moving rounds away from the bedside and inviting parents to participate in their infant's care planning.[65]

Parents may be more comfortable in the NICU if they are accompanied by a family member or friend.[67] A recent study showed that African-American teenage mothers establish a relationship with their infant by visiting regularly and learning how to care for their infant.[106] Parental visiting patterns may be categorized by care providers as visiting "too much"[66] or "too little."[67] Financial constraints (e.g., transportation costs, childcare, loss of work time), chaotic social situations and/or poor physical and mental maternal health may contribute to fewer visits.[67] Parents may fear that the infant will not survive, feel helpless or not feel their visits are important for their sick baby. Parents should be taught by

---

*References 17, 39, 43, 57, 71, 107, 110, 112, 127, 144.

example how important their presence and caretaking are to their baby's survival and recovery, as well as important infant cues and behaviors[112] (see Chapter 13). Maximizing every parental visit by scheduling care-by-parents[127,136] (e.g., bathing the baby, breastfeeding, kangaroo care, nipple feeding) communicates the importance of parent care and enables them "to be an expert on how to care for your baby by the time she's ready to go home."

Sibling Relationships

The inclusion of other children in the events surrounding the birth of a sick newborn is important.[114] From a sibling's viewpoint the anticipated birth of a new infant is a stressful time of noticeable physical and psychologic changes within the family. In preparation for the impending birth, the child is told that the mother will be going to the hospital for a few days and will return with a baby brother or sister. With the birth of a premature or ill infant the mother may go to the hospital unexpectedly, stay a long time, and not return home with the anticipated playmate. Instead of a celebration of the expected happy event, parents are grieving the loss of the normal newborn and the current crisis of their sick infant.

Parents are often unsure what to tell the other children and whether or not the children should see the infant. The siblings themselves may feel left out, rejected, or worried that they, too, may get sick. They may feel they are to blame and that their jealous feelings about their new rival may have caused this tragedy. Confused by their parents' distress, the other children may speculate that it is related to them and their "bad" behaviors. They may be disappointed and angry that they did not get the "playmate" they had wanted. Because parents are unsure and confused about how to manage these issues, it is often helpful for the staff to introduce the topic.

Because children will make up an explanation for the infant's illness, it is better to have it based on accurate information. Before explaining the infant's condition to siblings, elicit their ideas and perceptions about "what is the matter." Any fears, fantasies, misconceptions, or proper information is thus used to begin the explanation of "where the baby is." Explanations must be tailored to the individual child's cognitive and developmental level. The child should be told that the infant is sick but in a way that is different from his or her illnesses; the infant's illness is not "catching," and it is not like any of the illnesses that child has experienced. To allay the siblings' fears about medical personnel, they should

also be told that the nurses and physicians are trying to help the infant "get better." Because children between 2 and 6 years are involved in magical thinking, they should be told they are not to blame and that they did not cause the infant's problem. If the infant is premature, a team member might say to the child, "The baby came out too early or too soon; he needed more time to grow inside." If the infant has spina bifida, a staff member might say, "The baby's spine did not grow right, so he may have trouble lifting his legs or walking."

A child of 3 years or younger usually does not understand much about the coming infant. More important to this age group is the separation from parents who are frequently at the hospital. To ameliorate the separation, childcare arrangements should be structured so that the child is cared for by familiar people in a familiar environment. The best care arrangement would be with a familiar person in the child's own home; second best would be a familiar person in the caregiver's home; and third best, an unfamiliar person in the child's own home. Least favorable, of course, would be an unfamiliar person in an unfamiliar setting. Many hospitals have a childcare facility run by volunteers that allows the child the opportunity to go to the hospital to "see where Mommy and Daddy are going" yet allows the parents the chance to see their infant without having to care for their older child or children. Parents may also choose to include the young child in all or selected visits.

Children of age 3 and older have more interest in babies and a better grasp about the physical meaning of life. Sometimes a picture of the baby or a look into the nursery through the windows is helpful to the other children. Many children benefit from visits to the nursery to see their brother or sister. The natural curiosity of the child about "what is going on" in the family is answered when the child actually sees the baby. Behavior problems such as bedwetting, sleeping and eating difficulties, and difficult separations from parents may be prevented or reduced by the reassurance of a visit that decreases the sibling's worry about the baby.[5] Sibling visitation must be individualized for every family.[65]

Sibling Visits

The decision to include siblings in the NICU depends to a great extent on the views, beliefs, and attitudes of the hospital staff.[44,114] Generally, the staff's concerns about and resistance to sibling visitation focus on a fear of an increase in nosocomial infection, disruption of unit routine and order, and potential harm to young children from exposure to the NICU environment. Infection control is the responsibility of parents and professionals. Parents must be educated about the dangers of infection and instructed on how to screen their children for symptoms such as fever, cough, or diarrhea. Professional staff must inquire about the health of visiting siblings, including their exposure to communicable diseases. Both parents and children must wash their hands before entering the nursery; small stools for children to reach the sink are helpful. Cover gowns are no longer used by parents, siblings or professionals. With vigilance, no increased bacterial colonization and no increased incidence of infection occur with sibling visits.[14,145]

Because sibling visitation may be beneficial, each NICU must evaluate the center's situation and consider instituting a sibling visitation policy.[65,114,139] The following general principles may be used in developing this policy:

- Communication and coordination between staff and family are necessary to promote successful sibling visitation.
- Children must be prepared, according to their age and development, for what they will see, hear, and feel in the NICU.[44] Language should be simple and honest; pictures of the infant or other infants can be helpful.
- Parents and staff screen the visiting sibling for signs of illness that would exclude the child from visiting.
- Parents and child must scrub.
- The initial visit should be held at a relatively quiet time in the nursery when a care provider is able to stay with the family. If the infant can be moved to a private room or family room area, this is preferable.

At the bedside the child is introduced to the infant and seated on a chair or stool at eye level with the infant. The care provider then again explains the equipment the child sees and any of the infant's "interesting" behaviors such as crying because of hunger, sucking on a pacifier, or eyes open "looking at you." Children may even be included in age-appropriate caregiving tasks. Choosing clothes, handling diapers and blankets, holding the bottle, or touching and talking to the infant are all ways "to help." The child may bring a present to the infant such as a simple toy, music box, or handmade picture or photograph of the family. After a visit, both parents and staff should be available to talk about

the visit or answer any questions. Some children, however, will not discuss the visit or ask questions until some later time. A method for enabling children to express their feelings in a nonverbal way is through play or books. A child who receives a book about physicians and hospitals or a "doctor" or "nurse" doll may "play out" feelings about the brother or sister and the hospital experience.

Creating a comfortable environment in which children feel free to ask questions is essential when siblings visit.[94] Every question deserves an answer, even "I don't know," when appropriate. Children are often quite unrestrained in their remarks and questions. Comments such as, "He's sure ugly!" or "Is he going to die?" or "Why is she tied up (restrained)?" are common. These may be embarrassing to parents who hesitate to make the same remarks or ask the same questions.

If the infant is hospitalized for a long time, the other children may lose interest or even wish it were all over. This response may upset parents who themselves may be struggling with the same feelings. The longer the infant is hospitalized, the greater the pressure on time and financial resources. Family routines are disrupted by continuing hospitalization, and the disruption may strain family relationships.

Staff and parent response to sibling visitation has been positive in hospitals where the policy has been implemented. Such a policy may facilitate family integrity and promotes mutual support during the stressful time of hospitalization.[14] Another advantage of visitation is that the older siblings do not endure repeated separations caused by parental visits to the hospital but are included as important and special family members. The presence of siblings in a nursery can be a rewarding experience for family and staff alike and perhaps is the ideal example of providing safe yet comprehensive family-centered care.

Although a flexible sibling visitation policy is viewed as the best possible situation, some alternatives such as coloring books and children's books should be considered (see Resource Materials for Parents). Staff should be sensitive to the needs of the siblings and understand that the parents must deal with both time and financial constraints.

Psychosocial Conferences

Psychosocial conferences for staff members to discuss the dynamics of family functioning and the effect of a seriously ill newborn on the family can be quite useful. These conferences, usually led by perinatal social workers, can give staff the opportunity to discuss and better understand their own feelings and reactions to families, infants, and the many stresses related to working in an NICU. In addition, weekly rounds with the entire multidisciplinary team (physicians, nurses, home health nurse coordinator, social workers, and financial counselors) are an effective vehicle to discuss and develop medical discharge and psychosocial care plans about each infant and family. The involvement of perinatal social workers to assess and evaluate the psychosocial functioning of families, to provide support and counseling services, and to coordinate the discharge planning and follow-up care for the infant and family is essential. Social workers need to evaluate all high-risk cases in addition to providing support in complicated medical conditions, including death of the infant[12] (Box 29-3).

Box 29-3	**HIGH-RISK FACTORS NEEDING SOCIAL WORK INTERVENTION**

1. Teenage pregnancy (ages 11 to 18)[2,20,32]
2. Single parent
3. Substance abuse[20,36,137]
4. Psychiatric history of present problem that interferes with appropriate functioning, especially as related to parenting abilities
5. Mother or father with a history of being physically and/or sexually abused or early deprivation by own family, or history of having abused or neglected own children
6. Battered women/domestic violence
7. Mental retardation, borderline intelligence, or significant physical handicaps
8. History of loss with previous pregnancy[11,130] or child because of stillbirth, birth defect, prematurity, abortion, custody case, or death
9. Rejection or ambivalence of current pregnancy as manifested by requests for termination of pregnancy, attempted abortion, or relinquishment
10. No prenatal care with previous or current pregnancies
11. Pregnancy exacerbating extreme depression, anxiety, or suicidal thoughts
12. Stressful home or personal situation because of marital or financial problems or lack of support
13. Long-term hospitalization during pregnancy requiring intervention in helping family adjust by arranging for younger children at home or for financial assistance
14. Other children with physical or mental handicaps
15. Attachment difficulties with the infant
16. Prior history with social services

Transfer Back to the Referring Hospital

Transfer of the infant from a tertiary center back to the referring or local community center for convalescent care and discharge is a frequent occurrence. This can be helpful in facilitating the relationship between the infant and parents, because the infant will be more accessible. Parents generally view the transfer as positive if the hospital is closer to home and if they feel comfortable with the level of care provided. Transfer is stressful, and there is always an adjustment period any time a transfer occurs.[50,88] Parents must adapt to different personalities of medical personnel and different procedures and visiting policies. Preparing the parents for the transfer, orienting them to the new hospital, and talking to the staff of the referral hospital about the infant and the parents is important to help ease the transition.[4,50,88,121,140]

Preparation to Take the Infant Home

The sixth psychologic task for parents concerns preparations for taking the infant home. Parents must understand their infant's individual needs and personality characteristics in addition to feeling a sense of competency in relating to their infant. Discharge is an anxiety-provoking event and ushers in the "crisis" of homecoming, which parents must face and master. The unsuccessful resolution of the previously discussed five psychologic tasks can contribute to maladaptive parenting and a poor outcome for the infant, including the possibilities of attachment difficulties, overprotectiveness, failure to thrive, vulnerable child syndrome, emotional deprivation, and battering.[81] To achieve a positive parent-child relationship after the hospitalization and through the transitional period that ensues, provision of appropriate follow-up support through the home adjustment period is crucial.[54,81,99,154]

Several behaviors demonstrate that parents are trying to understand the infant's care in preparation for discharge. First, parents may ask questions verbalizing a variety of concerns. For a premature infant, they might ask, "Do I need an apnea monitor at home?" or "Can the baby have visitors?" or "Do I need to wash my hands when handling the baby?" For a child with a congenital defect such as spina bifida, the parents might ask, "Can I lay the baby on his back?" or "Can I bathe him?" or "Do I need to pump the shunt?" For a child with a heart defect the staff might be asked, "Do I need oxygen?" or "Do I need to handle him differently?" or "What about going to higher altitudes?" All of these questions on the part of parents are typical and normal and represent the parents' working through their fears and anxieties.

On the other hand, parents who are highly anxious, extremely overprotective, or very indifferent should be a concern to the health care personnel. The inability to deal with the task of taking the infant home may indicate some unresolved feelings related to the previous psychologic tasks. Although most parents whose infants have been in a NICU do admit to initially treating their infant differently until they "got to know their child," a group of parents who are excessively overprotective does exist. This type of behavior often stems from parents who are struggling with intense feelings of guilt and failure. These parents either protect their child from everything because they feel so responsible for having caused the infant's initial problem or they demonstrate an indifference or lack of concern for the infant and the infant's welfare. Such parents may have an ambivalent attachment to their infant, who may continue to represent the threat of death or the parents' personal failure. This group of parents should be considered high risk for potential parent-child relationship difficulties and should be evaluated to determine an appropriate intervention.

At discharge there are infants whose medical conditions are still fragile, a substantial indication that these infants may not be normal and have long-term problems. These infants may be temperamentally difficult to manage, and parents understandably treat them differently.[15] Both parents and infants need additional support and appropriate intervention.[38,99,107]

There are many interventions that the perinatal health care team can employ to assist parents with discharge and through the transitional period that follows. In the hospital, adequate teaching of caregiving skills that enable the parent to develop a sense of mastery and competence is of paramount importance. In addition to tasks of care, parents should participate in planning and providing developmentally appropriate care and be able to read and respond to their infant's cues[154] (see Chapter 13). Maternal concerns about neonatal care center on elimination, feeding, and the infant's health.[78] If parents do not feel comfortable with their infant, their anxiety can cause adverse interactions with the infant. The parent needs to know the infant's mannerisms and behaviors; otherwise the parent may feel exhausted and resentful and then guilty. Teaching caregiving skills can often be facilitated in an environment that is less intense and crisis oriented than the NICU. Whenever possible, an infant should be transferred to a setting that is more conducive to the parents' initiation of the primary caregiving role; a more conducive setting might be a special care or transitional nursery,[13,55] a level II unit, or a general pediatric ward. Care by parents before discharge enables parents to assume full responsibility for their infant's care, tests the reality of caregiving, helps them learn caregiving activities and their infant's behavioral patterns, and confirms their readiness for independent parenting and the infant's readiness for discharge.[37]

Adequate discharge planning and follow-up arrangements[128] should include general pediatric care, home health care, nurse and paraprofessional home visitors, and parenting classes, especially for young or psychosocially high-risk parents.[35,100] Recent studies document positive effects of home visitation programs.[47,79,86,119,120] Referrals to county social service departments should be made for single mothers who are eligible for Temporary Assistance to Needy Families, Title 19 Medicaid, and state child health insurance programs. For infants with special problems (spina bifida, cerebral palsy, or Down syndrome), referrals should be made for special programs that provide services for the infants and support groups for parents. Parents whose infants have special medical needs (gavage feedings, tracheostomy or colostomy care, oxygen or ventilators) should be evaluated by the medical and nursing personnel to determine helpful community resources (equipment, supplies, respite or emergency care) and to make appropriate referrals. Home nursing care and homemaker services are sometimes covered by medical insurance and may be necessary to provide actual nursing activities and to relieve parents from the emotional burden inherent in caring for an infant with medical problems.[34] For infants who are developmentally and physically disabled, developmental intervention programs and follow-up programs provided by many hospitals that have NICUs are extremely valuable. These infants are eligible for Part C of the Individuals with Disabilities Education Act (IDEA). Locating babysitters who will care for a child with special problems can be an overwhelming task for parents; cultivating a resource list for parents and suggesting that parents exchange services with each other can also be helpful. Graduate parents, neonatal nurses, or respite care organizations can provide a useful service to parents in this situation. Last, parents should be referred to appropriate funding agencies (Health Care Programs for Children with Special Needs, Title 19 Medicaid, state child health insurance programs, or Social Security Disability) that provide financial assistance.

REFERENCES

1. Able-Boon H, Dokecki P, Smith M: Parents and health care providers communication and decision making in the intensive care nursery, *Child Health Care* 18:133, 1989.
2. Adams D, Kocik S: Perinatal social work with childbearing adolescents, *Soc Work Health Care* 24:85, 1997.
3. Affonso D: Missing pieces: a study of post-partum feelings, *Birth Fam J* 4:159, 1977.
4. Affonso DD, Hurst I, Mayberry LJ et al: Stressors reported by mothers of hospitalized premature infants, *Neonatal Netw* 11:63, 1992.
5. Affonso DD, Wahlberg V, Persson B: Exploration of mother's reactions to the kangaroo method of prematurity care, *Neonatal Netw* 7:43, 1989.
6. Affonso D, Bosque E, Wahlberg V et al: Reconciliation and healing for mothers through skin-to-skin contact provided in an American tertiary level intensive care nursery, *Neonatal Netw* 12:25, 1993.
7. Aguilera D, Messick J: *Crisis intervention theory and methodology,* ed 3, St Louis, 1978, Mosby.
8. American Academy of Pediatrics: The initiation or withdrawal of treatment for high-risk newborns, *Pediatrics* 96:362, 1995a.
9. American Academy of Pediatrics and American College of Obstetricians and Gynecologists: Perinatal care at the threshold of viability, *Pediatrics* 96:974, 1995b.
10. American Academy of Pediatrics and American College of Obstetricians and Gynecologists: *Guidelines for perinatal care,* ed 4, Elk Grove, Ill, 1997, The Academy.
11. Armstrong D, Hutti M: Pregnancy after perinatal loss: the relationship between anxiety and prenatal attachment, *J Obstet Gynecol Neonatal Nurs* 27:183, 1998.
12. Bachman D, Lind R: Perinatal social work and the family of the newborn intensive care infant, *Soc Work Health Care* 24:21, 1997.
13. Bachrach S et al: A model transitional-care program for premature infants, *J Perinat Neonatal Nurs* 9:31, 1985.
14. Ballard JL, Maloney M, Shank M et al: Sibling visits to a newborn intensive care unit: implications for siblings, parents and infants, *Child Psychiatry Hum Dev* 14:203, 1984.
15. Barnard K, Kelly J: Assessment of parent-child interaction. In Meisels S, Shankoff J, eds: *Handbook of early childhood intervention,* Cambridge, Mass, 1990, Cambridge University Press.
16. Barnett CR, Leiderman PH, Grobstein R et al: Neonatal separation: the maternal side of interactional deprivation, *Pediatrics* 54:197, 1970.
17. Bell P: Adolescent mothers' perceptions of the NICU, *J Perinat Neonatal Nurs* 11:77, 1998.
18. Benfield D, Leib S, Vollman J: Grief responses of parents to neonatal death and parental participation, *Pediatrics* 62:171, 1978.
19. Benfield DG, Leib S, Reutor J et al: Grief response to parents after referral of the critically ill newborn to a regional center, *N Engl J Med* 294:975, 1976.
20. Bialoskurski M, Cox C, Hayes J: The nature of attachment in a neonatal intensive care unit, *J Perinat Neonat Nurs* 13:66, 1999.
21. Bibring G, Dwyer T, Huntington D et al: A study of the psychological processes in pregnancy and of the earliest mother-child relationship: some propositions and comments, *Psychoanal Study Child* 16:9, 1961.
22. Bloom K: Perceived relationship with the father of the baby and maternal attachment in adolescents, *J Obstet Gynecol Neonatal Nurs* 27:420, 1998.
23. Bracht M, Ardal F, Bot A et al: Initiation and maintenance of a hospital-based parent group for parents of premature infants: key factors for success, *Neonatal Netw* 17:33, 1998.
24. Browne J, Smith-Sharpe S: The Colorado consortium of intensive care nurseries: spinning webs of support for Colorado infants and families, *Zero to Three,* June/July, 1995.
25. Buus-Frank M: Nurse versus machine: slaves or masters of technology? *J Obstet Gynecol Neonatal Nurs* 28:433, 1999.
26. Campbell S, Taylor P: Bonding and attachment: theoretical issues, *Semin Perinatol* 3:3, 1979.
27. Caplan G: Patterns of parental response to the crisis of premature birth, *Psychiatry* 23:365, 1960.
28. Caplan G, Mason EA, Kaplan DM: Four studies of crisis in parents of prematures: 1965, *Community Ment Health J* 1:149, 2000.
29. Catletta A, Miles M, Holditch-Davis D: Maternal perceptions of illness severity in premature infants, *Neonatal Netw* 13:45, 1994.
30. Chernick L, Cockrell T, Frech C et al: Current staff attitudes regarding parental visitation within NICU's, *Pediatr Res* 47:391c, 2000.
31. Christensson K, Cabrera T, Christenson E et al: Separation distress call in the human neonate in the absence of maternal body contact, *Acta Paediatr Scand* 84:468, 1994.
32. Christopher S, Baumann K: Measurement of affectionate behaviors adolescent mothers display toward their infants in neonatal intensive care, *Iss Compr Pediatr Nurs* 22:1, 1999.

33. Clark F: Making sense of *State v Messenger,* *Pediatrics* 97:579, 1996.

34. Colt D, Beyers J: Baby Saige goes home, *Continuing Care* 12:25, 1993.

35. Community Caring Project, C Henry Kempe, National Center for the Prevention and Treatment of Child Abuse and Neglect, Denver, Colo, 1991.

36. Cook C: Role of the social worker in perinatal substance abuse, *Soc Work Health Care* 24:65, 1997.

37. Costello A, Chapman J: Mothers' perceptions of the care-by-parent program prior to hospital discharge of their preterm infant, *Neonatal Netw* 17:37, 1998.

38. Cronin CM, Shapiro CR, Casiro OG et al: The impact of very-low-birth-weight infants on the family is long lasting, *Arch Pediatr Adolesc Med* 149:151, 1995.

39. Cuttini M, Rebagliato M, Bortoli P et al: Parental visiting, communication, and participation in ethical decisions: a comparison of neonatal unit policies in Europe, *Arch Dis Child Fetal Neonatal Educ* 81:F84, 1999.

40. Davis JA et al: *Parent-baby attachments in premature infants,* New York, 1983, St Martin's Press.

41. DeChateau P: The importance of the neonatal period for the development of synchrony in the maternal-fetal dyad: a review, *Birth Fam J* 4:10, 1977.

42. Doering L, Dracup K, Moser D: Comparison of psychosocial adjustment of mothers and fathers of high-risk infants in the NICU, *J Perinatol* 19:132, 1999.

43. Doering L, Moser D, Dracup K: Correlates of anxiety, hostility, depression and psychosocial adjustment in parents of NICU infants, *Neonatal Netw* 19:15, 2000.

44. Doll Speck L, Miller B, Rohrs K: Sibling education: implementing a program for the NICU, *Neonatal Netw* 12:49, 1993.

45. Doroshow RW, Hodgman JE, Pomerance JJ et al: Treatment decisions for newborns at the threshold of viability: an ethical dilemma, *J Perinatol* 20:379, 2000.

46. Drake E: Internet technology: resources for perinatal nurses, *J Obstet Gynecol Neonatal Nurs* 28:115, 1999.

47. Eckenrode J, Ganzel B, Henderson CR Jr et al: Preventing child abuse and neglect with a program of nurse home visitation, *JAMA* 284:1385, 2000.

48. Eidelman A, Hoffman N, Kaitz M: Cognitive deficits in women after childbirth, *Obstet Gynecol* 81:764, 1993.

49. Fantz RL, Fagan J, Miranda S et al: Early visual selectivity as a function of pattern variables, previous exposure, age from birth and conception and expected cognitive deficit. In Cohen L, Salapatic P, eds: *Infant perception,* vol. 1, New York, 1975, Academic Press.

50. Flanagan V, Slattery MJ, Chase NS et al: Mothers' perception of the quality of their infant's back transfer: pilot study results, *Neonatal Netw* 15:27, 1996.

51. Fromm E: *The art of loving,* New York, 1965, Harper & Row.

52. Gardner SL: Mothering: the unconscious conflict between nurses and new mothers, *Keep Abreast J* 3:192, 1978.

53. Gennaro S: Facilitating parenting of the neonatal intensive care unit graduate, *J Perinat Neonatal Nurs* 4:55, 1991.

54. Goldberg S: Prematurity: effects on parent-infant interaction, *J Pediatr Psychol* 3:137, 1978.

55. Goldson E: The family care center: a model for the transitional care of the sick infant and his family, *Child Today* 10:51, 1981.

56. Goldson E: The neonatal intensive care unit: premature infants and parents, *Infants Young Child* 4:31, 1992.

57. Gordon P, Johnson B: Technology and family-centered perinatal care: conflict or synergy? *J Obstet Gynecol Neonatal Nurs* 28:401, 1999.

58. Gottfried AW, Gaiter JL: *Infant stress under intensive care,* Baltimore, 1985, University Park Press.

59. Grace J: Development of maternal-fetal attachment during pregnancy, *Nurs Res* 38:228, 1989.

60. Grant P, Siegel R: Families in crisis: birth of a sick infant. Presented at the Perinatal Section Meeting of the American Academy of Pediatrics, Scottsdale, Ariz, April, 1978.

61. Gray J, Cutler C, Dean J et al: Perinatal assessment of mother-baby interaction. In Helfer B, Kempe CH, eds: *Child abuse and neglect: the family and the community,* Cambridge, Mass, 1976, Ballinger Publishing.

62. Gray J, Pompilio G, Pursley D et al: Baby CareLink: improving NICU care with telemedicine technologies, *Pediatr Res* 47:400a, 2000.

63. Green M, Solnit A: Reactions to the threatened loss of a child: a vulnerable child syndrome, *Pediatrics* 34:58, 1964.

64. Griffin T: Nurse barriers to parenting in the special care nursery, *J Perinat Neonatal Nurs* 4:56, 1990.

65. Griffin T: The visitation policy, *Neonatal Netw* 17:75, 1998a.

66. Griffin T: Visitation patterns: the parents who visit "too much," *Neonatal Netw* 17:67, 1998b.

67. Griffin T: Visitation patterns: the parents who visit "too little," *Neonatal Netw* 18:75, 1999.

68. Hagedorn M, Gardner S: Accountability for professional nursing practice. In Gardner S, Hagedorn M, eds: *Legal aspects of maternal-child nursing practice,* Menlo Park, Calif, 1997, Addison-Wesley Longman.

69. Haines C, Perger C, Nagy S: A comparison of the stressors experienced by parents of intubated and extubated children, *J Adv Nurs* 21:350, 1995.

70. Harmon RJ: The perinatal period: infants and parents. In Spittell JA, Brody E, eds: *Clinical medicine,* vol. 12, Hagerstown, Md, 1981, Harper & Row.

71. Harrison H: The principles of family-centered neonatal care, *Pediatrics* 92:643, 1993.

72. Heidrich S, Cranley M: Effect of fetal movement, ultrasound scans, and amniocentesis on maternal-infant attachment, *Nurs Res* 38:81, 1989.

72a. Helper B, Kempe CH, eds: *Child abuse and neglect: the family and the community,* 1976, Ballinger.

73. Hofer M: Early relationships as regulators of infant physiology and behavior, *Acta Paediatr Scand* 397(suppl):9, 1994.

74. Holditch-Davis D, Miles M: Mothers' stories about their experiences in the NICU, *Neonatal Netw* 19:13, 2000.

75. Jordan B: *Birth in four cultures,* St Albans, Vt, 1978, Eden Press.

76. Kaplan DM, Mason EA: Maternal reactions to premature birth viewed as an emotional disorder, *Am J Orthopsych* 30:539, 1960.

77. Kennell JH, Jerauld R, Wolfe H et al: Maternal behavior one year after early and extended post-partum contact, *Dev Med Child Neurol* 16:172, 1974.

78. Kenner C, Lott JW: Parent transition after discharge from the NICU, *Neonatal Netw* 9:31, 1990.

79. Kitzman H, Olds DL, Sidora K et al: Enduring effects of nurse home visitation on maternal life course, *JAMA* 283:1983, 2000.

80. Klaus MH, Kennell JH: Mothers separated from their newborn infants, *Pediatr Clin North Am* 17:1015, 1970.

81. Klaus MH, Kennell JH: *Parent-infant bonding,* ed 2, St Louis, 1982, Mosby.

82. Klaus MH, Jerauld R, Kreger NC et al: Maternal attachment: importance of the first postpartum days, *N Engl J Med* 286:460, 1972.

83. Koh THHG: Audiotaping of parentsneonatalogist conversations in NICUs, *Int J Clin Pract* 52:27, 1998.

84 Koh THHG, Casey A, Harrison H: Use of an outcome by gestation table for extremely premature babies: a cross-sectional survey of the views of parents, neonatal nurses and perinatalogists, *J Perinatol* 20:504, 2000.

85. Koh THHG, Harrison H, Morley C: Gestation versus outcome table for parents of extremely premature infants, *J Perinatol* 19:452, 1999.

86. Korfmacher J, O'Brien R, Hiatt S et al: Differences in program implementation between nurses and paraprofessionals providing home visits during pregnancy and infancy: a randomized trial, *Am J Pub Health* 89:1847, 1999.

87. Krahn G, Hallum A, Kime C: Are there good ways to give "bad news"? *Pediatrics* 91:578, 1993.

88. Kuhnly J, Freston M: Back transport: exploration of parents feelings regarding the transition, *Neonatal Netw* 14:69, 1995.

89. Leifer AD, Leiderman PH, Barnett CR et al: Effects of mother-infant separation on maternal attachment behavior, *Child Dev* 43:1203, 1972.

90. LeMasters EE: Parenthood as crisis, *Marriage Family Living* 19:352, 1957.

91. Lemons J, Schreiner R, Weiner G: The good doctor: a neonatologist's perspective, *J Perinatol* 19:189, 1999.

92. Leung J, Spear M, Locke R et al: Developmental changes in family reactions during their infant's prolonged hospitalization in the NICU, *Pediatr Res* 45:207a, 1999.

93. Levick J, Lindsay J: Parent-to-parent support: enriching traditional prenatal and NICU care, *Natl Assn Perinat Workers Forum* 12:9, 1992.

94. Levick J, Munch S: "I'm special too.": psychosocial aspects of sibling adjustment in the NICU, *Natl Assn Perinat Soc Workers Forum* 13:1, 1993.

95. Liederman PH, Seashore MJ: Mother-infant neonatal separation: some delayed consequences, Ciba Foundation Symposium 33, Amsterdam, 1975, Elsevier.

96. Lindsay JK, Roman L, DeWys M et al: Creative caring in the NICU: parent-to-parent support, *Neonatal Netw* 12:37, 1993.

97. Liu D, Diorio J, Tannenbaum B et al: Maternal care, hippocampal glucocorticoid receptors, and hypothalamic-pituitary-adrenal responses to stress, *Science* 277:1659, 1997.

98. Macnab AJ, Sheckter LA, Hendry NJ et al: Group support for parents of high-risk neonates: an interdisciplinary approach, *Soc Work Health Care* 10:63, 1985.

99. Marony D: Realities of a premature infant's first year: helping parents cope, *J Perinatol* 15:418, 1995.

100. McKim E: The difficult first week at home with a premature infant, *Neonatal Netw* 12:72, 1993.

101. McLennan J, Kotelchuck M: Parental preventive practices for young children in the context of maternal depression, *Pediatrics* 105:1090, 2000.

102. Mead M, Newton N: Cultural patterning of perinatal behaviors. In Richardson S, Guttmacher A, eds: *Childbearing: its social and psychological aspects,* Baltimore, 1957, Williams & Wilkins.

103. Meyer EC, Gracia Coll CT, Seifer R et al: Psychological distress in mothers of preterm infants, *J Dev Behav Pediatr* 16:412, 1995.

104. Miles M, Carlson J, Funk S: Sources of support reported by mothers and fathers in infants hospitalized in an NICU, *Neonatal Netw* 15:45, 1996.

105. Miles M, Funk S, Kaspan M: The stress response of mothers and fathers of preterm infants, *Res Nurs Health* 15:261,1992.

106. Miles M, Wilson S, Docherty S: African American mothers' responses to hospitalization of an infant with serious health problems, *Neonatal Netw* 18:17, 1999a.

107. Miles M, Holditch-Davis D, Burchinal P et al: Distress and growth in mothers of medically fragile infants, *Nurs Res* 48:129, 1999b.
108. Minde K: The impact of prematurity on the later behavior of children and their families, *Clin Perinatol* 11:227, 1984.
109. Minton C: Uses of photographs in perinatal social work, *Health Soc Work* 8:121, 1983.
110. Montalvo N, Vila B: Parent's grand rounds speech on neonatal intensive care unit experience, *J Perinatol* 19:525, 1999.
111. Murphy K: Threatened perinatal loss: defining and managing strategies used by parents of critically ill infants, Dissertation, Chicago, University of Illinois, 1989.
112. National Association of Neonatal Nurses: *Infant and family care developmental care guidelines,* Petaluma, Calif., 1995, The Association.
113. Neufeld M, Woodrum D, Tarczy-Hornoch P: Prenatal and postnatal counseling for parents of infants at the limits of viability, *Pediatr Res* 47:420A, 2000.
114. Newman CB, McSweeney M: A descriptive study of sibling visitation in the NICU, *Neonatal Netw* 9:27, 1990.
115. Newton N, Newton M: Mothers' reaction to their newborn babies, *JAMA* 181:206, 1962.
116. Noble DN, Hamilton AK: Families under stress: perinatal social work, *Health Soc Work* 6:28, 1981.
117. O'Brien M, Solidy E, McClusky-Fawcett K: Prematurity and the neonatal intensive care unit. In Roberts M, ed: *Handbook of pediatric psychology,* ed 2, New York, 1995, Guilford Press.
118. Oehler J, Hannan T, Catlett S: Maternal views of preterm infants' responsiveness to social interaction, *Neonatal Netw* 12:67, 1993.
119. Olds D, Korfmacher J: Maternal psychological characteristics as influences on home visitation contact, *J Community Psychol* 26:23, 1998.
120. Olds D, Henderson C, Eckenrode J et al: Theoretical and empirical foundations of a program of home visitation for pregnant women and parents of young children, *J Community Psychol* 25:9, 1997.
121. Page J, Lunyk-Child O: Parental perceptions of infant transfer from an NICU to a community nursery: implication for research and practice, *Neonatal Netw* 14:69, 1995.
122. Paul D, Leef K, Epps S et al: Usefulness of the prenatal consult: mothers' response, *Pediatr Res* 45:218A, 1999.
123. Perehudoff B: Parent's perceptions on environment stressors in the special care nursery, *Neonatal Netw* 9:39, 1990.
124. Perrin EC, West PD, Culley BS et al: Is my child normal yet? Correlates of vulnerability, *Pediatrics* 83:355, 1989.
125. Phillips C, Anzalone J: *Fathering: participation in labor and birth, ed* 2, St Louis, 1982, Mosby.
126. Plunkett JW, Meisels SJ, Stiefel GS et al: Patterns of attachment among preterm infants of varying biological risk, *J Am Acad Child Psychiatry* 25:794, 1986.
127. Raines D: Values of mothers of LBW infants in the NICU, *Neonatal Netw* 17:41, 1998.
128. Ramey C, Shearer D: A conceptual framework for interventions with low birth weight premature children and their families. In Goldson E, ed: *Nurturing the premature infant,* New York, 1999, Oxford University Press.
129. Rice RD: Maternal-infant bonding: the profound long-term benefits of immediate continuous skin and eye contact at birth. In Stewart D, Stewart L, eds: *21st century OB: now,* Marble Hill, Mo., 1977, NAPSAC.
130. Robertson P, Kavanaugh K: Supporting parents during and after a pregnancy subsequent to a perinatal loss, *J Perinat Neonat Nurs* 12:63, 1998.
131. Rosenblatt J: Psychobiology of maternal behavior: contribution to the clinical understanding of maternal behavior among humans, *Acta Paediatr Scand Suppl* 3978:3, 1994.
132. Rosenblum L, Andrews M: Influences of environmental demand on maternal behavior and infant development, *Acta Paediatr Scand Suppl* 397:57, 1994.
133. Rostow P: The family's perspective. In Jones MJ, Gleason C, Lipstein S et al, eds: *Hospital care of the recovering NICU infant,* Baltimore, 1991, Williams & Wilkins.
134. Ruiz A, Cravedi V, Cernadas J: Stress and depression in mothers of premature infants: evaluation of a psychosocial intervention model in the NICU: a randomized controlled study, *Pediatr Res* 45:222A, 1999.
135. Scharer K, Brooks G: Mothers of chronically ill neonates and primary care in the NICU: transfer of care, *Neonatal Netw* 13:37, 1994.
136. Scott L: Perceived needs of parents of critically ill children, *J Soc Pediatr Nurs* 3:4, 1998.
137. Seifer R, Lester B, LaGasse L et al: The maternal lifestyle study (MLS): attachment classification at 18 mo corrected age in infants exposed to cocaine/opiates, *Pediatr Res* 45:255A, 1999.
138. Sharp M, Strauss R, Lorch S: Communicating medical bad news: parents' experiences and preferences, *J Pediatr* 121:539, 1992.
139. Shea-McAleavey C, Janusz H: Sibling visiting—a plan for change, *Dimens Crit Care Nurs* 10:218, 1991.
140. Shellbarger S, Thompson T: The critical times: meeting parental communication needs throughout the NICU experience, *Neonatal Netw* 12:39, 1993.
141. Shields-Poe D, Pinelli J: Variables associated with parental stress in neonatal intensive care units, *Neonatal Netw* 16:29, 1997.

142. Siegel R: A family-centered program of neonatal intensive care, *Health Soc Work* 7:50, 1982.
143. Sieratzki J, Woll B: Why do mothers cradle babies on their left? *Lancet* 347:1746, 1996.
144. Singer L, Davillier M, Bruening P et al: Social support, psychological distress and parenting strains in mothers of VLBW infants, *Fam Relations* 45:343, 1996.
145. Solheim K. Spellacy C: Sibling visitation: effects on newborn infection rates, *J Obstet Gynecol Neonatal Nurs* 17:43, 1988.
146. Solnit AJ, Stark MH: Mourning and the birth of a defective child, *Psychoanal Study Child* 16:523, 1961.
147. Stainton M: Parents' awareness of their unborn infant in third trimester, *Birth* 17:92, 1990.
148. Stark M: Is it difficult to concentrate during the 3rd trimester and postpartum? *J Obstet Gynecol Neonatal Nurs* 29:378, 2000.
149. Stratmoen J: Poor communication a risk, *Aust Doctor,* March 2, 1995.
150. Sullivan J: Development of father-infant attachment in fathers of preterm infants, *Neonatal Netw* 18:33, 1999.
151. Taylor PM, Hall BL: Parent-infant bonding: problems and opportunities in a perinatal center, *Semin Perinatol* 3:73, 1979.
152. Thomson M, Westreich R: Restriction of mother-infant contact in the immediate postnatal period. In Chalmers I, Enkin M, Keirse M, eds: *Effective care in pregnancy and childbirth,* Oxford, England, 1989, Oxford University Press.
153. Tyson J: Evidence-based ethics and the care of premature infants, *Future Child* 5:197, 1995.
154. Vandenberg K: What to tell parents about the developmental needs of their baby at discharge, *Neonatal Netw* 18:57, 1999.
155. Wereszczak J, Miles M, Holditch-Davis D: Maternal recall of the neonatal intensive care unit, *Neonatal Netw* 16:33, 1997.
156. Widstrom AM, Ransjo-Arvidson AB, Christensson K et al: Gastric suction in newborn infants: effects on circulation and developing feeding behaviors, *Acta Paediatr Scand* 76:566, 1987.
157. Younger J, Kendall M, Pickler R: Mastery of stress in mothers of preterm infants, *J Soc Pediatr Nurs* 2:29, 1997.

RESOURCE MATERIALS FOR PARENTS

Brazelton TB: *On becoming a family: the growth of attachment,* New York, 1981, Delacorte Press.
Colorado Collective for Medical Health Care Decisions: *You are not alone* [film], Denver, Colo, 1999, Nickel's Worth Publications. NICKELWRTH@aol.com.
Harrison H, Kositsky A: *The premature baby book: a parent's guide to coping and caring in the first years,* New York, 1990, St Martin's Press.
Hatcher D, Lehman K: *Baby talk for parents who are getting to know their special care baby,* Omaha, Neb, 1985, Centering Corp.
Hawkins-Walsh E, Borum S: *Kate's premature brother,* Omaha, Neb, 1985, Centering Corp.
Johnson B: Institute for Family-Centered Care, 7900 Wisconsin Ave., Suite 405, Bethesda, Md, 20814.
Johnson J, Johnson M, Hatcher D: *Special beginnings,* Omaha, Neb, 1994, Centering Corp.
Kahn R, Green R, Little G: *Dreams and dilemmas: parents and the practice of neonatal care* [video], Trustees of Dartmouth College and Richard Kahn, 1998.
Lafferty L, Flood B: *Born early: a premature baby's story for children,* Grand Junction, Colo, 1994, Songbird Publishing.
Linden D, Paroli E, Doron M: *Preemies: the essential guide for parents of premature babies,* New York, 2000, Pocket Books.
O'Brien M et al: *An introduction to the NICU* and *Caring for your NICU baby* [videos], Baltimore, Md., 1994, Brookes.
Oehler J: *The frogs have a baby, a very small baby* [a coloring book for children], Durham, NC, 1979, Duke University Medical Center.
Sammons WAH, Lewis J: *Premature babies: a different beginning,* St Louis, 1985, Mosby.
Smith T: *Miracle birth stories of very premature babies: little thumbs up!* Westport, Conn, 1999, Bergin & Garvey.
Special care for your baby, Columbus, Ohio, 1982, Ross Laboratories.
The intensive care infant communicator: a different start, Philadelphia, 1988 and 1989, Wyeth-Ayerst Laboratories.
Websites for parents of premature infants: Parent-to-parent support and discussion: Preemie Child-for parents of preemie survivors of school-age, adolescents, and adults, Subscription address: LISTSERV@MAELSTROM.STJOHNS.EDU Website: http://www.comeunity.com; Preemie List—for parents of preterm babies, infants and young children; Preemie-L: homepage—http://www.preemie-l.org/; Resources for Parents of Preemies—http://members.aol.com/mariam/preemie.htm.
Your special newborn, Evansville, Ind, 1982, Mead Johnson Nutritional Division.
Zaichkin J: *Newborn intensive care: what every parent needs to know,* Petaluma, Calif, 2000, NICU Ink Book Publishers.

30 | Grief and Perinatal Loss

Sandra L. Gardner, Peggy Hauser, Gerald B. Merenstein

As a life passage, pregnancy and birth are associated with hopes and expectations, and joy and happiness for the future. Even though pregnancy and birth constitute a developmental crisis and major life change, expectant parents believe the gains of a healthy, happy child and family life offset any losses. Unfortunately, not all perinatal events have a happy ending. When pregnancy fails to produce a normal, healthy infant, it is a tragedy for the parents whose expectations of childbearing have not been fulfilled. Perinatal loss also affects their friends, family, and professional care providers.

Perinatal loss may be the first time a young adult has had the experience of coping with the illness or death of a loved one. Perinatal loss is especially significant because (1) it is sudden and unexpected, the most difficult loss to resolve[13]; (2) it interrupts the significant developmental stage of pregnancy and the situational crisis of pregnancy[13]; (3) it is the loss of a child who did not have the opportunity to live a full life[25,76]; and (4) it prevents progression into the next developmental stage of parenting that has been anticipated and rehearsed (at least in fantasy) during the pregnancy. Perinatal loss also often means interpersonal exclusion from the activities of childbearing friends and siblings.[51]

Unfortunately, loss and grief are often only thought of in relation to death. However, as final and irreversible as death is, it is just one form of separation and loss. Although less obvious, other loss situations may have an equally crucial effect. Loss comes in many forms—and during the perinatal period may occur without necessarily resulting in death. Circumstances of perinatal loss are at the same time parallel and different, because they all entail grief and mourning, and yet each has unique dimensions and characteristics.

The process of grief, its stages, and its symptoms are reviewed as a framework for understanding one's own feelings and those of others experiencing a loss. A desire to help and an idea of what is helpful and what is not helpful are presented as a basis for effective intervention by professionals.

THE GRIEF PROCESS

Grief, the characteristic response to the loss of a valued object, is not an intellectual and rational response.[26] Rather, it is personally experienced as the deep emotion of sadness and sorrow. To the individual, grief feels overwhelming, irrational, out of control, "crazy," and all-consuming. Mourning occurs in phases over time. After acknowledging that the loved object no longer exists, gradual withdrawal of emotion and feeling occurs, so that eventual psychologic investment in a new relationship is possible.

For grief to occur, the object must have been valued by the individual, so that its loss is perceived as significant and meaningful.[5] Because prenatally there is an investment of love in the fetus or newborn, the neonate is a valued object. To the extent the prenatal attachment has occurred, grief should be expected and felt at the loss of the fetus or newborn. Therefore loss at birth is a significant loss of a valued (although as yet only fantasized) person.

Loss, whether real or imagined, or actual or possible, is traumatic. The individual is no longer self-confident or confident about the surroundings, because both have been altered. Mourning and grief are forms of separation reactions. Fears of separation and abandonment are the universal fears of childhood regardless of age or developmental stage. Perhaps loss of a significant other awakens these childhood fears and reminds us of the basic "insecurity of all our attachments."[56]

Life changes are stressful to the individual because they threaten to disrupt continuity and a state of equilibrium.[70] Significant changes in the family configuration, such as accession of a new member, are normally a stressful occasion for family members. Perinatal complication or loss is even more of a stressful event for which the family has little or no preparation. The results of a crisis may be personal growth, maintaining the status quo, regression, or mental illness.[13,71] Often outcome depends on the type of help received during the crisis.

Decreasing the element of surprise through preparation for the situation to be encountered may modulate the effect of the event. Anticipatory grief[55,62,77,95] functions both to prepare and to protect the individual from the pain of impending loss. Prenatal diagnostic procedures, such as ultrasonography, amniocentesis, and fetoscopy, can now detect a variety of severe or lethal birth defects. When there is forewarning that the pregnancy or newborn is not healthy, the parents may begin a process of anticipatory grief and psychologically prepare for the loss of their child while simultaneously hoping for the neonate's survival.[4]

Parental withdrawal from the relationship established during pregnancy accompanies the intense emotions of anticipatory grief. Detachment protects and defends the parent from further painful feelings associated with the investment of self in a doomed relationship. If anticipatory grief proceeds, the parent may detach to the point of being unable to reattach to the infant if he or she survives. In this situation, the infant survives but the relationship with the parents may be significantly impaired. Maintaining even a remote hope that the fetus or newborn will survive protects the parents from the full experience of grief and total detachment from the child.

The degree of parental anticipatory grief is correlated with positive feelings about the pregnancy and the mode of delivery but not with the severity of the infant's illness. The more the parental investment and the higher the expectations for the pregnancy, the more anticipatory grief is associated with the development of a perinatal complication. The relative severity of the medical problem is not associated with the degree of anticipatory grief.

PERINATAL SITUATIONS IN WHICH GRIEF IS EXPECTED

Loss is a fact of life, not just of death. Every stage of development requires a loss of the privileges of the preceding stage and movement into the unknown of the next stage. Any life event involving change or loss is accompanied by grief work, including moving, divorce, separation, death of a spouse or family member, injury or illness, retirement, job change, menopause, and even success.[14,70] The concept of loss is even applicable to the physiologic and psychologic events of normal pregnancy and birth. Certainly, when pregnancy fails to produce a live, healthy infant, a perinatal loss situation exists (Box 30-1). These perinatal losses, including

Box 30-1	PERINATAL SITUATIONS IN WHICH GRIEF REACTION IS EXPECTED

I. Pregnancy
II. Birth
  A. Normal
  B. Cesarean section
  C. Forceps
  D. Episiotomy
  E. Medicated
  F. Prolonged or short labor
  G. Place of birth
III. Postpartum
  A. "Postpartum blues"
  B. Depression
  C. Psychosis
IV. Abortion
  A. Spontaneous
  B. Therapeutic
  C. Elective
  D. Selective
  E. Selective reduction (for multiple gestation)[20,66]
V. Stillbirth
VI. Loss of the perfect child
  A. Premature
  B. Deformed or anomalied baby
  C. Sick newborn
  D. "Wrong" sex
VII. Neonatal death
VIII. Relinquishment

stillbirth, loss of the perfect child, and neonatal death, are discussed in detail in this chapter.

Stillbirth

Stillbirth is the demise of a viable fetus that occurs after fetal movement when the infant is invested by the parents with a personality and individuality. Because stillbirth occurs later in pregnancy than most abortions, there are increased parental expectations about the baby and the birth process. Selective abortions for genetic indications often occur in the second trimester of pregnancy and involve the death of a wanted child. Even though parents understand the validity of the reason for terminating the pregnancy, sadness, guilt, and self-doubt often accompany the decision to abort. The anxieties related to termination procedures that include labor and birth, and the feelings of helplessness, isolation, and depression should be acknowledged and handled as in a stillbirth.

Fetal demise in utero happens either prenatally or in the intrapartum period. For 50% of stillbirths, death was sudden, without warning, and from unexplainable causes.[21] The majority of women whose fetus has died in utero spontaneously begin labor within 2 weeks of fetal demise.[21] Carrying the dead fetus and waiting for spontaneous labor or induction is sad and difficult for the woman and her entire family. Feelings such as helplessness, disbelief, and powerlessness characterize this period.[41] There is often an uncontrollable urge to flee and escape the unpleasant situation.[15,41]

For the family who experiences an intrapartum demise, the joyous expectations of labor and birth suddenly change to fear, anxiety, and dread that the "worst" could have possibly happened to them. The suddenness of fetal demise in labor and birth affects both parents and professionals with feelings of shock, denial, and anxiety. Whether the loss is an early or late fetal loss, the woman and her family maintain hope by believing that the professional has made a mistake and that the infant is still alive.[75] The onset (or continuation) of labor is approached with both hope and dread—hope that the infant may be born alive and dread that the infant's death will soon be a stark reality.

The discomfort of labor and birth is particularly difficult for the woman whose infant has died, because her work will not be rewarded with a healthy infant.[80] However, oversolicitous use of drugs at birth is not recommended, because they relegate the experience to unreality and give it a dreamlike quality.[96] Keeping parents together through this crisis is important for mutual support and sharing of the birth.[80,93] The deadening (and deafening) silence of a stillbirth forces the reality of the infant's death on both the parents and the professionals present at birth.[80]

In the past at the birth of a stillborn, the mother was heavily sedated or anesthetized and the infant was hidden and whisked away immediately. These women were often left with fears and fantasies: "Was the baby normal?" "What was the sex?" "What did the baby look like?" Seeing, touching, and holding the infant promote completion of the attachment cycle, confirm the reality of the stillbirth for both parents, and enable grief to begin.[8,75,96] Because it is easier to grieve the reality of a situation than a mystical and dreamlike fantasy, contact with the stillborn enables parents to grieve the infant's reality rather than their most frightening fantasies about the infant.[48,53,54,93]

After confirming the reality of the infant's death, a search for the cause, characterized by the universal question, "Why did the baby die?" begins. Either or both parents may blame themselves or feel guilty about real or imagined acts of omission or commission. An autopsy may determine the cause of death, but most often the cause is unknown, even after an autopsy; however, an autopsy may be useful in reducing parental guilt and uncertainty about future pregnancies, as well as in aiding the recovery from the loss.[41,96] The "empty tragedy"[54] of stillbirth forces the mother to deal with both the inner loss of the fetus and the outer loss of the expected newborn.

Loss of the Perfect Child

Even though pregnancy ends in the birth of a live child, the pregnancy outcome may not be what the parents had anticipated. Birth of an infant who does not meet parental expectations represents the realization of the parents' worst fears: a damaged child. Newborns who are preterm, anomalied, sick, or the "wrong" sex, or who ultimately die represent the loss of the fantasized perfect child.

After the birth of such a child, parental reactions include grief and mourning for the loss of the loved object (the perfect child) while simultaneously adapting to the reality and investing love in the defective child.[83,87] This reaction is analogous to parental mourning at the death of a child.[83] However, unlike the finality of death, birth of a living, defective child entails a persistent, constant reminder of the feelings of loss and grief because of parental investment of time, attention, and care for either a short time (preterm or sick newborn) or a lifetime (physically or mentally afflicted child).[83]

The psychic work involved in coping with the reality of the imperfect child and the inner feelings of loss is slow and emotionally painful.[87] The process is gradual and proceeds at an individual pace that cannot be hurried but can be facilitated and supported. Detachment from and mourning the loss of their fantasized child is necessary before parents are able to attach to the actual child.

Birth of an imperfect child represents multiple losses for parents. A primary narcissistic injury, a threat to the female's self-concept as a woman and mother and the male's self-concept as a man and a father, occurs when a less-than-perfect child is born.* Because the child is an extension of both parents, a less-than-perfect (i.e., deformed) child is equated with the perceived less-than-perfect part of the parental self.[87] In the mind of the parent, the

---

*References 18, 19, 45, 50, 51, 87.

imagined inadequate self has failed and caused the birth of the damaged child.[45]

Prematurity

Every woman expects to deliver a normal, healthy infant at term. Therefore the onset of premature labor is both physiologically and psychologically unexpected. Premature birth is a crisis and an emergency situation characterized by an increased concern for the survival of the infant and often the mother. Premature labor and birth are accompanied by feelings of helplessness, isolation, failure, emptiness, and no control.[45,83] The negative and dangerous atmosphere surrounding the premature birth experience may influence the relationship with the premature infant, who may also be perceived as dangerous and negative.

Normal adaptations to pregnancy are abruptly terminated by the birth of a premature infant.[45] Prenatal fantasies about the infant and the new roles of mother and father are interrupted by a premature birth. This forces parents who are "not ready to not be pregnant" to grieve the loss of a term infant and imposes premature parenting on individuals not yet ready for the experience.

As discussed in Chapter 29, anticipatory grief is one of the normal psychologic tasks accompanying premature birth. Anticipatory grief may be decreased by early contact between parents and infant and conversely increased by separation of parents from preterm infants.[45] Prolonging anticipatory grief with failure to progress through the other tasks results in altered relationships with the parents if the preterm infant survives.

Deformed or Anomalied Infants

In approximately 2 of every 100 births,[45] an infant is born with a birth defect. Because society values physical beauty, intelligence, and success, the birth of a physically or mentally defective child is seen as a catastrophe in our culture.[87,94]

Recent medical advances now make it possible to identify potential fetal problems in utero. As parents receive the information antenatally, they begin the process of anticipatory grief. They experience feelings of shock, anger, guilt, and hope. At the birth of their infant, there usually is the confirmation of the anomaly, and parents must deal with the reality of the situation. Whether anticipated or not, however, the birth of a child with a congenital defect is accompanied by ambivalent feelings for all concerned (parents, relatives, friends, and profession-

als). The first reactions to the reality of the situation are feelings of disbelief and shock. Feelings of shame, revulsion, and embarrassment at creating a damaged and devalued child are common.[80] Guilt, self-blame, and a search for a cause or reason for the tragedy are intermixed with feelings of anger.

The severity of loss and feelings of disappointment heavily burden the parents, a burden they feel no one else has experienced.[45] Their loneliness and isolation may be intensified by their self-imposed withdrawal from others. Unlike the birth of a healthy infant, the birth of an anomalied or sick child is not celebrated by society with announcements, visits, and gifts from friends and family. The negative responses of society's representatives (family, friends, acquaintances, and professionals) may increase the parents' negative feelings for a defective child.[94]

The extent of the infant's anomaly cannot be used as a criterion for the degree of parental grief reaction,[50] although a gross, visible anomaly may elicit more emotional reaction than a hidden or more minor one.[45] A seemingly "minor" anomaly as defined by the professional may represent a severe impairment to individual parents. The professional, who has had more contact with infants with a wide range of anomalies, views the individual infant's anomaly in a different context than do the parents, who may have limited or no experience with a deformed child or adult. The professional also views the infant's defect from a less personal, more objective, and less narcissistic position than the new parents.

When the newborn is sick, the degree of mourning and parental feelings of grief and loss are not equated with the severity of the neonate's illness.[4] Even seemingly "minor" illnesses such as jaundice or respiratory difficulty requiring phototherapy or minimal oxygen supplementation are associated with parental concern for survival and feelings of grief and loss. These feelings are often not acknowledged by the parents or professional care providers because of the nonserious medical nature of the condition. In the mind of the care provider, self-limiting and treatable conditions are compared with more serious and often fatal neonatal illnesses. The care provider feels relieved about the "minor" nature of the neonate's condition and conveys this to the parents. "This is an easy condition to remedy. You don't have anything to worry about. The baby will go home in a few days."

Thus only the medical aspects of the newborn's illness are dealt with, whereas parental feelings remain unspoken and unresolved. In an altruistic attempt to reassure and comfort the family about the newborn's complete recovery, the professional unwittingly may discount the parents' real feelings. If the care provider is not concerned, parents may feel that they, too, should not be concerned and thus distrust and discount their own feelings.

Neonatal Deaths

The reactions accompanying neonatal illnesses are similar to the grief reactions experienced by parents whose infant dies.[4] Failure to acknowledge (even minor) neonatal illness as a loss situation and to work through the associated grief prevents parents from detaching from the image of the perfect child and taking on the sick newborn as a person to love. This may result in an aberrant parent-infant attachment. The liveborn infant who is critically ill or has a severe anomaly represents a "painful time of waiting"[8] for the family. They must deal with the uncertainty of whether their child will live and be healthy, live and continue to need extensive medical or special care, or die.

More deaths occur in the first 24 hours of life than in any other period of life. Yet death of a newborn is not the expected outcome of pregnancy. The majority of neonatal losses are caused by prematurity (80% to 90%) and congenital anomalies that are incompatible with life (15% to 20%). Regardless of the cause of death, even infants who live only a short time are mourned by their parents.[43] Prenatal attachment and investment of love in the newborn result in a classic grief reaction at the newborn's death.[46]

Even a short period of life between birth and death gives parents an opportunity to know their child. Completion of the attachment process enables parents to psychically begin the next process of detachment. Attachment to the child's reality encourages detachment from that reality, rather than from the parents' most dreaded fears and fantasies about their infant. Parental contact with the child before death enables them to share life for a brief time.

In the case of multiple births, when one child or more dies and the others live, parents simultaneously grieve the loss of the dead infant while attaching to the survivor. In many situations of multiple birth, the surviving infant (or infants) are in an intensive care nursery. The diametrically opposite feelings of love and attachment and grief and detachment, as well as the anxiety associated with the care and well-being of the surviving infant are emotionally draining for

new parents. The process of grief may slow the parents' ability to become intimately involved with their surviving infant(s).[91] They may have ambivalent feelings toward the infant(s) who survives or toward the infant(s) who dies. With the loss of one of a multiple birth, there is less support for the grieving parents, because the frequent response by everyone is that they should be thankful for the survival of one (or more) of their infants.

Generally, death of a newborn occurs despite everything done to prevent it. This provides parents with some measure of comfort in knowing "that we did everything that could have been done." Yet when the neonate is so severely ill or deformed that a decision about initiating or continuing life support is necessary, the parents have an extra burden. The situation may involve conflicts between physicians, nurses, and family wishes, causing significant personal anguish. As part of the federal Baby Doe regulations, most hospitals now have ethics committees that address the medical, legal, and ethical controversies (see Chapter 32). Regardless of who makes this decision, it is first and foremost the parents who will live with the ramifications of that decision. When parents are involved in the decision-making process, they wonder if theirs was the right decision regardless of what the decision is. If the child lives or dies, they wonder how a different decision would have changed their lives.

STAGES OF GRIEF

The experience of grief is a staged process that occurs over time. To detach both externally and internally from the lost loved object, emotional investment is withdrawn so that it may be invested in new love relationships.[55] Each stage of grief represents a psychologic defense mechanism used to help the individual to adapt slowly to the crisis. This slow adaptation is purposeful, because it prevents the individual psyche from being overwhelmed by the pain and anguish of loss.[57,64]

Although the stage of grief is recognizable, the process of grief is dynamic and fluid rather than static and rigid. Parents, families, and professionals progress cyclically through the stages of grief rather than in an orderly progression from beginning to end. However, each person experiences the process of grief uniquely and at an individual rate. Knowledge of each stage is necessary to assess where an individual family member, the family as a unit, and the staff are in their grief process. This information is then used to support individuals when they are in their particular stage of grief (rather than attempting to maneuver them from stage to stage), contributing to the defense, or stripping the individuals of their defenses. Regardless of the type of perinatal loss, the experience of that loss through staged grief work closely parallels the grief stages of Elisabeth Kübler-Ross.[49]

The feelings of *disbelief* and *rejection* of the news are reflected in the responses "No! This couldn't happen to me!" "It isn't true! They've made a mistake!" This immediate response protects the individual from the shocking reality of loss by postponing the full effect of reality until the psyche is able to handle it.[75] By holding on to the fantasy of a positive outcome (e.g., the loss of the heartbeat is only temporary or the dead infant belongs to someone else), facing the awful truth and the grief associated with it is delayed at least temporarily.[57,75,80]

The initial stage of grief is characterized by overwhelming feelings of being stunned and surprised—often seen as emotional numbness, flat affect, or immobility.[94] Emotional detachment is often expressed as an inability to cope or respond with activities of daily living, an inability to remember what others have said, and a tendency to repeat the same question.[26,45,49,57,94] For the tragedy to be handled in manageable pieces without overwhelming the individual, the mind may acknowledge the event only intellectually, and there is a corresponding lack of emotional reaction,[57,94] or the event may be compartmentalized so that only a part of the situation rather than the whole becomes the focal point of attention.

Anger is the result of a gradually developing awareness of the situation's reality. As the significance of their perinatal loss begins to dawn on them, parents (and significant others) experience the diffuse emotions of anxiety and anger.[45] With the full effect of their loss comes more focused feelings of bitterness, resentment, blame, rage, and envy of those with normal pregnancy outcomes.[49]

Social prohibitions against the expression of anger, especially for women, encourage this powerful emotion to be turned inward toward the self. Anger directed inward results in depression and a deepening sense of guilt. "Why?" "What did I do wrong or not do right to have caused this to happen?" are the hallmarks of the self-examination and self-blame that accompany perinatal loss.[45,57,94] Answers are often irrational and have no cause-and-effect relationship with the reality of the circumstances. Irrational, feared causes include sexual intercourse (common worry of both men and women), career (of the mother) outside the home, superstitions, dietary habits, or lifting of heavy objects.[96] Ideas of punishment (for past wrongs, for negative or ambivalent feelings, or for an unwanted pregnancy)[6,87] are often thought to be the reason for the failed outcome. The search for a reason to answer the question "Why me?" requires correct information to dispel unrealistic fantasies of causation. However, the question does not require a literal answer (often no concrete answer exists) but is merely a wish for a change in the situation.[6]

Anger directed outward is usually expressed as overt hostility to those in the immediate environment (family, children, care providers, and infant)[52,57,94] or toward God.[52,64] Fathers exhibit more anger than mothers.[32] Blame and anger may be a destructive force in the relationships among family members and prevent these relationships from being a source of comfort and support.[57] Venting of angry feelings toward professional care providers protects these family relationships for more positive interactions. Anger moves the grieving process along, but persistence of anger may prevent grief work from progressing to subsequent stages.

Bargaining may occur concomitantly with denial and shock as an attempt to prevent or at least delay the loss.[63,90] Bargaining usually occurs with whomever the parents (family or staff) believe the supreme being to be. The "Yes, but" of this stage is a form of "conditional acceptance," while still attempting to make the reality other than what it is.[6,49] With the defective child, bargaining may take the form of shopping for a physician or searching for the magic cure.[94]

The onset of depression and withdrawal marks the stage of a greater level of acceptance of the tragedy. With the true realization of the effect of the loss, the individual acknowledges that indeed there is a reason to be sad. The predominant feelings of this stage are overwhelming sorrow and sadness[57] evidenced by tearfulness, crying, and weeping.[75,80] Feelings of helplessness, worthlessness, and powerlessness contribute to the sense that life is empty and futile. Withdrawal may be evidenced by requests to be left alone, by decreased or complete cessation of visits to the infant, and by silence.[49,63] The degree of withdrawal may be indicative of the depth of depression and the extent to which there is guilt and self-blame.[75]

Acceptance is the resolution stage of the grief process that is heralded by resumption of usual daily activities and a noticeable decrease in preoccupation with the image of the lost infant.[55] This stage most often is not witnessed by the perinatal professionals. The acceptance stage is characterized by emotional detachment of life's meaning from the lost relationship and reestablishing it independent of the lost object.[49,56] The lost relationship is seen in a new light—as giving meaning to the present.[56] The aggrieved person relinquishes that part of himself or herself that was defined in the lost relationship and establishes a new identity that is emotionally free to attach in another relationship.

For the family of a deformed child, acceptance is not an all-or-nothing proposition, but rather a daily adaptation and coping with the child and the defect.[79] For the family, periods of frustration and sorrow alternate with periods of delight and enjoyment of the child.[52] Because of the chronic sorrow experienced throughout the life of a defective child, the final stage of resolution of the family's grief is only possible after the child's death.[62,94]

The acceptance stage represents the ability to remember both the joys and sorrows of the lost relationship without undue discomfort.[26] With gradual integration of the loss, there are progressively fewer attacks of acute, all-consuming pain.[56] When recalling the lost infant, there are fewer feelings of devastation and more a feeling of sadness. The ability to "celebrate the loss" also identifies grief resolution. Celebration of the loss does not mean recall without sadness and sorrow but with an ability to find some meaning, some good, and some positive aspects in the situation (e.g., "At least we had our child for a time, even though it was a short time").

SYMPTOMS OF GRIEF

Although each person copes with grief in individual ways, there are expected reactions to loss situations. Knowledge of the differences and commonalities of the grief experience enables care providers to understand their own reactions as well as to share their thoughts and feelings with the grieving family. The professional care provider must learn to "hear" what the family says about how and where each member is in the process of grief resolution. Often the "message" is not a direct reference to the loss or one's feelings, but rather nonverbal communication. The professional must learn to recognize that individuals often communicate more by what they do and what they omit than by what they say.

The signs and symptoms of acute grief have been well described and include both somatic and behavioral manifestations of the emotional experience of the loss (Box 30-2). The behavior of the bereaved is characterized as ambivalent.[56] In perinatal situations, parents simultaneously hope that the infant will live and wish for the infant to die; they want to love and care for the child while at the same time wish to reject the child.[45,52] These feelings are frightening and socially unacceptable, and therefore often remain unspoken.

Often the intensity of grief is greater when the relationship and feelings of the lost person are ambivalent.[56] Even with the most positive of pregnancy outcomes, taking a new infant into the family results in ambivalent feelings for all family members. The degree of disruption that a perinatal loss brings to the family is equated with the severity of grief, especially because reproduction and a healthy perinatal outcome are highly valued in our society.[56]

Male-Female Differences

Although members of both sexes have the same grief reactions, women express more symptoms (crying, sadness, anger, guilt, and use of medications)[18,19,58] than men. This difference in symptomatology does not represent a different experience of grief, but merely a different expression of it. Understanding these differences and the reasons for them are crucial for care providers working with parents at the time of perinatal loss.

The father's degree of investment in the pregnancy, impending parenthood, and the circumstances of birth all affect his feelings of loss. Because the father's body does not directly experience the changes of pregnancy, the pregnancy may initially be less of a reality to him than to the pregnant woman. This lag in the physiologic reality contributes to a lag in the psychologic investment of the father in the child. The father's lag in psychologic investment often contributes to incongruent grieving,[65] a difference in mother's and father's grief reactions. Fathers often comment that the infant became real when he felt the fetus move in the mother or at first sight of the new infant. Fathers who form an early attachment to the child feel sadness, disappointment, and often anger at being denied the expected son or daughter.[32,80] Conversely, fathers who have been normally ambivalent or overtly negative about the pregnancy may feel guilt and responsibility for the failed outcome.[80]

Box 30-2	**SIGNS AND SYMPTOMS OF GRIEF**

I. Somatic (physiologic)
  A. Gastrointestinal system
    1. Anorexia and weight loss
    2. Overeating
    3. Nausea or vomiting
    4. Abdominal pains or feelings of emptiness
    5. Diarrhea or constipation
  B. Respiratory system
    1. Sighing respiration
    2. Choking or coughing
    3. Shortness of breath
    4. Hyperventilation
  C. Cardiovascular system
    1. Cardiac palpitations or "fluttering" in chest
    2. "Heavy" feeling in chest
  D. Neuromuscular system
    1. Headaches
    2. Vertigo
    3. Syncope
    4. Brissaud's disease (tics)
    5. Muscular weakness or loss of strength
II. Behavioral (psychologic)
  A. Feelings of
    1. Guilt
    2. Sadness

    3. Anger and hostility
    4. Emptiness and apathy
    5. Helplessness
    6. Pain, desperation, and pessimism
    7. Shame
    8. Loneliness
  B. Preoccupation with image of the lost infant
    1. Daydreams and fantasies
    2. Nightmares
    3. Longing
  C. Disturbed interpersonal relationships
    1. Increased irritability and restlessness
    2. Decreased sexual interest and drive
    3. Withdrawal
  D. Crying
  E. Inability to return to normal activities
    1. Fatigue and exhaustion or aimless overactivity
    2. Insomnia or oversleeping
    3. Short attention span
    4. Slow speech, movement, and thought process
    5. Loss of concentration and motivation

*Modified from Lindemann E: Symptomatology and management of acute grief, *Am J Psychiatry* 101:144, 1944; Marris P: *Loss and change,* New York, 1974, PantheonBooks; and Colgrove M: *How to survive the loss of a love,* New York, 1976, Lion Publishing.

Participation of the father in the events of labor and birth also influences his attachment and ultimately his feelings of loss. Exclusion decreases his involvement in these life-crisis events, whereas inclusion has many advantages for the mother, infant, and self (see Chapter 29). If the infant is ill, the father may initially have more and closer contact than the mother.[4,63] In the birth place, the father may see, touch, or hold the infant before the mother. The father observes the initial resuscitation and stabilization and may accompany the infant to the nursery and on transport to a regional center. Often the father receives the first information and support[60] about the infant's condition and returns to the hospitalized mother with the news. This early, prolonged contact coupled with the father's increased responsibility often contributes to the development of a closer and earlier bond between father and child than between mother and child. The initial lag in prenatal investment may be offset after birth by concentrated contact between the father and child, so that a loss is highly significant to the father.

Societal expectations about masculinity and femininity markedly influence the expression of grief. Society's message to men starts early in life: "Big boys don't cry" and "Don't cry, you'll be a sissy" (i.e., girl). The preferred male image in our society is the autonomous, independent achiever who is always strong and in control, even in the face of disaster.[33] In keeping with this image, the father may feel that he must make all the decisions and have all information filtered through him to protect the mother. However, this altruistic gesture prevents full disclosure and involvement of the mother. Assuming the role of strong protector also involves a heavy price for the father in suppression of his own feelings and delay of his own grief work. The role of "tower of strength" often engenders feelings of resentment from the mother. Although he attempts to live up to his (and society's) expectations of himself, the woman views his lack of feelings and emotions, especially crying, as "He doesn't care."

Many men have difficulty dealing with irrational behaviors as well as with the normal ambiguity and conflict of life. This difficulty makes the emotional response of grief and its accompanying ambivalent feelings and conflicts produce discomfort and anxiety in many men. The expression of appropriate human emotions becomes threatening and makes them feel vulnerable. To decrease the anxiety associated with grief and its expression, men often deal with feelings by denying them, increasing their work load, or withdrawing from the situation and refusing to discuss it.

The father's attitude and ability to communicate about the loss may help or impede the mother's grief work.[75] Lack of communication between a couple may contribute to intense mourning, psychiatric disturbances, and severe family disruption.[17,43] Synchrony of grieving between the mother and father is important in an ultimate healthy resolution for the family.[15] If the father denies and suppresses his own feelings of loss and grief, he may react to the normal signs and symptoms of grief in his partner as if they were abnormal. Often the father is able to resolve his grief faster than the mother, and he may become impatient with her continual "dwelling" on the loss.[58] Sometimes fearing the woman's prolonged grief, the man decides to "spare her" from his feelings and does not discuss them with her. Instead of being comforting as intended, failure to share grief leads to isolation and alienation within the relationship.[45]

In some situations the man may experience intense emotions, not unlike those his partner experienced at the time of the crisis, several months after the death. Because these intense emotions occur so long after the crisis, he may not even associate them with the death.[45]

TIMING OF GRIEF RESOLUTION

Parents

Emotional recovery from the pain of perinatal loss occurs with time. There is no complete agreement on the length of time necessary for the individual to resolve grief. Indeed, a specific timetable for mourning may be impossible to establish.[6,17] However, some general time frames are available for the duration of a normal grief reaction.

Acute grief reactions are the most intense during the first 4 to 6 weeks after the loss,[55,56,64] with some improvement noted 6 to 10 weeks later. Normal grief reactions may be expected to last from 6 months to 1 year[26,45,64] or 2 years.[56] Indeed, significant losses of a spouse or child may never be completely resolved.[57,88] "I'll never get over it."

One parameter for differentiating normal from pathologic grief has been the length of time for grief to be resolved. Grief work may still be categorized as normal even if it lasts longer than 1 year, especially if the person is working through unresolved grief from the past. Grief work is normally energy draining. Dealing with more than one grief or loss situation compounds the intensity of mourning and may prolong the grief reaction. Because perinatal loss represents more than the loss of the child (loss of the perfect child, loss of plans for the future, and loss of self-esteem),[51] feelings of sadness and depression may still be evident for a year or longer.[45,96]

Sorrow and grief may even last a lifetime. For families of defective children, "chronic sorrow"[27,39,62,83] is experienced as long as the child lives. These parents live with the constant reminder of what is not and what the child will never be and can never do. The grief of death is final—parents do the work and go on; chronic sorrow is grieving on a daily basis. Expecting the parents to "adjust to" or "accept" their child's defect without any elements of lingering sadness is unrealistic. Chronic sorrow is a justifiable reaction to the daily stresses and coping necessary when a child is defective. The final stage of grief resolution is only possible with the finality of the death of the child.

Even when grief has been resolved, anniversary grief reactions are normal. Renewal of sadness, crying, and normal grieving behaviors may be reactivated at certain times. These anniversary reactions may not be limited to the infant's date of death but may also be felt on the expected date of delivery, on the actual birthday, or when seeing an infant of the same age and sex as the lost child. Holidays may also reactivate grieving behaviors, especially those that bring together family and friends and recall memories of joy and happiness.

Staff

Those sharing a crisis (complication, illness, or death) often become closely attached, so that the loss is felt not only by the family but also by the professional care providers.[24,30] Repeatedly dealing with death and deformity increases the professional's exposure to personal feelings of grief and loss. This may be perceived either as a threat or a personal opportunity for growth.

The critical variable in the ability to face or assist others in handling loss is the manner in which the care providers have been able to resolve their own personal losses.[92,93] Unless the care providers are able to cope with personal feelings of loss and grief, they may not be able to give of the "self" to others. Care given without genuine involvement and responsiveness to the family's feelings does not facilitate and may actually impede the mourning process. Professionals who are able to deal honestly with their own feelings will be able to help others cope with theirs.

Helping parents deal with their grief may be difficult for professionals because of their attitudes and feelings about perinatal loss. For professionals trained to preserve life, loss of the best pregnancy outcome or death itself represents both a personal and professional failure.[45] When success is equated with life, the failure of death (or loss) is associated with feelings of guilt, anger, depression, and hostility.[57,84,96] Just when professionals are expected to be supportive and therapeutic, they may be overwhelmed with their own feelings. Professionally, the care providers may feel helpless when all efforts inevitably result in no change in the outcome.

The feelings and stages of grief experienced by the family are the same ones felt by the staff who are attached to the parents and their newborn. Many professionals working in perinatal care are of childbearing age, so that identifying with the parents and their plight is relatively easy. Because the sick, deformed, or dead infant could easily be that of the staff, they share with the parents the special stress of the loss of a child. The care provider often experiences the same fantasies of blame as the parents. "What did I do (or not do) to cause this?"

Repetitive contact with loss situations and death exposes the staff to recurring feelings of frustration, guilt, self-doubt, depression, anger, classic grief reactions, helplessness, sadness, hopelessness, loneliness, and relief.[24] Such uncomfortable feelings often lead to behaviors of avoidance and withdrawal as a means of self-protection.[17,30,31] Adequate medical care may be given, but psychologic care of the family may be neglected. The involved primary care providers may decrease their attachment to both parents and infant when an unfavorable outcome is

inevitable. Withdrawing emotional support and involvement may spare the professional but only adds to parental feelings of isolation, inadequacy, and worthlessness. Professionals who have risked family attachment and shared grief work may be more cautious in future involvements to protect themselves from the pain of loss.

Asynchrony and individual differences in handling grief reactions may also cause problems among the professional staff. Constant exposure to perinatal loss may desensitize some individuals until they are blasé or even callous about the crisis, whereas others have grief reactions that parallel the family's reaction. Some staff members may have reached the stage of acceptance, while others who are unable to let the infant go persist in the idea of a magical cure,[17] a characteristic of denial. The rationale of prolonging the child's life may in reality be prolonging death, and inevitably one needs to accept death's finality.

The staff cannot offer support to families experiencing loss unless they receive support in dealing with their own grief reactions. Those who receive support learn about their feelings and how to handle them and so have no need to displace their pain to others. The three most effective ways that NICU nurses have identified to manage their stress after a neonate's death are (1) discussion with co-workers, (2) supporting and comforting the grieving family, and (3) talking with their own families.[24] Various formats are available for meeting staff needs, such as mutual support of colleagues or group sessions involving peer counseling on a long-term or short-term basis.[24,45,59,92] Group meetings provide a vehicle for support and for sharing information and feelings among staff members.[24,30,45,92] Facilitated by an objective person with expertise in group process and the concepts of grief, the goal is to help the staff deal with their reactions so they will be better equipped to help the parents. Group sessions also serve to decrease stress, increase job satisfaction, and ultimately help prevent burnout. Staff members are encouraged to retain their humanity when an environment is created in which emotions are valued and their healthy expression facilitated, both at the time of loss and in its resolution.[42]

Sharing grief work with a family gives the care provider a chance for personal growth, to review past personal losses, and to evaluate the adequacy of their resolution. Helping others with loss or grief provides the professional with the opportunity to contemplate present and future losses, including one's own mortality. By working with those who have suffered a significant loss or death, a health care provider may gain a deeper perspective about life.

INTERVENTIONS

Those in a crisis feel an openness to help and assistance from others, so that those in the crisis emerge either stronger or weaker, depending on the help they receive.[10,71] This increased openness also makes those in a crisis more vulnerable to the reactions of others—to their facial expression, tone of voice, and choice of words. Helpful professional interventions provide psychologic assistance during a highly vulnerable period of personal development. The goal of intervention is to maintain the precrisis level of functioning and improve coping and problem-solving skills beyond the precrisis level (i.e., to facilitate personal growth). Effective intervention is characterized by helping grief work get started, by supporting those who are grieving adaptively, and by intervening with individuals who display maladaptive reactions.[15]

Nonhelpful Interventions

Caring for pregnant women and their infants is supposed to be a "happy" job. Birthing and caring for infants are supposed to be times of joy and celebration. Because no one expects death or loss to occur in maternity or nursery areas, when it does, both staff and families are shocked. To protect themselves from the reality of the situation or to "spare" the family, professionals may engage in interventions that do not help themselves or their patients.[35] Such interventions may be meant altruistically, but do not have the characteristics of effective intervention.

Maintaining the state of denial arrests grief work by preventing or delaying the acceptance of the reality of the loss situation. Progress toward resolution is not begun until the stage of disbelief is relinquished. Using drugs, not talking or crying about the loss, and using distraction all contribute to maladaptive reactions by maintaining the state of denial. The use of tranquilizers, sedatives, and other drugs does not help the recipient, but rather the giver. Excessive use of these medications prolongs the denial stage by making the feelings and emotions foggy and dreamlike.[31,43,50] The energy needed to begin the grief work is dissipated by the effect of the medications. Avoiding the reality of the situa-

tion becomes easier when mind-altering drugs make the tragedy even more unbelievable.

Not talking about the loss is a powerful way of denying that it ever existed. The inability of professionals to acknowledge that the loss has occurred and that the family is in pain maintains denial and repression.[48,57,93] Not discussing the loss prevents parents from learning the facts and facing its reality. Because a fantasy will be created to substitute for the unknown, the fantasy of what happened and why will be worse than the reality. By receiving truthful, honest communication, parents are not left to spend energy dealing with frightening fantasies.

Professional avoidance and unwillingness to talk with parents after a loss communicates other powerful messages that impede grief work. If the loss is not important enough to discuss, then perhaps it is not important at all. Not talking about the loss serves to reduce it and communicates to the parents, "I don't care; therefore neither should you." Avoidance of the topic or a hurried, businesslike or social communication that skirts the issue tells the parent that grief work is dangerous, that grief emotions are dangerous, and that others are afraid of grief and those experiencing it. In essence, not discussing the loss gives a loud and clear nonverbal message to not grieve.

An inability to cry in response to a significant loss is not helpful and impedes grief work. The prohibition against crying may have been learned early in life or may be the result of unresolved grief work. Parents may feel the need to be strong for each other, their family, or the staff and thus do not cry. Sometimes role reversal occurs, so that the grieving person feels the need to support others rather than be the recipient of support. Often the significance of parental loss is neither recognized nor acknowledged by the professional for fear that "she or he will cry." Rather than talking about the loss as a technique to facilitate tears, no one says anything so no one will cry, and no one's grief progresses through the grief stages.

Distraction is another way of denying the loss or its significance. Professionals, a spouse, or other family members try to distract parents from the feelings and emotions of acute grief by engaging in light, social conversation or by keeping them busy with work or recreation. Dealing only with the physical care and not the need for psychologic care after birth is a form of distraction used by care providers.[35] Parents are preoccupied with their shattered expectations of the past and the stark reality of the present, and they are not interested in distractions.

After an unfavorable perinatal outcome, there is often confusion by the couple about their status: "Am I a mother or father . . . or not?" Failure to acknowledge the newly acquired role of mother or father (even if the fetus or newborn dies) discounts their psychologic investment in the pregnancy, fetus, and newborn. Quickly removing the infant from the maternity or nursery areas or removing all the baby items from the home negates the infant's existence.[45] This is not helpful for grief resolution and prevents parents from making choices and decisions and thus maintaining control over the reality of the situation.[40]

Isolation of the grieving family prevents the development of dependent relationships with others who might potentially provide support and comfort. Without others, parents are unable to share their grief and may thus increase their feelings of guilt, anger, blame, and lack of self-worth at their failed pregnancy. Those directly experiencing a perinatal loss may be isolated from the rest of society, including their families, who do not view loss of a pregnancy or neonate as significant.[8,45] Empathy with the parents' definition of the loss as important is necessary for society to be supportive. The goal of recent research, professional literature, and education has been to sensitize the care provider to the effect of perinatal loss. Only recently have books specifically about perinatal loss become available to give information and assistance to parents.

To decrease contact with the grieving mother, the staff may neglect her or perform cursory physical care, or there may be overconcern for providing physical care.[57] Assigning a room at the end of the hall, not going into the room, delay in answering requests, or placing the mother on another floor are ways of avoiding families. Use of private rooms and room assignments off the maternity floor may be helpful but may be used by staff to remove the unpleasant and uncomfortable situation. Early discharge to a supportive environment may be helpful, but without plans for follow-up may merely be a way to remove the constant, painful reminder.

Keeping the childbearing couple together throughout the perinatal events facilitates a shared experience of the reality of the situation.[48,93] Separation of the mother and father or of the couple from friends, family, and other children is not helpful. Exclusion of family members from the experience also excludes them from providing support for the mother and the couple. Relaxed visiting policies and as much contact as possible between the hospitalized mother and father (and other family members) are important.[93]

Prohibiting contact between the parents and the infant allows for fearful fantasies of the truth that are always more frightening than the reality of the situation. Delayed contact prolongs the state of disbelief and denial.[15] Restrictive visiting policies in the nursery, institutionalizing an infant without looking at all alternatives, or any other policy that separates parents from their infant, does not facilitate grief. Especially in the case of a deformed, stillborn, or dead infant, the message of delayed or no contact is that the infant is too horrible and too unacceptable to be seen or touched. Because parental egos are so symbiotically attached to their offspring, an unacceptable child is equated with an unacceptable and unworthy self. The fantasy that the damaged or dead child is representative of the damaged and defective self is borne out in the behavior and separation policies of the care providers.

In an attempt to offer the grieving family comfort, friends, relatives, and even professionals often make comments that are nonsupportive and nonhelpful[41,45,84]:

"Well, you're young. You can have more babies."

"Just have another baby right away."

"Well, at least you have others at home."

"It's better to lose her now when she's a baby than when she's 4 years old."

"He never would have been totally normal anyway."

"He was born dead. You didn't get a chance to know or get attached to him anyway."

"It's God's will."

Cliches and platitudes such as these do not help because of the message they give about the parents and the infant.[59,75] These comments at best reduce and at worst negate the effect of prenatal attachment to the fetus. The importance of psychologic investment and attachment by the parents to this fetus or newborn is said to be basically unimportant and essentially nonexistent.[45] Because infants are viewed as an extension of the parents' self, "by a not very subtle process of identification, the parents see a part of themselves in the baby, and nobody likes to be told that part of them is better off dead."[75] Also, comforting parents whose infant has died with the information that the child was not perfect and never would have been normal and healthy reinforces their belief that they are as defective and unsatisfactory as their dead child.[45]

Such comments also convey a message about the importance of an individual life.[48] Essentially, they say that one fetus or newborn is fairly interchangeable with another. They negate the importance of and indeed the existence of the infant for the parents, siblings, family, and society. The life of the individual is devalued, because he or she is easily replaced by "another baby." Comparing one infant's illness or deformity with another's is not helpful for parents whose own infant's deformity is certainly more important than any other infant's problem.[59]

The power of words to help during grief is outweighed only by their power to not help. Because parents are increasingly open during a perinatal crisis, they are sensitive not only to what is said and how it is said but also to the nonverbal message. Giving premature or false reassurance may be more for relief of the professionals than for the parents.[10,41,59] Comments such as "It's okay" and "Everything's going to be all right" must be genuine and timed appropriately for the parent. Telling parents that they have a child with Down syndrome and then saying, "But everything will be all right" is hardly helpful. Giving reassurance that subsequent pregnancies and infants will be all right or unaffected is not helpful before the parents are ready to think about and project into the future.

The basic terminology accompanying perinatal grief situations may be upsetting to parents. Instead of "dead," professionals substitute less frightening and less final words. The use of "loss" when "death" is appropriate may be misinterpreted (especially by children). The terms "lose, loss, and lost" connote misplacing, so that comments such as "I'm sorry you lost your baby" may be responded to by "I didn't lose (misplace) my baby. My child died." Medical professionals skirt the use of the words "dead, died, and die." Care providers are taught as students to use the word "expired" when referring to a patient who has died. Meant to soften the effect of "dead," the word "expired" may have its own effect, as a mother whose infant son died wrote in a poem: "The baby expired they said, as if you were a credit card."[85]

Other situations that do not facilitate grief work include dealing with multiple losses or stresses and ambivalence or mental illness.[96] The reaction to the loss of a significant relationship is intensified in the context of multiple losses, stresses, and problems.[5,96] Because perinatal losses represent not only a loss of the wished-for perfect child, but a threat to the parental self, self-concept, and self-worth, they represent situations of multiple loss.

Helpful Interventions

Professionals have an opportunity to make a significant difference in the outcome after the crisis of perinatal loss for the individual, the couple, and the family. A care provider who is knowledgeable about the grief process and comfortable in sharing another's grief is equipped to assist the family and its members toward a long-term healthy adjustment rather than a dysfunctional and pathologic one. Interventions that are helpful for family members also assist staff members in their own grief work.

Factors that influence an individual's personal experience of grief (and ultimately appropriate interventions) are outlined in Box 30-3. Care for the grieving is individualized through assessing these factors, planning, and continually evaluating the individual. Eliciting such personal information may not be as difficult as it first seems. Those in crisis often spontaneously share crucial data with little prompting. The importance of active listening to questions and comments or a more formalized therapeutic interview process may provide the needed encouragement and permission to begin communication.

A history of previous losses and their type and timing in the life cycle are important data for the care provider dealing with the current loss. Past experiences with a crisis or loss influence an individual's behavioral and coping style with current problems. Experiencing a previous perinatal loss affects a subsequent pregnancy.[2,16,73] These pregnancies are characterized by guarded emotions, marking the progress of the pregnancy and seeking out or avoiding various behaviors.[16] A previous perinatal loss may compound the individual's reaction to a current loss. Dealing with problems alone, with help and support from others, or withdrawing altogether are possible ways of coping with the loss.

The degree of attachment and the meaning of the pregnancy and impending parenthood to the family define expectations and influence reactions if an optimal outcome does not occur. The experience of grief depends on whether the loss situation was sudden and unexpected or if there was forewarning about a problem or complication. The definition and meaning of the crisis (i.e., the nature and severity of a deformity, the finality of death, or the chronic sorrow of a defective infant) reflect the individual's and family's value system and previous crisis experience. The process of grief is affected by the event itself, the previous and current coping mechanisms, and the family's definition of the event.[38] Consideration of all these factors is crucial in instituting appropriate intervention.

Box 30-3	FACTORS TO EVALUATE IN INDIVIDUALIZING GRIEF INTERVENTIONS

I. Previous losses
   A. Type
      1. Separation
      2. Divorce
      3. Death
      4. Spontaneous abortion (miscarriage)
      5. Elective or selective abortion
      6. Period of infertility
      7. Relinquishment of child
      8. Perinatal loss
   B. Timing in the life cycle
      1. Distant
      2. Recent
   C. Coping styles (of each individual and the family as a unit)
   D. Grief work
      1. Resolved
      2. Unresolved
II. Prenatal attachment
   A. Degree of psychologic investment in relationship with fetus or newborn
   B. Decision making about pregnancy and infant
      1. Planned or unplanned
      2. Wanted or unwanted
   C. Meaning of pregnancy and infant to individual and family
   D. Parental expectation about child-bearing

III. Nature of the current loss
   A. Timing
      1. Sudden and expected
      2. Anticipatory grief
   B. Definition and meaning of the event (death, deformity) to individual members of the family
   C. Multiple losses
      1. Self
      2. Perfect child
   D. Nature and severity
      1. Of loss
      2. Of defect
IV. Cultural influences
   A. On experience and the expression of grief
   B. Societal expectations dictate acceptable and unacceptable behaviors of mourning
V. Strengths (individual and family)
   A. Support system (family, friends, religious, community, or social agencies) mobilized when necessary
   B. Stable relationships—couple supportive of each other
   C. Financial stability
   D. Coping abilities—can evaluate, plan, and adjust to novel situations
   E. Good health
   F. Receptive and intelligent
   G. Realistic expectations about childbearing and child rearing

Cultural practices among families and professionals may sometimes differ. For example, in some cultures, it may not be acceptable to see or hold your baby (as in some Native American cultures). In the Muslim culture, the family is the primary system of support, and it is rare to see a Muslim family emote publicly.[37] It is critical for health care practitioners to recognize cultural and religious differences to minimize misinterpretations and conflicts with families. With increasing immigration, practitioners must be able to respond with a more ethnic-sensitive approach.[37] It is essential to be creative and flexible thus respecting families' cultural and religious belief systems.[61]

The national association SHARE: Pregnancy and Infant Loss Support has revised the Rights of Parents When a Baby Dies and Rights of the Baby (Box 30-4). These documents serve as (1) guidelines for creation of protocols, checklists, and bereavement programs,[74] (2) affirmation and empowering tools for bereaved parents, and (3) communication points for parents and care providers initiating the grief process.[69]

Environment

The first step in facilitating grief work is to create an environment that is supportive, permissive, and conducive to the expression of feelings. This type of environment does not depend on physical surroundings but rather is created and maintained by a warm, receptive, accepting, and caring staff. Such an environment centers its concern more on the people giving and receiving care than on the tasks of care.[45] This type of environment is nonjudgmental and is characterized by an attitude of openness and freedom.[75] People feel safe enough to ventilate a full range of feelings—sadness, anger, despair, and even humor—without the fear of condemnation or rejection. The staff become role models of open communication, facing grief and feeling comfortable in an uncomfortable situation. The safety of such an environment generates feelings of acceptance and understanding so that grieving and healing may proceed.

Professional presence and support is essential to families in crisis because of the increased dependency needs that accompany grief and loss. Yet certain

Box 30-4	RIGHTS OF PARENTS AND INFANT WHEN AN INFANT DIES

Rights of Parents

1. To be given the opportunity to see, hold, and touch their baby at any time before and/or after death, within reason
2. To have photographs of their baby taken and made available to the parents or held in security until the parents want to see them
3. To be given as many mementos as possible (i.e., crib card, baby beads or bracelet, ultrasound and/or other photographs, lock of hair, feet and hand prints, and record of weight and length)
4. To name their child and bond with him or her
5. To observe cultural and religious practices
6. To be cared for by an empathetic staff who will respect their feelings, thoughts, beliefs, and individual requests
7. To be with each other throughout hospitalization as much as possible
8. To be given time alone with their baby, allowing for individual needs
9. To be informed about the grieving process
10. To request an autopsy; in the case of a miscarriage, to request to have or not have an autopsy or pathology examination as determined by applicable law
11. To plan a farewell ritual, burial, or cremation in compliance with local and state regulations and according to their personal beliefs, religion, or cultural tradition
12. To be provided information on support resources that assist in the healing process (i.e., support groups, counseling, reading material, and perinatal loss newsletters)

Rights of the Infant

1. To be recognized as a person who was born and died
2. To be named
3. To be seen, touched, and held by the family
4. To have life-ending acknowledged
5. To be put to rest with dignity

From SHARE: Pregnancy and infant loss support, St. Joseph's Health Center, St. Charles, Mo, 1995.

that you can be alone with your baby?" offers both support and privacy. Many parents later regret not having time alone and not thinking to ask to be alone with their infant.

A quiet place away from the hustle and bustle of the routine may facilitate both attachment and detachment. The mother of a stillborn child who is quickly shown her infant in the delivery room as her episiotomy is being repaired is not in an optimal physical (or psychologic) environment. Attaching to and saying good-bye to her infant is better accomplished in a quieter and more private setting with significant others present. Active participation of parents at the death of their newborn may not optimally occur in a busy intensive care unit. Rather, adaptation of hospice concepts to neonatal care provides a private, homelike room and more palliative care than cure to the dying newborn and the family.[90] In very rare situations (e.g., chromosomal anomalies), parents and professionals may opt to provide end-of-life care ideally with hospice care at home.

Supportive, Trusting Relationships

A relationship with a caring individual who offers consistency and support is the foundation of a therapeutic environment. During periods of crisis, when there is a temporary increase in dependency needs and feelings of loneliness, it is an adaptive behavior to seek emotional support from family, friends, and professionals.[56,57,60] Even the crisis of normal childbearing prompts many cultures to provide a "doula"[72] to teach the new mother and give her emotional support. For a mourning family, the relationships established with helpful professionals are more important than the physical care given.[30]

Support, "sharing one's ego strength with another in a time of need,"[34] is particularly helpful in perinatal loss because of the threat to self-concept and self-esteem suffered by parents. Support may be as simple as remaining with the parents. "Being there" indicates not merely physical presence, but an emotional availability and willingness to share their experience of loss. Often professionals, family, and friends are hampered by "not knowing what to say." Usually words are initially unnecessary or do not adequately describe the moment, and silent presence may better convey the message. Often it is not what is said but the mere presence of loving others that conveys empathy and support to parents and colleagues. Yet presence is not enough; meaningful interaction between parents and professionals is also necessary for a trusting relationship to develop.

aspects of a conducive environment such as privacy, quiet, and comfort may be difficult to obtain in a noisy and busy perinatal setting. The recommendation to never leave the family alone must be balanced with their need for privacy and personal time alone with their infant (stillborn, ill, or dying).[93] Simply saying, "I will stay with you unless you ask me to leave so that you can have some private time alone with your child" or "Would you like me to leave for a while so

The initial meeting with the professionals, including verbal and nonverbal cues, leaves a lasting impression on the family. Addressing family members by name personalizes the encounter, and a brief touch or handshake represents an extension of self, a gesture of warmth, concern, and acceptance from professional to parents. An introduction that includes a brief explanation of the professional's role in relation to them and their infant helps to orient them: "Good morning, Mr. and Mrs. Black. I'm Sue, your baby's primary nurse. That means that I will be caring for Jason while he is here and working with you." Orientation to the physical surroundings and technical equipment eases the transition to an unfamiliar and often intimidating hospital environment. Providing physical comfort such as rocking chairs, privacy for interaction, and sleeping facilities for parents demonstrates the philosophy of the parents' worth and importance to their infant.

Empathy, an emotional understanding and identification with the plight of another, characterizes a helping relationship. In such a relationship, "How are you?" is asked with the emphasis on you and a genuine interest in the answer—unlike a social inquiry in which an automatic "Fine" is expected. Recognition of verbal and nonverbal cues of parental feelings (e.g., "You look tired" and "I hear that you are frustrated") communicates that these emotions are legitimate, understood, and accepted. A willingness to help, listen, console, and give encouragement and positive feedback establishes the professional as a sensitive, responsive person whom parents will trust. Supporting any and all parental involvement, supporting damaged parental egos, and helping parents to succeed in the tasks of attachment and detachment are goals of effective intervention.

The tone of in-hospital perinatal settings is often determined by the nursing staff. Generally, residents, interns, and specialists remain for short periods, and the private physician or permanent medical staff are not available on a minute-to-minute basis. Development of a safe, trusting environment depends on viewing parents as essential and not as visitors or "disruptors" of the ward routine.[35] Pleasant and relaxed surroundings convey the message of hospitality and "You are welcome here."

Both professional and nonprofessional support systems are available in the crisis of perinatal loss. Yet relating to many people during crisis is difficult for parents. Primary care (both medical and nursing) provides the same care provider for both the physiologic and psychologic care of the infant and the family. Thus the family is able to relate to as few professionals as possible. This special caring reassures parents that a few special people love, know, and are invested in their infant. Primary care providers share with the parents the joys of even small gains and the sorrows and tears of complications or death. Professionals and parents benefit from primary care systems in the emotional and psychologic satisfaction of such involvement. Yet this involvement is not without a price of vulnerability to an individual's feelings of loss and grief. Peer support on an individual basis or in a group setting is essential in dealing with the stress of continual attachment and loss.[24]

Normal grief reactions may be facilitated by nursing and medical professionals using others (social workers or counselors) when necessary.[4] Collaboration and consultation with these professionals help the staff gain insight into parental and personal behaviors and appropriate intervention strategies. The staff may also benefit from the expertise of a trained counselor in dealing with their own feelings of loss and grief.[46]

Pathologic Grief

Maladaptive responses to perinatal loss are indications for referral for specialized care.[94] The following may be indicators of a pathologic grief state[55]:

- Overactivity without a sense of loss
- Acquisition of symptoms belonging to the last illness of the deceased
- Psychosomatic conditions
- Altered relationships to friends and relatives
- Furious hostility against specific others
- Formal manner resembling schizophrenia
- Lasting loss of social interaction patterns
- Assuming activities detrimental to social and economic existence
- Agitated depression

Involvement of clergy and religious organizations is often comforting and supportive to the family.[9] Religious rituals (i.e., baptism, prayer service, or anointing) may be advocated by certain denominations and provide a measure of comfort and hope. Often parents in crisis do not think to request infant baptism or calling their priest, minister, or rabbi. Offering to call a clergy member of their choice or the hospital chaplain may be helpful.[9,12] Primary care providers who have shared intimately with the parents the experience of their child's life and death may be invited to attend the funeral or memorial service. For both care providers and parents, this may represent the final act of caring for the infant.[24]

Nonprofessional support systems such as the couple, family, friends, and parent groups are often forgotten as sources of potential help to grieving parents. In our society of isolated, mobile, nuclear families, it may be erroneous to assume that a support system exists. On the other hand, it may be unrecognized because it does not fall into a traditional definition, such as the next-door neighbor or other friend who may be more supportive (and available) than the grandparents. Biologic kinship is not the only valid criterion for a support system; an emotional kinship is the most important factor.

Because professional availability and involvement with the parents is not lasting, the professional has a responsibility to identify, foster, and facilitate a nonprofessional (social) support system. Simply identifying supportive others and expecting them to automatically help in a perinatal loss situation may not be realistic. Unless those who constitute the support system are as well informed and instructed as the parents about the situation, they will not be able to offer emotional comfort. For example, if the parents wish to talk about their loss but the support system empathically wishes to spare them by not discussing it, no help will be given or received.

The quality and quantity of ties one has with a social network is associated with improved health status and life satisfaction.[36] For parents experiencing a perinatal loss, the quality and quantity of ties with their social network (i.e., extended family, friends, and colleagues) may be profoundly affected. In one study, most families suffered permanent loss of relationships because others were unsure of how to react, avoided talking about the baby or made comments that diminished the intensity of the loss.[23] Fathers especially receive little personal attention as friends and colleagues focus their attention on the mother's grief.[23] Because grandparents grieve for their grandchild, and may feel guilt and grief for their own child,[22] they may be emotionally unavailable to support the grieving parents. To prevent social network disruption for grieving families, health care providers can (1) share information with families about reactions to expect and reasons for these reactions, (2) support families and enable them to rebuild their networks, and (3) emphasize and support the family's belief in their strengths and capacities.[23]

Open communication between the parents is essential in preserving and fostering a close relationship by the giving and receiving of mutual support.

Sharing the experience presents the couple with the opportunity for personal growth and growth as a couple. Yet the individual experience of grief within the context of a couple is all too often fertile ground for misunderstanding and resentment. One study showed that disruption of a couple's sexual relationship occurred after the death of a child.[78]

Parental support groups offer their members an opportunity to discuss their feelings with others who have been through similar traumas. Knowing how others who have experienced perinatal loss have felt and dealt with similar situations is emotionally comforting and stabilizing to parents experiencing their own loss. Parents provide each other with validation for their feelings and a sense that they are not alone in their pain.

Each individual has different needs, different ways of adapting to crisis, and different ways of giving and receiving support. It is essential that professionals use techniques that are real and spontaneous and not adopt words or actions that are foreign to one's own self. Interventions must also be gauged to the parents' needs and pace.

In one study[88] and from clinical experience, fathers state that they receive most of their support from their spouse. They report that little attention is paid to fathers by hospital staff, causing more denial and difficulty expressing their grief. It is critical for hospital staff to address father's feelings when addressing parental grief. Suggestions to assist fathers in their grief include implementation of all-male support groups, validation of their feelings, and asking direct open-ended questions. These may include "What are you feeling right now?" "Tell me how your day is going?" and "Tell me about your coping strategies." Health care providers can help fathers by reflecting his statements, using his name, and assisting him with expressing his feelings. Fathers need to be included and acknowledged in all discussions with staff.[89]

Information

Information aids in intellectually understanding the crisis, thus facilitating a sense of control over it. Actively seeking and using information enables confrontation and mastery of the crisis. Knowledge about a situation strengthens the ego, because it enables "worry work" and psychologic preparation for expected events. Because "the void of the unknown is more frightening than the known; facts are more reassuring than awesome speculations,"[10] a major role of the professional is to provide and clarify facts and information relevant to the perinatal loss situation. In the search for meaning that always accompanies loss, medical facts may help alleviate some parental guilt about causing the tragedy. Repeating to the parents that "Nothing you did or did not do could have caused this problem" is reassuring. Sketchy or no information only serves to contribute to parental denial of the reality or to their fantasies of causation.[59,75] Confronting the crisis and realizing its real element of danger and trouble starts the process of grief by giving permission for the expression of feelings of fear, sadness, and loss.

Because the family as a unit, composed of each individual member, must deal with perinatal loss, it is important to encourage and support open, interfamily communications. Keeping secrets, especially between the parents, should be discouraged because this eventually undermines trust and promotes asynchronous grief work. When parents are given the same information and talk with each other about their loss and their feelings, more synchronous grief reactions develop.[45,59] Telling parents together with the infant present prevents misunderstanding, misinterpretations, and "shading" of information to one parent.[45] Informed parents are better able to share their experience with each other and to participate in joint decision making with the professional.

The question often arises, "When to tell?" and "How much to tell?" the parents. Parents should be told as soon as possible about perinatal complications or problems.[45,59] Receiving this information at the earliest possible time helps parents establish trust in the care provider, appreciate the reality of the situation, begin the grief process, and mobilize both internal and external support. Information must be given in its entirety, because attempts "to spare" parents by staging the truth only serve to undermine their trust in professional credibility. The couple's relationship may also suffer if one parent colludes with the professional in a conspiracy of silence. This is best illustrated by the following incident:

> To spare a diabetic mother from the truth about her infant's congenitally absent limbs, the physician and father decided to tell her about his missing legs, but not the missing arm. On arriving to transport the baby, the nurse asked if the mother had been told. "Yes" was the response, so she took the infant to the mother's room before transport. As she uncovered the infant, the mother gasped and looked at the physician and father and said, "You lied to me. You didn't tell me about his arm, too."

When given the unedited truth, parents are able to face reality and begin the grief process without fear that "something else is the matter that they aren't telling me about."

The individual's stage of grief influences not when or what will be said, but how the information will be given and received. During the initial stage of shock, information—if processed—is processed slowly.[45] Often events take on a foggy, dreamlike quality so that sensory information remembered is not believed. Yet to give no information only perpetuates this frightening feeling. Communication to those in shock and denial must proceed simply, slowly, and with much repetition and reinforcement. Giving information once does not ensure that it will be either retained or understood. Repetition by the professionals is necessary for gradual acceptance of the reality of the situation. This may be a nuisance for the professional who "has already told her that. Why can't she remember it?" Parents are so shocked they do not hear what is said and information must be patiently repeated.

Even though an early contact with parents almost ensures they will be in a state of shock, the tone and content of the first meeting is not forgotten.[45] Initial information about the infant and his or her condition may have long-term effects on the parents' ability to attach or detach. In the past, parents were given a pessimistic outlook with the belief that "It will be easier for them. They won't get so involved." Negative descriptions and initial pessimism only increase the amount of grief and detachment while effectively blocking attachment behaviors. Should the sick or defective infant survive, the parents may have detached to the point of at least emotionally burying the infant. Knowledge of better survival rates and the quality of survival enables a truthfully optimistic outcome for many sick neonates. Therefore information must be given clearly (not medical jargon) with a minimum focus on possible complications and medical odds.[45,94]

Volunteering information to parents is essential, but encouraging their questions is equally important. As the normal mechanism for adapting to crisis and gaining mastery over a situation, questions help the professional "to start where the parents are" and to begin communication with their concerns. Questions and comments unrelated to the discussion may indicate either failure to comprehend or failure to send the information clearly.[94]

Direct questions deserve direct answers, because they indicate a readiness and desire for information. Indirect questions or comments by the parents may indicate concern about their own infant that cannot be directly expressed. "Baby Stevie (who died yesterday) had severe respiratory distress syndrome, didn't he?" The parents want to be reassured that their infant is not going to die, too.

During the crisis of perinatal loss, interpersonal communication is difficult. Therefore it is important that as few professionals as possible relay information to the parents. Primary care providers (nurse and physician) should coordinate and provide continuity in giving information to parents because individual care providers will supply information about the same topic in different ways. The use of varied terms, inflections, and attitudes by a multitude of professionals becomes a monumental source of confusion and anxiety for parents. A trusted relationship with a primary nurse and physician through whom all communication flows minimizes unnecessary anxiety and concern for parents.

It is absolutely essential that the nurse (or primary nurse) be present and assist the physician in communication with the parents. Any anxiety-producing information (poor prognosis, complication, or impending death) may not be heard or understood initially by the parents. The nurse must know exactly what information was given and how the parents were given this information. After the physician departs, the nurse must be able to offer clarification, explanation, and support to the distraught parents. Nothing is more distressing than finding a crying, upset mother who is unable to relate what the physician said, why she is upset, or even if she understood what was said.

No family or parent should have to wonder and worry about a dreaded or feared outcome without being given the proper information. If the primary care physician is unavailable to speak with the family, then someone from the health care team must assume this responsibility. No mother whose infant is ill, deformed, or dead should awaken from an anesthetized birth to find her physician absent and the nurses unable to answer "How's my baby?" A plan of action for telling individual parents must be decided and agreed on by all care providers.

Parents are interested in the daily (or hourly) progress of their infant, including both positive and negative developments. A crisis or negative development in an infant's condition is important for parents to know about as soon as possible. They are then able to participate and care for their infant through the difficulty and to trust professional communication. Parents should have unlimited access to phone and/or personal contact with the staff in the perinatal care setting. Phone calls into the hospital from concerned parents should be possible any time of the day or night. The knowledge that information about their infant and access to a caring professional are available at any hour often is enough to comfort parents of a critically ill infant.

Encouraging Expression of Emotions

Because grief is an emotional reaction to loss, expression of these emotions is necessary for grief work to begin and proceed. Verbalizing thoughts and feelings provides an outlet for the intense emotions accompanying grief and signifies to others that emotional support is needed.[57] For some the open expression of emotions may be difficult because of influence from their culture, sex roles, and social status. Yet the containment of intense feelings uses a great deal of emotional and physical energy that could be more productively used in "moving on" with the grief work. Those who are stoic and noncommunicative have symptoms of grief for a longer period of time than those who freely express their feelings and emotions.[7]

Talking about the loss helps parents to validate and assimilate the experience. Timing and events are clarified, including forgotten details, by discussion with each other and with their care providers. Confronting the reality enables them to work through the shock and disbelief, verbalize their fears and disappointments, and begin to cry and grieve. Expression of feelings gradually permits a clarification of the meaning of the loss to the parents.[93] Talking lightens the burden of loss, because every time the experience is shared with another, half of the experience and the accompanying emotions are given away. Telling, retelling, reviewing, and reliving the experience are all necessary ways to understand and gain mastery over a frightening and most often unexpected situation.[52,63,80,84]

Verbal and nonverbal cues tell professionals "where the parents are" in their grief process. To elicit feelings, the professional may verbalize his or her own perceptions and observations:

"Mrs. Green, you sound tense (upset, tired) today."

"Mr. Brown, you look worried today."

"I'm sorry that your baby died."

These statements indicate the listening ear and observing eye of one who cares. They set the stage for communication: "It's okay to talk with me about how you are feeling, because I acknowledge your pain."

Feeling scared, alone, and out of control, parents often deny their feelings under direct questioning. Thus "Do you think you did or didn't do something to cause your baby's problem?" may be answered negatively, even though parents are consumed with guilt. Direct questioning places parents in an awk-ward and vulnerable position of revealing their most personal doubts and fears. Direct questions may be reworded with safer and more indirect statements:

"Most parents feel overwhelmed and sad when their baby is sick."

"Many parents wonder if the cause of their baby's death is something they did or didn't do."

"It is helpful to many parents to talk about their doubts and fears. These feelings are common and normal in such a difficult situation."

The professional gives parents information about the feelings and emotions commonly felt in similar situations. Because there is safety in numbers, if "most" or "many" parents feel this way and it is ex-pected, then it might be safe to share their feelings. Validating parents' reactions as appropriate reas-sures them that they are not crazy. With this type of invitation, the feelings may be free to come spilling forth or the parents may need time to establish a re-lationship with this professional before they are ready to talk about such personal emotions.

Empathetic actions and comments may open communication pathways with parents. A profes-sional presence that is warm and caring may facili-tate more communication than any words. Touching or holding grieving parents may help feelings be ex-pressed. Nonverbal cues such as nodding, direct eye contact, uninterrupted attention, and the physical closeness of pulling up a chair and sitting down gives positive feedback to verbal communication and indicates active listening by the professional.

Crying is the expression of feelings of sadness, sorrow, and intense longing that accompany the pain of loss.[55,96] A healthy catharsis, crying should be expected and encouraged in any loss situation. Yet the cultural, sexual, and professional taboo against crying has defined it as an unacceptable and inappropriate response, and one that should be sup-pressed. Because tears are healing and therapeutic, professionals must learn to be comfortable with the crying of others. "Don't cry" is often heard from those attempting to comfort grieving parents (or col-leagues). This is an admonition against the behavior rather than an empathetic comment. "It's okay to cry," or "Go ahead and cry—let it out" gives per-mission and acceptance to the behavior and the need for it.

By expecting tears, providing a safe environment for their expression, and encouraging the behavior by words and actions, the professional may facilitate crying in both mothers and fathers. All too often, tears are blocked in a relationship in which one part-ner (usually the man) is expected to be stoic and in control, while the other's (usually the woman's) tears are defined as too upsetting or difficult. Be-cause the ability to cry is a healthy response, the cou-ple must be encouraged to use this outlet together.

In the past, crying in the presence of patients and their families was defined as "unprofessional." Yet the cool, controlled exterior defined as "profes-sional" was seen by others as noncaring and non-feeling. When the professional cries with the par-ents, it is an acceptable expression of genuine emotion, a demonstration of empathy, and a role model of the appropriateness of tears given the sit-uation. Parents do not define the tears of care providers as weak or unprofessional. Rather, they feel a special bond of love and care with profes-sionals who have been free enough to share their grief. Instead of relearning that crying is acceptable, many parents and care providers must learn for the first time.

Talking and crying about the loss are easier to fa-cilitate than the expression of anger. Because of the social expectations of dependency of the patient role and real or imagined consequences of retaliation (against the infant or against job status), perinatal care settings are not safe environments for the ex-pression of anger. Parents (and colleagues) will only be able to vent anger in an environment free of pun-ishment or retaliation for their behaviors. It is the responsibility of the professionals to create an en-vironment that allows open expression of negative criticism and anger.

Seeing and Touching

Seeing and touching are as important to the parents of a sick, deformed, or dead infant as they are to the parents of a normal, healthy one. In the past, fear that seeing a deformed or dead infant would intensify grief and be overly upsetting resulted in no contact between parents and their newborn. Despite the fact that many mothers wished to see their infants, the prevailing practice was to discourage and prevent it. Often no information, including sex or physical characteristics, was given to grieving parents, who were left to fantasize about their newborn's prob-lems or cause of death. More recently, research and practice indicate that parental contact with the infant does not cause "unduly upsetting immediate reac-tions or appear to result in pathologic mourning."[43]

The decision to see and touch their infant is ulti-mately a parental one.[48,96] Making decisions *for* clients is not the professional's role; making deci-sions *with* clients is. Each parent must make the decision for himself or herself; neither may decide for the other. Altruistic others, such as professionals, spouse, or other family members, must not usurp the right to individual decision-making. Often, in an attempt to protect the mother, the father or professional decides that she should not have contact with her infant. They either actually discourage it or do nothing to facilitate it. Mothers who have not seen their infants always know who prohibited it. The couple's relationship may suffer irreparable damage if one decides for the other, even if the motive is altruistic. The professional's role is to facilitate a healthy decision by each parent so that their individual needs to see or not to see the infant are met.

Parents may not realize that seeing and touching their infant is an option,[93] or they may just be too overwhelmed or afraid to ask if it is possible. Instead of waiting for parents to ask, the professional care provider takes a more active role by offering the possibility to the parents: "Would you like to hold your baby?"

Time is often required to make the decision, because initially parents are ambivalent about seeing and holding a deformed or dead infant. Most mothers and fathers want to see their child, but fear what they might see and how they may feel.[80] The care provider may alleviate the parents' ambivalence by acknowledging that being with the infant will be difficult but that the professional will remain with them unless asked to leave. The emotional support of the physical presence of an empathetic professional may allay the fear of becoming out of control. The professional can reassure the family by explaining what they will see before they hold their infant. Making such a crucial decision in the initial stages of loss is difficult. Giving parents information about the positive aspects of seeing and holding the infant in facilitating their grief process helps make their decision an informed one.[12,96]

Seeing the infant brings the dreaded impossibility of perinatal loss into stark reality.[59,96] Parents confirm with their own eyes that the infant is alive or dead, or normal or abnormal. Contact enables claiming behaviors and identification of the infant as their own. While holding their infant, parents examine it and begin to recognize familiar family characteristics: "She has my long fingers and her father's red hair." Even small, severely deformed, or macerated infants are able to be recognized and claimed by the parents as part of their family.[48] The normal, endearing characteristics that identify the child as "mine" are remembered.

Parental contact confirms the infant's own reality and eliminates the prenatal fantasy of the expected child. For the parents of infant with an anomaly, grief work about the fantasized perfect child may begin, so that the actual child may become the object of love. Early and frequent contact between the parents and the infant encourages a realistic perspective of the infant's problems. A stillborn or aborted fetus may be physically normal rather than the deformed infant imagined by the parents. Seeing the infant allays doubts and fears about the infant's normal state and about the parents' ability to subsequently have a normal child.[53,54,75] Seeing and touching enables parents to grieve the infant's reality rather than a feared and dreaded, thus more frightening, fantasy. It is easier to grieve a real infant than a mystical dreamlike fantasy of the infant.[45,48,53,54]

Whether the ultimate decision is to see or not see the infant, the professional must honor and respect that choice.[96] Cultural taboos against viewing dead bodies may preclude some parents from seeing and touching their infant. Yet many such cultures support their members by formalizing the grief process in sanctioned ritual and ceremony. For those parents who decide not to see and touch, it is important for the professional to reassure them of their infant's normal condition (e.g., "He had 10 fingers and toes"). Describe the infant in as much detail as necessary to give parents a mental picture. Include sex, size, hair color, skin, weight, and distinguishing characteristics. A simple, realistic description of any anomaly is also helpful, because the fantasy of the defect is worse than its reality.

Adequate preparation for the first encounter with their infant includes a description of everything parents will see, hear, and feel.[48,96] Verbal preparation for viewing an infant with a congenital anomaly includes not only a simple description of the abnormality, but also the infant's normal characteristics. Seeing a picture of the abnormality first may help parents prepare for seeing their infant. Remaining with the parents at the initial visit, the professional describes the anomaly and points out normal findings. Focusing by parents on the normal familial characteristics helps in attaching to the less-than-perfect child. Although parents of a dead, deformed child view the abnormality, they often focus on the normal traits and remember the infant not as "monstrous" but as beautiful.

For those who have never seen a dead body, the mind may invent frightening images and sensations. Certainly, "dead" is associated with the temperature sensation of cold. However, a newborn who has been placed under a radiant warmer or in an incubator may feel warm rather than cold shortly after death. Hence the statement by a mother, "You couldn't be dead. You feel so warm." The professional must touch the infant and prepare the parents for the tactile sensation of warm or cold: "The baby will feel warm to you because she (or he) has been under the radiant warmer."

To prepare parents for seeing their infant, the professional must observe the child. Color, skin condition, and size must all be described: maceration, "peeling of the skin," peripheral shutdown, "the blue-white discoloration," and the small size, "as long as the length of my hand" are not shocking with adequate preparation. Any equipment that must remain on the body should be described and explained before viewing. Even an umbilical cord clamp may cause concern in a parent who has never seen one. The reason for not removing equipment must also be explained. Respectful care of the infant's body after death shows respect for the person of the infant and for the grieving parents. Attention to details such as wrapping the infant in a blanket rather than a surgical drape or towel, cleaning the infant, and holding the infant in a cuddling position indicate care and concern.

Parents whose infant has died, is deformed, or is ill proceed with attachment behaviors of seeing and touching in the same manner as parents of normal, healthy infants.[45,48] Touching is important, but the distinction must be made between touching and holding. Cradling one's infant is quite different from merely touching with a hand. Holding the infant, whether healthy, sick, or dead, for the first time is a momentous event. Touching the infant who has died is not sufficient; parents must be given the opportunity to hold and cuddle the child before, during, and after death. Other parenting behaviors, such as bathing and dressing their infant, should also be offered to parents.[12]

Parents of a dead infant may need more than one chance to see and touch the infant. The first time, they attach to the reality of their infant. Subsequent encounters allow a final chance to see and hold their child. Parents have described the initial encounter as saying "Hello" and the subsequent one as saying "Good-bye." Some parents may be able to accomplish closure with one visit, whereas others who might benefit from a final visit may not ask or think to ask. Offering another contact with their infant leaves the decision with the parents.

The emotional effect of seeing the infant requires support, time, and permission to cry. Attaching is a process that occurs over time. Providing parents sufficient time with their infant takes precedence over paperwork, ward routine, or taking the infant to the morgue. Parents have indicated a need to hold their infant for a "longer" time and not feel pushed by care providers.[12] Even infants who have been removed to the morgue may be returned if parents need more time and contact for detachment.

When an infant dies, there are limited opportunities for memories. Professionals have the responsibility of helping parents make memories so that they will have a tangible person to mourn. Encouraging parents to name their infant gives the child a separate identity, which helps facilitate the grieving process. Tangible mementos may include photographs, handprints and footprints, a lock of hair, measurements of the infant, identification bands, the blanket the infant was wrapped in, a blessing or baptismal certificate, and birth and death certificates. Parents find most beneficial the interventions that acknowledged the infant (e.g., photographs, holding the infant, and receiving personal mementos).[12,40,69,81] Even when parents say they do not want mementos, they should be kept in hospital files and the parents made aware that they will be available to them in the future if they want them. Taking pictures of the infant, obtaining other mementos, and telling the parents that they will be available to them on request respects their immediate decision not to see or have information on the infant, but also provides a mechanism for them to "know" their infant at a later date if they wish to do so.

Before an infant is transported to a newborn special care unit, photographs should be taken and given to the parents to promote bonding. If the infant remains hospitalized for a long time or requires surgery, pictures taken at weekly intervals or before and after surgery can help confirm the reality of the child's condition and progress and assist with bonding as well as the grief process. Despite the outcome, parents will appreciate some lasting record of their child's life.

The staff who provide emotional support for parents must also receive support from each other. Expecting the staff to immediately return to work is unrealistic. Such an emotional experience takes time and space for decompression, which is facilitated by the use of exercise, crying, and being alone for quiet time.[24]

Open Visiting and Caretaking Policies

Perinatal care settings with open visiting and caregiving policies foster a shared family experience and support from others. Regardless of the type of perinatal loss, no mother should experience it alone—a spouse, friend, family member, or identified supportive other should remain with her.[12,48] Members of the mother's support system will also need an outlet for the expression of their grief.

Women suffering the grief of perinatal loss should be given a choice about their room assignment. Arbitrary removal from the obstetric unit may deny the mother's maternity: "Am I a mother or not?" It may also escalate her feelings of failure, guilt, and worthlessness as a woman and a mother. Because she did not produce a normal, healthy infant, she may feel punished and banished from the maternity area by isolation on another floor. Her care may be entrusted to those without expertise in the physiologic and psychologic care of the normal postpartum period, much less a postpartum complicated by loss. Placement at the end of the hall far from the nurse's station, with the door closed and no company from staff and family, only increases her feelings of loneliness and isolation. Yet being on a happy maternity floor with normal, healthy infants and their mothers may be an exceedingly difficult and constant reminder of her loss and even complicate her recovery.[43,93] Information about the advantages and disadvantages of staying or leaving the maternity ward should be given by the professional. The mother, knowing what will be helpful, makes the decision.[96]

The alternative to maternal hospitalization is early discharge as soon as medically possible so the mother may join her infant when the infant has been transported to another hospital. Early discharge also facilitates an easier mobilization of supportive others in the familiar surroundings of home. Removal from the constant reminder of one's failure (i.e., other healthy infants) may let the grief work begin.[96] Early discharge is not therapeutic when the professional assumes there is a support system to provide care and no one is available. Without a plan for follow-up care and contact, early discharge merely relocates the problem.

Caregiving is as important for the parents of a sick deformed, or dead infant as it is for the parents of a normal infant. Open visiting and caregiving policies increase interaction between the parents and their infant by actively involving them in the reality of their child's illness, deformity, or im-

pending death. Even if the child lives only a short time, parental access and taking care of the infant complete the attachment process and enable them to begin the detachment of grief work. Even minimal caregiving helps parents overcome their sense of helplessness and be comforted by "We did all that we could have done. We cared, we made a difference to our baby." Active parental involvement decreases poor outcomes such as aberrant parenting styles, attachment problems, and unresolved grief.[45]

The loneliness and isolation of death is decreased for both parents and infant when they are together at the time of death. Parents are often comforted and relieved that their fantasy of the agony of the death scene is not borne out in the quiet, peaceful reality of death.[45,92] Having experienced the beginning of life together, experiencing the ending of life as a family symbolizes closure and completion. Parents who are able to share even a brief life with their child and the moment of death are able to face death's finality knowing they did not abandon their child but provided the infant with love and care. Parents who are not present at death may take care of the infant afterward by seeing and holding their infant.

Parents need to be given the opportunity to make final plans for their deceased infant. The planning will help them face the death and facilitate the grief process. For many parents this is their first experience with death and making final arrangements, and they are not aware of the options. It is helpful to provide the family with detailed, specific verbal and written information about cremation, burial, funeral, or hospital disposal.[12,40]

A funeral may be chosen for religious reasons or as a declaration of the fetus or newborn as a person befitting burial rather than disposal. Burial leaves a specific place of remembrance that this infant lived. Care for the infant after death may include funeral arrangements, such as choosing the clothes, bathing, and even dressing the infant.[12,92] If parents choose not to have a funeral, they may wish to have a memorial service or do something special, such as plant a rosebush or tree, in memory of their infant. Regardless of their decision, the birth and death of their infant is a life event for the family, and it is important to recognize it.

Autopsy

For parents who experience a stillbirth, spontaneous abortion, or neonatal death, knowing why the infant was deformed or died eases their recovery from grief.[45] In the search for a cause, many parents blame themselves for doing too much or too little to favorably influence the outcome. Knowing why the infant died or the converse, that not even the "experts" know why the infant died, may help assuage their personal feelings of guilt and failure.

Approaching the family for permission for an autopsy must be done by the primary care providers (physician and nurse) with the utmost of tact and respect for the family's feelings.[92] Too often the permission for autopsy is denied because of the way the subject is broached by professionals. Telling the family about their infant's death in one breath and asking for an autopsy with the next breath is not appropriate. Parents need time to deal with the reality of the death, including seeing and holding their infant and being with each other and supportive others before they are even ready to think about an autopsy. Consideration of the family's feelings and stage of grief greatly enhances communication with the professional.[92] Reasons for the autopsy, including a possible answer to the question of "Why?" their infant died or was deformed, are important to discuss in a relaxed and unhurried manner.[1] Parents may feel rushed to make a decision without clearly understanding the advantages and disadvantages and resist the emotional topic of a postmortem examination. Time for discussion with an empathetic professional as well as between themselves facilitates an informed parental decision.

The professional who receives permission for an autopsy is then obliged to discuss with the parents all findings.[1,31,43] This may entail more than one meeting with the parents, because they should be informed of the findings as soon as they are available. Therefore the professional may meet with them within 24 hours of completing the autopsy to discuss gross and preliminary findings and again 6 to 8 weeks later to discuss microscopic results.[45,92] Autopsy data may indicate either a condition that has implications for subsequent pregnancies or one that has little chance of recurrence.[1] The need for genetic counseling for future pregnancies may be evident from autopsy results. Discussing the results with the report in hand and offering parents a copy for future reference is also important.

Anticipatory Guidance

Encounters with parents after the death of their infant give professionals the opportunity for anticipatory guidance—information about what to expect from themselves and from others. Reactions to peri-

natal loss differ markedly, so that family, friends, and acquaintances may not act as parents might expect. Some will be supportive and emotionally empathetic, especially if they have suffered a perinatal loss. Others will be uncomfortable and, not knowing what to say or do, may choose to avoid the couple and never mention the loss, even in future conversations. Those who are unaware of the loss may question the newly nonpregnant parents about the new infant. These inquiries are both awkward and painful.

Knowledge of the universal feelings and behaviors associated with grief gives comfort and relief to parents. Knowing what to expect from grief (i.e., how it progresses and how long it takes) is valuable to those who are or will be experiencing it.[45,81,96] Knowing the stages of grief and that the accompanying behaviors and emotions are normal decreases the feeling of "going crazy." Recovery from the loss takes time and cannot be hurried or ignored. The most difficult time is immediately after birth and the first few months after the loss (2 to 4 months).[82] The emotions of grief begin to lessen toward the end of the first year.

Parents should be encouraged to support and care for each other in their time of loss. Professionals should advocate mutual support by a free expression of feelings and emotions between the parents. Although parents need each other during grief, they also need an identified support system with whom to talk and cry. The ability to reach outside of the nuclear family to friends, extended family, and professionals should be encouraged. Professionals have a responsibility to ask whom parents turn to for help and support in a crisis. If there are no identified supportive others, parents must know whom to call for help in the initial bereavement period.

Anticipatory guidance is also essential at the discharge of an anomalied, preterm, or previously ill newborn. Knowing what to expect when going home with an infant with a defect or an infant who has been hospitalized for months makes the transition from hospital to society easier for parents. Evaluation of the grief process and the attachment level of the parents to a less-than-perfect infant is vital.

Long-Term Follow-up Care

Follow-up care and contact with professionals are needed by grieving parents.[30,40] Follow-up meetings function as a catharsis for parents, as well as an opportunity for assessment, counseling, and possibly referral. Primary care providers (physicians, nurses, and social workers) from the perinatal care setting may provide follow-up. One study documented a significant decrease in the intensity of a mother's grief after stillbirth when she received one telephone call from the physician.[44] For the family, relating to providers with whom a relationship has been established may be easier than establishing a new relationship with a stranger.[40] However, being with those who are associated with the loss event may be uncomfortable for the parents at the height of their grief. For the professional, the ability to continue to be a source of help and comfort to families with whom one has established a relationship may help complete their grief reactions. Maintaining contact with the family may be painful as the professional relives the feelings of grief and loss associated with sharing their tragedy. Although painful, this reexperience of intense feelings gives both parents and professionals another opportunity to work toward grief resolution.

When and where to provide continuing care for families are crucial questions. Contact in the perinatal care setting both at the time of death and daily until discharge provides immediate care. However, when discharged, all too often the family returns home alone to face weeks and months of unsupported and lonely grief. Without feedback about their normal reaction and society's expectation that they will shortly be "back to normal," they are abandoned to their emotions. They suffer in silence and often drift apart in their misery. With their support system withdrawn but still feeling overwhelmed with grief, parents describe the period between 2 and 4 months after the loss as the most difficult time.[43,82,92] At 2 months after perinatal loss, parents show increased symptoms of anxiety and depression that are reduced by 8 months but still higher than in parents not experiencing perinatal loss.[86] Follow-up care from professionals is most meaningful and needed by parents during this period when they feel deserted by previously supportive others. Parents experience a need for spiritual support weeks and months after the loss. Meeting with families sooner (within weeks of their loss) may alleviate the effect of decreasing support as the months go by.[92] The professional who acknowledges the withdrawal of others but can be relied on to be available provides the parents with the emotional anchor of long-term care and support.

Breaking appointments or continually not being available may be resistance to follow-up contact with the professionals but also represents a reluctance to return to the perinatal care setting with its painful memories. A visit from the professional in the home provides a nonthreatening, familiar environment for follow-up care. The more comfortable home environment enables assessment of family interactions and facilitates communication at the "feeling" level.

Each family member and the family as a unit must be assessed for their place in the grief process:

- In what stage of grief is each family member?
- Is anyone "stuck" in a stage of grief?
- Are behaviors appropriate for normal grief reactions, or do altered behaviors represent pathologic grief reactions?
- Do altered behaviors warrant referral for further treatment and evaluation?
- Do the caregiving and attachment behaviors of the parents reflect resolution of grief over loss of the perfect child and adoption of the less-than-perfect child as the love object?

Just because everything was progressing normally at previous encounters does not mean that it should be assumed to still be so. As the flood of initial grief subsides, problems and questions that were not considered suddenly become of great concern. For the first time in months, the regressive behavior of siblings may not only be noticed but may be extremely annoying to parents. The beginning of grief resolution may allow future projections such as "When can I have another baby?" or the dread of the painful anniversary of the loss.[92]

Referral to public health nurses or visiting nursing services in the community for follow-up care is appropriate. However, a written referral alone is not enough. Involving them in the hospital care and discharge planning is essential for a smooth transition to home care. Having the new professional meet the family in the hospital with the primary care providers facilitates trust transference from the familiar to the unfamiliar. Traditionally, home care providers have been involved in care of normal mothers and infants in the community. Involvement in perinatal loss situations requires knowledge about the process of grief and willingness to share the grief of the parents. Because these may be new skills for many, continuing education programs that teach the theory and skills of effective intervention help the professional be more comfortable with a perinatal loss situation.

Additional expertise may be warranted when the professional recognizes signs and symptoms of pathologic grief, delayed or absent grief, or concurrent multiple stresses or losses. Parents may not be ready for genetic counseling, infant stimulation programs, or financial programs until months later. Between 3 and 6 months after their loss, parents may be ready to reach outside of the nuclear and extended family for help and support for the first time. Suggesting a local hospital support group or the local chapter of a national support organization may at first be met with resistance. Leaving the names and phone numbers of such organizations ensures that the parents have the information at their disposal when they are ready to use it. Until their own support system has withdrawn, parents may not be ready for a support group of other parents.

Throughout this section, examples of "what to say" and "how to say it" have been used to illustrate helpful interventions for grieving families. It is essential to state that "there are no scripts." Parents do not say one thing and the professionals answer with a parroted response. Each encounter is a unique situation consisting of distinct parental and professional personalities. Each situation must be evaluated separately and individual interventions instituted.[40] It is recommended that the professional learn by observing an experienced colleague with grieving families and that the professional "practice" with role playing and situation solving before actually attempting to intervene with the parents.

CHILDREN AND GRIEF

Explaining and helping a surviving child to understand the loss of an infant is an enormous task for parents. Facilitating the child's normal feelings of sadness, worry, and anger after a loss may be difficult for parents who fear being flooded with their own emotions. Unresolved grief from the parents' own childhood may prevent the expression of grief by their children.

To maintain the myth of childhood (innocent happiness), children are often shielded from any knowledge about death, even when it is an inevitable event in their lives. Thus children are prevented from full realization, validation, and expression of their feelings and emotions. They are not able to formalize and express their grief over the loss of a significant person.

Even though adults are encouraged to cry, talk, and gradually understand and integrate their feelings of grief, no one helps the child deal with the same frightening feelings. No one discusses the loss with the child, because "He might cry" and because of the adult's inadequacy and lack of understanding of how and what to say. No amount of secrecy or denial of the situation will hide the fact that the child is being excluded from an important family event.

Attempts to protect children from feelings of grief and mourning because of death or other important losses isolate the child. Age and developmentally appropriate explanations include the child in the family's experience, rather than separating and excluding him from "what is going on." Shielding children from the knowledge of death denies them the reality of life and the opportunity for personal growth and mastery of the experience. Like the subject of sex, death is taboo for children.

A child's grief and mourning in response to perinatal loss depend on his cognitive and developmental level, the extent of prenatal attachment and expectation about the infant, the degree of ambivalent feelings, and the response of his or her parents to the death. Because the child's understanding of death differs from that of adults, knowledge of the stages of growing awareness is essential for both parents and professionals working with children experiencing grief[46,47] (Table 30-1). Regardless of age or developmental stage, the universal fear of childhood is the fear of separation and abandonment. For a young child (under age 5), the loss of the infant is experienced indirectly through parental grief. A young child reacts to the emotional withdrawal of grieving parents and fears loss of them (and their love).

Although children at different developmental stages have their own conceptions of death, adults must provide them with the facts about the situation in language that they are able to understand. They may benefit from guidance by the nurse, social worker, or other health professional regarding beneficial approaches to facilitate the child's grief work. The professional serves as a resource, role model, and support system to parents caring for their surviving children. Printed materials are also available to assist parents in helping their other children understand death (see Resource Materials for Parents at the end of this chapter). Age-appropriate story books concerning death can facilitate grief discussion and elicit questions and feelings from children.

Just as grieving adults need repetition, children need repeated explanations and discussions about the loss. Constantly in a state of developmental flux, the child attempts to view the loss in new ways as a result of increasing maturation. Asking questions

Table 30-1	A CHILD'S DEVELOPING CONCEPT OF DEATH	
AGE	**COGNITIVE UNDERSTANDING**	**HOW EXPERIENCED**
Infant (to 12 mo)	None	Indirectly through parental grief expressed in: Emotional withdrawal Inability to provide concern and continuity in caregiving behaviors Overconcern because of fear of recurrent loss
Toddler (1-3 yr)	Little understanding of cause and effect Death may be confused with sleeping or being away	React to changes in behavior of grieving parents and reflect their feelings and anxiety
Preschooler (3-6 yr)	View death as a temporary state and not an inevitable occurrence Believe that they are the center of the universe and can do anything, and that thinking is doing (thoughts have the power of actions)	Expect the dead to return—ask questions about "when?" Fear (and feel guilty) that negative thoughts or actual death wishes caused the death
School age (6-12 yr)	Understand that death is inevitable and irreversible 6-9 year olds: personify death as a separate person (skeleton, boogey man) About 8 years old: "death phobia," a normal developmental stage characterized by preoccupation with thoughts of own death or that of a loved one Reasons concretely with ability to see cause-and-effect relationships	Realize death occurs in adults like parents and even in children; realize death is permanent, not temporary, state May show interest in biological aspects of death and details of funeral
Adolescents (12 yr)	Able to think abstractly about death like the adult; philosophic reasoning	Similar to adult

Modified from Gardner SL, Merenstein GB: Helping families deal with perinatal loss, *Neonatal Netw* 5:17, 1986; American Academy of Pediatrics Committee on Psychosocial Aspects of Child and Family Health: The pediatrician and childhood bereavement, *Pediatrics* 105:445, 2000.

(usually at inopportune times) and making comments about the infant are ways the child continues to process the experience, often long after the parents have completed it. These questions and comments may seem endless and resurrect the parent's own grief. The child's inquiries must be encouraged and supported so that he or she knows that talking about the loss or death is acceptable. Exploring the child's feelings for fears of causation, guilt, or the wonder if "death is catching" enables them to be dealt with appropriately. Truthful discussion with the child dispels the worst fears and fantasies and replaces them with reality that is "not too horrible to discuss" with parents. If the cause of the infant's death is known, it is explained to the child in simple, direct terms: "Baby Bobby couldn't breathe by himself because his lungs were sick. His sick lungs only happen to little babies."

A subsequent illness may precipitate worry by the child that he or she, too, will die. Often this fear is not verbalized but acted out by significant behavioral changes such as withdrawal, clinging and whining, or overactivity that are uncharacteristic for the child. Verbal reassurance that the child is not going to die and a reminder that "the baby died of a sickness that only little babies get; big boys and girls can't get it" are helpful.

The normal feelings that accompany grief should be acknowledged and explained to the child. "Mommy and Daddy feel sad that Baby Jean died. Sometimes we will cry because we feel sad. It's okay to cry when you feel sad." Permission for the expression of the child's feelings should also be given verbally: "You might feel sad, too. It's okay for you to cry when you're sad. Then we will talk about how you are feeling." Encouraging children to draw or write their feelings is another way of giving them permission to express their grief.

Using words such as "went away," "expired," "lost," or "went to sleep" is dangerous in describing death to children. Because young children are concrete and literal, they think they might die if they "go to sleep," or that anyone who leaves them is in danger of dying. Children also relate current experiences to past ones and interpret "lost" quite literally. In the mind of the child, if the parent only searched well enough, the misplaced (i.e., "lost") child would be found.

Including children at funeral or memorial services facilitates their grief and prevents exclusion from a significant family event. Consideration of the family value system, age of the child, and religious custom must enter into the decision to include the child. Adequate preparation includes a discussion of everything the child will see, hear, and feel, including the normal adult emotions of crying and sadness. An adult besides the grieving parents should accompany the child to reiterate what is happening and to meet the child's physical and psychologic needs. Adult support is necessary so that the child is able to express and deal with his or her feelings.

Helping children with their grief is also therapeutic for parents. Assisting children to master the crisis of loss ultimately augments the parents' self-esteem and restores confidence in their parenting skills.[45] Parents are able to deal in a healthy way with their own grief when they are able to facilitate the grief of their other children.

PATHOLOGIC GRIEF

The absence of grief when it would be expected is not a healthy sign but rather a cause for concern. The emotions of grief and their expression are healing. Early and full expression of grief is associated with an optimal outcome.[45] However, many people in grief-producing situations attempt to avoid the pain of grief and the expression of emotions, the result of which prolongs mourning, delays a return to the previous lifestyle, prevents the creation of new attachments and relationships, and ultimately results in pathologic grief (see the list on p. 769).[17,45,55]

Not grieving precludes opportunities for growth and change. No new coping styles will be attempted. No novel alternatives to problem solving and adapting to a crisis will be added to the repertoire of behavior for future use. In other words, those who choose not to do grief work say "no" to their own potential and remain frozen in development.[42] Under the stress of not resolving their grief, some may even regress in their development.

Reproductive loss is a blow to self-concept and self-esteem, as well as loss of the infant. Blocking appropriate feelings of loss, grief, and anger results in a significant decrease in one's sense of self-esteem.[19] After death of their neonates, 33% of mothers suffered severe and tragic outcomes (including psychoses, phobias, anxiety attacks, and deep depression).[17,45,96] Those who are unable to effectively resolve their grief may suffer lifelong emotional damage.[56]

Not working through grief associated with repetitive contact with perinatal loss also affects the staff. To cope with feelings, they may hide behind a "professional" demeanor characterized by decreased spontaneity and withdrawal. Such a provider defends against the repeated pain of loss by emotional dissociation from the situation; the real self does not respond, but the role of the omnipotent, unemotional physician or nurse responds. The result, self-alienation, eventually desensitizes the professional to the experience and ultimately prevents any empathy with the experience of others.[42] Emotions that are unable to be acknowledged or expressed healthily are vented in ways that may be destructive to relationships in personal and professional life.

Unresolved grief does not disappear and is not dissipated. The emotions accompanying grief may never be expressed but are not forgotten by the unconscious mind. Containment of these emotions through repression or suppression takes psychic energy. A conscious, intentional decision to postpone or dismiss grief to meet others' needs or to meet immediate demands of the loss situation (e.g., funeral arrangements) is called delayed grief.[55,56] For a period of time (days, weeks, or longer), there is little or no grief response when such a reaction would be expected and appropriate. Delayed grief may also be the result of repression, the unconscious contents that seem to have a life and energy of their own that become the sources of later emotional conflict.

Grief that is inhibited and never resolved is called abortive.[56] Those who have aborted their grief work often live bereft of "joie de vivre" with no interest, concern, or enthusiasm for life. Chronic grief is characterized by an indefinite prolonging of the acute stage of depression.[56] Indeed, chronic depression may be traceable to unresolved grief from the past.

Grief that is not resolved remains buried in the psyche, waiting for an opportunity to "rear its ugly head." A current loss may remind the psyche of the unmourned grief from a previous loss or losses.[25,57] As the two (or more) losses become intertwined and are experienced as one and the same, repressed emotions of unresolved grief pour forth.[57,84] Grieving more than one loss or a lifetime of losses is more difficult and emotionally draining than grieving one event at a time.[25] Cumulative grief work may also be occurring when a current loss of seemingly little importance overwhelms the person with intense emotions.[25,56] This flood of emotions seems disproportionate to the current loss and is only peripherally related to it. The unconscious, unresolved grief is finally uncovered when the individual is flooded with emotions. Thus the emotional components of any grief reaction may be influenced by aspects of unresolved grief from the past.[57]

Grief and loss events of the perinatal period have only been equated for a relatively short time (approximately 25 years). Because loss during the perinatal period is a common experience, many childbearing and older women (and men) have never grieved over their spontaneous abortion, stillbirth, or neonatal death, even 10 to 20 years after its occurrence. Parents in a current perinatal loss may also be dealing with unresolved grief from a previous perinatal loss. Unresolved grief (whether from perinatal or other loss events of life) may become available for resolution in subsequent crisis events. A mother who delivers a normal healthy newborn, yet is depressed postpartally, may not have postpartum depression. Instead she may be grieving the unresolved loss of a spontaneous abortion, therapeutic abortion, or other perinatal loss.[80,84] The normal grief reaction accompanying relinquishment may persist and often leads to chronic unresolved grief that may present itself during and after a subsequent pregnancy.[3] Her depressed mood could also be resulting from unresolved grief from the loss of a parent, spouse, or child. Depressed menopausal women may be experiencing the cumulative effects of a lifetime of unresolved grief. The symptomatology of unresolved grief is as follows[84]:

- Vivid memory for the details of the perinatal loss event
- Flashback to the event
- Anniversary grief (date of birth or expected date of delivery)
- Emotions of grief (sadness, anger, or crying) when talking about loss
- Intense emotions with subsequent loss or crisis

Recognizing unresolved grief has implications for facilitating grief work in a current loss, episodic care, and health maintenance. The energy to keep unresolved emotions restrained could better be used

in personal growth and development, grieving, and maintaining and establishing relationships.[29] The lifelong stress of unresolved grief contributes to both psychologic and physical illness, including increased death rates and an earlier death.[70,92]

Not grieving a perinatal loss affects the individual involved and the relationships with significant others, including present and future children. Asynchronous grief and the absence of grief in one or more family members weaken and strain family relationships.[45] The irritability and preoccupation of normal grief may overly disrupt the family. Differences may be magnified to the extent that major rifts and disruptions in the relationship occur, resulting in increased incidence of separation and divorce.[45]

Exclusive dedication to the care of a deformed or ill child to the detriment of other family relationships is symptomatic of a pathologic grief reaction.[45,83,94] The parent who neglects other children, the couple's relationship, and social outlets is so overwhelmed with guilt about having caused the child's defect that nothing else in life matters. This guilty attachment and exclusive dedication are ways of avoiding grief work.[83] Other forms of pathologic reactions include parental rejection and intolerance of the deformed or ill child.[45]

The parent who is emotionally withdrawn and unavailable to the family because of chronic grief and depression is not able to attach and care for present or subsequent children. Aberrant parenting styles (resulting in a vulnerable, battered, or failure-to-thrive child) may be the result of prolonged separation, unresolved grief, or grief that has progressed beyond the anticipatory phase, so that emotional ties with the infant have been severed.[45] These difficulties with caring and parenting may affect the deformed or ill child and all the children in the family. In turn, these children may grow up unable to parent subsequent generations because of the type of ineffectual parenting they received. Parents who grieve inappropriately may leave their children a legacy of psychosocial problems such as difficulty with separation, independence, and control (e.g., school phobia and toilet training); a failure to thrive; and sleep disturbances.

Because detachment is necessary before a healthy attachment may again occur, unresolved grief affects future children. It is necessary to first complete the grief work over the loss of one child to be optimally ready to emotionally invest in a new infant.[45] The replacement child, a well-documented psychiatric syndrome, is associated with unresolved parental grief after the death (or loss) of a child.[25,67] Without withdrawing their emotional attachment to the lost child, parents plan, conceive, and bear another to replace their loss and alleviate their grief. Parental hopes, desires, and fantasies invested in the lost child are not relinquished but merely transferred to the replacement child. Planning for a new pregnancy and another child should begin only after the grief process for the lost child is completed.[45,84] Generally, 6 months to 1 year is the earliest that grief will be resolved so that the ego is free to invest in a relationship with another fetus and newborn.

REFERENCES

1. American Academy of Pediatrics and The American College of Obstetricians and Gynecologists: *Guidelines for Perinatal Care,* ed 4, Elk Grove, Ill, 1997, The Academy.
2. Armstrong, D, Hutti, M: Pregnancy after perinatal loss: the relationship between anxiety and prenatal attachment, *J Obstet Gynecol Neonatal Nurs* 27:183, 1998.
3. Askren, H, Bloom, K: Post adoptive reactions of the relinquishing mother: a review, *J Obstet Gynecol Neonatal Nurs,* 28(4):395, 1999.
4. Benfield D, Leib S, Reuter J et al: Grief response of parents after referral of the critically ill newborn to a regional center, *N Engl J Med* 294:975, 1976.
5. Benoliel JQ: Assessment of loss and grief, *J Thanatology* 1:182, 1971.
6. Berezin N: *After a loss in pregnancy, help for families affected by a miscarriage, a stillbirth, or the loss of a newborn,* New York, 1982, Fireside Books.
7. Bibring GL: The death of an infant: a psychological study, *N Engl J Med* 283:370, 1970.
8. Borg S, Lasker J: *When pregnancy fails: families coping with miscarriage, stillbirth, and infant death,* Boston, 1981, Beacon Press.
9. Burke S, Matsumoto A: Pastoral care for perinatal and neonatal health care providers, *J Obstet Gynecol Neonatal Nurs* 28:137, 1999.
10. Cadden V: Crisis in the family. In Caplan G, ed: *Principles of preventive psychiatry,* New York, 1964, Basic Books.
11. Cain A, Cain B: On replacing a child, *J Am Acad Child Psychiatry* 3:443, 1964.
12. Calhoun LK: Parents' perceptions of nursing support following perinatal loss, *J Perinat Neonatal Nurs* 8:57, 1994.
13. Caplan G: *Principles of preventive psychiatry,* New York, 1964, Basic Books.
14. Colgrove M, Bloomfield H, McWilliams P et al: *How to survive the loss of a love,* New York, 1976, Lion Books.
15. Costello AC, Gardner SL, Merenstein GB: Perinatal grief and loss, *J Perinatol* 8:41, 1988.
16. Cote-Arsenault D, Mahlangu, N: Impact of perinatal loss on the subsequent pregnancy and self: women's experiences, *J Obstet Gynecol Neonatal Nurs* 28:274, 1999.
17. Cullberg J: Mental reactions of women to perinatal death. In Morris N, ed: *Psychosomatic medicine in obstetrics and gynecology,* New York, 1972, S Karger.
18. Cummings ST: The impact of the child's defect on the father, *Am J Orthopsychiatry* 46:246, 1976.
19. Cummings ST, Bayley HC, Rie HE: Effects of the child's deficiency on the mother: a study of mothers of mentally retarded, chronically ill, and neurotic children, *Am J Orthopsychiatry* 36:595, 1966.
20. D'Alton M: Meeting the multiple challenges of multiple gestation, *Contemp OBGYN* July, 1996, p. 96.
21. Danforth DN: *Obstetrics and gynecology,* Philadelphia, 1990, Lippincott.
22. de Frain J, Jakub D, Mendoza B: The psychological effects of sudden infant death on grandmothers and grandfathers, *Omega* 24:165, 1992.
23. de Montigny F, Beaudet L, Dumas L: A baby has died: the impact of perinatal loss on family social networks, *J Obstet Gynecol Neonatal Nurs* 28:151, 1999.
24. Downey V, Bengiamin M, Heuer L et al: Dying babies and associated stress in NICU nurses, *Neonatal Netw* 14:41, 1995.
25. Eason WM: *The dying child,* Springfield, Ill., 1970, Charles C. Thomas.
26. Engel GL: Grief and grieving, *Am J Nurs* 64:93 1964.
27. Fraley A: Chronic sorrow in parents of premature children, *Child Health Care,* 15:114, 1986.
28. Gardner SL, Merenstein GB: Helping families deal with perinatal loss, *Neonatal Netw* 5:17, 1986.
29. Garland KG: Unresolved grief, *Neonatal Netw* 5:29, 1986.
30. Geis DP: Mothers' perceptions of care given their dying child, *Am J Nurs* 65:103, 1965.
31. Giles PFH: Reactions of women to perinatal death, *Aust NZ J Obstet Gynaecol* 10:207, 1970.
32. Goldbach KR, Dunn DS, Toedter LJ et al: The effects of gestational age and gender on grief after pregnancy loss, *Am J Orthopsychiatry* 61:461, 1991.
33. Goldberg H: *The hazards of being male,* New York, 1976, Sanford J. Greenberger.
34. Gonzalez MT: Nursing support of the family with an abnormal infant, *Hosp Top* 15:68, 1971.
35. Griffin T: Nurse barriers to parenting in the special care nursery, *J Perinat Neonatal Nurs* 4:56, 1990.
36. Hanson S, Boyd S: *Family health care nursing,* Philadelphia, 1996, FA Davis.
37. Hebert M: Perinatal bereavement in its cultural context, *Death Stud* 22:61, 1998.
38. Hill R: Generic features of families under stress. In Parad H, ed: *Crisis intervention,* New York, 1965, Family Service Assn. of America.

39. Humel P, Eastman D: Do parents of preterm infants suffer chronic sorrow? *Neonatal Netw* 10:59,1991.

40. Jack A: Current Canadian neonatal research: memories of a gentle presence, *Neonatal Netw 14:49, 1995.*

41. Johnson JM: Stillbirth: a personal experience, *Am J Nurs* 72:1595, 1972.

42. Jourard S: *The transparent self,* rev ed, New York, 1971, Van Nostrand Reinhold.

43. Kennell JH, Slyter H, Klaus MH: The mourning response of parents to death of a newborn infant, *N Engl J Med* 283:344, 1970.

44. Klass D, Marrwit S: Toward a model of parental grief, *Omega* 19:31, 1988.

45. Klaus M, Kennell J: *Parent-infant bonding,* ed 2, St Louis, 1982, Mosby.

46. Koocher GP: Children, death, and cognitive development, *Dev Psychobiol* 9:369, 1973.

47. Koocher GP: Talking to children about death, *Am J Orthopsychiatry* 44:404, 1974.

48. Kowalski K, Osborn M: Helping mothers of stillborn infants to grieve, *MCN Am J Matern Child Nurs* 2:29, 1977.

49. Kübler-Ross E: *On death and dying,* New York, 1969, Macmillan.

50. Lax RF: Some aspects of the interaction between mother and impaired child: mother's narcissistic trauma, *Int J Psychoanal* 53:339, 1972.

51. Leon I: The psychoanalytic conceptualization of perinatal loss: a multidimensional model, *Am J Psych* 149:1464, 1992.

52. Lepler M: Having a handicapped child, *MCN Am J Matern Child Nurs* 3:32, 1978.

53. Lewis E: The management of stillbirth: coping with an unreality, *Lancet* 18:619, 1976.

54. Lewis E, Page A: Failure to mourn a stillbirth: an overlooked catastrophe, *Br J Med Psychol* 51:237, 1978.

55. Lindemann E: Symptomatology and management of acute grief, *Am J Psychiatry* 101:141, 1994.

56. Marris P: *Loss and change,* New York, 1974, Pantheon Books.

57. McCollum A, Schwartz H: Social work and the mourning parent, *Social Work* 17:25, 1972.

58. Menke J, McClead R: Perinatal grief and mourning, *Adv Pediatr* 37:261, 1990.

59. Mercer R: Crisis: a baby born with a defect, *Nursing 77* 7:45, 1977.

60. Miles M, Carlson J, Fink S: Sources of support reported by mothers and fathers of infants hospitalized in NICU, *Neonatal Netw* 15:45, 1996.

61. Miles M, Wilson S, Docherty S: African-American mothers' responses to hospitalization of an infant with serious health problems, *Neonatal Netw* 18:17, 1999.

62. Ohlshansky S: Chronic sorrow: a response to having a mentally defective child, *Soc Case* 43:190, 1962.

63. Opirhory GJ: Counseling the parents of a critically ill newborn, *J Obstet Gynecol Neonatal Nurs* 8:179, 1979.

64. Parkes CM: *Bereavement: studies of grief in adult life,* New York, 1972, International Universities Press.

65. Peppers L, Knapp R: *Motherhood and mourning perinatal death,* New York, 1980, Preager.

66. Porreco R, Harmon R, Murrow N et al: Parental choices in grand multiple gestations: psychological considerations, *J Mat Fetal M* 4:111, 1995.

67. Pozanski E: The replacement child: a saga of unresolved parental grief, *J Pediatr* 81:1190, 1972.

68. Primeau M, Lamb J: When a baby dies: rights of the baby and parents, *J Obstet Gynecol Neonatal Nurs* 24:206, 1995.

69. Primeau M, Recht C: Professional bereavement photos: one aspect of a perinatal bereavement program, *J Obstet Gynecol Neonatal Nurs* 23:22, 1994.

70. Rahe R, Meyer M, Smith M et al: Social stress and illness onset, *J Psychosom Res* 8:35, 1964.

71. Rapaport L: The state of crisis: some theoretical considerations. In Parad H, ed: *Crisis intervention,* New York, 1965, Family Service Assn. of America.

72. Raphael D: *The tender gift: breastfeeding,* New York, 1973, Schoken Books.

73. Robertson P, Kavanaugh K: Supporting parents during and after a pregnancy subsequent to a perinatal loss, *J Perinat Neonatal Nurs* 12:63, 1998.

74. Ryan P, Cote-Arsenault D, Sugarman L: Facilitating care after perinatal loss: a comprehensive checklist, *J Obstet Gynecol Neonatal Nurs* 20:385, 1991.

75. Saylor D: Nursing response to mothers of stillborn infants, *J Obstet Gynecol Neonatal Nurs* 8:39, 1977.

76. Schoenberg BA, Carr A, Perety D et al: *Loss and grief: psychological management in medical practice,* New York, 1970, Columbia University Press.

77. Schoenberg BA et al: *Anticipatory grief,* New York, 1974, Columbia University Press.

78. Schwab R: Effects of a child's death on the marital relationship: a preliminary study, *Death Stud* 16:141, 1992.

79. Seidman R, Kleine P: A theory of transformed parenting: parenting a child with developmental delay/mental retardation, *Nurs Res* 44:38, 1995.

80. Seitz P, Warrick L: Perinatal death: the grieving mother, *Am J Nurs* 74:2028, 1974.

81. Sexton P, Stephens S: Postpartum mother's perceptions of nursing interventions for perinatal grief, *Neonatal Netw* 9:47, 1991.

82. Siegel R et al: The impact of neonatal loss, *Pediatr Res* 16:93A, 1982.

83. Solnit A, Stark M: Mourning and the birth of a defective child, *Psychoanal Study Child* 16:523, 1961.

84. Stack J: Spontaneous abortion and grieving, *Am Fam Pract* 21:99, 1980

85. Traxler P: *Poem for my son, blood calendar,* New York, 1975, William Morrow.

86. Vance JC, Najman JM, Thearle MJ et al: Psychological changes in parents eight months after the loss of an infant from stillbirth, neonatal death, or SIDS: a longitudinal study, *Pediatrics* 96:933, 1995.
87. Waechter E: The birth of an exceptional child, *Nurs Forum* 9:202, 1970.
88. Wagner T, Higgins P, Wallerstedt C: Perinatal death: how fathers grieve, *J Perinatal Educ* 6:4, 1997.
89. Wallerstedt C, Higgins P: Facilitating perinatal grieving between the mother and the father, *J Obstet Gynecol Neonatal Nurs* 25:389, 1996.
90. Whitfield JM, Siegel RE, Glicken AD et al: The application of hospice concepts to neonatal care, *Am J Dis Child* 136:521, 1982.
91. Wilson AL, Fenton LJ, Stevens DC et al: The death of a newborn twin: an analysis of parental bereavement, *Pediatrics* 70:587, 1982.
92. Wooten B: Death of an infant, *MCN Am J Matern Child Nurs* J 6:257, 1981.
93. Yates SA: Stillbirth: what staff can do, *Am J Nurs* 72:1592, 1972.
94. Young RK: Chronic sorrow, parent's response to the birth of a child with a defect, *MCN Am J Matern Child Nurs* J 2:38, 1977.
95. Yu V, Jamieson J, Astbury J: Parents' reactions to unrestricted parental contact with infants in the intensive care nursery, *Med J Aust* 1:294, 1979.
96. Zahourek R, Jensen J: Grieving and the loss of the newborn, *Am J Nurs* 73:836, 1973.

RESOURCE MATERIALS FOR PARENTS

Balter L: *A funeral for Whiskers,* New York, 1991, Barron's Educational Services.

Bell J, Esterling LS: *What will I tell the children?* Omaha, Neb, 1986, American Cancer Society.

Berezin N: *After a loss in pregnancy,* New York, 1982, Fireside Books.

Borg S, Lasker J: *When pregnancy fails,* Boston, 1981, Beacon Press.

Brown L, Brown M: *When dinosaurs die: a guide to understanding death,* Boston, 1996, Little Brown.

Burns L, Ilse S: *Miscarriage: a shattered dream,* Maple Plain, Minn, 2000, Wintergreen Press.

Buscaglia L: *The fall of Freddie the leaf,* Thorofare, NJ, 1982, Slack.

Davis D: *Empty cradle, broken heart,* Golden, Colo, 2000, Fulcrum Publishing.

Eddy ML, Raydo L: *Making loving memories, a gentle guide to what you can do when baby your dies,* Omaha, Neb, 1990, Centering Corp.

Emswiler M, Emswiler J: *Guiding your child through grief,* New York, 2000, Bantam Trade.

Ferguson D: *A bunch of balloons,* Omaha, Neb, 1992, Centering Corp.

Grollman E: *Talking about death: a dialogue between parent and child,* Boston, 1990, Beacon Press.

Grollman E: *Straight talk about death to teenagers,* Boston, 1993, Beacon Press.

Harrison H: *The premature baby book,* New York, 1983, St Martin's Press.

Isle S: *Empty arms,* Maple Plain, Minn, 1996, Wintergreen Press.

Leon IC: *When a baby dies: psychotherapy for pregnancy and newborn loss,* New Haven, Conn, 1990, Yale University Press.

Linden D, Paroli E, Doron M: *The essential guide for parents of premature babies,* New York, 2000, Pocket Books.

Mellonie B, Ingpen R: *Lifetimes: the beautiful way to explain death to children,* New York, 1983, Bantam Books.

Miller S: *Finding hope when a child dies,* New York, 1999, Simon & Schuster.

National Center for Education in Maternal and Child Health: *A guide to resources in perinatal bereavement,* 1988, National Maternal and Child Health Clearing House, 38th and R Streets NW, Washington, DC 20057.

Simon N: *The saddest time,* Chicago, 1986, Whitman.

Standucher C: *Men and grief,* Oakland, Calif, 1991, New Harbinger Publications.

Tracy A, Maroney D: *Your premature baby and child,* New York, 1999, Berkley Books.

Viorst J: *The tenth good thing about Barney,* New York, 1971, Macmillan.

Wass H, Coor C: *Helping children cope with death: guidelines and resources,* Washington, DC, 1984, Hemisphere.

Wise-Brown M: *The dead bird,* Reading, Mass, 1958, Addison-Wesley.

Woods JR, Esposito JL: *Pregnancy loss: medical therapeutics and practical considerations,* Baltimore, 1987, Williams & Wilkins.

Zaichkin J: *Newborn intensive care: what every parent needs to know,* Petaluma, Calif, 1996, NICU Inc.

VIDEOS

"*What do I tell my children?*" Newton, Mass, 1990, Lifecycle Productions.

When a baby dies, LaCrosse, Wisc, 1991, Resolve Through Sharing, LaCrosse Lutheran Hospital.

NATIONAL ORGANIZATIONS

American Academy of Pediatrics: The pediatrician and childhood bereavement, *Pediatrics* 105:445, 2000.

A place to remember, de-Ruyter-Nelson Publications, Inc., 1885 University Ave., Suite 110, St Paul, MN 55104, (800) 631-0973.

Bereavement Services/RTS, 1910 South Ave, La Crosse, WI 54601, (608) 791-4747. E-mail: berservs1:hl.gundluth.org.

Centering Corp., Box 3367, Omaha, NE 68103-0367, (402) 553-1200.

Climb, Inc., Center for Losing Multiple Births, PO Box 1064, Palmer, AK 99645, (907) 746-6123.

Parents of Stillborn, 5570 South Langston Road, Seattle, WA 98718, (206) 772-5338.

SHARE Pregnancy and Infant Loss, St Joseph's Health Center, 300 First Capitol Drive, St Charles, MO 63301, (800) 821-6819.

The Compassionate Friends, Inc, PO Box 3696, Oak Brook, IL 60522-3696, (630) 990-0010.

31 Follow-up of the NICU Infant

Marilee C. Allen, Pamela K. Donohue, Margaret Porter

Even during the acute illness of their child, parents of NICU infants have concerns about how their child will do through infancy, childhood and into adulthood. As their child's convalescence begins, so does discharge planning, which brings questions about outcome to the forefront. Unfortunately, it is impossible to know the outcome of an individual infant.

In this chapter we will describe health and neurodevelopmental outcomes of NICU infants and discuss perinatal risk for the disability. We will present an approach to discharge planning, neurodevelopmental follow-up, and counseling parents of NICU infants.

There are many reasons that infants require neonatal intensive care. The most common reason is preterm birth, with its subsequent complications. Much has been published about the outcome of VLBW infants with birth weights below 1500 g.* Since 1980 the focus has been on ELBW infants with birth weights below 1000 g.[18,36,39] More recent studies have focused on the survival and outcome of even more immature infants with birth weights below 750 g (we call these the incredibly low birth weight or ILBW infants), or on infants born at the lower limit of viability (i.e., 21 to 25 weeks' gestation).† Infants with intrauterine growth restriction (IUGR) are also vulnerable to a wide range of complications requiring neonatal intensive care, especially if they are also preterm.[3,25,28] Full-term infants with meconium aspiration (MAS), persistent pulmonary hypertension of the newborn (PPHN), infection, or hypoxic-ischemic encephalopathy (HIE) also require intensive care and are at risk for health and developmental sequelae.‡ Finally, there are a number of infants with significant congenital anomalies or multiple congenital anomalies who require surgery

and/or neonatal intensive care. We will not attempt to describe the outcomes of infants with congenital anomalies, because outcome predictions are specific for each anomaly or combination of anomalies and complications that occur.[11,33]

HEALTH OUTCOMES

Many NICU infants continue to be more vulnerable to respiratory and gastrointestinal infections throughout infancy.[11,22,29,37] Infants with chronic lung disease (CLD) resulting from prematurity, pneumonia, MAS, or PPHN are particularly vulnerable to respiratory infections, especially respiratory syncytial virus (RSV).[22,30,31] Respiratory infections may be so severe that the infant may require rehospitalization, including intubation and mechanical ventilation. Ear infections are also more common in infants with CLD. Many infants require multiple medications and/or durable medical equipment (e.g., apnea monitors, nebulizers, feeding pumps, and suction) in their homes after discharge from the NICU; these needs may persist for a year or more. Infants with complex medical problems often benefit from periodic home nursing visits, and a few need shift nursing (8 to 12 hours each day) to provide their parents with time to sleep.

Nutrition and growth are often major concerns in the NICU, and these concerns continue even after NICU discharge.[22,29,37] Normal postnatal head growth is associated with good neurodevelopmental outcome. Preterm infants born at the limit of viability, infants with significant CLD and severely IUGR infants have a higher risk of poor growth, and some remain small for their age. Some infants demonstrate poor growth despite adequate intake, probably because of increased metabolic needs. Inadequate intake can result from oromotor dysfunction or food refusal. Some infants have such severe feeding problems with poor growth or a dysfunctional swallow that they require gastrostomy feedings. (These are often infants born at the limit of viability, with severe CLD or with cerebral palsy.)

---

*References 3, 8, 17, 22, 38, 39.
†References 6, 16, 21, 26, 37, 43.
‡References 19, 24, 27, 32, 34, 40.

THE NEURODEVELOPMENTAL DISABILITIES

The World Health Organization (WHO) has differentiated among the words *impairment, disability,* and *handicap*[44]:

- A structural, psychologic, or physical abnormality is an **impairment.**
- An inability to perform normally or a restriction in daily activity is a **disability.**
- A disadvantage in society because of a disability is a **handicap.**

The neurodevelopmental disabilities are a group of chronic, nonprogressive disorders of central nervous system (CNS) function that occur as result of malformation of or insult to the developing brain.[12] There is a spectrum of neurodevelopmental disabilities, from the major disabilities, to sensory impairments, to the more subtle disorders of higher cortical functioning (Box 31-1).

Cerebral Palsy

Cerebral palsy (CP) is a motor impairment, a disorder of movement and posture that results from injury to or malformation of the developing brain.[12] It is difficult to diagnose CP with any degree of certainty before 6 to 12 months of age, and it sometimes takes until the child is 18 to 24 months before the diagnosis is certain. Diagnosis of CP is made when there are persistent neuromotor abnormalities on examination and impaired motor function. Delay in motor milestone attainment is a manifestation of motor impairment, as is deviant (i.e., nonsequential) motor milestone attainment.

CP can be classified as to physiologic type, topography (i.e., muscle groups involved), and severity[12] (see Box 31-1). Persistently increased muscle tone and increased deep tendon reflexes with persistence of pathologic reflexes (e.g., Babinski) are signs of spasticity. Joint contractures and hip dislocation are major problems seen in children with spastic CP. Variable tone with persistent primitive reflexes, often with involuntary movements, are signs of extrapyramidal CP. It may take until the child is 2 to 3 years old before involuntary movements are seen. Children who manifest signs of both spasticity and extrapyramidal CP have mixed CP. Extrapyramidal CP is generalized, but spasticity should be further typed according to which limbs are most significantly involved.

Spastic diplegia, the most common form of CP in preterm infants, is characterized by spasticity in both lower extremities, with mild or minimal involvement of the upper extremities.[12] Spastic hemiplegia is characterized by involvement of one side of the body, with the upper extremity more involved than the lower. Because intrauterine and perinatal strokes are usually unilateral, children who had strokes often demonstrate spastic hemiplegia. Quadriplegia is the most severe form of spastic CP, with both upper and lower extremities involved, the lower more than the uppers. Children who had HIE who develop CP are most likely to have spastic quadriplegia or severe mixed CP.

Physiologic and topographic forms of CP can be further classified as to severity.[12,44] The more severe the CP, the earlier it can be diagnosed. Children with profound CP are completely dependent on others for care. Children with severe CP may require power wheelchairs for mobility and other forms of adaptive technology. Children with moderate CP are generally able to sit without assistance but require assistance for mobility and self-help skills. Many outcomes researchers now report motor disability in terms of disabling CP, referring to children with moderate, severe or profound CP.

Children with mild CP have delay or deviant (i.e., nonsequential) motor milestones, and often benefit from physical and occupational therapy and other CP interventions (e.g., orthotics, botox injections, orthopedic surgery). Nevertheless, children with mild CP are often quite functional by midchildhood.[12] Because it is difficult to distinguish be-

---

Box 31-1	**NEURODEVELOPMENTAL DISABILITIES**

I. Major disability
   Cerebral palsy (CP)
   Mental retardation (MR)
II. Sensory impairment
   Hearing impairment
   Visual impairment
III. Subtle disorders of higher cortical function
   Language delay or disorder
      Expressive language delay
      Receptive and expressive language delay
   Minor neuromotor dysfunction
      Fine motor incoordination
      Sensorimotor integration problems
   Learning disability
      Variable cognitive abilities
      Visual-perceptual problems
   Behavior problems
      Attention deficit disorder (ADD)
      Attention deficit hyperactivity disorder (ADHD)
      Emotional lability

tween mild CP and minor neuromotor dysfunction (MND, mild motor impairment, sometimes called minimal CP), in younger children, many researchers report only disabling CP. Because of their increased risk for cognitive and other associated deficits, children who present with motor delay need a comprehensive evaluation that includes neuropsychologic testing.

Mental Retardation

Mental retardation (MR) is a global impairment of cognitive functioning resulting from injury to or malformation of the developing brain, which impairs the child's ability to adapt and function in society.[12,44] MR frequently presents with a delay in language and problem solving abilities, and its diagnosis MR requires a comprehensive evaluation of the child, with neuropsychologic testing and assessment of adaptive abilities. Although it rarely occurs, a child with a low score on an intelligence test but normal adaptive functioning would not be diagnosed with MR.

Neuropsychologic testing includes an assessment of a child's intelligence quotient (IQ), or in younger children, their developmental quotient (DQ) or mental developmental index (MDI). Intelligence is not one entity, but many different abilities, including auditory and visual memory, visual-perceptual abilities and understanding complex language concepts. The older the child is, the more abilities can be tested and therefore the more accurate the tests are in assessing intelligence. Intelligence tests for school-age children and adults consist of a variety of subtests. Most children with MR have lower abilities for age across the board, so that severity of MR is easily classified. Many preterm children have a significant variability in cognitive abilities, with high scores on some subtests and low scores on others, which makes them more difficult to classify and to teach.

MR is classified in terms of severity, from profound (IQ below 20), to severe (IQ 20 to 34), to moderate (IQ 35 to 49), to mild (IQ 50 to 70).[44] Children with severe to profound MR generally need assistance with basic self-help skills, whereas children with moderate MR can learn basic self-help skills and as adults work in sheltered workshops. Children with mild MR can learn basic academic skills and as adults may work in low level jobs. Children with an IQ of 70 to 80 or 85 have borderline intelligence, not MR. They are capable of academic learning, but may have trouble keeping up with their class. The most important quality that enhances adult functioning of children with cognitive impairments is their skill at interpersonal relationships and their ability to communicate.

Sensory Impairments

Hearing impairment occurs in 1% to 10% of NICU infants.[3,12,27] Many states require hearing screening for all newborns, using either auditory evoked responses or transient evoked otoacoustic emissions. All NICU infants should have their hearing screened before discharge. Because of the risk of progressive hearing impairment, infants with congenital cytomegalovirus (CMV) infection and infants with PPHN should have serial hearing evaluations during infancy and early childhood (as should infants with recurrent ear infections).[1,12,27,33]

Neonates demonstrate hearing thresholds similar to older children and adults. Even preterm infants as early as 24 to 25 weeks' gestation demonstrate an immature brainstem waveform in response to sound stimuli, although the pattern of the waveform matures to a normal waveform. Infants hear and process language throughout their first year, beginning at birth. Recognizing a hearing impairment early, with appropriate early interventions (e.g., hearing aides, total communication approach to language) is crucial for optimal language development in infants.

Retinopathy of prematurity (ROP) results from injury to the very immature developing retina, which causes abnormal proliferation of vessels. Ophthalmologists need to carefully examine the retinas (especially in the periphery) of preterm infants serially until their retina is fully vascularized. Severe ROP, which tends to occur in the most immature and sickest preterm infants, is treated with laser to try to prevent retinal detachment and blindness. Preterm infants may develop severe myopia (i.e., nearsightedness), strabismus, cataracts, and glaucoma.

Infants with congenital CMV or toxoplasmosis infection should be examined by ophthalmologists for chorioretinitis. Neonates symptomatic with congenital infection (i.e., CMV, rubella, or toxoplasmosis) have a high risk (e.g., 20% to 30%) of visual and/or hearing impairment.[1] If infants with HIE develop disability, they tend to have severe multiple disabilities, including cortical blindness and hearing impairment.[24] Cortical blindness is sometimes difficult to diagnose in infants with severe to profound MR. Failure to blink in response to a visual threatening gesture may be the result of a mental age below 2 to 3 months rather than visual impairment.

Subtle Disorders of Higher Cortical Function

Even if the NICU infant does not develop major disability or sensory impairment, he or she has an increased risk of the more subtle disorders of higher cortical function* (see Box 31-1). These disorders, because they are milder than the major disabilities, may not present in infancy or may present in infancy with nonspecific symptoms (e.g., irritability, posturing, feeding problems). Any given child may manifest only one dysfunction, or any combination of them. Diagnostic criteria, and even nomenclature, for these disorders vary so widely that preschool and school-age outcome studies require a comparison group followed and evaluated in the identical manner.

Language delay may present as early as 6 to 12 months as delay or deviance (i.e., nonsequential) in language milestone acquisition.[12,13] Expressive language delay, either alone or in combination with receptive language delay, is common in preterm and other NICU infants. Every child who presents with delayed language should have a hearing test and neuropsychologic testing to distinguish between language disorder, hearing impairment, and mental retardation. Even if the child appears to respond to the sound, he or she may not hear speech distinctly enough to be able to understand it or mimic it well.

Minor neuromotor dysfunction (MND) is generally manifested the earliest, presenting as mild delay or deviant motor milestone acquisition in conjunction with mild or transient neuromotor abnormalities.[3,12,14,41] These are children who sit by 1 year of age and walk by 2 years, although they may have an abnormal gait (e.g., toe-walking, persistent wide base, dragging one leg, significant overflow movements). This mild motor impairment has also been called *minimal CP* and the *clumsy child syndrome.* These children generally look normal by 3 to 5 years of age, although they may continue to have some balance or motor planning problems. Introducing these children to a variety of sports is beneficial, as long as performance in the sport is not valued above the child's self-esteem.

Fine-motor incoordination, visual-perceptual deficits, and sensorimotor inefficiencies may accompany MND, but they may not be recognized until preschool-age.[3,12,36,41] Visual-perceptual deficits, often in combination with fine-motor incoordination, are manifest by an inability or difficulty with recognizing and copying figures, letters and num-

bers, completing puzzles and mazes, and/or copying block designs. Fine-motor incoordination makes it difficult to button, zip, cut with scissors, draw, and write. Introducing these children early to a computer and keyboard helps them compensate if their writing is illegible. Sensorimotor inefficiencies are characterized by difficulty following directions that include demonstrating an action (e.g., tying shoelaces) and tolerating motion through space (e.g., swinging on a swing) or different tactile sensations (clothing or food textures). For children with MND, fine-motor incoordination and/or sensorimotor inefficiencies, failures in school and on the playground erode self-esteem and peer relationships. The greatest challenge for their parents and teachers is to help preserve the child's self-esteem.

Language disorder, visual-perceptual problems, MND, transient neuromotor dysfunction and variable cognitive abilities are all associated with later learning disability (LD) and other school problems.* LD means difficulty learning one or more academic subjects (reading, writing, arithmetic) in children with normal intelligence who have had adequate exposure to school. Some children have more of a *learning inefficiency,* in that they do well in the early grades of school, but they have a relative inefficiency in reading or writing that gets them into trouble as the work becomes more complex. Their intelligence and resiliency helps them to make adaptations in learning, but they become overwhelmed in situations in which speed and accuracy are viewed as important.

Behavior problems are more frequent in preterm and other NICU children.[3,12,21,34] Some children have attention deficit disorder (ADD), characterized by marked distractibility, short attention span, and impulsivity. ADD can occur with or without hyperactivity: the child may be restless, always on the move, constantly busy (i.e., ADHD) or may just demonstrate difficulty paying attention and impulsiveness (i.e., ADD). Other children demonstrate behavior problems characterized by noncompliance, aggression, opposition-defiance, or emotional lability. Emotional lability can be disabling: the child may be so moody that it interferes with peer relationships and school performance.

It is important to recognize these more subtle problems as soon as possible. Counseling parents and teachers can prevent the devastating effect these "mild" disabilities have on self-esteem, peer relationships, and performance at school and at home.[10] Early

---

*References 3, 12, 25, 28, 29, 31, 34, 39, 41.

*References 3, 12, 36, 38, 39, 41.

detection and intervention aims not only to improve the child's ability to function, but also to encourage activities that improve the child's self-esteem. The social and emotional complications can be prevented by improving the child's ability to cope with the demands of school and playground and by providing the child with a network of supports.

Diagnosis of Disability

CP and MND may be recognized and diagnosed in the first 2 years after birth. MR may present as language delay in infancy, but it may take 1 to 2 years to make a definitive diagnosis, especially if the child also has CP. The more severe the CP or MR, the sooner it may be recognized and diagnosed. Occasionally a child may have significant motor delay initially but seems to "catch up" by 1 to 2 years, with concomitant improvement in neuromotor abnormalities. These children are often children with ongoing health problems (e.g., chronic lung disease), and end up with just a diagnosis of MND. Language disorders, visual-perceptual difficulties and fine-motor incoordination are generally recognized and diagnosed during the preschool years (ages 3 to 5). LD can not be diagnosed until school-age. Mild LD or learning inefficiencies may not be recognized until middle school or high school.

Because there is so much overlap among the neurodevelopmental disabilities, whenever abnormality in one area is detected, the child should have a com-prehensive, multidisciplinary evaluation of all his or her abilities. The classic example of this is the child who presents with delayed walking and a tendency to be up on her toes. In the past, she might have been seen in an orthopedic clinic, and perhaps been referred for physical therapy and ankle-foot orthotics (AFOs). Once she was walking normally, her parents would be reassured that she is fine. Her mild motor impairment is a signal that she may have other disabilities (e.g., LD, ADD) that will prove to be far more handicapping in her life in school and in society.

PERINATAL RISK FACTORS FOR NEURODEVELOPMENTAL DISABILITY

Many conditions that require neonatal intensive care also increase risk for neurodevelopmental disability, including prematurity, persistent pulmonary hypertension of the newborn, hypoxic-ischemic encephalopathy, and IUGR.[2,3,12,42] Although many perinatal risk factors have been identified, none allows diagnosis of neurodevelopmental disability in the neonatal period. Perinatal and demographic risk factors can be used to identify NICU infants with a high risk of neurodevelopmental disability, so that they can be followed closely and referred for comprehensive evaluations and early intervention programs when appropriate (Box 31-2).[2,3,12,42]

Box 31-2	PERINATAL RISK FACTORS
Prematurity	Prolonged prenatal/perinatal/neonatal asphyxia
	Cardiopulmonary resuscitation
	Intraventricular hemorrhage (IVH)
	Intraparenchymal hemorrhage or infarction
	Intraparenchymal cysts/periventricular leukomalacia (PVL)
	Neonatal seizures or symptoms of hypoxic-ischemic encephalopathy (HIE)
	Intrauterine growth restriction (IUGR)
	Poor postnatal nutrition and growth
	Congenital anomalies
	Chronic lung disease (CLD)
	Sepsis or meningitis
	Abnormal neonatal neurodevelopmental examination
Intrauterine growth restriction (IUGR)	Early IUGR (beginning in second trimester or early in third trimester)
	Microcephaly
	Congenital anomalies
	Polycythemia/Hyperviscosity, especially if symptomatic
	Congenital infections symptomatic at birth (e.g., toxoplasmosis, cytomegalovirus [CMV], rubella)
	Maternal ingestions (e.g., alcohol, phenytoin, heroin, cocaine)
	Perinatal asphyxia with symptoms of hypoxic-ischemic encephalopathy (HIE)
	Abnormal neonatal neurodevelopmental examination

Continued

Box 31-2	PERINATAL RISK FACTORS—cont'd
Hypoxic-ischemic encephalopathy (HIE)	Prolonged prenatal/perinatal asphyxia Cardiopulmonary resuscitation Prolonged moderate (stage 2) or severe (stage 3) HIE[32,34] Neonatal seizures Congenital anomalies, especially developmental brain malformations (e.g., schizen- cephaly, lissencephaly) Encephalomalacia or other neuroimaging abnormalities Significantly abnormal EEG (e.g., burst-suppression or low voltage) Abnormal neonatal neurodevelopmental examination
Persistent pulmonary hypertension of the newborn (PPHN) and/or meconium aspiration syndrome (MAS)	Prolonged prenatal/perinatal/neonatal asphyxia Cardiopulmonary resuscitation Symptoms of moderate or severe HIE Congenital anomalies, especially congenital diaphragmatic hernia (CDH) Low birth weight/SGA/IUGR Chronic lung disease (CLD) Sepsis or meningitis Abnormal neuroimaging study Abnormal neurodevelopmental examination

Risk does not imply causation; it is merely a marker of brain injury. Intraventricular hemorrhage (IVH) is a marker of brain injury; therefore it is an important risk factor in preterm infants.[2,35,42] Brain plasticity in newborns allows another area of the brain to take over the function of the injured area. On the other hand, the IVH that is seen may be only a small part, with a large unseen area of brain injury.

There is a great deal of variability in how predictive individual risk factors are of neurodevelopmental outcome.* Very low Apgar scores, especially at 5 to 10 minutes or more after birth, are associated with later CP. These low Apgar scores are signs of severe perinatal depression. However, the signs and symptoms of HIE predict CP far better than low Apgar scores. Even within a risk factor category, the degree of risk can vary. Infants who are symptomatic with congenital cytomegalovirus (CMV) infection at birth are far more likely to develop CP, MR, and sensory impairment than infants who are asymptomatic at birth with congenital CMV infection.[1]

Multiple risk factors increase an infant's risk of neurodevelopmental disability, and the effects may be more than additive.† As a group, preterm infants or full-term infants with IUGR tend to have lower mean intelligence quotients than full-term AGA infants. Infants with both prematurity and IUGR are vulnerable to the complications of each condition. These effects of prematurity and IUGR on IQ are far more pronounced in children from lower socioeconomic status (SES) than in children of higher or moderate SES.

NEURODEVELOPMENTAL OUTCOMES

In this section we will summarize reported neurodevelopmental outcomes for some of the most frequent conditions that require neonatal intensive care. Box 31-2 lists some of the risk factors for neurodevelopmental disability that have been reported in each condition. This is only a partial list that focuses on the most important or studied risk factors. We have not attempted to describe the neurodevelopmental outcome of another frequent cause for neonatal intensive care—congenital anomalies or malformations. This is a very large and somewhat understudied group. For the most part, outcome for this group is viewed in terms of what combinations of anomalies an individual infant has, what complications the infant encountered, and whether brain injury was apparent while the child was in the NICU. There are only a few scattered reports of neurodevelopmental outcome for some of the major congenital anomalies (e.g., some types of congenital heart disease and congenital diaphragmatic hernia). Even when congenital anomalies occur in the absence of chromosomal abnormalities, recognized dysmorphic syndrome or identified brain injury or malformation, there is an increased risk of neurodevelopmental abnormalities, especially in preterm or IUGR children.[15]

---

*References 2, 3, 12, 15, 25, 28, 42.
†References 2, 3, 12, 15, 25, 28, 42.

Prematurity

For more than 50 years there have been reports in the medical literature that describe the neurodevelopmental outcome of preterm VLBW infants (birth weight less than 1500 g). With the beginning of neonatal intensive care in the mid-1960s, a number of tertiary care NICUs reported the incidence or prevalence of major disability (i.e., CP and MR) in their VLBW infants. A meta-analysis of 110 studies published between 1960 and 1990 reported a median incidence of CP in 7.7% of VLBW infants (with a range of 0% to 50%).[17] More recent studies report that 5% to 14% of VLBW infants develop CP and 4% to 8% develop MR.[3] Hearing impairment occurs in 0.1% to 5.4% and visual impairment in 0.1% to 5.5%. Multiple disabilities occur in 1.2% to 4.5% of VLBW infants and in 14% to 16% of infants with birth weights of less than 800 g. One reason for the variability in reported incidences (beyond the fact that different populations are studied and neonatal intensive care practices vary by location and time) is that different outcome studies use different definitions of disability (e.g., whether they include children with mild CP or children with borderline intelligence) and follow children to different ages.

Although the mortality rate rises with lower gestational age and birth weight, there does not seem to be a similar rise with incidence or prevalence of neurodevelopmental disability until the limit of viability.* There have been a few reported survivors born at 21 or 22 weeks' gestation or at 300 to 500 g birth weight. (Usually it is the bigger infant of 21 to 22 weeks' gestation and the more mature but severely IUGR infant who survive at these limits.) Few, if any, of the survivors at these extremes have been reported as demonstrating normal development. Most neonatologists consider 23 to 24 weeks of gestation and 500 to 600 g birth weight to be the lower limit of viability. Outcome studies on these infants have found a much higher incidence of major disability in infants born at the limit of viability than in VLBW infants. A recent outcome study of infants born at 21 to 25 weeks' gestation in Great Britain reported that approximately half had major disability on follow-up to 2 years.[43]

VLBW children demonstrate a normal range of intelligence, with some having above-average to superior IQs. A meta-analysis of cognitive outcomes published in 1989 found that preterm children (when all reported birth weight groups were included) had a mean IQ that was 6 points lower than that of full-term control children.[8] Although a difference of 6 IQ points is not clinically meaningful, they represent the fact that there are more preterm children with MR, borderline, and low-average intelligence than is found among full-term children. A number of studies of school-age outcomes have found that 5% to 48% of VLBW children had school problems, including learning disability, failed grades or requiring special education.[3,36] Studies that have compared the outcomes of normally intelligent VLBW children with full-term control subjects have found that VLBW children have more language delay, more visual-perceptual problems, lower reading quotients, greater difficulty with arithmetic, and more problems with attention and behavior.[3,36] More children with incredibly low birth weight (less than 750 g) have these disorders of higher cortical function than bigger preterm infants with birth weights 750 to 1500 g.[21]

Intrauterine Growth Restriction

The neurodevelopmental outcome of IUGR infants is determined by the cause of IUGR, by the timing, severity, and duration of the insult, and by perinatal complications the IUGR infant encounters.[1] Early severe IUGR often reflects a chromosomal anomaly, other severe genetic disorder, or congenital infection that occurred early to cause organ malformation or significant injury. Some causes of IUGR cause death (e.g., trisomy 18) or severe disability (e.g., Smith-Lemli-Opitz syndrome). Some carry a high risk of neurodevelopmental disability (e.g., fetal alcohol syndrome). Others are associated with only mild disability (e.g., an increased incidence of attention and behavior problems in infants born to mothers who took narcotics or cocaine during pregnancy). Infants who are small for gestational age because of small maternal size generally have normal neurodevelopmental outcome, although they may still be at risk for medical problems (e.g., hypertension, heart disease) in adulthood.

One of the most common causes of IUGR is uteroplacental insufficiency; this is generally a diagnosis of exclusion. The fetus responds in many adaptive ways when the supply of nutrients and/or oxygen is limited. There is first a decrease in subcutaneous tissue, resulting in lower birth weight, then a decrease in length, before head and brain growth are affected. Nevertheless, the problem may be severe enough to overwhelm these adaptations and lead to brain injury, then fetal death. In addition, a chronically compromised fetus, with decreased

---

*References 3, 6, 16, 18, 20, 26, 37, 43.

glycogen and nutrient stores, has more difficulty with the stresses of labor and delivery, leading to perinatal depression or asphyxia, cold stress, hypoglycemia and hypocalcemia. Polycythemia may result from chronic intrauterine hypoxia but may lead to the complications of hyperviscosity, with resulting brain injury.

Prospective studies of full-term IUGR infants do not show an increased risk for major disability, but retrospective studies of CP and MR have demonstrated that more disabled children were IUGR than expected.[1] Prospective studies of full-term IUGR school-age children compared with full-term AGA children showed that more IUGR children had language problems, learning disability, minor neuromotor dysfunction, hyperactivity, and attention and behavior problems.

Preterm IUGR children demonstrate the disadvantages of both prematurity and IUGR, and we can assume the IUGR is more severe because it occurred so early in gestation. When preterm IUGR infants are compared with AGA control subjects matched for gestational age, the IUGR children demonstrate more motor impairments, lower cognitive scores, and more attention problems.[1,25,28] Preterm IUGR infants have neurodevelopmental outcomes similar to preterm AGA infants matched for birth weights. This is especially important at the limit of viability: the preterm IUGR infant with gestational age of 28 weeks and birth weight of 550 g will have the same high incidence of neurodevelopmental disability as other preterm infants with birth weights of 500 to 600 g. Preterm IUGR infants without neurodevelopmental disability also have a high incidence of the more subtle disorders of higher cortical function.

Hypoxic-Ischemic Encephalopathy

The extent and nature of an asphyxiating insult cannot be determined for individual infants, so we rely on recognizable signs and symptoms of asphyxia to predict outcome.[3,24,34] Initial predictions were based on low Apgar scores (0 to 3 at 10 or 20 minutes), the need for positive pressure ventilation (for 1 minute or more), the need for cardiopulmonary resuscitation or the response to resuscitation (e.g., no heart rate at 5 minutes or no spontaneous respirations at 20 minutes). These risk factors carried a 2% to 25% risk of disability (usually severe multiple disabilities). The striking finding was that the majority (75% to 98%) of children with these severe risk factors did not develop major disability. Certain signs and symptoms of asphyxia (e.g., hypoto-

nia followed by extensor hypertonia) carried a higher risk of disability, especially when there were multiple signs and symptoms.

Many infants with congenital brain malformations or prenatal brain injury may present with perinatal depression: they do not breathe normally at birth and may require positive pressure ventilation or further resuscitation. These infants should be distinguished from the infants with HIE caused by an asphyxiating insult. In addition, infants with some inborn errors of metabolism may present with neurologic or nonspecific generalized symptoms that suggest asphyxia or infection.

In 1976 Sarnat and Sarnat published a landmark article that described three stages of HIE, and subsequent papers have shown these stages to be most predictive of outcome.[34] Infants with severe stage 3 HIE (coma, severe hypotonia or increased extensor tone, intermittent decerebration, decreased or absent reflexes, variable pupil reactivity, and abnormal EEG) either died or had severe multiple disabilities. Only 20% to 30% of infants with moderate stage 2 HIE (lethargy or coma, mild hypotonia, overactive reflexes, seizures, abnormal EEG and generalized parasympathetic function-constricted pupils, bradycardia, profuse secretions, and diarrhea) had severe multiple disabilities. The remainder had lower scores on tests of cognition, vocabulary, reading, spelling, arithmetic, and spelling than children with mild stage 1 HIE (hyperalert state, with jitteriness, overactive and easily elicited reflexes, increased sympathetic function, dilated pupils, and decreased gastrointestinal motility) or healthy control children.

Infants with symptoms of HIE should have both an EEG and neuroimaging study (e.g., head CT scan or MRI). Very low voltage EEG patterns (signifying little brain activity) and burst-suppression EEG patterns carry an extremely poor prognosis. Diffuse encephalomalacia is associated with a high risk of severe multiple disabilities. Mild HIE with only a subarachnoid hemorrhage carries a good prognosis.

Persistent Pulmonary Hypertension of the Newborn/Meconium Aspiration Syndrome

Persistent pulmonary hypertension of the newborn (PPHN) and meconium aspiration syndrome (MAS) often overlap clinically, and outcome studies report a high risk (13% to 24%) of major disability.[3,27,32,40] Up to 30% of children with PPHN have mild impairments, including minor neuromotor dysfunction, borderline intelligence and attention problems. Both CLD and hearing impairment are common sequelae: 7% to 35% of children had CLD and 20% to 50% had hearing impairment. Because the hearing impairment may be progressive, PPHN requires serial hearing evaluations during infancy and early childhood.

Many infants with PPHN and/or MAS require extracorporeal membrane oxygenation (ECMO) as a lifesaving intervention. Survivors of ECMO have a 2% to 26% incidence of major disability and a 3% to 21% incidence of hearing impairment.[3,32] Borderline intelligence, language delay, visual impairment, and minor neuromotor dysfunction occur in 8% to 49% of ECMO survivors. In a population of ECMO survivors evaluated at age 5, 5% had CP (most had mild CP) and 11% had MR (1% had severe MR). The mean IQ score for ECMO children was lower than that of 37 healthy control subjects (96 versus 115; $p <0.001$). CLD occurs in 7% to 40% of infants treated with ECMO, and in 63% with congenital diaphragmatic hernia requiring ECMO.[32]

NEURODEVELOPMENTAL FOLLOW-UP OF THE HIGH-RISK INFANT

Under ideal conditions parents of all NICU infants should be offered comprehensive, coordinated, developmentally based, family-oriented follow-up for their infant through infancy and childhood. Each NICU infant is unique, as is each infant's family. The primary goals of follow-up are (1) to counsel the child's family about their child's development so that they are empowered to optimize their child's health, growth, and development, (2) to recognize and diagnose significant health conditions and neurodevelopmental disabilities early, so as to facilitate appropriate referrals for community services and monitoring provision of those services, and (3) to anticipate future difficulties and needs so that optimal development can be promoted and secondary complications can be avoided or minimized. The ultimate goal is to promote the child's integration into the family, school, and community.

Follow-up resources are generally limited, however, and today insurance and managed care organizations frequently dictate who can be followed. Consequently, criteria for referral of high-risk NICU infants vary widely. Some high-risk infants are routinely referred to state-run early intervention programs without a recognition of the importance of monitoring the child's development, anticipating and planning for future needs, and counseling parents along the way. The dynamics of developmental follow-up are such that periodic assessments of the child's health and development are needed to determine whether current interventions are effective and sufficient. Parents often need guidance to better understand what to expect from their child, how to interpret their own observations of their child, and how health care and community services can support their child's development.

Developmental Milestone Attainment

In developmentally based follow-up, much of the information about the child's development comes from a careful interview of the parent regarding the child's health status and developmental milestone attainment.[3,9,12-14] Noting the age of acquisition of the gross-motor, fine-motor, language, and self-help milestones helps to determine developmental delay, as long as the interviewer asks the questions in a clear and defined (i.e., standard) manner. Parents are very good historians about their child's current functioning and recent accomplishments, which is why eliciting a history of developmental milestone attainment during serial clinic visits is so useful in assessing a child's rate of development. Sometimes additional explanation may be needed in order to determine age of milestone acquisition. For example, to the parent of a very young or delayed child, sitting independently may mean being propped up on a couch surrounded by pillows. Sitting independently actually means sitting in the middle of the floor for at least a minute without anything to aid the child.

Additional explanations or clarifications of the milestones are even more important for the language milestones.[9,13] The first (meaningful) word, an 11-month activity, is when the child says a word that the family understands to mean something (not including proper names). It does not matter if others do not understand the child , or even what the word is, as long as it is used to communicate an idea. Attainment of a social smile is not the first time the parents see their baby smile, but when they can elicit a smile by talking, playing with, or tickling the child (generally by 6 to 8 weeks). Cooing is distinguished from babbling: cooing is vocalization of the vowel sounds (a 3-month activity) and babbling (a 6-month activity) is the repetition of consonant sounds.

Delay in language and self-help milestones raises concerns about MR, language disorder, and/or hearing impairment.[3,12] Every child with delayed language should have his or her hearing evaluated and should receive a cognitive evaluation. Many developmental follow-up clinics rely on neuropsychologists to assess the cognition of high-risk infants, either with sequential assessments or with one assessment at a specific time (e.g., at 18 months). The most commonly used infant cognitive test is the Bayley Scales of Infant Development. Pediatricians tend to use the CAT/CLAMS or the Gesell Development Schedules. For preschool-age and school-age children, several cognitive tests are available, including the Wechsler Preschool and Primary Scale of Intelligence (WPPSI), the Wechsler Intelligence Scale for Children (WISC), the Stanford-Binet Intelligence Scale, the Kaufman Assessment Battery for Children (K-ABC), and the McCarthy Scales of Children's Abilities.

Correction for Degree of Prematurity

One controversy that arises when following preterm infants is whether to correct for degree of prematurity (i.e., whether to use the child's chronologic age, calculated from birth, or use age corrected for degree of prematurity, calculated from the date the infant was due to be born).[3,4,9,12] This problem is most significant in extremely preterm infants early in their first year. For example, if a 6-month-old child born at 27 weeks' gestation is developmentally at the 3-month level, she is demonstrating significant delay if she is viewed as a 6-month old, but is developing right on time if she is viewed as a 3-month-old. By the time she is 5 years old, it is less important: no one distinguishes between a 57-month-old and a 60-month-old.

The answer is most definitive for motor milestones.[5] When correcting for degree of prematurity, populations of normal VLBW infants attain motor milestones at the same ages as full-term infants. When using motor milestones in VLBW infants, using age corrected for degree of prematurity and using the criteria of 50% delay make the most effective screen for CP (i.e., better specificity and positive predictive values). Infants who demonstrate significant delay in motor milestone attainment should be referred for a comprehensive neurodevelopmental examination and multidisciplinary evaluation.

The question is more controversial for language milestone attainment and performance on cognitive testing in extremely preterm infants.[3,9,12] Most psychologists and neurodevelopmental pediatricians correct for degree of prematurity in early infancy, although some only partially correct (e.g., correct for half the difference between gestational age at birth and 40 weeks' gestation), and some correct for only one or two years because they are concerned that full correction overestimates the child's cogni-

tive abilities and fails to identify infants who would benefit from community services.

Neurodevelopmental Examination

For high-risk infants the neurologic examination is expanded to include a detailed assessment of posture, muscle tone, reflexes, postural reactions, and functional abilities.[12] Interpretation of the examination requires a thorough understanding of the normal pattern of development over time, the examiner's skill at assessing the infant's performance, recognizing deviations from the norm and determining the significance of these findings.

Abnormalities of posture, muscle tone, and reflexes are common in preterm and other high-risk NICU infants during the first year. These abnormalities include asymmetries, marked extensor tone through the neck and trunk with significant shoulder retraction or elevation, hypotonia, and lower extremity hypertonia and hyperreflexia, especially at the ankles. CP should be considered in infants with persistent neuromotor abnormalities and motor delay. Mild delay and neuromotor abnormalities suggest MND. For many preterm infants these findings can no longer be elicited at 1 year. Preterm children who demonstrated neuromotor abnormalities during their first year are at risk for school and behavior problems, whether or not the abnormalities persist.[38,42]

PARENT TEACHING

When a newborn requires intensive care hospitalization, the parents are typically overwhelmed and frightened. The same is true at discharge. Although parents may have asked since admission, "When can my baby come home?" the reality of assuming care for a child who has been surrounded by health care providers and high-technology equipment for several weeks can be daunting.

An organized, well-implemented discharge plan is the beginning of successful follow-up of a NICU graduate. A multidisciplinary team approach uses the expertise of many disciplines to formulate and implement the discharge and follow-up plan. The team can be composed of a variety of individuals, depending on the resources of the NICU.

Physicians, nurses, case managers, and social workers can all play an important part in the discharge process. The infant's hospitalization is more likely to be considered successful by the family if the discharge plan proceeds smoothly, even if the child had significant medical complications.[23]

The key to successful discharge and follow-up is early and active involvement by the family. Participation in the discharge process contributes to the parent's education about their child's medical condition and may give them more self-confidence in their ability to care for their child at home. It also gives them the opportunity to work with community agencies and/or providers who will care for their child after discharge.

Families may react to the impeding discharge in various ways. Some openly seek information and guidance from NICU caregivers; others do not. Regardless of communication style, parents need to appreciate the "big picture." Counseling parents in an open and truthful way about their child's past medical history, prognosis and ongoing needs will help them have realistic expectations.

Clearly defined discharge criteria provide both the family and staff a point of reference from which to judge the child's progress. Discharge criteria should be reviewed in a multidisciplinary team meeting with the family. Setting goals the child, parents, and staff must accomplish before discharge help keep everyone focused and prevents important components of the discharge process from being overlooked. Parents should be encouraged to invite family members and friends to this meeting. A support network for the family is crucial to a smooth transition for the child from the hospital to the home environment.

Before discharge parents need to consider health insurance coverage for the baby. They often need advice about how to add the baby to one or both parents' commercial policies or to apply for medical assistance. It is important to begin this process as soon as possible after the infant is born, to avoid missing any deadlines for enrollment (which vary by employer or payor). Also, the enrollment process may take several weeks to complete, and coverage will need to be in place before discharge, transfer, or home care arrangements can be made.

Once insurance coverage is settled, parents should be encouraged to identify a follow-up primary care pediatrician. Early identification of a pediatrician gives the NICU staff the opportunity to have ongoing communication with the physician, which allows for continuity of care once the child goes home. If parents need help choosing a pediatrician they should be encouraged to interview potential providers. During the interview process parents should ask questions concerning hours the pediatric practice is open (evenings and weekends), what happens if the child needs to be seen when the practice is closed, the availability of the pediatrician for telephone consultation, and with which hospital or hospitals the pediatrician is affiliated. Because a good working relationship between parents and pediatrician is invaluable, parents should choose a physician with whom they can develop a healthy rapport.

Some infants are not discharged from the NICU home but are transferred to another unit or facility for postacute care. In this era of managed care, it is often not considered an appropriate use of resources for an infant to remain hospitalized in a tertiary care unit until discharge. Although driven by reimbursement, transfer to postacute care may be beneficial to families. Postacute care facilities are often available closer to the parents' home (especially if the NICU is part of a regional referral center) and may provide a more homelike setting. Possible locations for postacute care should be discussed with the parents, as well as the criteria for transfer. Families are often reluctant to leave the NICU environment once a trusting relationship has been established with caregivers and the NICU routine has become familiar. Parents should be counseled about the infant's changing needs and how postacute care facilities can provide beneficial services that are not possible in an acute care setting (e.g., parents rooming-in with the child). Transfer to a lower level of care should be presented early in the hospitalization as an expected milestone along the way to going home. The primary care pediatrician can also help to alleviate parental fears concerning transfer, particularly if the child is being transported back to the home community.

All applicable screening and preventive care must be complete before discharge, and the dates and results should be communicated to the primary care pediatrician and the parents. The American Academy of Pediatrics (AAP) has policy statements concerning planning for NICU discharge and many recommendations regarding screening on their website: www.aap.org.

Metabolic Screening

Although healthy, full-term newborns are often not screened for metabolic disorders (such as phenylketonuria) until discharge from the hospital, initial screening of sick or premature infants should be performed as soon as possible after birth, before the administration of blood or antibiotics. Although it is common for these infants to have some relatively abnormal results—especially to thyroid function tests—compared with their healthy counterparts, early screening is recommended to identify, in a timely manner, those rare infants who truly have a metabolic disorder. Subsequent screenings should take place according to an established routine, depending on state requirements, to be sure that the infant is approaching normal values. If the infant is not on full feedings or is very ill when the last scheduled screening is performed, it may take longer for the values to return to normal. Additional specimens may be necessary to determine whether treatment is required.

Hearing Screening

All infants, especially those who have required NICU admission, should be screened for hearing loss using otoacoustic emissions (OAE) or auditory brainstem response (ABR) testing. This screening should be performed once the infant is medically stable and at least 33 weeks' postmenstrual age, preferably before discharge to home. Infants who do not pass this initial screening should be retested in approximately 1 month. Immaturity, poor testing conditions resulting from environmental noise, or an inexperienced technician may cause false-positive results. If an infant does not pass the initial screening, parents are often alarmed. They should be advised that the screening does not provide a definitive diagnosis of hearing loss; however, the importance of follow-up should be emphasized.

Vision Screening

Development of severe retinopathy of prematurity (ROP) may still be a concern at the time of NICU discharge for infants born at less than term. Any infant born at less than 28 weeks' gestation or less than 1500 g should have a retinal examination every 2 weeks, starting at 4 to 6 weeks of age, until full retinal vascularization occurs (about 40 weeks' postmenstrual age). Other premature infants felt to be at high risk should also be evaluated. Infants with ROP should be examined every 1 to 2 weeks. Follow-up with a pediatric ophthalmologist should be arranged before discharge. Parents should understand that premature infants are also at high risk for myopia, strabismus, and amblyopia. Periodic screening by an ophthalmologist throughout early childhood should be part of the routine care of a premature infant.

Immunizations

Former NICU infants should receive routine childhood immunizations. Many times, immunizations have been started in the NICU before discharge. In these cases parents should be given the standard immunization record book to take home. Immunizations administered in the NICU should also appear in the discharge summary.

RSV Prophylaxis

Respiratory syncytial virus (RSV) poses a risk of serious morbidity or even death for infants who were born prematurely. RSV prophylaxis should be initiated before discharge of these infants into the community setting during RSV season (see Chapter 23). Whether the infant is given RSV-IGIV or palivizumab should be coordinated with the follow-up pediatrician, because resources in the community may differ from those available in the NICU.[7,30]

Neurodevelopmental Follow-up

During the hospitalization parents may ask questions about outcome that simply cannot be answered. Although the infant's risk of cognitive and motor impairment should be discussed, parents must understand that the diagnosis of developmental disability cannot be made before 12 to 24 months of age. This need to "wait and see" creates an additional burden for families that the NICU staff should help the family anticipate. Referral to a multidisciplinary developmental follow-up clinic should provide the family with ongoing information about their child's progress and give parents the opportunity to speak with professionals about their concerns. These clinics often provide families with concrete, focused tasks to undertake with their child that may optimize infant development and help parents feel they are contributing to their child's success.

Any necessary durable medical equipment or supplies, such as an apnea monitor, feeding pump, or oxygen for home use, should be delivered to the family's home before discharge. The company supplying the equipment should provide training in its use. NICU nurses or respiratory therapists should verify the parents' understanding of the purpose of the equipment and its operation. It is helpful for any parents who will be taking home an infant with special equipment or complex needs to "room-in" with their infant before discharge and assume his care, while NICU staff is available for assistance.

Many infants do not achieve full breastfeeding before discharge, because their mothers are unable to be present for all feedings. At discharge, it is essential to provide clear verbal and written instruction to the breastfeeding mother about how to assess her infant's hydration status if the transition from partial to full breastfeeding is to occur at home. It is also important to ensure that the mother has access to medically sound breastfeeding support from the child's pediatrician or a qualified lactation consultant.

At the time of discharge the NICU staff must provide the primary care pediatrician and the parents with a complete and accurate history of the child's NICU course including recommendations for ongoing care. The parents should be advised to keep this summary *with the infant* (i.e., in the diaper bag) at all times; written documentation of the NICU hospital course could be invaluable if the child needs to be seen on an emergency basis shortly after hospital discharge by a health care provider who is unfamiliar with the child's history. The AAP provides a form for summarizing the history and current needs of children with special health care needs on their website.

Successful care of a former NICU infant after hospital discharge depends on the parents' ability to be advocates for their child. Parents need to be equipped with information not only about their child, but also about the medical care system that will be providing follow-up care. Parents who have adequate information can often anticipate and therefore avoid problems.

REFERENCES

1. Allen MC: Developmental outcome and follow-up of the small for gestational age infant, *Semin Perinatol* 8:123, 1984.
2. Allen MC: The high-risk infant, *Pediatr Clin North Am* 40:479, 1993.
3. Allen MC: Outcome and follow-up of high-risk infants. In Taeusch HW, Ballard RA, eds: *Avery's diseases of the newborn*, Philadelphia, 1998, WB Saunders.
4. Allen MC, Alexander GR: Using gross motor milestones to identify very preterm infants at risk for cerebral palsy, *Dev Med Child Neurol* 34:226, 1992.
5. Allen MC, Alexander GR: Screening for cerebral palsy in preterm infants: delay criteria for motor milestone attainment, *J Perinatol* 14:190, 1994.
6. Allen MC, Donohue PK, Dusman AE: The limit of viability: neonatal outcome of infants born at 22 to 25 weeks' gestation, *N Engl J Med* 329:1597, 1993.
7. American Academy of Pediatrics Committee on Infectious Diseases and Committee of Fetus and Newborn: Prevention of respiratory syncytial virus infections: indications for the use of palivizumab and update on the use of RSV-IGIV, *Pediatrics* 102:1211, 1998.
8. Aylward GP, Pfeiffer SI, Wright A et al: Outcome studies of low birth weight infants published in the last decade: a meta-analysis, *J Pediatr* 115:515, 1989.
9. Belcher HM, Gittlesohn A, Capute AJ et al: Using the clinical linguistic and auditory milestone scale for developmental screening in high-risk preterm infants, *Clin Pediatr* 36:635, 1997.
10. Bennett FCMJG: Effectiveness of developmental intervention in the first five years of life, *Pediatr Clin North Am* 38:1513, 1991.
11. Boyd PA, Bhattacharjee A, Gould S et al: Outcome of prenatally diagnosed anterior abdominal wall defects, *Arch Dis Child Fetal Neonatal Educ* 78:F209, 1998.
12. Capute AJ, Accardo PJ: *Developmental disabilities in infancy and childhood: neurodevelopmental diagnosis and treatment*, ed 2, Baltimore, 1996, Paul H Brookes Publishing.
13. Capute AJ, Palmer FB, Shapiro BK et al: Clinical linguistic and auditory milestone scale: prediction of cognition in infancy, *Dev Med Child Neurol* 28:762, 1986.
14. Capute AJ, Shapiro BK, Palmer FB et al: Normal gross motor development: the influences of race, sex and socio-economic status, *Dev Med Child Neurol* 27:635, 1985.
15. Drillien CM: The small-for-date infant: etiology and prognosis, *Pediatr Clin North Am* 17:9, 1970.
16. Emsley HC, Wardle SP, Sims DG et al: Increased survival and deteriorating developmental outcome in 23 to 25 week old gestation infants, 1990-4 compared with 1984-9, *Arch Dis Child Fetal Neonatal Educ* 78:F99, 1998.
17. Escobar GJ, Littenberg B, Petitti DB: Outcome among surviving very low birthweight infants: a meta-analysis, *Arch Dis Child* 66:204, 1991.
18. Finnstrom O, Otterblad OP, Sedin G et al: Neurosensory outcome and growth at three years in extremely low birthweight infants: follow-up results from the Swedish national prospective study, *Acta Paediatr* 87:1055, 1998.
19. Glass P, Wagner AE, Papero PH et al: Neurodevelopmental status at age five years of neonates treated with extracorporeal membrane oxygenation, *Pediatrics* 127:447, 1995.
20. Hack M, Fanaroff AA: Outcomes of children of extremely low birthweight and gestational age in the 1990's, *Early Hum Dev* 53:193, 1999.
21. Hack M, Taylor HG, Klein N et al: School-age outcomes in children with birth weights under 750 g, *N Engl J Med* 331:753, 1994.
22. Hack M, Weissman B, Breslau N et al: Health of very low birth weight children during their first eight years, *J Pediatr* 122:887, 1993.
23. Hurt H: Continuing care of the high-risk infant, *Clin Perinatol* 11:3, 1984.

24. Ishikawa T, Ogawa Y, Kanayama M et al: Long-term prognosis of asphyxiated full-term neonates with CNS complications, *Brain Dev* 9:48, 1987.

25. Kok JH, den Ouden AL, Verloove-Vanhorick SP et al: Outcome of very preterm small for gestational age infants: the first nine years of life, *Br J Obstet Gynaecol* 105:162, 1998.

26. Lorenz JM, Wooliever DE, Jetton JR et al: A quantitative review of mortality and developmental disability in extremely premature newborns, *Arch Pediatr Adolesc Med* 152:425, 1998.

27. Marron MJ, Crisafi MA, Driscoll JM, Jr et al: Hearing and neurodevelopmental outcome in survivors of persistent pulmonary hypertension of the newborn, *Pediatrics* 90:392, 1992.

28. McCarton CM, Wallace IF, Divon M et al: Cognitive and neurologic development of the premature, small for gestational age infant through age 6: comparison by birth weight and gestational age, *Pediatrics* 1996; 98:1167-1178.

29. McCormick MC, Brooks-Gunn J, Workman-Daniels K et al: The health and developmental status of very low-birth-weight children at school age, *JAMA* 267: 2204, 1992.

30. Meissner HC, Welliver RC, Chartrand SA et al: Immunoprophylaxis with palivizumab, a humanized respiratory syncytial virus monoclonal antibody, for prevention of respiratory syncytial virus infection in high risk infants: a consensus opinion, *Pediatr Infect Dis J* 18:223, 1999.

31. O'Shea TM, Goldstein DJ, deRegnier RA et al: Outcome at 4 to 5 years of age in children recovered from neonatal chronic lung disease, *Dev Med Child Neurol* 38:830, 1996.

32. Robertson CM, Finer NN, Sauve RS et al: Neurodevelopmental outcome after neonatal extracorporeal membrane oxygenation, *CMAJ* 152:1981, 1995.

33. Robertson CM, Cheung PY, Haluschak MM et al: High prevalence of sensorineural hearing loss among survivors of neonatal congenital diaphragmatic hernia. Western Canadian ECMO Follow-up Group, *Am J Otol* 19:730, 1998.

34. Robertson CMT, Finer NN, Grace MGA: School performance of survivors of neonatal encephalopathy associated with birth asphyxia at term, *J Pediatr* 114:753, 1989.

35. Roth SC, Baudin J, McCormick DC et al: Relation between ultrasound appearance of the brain of very preterm infants and neurodevelopmental impairment at eight years, *Dev Med Child Neurol* 35:755, 1993.

36. Saigal S, Szatmari P, Rosenbaum P et al: Cognitive abilities and school performance of extremely low birth weight children and matched term control children at age 8 years: a regional study, *J Pediatr* 118:751, 1991.

37. Sauve RS, Robertson C, Etches P et al: Before viability: a geographically based outcome study of infants weighing 500 grams or less at birth, *Pediatrics* 101:438, 1998.

38. Vohr BR, Garcia Coll CT: Neurodevelopmental and school performance of very low-birth-weight infants: a seven-year longitudinal study, *Pediatrics* 76:345, 1985.

39. Vohr BR, Msall ME: Neuropsychological and functional outcomes of very low birth weight infants, *Semin Perinatol* 21:202, 1997.

40. Walsh-Sukys MC, Bauer RE, Cornell DJ et al: Severe respiratory failure in neonates: mortality and morbidity rates and neurodevelopmental outcomes, *J Pediatr* 125:104, 1994.

41. Weisglas-Kuperus N, Baerts W, Fetter WP et al: Minor neurological dysfunction and quality of movement in relation to neonatal cerebral damage and subsequent development, *Dev Med Child Neurol* 36:727, 1994.

42. Weisglas-Kuperus N, Baerts W, Smrkovsky M et al: Effects of biological and social factors on the cognitive development of very low birth weight children, *Pediatrics* 92:658, 1993.

43. Wood NS, Marlow N, Costeloe K et al: Neurologic and developmental disability after extremely preterm birth, *N Engl J Med* 343:378, 2000.

44. World Health Organization: *International classification of impairments, disabilities and handicaps: a manual of classification relating to the consequences of disease,* Geneva, Switzerland, 1980, The Organization.

32 | Ethics in Neonatal Intensive Care

Julie Swaney, Nancy English, Brian S. Carter

Clinical decision-making is influenced by the values of the individuals involved. In the NICU, these values include preserving life, decreasing morbidity, and relieving pain and suffering. Sound clinical skills and judgment, combined with societal and personal values, result in the art of clinical practice.

Technologic advances in medicine have benefited many patients. We are better able to prolong life; at the same time, we are more often in a position to make deliberate decisions about when and how death will occur. Concomitantly, it has become necessary for society to reassess whether the value of prolonging life conflicts with other values, such as relieving pain and suffering, and reducing morbidity. In such cases, values of society, the family, and the health care professional necessarily enter into and influence the decision-making process.

Ethical reasoning insists that we understand the role of values as well as medical data in making decisions.

HISTORY

Historically, ethical concerns in neonatal care focused on the risks and benefits of available technology (Table 32-1). An example is oxygen therapy with the offsetting dilemma that treatment could cause degrees of blindness and/or residual lung damage, whereas nontreatment might result in death or brain damage (1960s). Treatment of premature infants and those with birth defects became technically possible in the 1950s with development of infant ventilators and refined surgical techniques. Because these new technologies not only failed to eliminate all bad outcomes and added new problems, controversies developed over when and how much to use them. Care of newborns with spinal cord defects is illustrative.

Zachary[70] and Shurtleff[55] advocated aggressive management, which increased survival rates but offered questionable quality of life for those more severely affected. Lorber[37,38] was less optimistic about the effects of aggressive management of infants

with meningomyelocele and is recognized for his selective nontreatment of some of these infants.

Discussion of treatment of seriously ill newborns was stimulated by the 1973 publication of Duff and Campbell.[21] Their seminal article described the selective nontreatment or withdrawal of treatment for 43 seriously ill newborns at Yale-New Haven Hospital (between 1970 and 1972) whose "prognosis for meaningful life was extremely poor or hopeless." According to Duff and Campbell[21]:

> Both treatment and nontreatment constitute unsatisfactory dilemmas for everyone. . . . When maximum treatment was viewed as unacceptable by families and physicians in our unit, there was a growing tendency to seek early death as a management option, to avoid that cruel choice of gradual, often slow, but progressive deterioration of the child.

They recognized that most survivors of NICUs are healthy; they also recognized that some infants remain severely disabled by congenital malformations that, until recently, would have resulted in premature death. They were legitimately concerned about the quality of life for these infants and their families.

The majority of newborns treated in NICUs do grow up to lead active, productive lives, but not all fare well with even the most aggressive of treatments.[38] Consequently, there is increasing concern over what is "appropriate" treatment of newborns, particularly seriously ill or disabled ones. Recognizing the risks and benefits of technology, Eisenberg[23] stated, "At long last, we are beginning to ask, not *can* it be done, but *should* it be done."

Baby Doe (1982) and Baby Jane Doe (1983) became the focus of controversy over the issue of withholding treatment and nutrition from handicapped infants.[9,17,48,62] Today, new issues require our attention. Recent advances in fetal surgery raise the question of whether interventions for nonlethal conditions warrant the attendant risks of preterm birth and treatment postnatally in the NICU. Assisted

Table 32-1	SELECTED ISSUES IN PERINATAL/NEONATAL HISTORY OF ETHICAL IMPORT		
TIME	**FETAL DIAGNOSIS**	**FETAL THERAPY**	**NEONATAL THERAPY**
1900s (early)			Temperature regulation, nutrition; limited survival in LBW and anomalied infants
			Recognition of congenital rubella syndrome
			Cardiovascular surgery in the newborn period
			Modern incubator developed
1950s		Tocolysis (ETOH)	Oxygen therapy for respiratory distress
			EBF (Rh) incompatibility recognized
			Oxygen toxicity recognized: RLF/blindness in treated infants; CP and mortality in those untreated
			Other iatrogenic diseases
			Antibiotic usage broadens
1960s	Placentocentesis	Intraperitoneal blood transfusion for EBF	Birth of "modern" NICUs
	Early ultrasonography		Field of teratology develops after thalidomide disaster
	FHR monitoring		Improved outcome for infants <2500 g
	Fetal scalp pH assessment		Surgical management of meningomyelocele becomes an issue
	Amniocentesis		
	Chromosomal analysis		
1970s	Fetoscopy	Intravascular blood transfusion for EBF	CPAP, modern neonatal ventilator
	Real-time ultrasonography	Beta-adrenergic agonists for tocolysis	Improved outcome for infants <1500 g
	Improved structural, chromosomal, and metabolic diagnostics	Corticosteroids for lung maturation	BPD recognized
			Problems of the VLBW infant: IVH, BPD, NEC
		Legalization of abortion	TPN/HAL becomes available
1980s	Chorionic villous sampling	Fetal surgery	Improved pediatric surgery
	Cordocentesis	Prophylactic penicillin for group B streptococcus infection	Newborn metabolic screening
	Doppler flow studies of placenta and umbilical vessels	Treatment of fetal dysrhythmias via maternal medications	High-frequency ventilation
	New reproductive technology		Surfactant replacement therapy
	AFP monitoring		Improved survival in infants <1000 g
			ECMO
			IV immunoglobulin
1990s	Fetal cell isolation in maternal blood		Liquid ventilation
	PCR (polymerase chain reaction) and genetic amplification		Recombinant erythropoietin
			Nitric oxide therapy
2000	First-trimester high-resolution ultrasonography	Further advances in fetal surgery (including that for nonlethal anomalies)	
2000-2010	Potential genetic testing	Potential genetic treatments	

reproduction technologies (ART) contribute to increasingly greater numbers of VLBW infants born as multiples (twins, triplets, and higher-order multifetal gestations) in NICUs. At what point these well-intended services should be restrained or curtailed in order to prevent prematurity and its associated morbidities pose new ethical questions.

Throughout this short but focused "history" of ethical issues in neonatal care, it has become increasingly apparent that there are significant issues regarding appropriate treatment and the limits of treatment. Not only numerous issues, but numerous individuals are involved in the decision-making process regarding treatment and nontreatment options.

More people become involved as technologic advances increase treatment options. Parents have always been presumed to be the best decision-makers on their child's behalf. Health care providers have also been committed to providing what is in the best interests of their patients. Historically, decisions were made privately between parents and their physician. In the modern NICU, treatment goals and decisions are made in the context of a health care team composed of professionals from various moral communities who offer specialized input into the care of the neonate and the family. Parents must be included in the team, because their values are of paramount importance in establishing goals and making decisions about their infant's care. Societal concerns have generally focused on protecting infants against decisions that are detrimental to their best interests by statutes on child abuse and neglect. Professional groups such as the American Academy of Pediatrics (AAP),[5,6] American College of Obstetrics and Gynecology (ACOG),[7] and the Canadian Pediatric Society (CPS)[16] have now addressed these concerns in published guidelines for care of critically ill infants. Community groups[20,22,66] are addressing limitations of care for high-risk newborns as well. Clinical decision-making is impacted by parents, the health care team, professional groups, and society. Respect for clinical decision-making, preferably made by parents and clinicians together, the appropriateness of care, and the protection of children against harm are constantly being balanced.

DEFINITION OF BIOETHICS

Ethics is the study of rational processes for determining the most morally desirable course of action in view of conflicting value choices. Ethics is a branch of philosophy that considers competing values to obtain the best possible outcome to a given situation. When values conflict and each value is morally justifiable, an ethical dilemma exists. For an ethical dilemma to exist, a real choice between possible courses of action must exist.

Bioethics seeks to determine the most morally desirable course of action in health care given the conflicting values inherent in varying treatment options.[8] Most often, when a conflict of values does not exist, moral conflict does not exist. That is, when the health care providers and parents all agree that it is most beneficial to an infant not to treat the infant aggressively and to allow the infant to die, no dilemma or conflict between them exists. Of course,

that they agree does not mean that conflict does not exist with moral views of outside parties or principles. Regardless, the goal is to determine the most morally desirable course of action under a given set of circumstances.

THEORIES OF ETHICS

An ethical theory provides a basis for making morally appropriate decisions. There are many theories or approaches to ethics to consider. **Principle-based ethics** identifies fundamental principles that form the foundation of ethical deliberation. This approach emphasizes the centrality of principles and rules to determine moral duty. Principles commonly recognized are autonomy, beneficence, nonmaleficence and justice.[12] **Virtue ethics** is character-based and as such identifies the virtues of the moral agents involved, rather than the applied principles, as essential to ethical outcome. Various views of the moral life emphasize different virtues as more primary than others. In modern bioethics, primary virtues include respect, fidelity, honesty, and benevolence. **Casuistry** is case-based ethics in which the claims, grounds, and warrants of a particular case are compared with similar cases. The basic question for moral casuistry is how a general moral precept is to be understood in similar sets of circumstances. **Narrative ethics** is story-based in which the narrative itself is a method of ethical reasoning. Every case has different "narratives" to consider, such as medical knowledge, personal identity, patient experience, and the doctor-patient relationship. Although the medical model may focus on disease, psychopathology, objectivity, and diagnosis, the narrative model may focus correspondingly on illness, "the person," subjective experience, and caring. **Feminist ethics** is relationship based and considers primarily the ethics of care. All of these approaches are important to consider. Deciding which moral theory is operative is important to proceeding.

CLINICAL DILEMMAS IN THE NICU

Personhood

Decision-making in the NICU often revolves around the concept of *personhood*. When is one a person? Determining what this means depends on which moral community is consulted. Designation of personhood is morally significant because it determines whether and what duties and obligations are owed to a particular newborn.

Some communities believe personhood is present at the moment of conception; they equate "human" with "person." Shelp[54] refers to this as the "genetic theory of personhood." Others believe personhood depends on the presence or absence of certain basic human qualities. Shelp calls this moral theory "property based." Although with the latter theory there is agreement that the concept of personhood is nongenetic, there are differences regarding which qualities qualify for "person" status.

Fletcher[27] and Engelhardt[24] support the "property-based" stance. They believe that there are human lives that are "subpersonal." Fletcher said, "It is not what is natural but what is personal which has the first-order value in ethics."[27] They believe that neocortical function is required for personhood. Engelhardt[24] related qualities such as self-consciousness, rationality, and self-determination to personhood. He distinguished between persons in a moral sense and persons in a social sense. Infants are deemed persons only in a social sense, not a strict sense by which societal rights are obligatory. The rights of the infant, according to Engelhardt, are held in trust by his or her parents; therefore "decision(s) about treatment . . . belong properly to the parents because the child belongs to them in a sense that it does not belong to anyone else, even to itself."[24]

Tooley[61] suggested that "The ability to see oneself as existing over time is a necessary condition for the possession of a right to life."[32] If Tooley's reasoning is correct, then no infant has a right to life, at least not for some time. Although the "pro-life" moral community assigns person status to all with potential life, Tooley denied that potential has anything to do with a right to life. He advocated a quality-of-life standard. When a life is full of intractable pain and suffering, death is seen as a morally acceptable option. In fact, it is sometimes considered a relatively better outcome than continuing life.

Ramsey[50] and Robertson[52] held a contrasting view. For them, death is never better than life; quality-of-life assessments are not part of their moral reasoning. Life is considered sacred—an absolute good. Both the fetus and newborn are considered a person with a right to live. Therefore "death must always be imposed nonhumanly by God or nature or some other cosmic arbiter."[27] This "pro-life" position supports the moral right of deformed fetuses and deformed newborns to whatever care would be given a normal infant, implying that abortion and infanticide are morally reprehensible. If antibiotics would be given to a normal infant, then they must also be administered to a newborn infant with trisomy 18.

If one is deemed a "person," then society owes one certain obligations and expects certain duties. If one is not deemed a "person," then it is morally reasonable for societal benefits to be withheld or withdrawn. Whatever justification is needed for a particular moral dilemma in the NICU extends from this beginning. Clearly, there is no final definition of personhood, and differing definitions must be considered.

Patienthood

A primary problem confronting a perinatal clinician is the fundamental question: Who is the patient? The adult patient is generally competent and worthy of respect as a moral agent. However, in the case of a newborn, the newborn, the family, and, in some circumstances, society have been variously considered the "patient." The accordance of rights to the newborn as an independent agent is a relatively recent occurrence. Neonatal cases are inextricably bound in the context of varying definitions of personhood and of complicated family and societal situations. The fundamental question remains: To whom is the moral duty owed? To the infant? To the family as "patient"? To society? If there are competing moral obligations, then it is essential to determine to whom the primary moral duty is owed.

Professional-Patient Relationship

The importance of the professional-patient relationship cannot be underestimated, because this is the human context in which decision-making occurs. With neonates this includes a relationship between parents as surrogates and the health care team.

When the four major principles—autonomy, beneficence, nonmaleficence, and justice—are applied to health care relationships, several moral rules can be derived. These moral rules include fidelity, truth telling, and confidentiality. The professional-patient relationship is considerably affected by the meaning and extent of these rules.

Fidelity, or promise-keeping, may be derived from the principle of autonomy. The duty to keep promises may promote the greatest good (utilitarian) or be seen as an obligation (formalist). Many relationships between professionals and patients (or surrogates) involve promises or contracts, whether implicitly or explicitly made. For example, once professionals have established a relationship with a patient, their duty of fidelity includes not abandoning or neglecting that patient. An obvious problem in dealing with surrogates may be conflicting duties to the surrogates and the patient. Promises made by professionals are binding except when they are superseded by stronger obligations.

Truth telling, like fidelity, can be derived from the principle of autonomy or respect for persons. It implies an implicit contract between parties that the truth will be told. At the heart of truth telling is trust, which gives professional-patient relationships their integrity. Lying violates implicit contracts, respect for persons, and trust. It also impedes informed consent.

Utilitarians and formalists may agree on the duty to tell the truth, although they may disagree on the duty not to deceive. Cases have been made for "benevolent deception," when intentional deception is morally justifiable if its primary intent is for the benefit of the patient. In such cases telling the truth may be a violation of **beneficence** and **nonmaleficence.** Others argue that deception, benevolent or not, is morally wrong, because it violates respect for persons and trust. Ultimately the professional-patient relationship erodes. Respect for persons involves acknowledging patient autonomy to know, or not to know, the truth of his or her particular situation.

It is generally agreed that **confidentiality** should prevail in professional-patient relationships. With minors, confidentiality extends to the parents or legal guardians. Part of the implied contract is that information gained by both parties will be kept confidential. From the earliest days of medicine, protecting the patient's privacy has been a fundamental tenet of clinical practice. There are, of course, instances where confidentiality is justifiably breached. It is at this point that many ethical dilemmas arise.

Breach of confidentiality may be morally and legally justified to protect the life of a patient or the lives of others who may be endangered. The value of human life overrides the relationship, but the professional should be able to demonstrate clear danger before violating a patient's privacy. This may also be seen as a violation of autonomy. "The health care professional's breach of confidentiality thus cannot be justified unless it is necessary to meet a strong conflicting duty."[12]

Obviously, health care professionals can be torn between conflicting moral obligations, such as between the patient and society. Such instances in which a breach may be justified include child abuse and neglect, and certain communicable diseases. But there is strong justification among both utilitarians and formalists for maintaining the privacy and confidentiality of patient information. Most important, the genuine integrity of the professional-patient relationship will be enhanced and preserved when confidentiality, like fidelity and truth telling, is respected and upheld. This integrity of relationship then becomes the basis of the decision-making process.

Informed Consent

The issue of valid informed consent is repeatedly raised in the environment of the NICU. All relevant information for a decision must be given. Voluntary consent, free of coercion, by competent persons must be obtained. Information given to parents may be poorly understood for many reasons, including the complex nature of the information; the emotional or physical state of the parents after the birth of a sick, premature, or anomalous infant; physical separation of the parents from their newborn; or feelings of bewilderment and intimidation leading to uncontested paternalism. Indeed, there are indications that valid informed consent is an ideal toward which we work but one that, within the realities of practice, may rarely be obtained. Consent should be sought, however, and open lines of communication and parental education established to facilitate some level of understanding and enable more than token participation in decision-making by the parents.

One standard that has been put forth in an effort to accomplish informed consent is the "reasonable person standard." It asks, "What would a reasonable person want in this circumstance?"

There are several ways in which the reasonable person standard might be enacted in the NICU, thus ensuring that more-valid informed consent is obtained. First, early contact should be made with the parents or family regarding the expected course of problems and special management needs of the newborn. This consultation may even be initiated before delivery. Second, information should be provided by the clinical staff in a factual, compassionate manner. Parents may need continued orientation or reorientation to the NICU environment. This may be especially necessary for parents who are geographically separated from their child. Third, phone calls and photographs are important means for parents to maintain emotional involvement with their child. Fourth, social workers, clergy, or other support resources should be contacted and utilized early to manage emotional distress and to facilitate communication. Fifth, regular patient care conferences with the parents should be scheduled. This will keep parents apprised of the newborn's status and will keep the staff informed about the parents' level of understanding, perspectives, and values. Additional efforts to communicate must be made at the time of special procedures, tests, or therapies to enhance everybody's understanding and the informed consent process.

An integral part of the informed consent process and one that directly affects decision-making is the principle of fidelity, commonly referred to as truth telling, as discussed above. Issues of what to tell, how and when to tell, and whom to tell become a daily part of the staff's interaction with each other and the families of affected newborns.

In practice, the issue of truth telling is considered an essential component of the professional-patient relationship. Information should be shared among staff members and presented to the family truthfully, compassionately, and without bias. However, it is often best for a single voice (e.g., the attending neonatologist or primary care clinician) consistently to relate information and interpret facts for families in order to minimize confusion or misinformation.

Double Effect

The principle of "double effect" asserts that an action may be considered good if the intent of the action is a positive value, even if the secondary effects of the action might be considered harmful if undertaken as the primary goal; further, the good effect should be commensurate with the harm. Double effect is used frequently in the NICU. An example is the use of narcotics in a dying newborn: the positive goal is reduction of suffering, even at the expense of shortening life.

Problems of Uncertainty

A major difficulty in ethical decision-making is the medical uncertainty that exists around such decisions. It is difficult to determine what may be in the best interest of the child when the prognosis remains unclear. Even when the prognosis seems clear, there are always those children who confound science, whose outcomes are far from expected.

Some of the most frequent problems in working with perinatal cases arise as a result of this uncertainty. Parents always ask, "Will my baby be okay when he (or she) grows up?" Answers are often unsatisfying or incomprehensible. In most cases with premature infants, "truth telling" may compel an answer that when reduced to its simplest form says, "I don't know." A statistical approach to answering the question may be: "Most babies like yours grow up to be normal," or "Some babies like yours have serious problems." These answers are often followed by a litany of statistical probabilities of each morbidity. Neither approach answers the mother's question of what her particular baby will be like. Such approaches serve to complicate the clinician's relationship with parents over issues such as expertise, veracity, and disclosure. The statistical approach may answer the NICU staff's question of quality of care, but few parents understand such statistics or are willing to apply them to a loved one. Nonetheless, uncertainty is a way of life in many perinatal cases, and this observation significantly compromises the resolution of ethical problems in the NICU.

In considering medical uncertainty, it may be helpful to recognize two general classes of perinatal cases. NICU patients can be generally classified as either (1) premature infants without known anomalies or (2) near-term infants with major anomalies, either syndromic or nonsyndromic. For infants with known syndromes or major anomalies, prognoses from the literature are describable with reasonable accuracy. Thus the prognosis for an infant with trisomy 18 can be given with a fairly high degree of accuracy, permitting reasonable application of these processes.

A detailed review of neonatal outcome is beyond the scope of this chapter, but several conclusions appear justified. First, infant mortality has declined rapidly since the establishment of NICUs, and the major mortality groups are in lower weight and younger gestational age–groups.[31,42] Second, coincident with the decline in mortality have come major improvements in neonatal morbidity (both neurodevelopmental and pulmonary) from nearly 50% in the pre-NICU era to current figures in the range of 15% from many institutions.[42] Third, the absolute number of normal premature survivors has increased dramatically, and the absolute number of moderately and severely affected survivors appears to have increased as well.[42]

"Extreme prematurity, on the other hand, is characterized by an enormous uncertainty. . . . In these cases predictions of outcome at birth are probabilistic at best."[51] Recognizing this, attempts have been made to establish guidelines for treatment of ELBW infants.[7,16,20,22,66] The morbidities in premature survivors are variable in nature, but CNS morbidities generally include visual impairment and blindness, speech and hearing impairment, neuromuscular impairment, and serious retardation. Few premature survivors require long-term institutional care.[42] The combined risk for one or more of these handicaps is in the range of 15% to 20%.[19,29,30,67] Most would agree that these are indeed serious handicaps, with major effect on the patient and family. However, do they justify withholding or withdrawing treatment? And if so, under what circumstances?

For perinatal clinicians who consider quality of life a major consideration, it remains an exceedingly difficult practical problem to predict which particular child will be significantly handicapped. The predictive value of nursery evaluations in estimating long-term handicap is low.

The intent of raising these questions is to underscore the complexity of ethical discussions as particularly applied to problems in the modern NICU. This in no way reduces the enormity of such problems for the patient, the family, health care providers, or society. Technologic advances may resolve old uncertainties but often seem to carry new uncertainties that are equally perplexing.

Setting Goals

Treatment goals need to be established so that incremental decisions can be made. Preferably, goals should be established by the parents based on their values for their child. Parents need to be involved, not just informed, in determining the overall goals of treatment. Decisions toward that end can then be made. Goals expressed by parents may be living a "normal" life, living with a debilitating outcome but without excruciating pain or suffering, existence without any notable "quality of life," and so on. Accordingly, treatment goals may be to improve an infant's health, help the infant to maintain the current state of health, or help the infant to die with maximum palliative care. All too frequently decisions are made before the treatment goal is established. The parents and health care team members may be working toward differing goals. The physician, health care team, and parents all need to be guided by established goals so that beneficial treatment can be offered. The AAP Committee on Fetus and Newborn has stated that although the role of parents in goal-setting and decision-making must be respected, "physicians should not be forced to undertreat or overtreat an infant if, in their best medical knowledge, the treatment is not in compliance with the standard of care for that infant."[6]

Treatment and Nontreatment

For parents to be involved in determining overall treatment goals and in the decision-making process, they must be fully informed to consent to or refuse treatment for their child. Infants should be treated humanely and with respect in an environment that is conducive to maximum comfort and healing. Humane judgments should be made in determining how infants can most benefit from treatment in any given situation. Palliative care should be provided to all infants at all times. As noted in Chapter 12, sufficient analgesia should be administered to infants having surgery because they can, indeed, experience physical and psychologic pain. Staff and parents should maximize the development of premature infants and offer every possible benefit to them. The nursery environment should be as free from excessive overstimulation as possible (see Chapter 13).

Other perplexing ethical questions arise when the benefit of treatment is unclear. Even the most perfunctory of decisions should be based on the patient's best interests, yet "best interests" are often difficult to determine. Should a child born with anencephaly be resuscitated or receive life-sustaining interventions solely for the purpose of organ transplantation? Should an ELBW infant receive aggressive ventilatory therapy? Medical and ethical decisions involve not only the question of what kind of treatment serves the patient's best interest but also of the appropriateness of treatment at all. Limited or non-treatment decisions are agonizing and regularly result in ethical discussions. **A nontreatment decision is sometimes incorrectly referred to as withholding or withdrawing** *care.* **Only** *treatment* **may be withheld or withdrawn.** *Care* **should always be provided, whether it be curative care or palliative care.**

"Nonbeneficial" Treatment

The concept of "nonbeneficial" medical treatment may be as perplexing as the concept of benefit. It does, however, deserve attention, because there are increasing circumstances in which treatment may be considered to be nonbeneficial and thus withheld or withdrawn. There is no ethical obligation to offer nonbeneficial treatment, yet there is no one definition of "nonbeneficial."

Most often, judgments about benefit are based on medical or physiologic data. It may be medically nonbeneficial to resuscitate an infant under certain conditions, because the treatment cannot alter the course of the illness or problem, yet there are psychologic, social, and religious reasons that such treatment might be offered. If, because of the treatment, the family has time to hold the infant and say goodbye, the resuscitation may not be considered by them to have been nonbeneficial. Of course, the opposite is also true; that is, what may not be physiologically nonbeneficial may be considered to be nonbeneficial by the family and/or surrogates based on religious or other reasons. Again, there is no ethical obligation to offer nonbeneficial treatment. It is possible to get a medical effect but not a medical benefit.[53] The distinction can be significant. Determination of the appropriateness of treatment should be based on medical benefit as determined by family goals for the patient, which include physiologic, psychologic, social, and religious data.[33] By attending to all of these aspects of care, which include staff and family input alike, a determination of what is nonbeneficial therapy, and thus what is beneficial therapy, can be made.

Research Ethics

A persistent, and controversial, issue in neonatal care has been the introduction of new therapies or procedural interventions into the NICU without appropriate research into their safety, efficacy or net benefit, and long-term outcomes for those critically ill infants who receive them. Appropriate studies in animal models ideally would be followed by randomized, controlled clinical trials in human newborns (see Chapter 1). The introduction of extracorporeal membrane oxygenation (ECMO), high-frequency ventilation, and recombinant erythropoetin all have been examples of interventions that crept into neonatal care before controlled trials were conducted. In recent years, the use of glucocorticoids either to enhance fetal lung maturity antenatally, or to prevent or treat bronchopulmonary dysplasia (BPD) postnatally is an example worth evaluating.

Although the benefits of a two-dose regimen of antenatal steroids was demonstrated in 1972,[36] the development of recent practice patterns in which multiple doses of steroids were used over successive weeks of pregnancy was unsubstantiated by randomized clinical trials designed to address the efficacy or safety of such practices. Subsequently the NIH held a Consensus Development Conference and published a statement advising that repeat courses of steroids not be routinely used.[40] Research conducted after these practice patterns were established demonstrated increased maternal infection and suppression

of the normal hypothalamic-pituitary-adrenal axis and both fetal and neonatal decreased somatic and brain growth, adrenal suppression, neonatal sepsis, chronic lung disease, and increased mortality. Additionally, neurodevelopmental outcome studies suggested an increase in psychomotor delay and behavioral problems (see Chapters 13, 23, and 32).

The acute, seemingly beneficial, effects of administering systemic steroids to newborns with lung disease, however, was not met with significantly improved mortality or long-term outcome. It is also associated with a number of acute side effects (e.g., gastrointestinal perforation, hypertension and hyperglycemia), and possible long-term consequences on lung and central nervous system function which are harmful.[11,43,57] Recent studies that caution about the poor postnatal brain growth among some ELBW NICU survivors raise additional concerns about the wisdom of adding risks associated with steroid treatment on top of an already predisposed at-risk newborn.[43,46] Research into the future use of steroids in premature infants should be well designed, adequately powered to provide answers, and should include an evaluation of long-term neurodevelopmental outcome.[25]

DECISION-MAKING IN THE NICU

In the NICU, decisions of serious proportion are encountered regularly, based on medical facts and nonmedical values. From the moment of birth, and in some cases even earlier, a foremost issue is that of determining the appropriate level of treatment (or nontreatment) of sick or anomalous newborns. Entire texts have been devoted to this issue.[32,65] Primary concerns are when to treat, when to limit treatment or not offer curative treatment at all, and who should be involved in the decision-making process.

A frequently encountered treatment problem requiring attention, other than the much-publicized anomalous infant, is the extremely premature or VLBW infant whose course is marked by slow or absent progress despite appropriate and seemingly heroic intervention. The development of complications from disease is of further concern. In concert, these may portend a guarded or very poor prognosis. Recognizing this, the CPS and the Society of Obstetricians and Gynecologists of Canada have published guidelines for the care of women at 22 to 25 weeks' gestation.[16]

These cases may prompt "quality of life" and "ordinary versus extraordinary treatment" discussions. The President's Commission[49] noted that "there is no basis for holding that whether a treatment is common or unusual, or whether it is simple or complex, is in itself significant to a moral analysis of whether treatment is warranted or obligatory"— a view that had been previously voiced by moral philosophers. The AAP has published a strategy for the initiation and withdrawal of treatment for high-risk newborns.[4] General recommendations include the importance of ongoing evaluation, parental participation, establishing the goals of humane care, and upholding the best interests standard seeking to benefit the infant: "It is inappropriate for life-prolonging treatment to be continued when the condition is incompatible with life or when the treatment is judged to be futile."[4] The AAP Committee on Bioethics further "supports individualized decision-making about life-sustaining medical treatment for all children, regardless of age. These decisions should be jointly made by physicians and parents."[4] If we are honest about our professions, we must realize that "quality of life" is what we are all about. Health care professionals are entrusted by society to advance the health and well-being of the mind and body of all persons, so that they can lead their lives and function as part of the human family, individually or collectively. No individual is capable of establishing what is an acceptable "quality of life" for all persons in all circumstances. Each case requires our collective efforts to facilitate the best decision for that particular patient.

Steps in Ethical Decision-Making

The approach should follow a method that clearly demonstrates the practice of applied clinical ethics. As stated by Pellegrino,[45] the goal of applied ethics is making right and good moral decisions for and with a particular patient. Such a decision requires first, that a decision-maker be determined. The decision-maker, whether that be a parent, health care provider, or other, must understand his or her own (1) philosophy of relationship to the patient (or family), (2) interpretation of ethical principles and values, (3) theoretic basis of ethics used (utilitarian, deontologic, and so on), and (4) source from which morality is derived. An ethical "workup" is then undertaken in which substantive issues are identified and worked through, resulting in a decision.[59] Implementing decisions requires determining who shall decide, by what criteria they shall be allowed to do so, and subsequently how the decisions or actions are to be implemented.

Box 32-1 presents the essential steps to decision-making in neonatal cases where a dilemma exists. Consider all involved values and possible solutions to the problem, realizing that alternative solutions may uphold different principles and result in different (positive or negative) consequences. Options that may appear acceptable to the family may be unacceptable to the health care team, or vice versa. There may be societal (legal) constraints on certain actions. In some instances, only one option will be consistent with the rules and principles to which the decision-maker subscribes. Other options may present apparent conflicts between competing values or result in unacceptable consequences. In a decision, there will more than likely be some give and take. Some priority must be assigned to a certain set of values, rules, principles, or resultant effects of any action or inaction. A decision should be made in light of these issues. This process need not always be invoked in full. Often, when the case is carefully dissected and medical facts, values, treatment alternatives, and expected prognoses are revealed, issues that at first seemed in question are clarified, and it becomes apparent that no real dilemma exists.

Good ethics, then, start with good facts and effective communication. All parties involved should be aware of all relevant facts, be they medical, social, human value, or legal in nature. Decisions should not be based on personal opinion or insufficient data. The

---

Box 32-1	**APPROACH TO ETHICAL DILEMMAS IN NEONATAL CARE**

1. Consider who is involved in making and implementing the decision (family, guardians, clinicians, society).
2. Decide who will make the final decision. Is referral to an ethics committee indicated?
3. Clarify all of the medical facts within the case; consider indications, alternatives, and consequences of each action or inaction.
4. Understand significant human factors and values (for patient, family, and health care team).
5. Identify the ethical dilemma or conflict.
6. Make a decision.
   a. List options as solutions to the problem.
   b. Weigh and prioritize values.
   c. Make a decision.
7. Check for moral and rational defensibility.

Modified from Brody H: *Ethical decisions in medicine*, Boston, 1981, Little Brown; and Francoeur RT: From then to now. In Harris CC, Snowden F, eds: *Bioethical frontiers in perinatal intensive care*, Natchitoches, La, 1985, Northwestern State University Press.

value placed on one's medical well-being may differ between the health care team and the patient and/or family, and discrepancy may lead to a perceived problem. This serves to remind us of the need for a formal approach to problem solving in hard cases.

A viable patient-professional relationship that clarifies facts (taking into account uncertainties and the difficulties of prognosticating), human values and feelings, and the interests of all relevant parties is essential to ethical decision-making. Decisions made should reflect a moral choice that is beneficial to the patient as determined by the established, informed decision-makers. We should all work toward achieving a position that is both morally congruent with the values deemed of greatest worth in an individual case and applicable within the moral community as a whole.

Although it may be arguable whether the patient is the neonate, the family, or another societal group, it is prudent to develop a consensus wherever possible and thus minimize conflict among the interested parties. Efforts should be made to involve the parents early in the care of their child and to listen carefully to their values, goals, and dreams. Clinical information should be presented sensitively and thoroughly. These efforts may help to minimize the stresses on the parents and prepare them to participate in decision-making regarding the care of their child. These efforts will also assist staff as they participate with the parents in the decision-making process. With careful attention to the needs of patients, families, and staff, many conflicts can be resolved at an early stage before positions are hardened and emotional investment is high.

In most cases, consensus is reached. In a minority of cases, conflict is unavoidable. In some cases, medical care raises issues that are highly controversial either within the group of clinicians providing care or in the broader context of societal problems. In many cases, the family is far from homogeneous in its expression of wishes. Many parents are young and in the process of achieving independent adulthood with well-developed values. Single-parent families are not uncommon. The birth of a critically ill infant may serve as a focus to crystallize disagreements between spouses or may aggravate conflicts between the parent (or parents) and the extended family. In such cases a more formal process, such as a formal conference between clinicians and the family, appeal to an ethics committee, or even involvement of the legal system, may help to resolve or minimize conflicts of values. It is preferable, however, that decisions be made by involved parties as close to the bedside as possible.

Proxy Decision-Makers

In dealing with newborns who are, by their very nature, incompetent and cannot make decisions for themselves, value conflicts must be resolved with the input of a proxy or surrogate decision-maker acting on the infant's behalf. This may be the parents, a family member, friend, guardian *ad litem,* or the physician. To be considered a valid surrogate, the person should be competent, knowledgeable of integral values of the patient or family, free from conflicting interests, and without serious emotional conflicts in dealing with the case.

Society has for many reasons allocated to the parents the primary authority role in collaboration with health care providers in making decisions about their newborn's care. In most instances the parents are best suited for such matters and have the infant's best interests in mind. They are usually present when possible, are concerned for their infant's well-being, and are willing to hear the facts of their infant's condition, as well as learn of needed therapies. Of all people, they also know best the values of the family culture or environment in which the infant will be raised.

Yet parents may be less than dispassionate decision-makers. They are understandably overwhelmed at times, both physically and emotionally exhausted, and baffled or intimidated by the high-tech environment of the NICU and the complexities of their infant's care. Amid feelings of grief, fear, anxiety, and wonderment over their premature or anomalied infant, they may be uncertain of their proper role and responsibilities as parents. Health care providers need to give daily updates on the infant's condition and anticipated course. Parents' needs for emotional support and avenues to both vent their frustrations and explore their concerns over economic, marital, family and/or sibling, and career effects of their predicament make resources such as nurses, social workers, and chaplains essential in providing assistance to allow them to participate in goal-setting and difficult decision-making. Occasionally it will be necessary to assess the level of parental competency in assuming the role of surrogate, recognizing when additional help or support for them is needed to fulfill this role.

Physicians as decision-makers, an often-cited traditional paternalistic role, are yet another option. They know and understand the complexities of the medical condition and treatment more than do parents, and should promote the patient's best interests in advocating treatment. They may be more objective about individual cases and are not emotionally overwhelmed, as the parents might be. Also, based on experience, they offer a perspective of effectiveness of treatments and can be consistent in treating similar cases.

However, physicians may also encounter problems when they act as the principal decision-makers. Although their knowledge of medical facts is the most complete of all persons, it is at the same time, unfortunately, incomplete. Accurate diagnoses and certainty in prognoses are at times elusive. Medical knowledge does have limits. Statistics are helpful for groups of similarly affected patients, but individual outcomes are difficult to predict. Further, while having the degree of specialized information and knowledge they do, physicians do not necessarily possess any more moral expertise than do parents or others.

Treatment versus nontreatment decisions are ultimately moral, not simply medical, decisions. These decisions are weightier than most clinical decisions that physicians make. There is more involved than a rote, rational process employed in isolation from the family or health care team. The physician must contend with his or her own values and emotions, as well as the medical facts, in each individual case. He or she must facilitate parental and health care team communication and interaction and ultimately order the provision or withdrawal of care.

Fortunately, physicians do not work in isolation from the health care team when making decisions about patients. Nurses, child life workers, social workers, and chaplains are vital members of the decision-making team. A potential problem with each of these clinicians as surrogates is that there may be a conflict of interest between them and the patients for whom they are deciding. Members of the health care team may be biased toward the prolongation of life, have preconceived and strong biases about euthanasia, or be influenced by issues unrelated to the patient, including advancement of care, financial issues, or societal issues. Hence they may not fully take into account the best interests of the patient or the values of the involved family. In contrast to parents, they do not live with the results of their decisions and actions. There may also be a lack of consistency in their application of principles to similar cases, and they may give in to strong pressures (real or perceived) exerted by the law or very assertive parents.

Various factors should contribute to minimizing the potential problems in parents and health care professionals reaching morally defensible decisions in the best interest of the premature or anomalous infant. The professionalism of health care team members who are committed to serving the health and interests of their patients is a foremost consideration that serves this purpose. A sense of duty leads these professionals to assist families in achieving their life goals through facilitating open communication and discussion of their varied concerns. A great sense of personal and professional satisfaction may be derived by helping families accept and deal with their emotions, questions, and concerns for their infant and their own circumstances. Professionals may benefit from the support afforded by each other and certainly will avoid problems if efforts are made to communicate well with each other.

In recent years, hospital ethics committees have been given an increasing role in facilitating ethical decision-making for sick neonates and have, in rare instances, actually functioned as proxy decision-makers. As more institutions are establishing committees, their roles are more focused on education, policy interpretation, and advisory functions than on decision-making. Decision-making by committees might be problematic in that it may threaten the traditional physician-patient and/or family relationship and usurp both the physician's authority and the parents' autonomy. Siegler[56] noted a number of ways in which a committee "can constrain and modify physician-patient decisions," including the imposition of administrative and regulatory burdens. The mechanics of the committee process, time, and distant relationship to the family and case have also been raised as problems in utilizing committees.

Weir[65] noted that a committee, especially an infant bioethics committee, may have the potential of meeting all of the criteria for a proxy decision-maker. Ethics committees are multidisciplinary in composition and have the goals of emotional stability, objectivity, impartiality, and consistency. Ideally they may facilitate the resolution of conflicts between parents and physicians in matters of treatment and be more capable of both addressing and working through the ethical or moral aspects of cases than parents, health care professionals, or other individuals. In reality, their most useful role seems to be one of improving effective communication between staff and families. Finally, they may prove to be a safeguard for infants where parents and professionals are working toward an end that may be perceived as contrary to the infant's best interests.

Surely, much reflective thinking should be invested in our decisions, as individuals, parents, or members of a committee. However, a small number of cases will proceed beyond institutional review to a court. Courts may present many of the criteria for being good proxies—they are disinterested parties, free of emotional involvement, and mostly consistent in reasoning from case to case. They can ensure that all relevant facts are presented and considered, and judges are capable of exercising unmatched control of data collection, investigation, questioning of experts, and seeking of alternative solutions. A judge can also appoint a guardian *ad litem* to be the patient's advocate when necessary.

Yet there are at least a few weaknesses in courts as proxies. They are removed from the NICU and have no contact with the case, patient, staff, or family whose problem they are deciding; hence they are more remote than other possible proxy decision-makers. Time may be consumed in working through cases, which may result in additional problems, changes in pertinent facts, or prolongation of suffering. Decisions rendered by judges may also reflect some bias based on personal considerations of the judge rather than consistent judicial decisions across lines of legal jurisdiction. Also, some would argue that courts are by design adversarial, using force to resolve conflict rather than promoting cooperation.

Standard of Best Interest

The best-interest standard has been advocated by the President's Commission and others seeking to accomplish valid moral decision-making in difficult neonatal cases.[49,64,65] We are obliged "to try to evaluate benefits and burdens from the infant's own perspective."[49] This standard is accepted in the case of newborns over the autonomy-promoting "substituted judgment," because substituted judgment can only be applied hypothetically to a never-competent newborn. This standard is accepted as the best method available to "reasonable" adults who have to make decisions for neonates.

The potential for self-seeking by the decision-maker is easy to understand and has been recognized. The interests of parents, siblings, physicians, hospital staff or administration, and society may all seem to compete with those of the newborn. But the interests of others—be they emotional, economic, or otherwise problematic—cannot justifiably override those of the patient[10] based on the actual or potential personhood of the critically ill neonate. Individual or societal problems or perceived burdens are generally not viewed on the same moral plane as a person's claim to life.

Certainly there will be cases that stretch the best-interest standard to its limits. Cases of protracted treatment with uncertain prognoses beg the question of quality of existence (in which nonmaleficence is the principle of concern) and will require consideration of more than mere suffering and pain. Indeed, in the words of Arras,[10] "Sometimes circumstances may be so extreme and the consequences so dreadful that the priority of justice can no longer be maintained." In this sense we need to find the best balance of beneficence, nonmaleficence, and justice.

We must also consider other morally relevant concerns of neonates who may be doomed to brief lives with less than recognizably "human" existence. Human capacities (ability to think, be aware of self, and relate to other people) may be different from biologic human life. The preservation of biologic human life bereft of the benefit of distinctly human capacities is controversial and has been challenged in quality-of-life decisions.[10,21,32,37,65] Walters has written of the "proximate personhood" model.[63] Arras[10] suggested the "relational potential standard"—Does this child have the ability, or potential, to relate to physical space and time and to communicate to others?—as a means to address these concerns more aptly than the "misapplied best interest standard," calling on society itself to inquire "into the conditions of valuable human life."

Priority should be given to attempts at effecting a cure in these ill infants; when a cure cannot be achieved, patient comfort should be sought. Some maintain that life itself may not always be an absolute good; thus it may be morally justifiable to withhold or withdraw futile treatment associated with inhumane risks or harms that would prolong dying. Mitchell,[39] a member of the American Nurses Association Committee on Ethics, has stated:

> Some infants are so premature and underweight, so profoundly impaired, so hopelessly diseased, or so severely asphyxiated that their foreshortened lives are full of misery for them and those around them. For infants who are so impaired that medical therapies are futile or . . . would only prolong suffering, invasive medical procedures and surgery are morally as well as medically inappropriate.

She calls on nurses to shift their focus in such cases to "seek primarily to provide comfort, relieve suffering and help a grieving family."

Creating an Ethical Environment

Ethical decisions do not happen in a vacuum. It is important that environments exist that promote ethical behavior and deliberation. Such environments should be institutional (the nursery, the hospital, the community, social and political structures) and attitudinal. Attitudes include those where families and staff are empowered to express their opinions and engage in the decision-making process, where all voices are valued, where information is openly and honestly shared (including uncertainties), where respect for all individuals is upheld, where the predominant concern is to benefit the patient, whether that be minimizing overstimulation of patients, administering appropriate analgesia, or providing appropriate palliative care. Routine ethics rounds or ethics committee and palliative care consults, along with family care conferences and generally good family communication are recognized means of enhancing such an environment in the NICU. Yet none of these replace the responsibility of all staff members consistently to promote an overall ethical milieu in the nursery in which ethical practice is the standard of care.

Some institutions hold weekly staff conferences for education, clarification, and open and informed communication among staff members. Information can be clarified and family care conferences can be arranged. When the NICU staff enter into these dialogs with parents, or when an ethics consultant joins in, the ability to clarify the goals of care and understand the present condition of the patient, and potential future concerns of all parties as they view the patient, is enhanced.

ETHICS COMMITTEES AND INFANT BIOETHICS COMMITTEES

It is preferable to keep the decision-making responsibility within the professional-patient relationship. In the vast majority of cases, members of the health care team and the parents do have the infant's best interests in mind. Yet in view of the vast dimensions and difficulties of some of these decisions, many people may consult with an Infant Bioethics Committee (IBC). Where there is agreement about a treatment plan, the committee might be consulted for confirmation of that plan; where there is a dispute about a proposed course of treatment, the committee might be consulted for clarification of ethical principles, values, and various treatment options that would be consistent with ethical and legal standards.

The stimulus to the establishment of IBCs in the United States was the controversy over and death of Baby Doe in Bloomington, Indiana, when society (and government) became acutely aware of the moral issues surrounding what many perceived to be wrongful nontreatment. This incident provided strong moral justification for a process of committee review of infant cases, particularly when treatment is being withheld or withdrawn to effect the termination of life. The government, in response, proposed a series of regulations to monitor the medical treatment of handicapped newborns.* There has been a longstanding regulation (Child Abuse Prevention and Treatment Act amendment)[2] written with the intent of protecting disabled infants with life-threatening conditions from medical neglect. These guidelines, along with the recommendations of the AAP, encourage hospitals to create IBCs or to have access to one for consultation. "The Academy believes the creation of infant bioethical review committees constitutes a direct, effective, and appropriate means of addressing the existing education and information gaps."[3] Members are necessarily from various disciplines and areas of expertise: physicians, nurses, lawyers, clergy, social workers, ethicists, administrators, and community representatives. It is intended that such an interdisciplinary group will represent both the practical knowledge that is crucial to total case management and the various values that enter into treatment decisions. Their purpose is to promote quality decisions regarding treatment of ill newborns.

IBCs are a resource for consultation and advice. They are not a decision-making body, although some groups are moving toward a consensus model. Different committees have different procedures.[26,34] Committee functions and responsibilities may include (1) offering counsel and ethical review in cases involving disabled infants, (2) educating hospital personnel and families of disabled infants with life-threatening conditions, (3) reviewing prospectively the components of federal and state guidelines regarding care and management of such infants, (4) reviewing retrospectively case management and any deviations from federal and state guidelines as they exist, and (5) developing any policy statements for the institution as they are appropriate or necessary.

---

*The original statute stated that no handicapped individual could be discriminated against solely on the basis of handicap.[1] See also articles by Angell[9] and Victoroff.[62]

Typically, anyone involved in a particular case may request a consultation from the IBC. The legal responsibility of all participants in case management and decision-making, including ethics committee members, is consistent with that of any surrogate.

COMMUNICATING WITH FAMILIES

The most important element in communicating with families is listening to them. Indeed, consistent, sensitive and thorough communication of clinicians with families is essential to good patient care. The more complex the medical situation, the more crucial it is that parents receive consistent information, perhaps from a single designated person on the health care team. Parents are often confused by the various prognostications offered by multiple subspecialists and are unable to synthesize the data into a "larger picture" of what is happening to their baby. Yet in the urgency to communicate information clinicians sometimes forget to listen to the grief, fears, and concerns of parents for their child. These feelings can profoundly influence decisions that are made and how they are made. Ethics as a rational process must also take into consideration the range of human emotions involved in life and death issues, not just clinical information. What parents would not be distraught over the premature birth of their infant? Overwhelmed by their severely disabled infant? The prospect of lifetime rehabilitation? The reality or prospect of suffering? The prospect of death of their newborn?

Good communication with parents is essential, because parents play a vital role in the decision-making process. They, along with the infant, are the most affected. No matter what their religious or sociocultural background, almost all parents experience shock and grief over their child's need for intensive care. They deal with this in better and worse ways. For many parents the ability to participate in ethical decision-making is impaired while they are in such an acute stage of shock. Usually, prenatal diagnosis of anomalies gives parents time to adjust to their child's condition before birth and/or before decisions have to be made. This adjustment time can be most valuable. To participate in ethical decision-making, particularly decisions about withholding or withdrawing treatment, parents must have achieved some degree of emotional reorganization and acceptance. Staff assistance in helping them move from emotional disorganization to reorganization is crucial to further decisions that need to be made. At this point, parents may be better able to absorb medical data, ethical values, and principles. Although there may not be a theoretic difference between withholding and withdrawing treatment, there is a large emotional difference. The sound clinician, as well as the ethicist, must be sensitive to this distinction.

Choices about treatment and nontreatment do affect the grieving process. Questions such as "Am I just prolonging suffering by keeping her alive?" are countered by "Am I not giving her a chance and playing God by allowing her to die?" Duff and Campbell[21] report families experiencing "a normal mourning for their losses" after allowing their seriously ill infants to die. What remains for many parents are doubts that their choice was correct. For some, decisions based on certain religious principles or other value criteria offer moral justification of behavior that assists in the mourning process. For others, the justification may be logically but not emotionally clear. In these instances, grieving can become more complex and difficult.

A valuable role of an IBC may be to offer input into, if not confirmation of, the parents' decision in a way that helps to allay guilt that can interrupt normal grieving. Ethics, while at once highly theoretic and intellectual, must consider that the situations with which it most intimately deals are highly emotional. For parents the psychologic trauma will affect their ethical considerations, and ethical decisions will have further psychologic effect.

A real value of an interdisciplinary health care team is the particular attention paid to the many complex aspects of a patient's living and dying. When parents are facing the death of their child, the entire team may be involved in assisting them. Nurses and physicians, social workers, clergy, and psychologists may all be intimately involved with monitoring the patient's comfort level and deteriorating course and with comforting grieving parents. Baptisms (when appropriate) and especially funerals are important ritualistic ways of organizing the meaning of the traumatic event. The entire staff should encourage parents to offer all that they can to their dying child. They should provide active palliative care—maximum comfort for the patient and maximum support to the family. Helping patients and families cope with death is a privilege. It can be personally and professionally satisfying, and ultimately immeasurably helpful to everyone involved, to enter emotionally into this process. Often care of the living means care of the dying.

Good communication between staff members is also important. The effect on the health care team members of helping an infant die should also be recognized because their concern and involvement with the infant are usually significant. Helping someone through the dying process can be a difficult, though rewarding, experience. In such instances professionals may agree with the decision (preferably the parents') to withhold or withdraw treatment. Professionals may also disagree with the decision but may place a higher value on the parents' autonomy to decide than on the decision itself. Respecting this, they may abide by the parents' wishes for their child. No one should be forced to compromise personal or professional integrity, however, and in cases in which one's ethics or integrity is being violated, the case may be transferred. Preferably, professionals can learn about the range of ethically defensible options and can support the parents in choices different from their own.

PALLIATIVE CARE

Palliative care is an emerging nursing and medical specialty encompassing a comprehensive approach to the needs of those with a life-limiting disease or condition. It is family-centered and interdisciplinary. Professionals, patients and their caregivers become partners in all decisions affecting the plan of care. The emphasis is on enabling the patients and their families to increase their options of care by stating their desires for end of life care through advance planning.

The World Health Organization (WHO)[68] defined palliative care as "the active, total care of patients whose disease is not responsive to curative treatment. . . . The goal of palliative care is achievement of the best possible quality of life for patients and their families." Palliative care, the WHO continued:

- Affirms life and regards dying as a normal process and neither hastens nor postpones death
- Provides relief from pain and other distressing symptoms
- Integrates the psychological and spiritual aspect of patient care
- Offers a support system to help a family cope during a patient's illness and during their bereavement

In the mid-1960s Dame Cicely Saunders, a nurse who later became a physician, initiated the palliative approach, which emphasizes quality of daily life for the patient and family. She advocated doing whatever is possible to relieve the patient's pain and suffering as a consequence of the disease. Her recognition that both family and patient need continual psychologic as well as spiritual support from the time of diagnosis, decline, and death is now an integral part of the continuum of care.[18]

Palliative care can and should occur from the earliest recognition of a life-threatening condition and can be concurrent with efforts to prolong life.[13,35] The focus is to provide all available resources that ensure the patient's comfort and offer support to the family and caregivers.

Death, like birth, is recognized as a rite of passage embracing the spiritual needs of the patient and family. Thus spiritual caregiving, along with cultural and religious rituals, is an integral part of the palliative care plan. At the time of death professionals make every attempt to create a sacred and spiritual space within the environment for patients and family. Often when death is impending the patient is moved to a special room where family gather to say their farewells. Professionals offer support at this critical period and continue to be available during the period following death.

The emerging palliative care model is holistic and centered on the needs of both the patient and family. Many medical centers now have palliative care consultation teams consisting of a palliative care physician, ethics consultant, nurse, chaplain, and social worker who are available to collaborate with hospital staff on the multifaceted issues in end of life care. Some hospitals even offer palliative care units.

The American Academy of Pediatrics (2000) issued a statement suggesting that a palliative care model, as described above, be integrated as a care option for children with a life-threatening or terminal condition. The goal of care is "to add life to the child's years not simply years to the child's life."[4]

The Phase Model

Palliative care for sick or dying newborns is most effective when it is part of the infrastructure of the NICU.[35,60] Palliative treatment protocols can be in place and initiated particularly when an infant's presenting condition may be life-threatening. **We propose a hypothetic[5] phase model for palliative care in the NICU based on the principles of interdisciplinary involvement, shared decision-making and comprehensive treatment,**[41] **as presented in Figure 32-1.**

In **phase I, the focus is on active symptom management** in accordance with current ethical

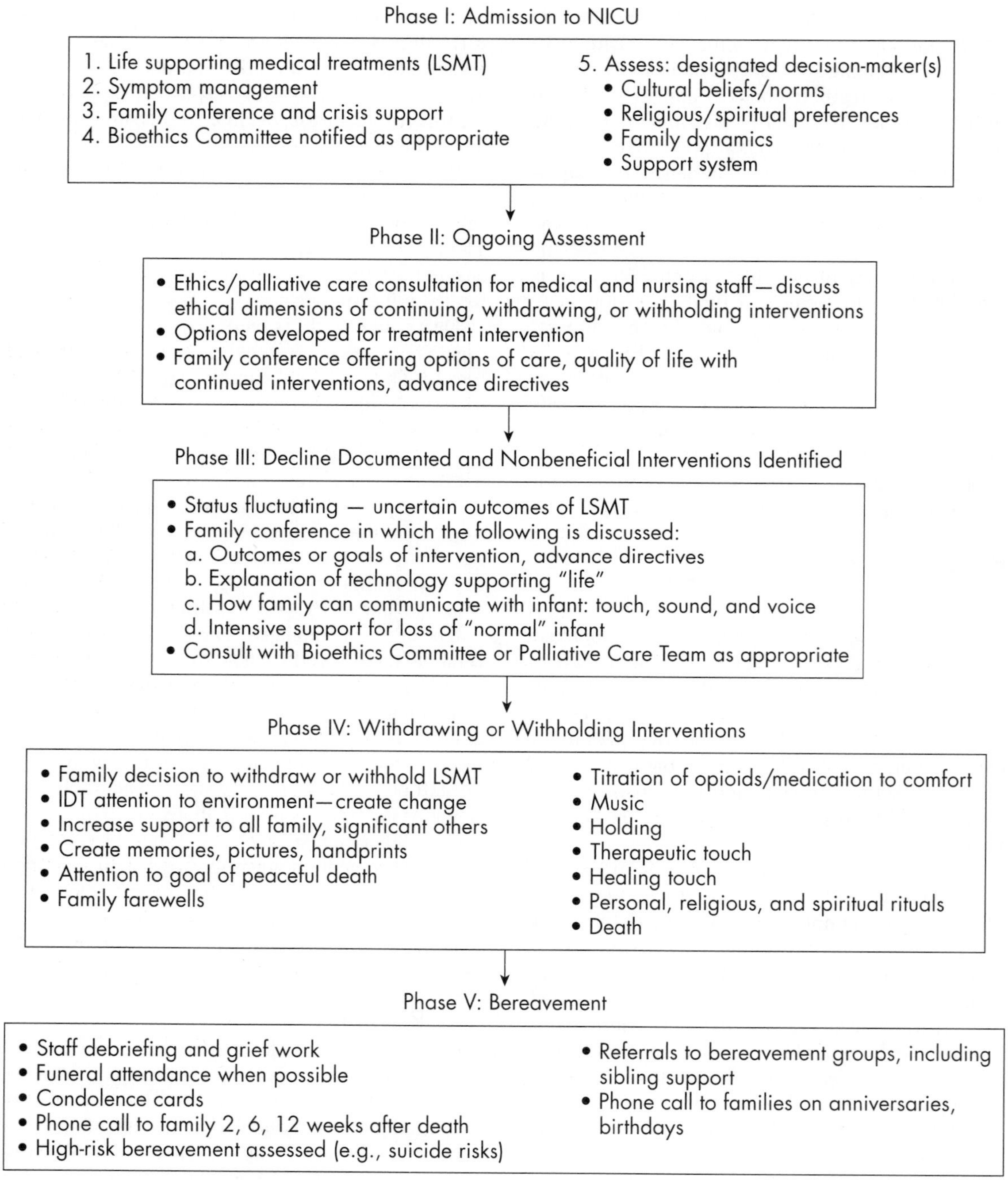

Phase I: Admission to NICU

1. Life supporting medical treatments (LSMT)
2. Symptom management
3. Family conference and crisis support
4. Bioethics Committee notified as appropriate

5. Assess: designated decision-maker(s)
   • Cultural beliefs/norms
   • Religious/spiritual preferences
   • Family dynamics
   • Support system

Phase II: Ongoing Assessment

• Ethics/palliative care consultation for medical and nursing staff—discuss ethical dimensions of continuing, withdrawing, or withholding interventions
• Options developed for treatment intervention
• Family conference offering options of care, quality of life with continued interventions, advance directives

Phase III: Decline Documented and Nonbeneficial Interventions Identified

• Status fluctuating — uncertain outcomes of LSMT
• Family conference in which the following is discussed:
   a. Outcomes or goals of intervention, advance directives
   b. Explanation of technology supporting "life"
   c. How family can communicate with infant: touch, sound, and voice
   d. Intensive support for loss of "normal" infant
• Consult with Bioethics Committee or Palliative Care Team as appropriate

Phase IV: Withdrawing or Withholding Interventions

• Family decision to withdraw or withhold LSMT
• IDT attention to environment—create change
• Increase support to all family, significant others
• Create memories, pictures, handprints
• Attention to goal of peaceful death
• Family farewells

• Titration of opioids/medication to comfort
• Music
• Holding
• Therapeutic touch
• Healing touch
• Personal, religious, and spiritual rituals
• Death

Phase V: Bereavement

• Staff debriefing and grief work
• Funeral attendance when possible
• Condolence cards
• Phone call to family 2, 6, 12 weeks after death
• High-risk bereavement assessed (e.g., suicide risks)

• Referrals to bereavement groups, including sibling support
• Phone call to families on anniversaries, birthdays

FIGURE 32-1   Integrating palliative care and bioethics in neonatal intensive care: an interdisciplinary approach.

considerations and guidelines outlined in this chapter. The family is made aware of the critical nature of the infant's condition. The physician, chaplain, and social worker are available and offer support, fully aware that the response of the parents to tragic news is often numbness, shock, and disbelief.[14,58] The chaplain and clinical social worker initiate the palliative care plan and clearly outline to all NICU staff and the ethics committee, if involved, the family dynamics, cultural beliefs and any other information that may help the caregiving team.

In **phase II, outcomes of life-sustaining treatment may still be uncertain.** In a palliative care model, physiologic data along with staff observations of the child's responsiveness or nonresponsiveness may be indicators of when the goals of care should change from curative to palliative treatment. In such situations, family conferences with all involved staff members present should be offered. At this point, treatment goals and advance directives can be discussed. Continuing support of the family is essential, including helping them to communicate with their baby.

In **phase III, the infant's decline is documented and the continuation of curative treatment increasingly appears to be nonbeneficial to the patient.** The ethics committee or palliative care team may be consulted. The family is requested to consider withdrawing and/or withholding all life-sustaining medical treatment. Clear and honest communication among all persons involved is critical. **The family should be reassured that comfort care will be maximized.**

In **phase IV, the infant's continuing decline is documented and life-sustaining medical treatment is withdrawn or withheld. Comfort care is of utmost importance.** This includes aggressive symptom management as well as emotional, spiritual, and cultural support to the patient and family. This phase involves a transition to a supportive care environment, where farewells are offered and tears can be shed. The emphasis of care is toward helping parents create memories of their infant's brief life and providing privacy for family farewells, baptisms, or rituals. Often a special area in the NICU has been designated for family members to gather. Memory books, photos, handprints, and music can help the parents realize that their child was a unique human being who spent a brief time on this earth. **The chaplain or social worker is available while life-sustaining treatment is withdrawn.**

Phase V is a time of bereavement. Often the staff as well as the family will need some time for debriefing and support for their roles in the death of the infant (see Chapter 30). Continuing contact with the family at various intervals by a designated staff member or bereavement coordinator is essential to assess the coping of the family, including the siblings of the infant who died. Indicators of complicated grief should be assessed and referrals to support groups or communities may be made. Periodic memorial services provided for the staff as well as for the families may assist in the ongoing grief process.

Palliative care, offered by an interdisciplinary team, promotes continuity of care from diagnosis to death. It allows the family time and support to make difficult decisions regarding quality of life and the quality of a good death. When palliative care is included in the infrastructure of the NICU, it may promote clear communication among staff members and family, especially during the transition from curative treatment to supportive care when life-sustaining treatment is deemed to be non-beneficial to the infant. Palliative care recognizes that a child's death can have profound and often long-term effects on the lives of surviving family members. Grief and bereavement support continues to be offered after the death of a child for an undetermined amount of time.

SOCIAL ETHICS

Moral judgments made in the hospital setting do not occur in isolation from the larger social context of which institutions and individuals are a part. Such judgments can be considerably affected by prevailing social values and perspectives. Further, while decisions in the nursery generally are interpersonal in nature, they may also have a significant effect on the larger community. Technologic advancements have enabled some severely disabled infants to survive and grow, albeit with mental and physical handicaps. Indeed, these are not the majority of newborns, but they often require numerous hospitalizations and costly rehabilitation. Society frequently bears the financial, physical, and social costs of these individuals.

Social ethics reflects on the sociocultural aspects of human life. It considers how individuals as moral agents are accountable for their behavior in social structures and public policy issues. It can also refer to shared patterns of moral judgment. Moreover, it focuses on how social contexts influence individual moral behavior and the range of moral responsibility.

In a pluralistic society such as ours, there is no one social ethic. Some believe in rugged individualism; others in equality of opportunity, worth, and treatment; still others believe that we bear mutual responsibility for one another. An underlying concern of most socioethical systems is concern for both the individual and the common good.

In NICUs, bioethics and social ethics converge. Treatment decisions have social implications; societal values influence treatment decisions. As described, government regulations highlight the paradox of societal values regarding the treatment of disabled infants. These federal guidelines advocate the use of "reasonable medical judgment" in treating disabled infants, yet their effect has been to increase the obligation to treat to the point of "unreasonable." Through government, society expresses the determination to treat; yet societal commitment to long-term care of these patients and families is wholly insufficient. Public funds for such care have been reduced, yet the urgency for treatment of these infants has increased. The values inherent in our public policy decisions regarding initial and long-term treatment are curiously disparate.

After comparing the health care and social policies of the United States with the seemingly more equitable policies of Great Britain and Sweden, Young[69] concluded, "We need to strive for a better balance between aggressive treatment in the neonatal intensive care units initially, and the resources currently allocated for the long-term care of the disabled." Such a balance might include being more selective about aggressive treatment, as well as learning more about prematurity and trying to prevent it. Young continued, "To the extent that society fails to ensure that seriously ill newborns have the opportunity for an adequate level of continuing care, its moral authority, to intervene on behalf of a newborn whose life is in jeopardy, is compromised."[69]

Recognizing this disparity, various community groups have attempted to establish guidelines for standards of care that are fiscally, morally, and medically responsible in order to guide parents and clinicians in goal-setting and decision-making. They have recognized the high cost, in every respect, of neonatal and pediatric intensive care. Their impetus has been to determine community "agreed upon" values for treatment and nontreatment of disabled infants to effect a standard of care for the extreme premature, severely disabled, and critically ill infant. Managed care organizations are also assessing the ethics of reasonable care and the limits of treatment to be offered. While not wholly able to determine "agreed upon" values for treatment and nontreatment standards of care, these community and professional groups have offered important social voices to the complexity of neonatal care.

GLOSSARY

Best Interest A standard used to determine the validity of proxy consent in decision-making. Treatment decisions are based on what most "reasonable persons" would assess as the burdens and benefits that would likely accompany the child's life. This standard leads clinicians to seek treatment resulting in a "net benefit" to the child.

Deontology (Formalism) A theory of ethics that holds that the moral rightness of an act must be decided totally independent of the consequences of that act. Duty is independent of consequential good, and certain moral commands (rules) operative under fundamental principles must be obeyed under all circumstances.

Dilemma A situation that exists when more than one possible course of action exists and differing values are held of each possible course of action by the parties involved. Moral dilemmas arise when an appeal to moral considerations can be made for opposing courses of action; when it is apparent that an act can be considered both morally right and morally wrong, and that on moral grounds there is a sense of "ought" and "ought not" to perform the act.

Double Effect A principle, often viewed within the larger context of nonmaleficence, that claims that an act having a harmful effect is not always morally prohibited. Any harmful effect of an act is viewed as indirect, unintended, or simply a foreseen effect but not as the direct and intended effect (e.g., if an act, as in treatment, brings about death, it is not always to be prohibited). Four conditions are often given to clarify this principle for specific acts:
- The action itself must be "good" or at least morally indifferent.
- The agent must intend only the good effect and not the harmful effect.
- The harmful effect cannot be a means to the good effect.
- There should be a favorable balance between the good and harmful effects of the action.

Ethics The study of moral conduct, systems, and ideas.

Morals The conduct and codes of conduct of individuals and groups. Three popular uses of the term exist: (1) in contrast to immoral (right versus wrong), (2) in contrast to nonmoral (actions that have no bearing or question of right and wrong), and (3) "morals" (the behavior pattern of an individual or group).

Nonbeneficial Treatment The notion that the efficacy of treatment is very low. There is no ethical obligation to offer nonbeneficial treatment. Nonbenefit may best be judged by the overall medical benefit, not just effect, that a given treatment has on a patient. Treatment is nonbeneficial if it is useless. Physiologic, psychologic, religious, and social data should be considered in making a determination of nonbenefit. Determination of nonbeneficial treatment should be based on medical benefit in consort with family goals for the patient.

Personhood A characteristic that may be used in decision-making that is based on the idea that possession of certain capabilities (typically higher brain functions such as consciousness, rationality, perception of space and time, and the ability to communicate) constitute personhood; and that only "persons" have any moral claim to life, treatment, and so on.

"Proxy" Decision-Maker (Surrogate) A designated person who will act on behalf of an individual who is incapable of making decisions.

Reasonable Person Standard A standard by which the validity of informed consent is measured. Information to be disclosed is determined by referring to a hypothetical "reasonable person" and determining whether such a person would see any significance in the information in assessing risk and deciding whether to submit to a treatment or procedure.

Rights Those things to which people have a just claim; a claim to a condition to which the individual is entitled.

Utilitarianism (Consequentialism) A theory in ethics that holds that an act is right when it brings about a good outcome for the greatest number of people, upholds the greatest balance of "good" over "evil," and seeks to effect "utility" or the most useful outcome. "The end justifies the means." This may be developed into rules that are adhered to in order to maximize benefits and minimize harms (rule utilitarian) or simply appealed to in individual actions (act utilitarian).

Values Those things that have worth or are desirable to an individual or group.

Virtues A habit, disposition, or trait that a person may possess or aspire to possess; specifically, a moral virtue upholds what is morally right or praiseworthy.

REFERENCES

1. Ajayi-Obe M, Saeed N, Cowan FM et al: Reduced development of cerebral cortex in extremely preterm infants, *Lancet* 356:1162, 2000.
2. Amendments to the Child Abuse Prevention and Treatment Act, 98 Stat 1749, 1984, 45 CFR PART 1340, April 15, 1985.
3. American Academy of Pediatrics: *Components of the American Academy of Pediatrics on proposed rule regarding nondiscrimination on the basis of handicap relating to health care for handicapped infants.* Undated manuscript.
4. American Academy of Pediatrics Committee on Bioethics: Ethics and the care of critically ill infants and children, *Pediatrics* 98:149, 1995.
5. American Academy of Pediatrics Committee on Fetus and Newborn: Perinatal care at the threshold of viability, *Pediatrics* 96:974, 1995.
6. American Academy of Pediatrics Committee of Fetus and Newborn: The initiation or withdrawal of treatment for high-risk newborns, *Pediatrics* 96:362, 1995.
7. American College of Obstetricians and Gynecologists Committee on Ethics: *Patient choice: maternal-fetal conflict,* ACOG committee opinion 55, 1987.
8. American Hospital Association: *Report of the Special Committee on Biomedical Ethics: values in conflict: resolving ethical issues in hospital care,* Chicago, 1985, American Hospital Publishing.
9. Angell M: The Baby Doe rules, *N Engl J Med* 314:642, 1986.
10. Arras JD: Toward an ethic of ambiguity, *Hastings Cent Rep* 14:25, 1984.
11. Bancalari E: Corticosteroids and neonatal chronic lung disease, *Eur J Pediatr* 157:S31, 1998.
12. Beauchamp T, Childress J: *Principles of biomedical ethics,* ed 2, New York, 1983, Oxford University Press.
13. Beltrin J, Coluzzi P: A model for comprehensive palliative care, *Talbot J Health Care,* Spring/Summer, 1997.
14. Board R, Ryan-Wenger N: State of the science on parental stress and family functioning in pediatric intensive care units, *Am J Crit Care* 9:2, 2000.
15. Brody H: *Ethical decisions in medicine,* Boston, 1981, Little Brown.
16. Canadian Pediatric Society and Society of Obstetricians and Gynecologists of Canada: Management of the woman with threatened birth of an infant with extremely low gestational age, *Can Med Assoc J* 155:547, 1994.
17. Caplan AL, Murray TH, eds: *Which babies shall live? Humanistic dimensions of the care of imperiled newborns,* Clifton, NJ, 1985, Humana Press.
18. Clark D: Palliative care history: a ritual process? *Eur J Palliative Care* 7:50, 2000.
19. Costeloe K, Hennessy E, Gobson AT et al: The EPICURE study: outcomes to discharge from hospital for infants born at the threshold of viability, *Pediatrics* 106:659, 2000.
20. Doroshow RW, Hodgman JE, Pomerance JJ et al: Treatment decisions for newborns at the threshold of viability: an ethical dilemma, *J Perinatol* 20:379, 2000.

21. Duff R, Campbell AGM: Moral and ethical dilemmas in the special care nursery, *N Engl J Med* 289:890, 1973.

22. ECHO: Extreme Care, Human Options: *Community recommendations for appropriate, humane medical care for dying or irreversibly ill patients,* Carmichael, Calif, 1997, Sacramento Health Care Decisions.

23. Eisenberg L: The human nature of human nature, *Science* 176:123, 1972.

24. Engelhardt HT Jr: Viability and use of the fetus. In Bondeson WB, eds: *Abortion and the status of the fetus,* Dordrecht, Netherlands, 1983, D Reidel Publishing.

25. Finer NN, Craft A, Vaucher YE et al: Postnatal steroids: short-term gain, long-term pain? *J Pediatr* 137:9, 2000.

26. Fleischman A, Murray T: Ethics committees for infants Doe? *Hastings Cent Rep* 13:5, 1983.

27. Fletcher J: *Humanhood: essays in biomedical ethics,* Buffalo, NY, 1979, Prometheus Books.

28. Francoeur RT: From then to now. In Harris CC, Snowden F, eds: *Bioethical frontiers in perinatal intensive care,* Natchitoches, La, 1985, Northwestern State University Press.

29. Hack M, Taylor G, Klein N et al: Functional limitations and special health care needs of 10- to 14-year-old children weighing less than 750 grams at birth, *Pediatrics* 106:554, 2000.

30. Hack M, Wilson-Costello D, Friedman H et al: Neurodevelopment and predictors of outcomes of children with birth weights of less than 1000g, *Arch Pediatr Adolesc Med* 154:725, 2000.

31. Koops BL, Morgan LJ, Battaglia FC: Neonatal mortality risk in relation to birth weight and gestational age: update, *J Pediatr* 101:969, 1982.

32. Kuhse H, Singer P: *Should the baby live?* New York, 1985, Oxford University Press.

33. Lantos JD, Singer PA, Walker RM et al: The illusion of futility in clinical practice, *Am J Med* 87:81, 1989.

34. Leiken S: Children's hospital ethics committees, *Am J Dis Child* 141:954, 1987.

35. Levetown M: Pediatric care: the inpatient/ICU perspective. In Ferrell, G, Coyle, N, eds: *Textbook of palliative nursing,* New York, 2001, Oxford University Press.

36. Liggins GC, Howie RN: A controlled trial of antepartum glucocorticoid treatment for prevention of the respiratory distress syndrome in premature infants, *Pediatrics* 50:515, 1972.

37. Lorber J: Results of treatment of myelomeningocele, *Dev Med Child Neurol* 13:279, 1971.

38. Lorber J: Early results of selective treatment of spina bifida cystica, *Br Med J* 4:201, 1973.

39. Mitchell C: Care of severely impaired infant raises ethical issues, *Am Nurse* 16:9, 1984.

40. National Institutes of Health NIH consensus statement *Antenatal corticosteroids revisited: repeat courses,* 2000, 17:1, 2000.

41. Nelson-Marten P, Braatan J, English NK: Critical caring: dying in the intensive care unit (adapted). In Thompson C, ed: *Nursing clinics of North America: evidenced based practice in critical care,* to be released Winter 2001.

42. Congress of the United States, Office of Technology Assessment: *Neonatal intensive care for low birth weight infants: costs and effectiveness,* Washington, DC, 1987, US Government Printing Office.

43. O'Shea TM, Kothadia JM, Klinepeter KL et al: Randomized placebo-controlled trial of a 42-day tapering course of dexamethasone to reduce the duration of ventilator dependency in very-low-birth-weight infants: outcome of study participants at 1-year adjusted age, *Pediatrics* 104:15, 1999.

44. American Academy of Pediatrics, Committee on Bioethics and Committee on Hospital Care: *Palliative care for children,* Pediatrics 106:2, 2000.

45. Pellegrino ED: The anatomy of clinical ethical judgments in perinatology, *Semin Perinatol* 11:202, 1987.

46. Peterson BS, Vohr B, Staib LH et al: Regional brain volume abnormalities and long-term cognitive outcome in preterm infants, *JAMA* 284:1939, 2000.

47. Pickett M, Cooley ME, Gordon DB: Palliative care: past, present and future perspectives in palliative care, *Semin Oncol Nurs* 14:2, 1998.

48. Pless JE: The story of Baby Doe, *N Engl J Med* 309: 663, 1983.

49. President's Commission for the Study of Ethical Problems in Medicine and Biomedical and Behavioral Research: Deciding to forego life-sustaining treatment, Washington, DC, 1983 U.S. Public Health Service, Health and Human Services.

50. Ramsey P: *Ethics at the edges of life,* New Haven, Conn, 1978, Yale University Press.

51. Rhoden NK: Treating Baby Doe: the ethics of uncertainty, *Hastings Cent Rep* 16:34, 1986.

52. Robertson JA: Involuntary euthanasia of defective newborns. In Mappes TA, Zembaty JS, eds: *Biomedical ethics,* ed 2, New York, 1986, McGraw-Hill.

53. Schneiderman LJ, Jecker NS, Jonsen AR: Medical futility: its meaning and ethical implications, *Ann Intern Med* 112:949, 1990.

54. Shelp EE: *Born to die? Deciding the fate of critically ill newborns,* New York, 1986, The Free Press.

55. Shurtleff D: Care of the myelodysplastic patient. In Green M, Haggerty R, eds: *Ambulatory pediatrics,* Philadelphia, 1986, WB Saunders.

56. Siegler M: Ethics committees: decisions by bureaucracy, *Hastings Cent Rep* 16:22, 1986.

57. Stark AR, Waldemar AC, Tyson JE et al: Adverse effects of early dexamethasone treatment in extremely-low-birth-weight infants, *N Engl J Med* 344:95, 2001.

58. Sumner L: Pediatric care: the hospice perspective. In Ferrell BR, Coyle N, eds: *Textbook of palliative nursing,* New York, 2001, Oxford University Press.
59. Thomasma DC: Training in medical ethics: an ethical workup, *Forum Med* 1:33, 1978.
60. Toce S: Applying hospice principles to the care of the high risk newborn, 2000, Compendium of Pediatric Palliative Care, National Hospice and Palliative Care Organization.
61. Tooley M: *Abortion and infanticide,* New York, 1983, Oxford University Press.
62. Victoroff M: The ballad of Baby Doe: parental discretion or medical neglect? *Prim Care* 13:271, 1986.
63. Walters JW: Approaches to ethical decision-making in the neonatal intensive care unit, *Am J Dis Child* 142:825, 1988.
64. Weil WB: Issues associated with treatment and nontreatment decisions, *Am J Dis Child* 138:519, 1984.
65. Weir RF: *Selective nontreatment of handicapped newborns,* New York, 1984, Oxford University Press.
66. Wisconsin Association for Perinatal Care: *Position statement: guidelines for the responsible utilization of neonatal intensive care,* Madison, Wisc, 1997, Lawrence University.
67. Wood NS, Marlow N, Costeloe K et al: Neurologic and developmental disability after extremely preterm birth, *N Engl J Med* 343:378, 2000.
68. World Health Organization: *Cancer pain relief and palliative care: report of a WHO expert committee,* Geneva, Switzerland, 1990, World Health Organization.
69. Young EWD: Caring for disabled infants, *Hastings Cent Rep* 13:15, 1983.
70. Zachary R: Ethical and social aspects of treatment of spina bifida, *Lancet* 2:274, 1968.

Drug Index

Index

A

Abdomen. *See also specific abdominal structures, e.g., Kidneys.*
  musculature of, absence of, 619t
  physical examination of, 88, 89
Abdominal distention, 336
Abdominal masses, 629-630, 630t
  as indicator of genitourinary abnormality, 619t
  of kidneys. *See* Renal mass(es).
  neuroblastomas as, 633
Abdominal wall defect, 66t
ABO hemolytic disease, 424, 445-446, 450
Abscess
  of breast, 466t
  interventional radiology in draining of, 146
Acceptance, as stage of grief, 759-760
Accutane, in utero exposure to, 694, 694f
Acetaminophen (Tylenol)
  excreted in breast milk, 404t
  for pain relief, 206t, 209
Acetate, in total parenteral nutrition, 349t
Acid-base homeostasis, 179-190
  compensation in, 182
  disturbances in
    complications of, 189-190
    correction of, 182, 189
    evaluation of, 188-189, 188b
    prevention of, 187-188
  kidney function in, 614-615
  metabolic contribution to, 180-182
  physiology of, 179-182
  respiratory contribution to, 180
Acidemia, 179
Acidosis, 179-180
  biophysical profile in, 24-25
  complications of, 189

Acidosis—cont'd
  and contraction-induced hypoxia, 21
  nonrespiratory (metabolic), 181-182, 182f
    arterial blood gas analysis in, 189
    causes of, 186
    from pain response, 204
  nonstress tests and, 24
  renal tubular, 633-634
  respiratory, 180, 181-182, 182f
    arterial blood gas analysis in, 189
    causes of, 186
    treatment of, 189
  treatment of, 189
Acne neonatorum, 360t
Acquired immunodeficiency syndrome (AIDS). *See* AIDS (acquired immunodeficiency syndrome).
Acrocyanosis, 87, 490
Acrodermatitis enteropathica, 403t
Active sleep, 225t
Activity of newborn, 72-73
  in congestive heart failure, 580
  during initial physical examination, 87
  motor, 74
Acute renal failure, 621-626
  etiology of, 621-622, 622t
  fluid and electrolyte management in, 296
  laboratory data in, 622
  pathophysiology of, 621
  prevention of, 622
  treatment of, 622-626
A-delta fibers, 193, 193t
Adenoma sebaceum, 618t
Adenosine, 583t, 605
Adenovirus
  infection control in, 472t-473t
  pneumonia due to, 541t
Adhesive dressings
  application and removal of, 366
  transparent, 368

Agitation and irritability
  indicators of, 198b
  pain vs, 198b, 200, 200f
Aicardi's syndrome, 646
AIDS (acquired immunodeficiency syndrome), 462-464
  breastfeeding with, 402t
  history in, 462-463
  infection control in, 472t-473t
  laboratory data in, 463
  maternal, 402t, 462-464
  parent teaching regarding, 463-464
  prevention of, 462
  signs and symptoms of, 463
  treatment of, 463
Air leak
  as respiratory disease complication, 511-515
  data collection in, 512
  etiologic factors in, 511
  physiology of, 511, 511f
  pneumothorax as, 65t, 512, 619t
  prevention of, 511-512
  treatment of, 512-515
Airway
  anomalies of, 65t
  clearing, 55
  suctioning of. *See* Suctioning.
Akinesia syndrome, 613
Albuterol, for bronchopulmonary dysplasia/chronic lung disease, 521t
Alcohol abuse, 16, 164-165
  and breastfeeding, 407t
  with cocaine abuse, 165
  congenital heart defects due to, 578t
Aldactone (spironolactone)
  as cardiac drug, 583t
  for bronchopulmonary dysplasia/chronic lung disease, 522t
Alertness, during nipple feeding, 258t
Alkalemia, 179
Alkali infusions, in persistent pulmonary hypertension of newborn, 546, 547

t denotes table, b denotes box, and f denotes figure.

829